Three-Dimension Colored Diagrams for Meridians and Acupoints

(Chinese-English Edition)

三维经络穴位全彩图集

（中英对照版）

编　著　（按姓氏笔画排序）

老中医养生堂　刘嘉瑶
许博捷　杨丽雯
余骏腾　张金金
张晓雯　张淑巧
陈谷超　林　芳
段牡薇　贾荣曼
高玉伟　郭修兵
曹柏川　曹琳琰

Male Meridians and Acupoints

男性经络穴位

编　著　（按姓氏笔画排序）

老中医养生堂
许博捷

海峡出版发行集团 | 福建科学技术出版社
THE STRAITS PUBLISHING & DISTRIBUTING GROUP | FUJIAN SCIENCE & TECHNOLOGY PUBLISHING HOUSE

图书在版编目（CIP）数据

三维经络穴位全彩图集：汉英对照 / 老中医养生堂等编著．—福州：福建科学技术出版社，2018.1
ISBN 978-7-5335-5356-2

Ⅰ．①三…　Ⅱ．①老…　Ⅲ．①经络－图集②穴位－图集　Ⅳ．①R224.4

中国版本图书馆 CIP 数据核字（2017）第 107350 号

书　　名　三维经络穴位全彩图集（中英对照版）
编　　著　老中医养生堂　等
出版发行　海峡出版发行集团
　　　　　福建科学技术出版社
社　　址　福州市东水路 76 号（邮编 350001）
网　　址　www.fjstp.com
经　　销　福建新华发行（集团）有限责任公司
印　　刷　中华商务联合印刷（广东）有限公司
开　　本　889 毫米 ×1194 毫米　1/16
印　　张　48.5
图　　文　776 码
版　　次　2018 年 1 月第 1 版
印　　次　2018 年 1 月第 1 次印刷
书　　号　ISBN 978-7-5335-5356-2
定　　价　598.00 元

目录 Contents

第二章　穴位分部图解 —— 86
Chapter 2：Diagrams of Acupoints in Different Divisions

第三章　超速效三步对症按摩法 —— 154
Chapter 3：Super Quick-acting Three-step Symptomatic Massage Manipulations

本书特色与使用说明

1. 本书以最新国家标准《腧穴名称与定位》为依据，穴位英文名由拼音与代码组成，图中的穴位中文名旁仅上代码。除在句子中出现的穴名拼音不上音调外，其余穴名拼音均上音调。

2. 结合 AR 技术展示十四经脉循行和部分穴位的取穴，形象直观。读者通过扫描并关注“健康乐读汇”微信公众号，按提示下载客户端，扫描识别码即可观看。

3. 经络腧穴内容全面，查找方便：先以十四经脉为纲，按经脉展示穴位，随图附穴位主治病症，并以“★”标出本经常用穴；接着再分五大部位分别解析各个穴位定位。从整体到局部帮您梳理相关腧穴知识。

4. 穴位应用不求人：收录 35 种常见病症的超速效对症按摩，简单实用疗效佳。

Features and Instructions

1. This book is based on the newest national standard proclaimed by ***Nomenclature and Location of Acupuncture Points***. The international acupuncture nomenclature consists of spelling and code, whereas only code is added to the acupoints of the Picture beside the Chinese name considering limited space. Each spelling is marked with tone except for those occuring in sentences.

2. Circulations of the fourteen meridians and locations of some acupoints are displayed vividly and straightforwardly combined with AR technology. Readers may scan the QR code in back cover and focus on WeChat public account of ***Happy Reading on Health***. Download the application under the instructions, then you can easily watch after scanning the identification code.

3. Overall contents of meridians collaterals and acupoints are contained, convenient for search: The contents first takes the fourteen meridians as main thread, displays respective acupoints according to meridians, encloses indications of points and marks the common-used acupoints with“ ★ ”, then analyzes the location of every point according to different divisions. Acupoints knowledge is arranged from the whole to the parts for better understanding.

4. Acupoints massage self-application: Super quick-acting symptomatic massage mampulations for 35 common syndromes are included. It is simple and practical with well curative effect.

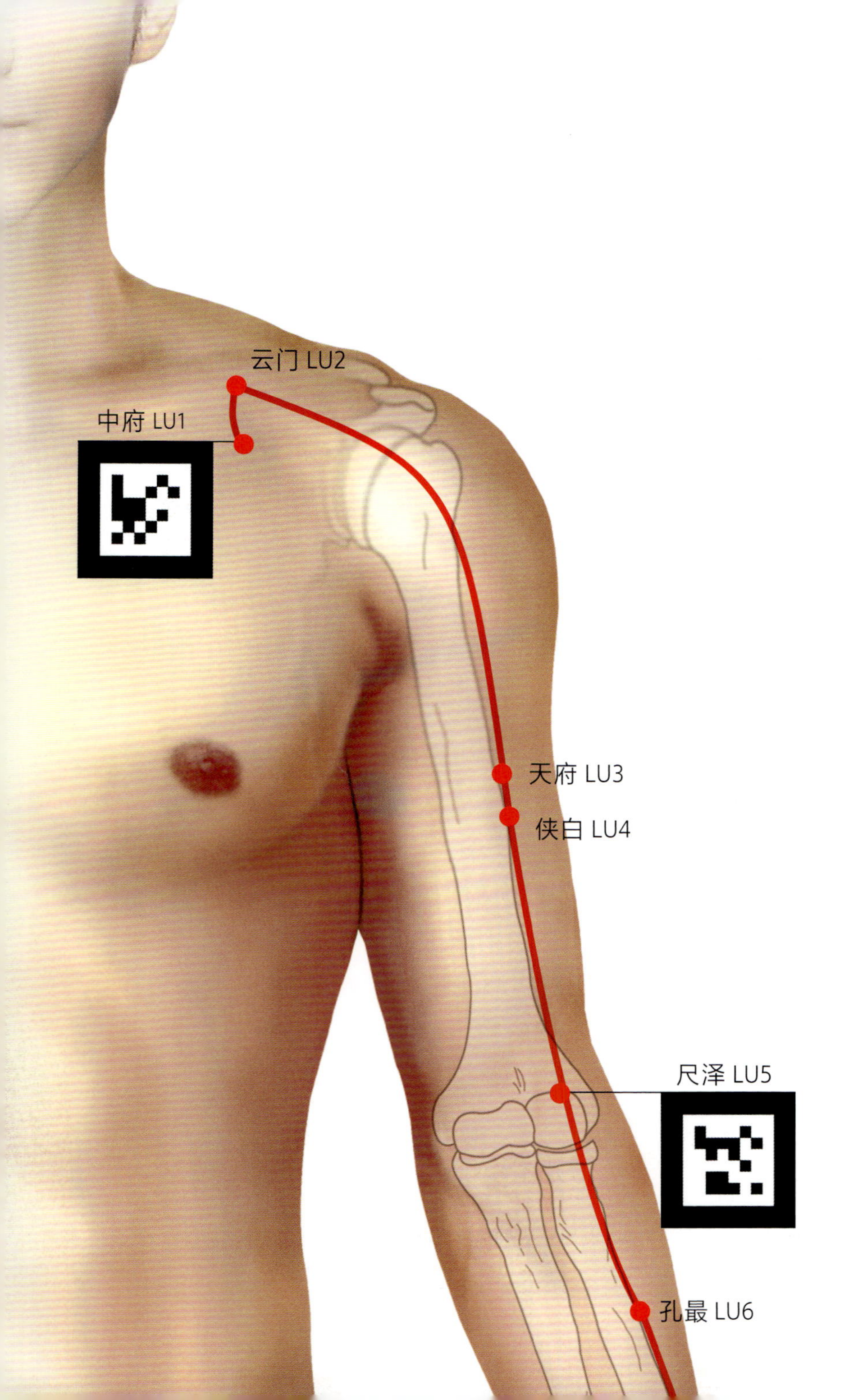

第一章　十四经穴图解

手太阴肺经

手太阴肺经从胸部走向手指，起于胸部的中府穴，经手臂内侧前缘，止于手拇指的少商穴，每侧 11 穴，共 22 穴。

肺经主治病症：①咳嗽、气急、喘息等呼吸系统疾病。②心烦、胸闷、上臂及前臂内侧疼痛不适等经脉循行部位的疾患。

LU	穴位	主治
★ 1	中府	咳嗽、气喘、胸痛、肩背痛
2	云门	咳嗽、气喘、胸痛、肩痛
3	天府	鼻出血、咳嗽、气喘、肩及上肢内侧疼痛
4	侠白	咳嗽、气喘、上肢内侧痛
★ 5	尺泽	咳嗽、气喘、咯血、潮热、胸部胀满、咽喉肿痛、急性腹痛、腹泻、肘臂痛
★ 6	孔最	咯血、鼻出血、咳嗽、气喘、咽喉肿痛、热病（一切外感引起的热性病如传染病、中暑等）无汗、痔血、肘臂痛
★ 7	列缺	外感头痛、咳嗽、气喘、咽喉肿痛、口㖞（口歪）、齿痛
8	经渠	咳嗽、气喘、胸痛、咽喉肿痛、手腕痛

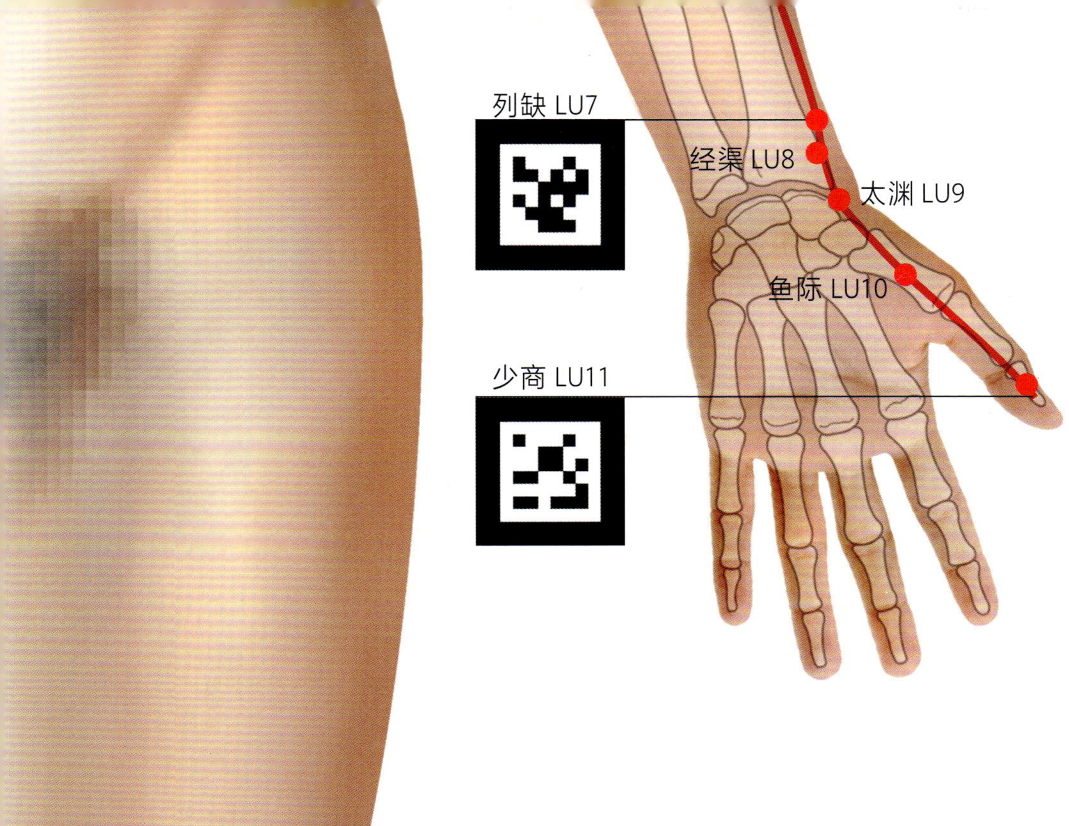

Chapter 1: Diagrams of Acupoints in the Fourteen Meridians

Lung Meridian of Hand-Taiyin, LU.

Lung Meridian of Hand-Taiyin from the chest to fingers. It emerges from Zhongfu acupoint, travels along the anterior-medial aspect of the arms and terminates at Shaoshang acupoint of the thumb. There are 11 acupoints in each side of Lung meridian and 22 acupoints in total.

Lung Meridian indications: ① Respiratory system diseases including cough, short breath and wheezing. ② Diseases of running courses of meridian including vexation, chest tightness and pain in medial side of upper arm and forearm.

LU	Acupoints	Indications
★ 1	Zhōngfǔ	Cough; asthma; chest pain; pain in the shoulder and the back
2	Yúnmén	Cough; asthma; chest pain; shoulder pain
3	Tiānfǔ	Nose bleeding; cough; asthma; pain in the shoulder and medial upper limbs
4	Xiábái	Cough; asthma; pain in medial upper limbs
★ 5	Chǐzé	Cough; asthma; hemoptysis; hot flash; fullness in chest; swelling and pain in the throat; acute abdominal pain; diarrhea; pain in the elbow and the arm
★ 6	Kǒngzuì	Hemoptysis; nose bleeding; cough; asthma; swelling and pain in the throat; fever (any heat disease caused by exogenous pathogenic factors such as heat stroke and infectious disease); adiapneustia; hemorrhoidal bleeding; pain in elbow and arm
★ 7	Lièquē	Exogenous headache; cough; asthma; swelling and pain in the throat; deviation of mouth; toothache
8	Jīngqú	Cough; asthma; chest pain; swelling and pain in the throat; wrist pain

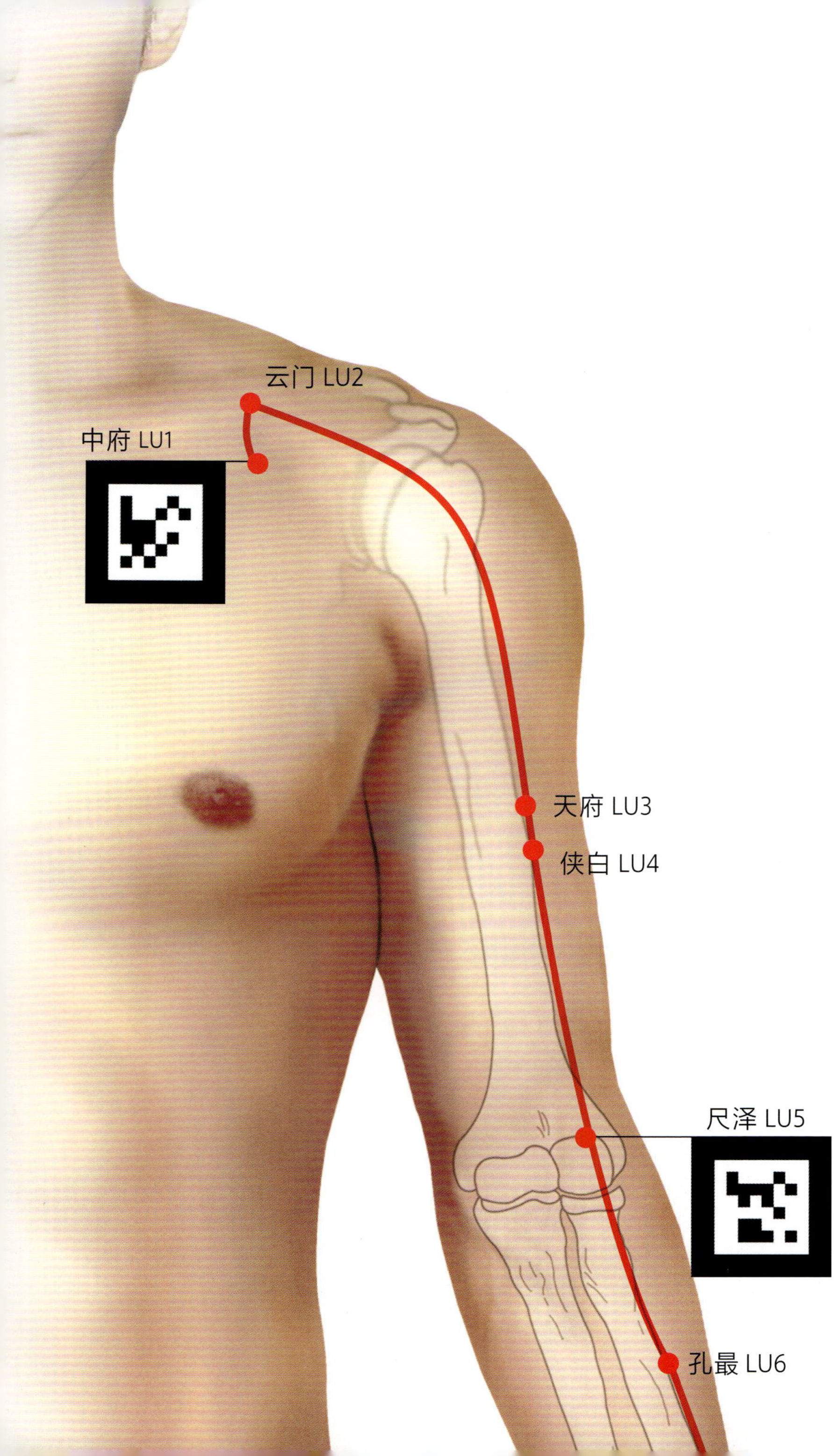

续表

LU	穴位	主治
9	太渊	感冒、咳嗽、气喘、咽喉肿痛、胸痛、无脉症、腕臂痛
★ 10	鱼际	咳嗽、哮喘、咯血、咽喉肿痛、失音、发热
11	少商	咽喉肿痛、发热、咳嗽、失音、鼻出血、昏迷、癫狂（指以情绪改变为主要症状的一类疾病）、指肿、麻木

★为本经常用穴

中府

用拇指按压中府穴，停留片刻后放松，反复 5~6 下，力度稍轻。同法按压对侧中府穴。每日 2 次。

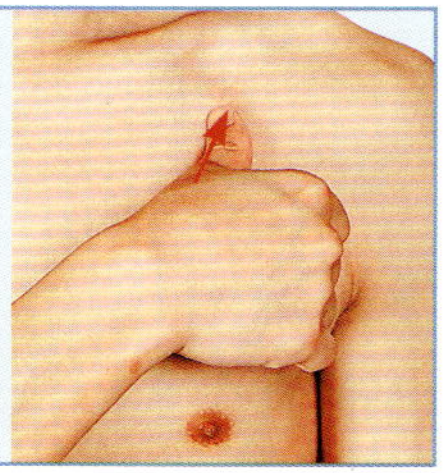

孔最

用拇指稍用力按压孔最穴，停留片刻后放松，反复 5~6 下。同法按压对侧孔最穴。每日 2 次。

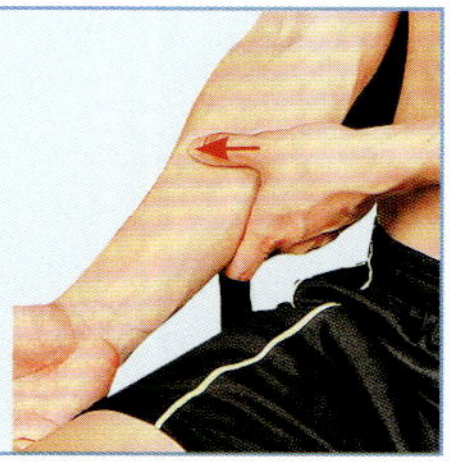

列缺

用拇指指腹按揉列缺穴 2 分钟，力度稍重，至有酸胀感。同法按揉对侧列缺穴。每日 2 次。

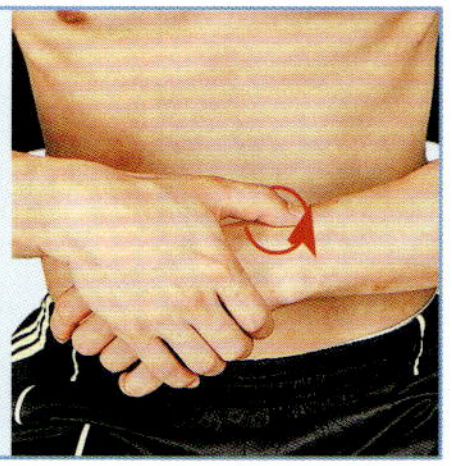

鱼际

用拇指按揉鱼际穴 2 分钟，力度稍重。同法按揉对侧鱼际穴。每日 2 次。

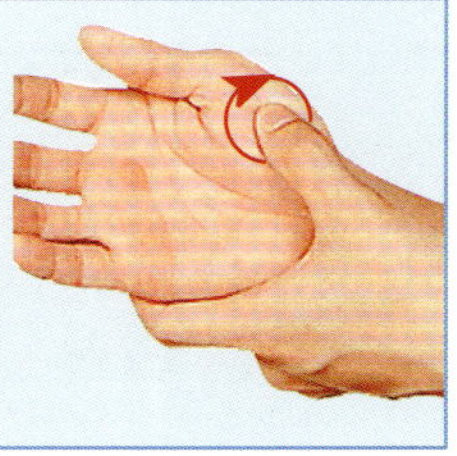

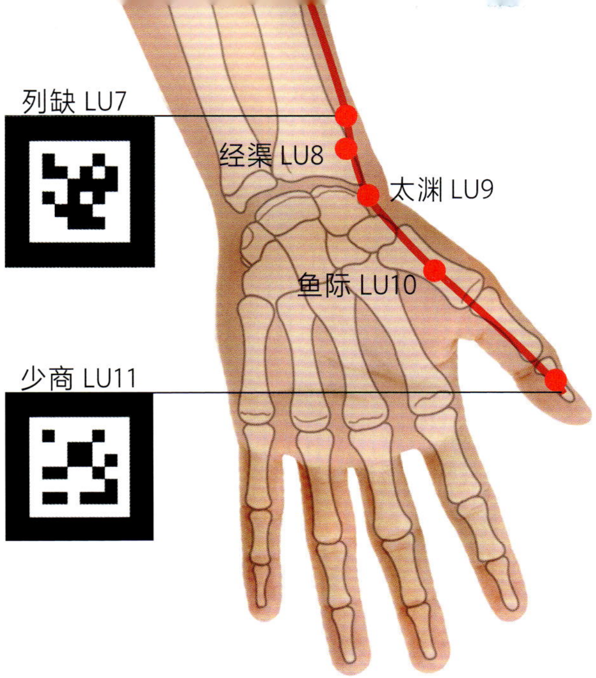

Continued

LU	Acupoints	Indications
9	Tàiyuān	Cold; cough; asthma; swelling and pain in the throat; chest pain; pulseless disease; wrist and arm pain
★ 10	Yújì	Cough; asthma; swelling and pain in the throat; hemoptysis; fever; aphonia
★ 11	Shàoshāng	Swelling and pain in throat; fever; cough; aphonia; nose bleeding; coma; manic-depressive psychosis(a kind of disease of which the main symptoms mood change); finger edema; numbness

★ Common acupoint used in treatment

Zhōngfǔ (LU1)

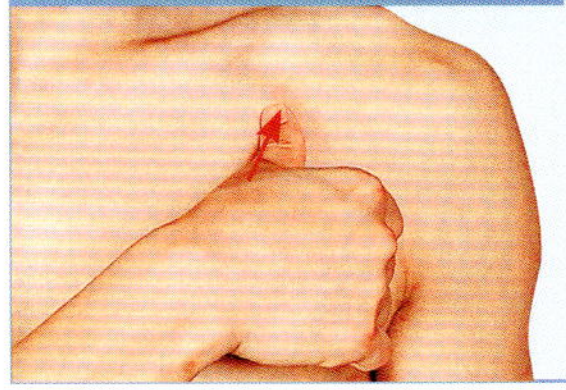

Use the thumb to press the Zhongfu acupoint for a minute and then relax, repeat 5~6 times with slight strength. Press the contralateral acupoint with the same method. Twice a day.

Kǒngzuì (LU6)

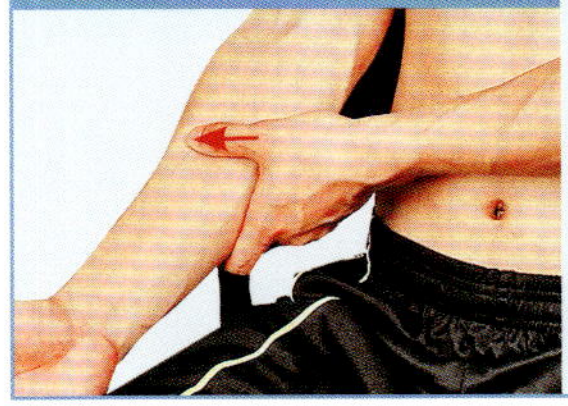

Use the thumb to press the acupoint with a little heavy strength for a minute, then relax. Press the contralateral acupoint with the same method. Twice a day.

Lièquē (LU7)

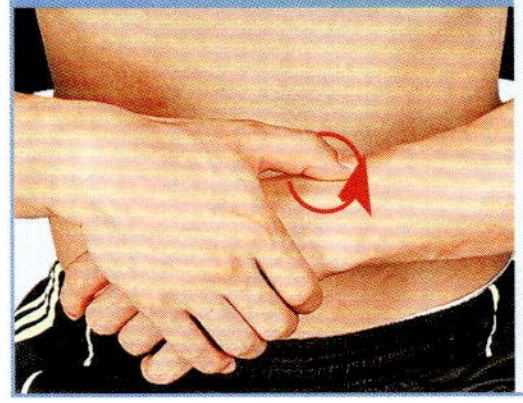

Use the finger pulp of the thumb to knead the acupoint for 2 minutes with a little heavy strength till feeling soreness. Knead the contralateral acupoint. Twice a day.

Yújì (LU10)

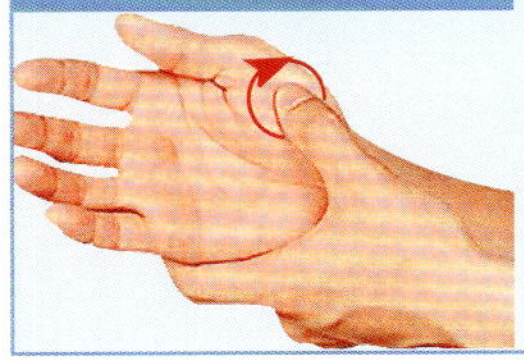

Use the thumb to knead the acupoint for 2 minutes with a little heavy strength. Knead the contralateral acupoint with the same method. Twice a day.

手阳明大肠经

手阳明大肠经起于食指末端的商阳穴，沿手臂外侧经过肩头，止于脸部鼻子旁的迎香穴。本经一侧 20 穴，左右两侧共 40 穴。

大肠经主治病症：①目赤、咽喉肿痛、齿痛、口㖞（口歪）、耳鸣、耳聋等头面五官疾患。②中暑、发热等热病。③腹痛、腹泻、便秘等肠胃病。④上臂部疼痛等经脉循行的疾患。

LI	穴名	主治
★ 1	商阳	咽喉肿痛、齿痛、耳聋、热病、手指麻木
2	二间	咽喉肿痛、齿痛、目痛、鼻出血、热病
3	三间	目痛、咽喉肿痛、齿痛、身热、手背肿痛
★ 4	合谷	头痛、齿痛、咽喉肿痛、口㖞、突发性耳聋、难产、闭经、便秘、上肢疼痛不遂
5	阳溪	头痛、目赤肿痛、齿痛、咽喉肿痛、手腕痛
6	偏历	目赤、耳聋、鼻出血、喉痛、水肿、手臂酸痛
7	温溜	头痛、面肿、咽喉肿痛、腹痛、肩背酸痛

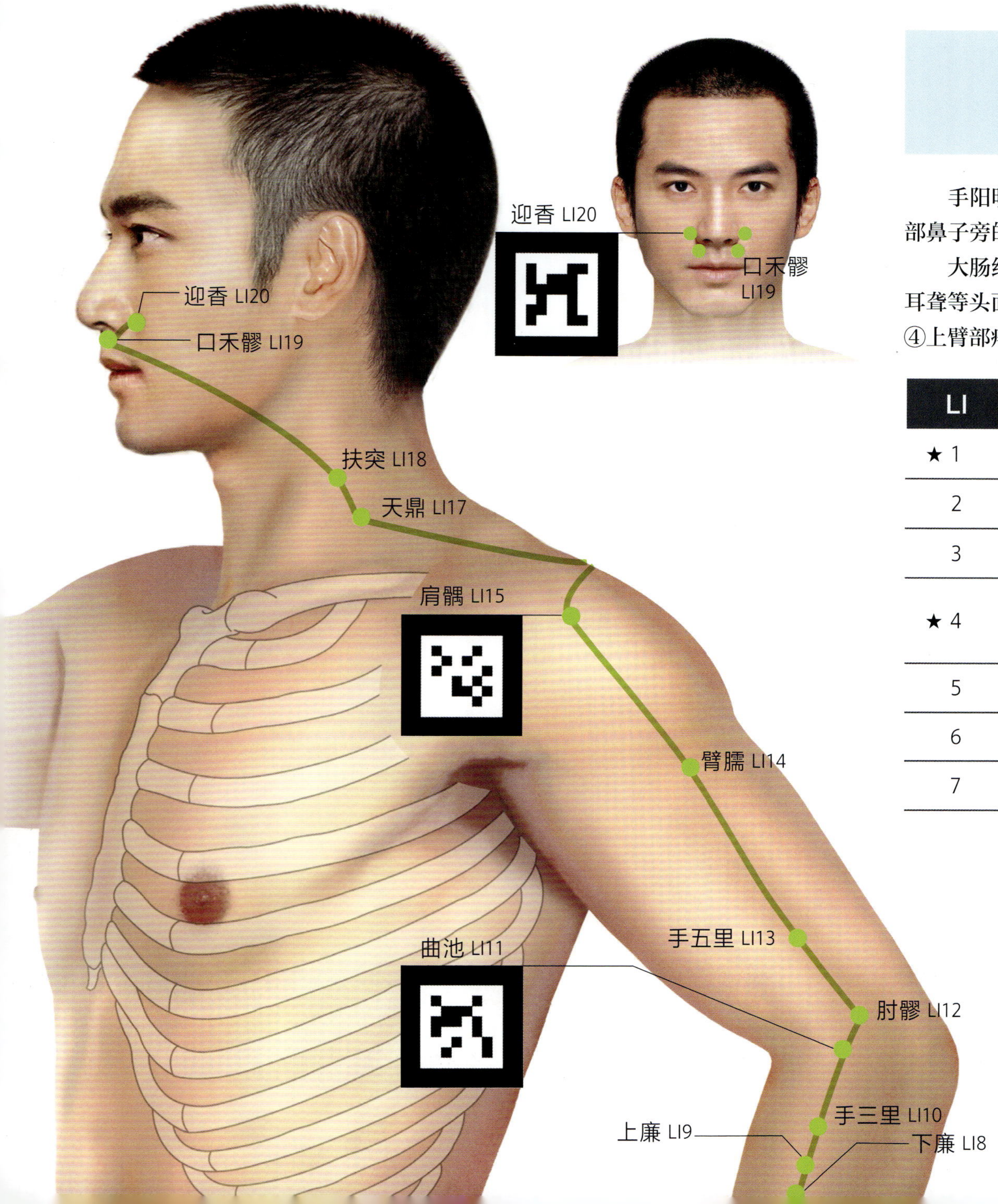

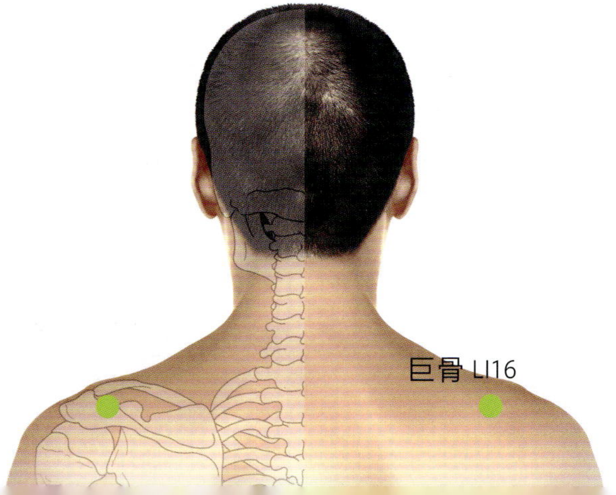

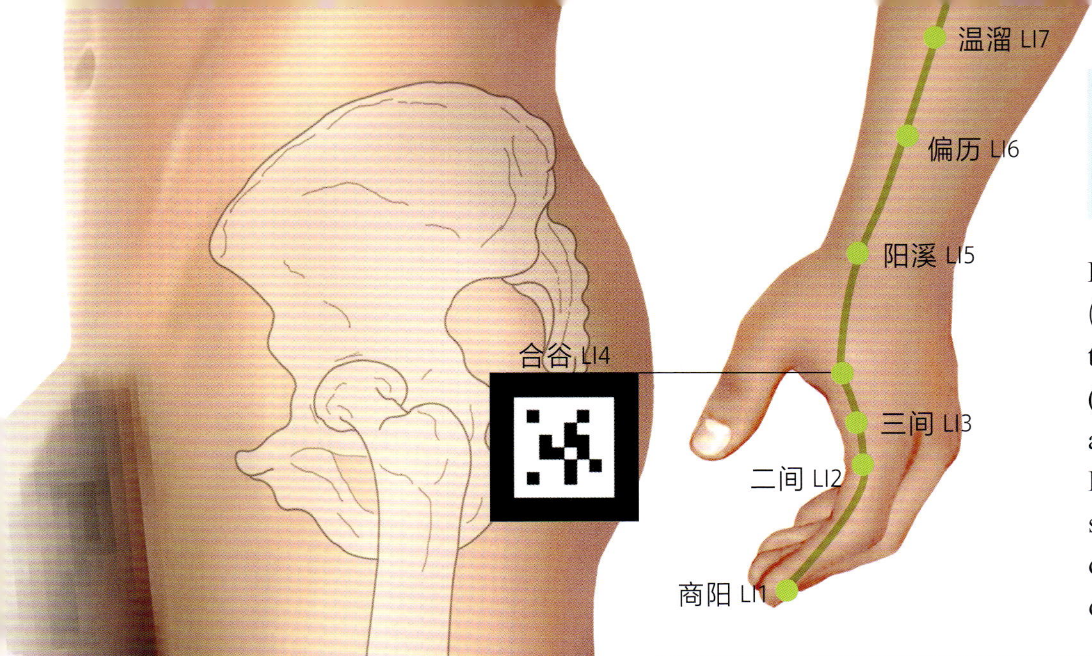

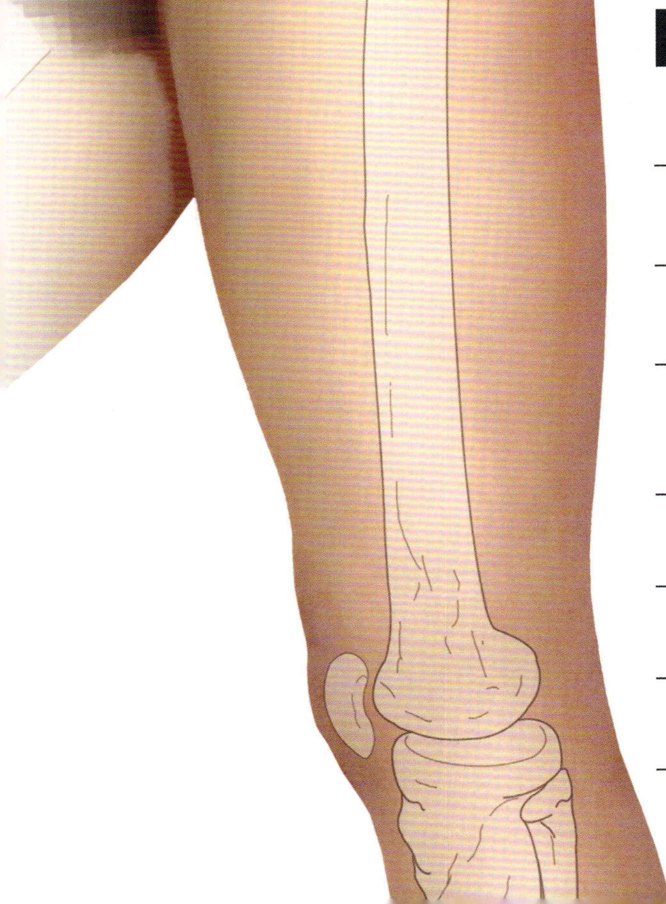

Large Intestine Meridian of Hand-Yangming, LI.

Large Intestine Meridian originates from the tip of the index finger (Shangyang acupoint), proceeds along the lateral side of the arm, passes through the highest point of the shoulder and ends at the side of the nose (Yingxiang acupoint). There are 20 acupoints in each side of the meridian and 40 acupoints in total.

Large Intestine Meridian indications: ①HEENT diseases including red eye, swelling and pain in the throat, toothache, deviation of mouth, tinnitus and deafness. ② Heat diseases including heat stroke and fever. ③ Any pain or discomfort on pathway of the meridian.

LI	Acupoints	Indications
★ 1	Shāngyáng	Swelling and pain in the throat; toothache; tinnitus; heat disease; finger numbness
2	Èrjiān	Swelling and pain in the throat; toothache; eyes pain; nose bleeding; heat disease
3	Sānjiān	Eyes pain; swelling and pain in the throat; toothache; fever; swelling and pain on the dorsum of the hand
★ 4	Hégǔ	Headache; toothache; swelling and pain in the throat; deviation of mouth; sudden deafness; dystocia; amenorrhea; constipation; pain and motor impairment in upper limbs
5	Yángxī	Headache; redness, swelling and pain of eyes; toothache; swelling and pain in throat; wrist pain
6	Piānlì	Red eye; deafness, nose bleeding; pain in the throat; edema; arm soreness and pain
7	Wēnliū	Headache; facial edema; swelling and pain in the throat; abdominal pain; soreness and pain in the shoulder and the back

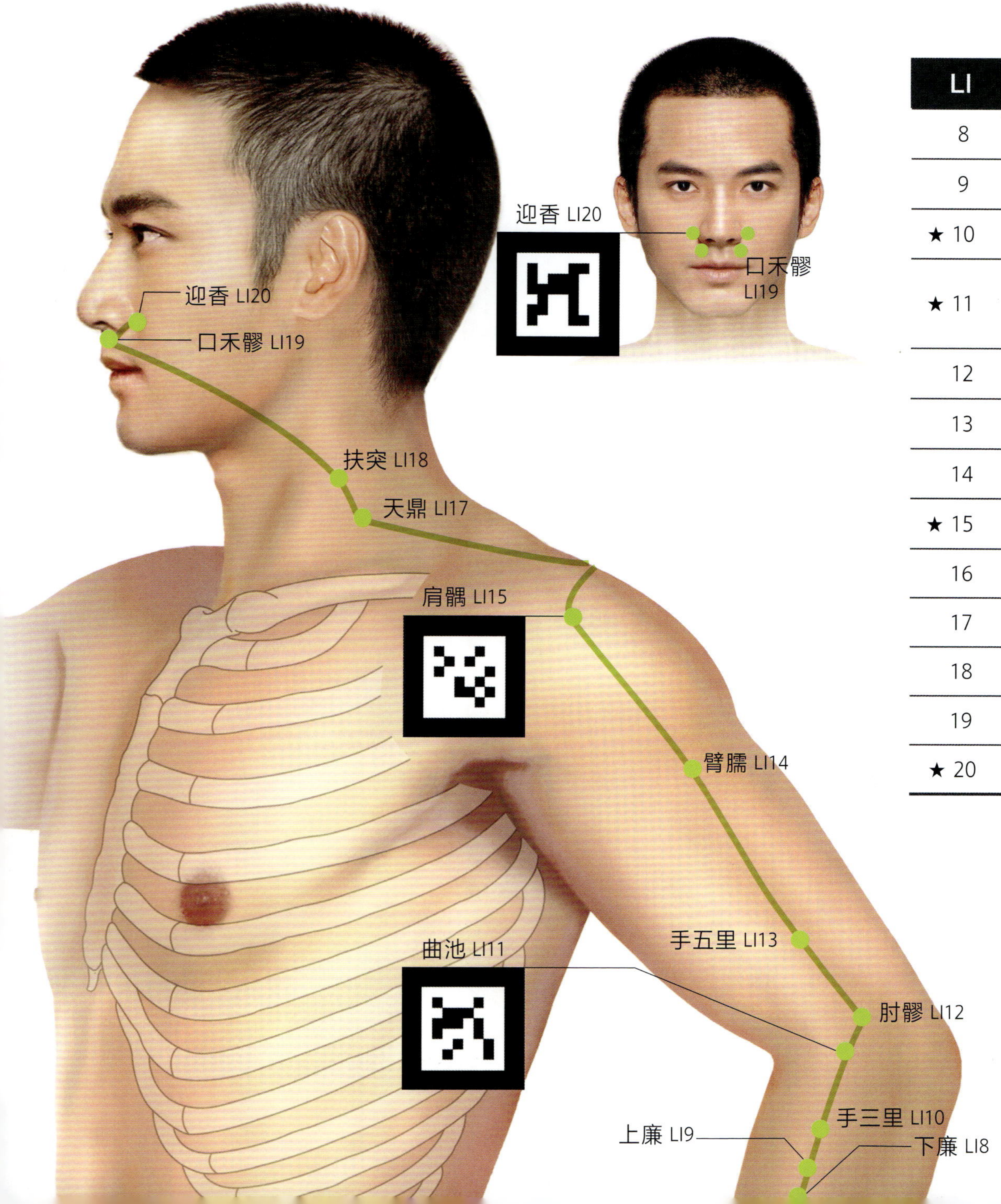

续表

LI	穴名	主治
8	下廉	头痛、眩晕、目痛、腹胀、腹痛、肘臂痛
9	上廉	手臂麻木、肩臂酸痛、半身不遂、腹痛肠鸣
★ 10	手三里	肩臂麻痛、上肢不遂、腹痛、腹泻、齿痛颊肿
★ 11	曲池	热病、咽喉肿痛、齿痛、目赤痛、头痛、眩晕、癫狂、肘臂疼痛、腹痛、青春痘（痤疮）
12	肘髎	肘臂酸痛、麻木、挛急
13	手五里	肘臂挛痛
14	臂臑	肩臂痛
★ 15	肩髃	上肢不遂、肩周炎
16	巨骨	肩臂挛痛不遂
17	天鼎	咽喉肿痛、失音
18	扶突	咽喉肿痛、失音、咳嗽气喘
19	口禾髎	鼻塞、鼻出血、口㖞
★ 20	迎香	鼻炎、口㖞、胆道蛔虫病

★为本经常用穴

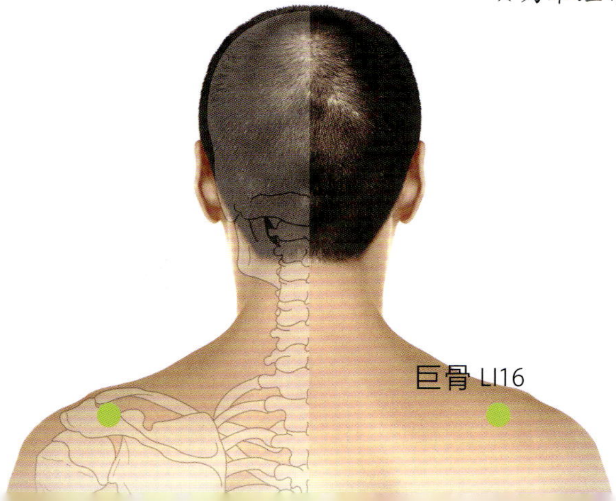

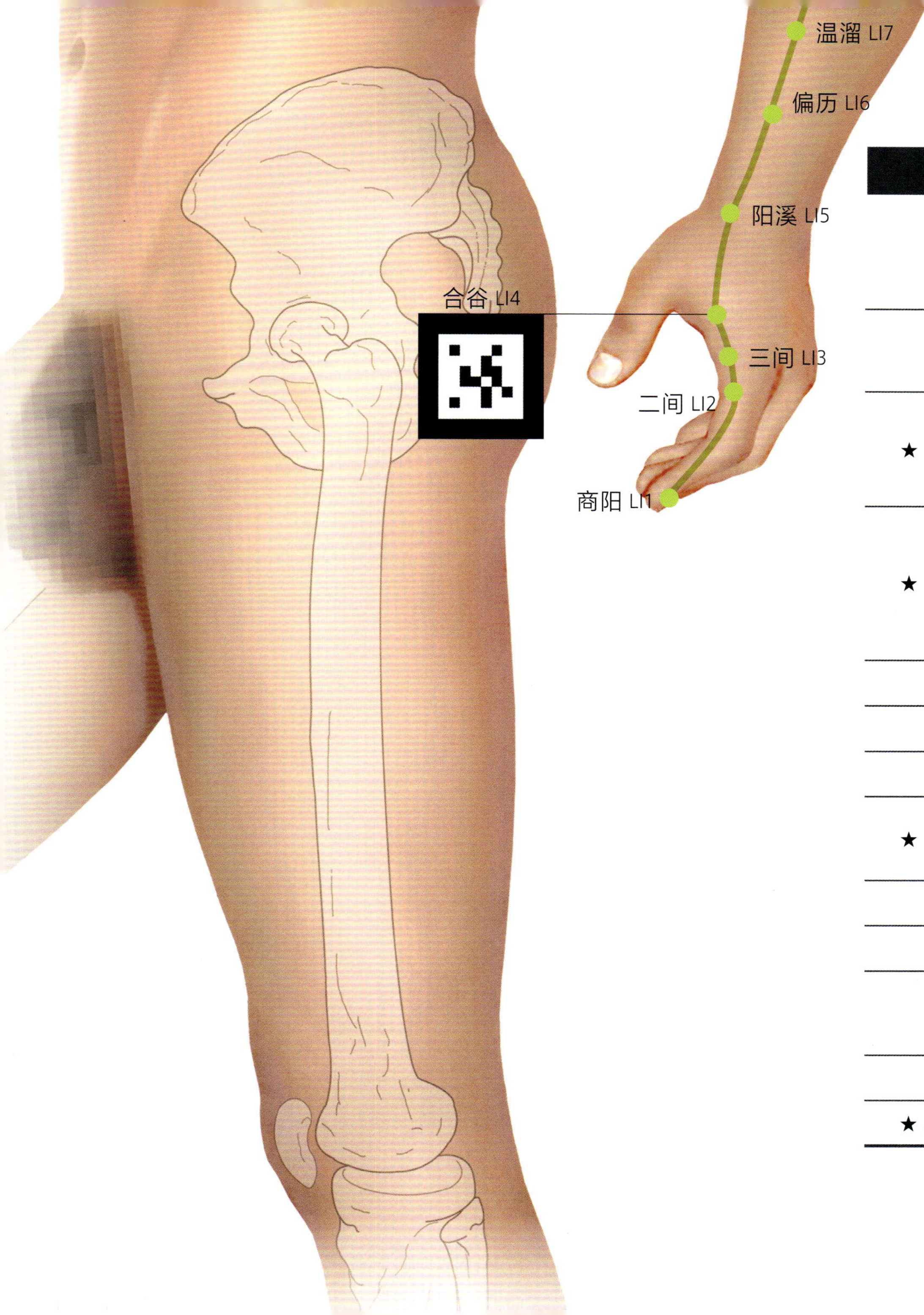

Continued

LI	Acupoints	Indications
8	Xiàlián	Headache; dizziness; eyes pain; abdominal distension; abdominal pain; pain in the elbow and the shoulder
9	Shànglián	Arm numbness; shoulder soreness; hemiplegia; abdominal pain and borborygmus
★ 10	Shǒusānlǐ	Shoulder numbness and pain; motor impairment in upper limbs; abdominal pain; diarrhea; toothache and facial swelling
★ 11	Qūchí	Heat disease; swelling and pain in the throat; toothache; redness and pain in eyes; headache; dizziness; manic-depressive psychosis; elbow pain; abdominal pain; acne
12	Zhǒuliáo	Soreness and pain in elbow; numbness; spasm
13	Shǒuwǔlǐ	Spasm and pain in elbow and arm
14	Bìnào	Pain in shoulder and upper limbs
★ 15	Jiānyú	Motor impairment in upper limbs; periarthritis of shoulder
16	Jùgǔ	Spasm and pain in the shoulder
17	Tiāndǐng	Swelling and pain in the throat; aphonia
18	Fútū	Swelling and pain in the throat; aphonia; cough and asthma
19	Kǒuhéliáo	Rhinobyon; nose bleeding; deviation of mouth
★ 20	Yíngxiāng	Rhinitis; deviation of mouth; biliary ascariasis

★ Common acupoint used in treatment

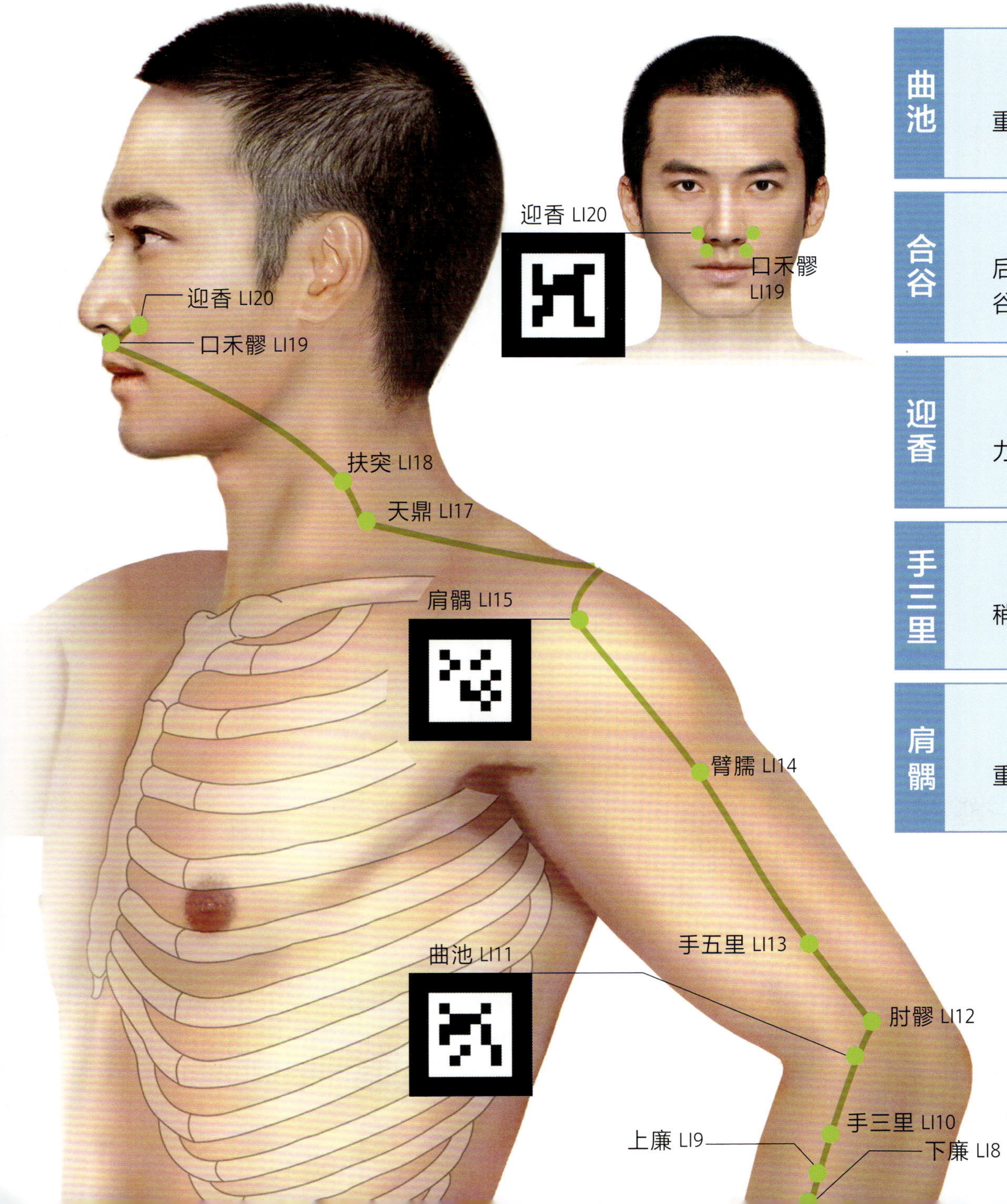

曲池

用拇指按揉曲池穴 2 分钟，力度稍重。同法按揉对侧曲池穴。

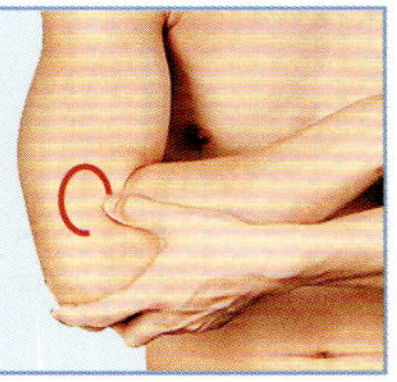

合谷

用拇指用力按压合谷穴，停留片刻后放松，反复 5~6 下。同法按压对侧合谷穴。

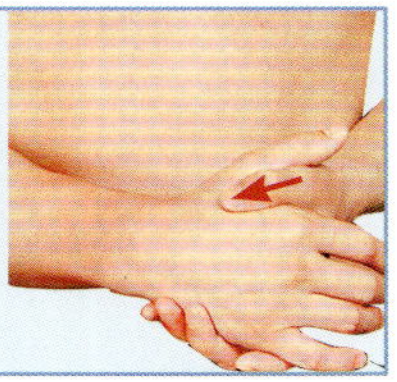

迎香

用两手食指按揉两侧迎香穴2分钟，力度稍重。

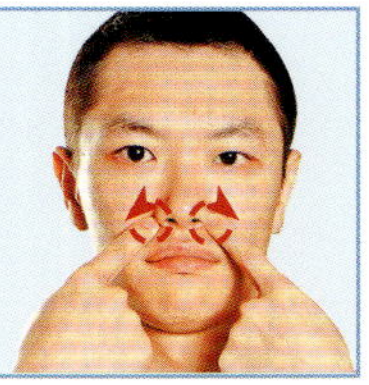

手三里

用拇指按揉手三里穴 2 分钟，力度稍重。同法按揉对侧手三里穴。

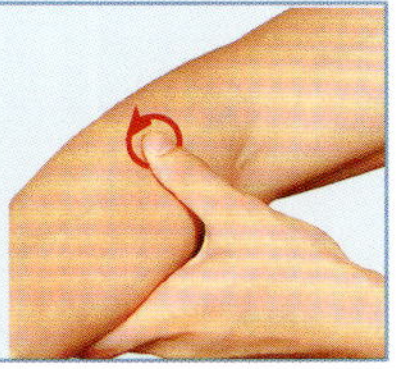

肩髃

用拇指按揉肩髃穴 2 分钟，力度稍重。同法按揉对侧肩髃穴。

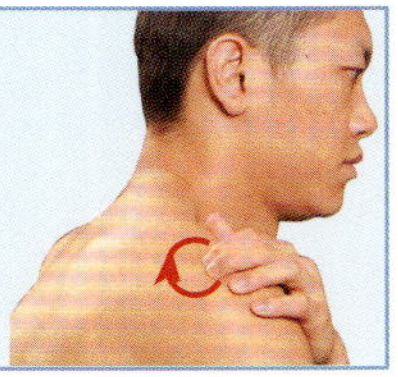

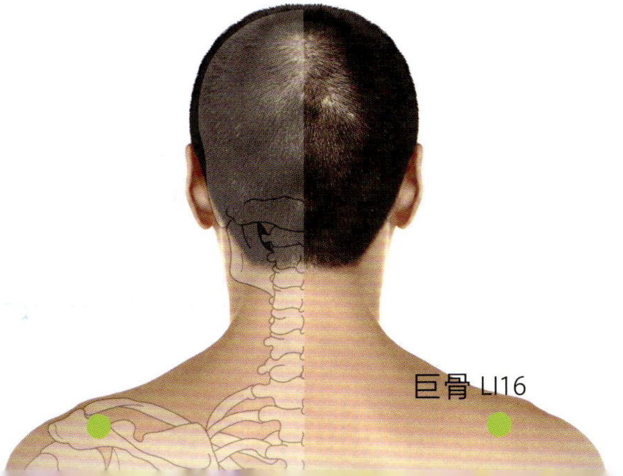

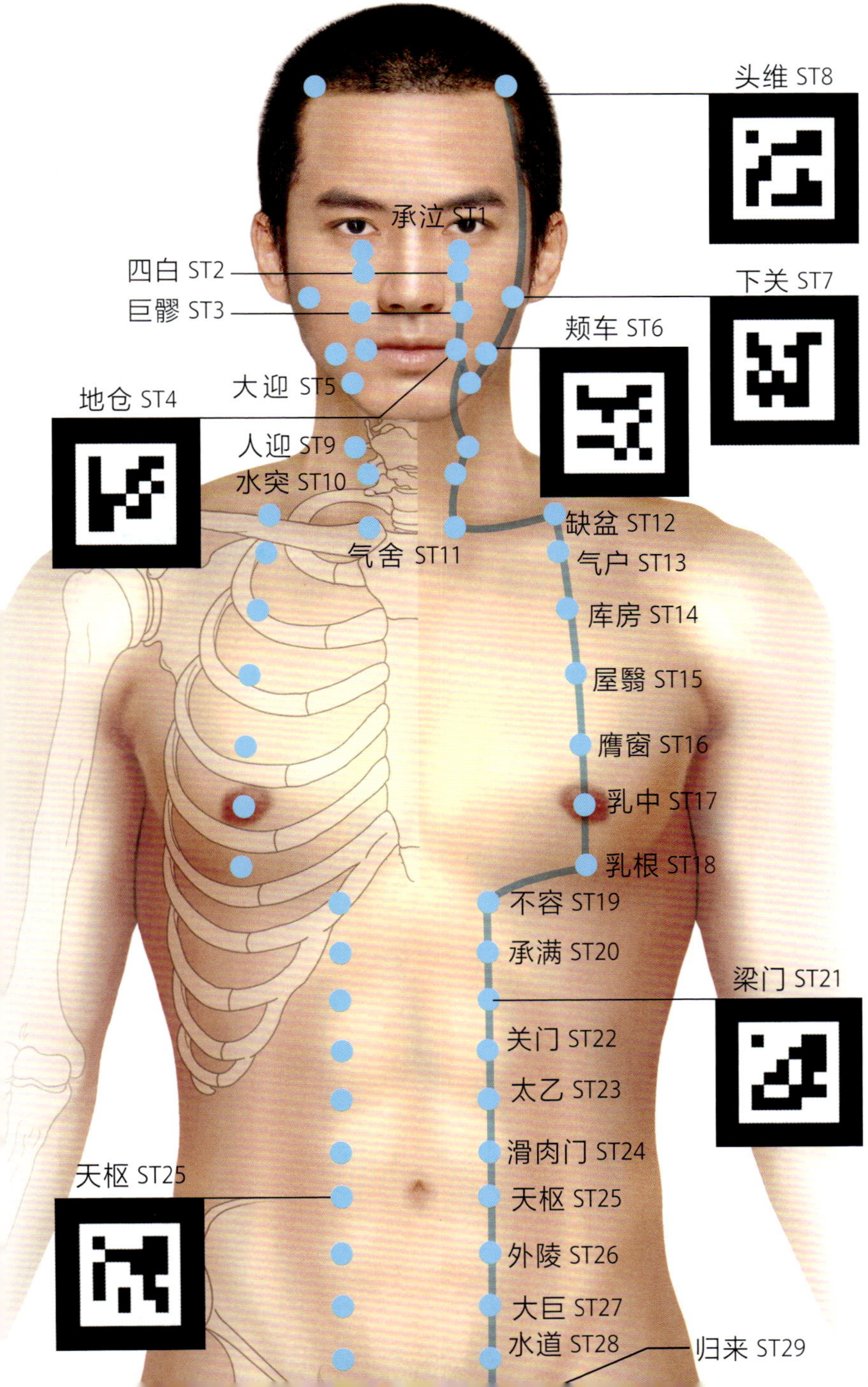

足阳明胃经

足阳明胃经起于头部，往下经过胸部、腹部、下肢外侧前缘达到脚背。本经一侧 45 穴，左右两侧共 90 穴。

胃经主治病症：①呕吐、腹胀、腹痛、水肿、食欲不振等肠胃疾病。②目赤、咽喉肿痛、齿痛、口歪、耳鸣、耳聋等头面五官疾患。③昏厥（昏迷）、癫狂、中风等神经精神系统疾病。④咳嗽、气喘、膝关节肿痛等经脉循行部位的疾患。⑤部分腧穴有强身健体的作用，常用于日常保健。

ST	穴名	主治
1	承泣	目赤肿痛、流泪、近视、眼睑抽动、面瘫、面肌痉挛
2	四白	目赤肿痛、眼睑瞤动（跳动）、近视、面瘫、胆道蛔虫病、头痛、眩晕
3	巨髎	面痛、齿痛、眼睑瞤动、面瘫
★ 4	地仓	面瘫、面肌痉挛、眼睑瞤动
5	大迎	颊肿、齿痛、面瘫、口噤
★ 6	颊车	面瘫、颊肿、齿痛、口噤不语、颞下颌关节炎
★ 7	下关	耳鸣、耳聋、齿痛、面瘫、颞下颌关节炎
★ 8	头维	头痛、眩晕、目痛、眼睑瞤动、老年痴呆（现代医学称“阿尔茨海默病”）

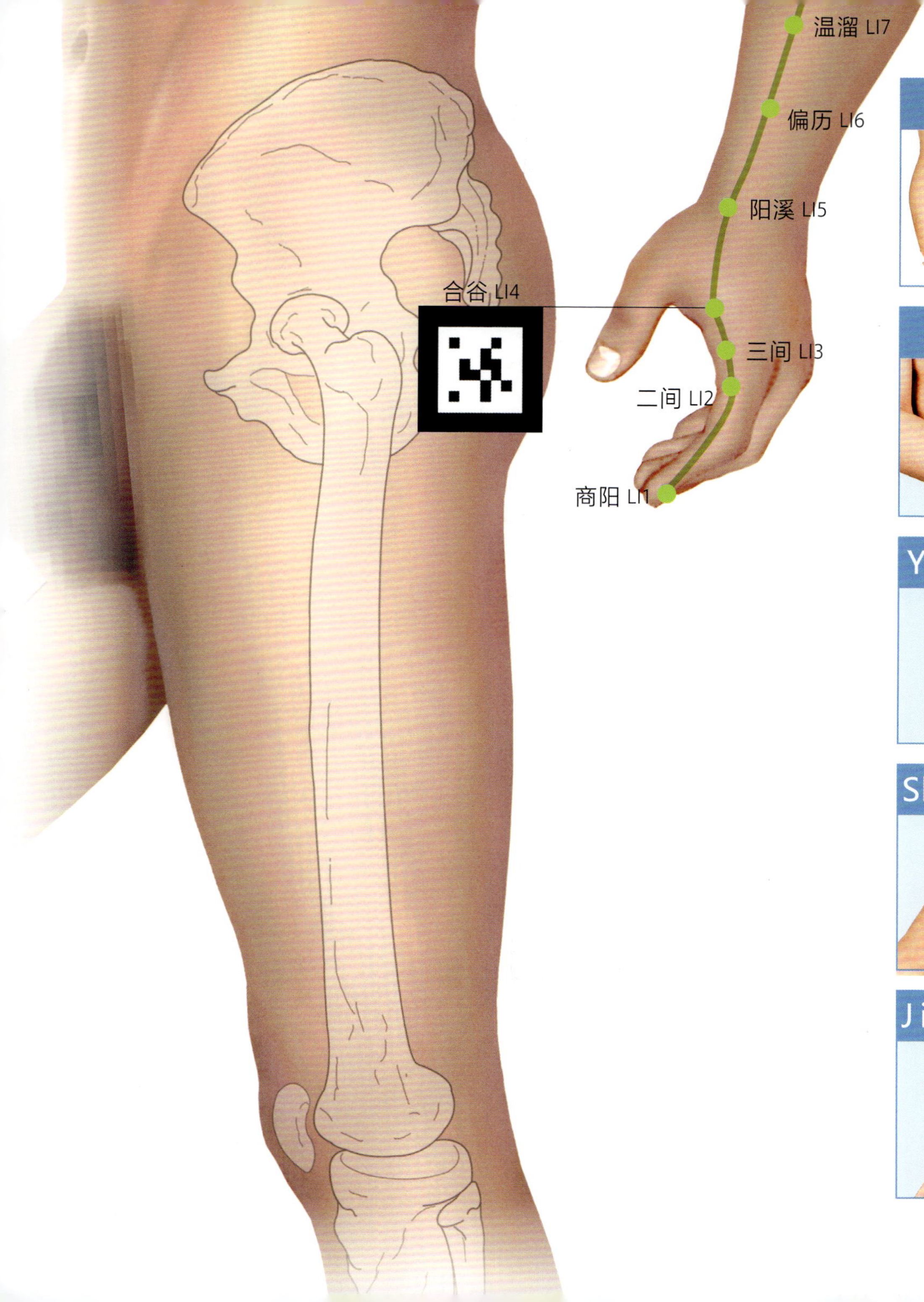

Qūchí(LI11)

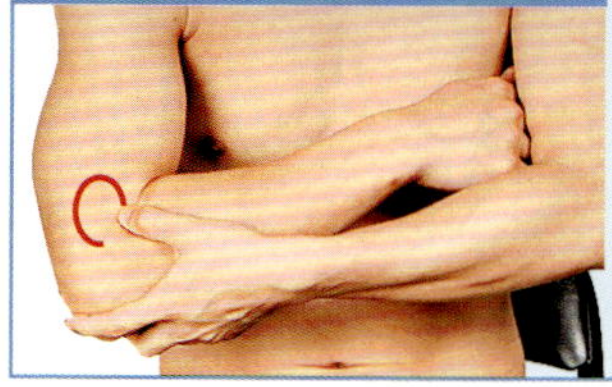

Use the thumb to knead the acupoint for 2 minutes with a little heavy strength. Knead the contralateral acupoint with the same method.

Hégǔ(LI4)

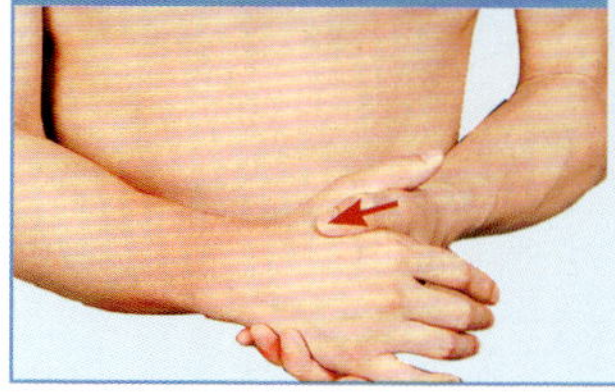

Use the thumb to press the acupoint for a minute and then relax, repeat 5~6 times. Press the contralateral acupoint with the same method.

Yíngxiāng(LI20)

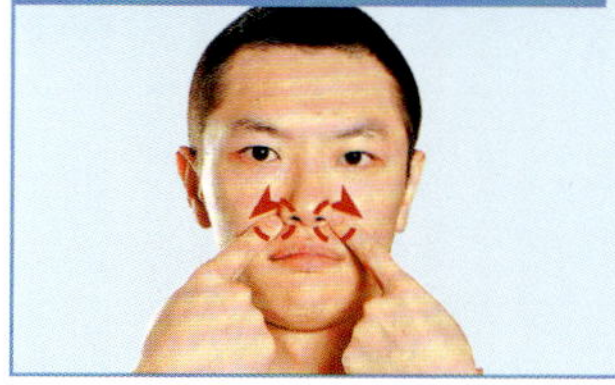

Use both index fingers to knead the acupoints of both sides with a little heavy strength for 2 minutes. Knead the contralateral acupoint with the same method.

Shǒusānlǐ(LI10)

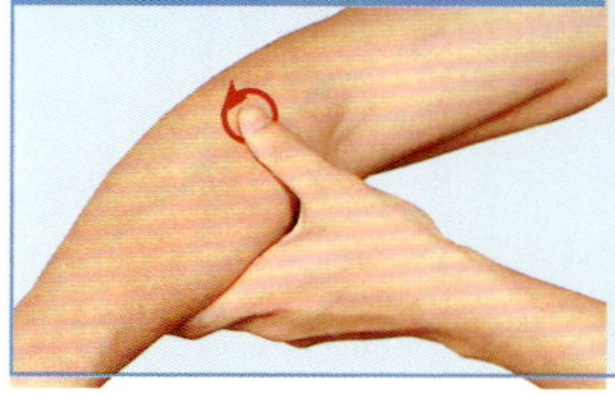

Use the thumb to knead the acupoint for 2 minutes with a little heavy strength. Knead the contralateral acupoint with the same method.

Jiānyú(LI15)

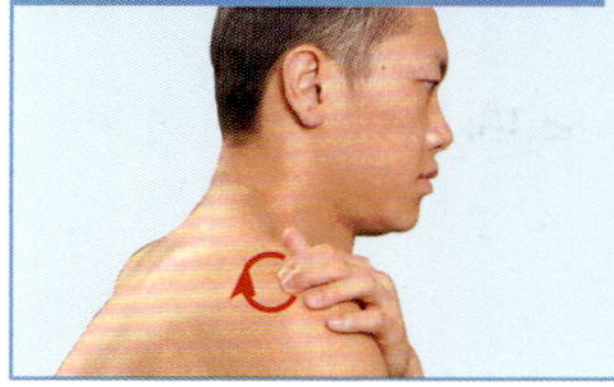

Use the thumb to knead the acupoint for 2 minutes with a little heavy strength.Knead the contralateral acupoint with the same method.

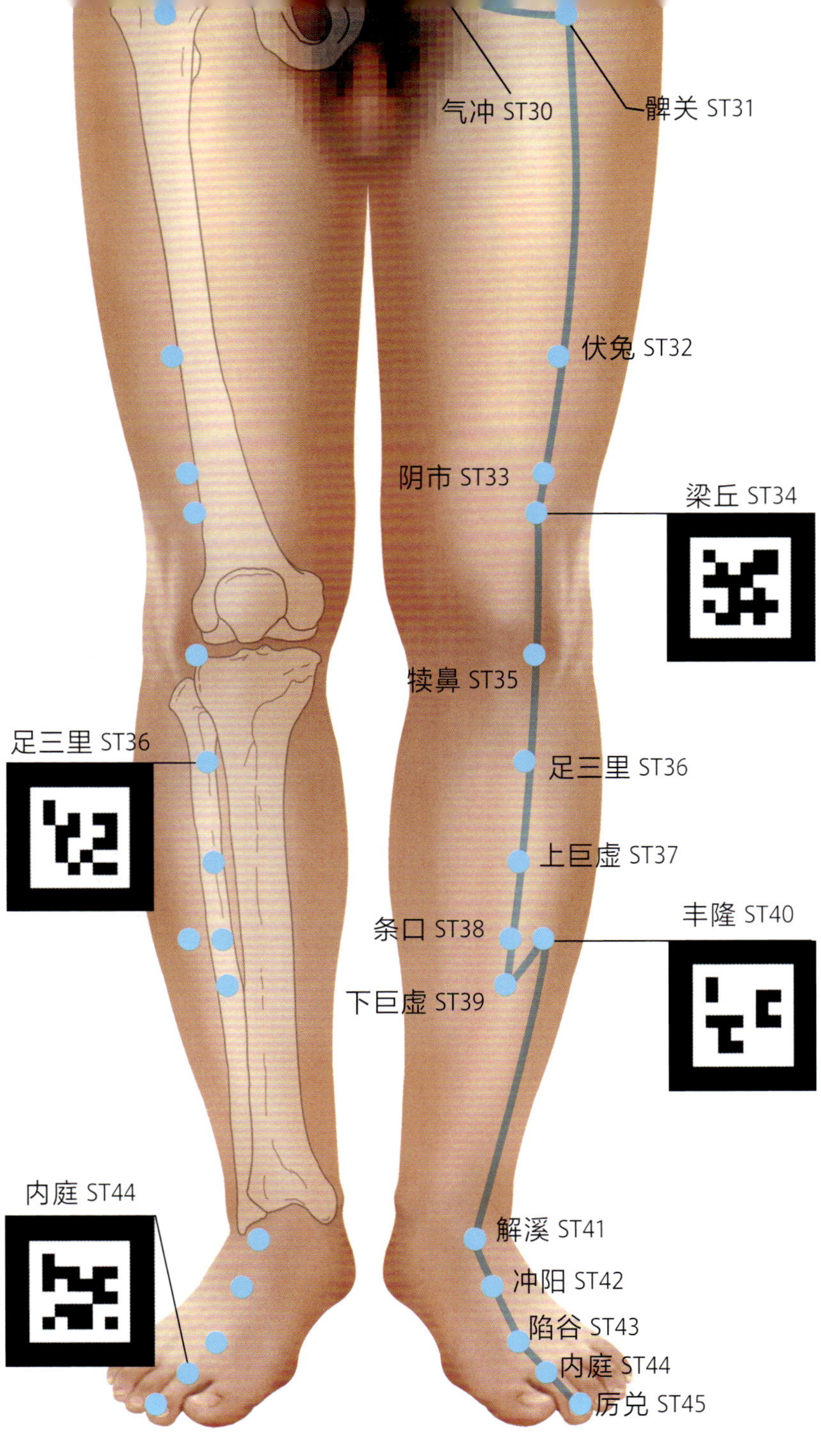

Stomach Meridian of Foot-Yangming,ST.

Stomach Meridian of Foot-Yangming originates from the head, it passes downward through the chest, abdomen and anterolateral aspect of the lower limb and ends on the dorsum of the foot. There are 45 acupoints in each side of the meridian and 90 acupoints in total.

The Stomach Meridian indications: ① Gastrointestinal diseases including vomiting, abdominal distension, abdominal pain, edema and poor appetite. ② HEENT diseases including red eye, swelling and pain in the throat, toothache, deviation of mouth, tinnitus and deafness. ③ Nervous system diseases including coma, manic-depressive psychosis and wind stroke. ④ Any disease on the pathway of the meridian including cough, asthma, swelling and pain of knees. ⑤ Some acupoints have the function of keeping health to the body.

ST	Acupoints	Indications
1	Chéngqì	Redness, swelling and pain in eyes; lacrimation; myopia; eyelid twitching; facial paralysis; spasm of the facial muscle
2	Sìbái	Redness, swelling and pain in eyes; eyelid twitching; myopia; facial paralysis; biliary ascariasis; headache; dizziness
3	Jùliáo	Facial pain; toothache; eyelid twitching; facial paralysis
★ 4	Dìcāng	Facial spasm; facial paralysis; eyelid twitching
5	Dàyíng	Cheek swelling; toothache; facial paralysis; lockjaw
★ 6	Jiáchē	Facial paralysis; cheek swelling; toothache; lockjaw; arthritis of temporomandibular joint
★ 7	Xiàguān	Tinnitus; deafness; toothache; facial paralysis; arthritis of temporomandibular joint
★ 8	Tóuwéi	Headache; dizziness; eyes pain; eyelid twitching; alzheimer's disease

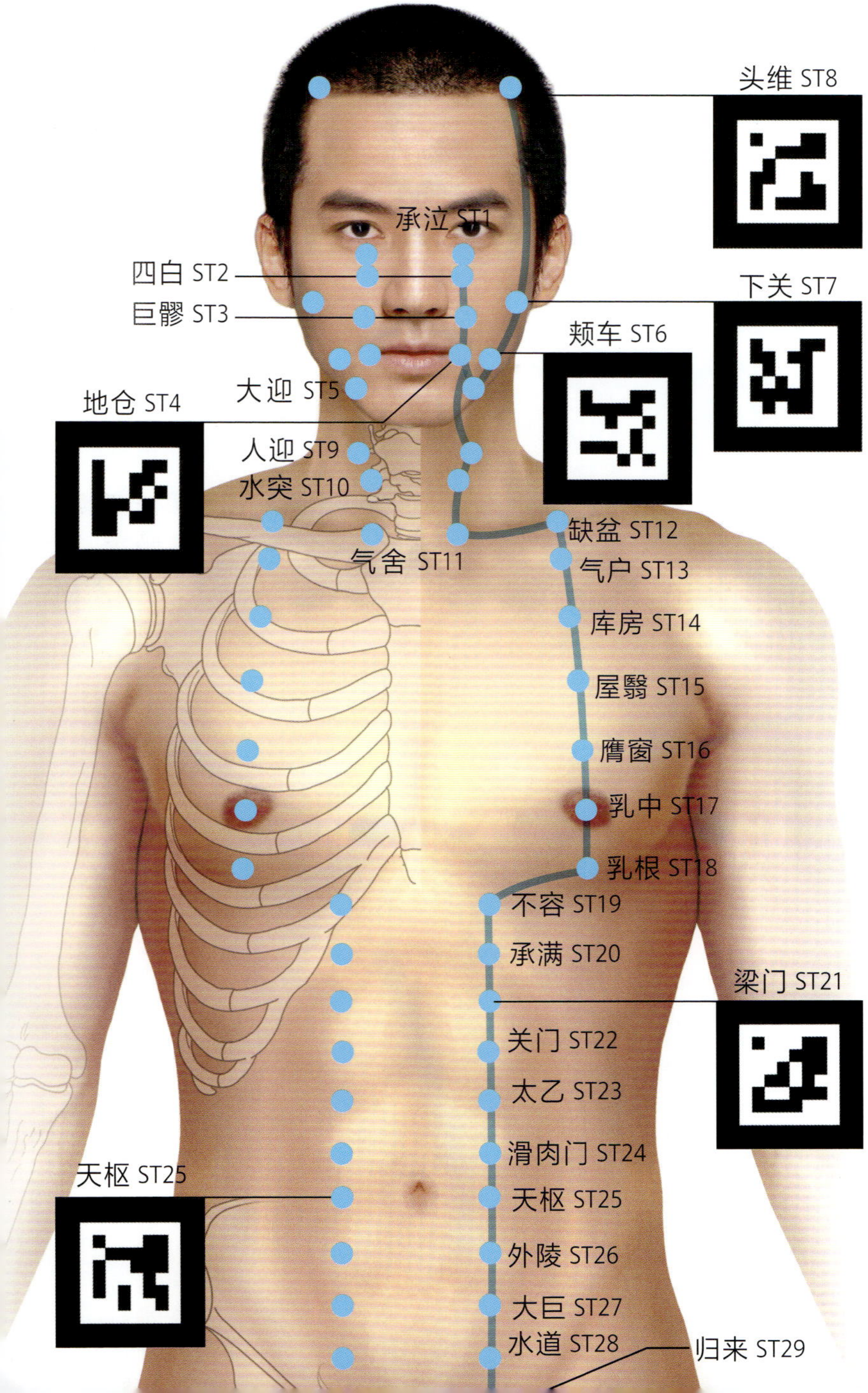

续表

ST	穴名	主治
9	人迎	咽喉肿痛、胸满喘息、头痛、眩晕、高血压、低血压
10	水突	咳嗽、气喘、咽喉肿痛
11	气舍	咳嗽、气喘、呃逆（胃气冲逆而上、呃呃有声）、咽喉肿痛、颈项强痛（僵硬疼痛）
12	缺盆	咳嗽、气喘、咽喉肿痛、颈肿
13	气户	咳嗽、气喘、呃逆、胸胁胀满
14	库房	咳嗽、气喘、呃逆、胸胁胀满
15	屋翳	咳嗽、气喘、呃逆、胸胁胀满、乳腺炎
16	膺窗	咳嗽、气喘、呃逆、胸胁胀满、乳腺炎
17	乳中	只作为定位标志，不宜施针法、灸法
18	乳根	咳嗽、气喘、胸闷、胸痛、乳腺炎、乳少
19	不容	呕吐、胃痛、腹胀、食欲不振
20	承满	呕吐、胃痛、腹胀、食欲不振、吐血
21	梁门	胃痛、呕吐、腹胀、食欲不振、泄泻

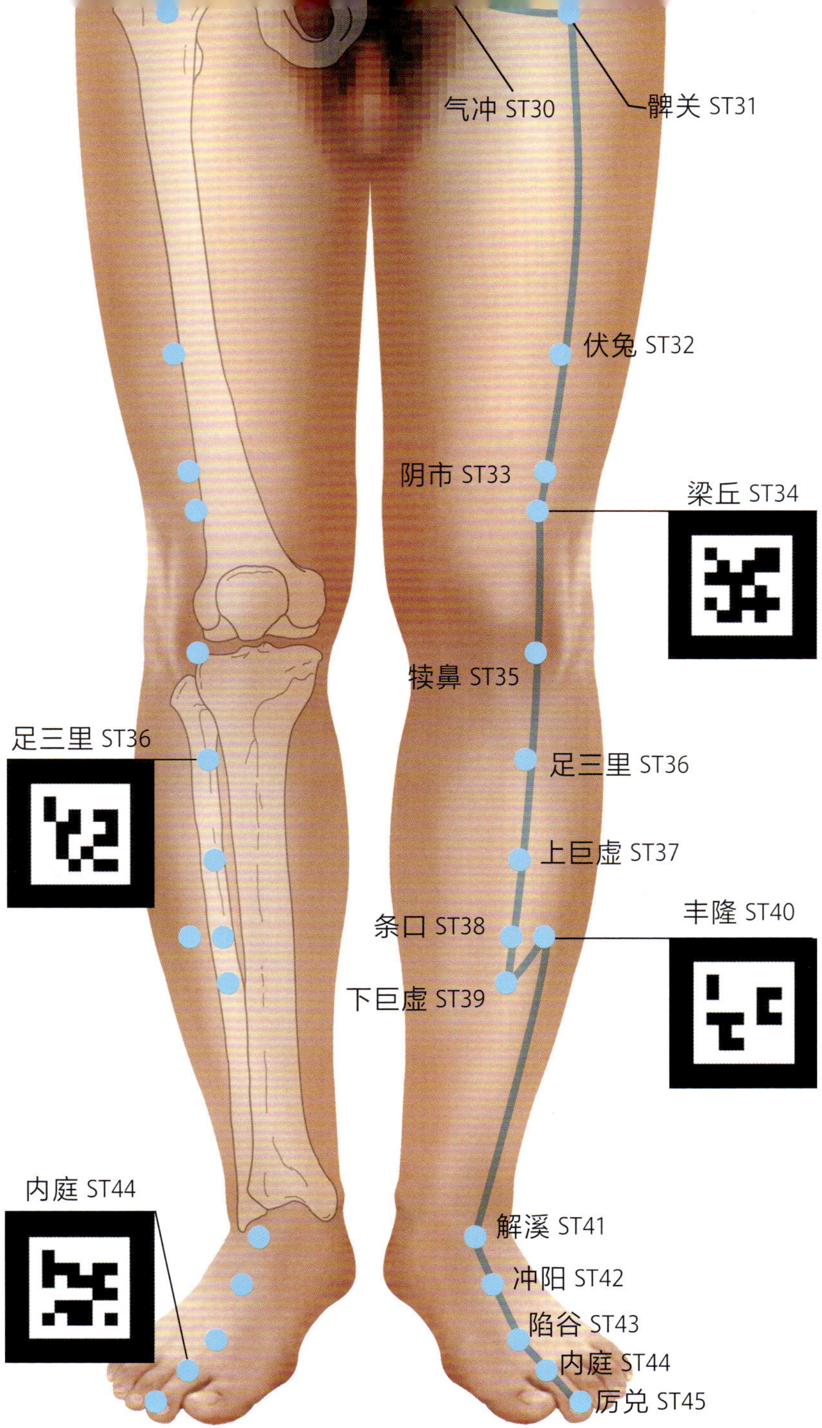

Continued

ST	Acupoints	Indications
9	Rényíng	Swelling and pain in the throat; fullness in the chest and asthma; headache; dizziness; hypertension; hypotension
10	Shuǐtū	Cough; asthma; swelling and pain in the throat
11	Qìshè	Cough; asthma; hiccup; swelling and pain in the throat; neck stiffness and pain
12	Quēpén	Cough; asthma; swelling and pain in the throat; neck swelling
13	Qìhù	Cough; asthma; hiccup; distension in the chest and the hypochondrium
14	Kùfáng	Cough; asthma; hiccup; distension in the chest and the hypochondrium
15	Wūyì	Cough; asthma; hiccup; distension in the chest and the hypochondrium; mastitis
16	Yīngchuāng	Cough; asthma; hiccup; distension in the chest and the hypochondrium; mastitis
17	Rǔzhōng	Only used for locating other acupoints,not for acupuncture and moxibustion
18	Rǔgēn	Cough; asthma; chest tightness; chest pain; mastitis; hypogalactia
19	Bùróng	Vomiting; stomachache; abdominal distension; poor appetite
20	Chéngmǎn	Vomiting; stomachache; abdominal distension; poor appetite; hematemesis
21	Liángmén	Stomachache; vomiting; abdominal distension; poor appetite; diarrhea

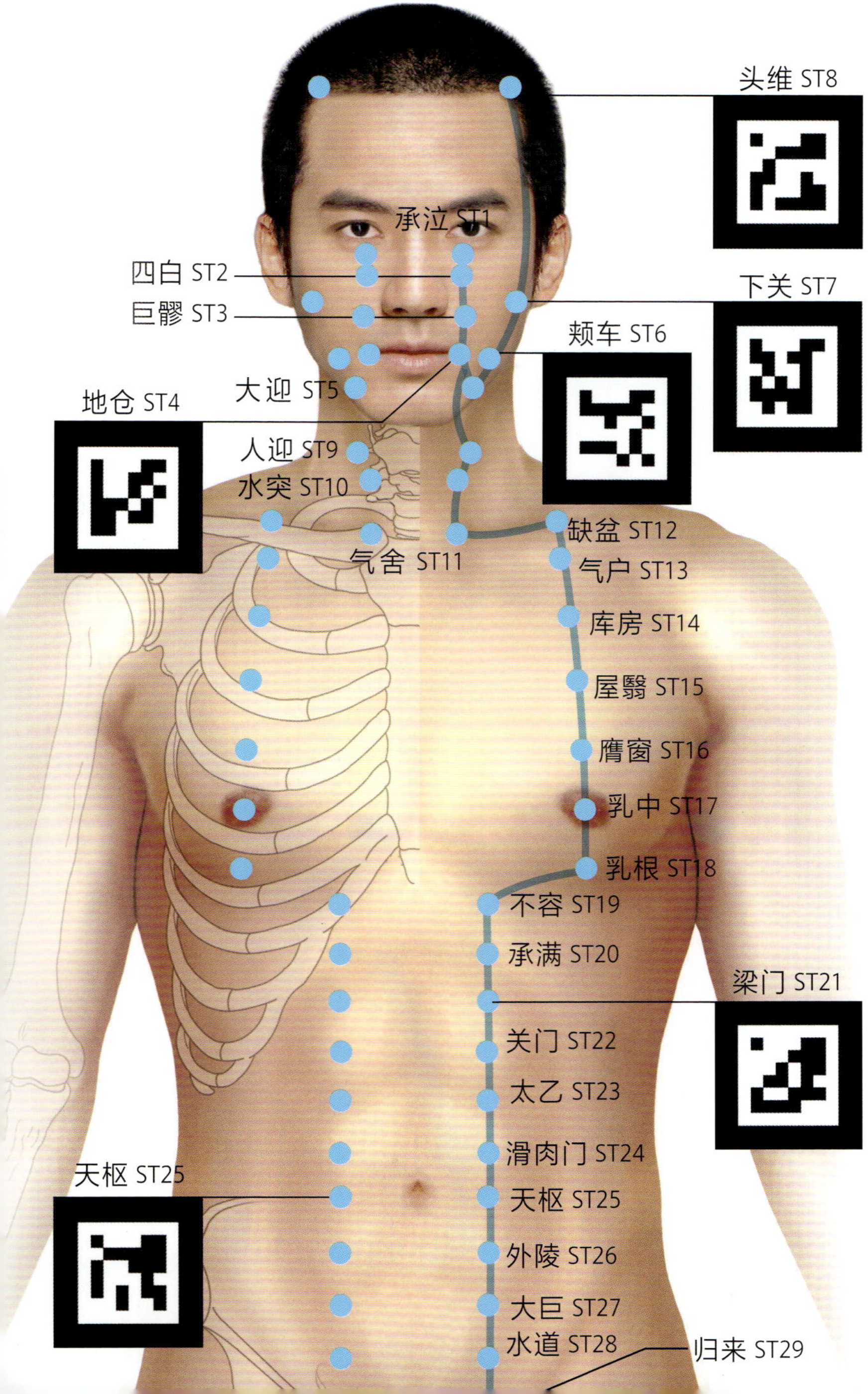

续表

ST	穴名	主治
22	关门	腹痛、腹胀、肠鸣、泄泻、水肿
23	太乙	胃痛、癫狂、心烦
24	滑肉门	胃痛、呕吐、癫狂
★ 25	天枢	腹胀肠鸣、绕脐腹痛、便秘、泄泻、月经不调、痛经、肥胖症
26	外陵	腹痛、痛经、疝气
27	大巨	小腹胀、小便不利、疝气、遗精、早泄
28	水道	水肿、小便不利、小腹胀满、痛经、不育、疝气
29	归来	腹痛、疝气、闭经、月经不调、带下
30	气冲	腹痛、阳痿、疝气、月经不调、不育
31	髀关	下肢痿痹（无力、麻木、疼痛、活动不利）、腰膝冷痛、腹痛
32	伏兔	下肢痿痹、腰膝冷痛、疝气、股外侧皮神经炎
33	阴市	腹胀、腹痛、腿膝冷痛及屈伸不利
★ 34	梁丘	急性胃痛、乳腺炎、膝关节肿痛、下肢不遂
★ 35	犊鼻	膝肿痛

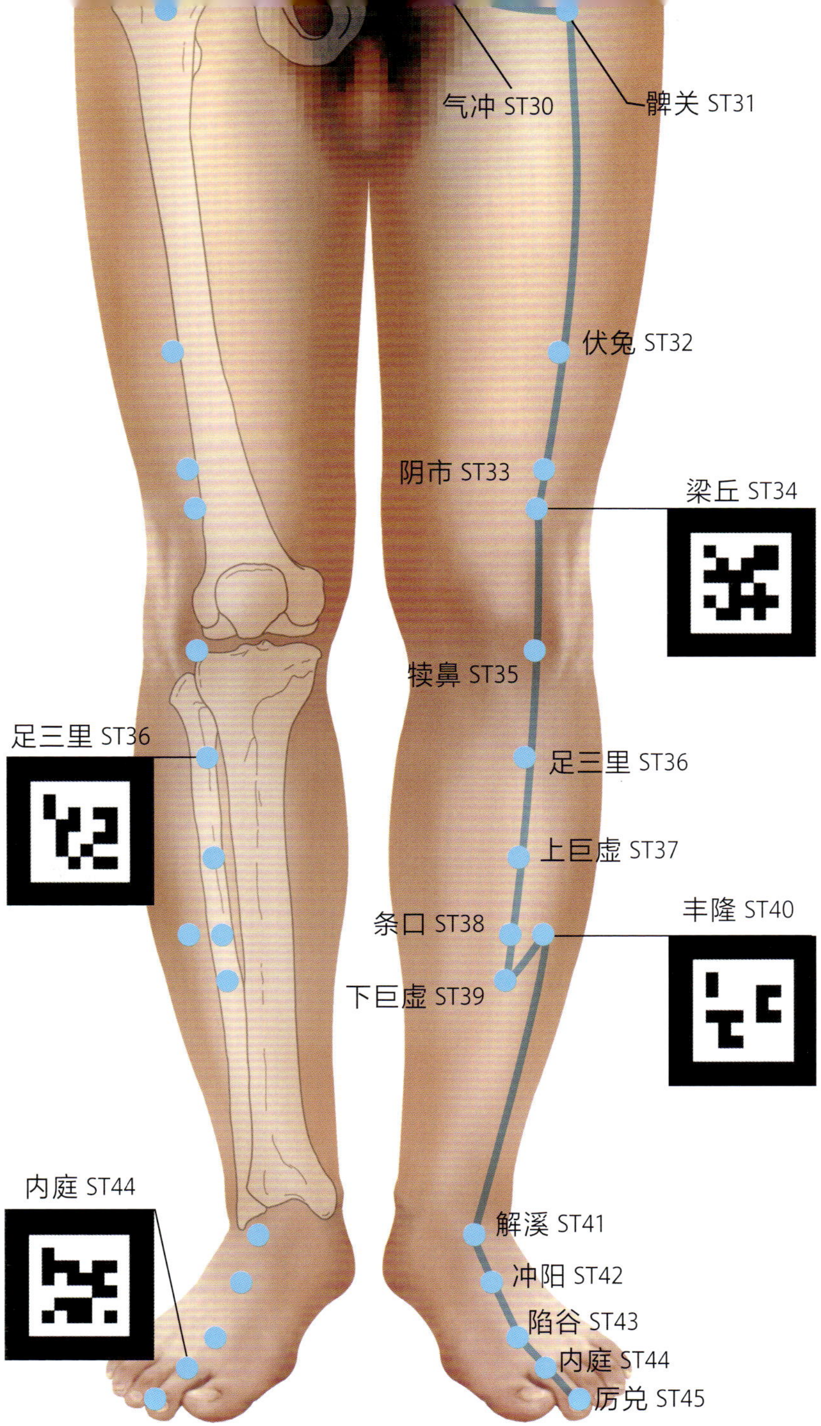

Continued

ST	Acupoints	Indications
22	Guānmén	Abdominal pain; abdominal distension; borborygmus; diarrhea; edema
23	Tàiyǐ	Stomachache; manic-depressive psychosis; vexation
24	Huáròumén	Stomachache; vomiting; manic-depressive psychosis
★ 25	Tiānshū	Abdominal distension and borborygmus; paraumbilical pain; constipation; diarrhea; irregular menstruation; dysmenorrhea; obesity
26	Wàilíng	Abdominal pain; dysmenorrhea; hernia
27	Dàjù	Lower abdomen distension; dysuria; hernia; spermatorrhea; prospermia
28	Shuǐdào	Edema; dysuria; lower abdomen distension; dysmenorrhea; infertility; hernia
29	Guīlái	Abdominal pain; hernia; amenorrhea; irregular menstruation; leukorrheal diseases
30	Qìchōng	Abdominal pain; erectile dysfunction; hernia; irregular menstruation; infertility
31	Bìguān	Flaccidity and motor impairment in the lower limb (numbness,pain,atony); coldness and pain of the waist and the knee,abdominal pain
32	Fútù	Flaccidity and motor impairment in the lower limb; coldness and pain of the waist and the knee; hernia; lateral femoral cutaneous neuritis
33	Yīnshì	Abdominal pain; abdominal distension; coldness and pain of knees and legs; difficulty in bending and stretching
★ 34	Liángqiū	Acute stomachache; mastitis; swelling and pain of knee joint; motor impairment in lower limbs
★ 35	Dúbí	Swelling and pain of knee joint

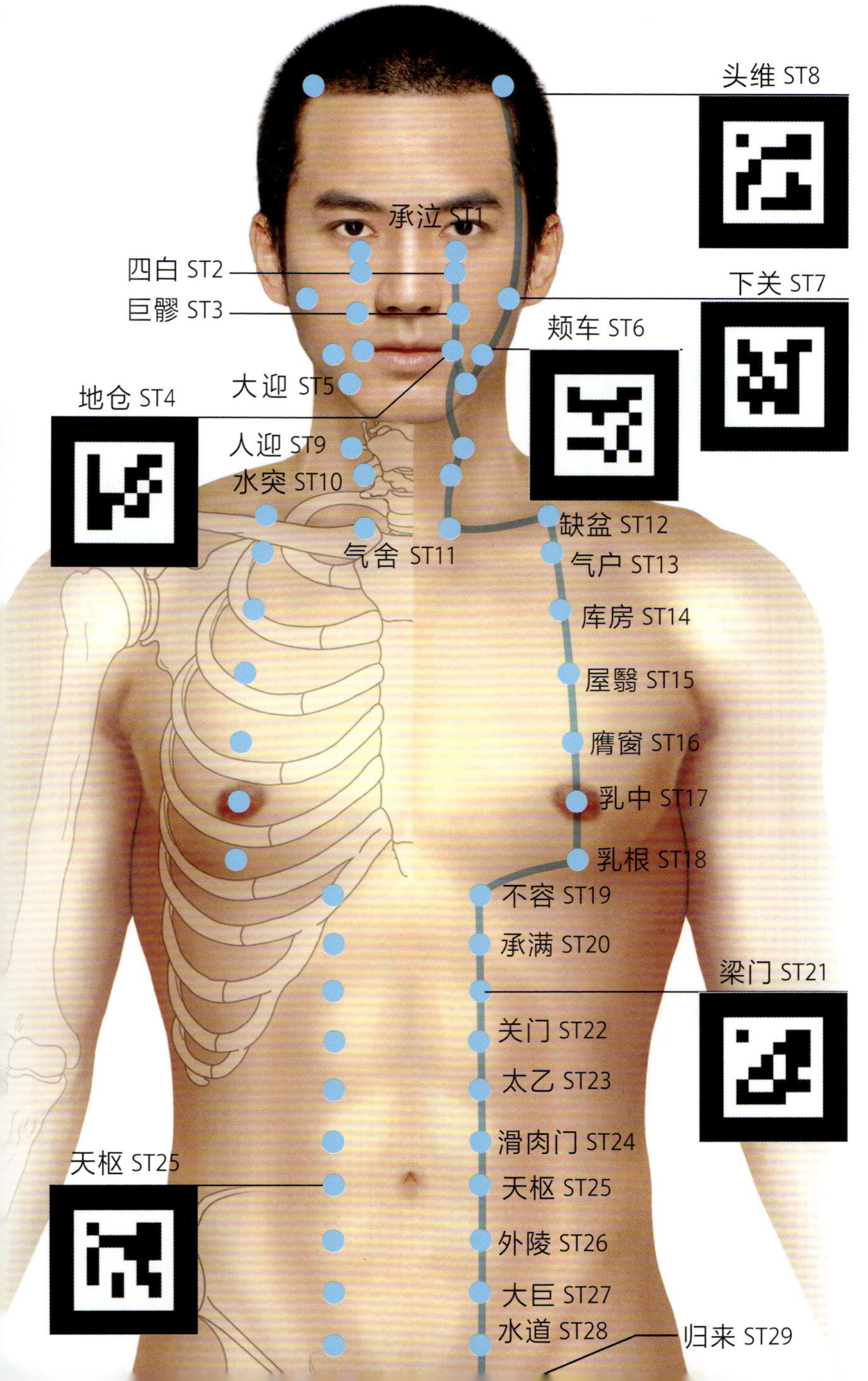

续表

ST	穴名	主治
★ 36	足三里	胃痛、呕吐、呃逆、腹胀腹痛、肠鸣、消化不良、泄泻、便秘、胃下垂、体虚、咳嗽气喘、心悸气短、头晕、失眠、癫狂、膝痛、下肢痿痹、水肿
37	上巨虚	腹胀、腹痛、泄泻、便秘、下肢痿痹
★ 38	条口	下肢痿痹、下肢浮肿、肩臂痛
39	下巨虚	小腹痛、泄泻、乳腺炎、下肢痿痹
★ 40	丰隆	咳嗽、气喘、哮喘、头痛、眩晕、癫狂、下肢痿痹
41	解溪	头痛、眩晕、癫狂、腹胀、便秘、下肢痿痹、足踝肿痛
42	冲阳	胃痛、腹胀、面瘫、足背肿痛无力
43	陷谷	目赤肿痛、面部浮肿、足背肿痛
★ 44	内庭	齿痛、咽喉肿痛、面瘫、热病、腹痛、腹胀、便秘、足背肿痛
45	厉兑	齿痛、咽喉肿痛、面瘫、热病、癫狂、鼻出血、足背肿痛

★为本经常用穴

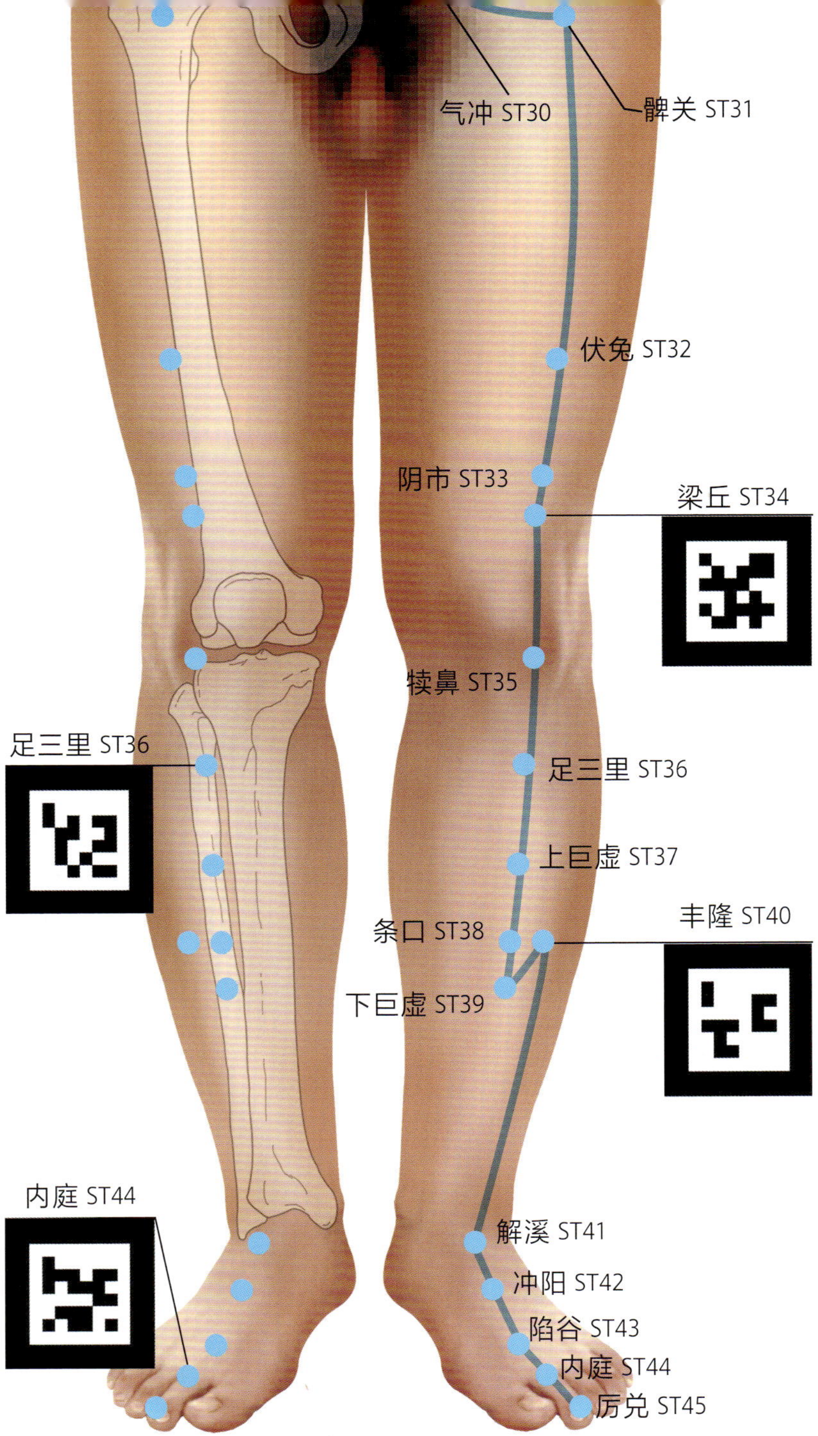

Continued

ST	Acupoints	Indications
★ 36	Zúsānlǐ	Stomachache; vomiting; hiccup; abdominal distension and pain; borborygmus; dyspepsia; diarrhea; constipation; gastroptosis; weakness; cough and asthma; palpitation and short-breath; dizziness; insomnia; manic-depressive psychosis; knee pain; flaccidity and motor impairment of lower limbs; edema
37	Shàngjùxū	Abdominal pain and distension; diarrhea; constipation; plegia of lower limbs
★ 38	Tiáokǒu	Flaccidity and motor impairment of lower limbs; edema of lower limbs; pain in the shoulder and arm
39	Xiàjùxū	Lower abdominal pain; diarrhea; mastitis; flaccidity and motor impairment of lower limbs
★ 40	Fēnglóng	Cough; asthma; headache; vertigo; manic-depressive psychosis; flaccidity and motor impairment of lower limbs
41	Jiěxī	Headache; dizziness; manic-depressive psychosis; abdominal distension; constipation; flaccidity and motor impairment of lower limbs; swelling and pain in the ankle
42	Chōngyáng	Stomachache; abdominal distension; facial paralysis; swelling, pain and atony on the dorsum of the foot
43	Xiàngǔ	Redness, swelling and pain in eye; facial swelling; swelling and pain on the dorsum of foot
★ 44	Nèitíng	Toothache; swelling and pain of the throat; facial paralysis; heat disease; abdominal pain; abdominal distension; constipation; swelling and pain on the dorsum of the foot
45	Lìduì	Toothache; swelling and pain of the throat; facial paralysis; heat disease; manic-depressive psychosis; nose bleeding; swelling and pain on the dorsum of the foot

★ Common acupoint used in treatment

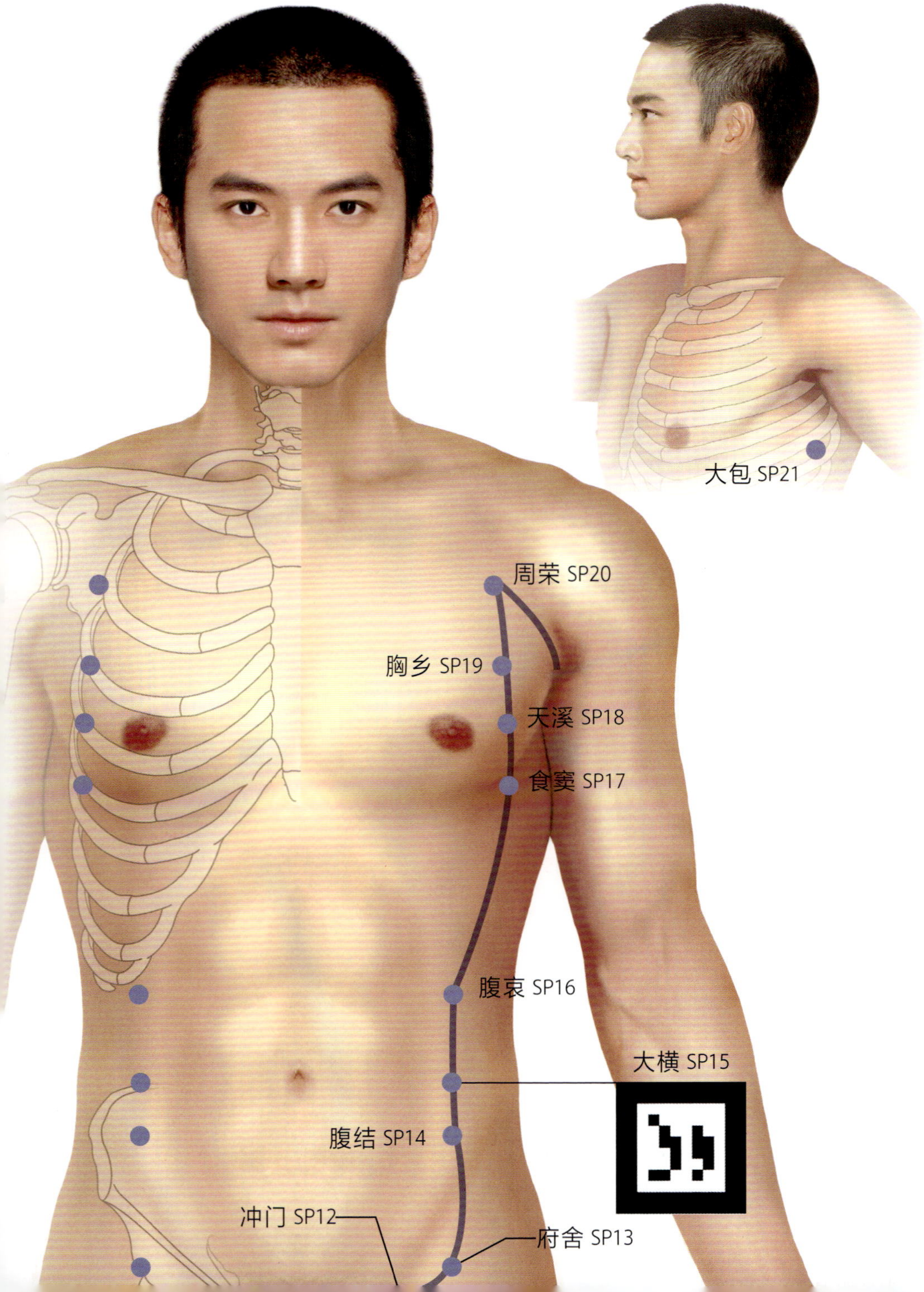

足太阴脾经

足太阴脾经起于脚拇趾内侧隐白穴，经过腿部内侧，止于胸部的大包穴。本经一侧 21 穴，左右两侧共 42 穴。

脾经主治病症：①腹胀、腹痛、泄泻、便秘等消化系统疾病。②咳喘、胸胁胀痛、腰腿痛等经脉循行部位的疾患。③本经还可治疗月经不调、痛经、带下、崩漏、不孕等妇科疾病。

SP	穴名	主治
1	隐白	崩漏（突然阴道大量出血或持续淋漓不断地出血）、月经过多、尿血、便血、腹胀、多梦
2	大都	腹胀、胃痛、泄泻、便秘、热病无汗
3	太白	胃痛、腹胀、腹痛、泄泻、便秘、纳呆（食欲不振）、足趾关节痛
★ 4	公孙	胃痛、呕吐、腹胀、腹痛、泄泻、便秘、心痛、胸闷
5	商丘	腹胀、泄泻、便秘、足踝肿痛、舌强肿痛（舌头僵硬疼痛）
★ 6	三阴交	月经不调、带下、难产、疝气、小便不利、遗尿、水肿、腹胀、泄泻、便秘、失眠、眩晕、下肢痿痹
7	漏谷	腹胀、肠鸣、小便不利、遗精、下肢痿痹

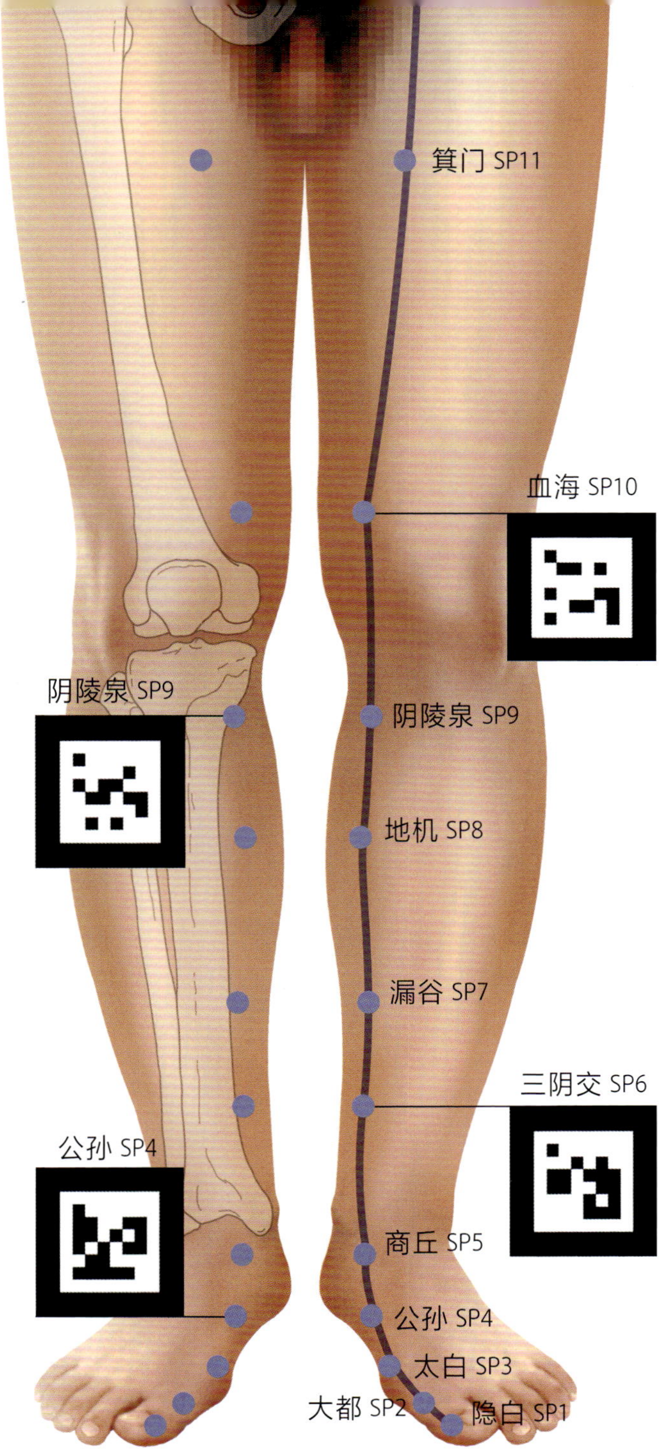

Spleen Meridian of Foot-Taiyin,SP.

Spleen Meridian of Foot-Taiyin originates from the medial aspect of the foot thumb (Yinbai acupoint). It travels along the medial aspect of the foot and ends in the chest (Dabao acupoint). There are 21 acupoints in each side of the meridian and 42 acupoints in total.

The Spleen Meridian indications: ① Digestive system diseases including abdominal distension and pain, diarrhea, constipation. ② Diseases on the pathway of the meridian including cough, distension in the chest and hypochondrium, pain in the waist and leg. ③ Gynaecological diseases including irregular menstruation, dysmenorrhea, sterility, metrorrhagia and leukorrheal diseases,etc.

SP	Acupoints	Indications
1	Yǐnbái	Metrorrhagia(acute massive bleeding or constant bleeding from vagina) and metrostaxis; menorrhagia; hematuria; bloody stool; abdominal distension; dreaminess
2	Dàdū	Abdominal distension; stomachache; diarrhea; constipation; heat disease with anhidrosis
3	Tàibái	Stomachache; abdominal distension; abdominal pain; diarrhea; constipation; poor appetite; pain in the toe joint
★ 4	Gōngsūn	Stomachache; vomiting; abdominal distension; abdominal pain; diarrhea; constipation; cardiac pain; chest tightness
5	Shāngqiū	Abdominal distension; diarrhea; constipation; ankle swelling and pain; swelling and stiffness of the tongue
★ 6	Sānyīnjiāo	Irregular menstruation; leukorrheal diseases; dystocia; hernia; dysuria; enuresis; edema; abdominal distension; diarrhea; constipation; insomnia; dizziness; flaccidity and motor impairment in the lower limb
7	Lòugǔ	Abdominal distension; borborygmus; dysuria; spermatorrhea; flaccidity and motor impairment in the lower limb

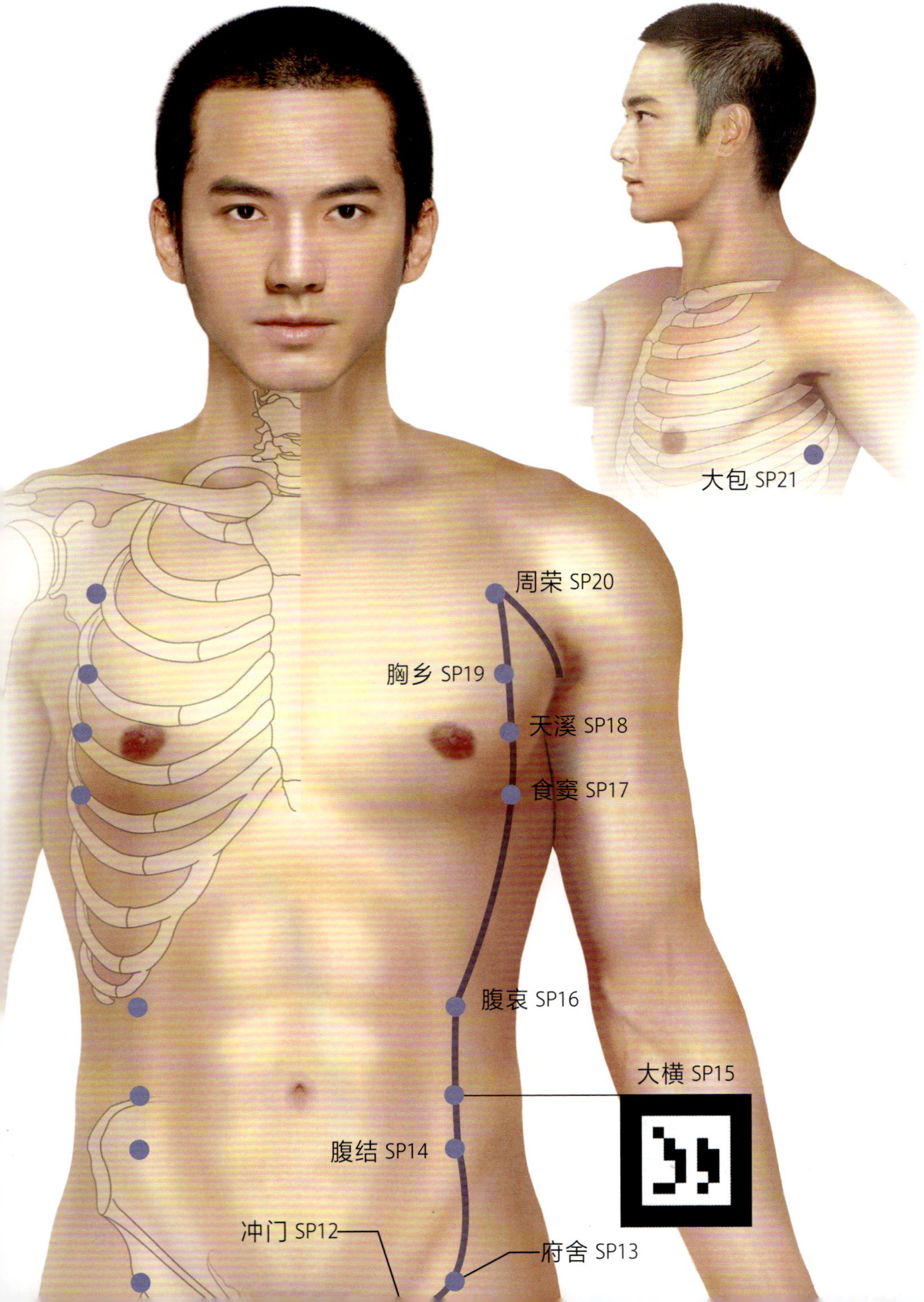

续表

SP	穴名	主治
★ 8	地机	腹胀痛、泄泻、水肿、小便不利、月经不调、痛经、遗精、腰痛、下肢痿痹
★ 9	阴陵泉	腹胀、水肿、黄疸、泄泻、小便不利或失禁、遗精、带下、膝痛
★ 10	血海	月经不调、经闭、崩漏、湿疹、荨麻疹
11	箕门	小便不通、遗尿、腹股沟肿痛
12	冲门	腹痛、崩漏、带下、疝气
13	府舍	腹痛、积聚（腹内结块或胀或痛）、疝气
14	腹结	腹痛、便秘、泄泻、疝气
15	大横	腹痛、便秘、泄泻
16	腹哀	腹痛、便秘、泄泻、消化不良
17	食窦	腹胀、食入即吐、水肿、胸胁胀痛
18	天溪	胸胁胀痛、咳嗽、乳腺炎、乳少
19	胸乡	胸胁胀痛
20	周荣	咳喘、不思饮食、胸胁胀满疼痛
21	大包	咳喘、胸胁胀痛、全身疼痛、四肢无力

★为本经常用穴

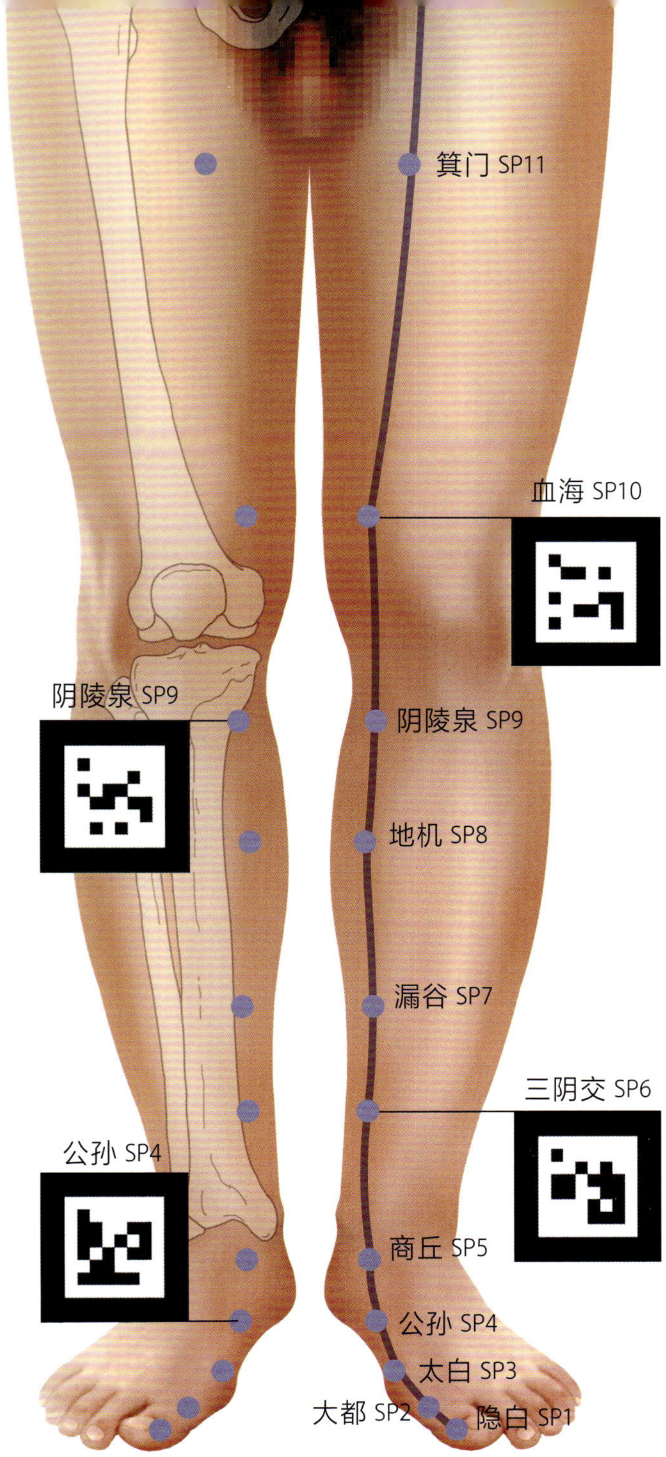

Continued

SP	Acupoints	Indications
★ 8	Dìjī	Abdominal distension and pain; diarrhea; edema; dysuria; irregular menstruation; dysmenorrhea; spermatorrhea; waist pain; flaccidity and motor impairment
★ 9	Yīnlíngquán	Abdominal distension; edema; jaundice; diarrhea; dysuria or enuresis; spermatorrhea; leukorrheal diseases; knees pain
★ 10	Xuèhǎi	Irregular menstruation; amenorrhea; metrorrhagia and metrostaxis; eczema; urticaria
11	Jīmén	Dysuria; enuresis; swelling and pain in the groin
12	Chōngmén	Abdominal pain; metrorrhagia and metrostaxis; leukorrheal diseases; hernia
13	Fǔshè	Abdominal pain; abdominal mass(lump which cause distension or pain); hernia
14	Fùjié	Abdominal pain; constipation; diarrhea; hernia
15	Dàhéng	Abdominal pain; constipation; diarrhea
16	Fù ‘āi	Abdominal pain; constipation; diarrhea; dyspepsia
17	Shídòu	Abdominal distension; vomiting right after eating; edema; distension and pain in the chest and the hypochondrium
18	Tiānxī	Distension and pain in the chest and the hypochondrium; cough; mastitis; hypogalactia
19	Xiōngxiāng	Distension and pain in the chest and the hypochondrium
20	Zhōuróng	Cough and asthma; poor appetite; distension and pain in the chest and the hypochondrium
21	Dàbāo	Cough and asthma; distension and pain in the chest and the hypochondrium; pain all over the body; flaccidity of limbs

★ Common acupoint used in treatment

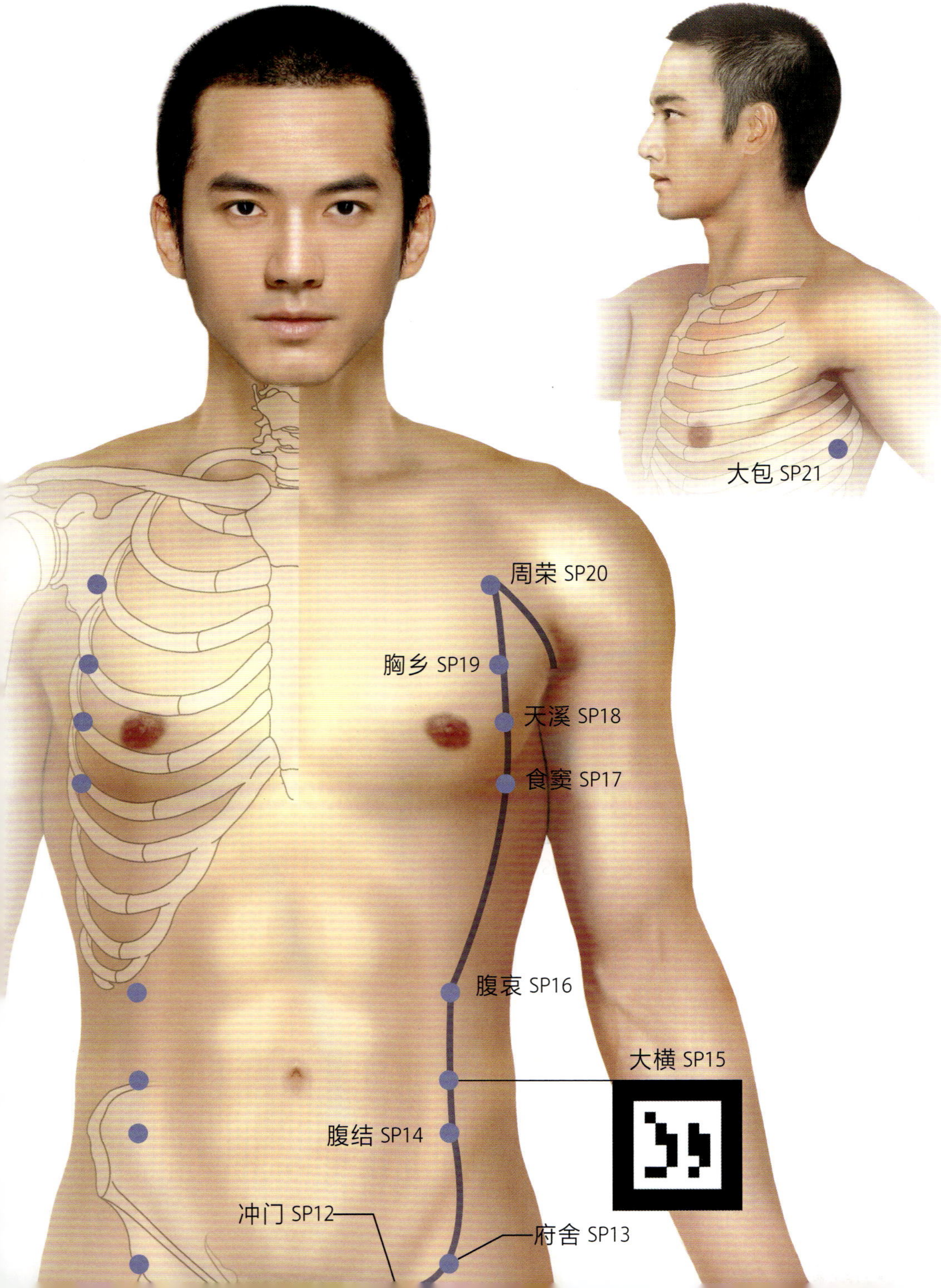

血海

用拇指按揉血海穴 2 分钟，力度稍重。同法按揉对侧血海穴。

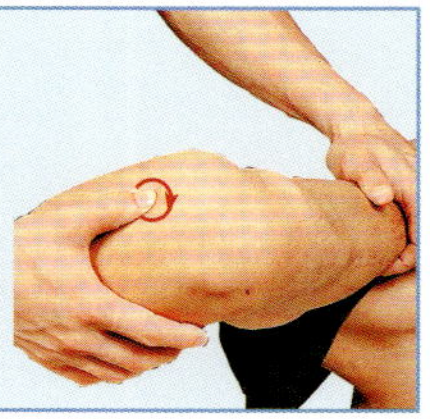

三阴交

用拇指用力按压三阴交穴，停留片刻后放松，反复 5~6 下。同法按压对侧三阴交穴。

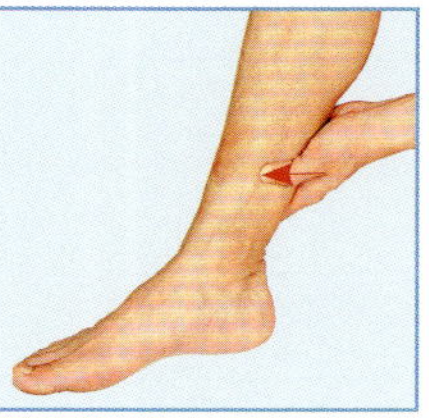

阴陵泉

用拇指按压阴陵泉穴，停留片刻后放松，反复 5~6 下。同法按压对侧阴陵泉穴，每次 2 分钟。

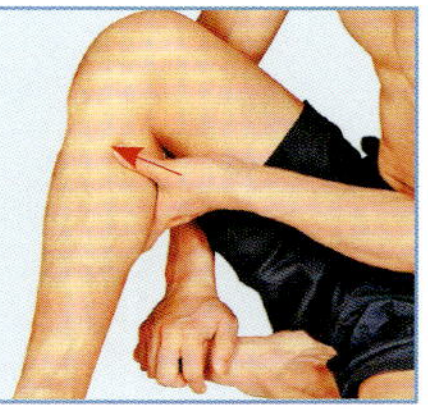

公孙

用拇指按揉公孙穴 2 分钟，力度稍重。同法按揉对侧公孙穴。每日 2 次。

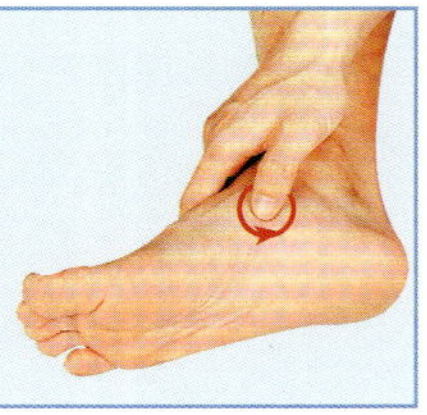

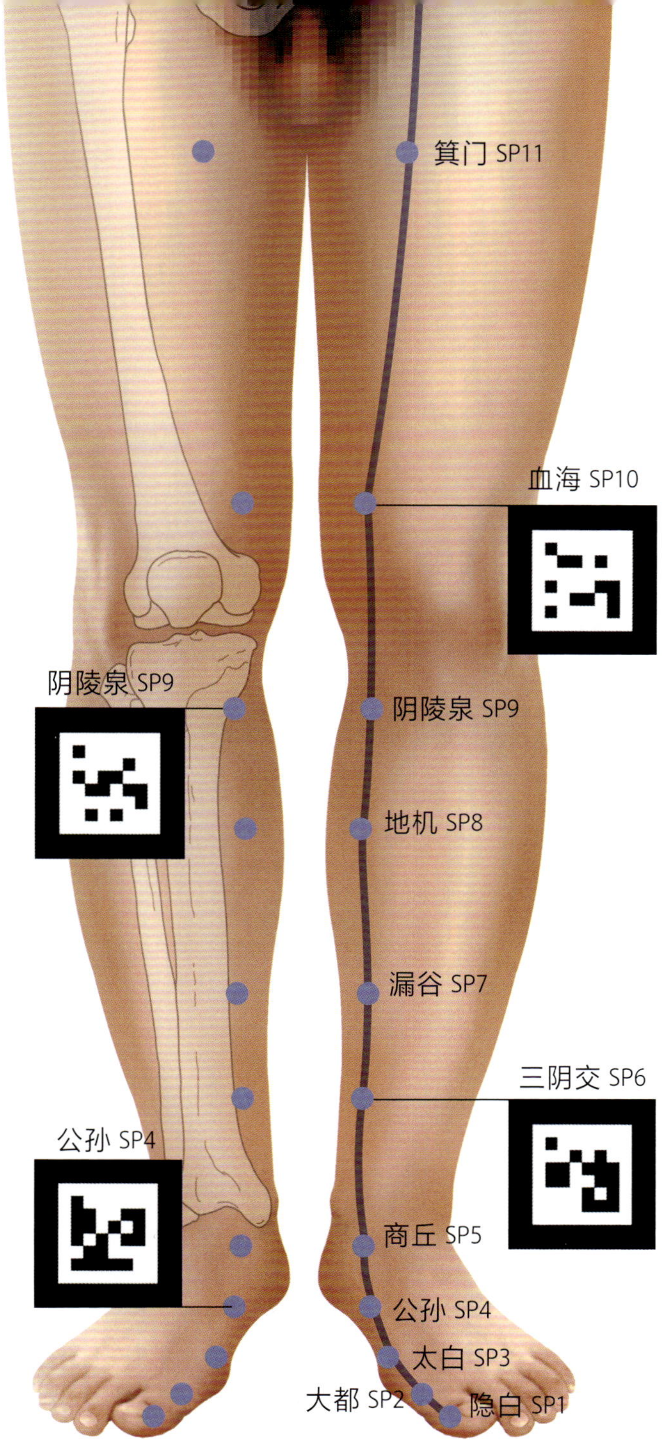

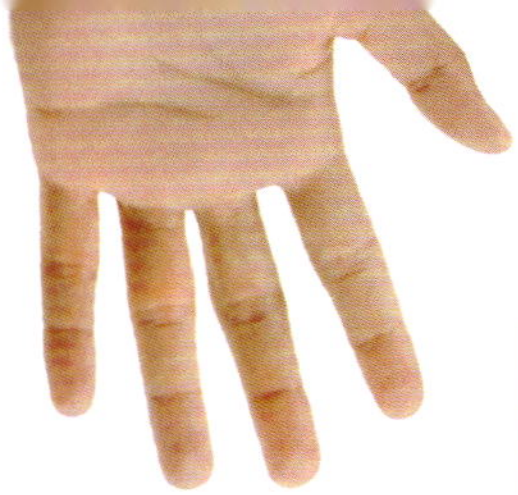

Xuèhǎi(SP10)

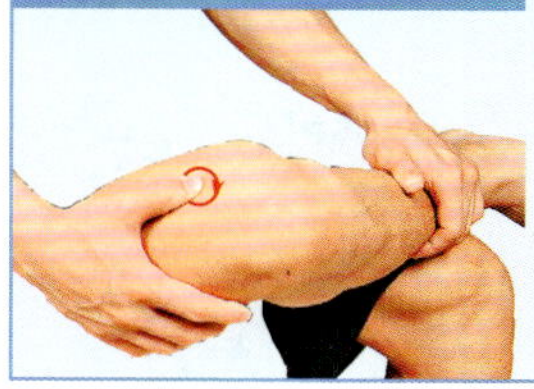

Use the thumb to knead Xuehai acupoint for 2 minutes with a little heavy strength. Knead the contralateral Xuehai acupoint with the same method.

Sānyīnjiáo(SP6)

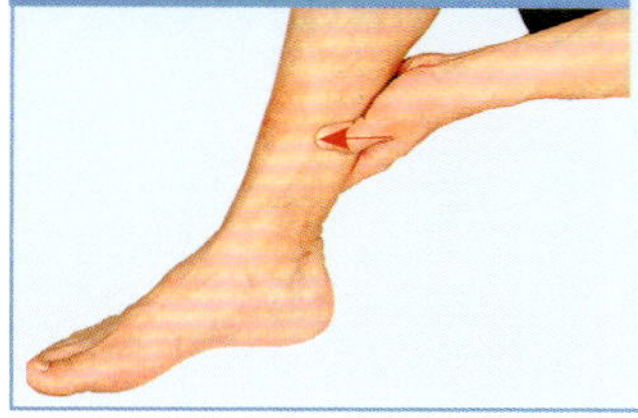

Use the thumb to press Sanyinjiao acupoint for a while, then relax, repeat 5~6 times. Press the contralateral Sanyinjiao acupoint with the same method.

Yīnlíngquán(SP9)

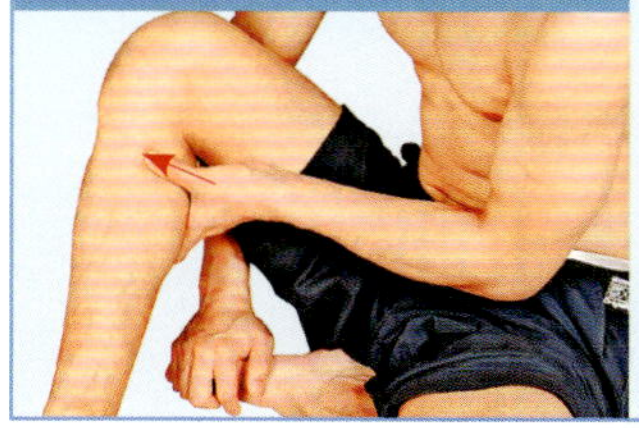

Use the thumb to press Yinlingquan acupoint for a while,then relax,repeat 5~6 times. Press the contralateral Yinlingquan acupoint with the same method. It takes 2 minutes for every time.

Gōngsūn(SP4)

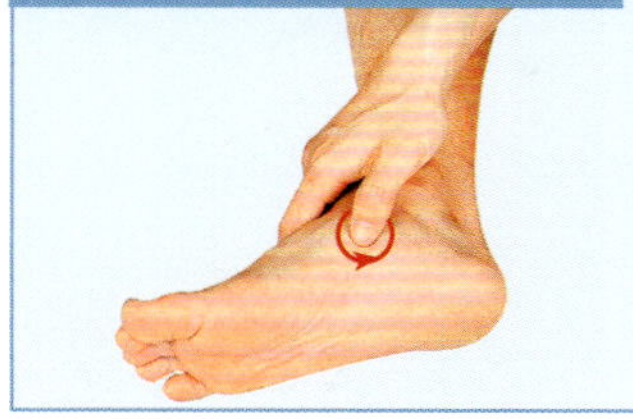

Use the thumb to knead Gongsun acupoint for 2 minutes with a little heavy strength, then knead the contralateral Gongsun acupoint with the same method twice a day.

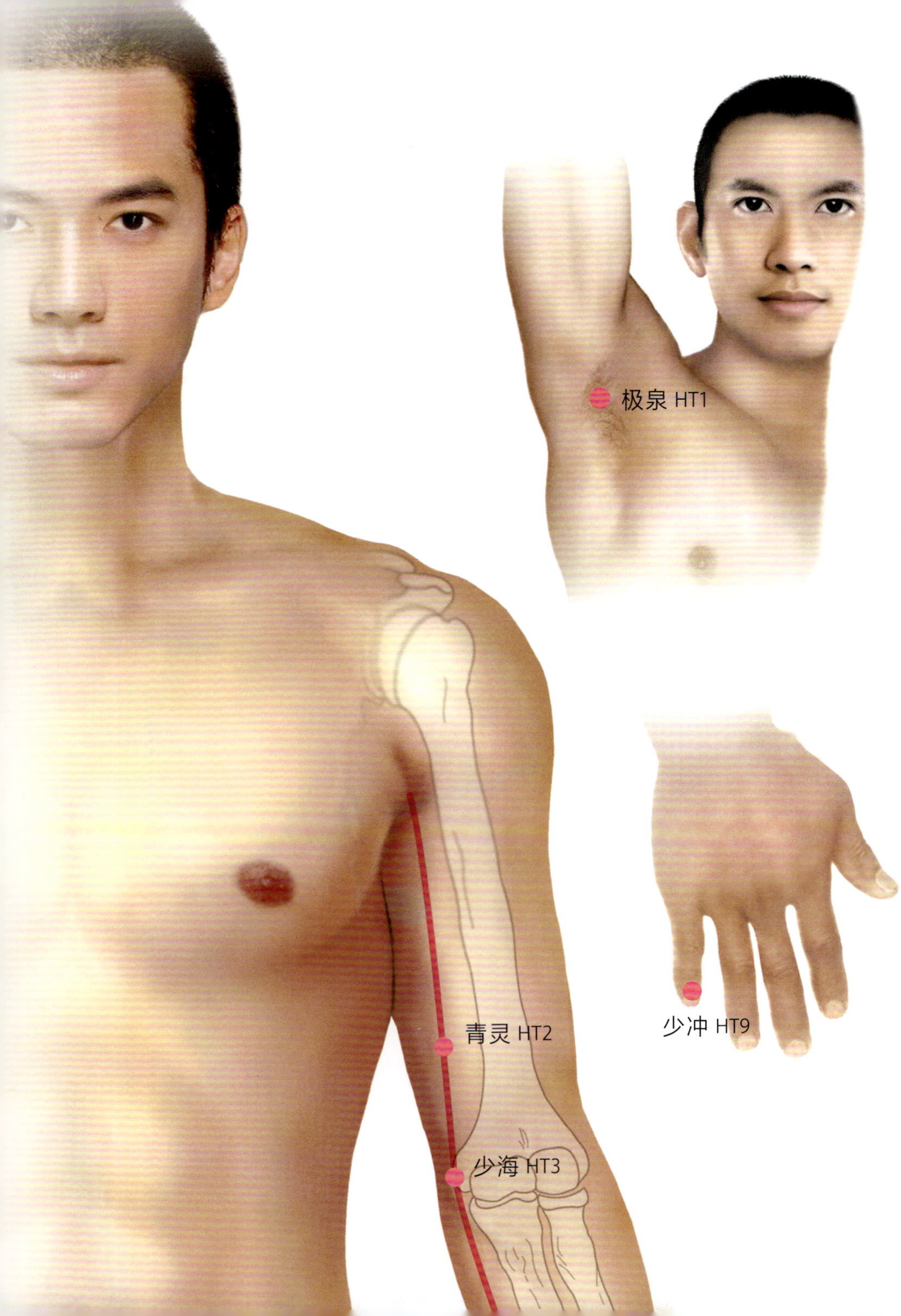

手少阴心经

手少阴心经起于腋窝中央的极泉穴，沿手臂内侧走到手小指内侧的少冲穴。本经一侧 9 穴，左右两侧共 18 穴，1 穴分布在腋窝部，8 穴分布在上肢掌侧面的尺侧。

心经主治病症：①心烦、胸闷、心悸、心痛等心胸疾病。②前臂痛、肘部痛等经脉循行部位的疾患。

HT	穴名	主治
1	极泉	心痛、心悸、胁肋疼痛、肩臂疼痛、上肢不遂
2	青灵	头痛、胁痛、肩臂疼痛
3	少海	心痛、肘臂挛痛麻木、胸胁痛
4	灵道	心痛、心悸、暴喑（突然失音）、肘臂挛痛、手指麻木
★ 5	通里	暴喑、舌强不语、心悸怔忡、腕臂痛
6	阴郄	心痛、惊悸、暴喑
★ 7	神门	失眠、健忘、痴呆、心痛、心悸
★ 8	少府	心悸、胸痛、小便不利、遗尿、小指挛痛
9	少冲	心悸、心痛、癫狂、昏迷、热病、胸胁痛

★为本经常用穴

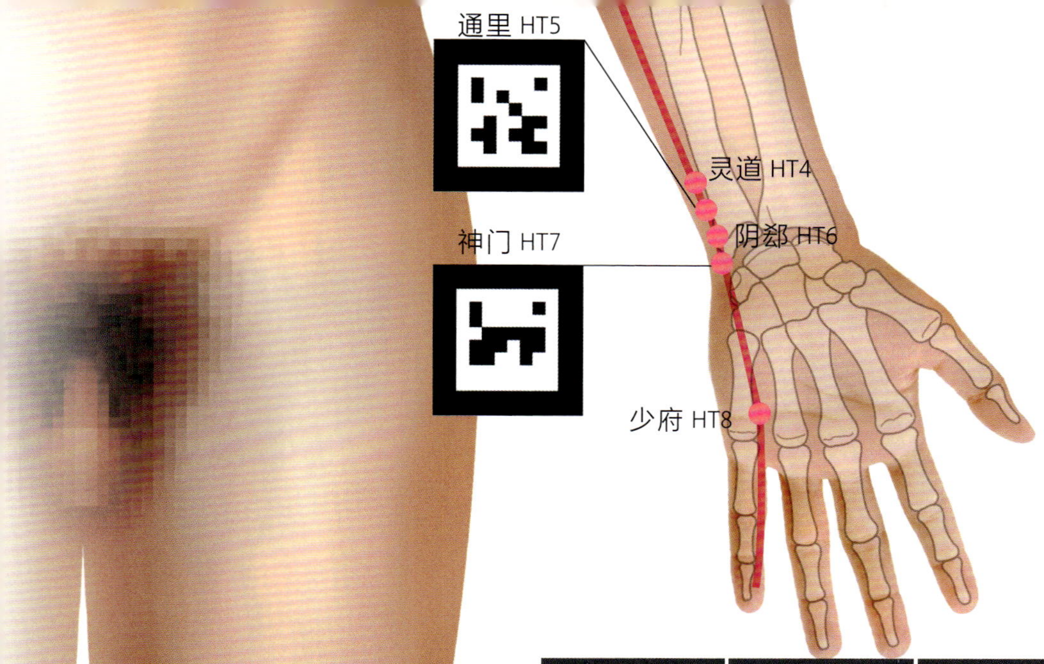

Heart Meridian of Hand-Shaoyin,HT.

Heart Meridian of Hand-Shaoyin starts in the center of axilla (Jiquan acupoint). It goes along the medial aspect of arm and terminates at the medial aspect of the little finger (Shaochong acupoint). There are 9 acupoints in each side of the meridian and 18 acupoints in total. There is an acupoint in the axillary region, the other 8 acupoints are on the palmar ulnar aspect of the upper limb.

Heart Meridian indications: ① Cardiac thoracic diseases including vexation, chest tightness, palpitation and cardiac pain. ② Diseases on the pathway of the meridian including pain in the forearm and elbow pain, etc.

HT	Acupoints	Indications
1	Jíquán	Cardiac pain; palpitation; pain in chest and the hypochondrium; pain in the shoulder and arm; motor impairment in upper limbs
2	Qīnglíng	Headache; pain in the hypochondrium; pain in the shoulder and arm
3	Shàohǎi	Cardiac pain; spasm, pain and numbness in the shoulder and elbow; pain in the chest and hypochondrium
4	Língdào	Cardiac pain; palpitation; aphonia; pain and spasm in the shoulder and elbow; finger numbness
★ 5	Tōnglǐ	Aphonia; voice loss due to tongue stiffness; palpitation and severe palpitation; pain in the wrist and the arm
6	Yīnxì	Cardiac pain; palpitation due to fright; aphonia
★ 7	Shénmén	Insomnia; amnesia; dementia; cardiac pain; palpitation
★ 8	Shàofǔ	Palpitation; pain in the chest; enuresis; spasm and pain in the little finger
9	Shàochōng	Palpitation; cardiac pain; manic-depressive psychosis; coma; heat disease; pain in the chest and the hypochondrium

★ Common acupoint used in treatment

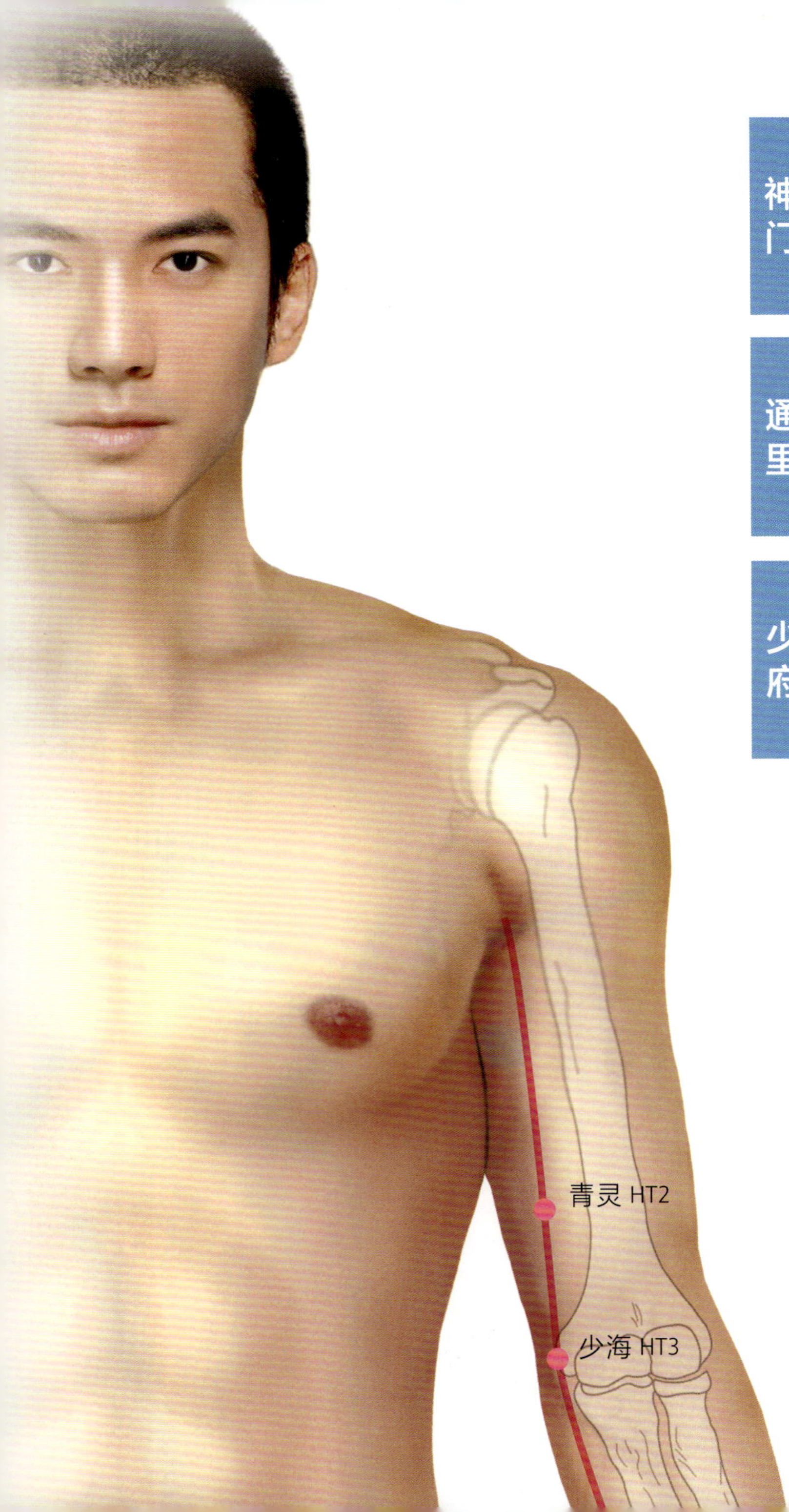

神门

用拇指稍用力按压神门穴，停留片刻后放松，反复 5 ~ 6 下。同法按压对侧神门穴。每日 2 次。

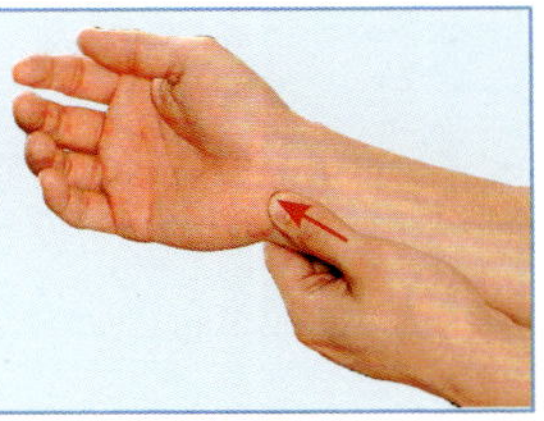

通里

用拇指按揉通里穴 2 分钟，力度适中。同法按揉对侧通里穴。每日 2 次。

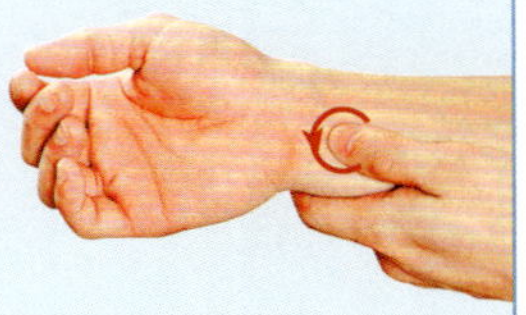

少府

用拇指稍用力按压少府穴，停留片刻后放松，反复 5~6 下。同法按压对侧少府穴。每日 2 次。

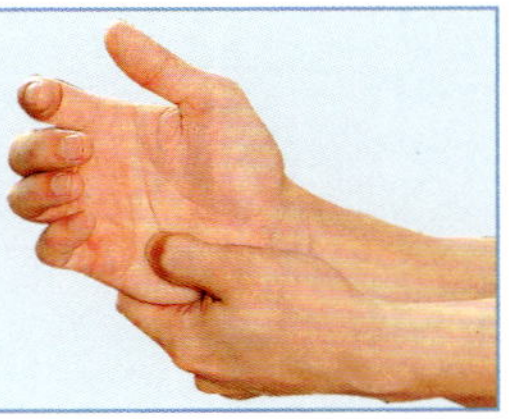

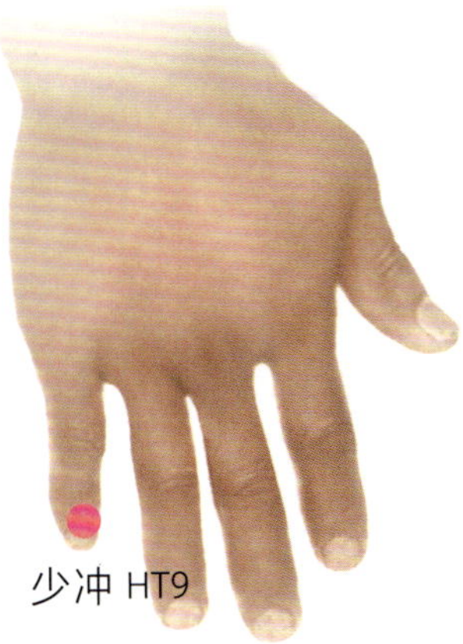

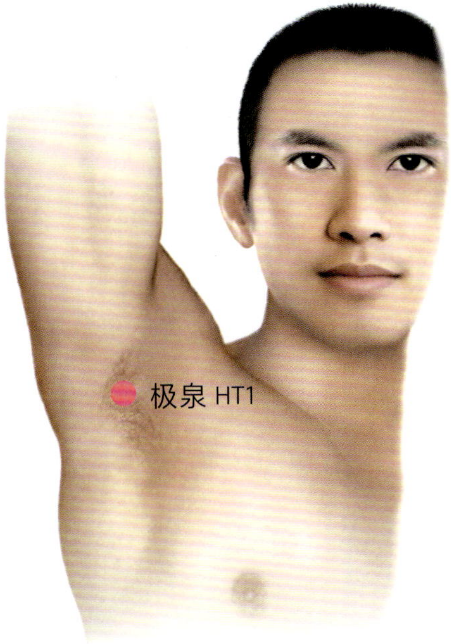

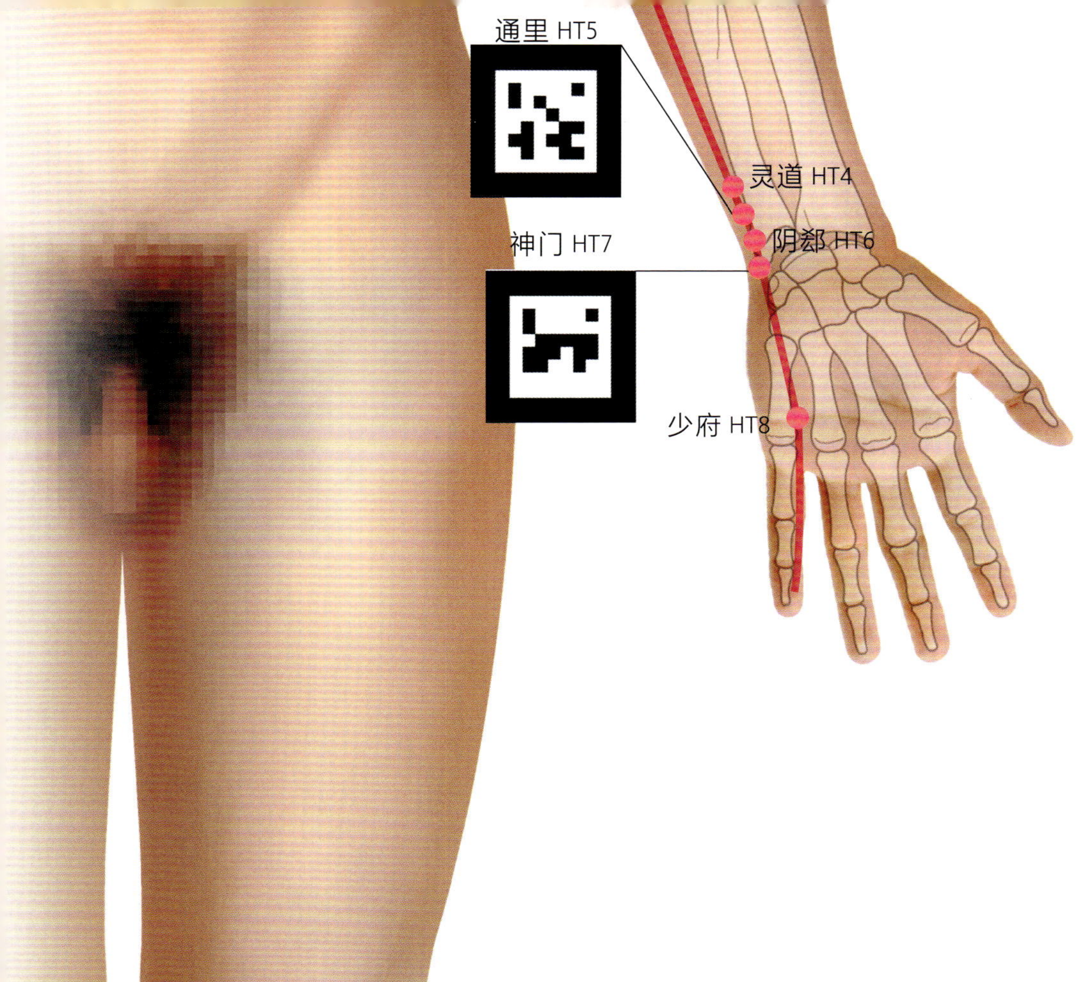

Shénmén(HT7)

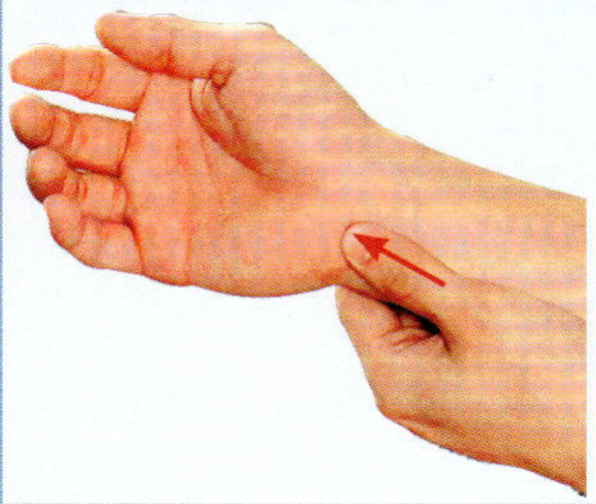

Use the thumb to press the Shenmen acupoint for a while, then relax, repeat 5~6 times with slight strength. Press the contralateral Shenmen acupoint with the same method.

Tōnglǐ(HT5)

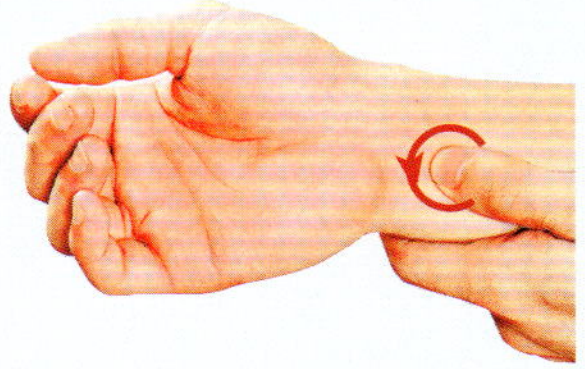

Use the thumb to press the Tongli acupoint with appropriate strength for 2 minutes, then relax, repeat 5~6 times a day. Press the contralateral Tongli acupoint.

Shàofǔ(HT8)

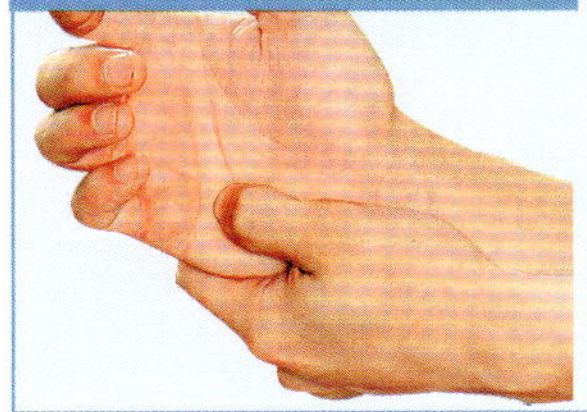

Use the thumb to press the Shaofu acupoint for a while, then relax, repeat 5~6 times with a little heavy strength. Press the contralateral Shaofu acupoint. Twice a day.

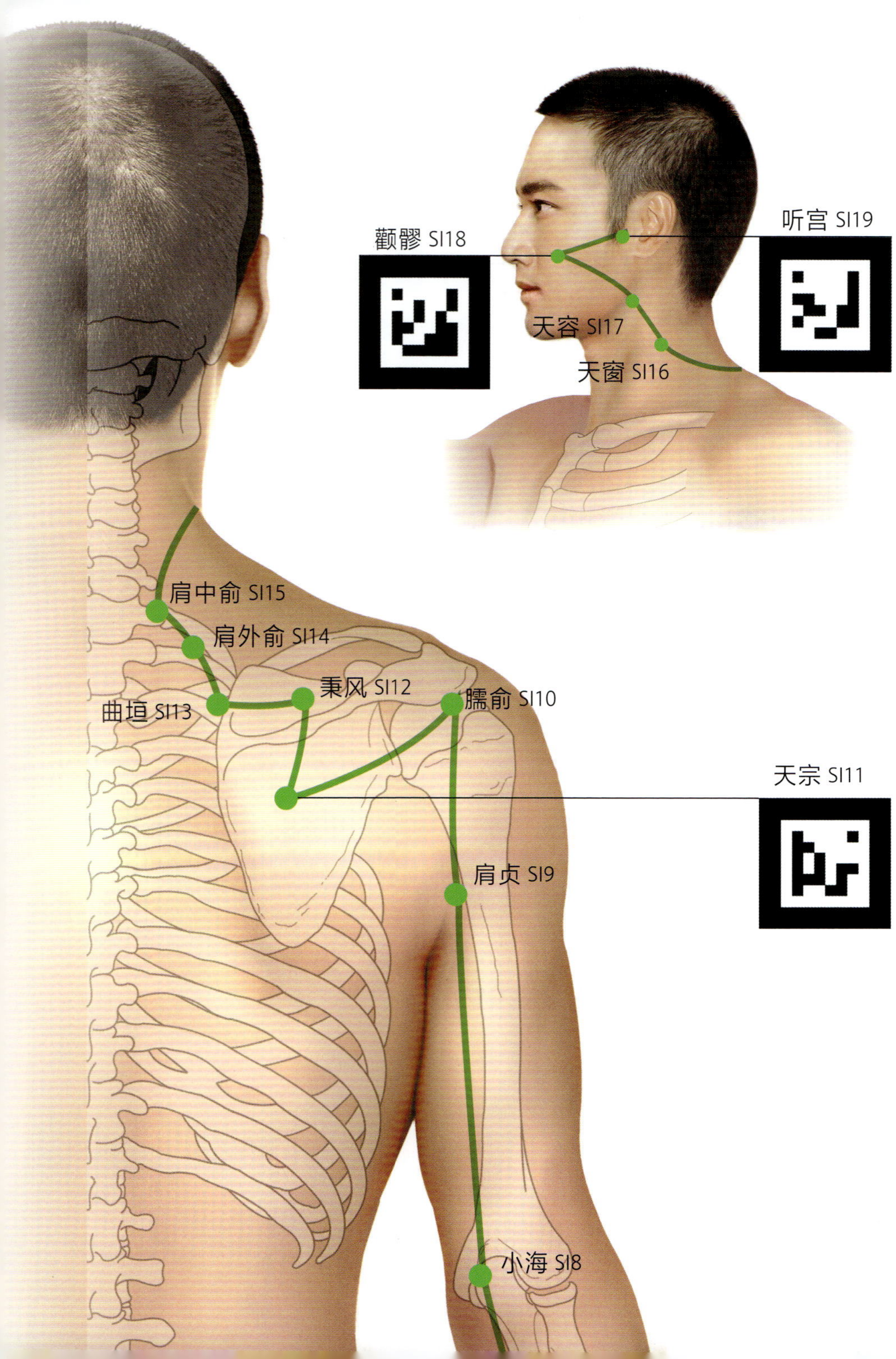

手太阳小肠经

手太阳小肠经起于手小指少泽穴，从手臂外侧到颈部，止于耳朵的听宫穴。本经一侧 19 穴，左右两侧共 38 穴。

小肠经主治病症：①头痛、目翳（眼内生遮蔽视线的目障）、咽喉肿痛、耳鸣、耳聋、口喎等头面五官疾病。②热病以及癫狂等精神疾病。③腕臂痛、头项强痛、腰背痛等经脉循行部位的疾患。

SI	穴名	主治
1	少泽	头痛、昏迷、热病、咽喉肿痛、耳聋耳鸣、乳少、乳腺炎
2	前谷	头痛、耳鸣、咽喉肿痛、热病、乳少
★3	后溪	头项强痛、眩晕、腰背痛、耳聋、咽喉肿痛、急性腰扭伤、手指及肘臂挛痛
4	腕骨	头项强痛、耳鸣、热病、指挛腕痛
5	阳谷	头痛、目眩、耳鸣、耳聋、热病、癫狂、腕臂痛
6	养老	头痛、面痛、急性腰痛、项强（颈项僵硬疼痛）、肘腕部痛
7	支正	头痛、目眩、热病、癫狂、项强、肘臂疼痛
8	小海	肘臂疼痛、癫狂
9	肩贞	肩背疼痛、手臂麻痛

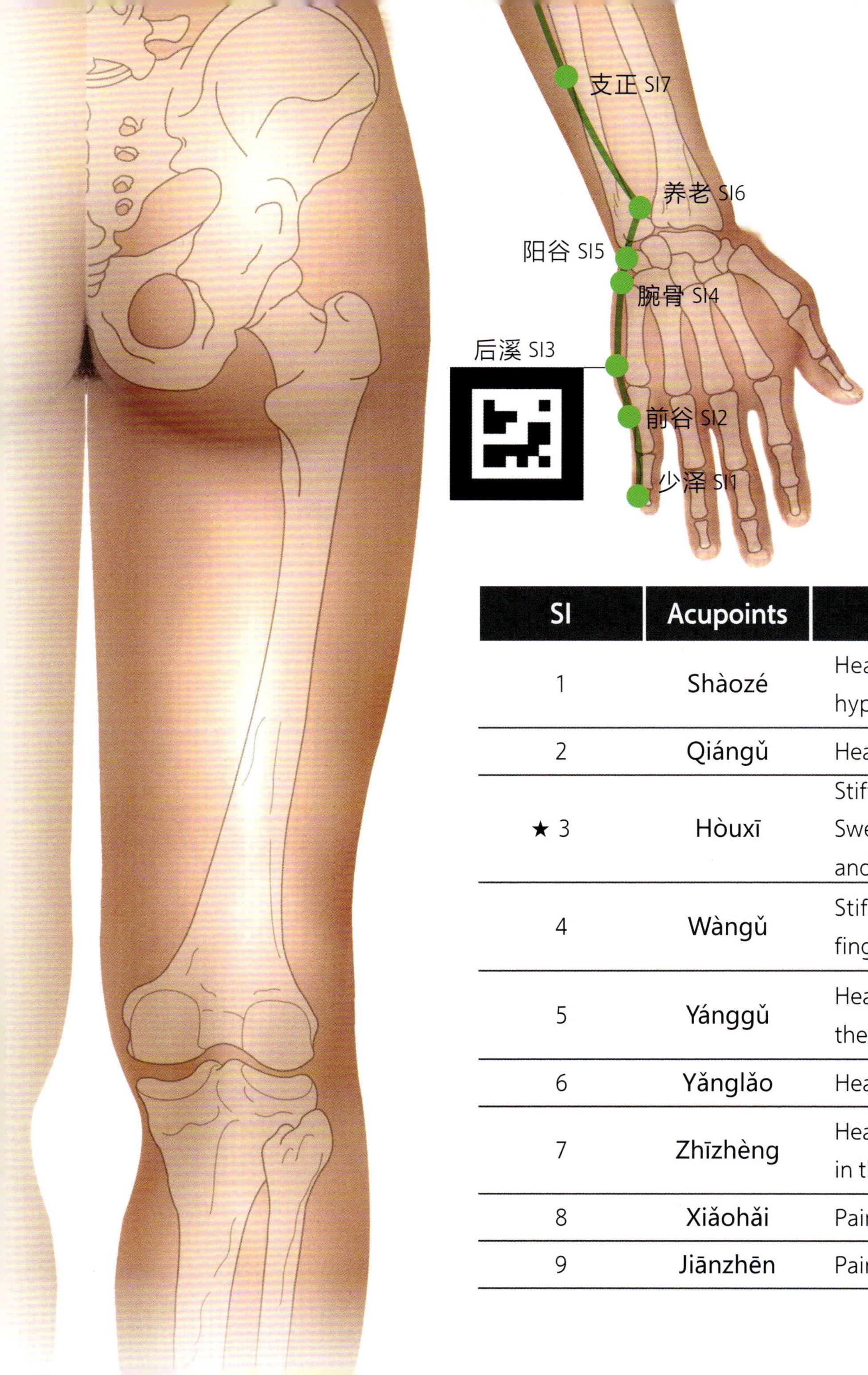

Small Intestine Meridian of Hand-Taiyang,SI.

Small Intestine Meridian of Hand-Taiyang starts at the little finger (Shaoze acupoint). It travels along the lateral aspect of the arm to the neck and ends in the ear (Tinggong acupoint).There are 19 acupoints in each side of the meridian and 38 acupoints in total.

The Small Intestine Meridian indications: ① HEENT diseases including headache, nephelium, swelling and pain in the throat, deviation of the mouth, tinnitus, deafness. ② Heat diseases and mental diseases including manic-depressive psychosis. ③ Diseases on the pathway of the meridian including pain in the arm, elbow pain, stiffness and pain in the neck and head, pain in the waist and back.

SI	Acupoints	Indications
1	Shàozé	Headache; coma; heat disease; swelling and pain in the throat; tinnitus and deafness; hypogalactia; mastitis
2	Qiángǔ	Headache; tinnitus; swelling and pain in the throat; heat disease; hypogalactia
★ 3	Hòuxī	Stiffness and pain in the neck and head; dizziness; pain in the waist and back; deafness; Swelling and pain in the throat, acute waist sprain spasm and pain of the finger, the elbow and the arm
4	Wàngǔ	Stiffness and pain in the neck and the head; tinnitus; heat disease; spasm and pain of fingers
5	Yánggǔ	Headache; dizziness; tinnitus; deafness; heat disease; manic-depressive psychosis; pain in the wrist and the arm
6	Yǎnglǎo	Headache; facial pain; acute waist pain; stiffness in the neck; pain in the elbow and wrist
7	Zhīzhèng	Headache; dizziness; heat disease; manic-depressive psychosis; stiffness in the neck; pain in the arm and the elbow
8	Xiǎohǎi	Pain in the arm and the elbow; manic-depressive psychosis
9	Jiānzhēn	Pain in the shoulder and the back; numbness and pain in the arm and the hand

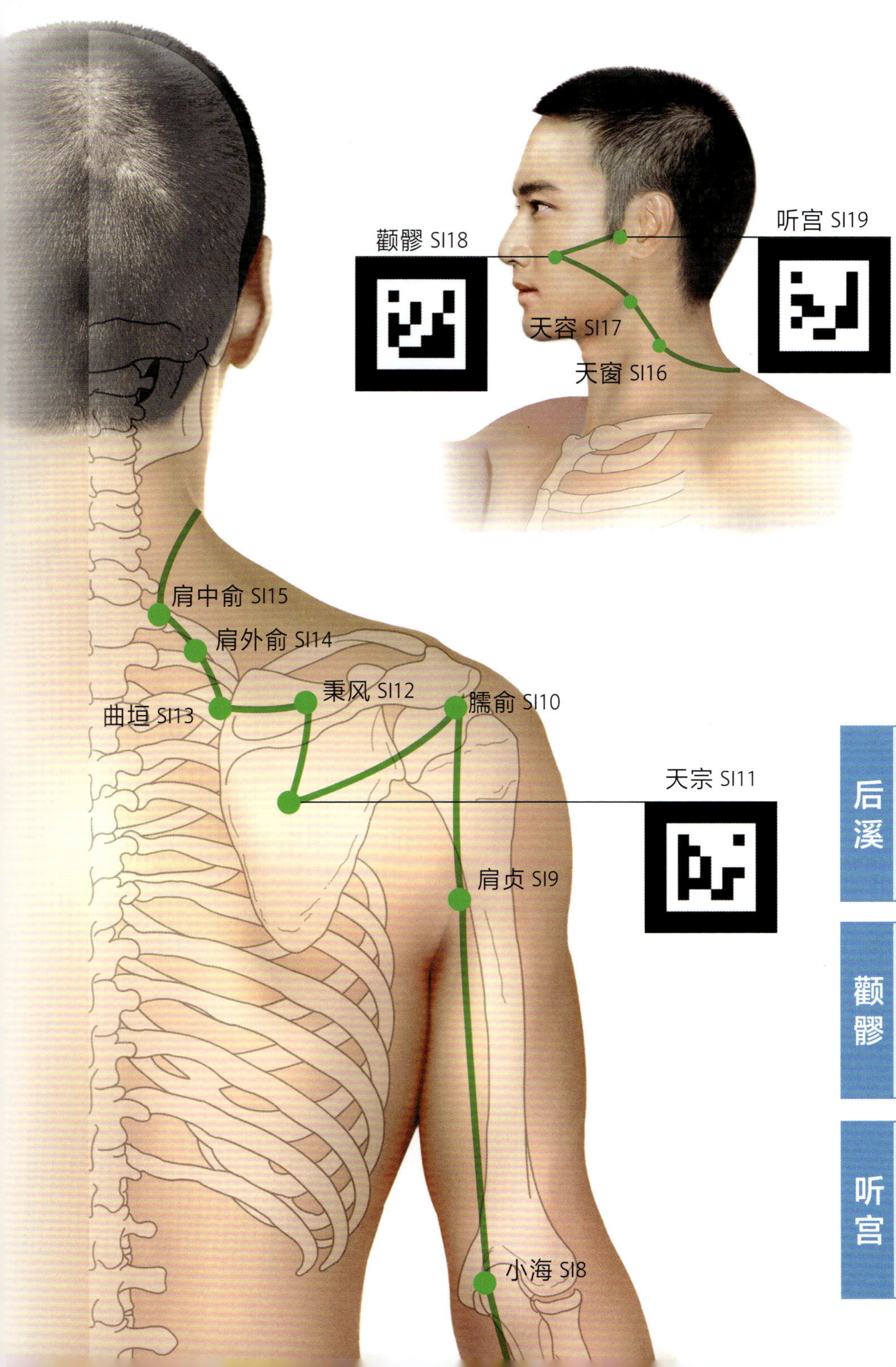

续表

SI	穴名	主治
10	臑俞	肩臂疼痛
★ 11	天宗	肩胛疼痛、乳腺炎、气喘
12	秉风	颈项及肩胛疼痛、手臂酸麻
13	曲垣	肩胛背项疼痛
14	肩外俞	肩背疼痛、颈项强急
15	肩中俞	肩背疼痛、咳嗽、气喘、目视不明
16	天窗	咽喉肿痛、暴喑、耳鸣、耳聋、颈项强痛
17	天容	咽喉肿痛、暴喑、耳鸣、耳聋、颈项强痛
★ 18	颧髎	口喎、眼睑瞤动、齿痛、颊肿
★ 19	听宫	耳鸣、耳聋、癫狂

★为本经常用穴

后溪

用拇指稍用力按压后溪穴，停留片刻后放松，反复 5~6 下。同法按压对侧后溪穴。每日 2 次。

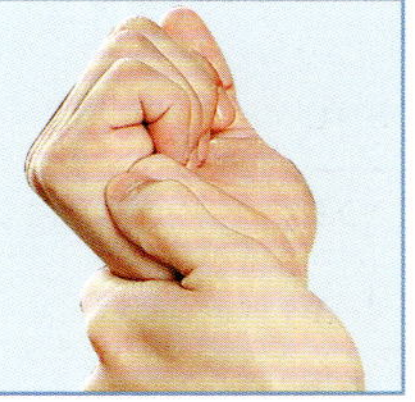

颧髎

用食指稍用力按压颧髎穴，停留片刻后放松，反复 5~6 下。同法按压对侧颧髎穴。每日 2 次。

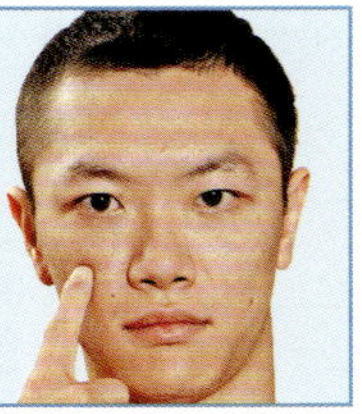

听宫

用中指稍用力按压听宫穴，停留片刻后放松，反复 5~6 下。同法按揉对侧听宫穴。每日 2 次。

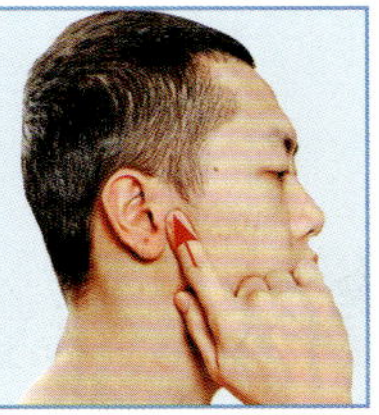

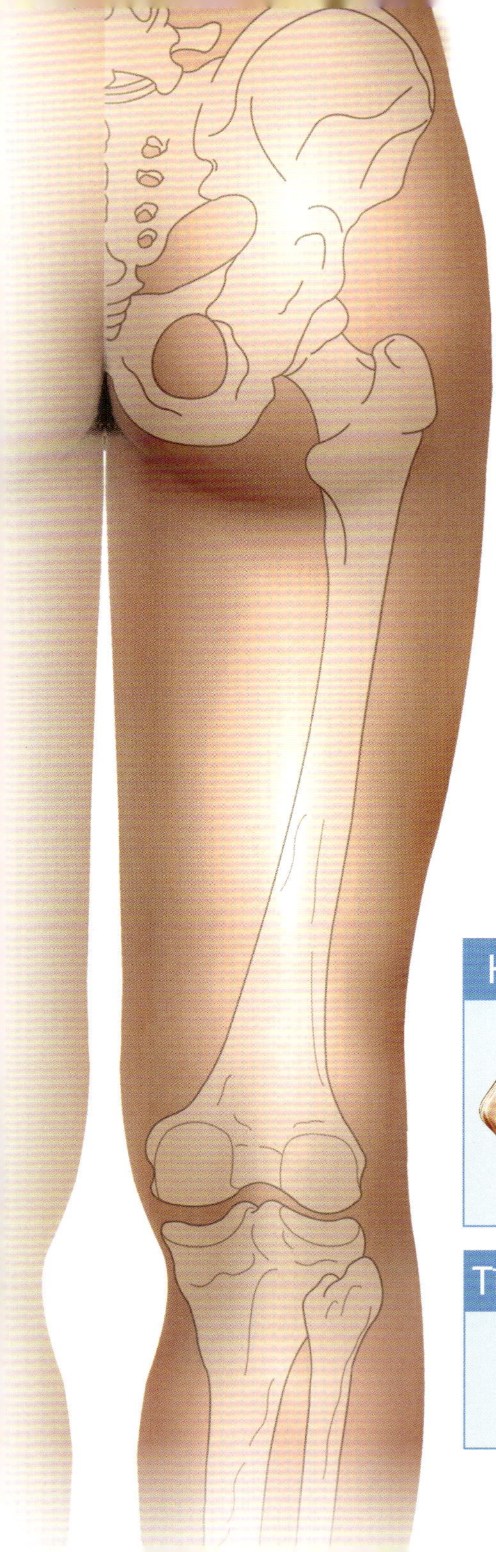

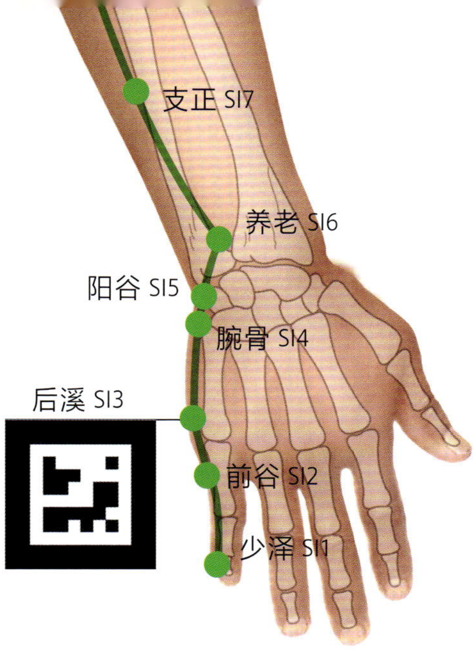

Continued

SI	Acupoints	Indications
10	Nàoshū	Pain in the shoulder and the arm
★ 11	Tiānzōng	Shoulder pain; mastitis; asthma
12	Bǐngfēng	Pain in the neck and the shoulder; numbness and soreness in the arm and the hand
13	Qūyuán	Pain in the back, the neck and the shoulder
14	Jiānwàishū	Pain in the shoulder and the back; neck stiffness
15	Jiānzhōngshū	Pain in the shoulder and the back; cough; asthma; blurry vision
16	Tiānchuāng	Swelling and pain in the throat; aphonia; tinnitus; deafness; stiffness and pain of the neck
17	Tiānróng	Swelling and pain in the throat; aphonia; tinnitus; deafness; stiffness of the neck
18	Quánliáo	Deviation of the mouth; eyelid twitching; toothache; swollen cheek
★ 19	Tīnggōng	Tinnitus; deafness; manic-depressive psychosis

★ Common acupoint used in treatment

Hòuxī(SI3)

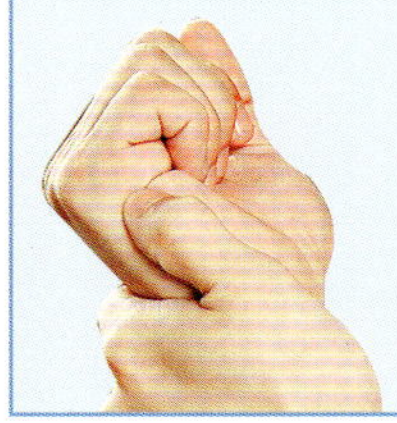

Use the thumb to press the Houxi acupoint for a minute,repeat 5~6 times with a little heavy strength. Press the contralateral Houxi acupoint with the same method. Twice a day.

Quánliáo(SI18)

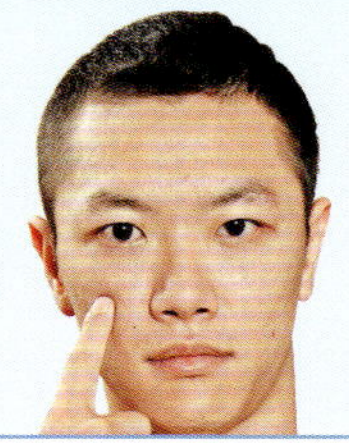

Use the thumb to press the Quanliao acupoint for a minute,repeat 5~6 times with a little heavy strength. Press the contralateral Quanliao acupoint with the same method. Twice a day.

Tīnggōng(SI19)

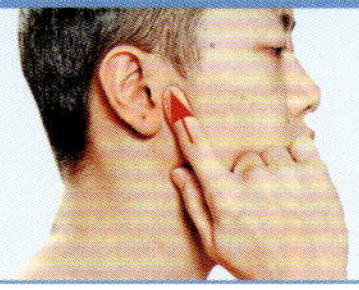

Use the thumb to press the Tinggong acupoint for a minute, repeat 5~6 times with a little heavy strength. Press the contralateral Tinggong acupoint with the same method. Twice a day.

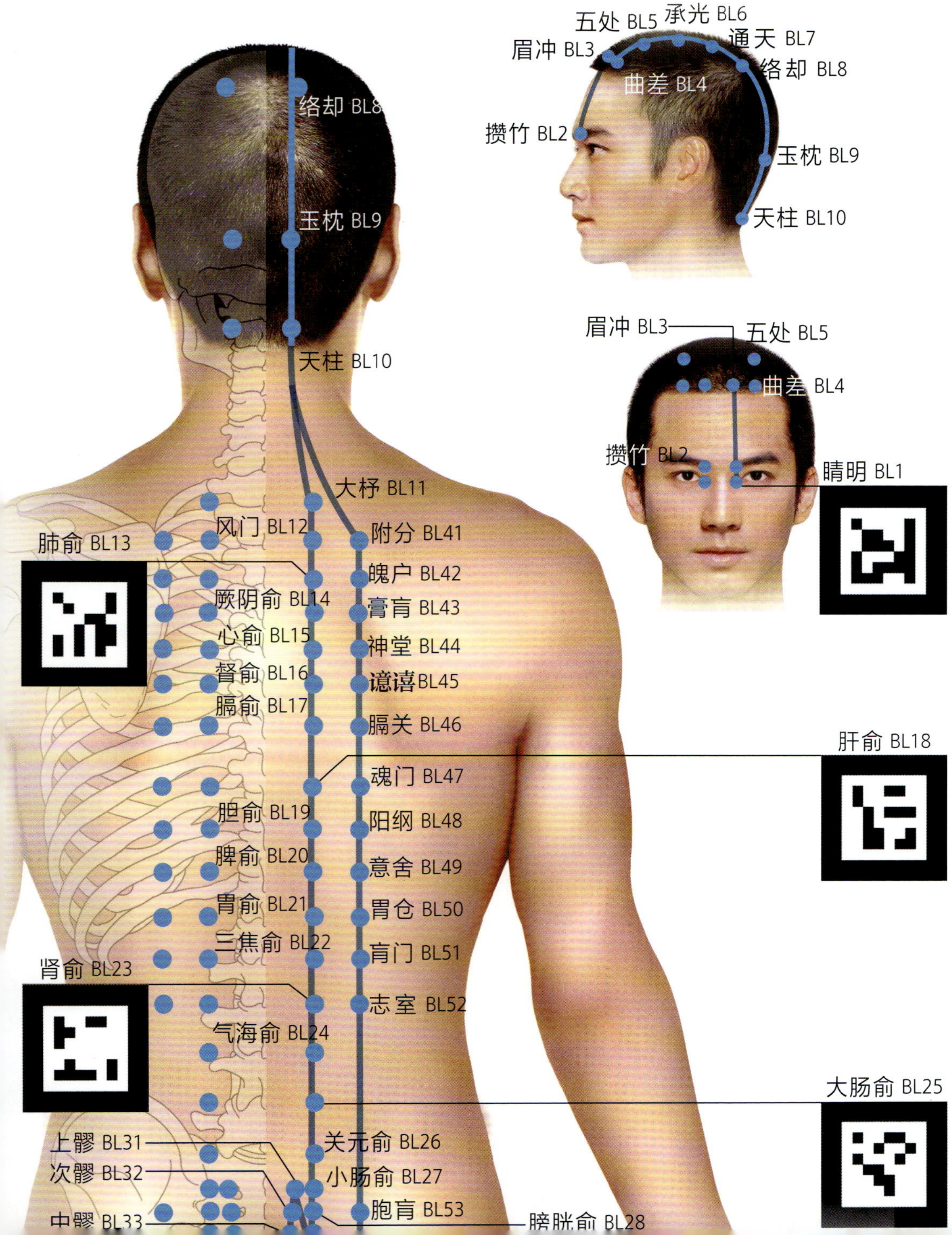

足太阳膀胱经

足太阳膀胱经起于眼睛内侧的睛明穴，经头顶、颈椎至脚小趾外侧的至阴穴。本经一侧 67 穴，左右两侧共 134 穴。

膀胱经主治病症：①头痛，口、眼睑瞤动，眉棱骨痛等头面五官疾病。②癫痫、失眠等神经精神系统疾病。③颈、背、腰、下肢疾患。④位于背部两条侧线的背俞穴主治其相应的脏腑疾患和有关的组织器官病症。⑤部分腧穴有强身健体作用，可用于日常保健。

BL	穴名	主治
★ 1	睛明	近视、目赤肿痛、目视不明、夜盲、目翳、急性腰痛
★ 2	攒竹	头痛、面瘫、腰痛、目视不明、眼睑瞤动、眼睑下垂、眉棱骨痛
3	眉冲	头痛、眩晕、鼻塞、癫痫
4	曲差	头痛、目视不明、鼻塞
5	五处	头痛、目眩、目视不明、癫痫
6	承光	头痛、眩晕、目视不明、鼻塞、癫痫
7	通天	鼻塞、鼻炎、头痛、眩晕
8	络却	头痛、耳鸣、鼻塞、目视不明、癫狂
9	玉枕	头项痛、目视不明
★ 10	天柱	头痛、眩晕、项强、肩背痛、目视不明、鼻塞
11	大杼	咳嗽、发热、头痛、肩背痛

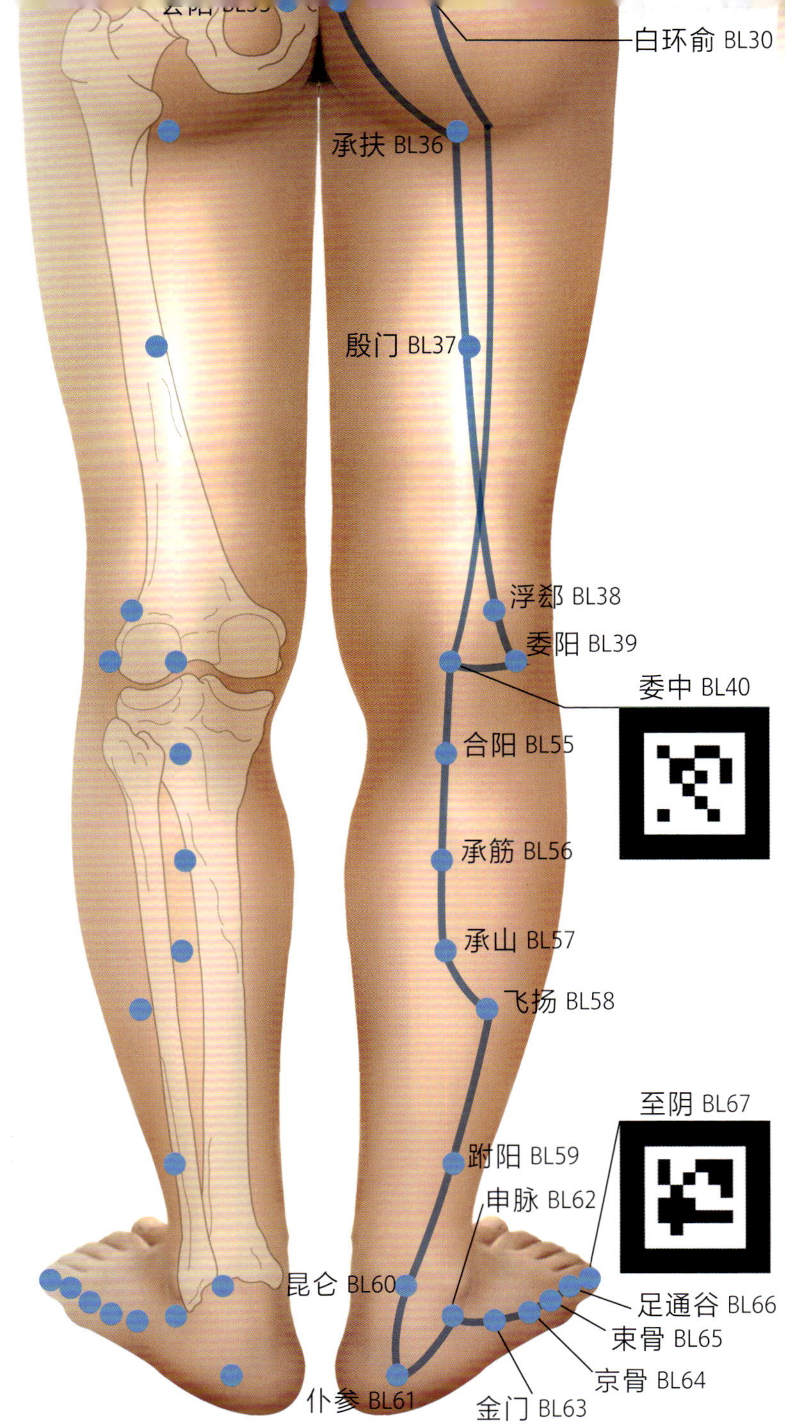

Bladder Meridian of Foot-Taiyang,BL.

Bladder Meridian of Foot-Taiyang originates from the inner canthus of the eye (Jingming acupoint). It runs through the top of the head and cervical vertebra and ends at the lateral side of the little toe (Zhiyin acupoint). There are 67 acupoints in each side of the meridian and 134 acupoints in total.

The Bladder Meridian indications: ① HEENT diseases including headache,mouth and eyelid twitching,supraorbital ridge pain. ② Nervous system diseases including manic-depressive psychosis, insomnia, etc. ③ Diseases in the neck, back, waist, lower limb. ④ Diseases of the tissue and organ on the pathway of the meridian. ⑤ Some acupoints of the meridian have the function of keeping health which can be used in daily life.

BL	Acupoints	Indications
★ 1	Jīngmíng	Myopia; redness, swelling and pain of the eye; blurry vision; nyctalopia; nepheliun; acute waist pain
★ 2	Cuánzhú	Headache; facial paralysis; waist pain; blurry vision; eyelid twitching; blepharoptosis; pain in the supraorbital ridge
3	Méichōng	Headache; dizziness; rhinobyon; epilepsy
4	Qūchā	Headache; blurry vision; rhinobyon
5	Wǔchù	Headache; dizziness; blurry vision; epilepsy
6	Chéngguāng	Headache; dizziness; blurry vision; rhinobyon; epilepsy
7	Tōngtiān	Rhinobyon; rhinitis; headache; dizziness
8	Luòquè	Headache; tinnitus; rhinobyon; blurry vision; epilepsy
9	Yùzhěn	Stiffness and pain in the neck and the head; blurry vision
★ 10	Tiānzhù	Headache; dizziness; stiff neck; pain in the shoulder and the back; rhinobyon
11	Dàzhù	Cough; fever; headache; pain in the shoulder and the back

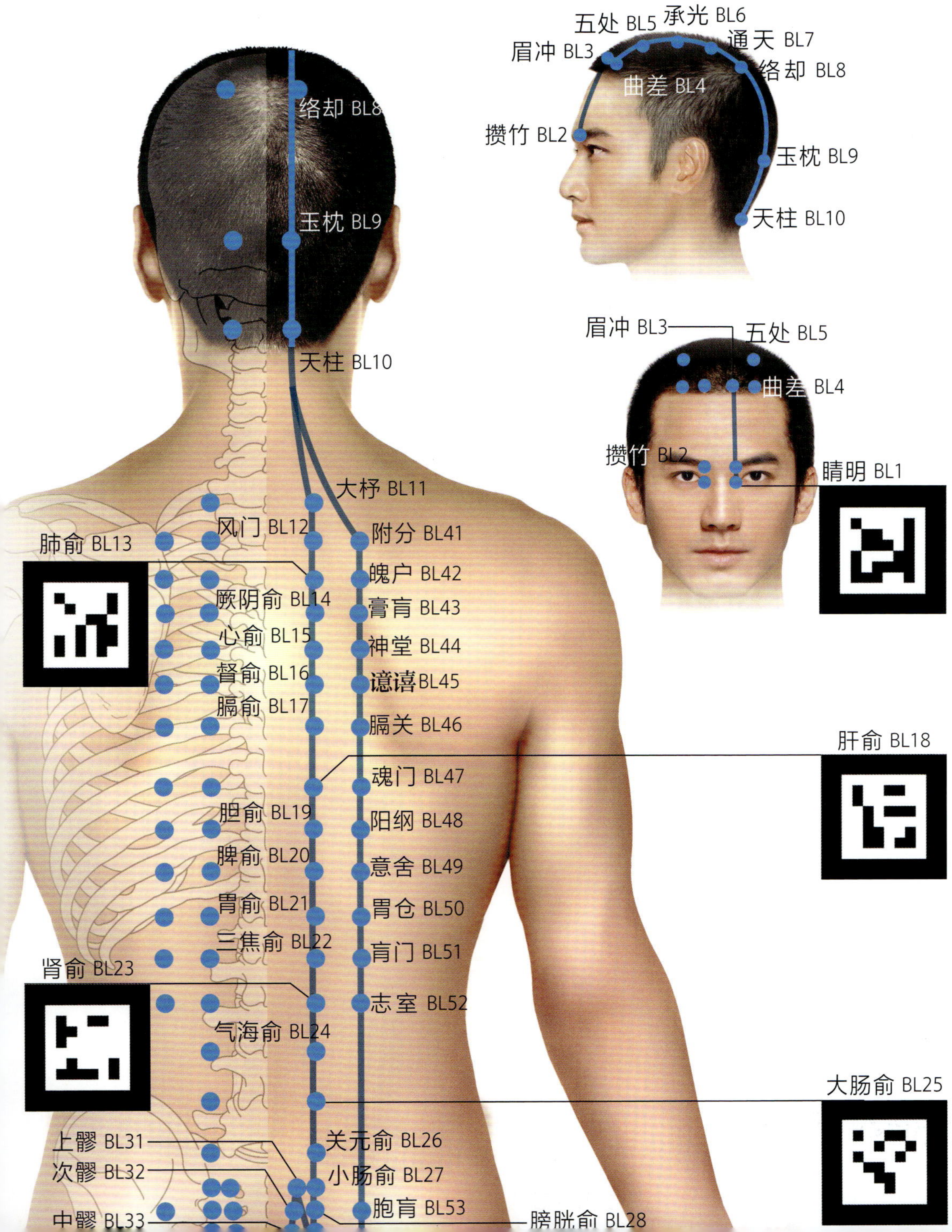

续表

BL	穴名	主治
12	风门	咳嗽、发热、头痛、胸背痛
★ 13	肺俞	咳嗽、气喘、鼻塞、盗汗、皮肤瘙痒、荨麻疹
14	厥阴俞	心痛、心悸、咳嗽、胸闷、呕吐
15	心俞	心痛、心悸、心烦、失眠、健忘、咳嗽、吐血
16	督俞	心痛、胸闷、气喘、胃痛、腹痛、腹胀
★ 17	膈俞	胃脘痛、呕吐、饮食不下、呃逆、咳嗽、气喘、荨麻疹
★ 18	肝俞	黄疸、胁痛、目视不明、夜盲、吐血、眩晕、呃逆、癫狂
19	胆俞	黄疸、口苦、呕吐、肺痨（肺结核）、潮热
20	脾俞	腹胀、呕吐、泄泻、便血、消化不良、水肿、黄疸、背痛
★ 21	胃俞	胃脘痛、腹胀、呕吐、胸胁痛
22	三焦俞	水肿、小便不利、腹胀、肠鸣、泄泻、腰背强痛
★ 23	肾俞	遗精、阳痿、月经不调、带下、遗尿、小便不利、水肿、耳鸣、耳聋、气喘、腰痛
24	气海俞	腰痛、痛经、腹胀肠鸣、胃下垂
★ 25	大肠俞	腰痛、腹胀、泄泻、便秘
26	关元俞	腹胀、泄泻、小便频数或不利、遗尿、腰痛

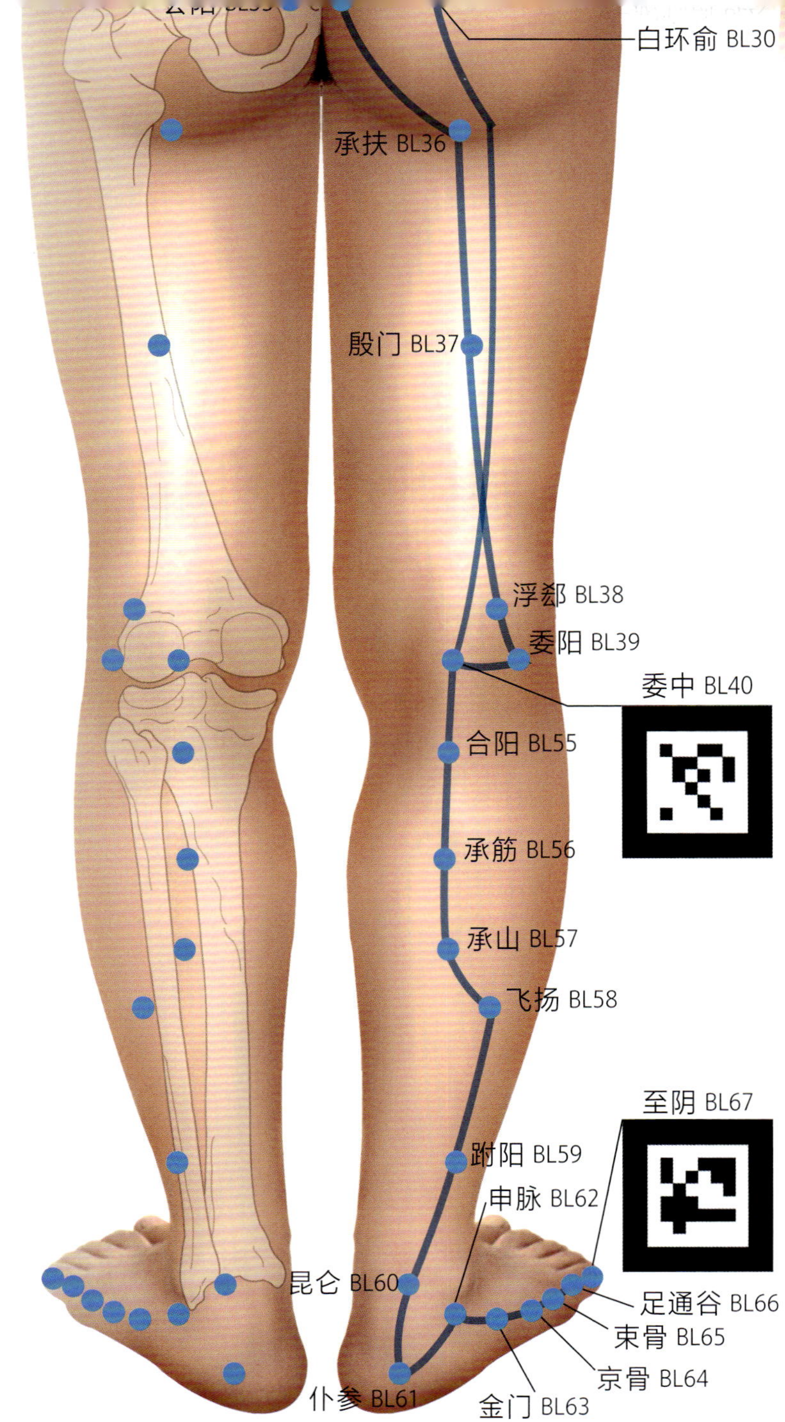

Continued

BL	Acupoints	Indications
12	Fēngmén	Cough; fever; headache; pain in the shoulder and the chest
★ 13	Fèishū	Cough; asthma; rhinobyon; night sweating; skin itching; urticaria
14	Juéyīnshū	Cardiac pain; palpitation; cough; chest tightness; vomiting
15	Xīnshū	Cardiac pain; palpitation; vexation; insomnia; amnesia; cough; hematemesis
16	Dūshū	Cardiac pain; chest tightness; asthma; stomachache; abdominal pain; abdominal distension
★ 17	Géshū	Stomachache; vomiting; swallowing incompetence; hiccup; cough; asthma; urticaria
★ 18	Gānshū	Jaundice; hypochondriac pain; blurry vision; nyctalopia; hematemesis; hiccup; manic-depressive psychosis
19	Dǎnshū	Jaundice; bitter taste in mouth; vomiting; phthisis; tidal fever
20	Píshū	Abdominal distension; vomiting; diarrhea; hematochezia; dyspepsia; edema; jaundice; backache
★ 21	Wèishū	Stomachache; abdominal distension; vomiting; pain in the chest and the hypochondrium
22	Sānjiāoshū	Edema; dysuria; abdominal distension; borborygmus; diarrhea; stiffness and pain in the waist and the back
★ 23	Shènshū	Spermatorrhea; erectile dysfunction; irregular menstruation; leukorrhea; enuresis; dysuria; edema; tinnitus; deafness; asthma; waist pain
24	Qìhǎishū	Waist pain; dysmenorrhea; abdominal distension and borborygmus; gastroptosis
★ 25	Dàchángshū	Waist pain; abdominal distension; diarrhea; constipation
26	Guānyuánshū	Abdominal distension; diarrhea; dysuria or frequent urination; enuresis; waist pain

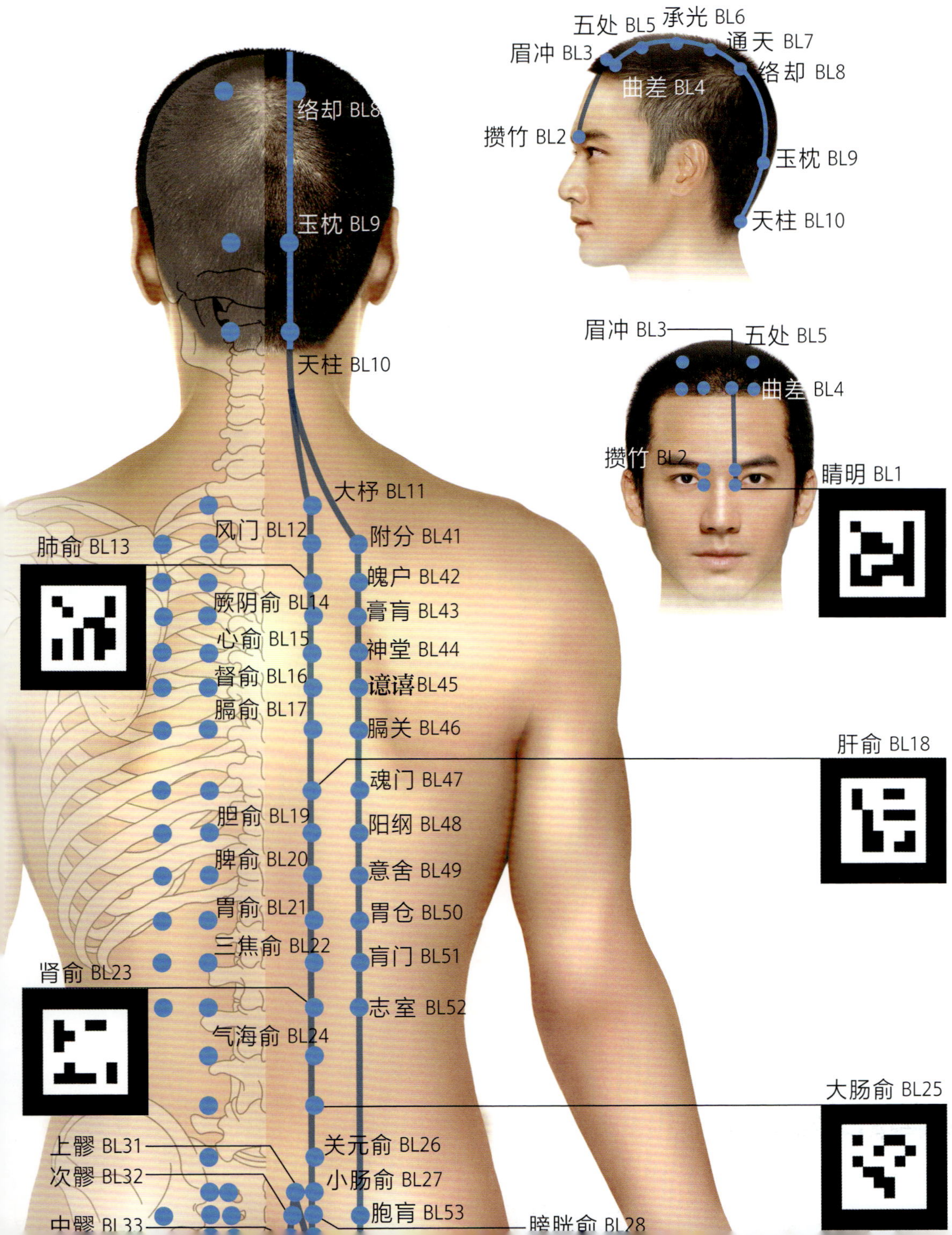

续表

BL	穴名	主治
27	小肠俞	遗精、遗尿、尿血、带下、腹痛、泄泻、腰痛
28	膀胱俞	小便不利、尿频、遗尿、遗精、泄泻、便秘、腰脊强痛
29	中膂俞	疝气、腰脊强痛
30	白环俞	遗精、带下、月经不调、遗尿、腰骶疼痛
31	上髎	月经不调、带下、遗精、阳痿、大小便不利、腰脊痛
★ 32	次髎	月经不调、痛经、带下、遗精、阳痿、小便不利、腰脊痛、下肢痿痹
33	中髎	月经不调、带下、小便不利、便秘、泄泻、腰痛
34	下髎	小腹痛、腰骶痛、小便不利、带下、便秘
35	会阳	泄泻、阳痿、带下
36	承扶	腰腿痛、下肢痿痹
37	殷门	腰腿痛、下肢痿痹
38	浮郄	膝腘痛麻挛急、便秘
39	委阳	腹痛、水肿、小便不利、腰脊强痛、下肢挛痛
★ 40	委中	腰痛、下肢痿痹、腹痛、吐泻、小便不利、遗尿、荨麻疹、皮肤瘙痒

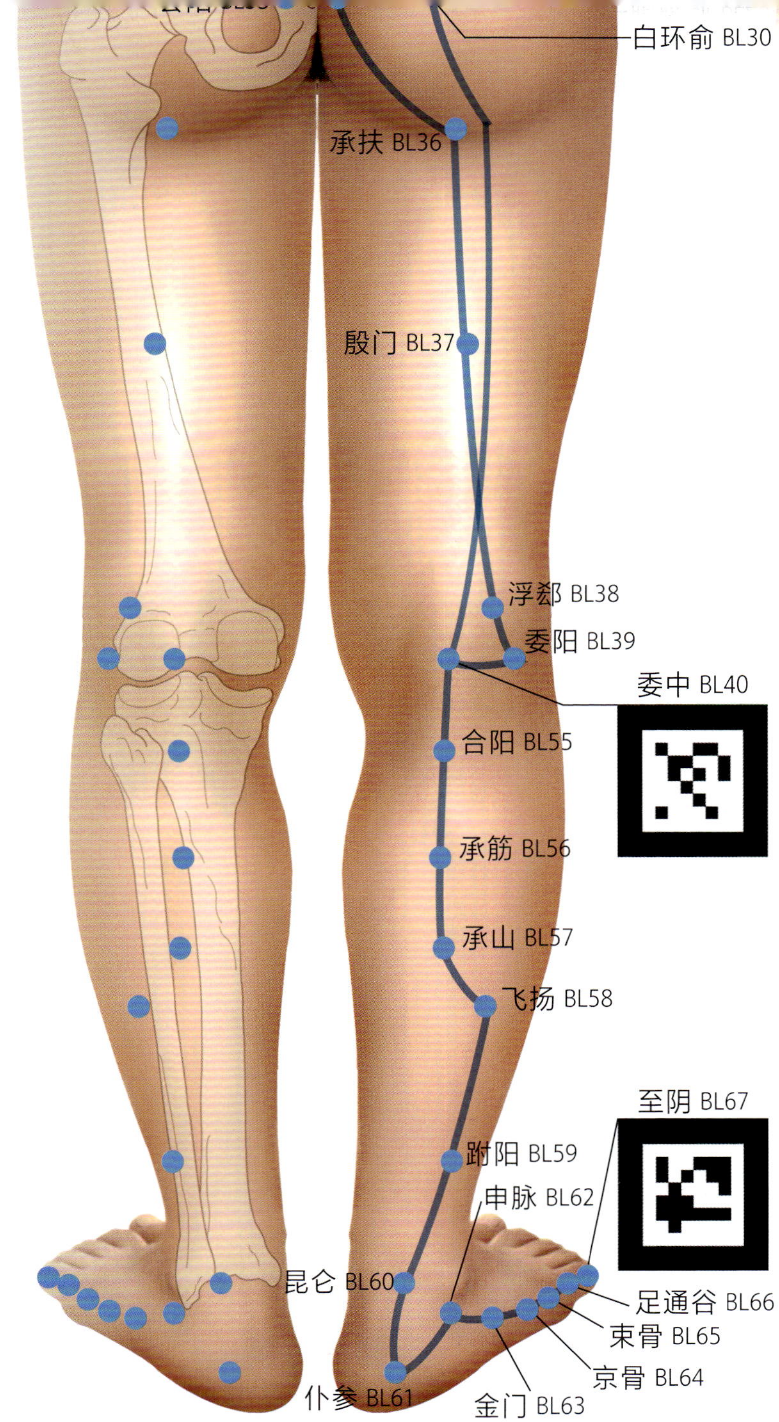

Continued

BL	Acupoints	Indications
27	Xiǎochángshū	Spermatorrhea; enuresis; hematuria; leukorrheal diseases; abdominal pain; diarrhea; waist pain
28	Pángguāngshū	Dysuria; frequent urination; enuresis; spermatorrhea; diarrhea; constipation; waist pain and backache
29	Zhōnglǚshū	Hernia; waist pain and backache
30	Báihuánshū	Spermatorrhea; leukorrheal diseases; irregular menstruation; enuresis; lumbosacral pain
31	Shàngliáo	Irregular menstruation; leukorrheal diseases; spermatorrhea; erectile dysfunction; constipation and dysuria; waist and spine pain
★ 32	Cìliáo	Irregular menstruation; leukorrheal diseases; spermatorrhea; dysmenorrhea; erectile dysfunction; dysuria; waist and spine pain; flaccidity and motor impairment of the lower limb
33	Zhōngliáo	Irregular menstruation; leukorrheal diseases; dysuria; waist pain; constipation; diarrhea
34	Xiàliáo	Lower abdomimal pain; lumbosacral pain; dysuria; leukorrheal diseases; constipation
35	Huìyáng	Diarrhea; erectile dysfunction; leukorrheal diseases
36	Chéngfú	Pain in the waist and lower limbs; flaccidity and motor impairment of the lower limb
37	Yīnmén	Pain in the waist and lower limbs; flaccidity and motor impairment of the lower limb
38	Fúxì	Pain, numbness and spasm in the knee; constipation
39	Wěiyáng	Abdominal pain; edema; dysuria; waist and spine pain; spasm and pain in the lower limb
★ 40	Wěizhōng	Waist pain; flaccidity and motor impairment of the lower limb; abdominal pain; vomiting and diarrhea; dysuria; enuresis; urticaria; skin itching

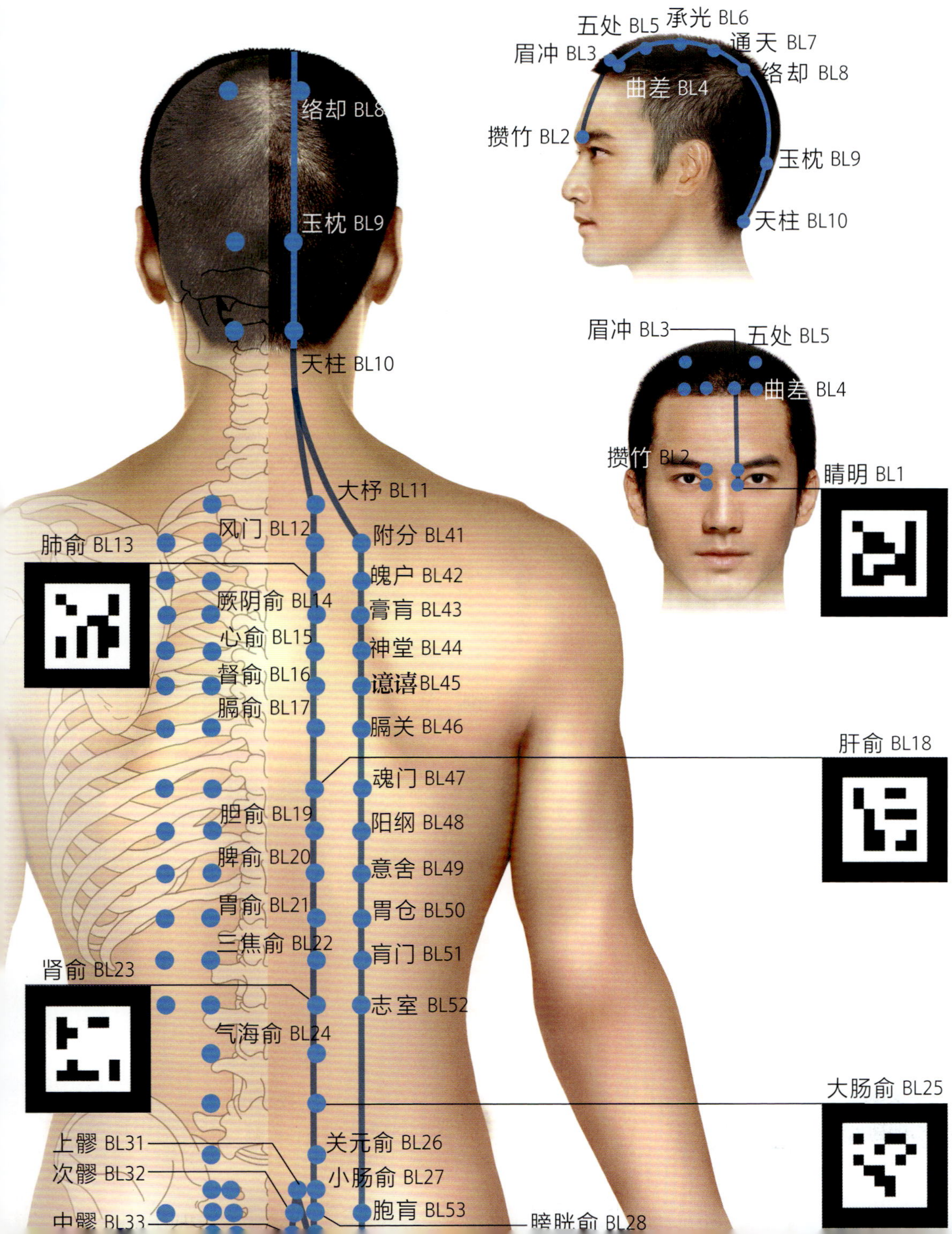

续表

BL	穴名	主治
41	附分	颈项强痛、肩背挛急、肘臂麻木
42	魄户	咳嗽、气喘、肺痨、肩背痛、项强
43	膏肓	咳嗽、气喘、肺痨、健忘、遗精、虚劳（脏腑气血虚损所致的病症）
44	神堂	心痛、心悸、咳嗽、气喘、胸闷、背痛
45	譩譆	咳嗽、气喘、热病、肩背痛
46	膈关	呕吐、呃逆、嗳气、消化不良、肩背痛
47	魂门	胸胁痛、呕吐、泄泻、黄疸、背痛
48	阳纲	肠鸣、泄泻、腹痛、黄疸、消渴（糖尿病）
49	意舍	腹胀、肠鸣、泄泻、呕吐
50	胃仓	胃脘痛、腹胀、水肿
51	肓门	腹痛、痞块（腹腔内结块）、便秘
52	志室	遗精、阳痿、遗尿、小便不利、水肿、月经不调、腰脊强痛
53	胞肓	肠鸣、腹胀、便秘、小便不利、腰脊痛
★ 54	秩边	腰腿痛、下肢痿痹、便秘、小便不利、遗精、阳痿

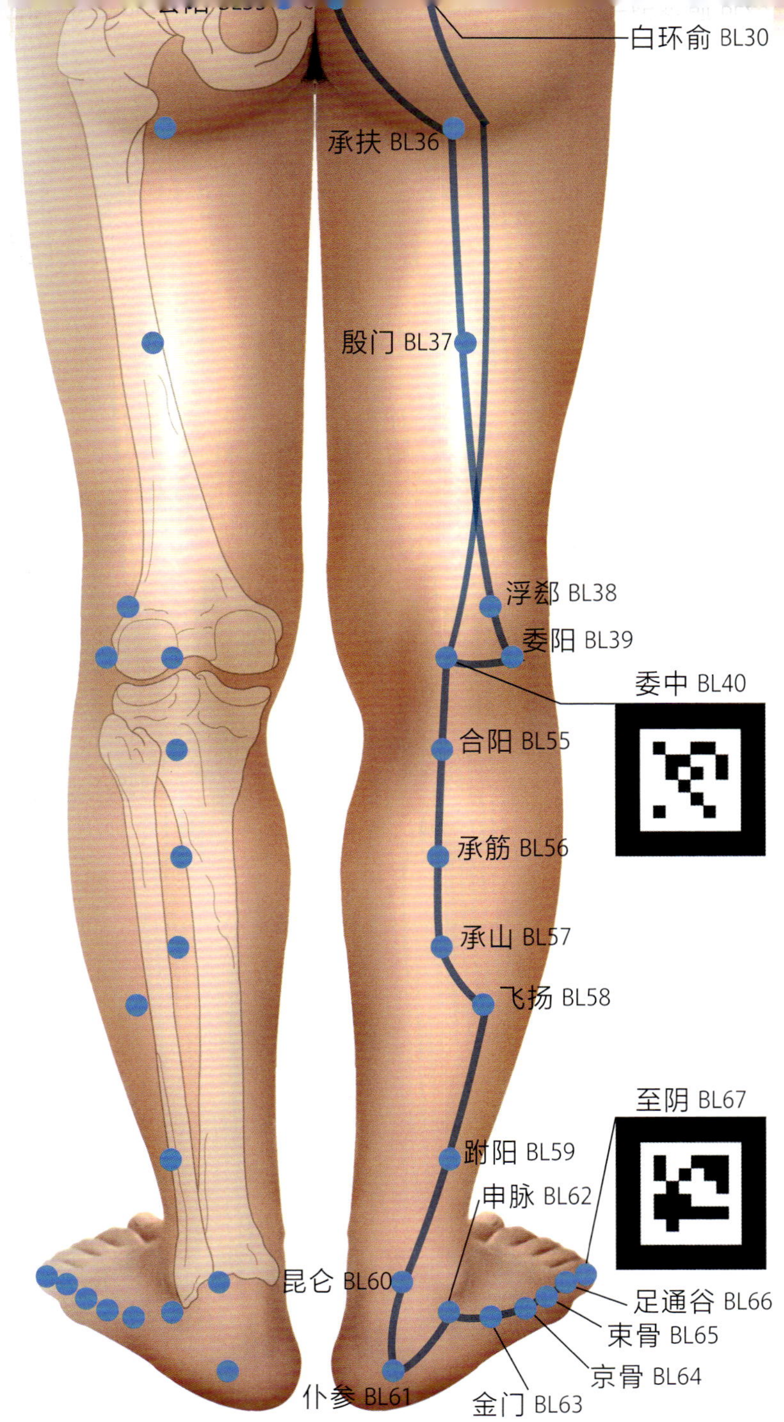

Continued

BL	Acupoints	Indications
41	Fùfēn	Stiffness and pain in the neck; spasm in the shoulder and the back; numbness in the elbow and the arm
42	Pòhù	Cough; asthma; phthisis; pain in the shoulder and the back; stiffness in the neck
43	Gāohuāng	Cough; asthma; phthisis; amnesia; spermatorrhea; consumptive disease (deficiency of Qi, blood and organs)
44	Shéntáng	Cardiac pain; palpitation; cough; asthma; chest tightness; backache
45	Yìxǐ	Cough; asthma; heat disease; pain in the shoulder and the back
46	Géguān	Vomiting; hiccup; belching; dyspepsia; pain in the shoulder and the back
47	Húnmén	Pain in chest and the hypochondrium; vomiting; diarrhea; backache; jaundice
48	Yánggāng	Borborygmus; diarrhea; abdominal pain; jaundice; diabetes mellitus
49	Yìshè	Abdominal distension; borborygmus; diarrhea; vomiting
50	Wèicāng	Stomachache; abdominal distension; edema
51	Huāngmén	Abdominal pain; abdominal lump; constipation
52	Zhìshì	Spermatorrhea; erectile dysfunction; enuresis; dysuria; edema; irregular menstruation; stiffness and pain of the waist and the spine
53	Bāohuāng	Borborygmus; abdominal distension; constipation; dysuria; waist and spine pain
★ 54	Zhìbiān	Waist and lower limb pain; flaccidity and motor impairment of the lower limb; constipation; dysuria; spermatorrhea; erectile dysfunction

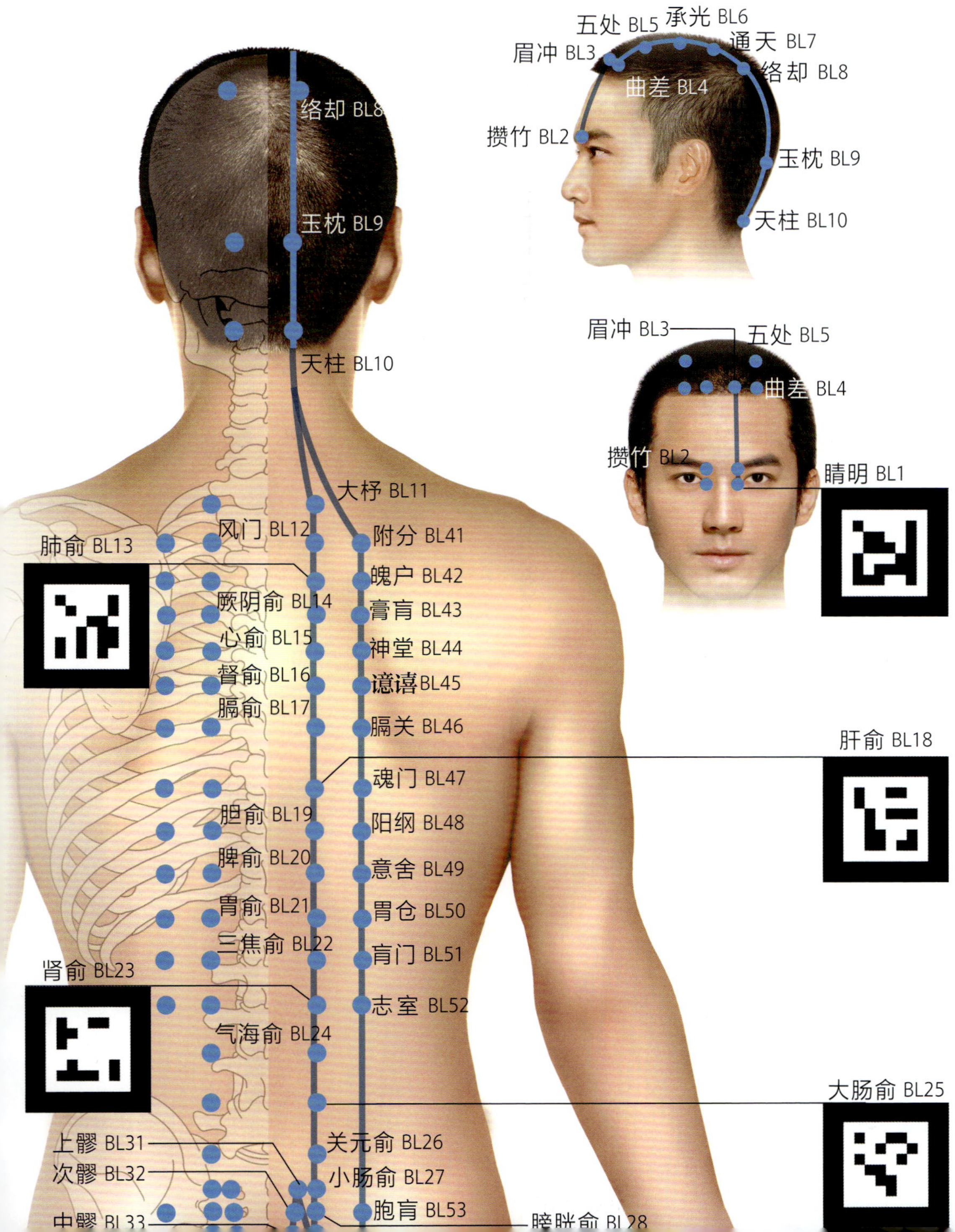

续表

BL	穴名	主治
55	合阳	腰腿痛、下肢痿痹、崩漏
56	承筋	腰腿拘急疼痛
★ 57	承山	腰腿拘急疼痛、便秘
58	飞扬	头痛、目眩、鼻塞、鼻出血、腰背痛、腿软无力
59	跗阳	头痛、腰腿痛、下肢痿痹、外踝肿痛
★ 60	昆仑	头痛、项强、目眩、鼻塞、腰痛、足跟痛
61	仆参	下肢痿痹、足跟痛、癫痫
★ 62	申脉	头痛、眩晕、失眠、目赤痛、眼睑下垂、腰腿痛、项强、足外翻
63	金门	腰痛、下肢痿痛、头痛、外踝肿痛
64	京骨	头痛、项强、目翳、癫痫、腰腿痛
65	束骨	头痛、项强、目眩、癫痫、腰腿痛
66	足通谷	头痛、项强、目眩、癫痫、腰腿痛
★ 67	至阴	胎位不正、难产、头痛、目痛、鼻塞、鼻出血

★为本经常用穴

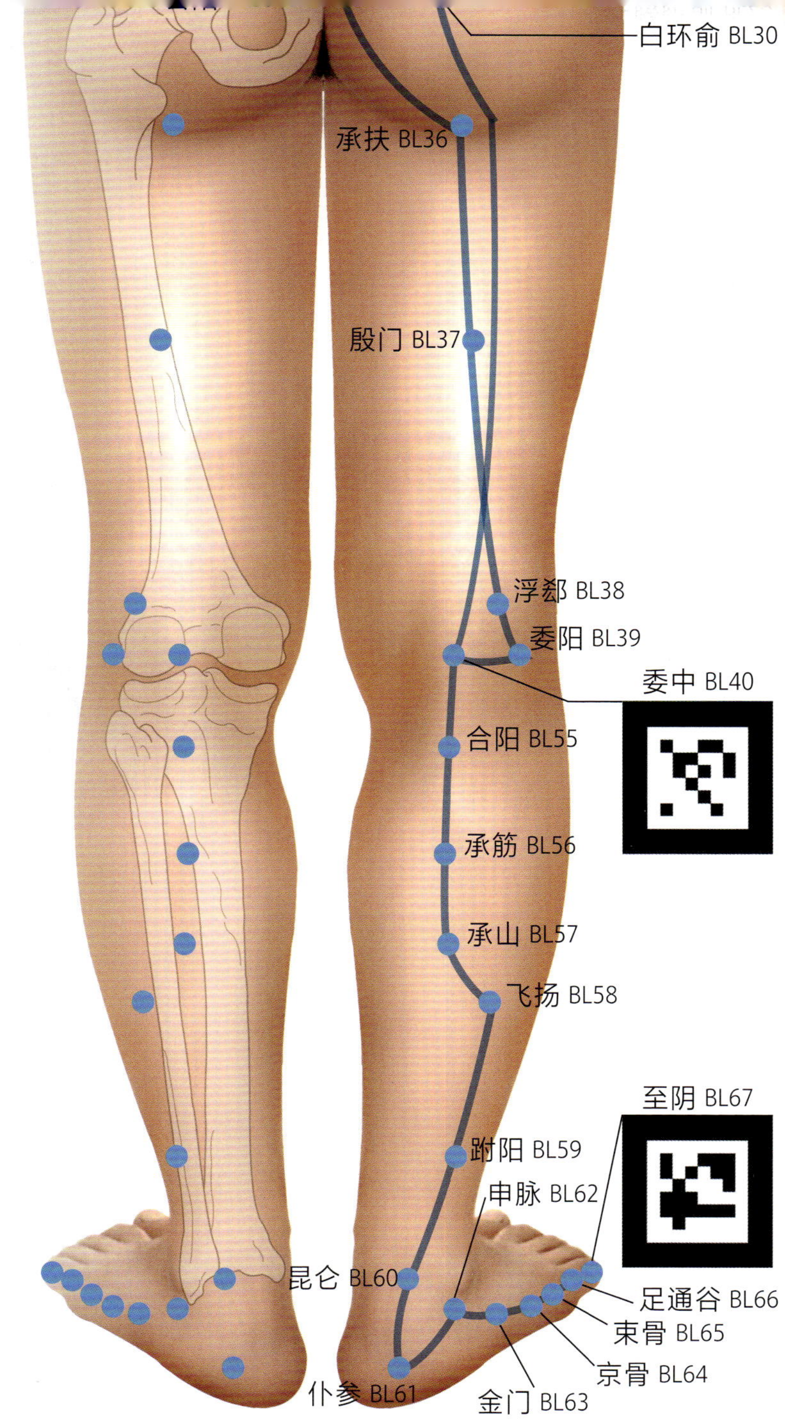

Continued

BL	Acupoints	Indications
55	Héyáng	Waist and lower limb pain; flaccidity and motor impairment of the lower limb; metrorrhagia and metrostaxis
56	Chéngjīn	Spasm and pain in the waist and lower limb
★ 57	Chéngshān	Spasm and pain in the waist and lower limb; constipation
58	Fēiyáng	Headache; dizziness; rhinobyon; nose bleeding; waist and back pain; softness and flaccidity in the leg
59	Fūyáng	Headache; waist and lower limb pain; flaccidity and motor impairment of the lower limb; swelling in the ankle
★ 60	Kūnlún	Headache; stiffness in the neck; dizziness; rhinobyon; waist pain; heel pain
61	Púcān	Flaccidity and motor impairment of the lower limb; heel pain; epilepsy
★ 62	Shēnmài	Headache; dizziness; insomnia; redness and pain in eyes; blepharoptosis; stiffness in the neck; strephexopodia
63	Jīnmén	Waist pain; flaccidity and pain of the lower limb; headache; swelling and pain in lateral malleolus
64	Jīnggǔ	Headache; stiffness in the neck; nephelium; epilepsy; waist and lower limb pain
65	Shùgǔ	Headache; stiffness in the neck; dizziness; epilepsy; waist and lower limb pain
66	Zútōnggǔ	Headache; stiffness in the neck; dizziness; epilepsy; waist and lower limb pain
★ 67	Zhìyīn	Malposition; dystocia; headache; eyes pain; rhinobyon; nose bleeding

★ Common acupoint used in treatment

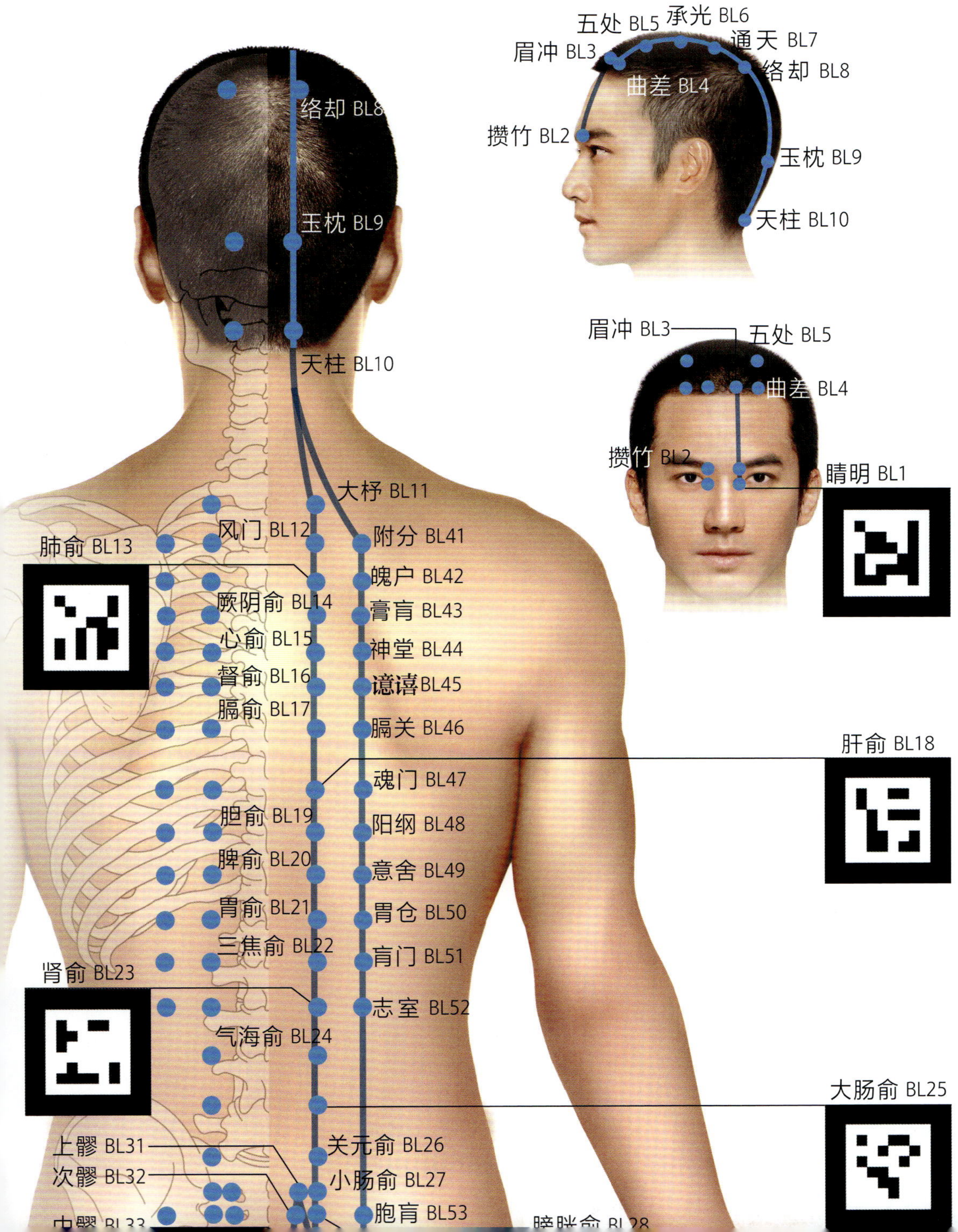

肾俞

两手握拳绕于背后腰部，用掌指关节稍用力按揉两侧肾俞穴 2 分钟。

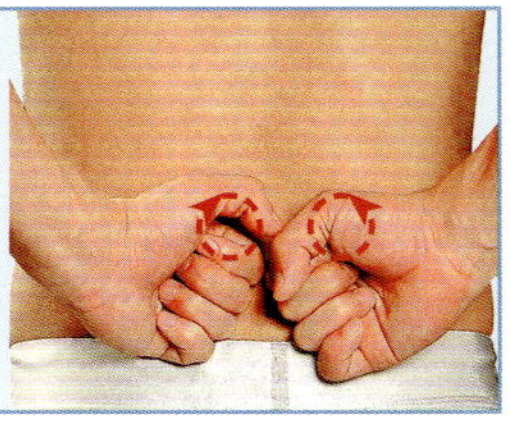

委中

用拇指用力按压委中穴，停留片刻后放松，反复 5 ~ 6 下。同法按压对侧委中穴。每日 2 次。

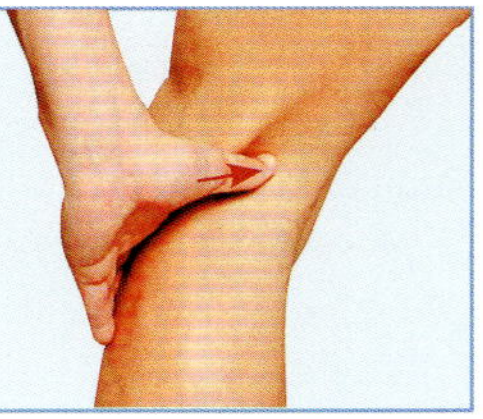

睛明

用双手拇指按揉两侧睛明穴 2 分钟，力度稍轻。

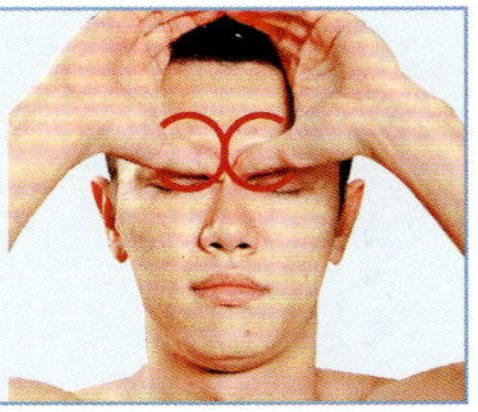

肝俞

一手握拳绕于背后，用掌指关节按揉肝俞穴 2 分钟，力度稍重。同法按揉对侧肝俞穴。

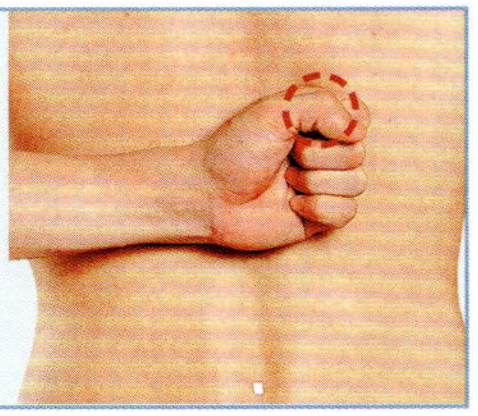

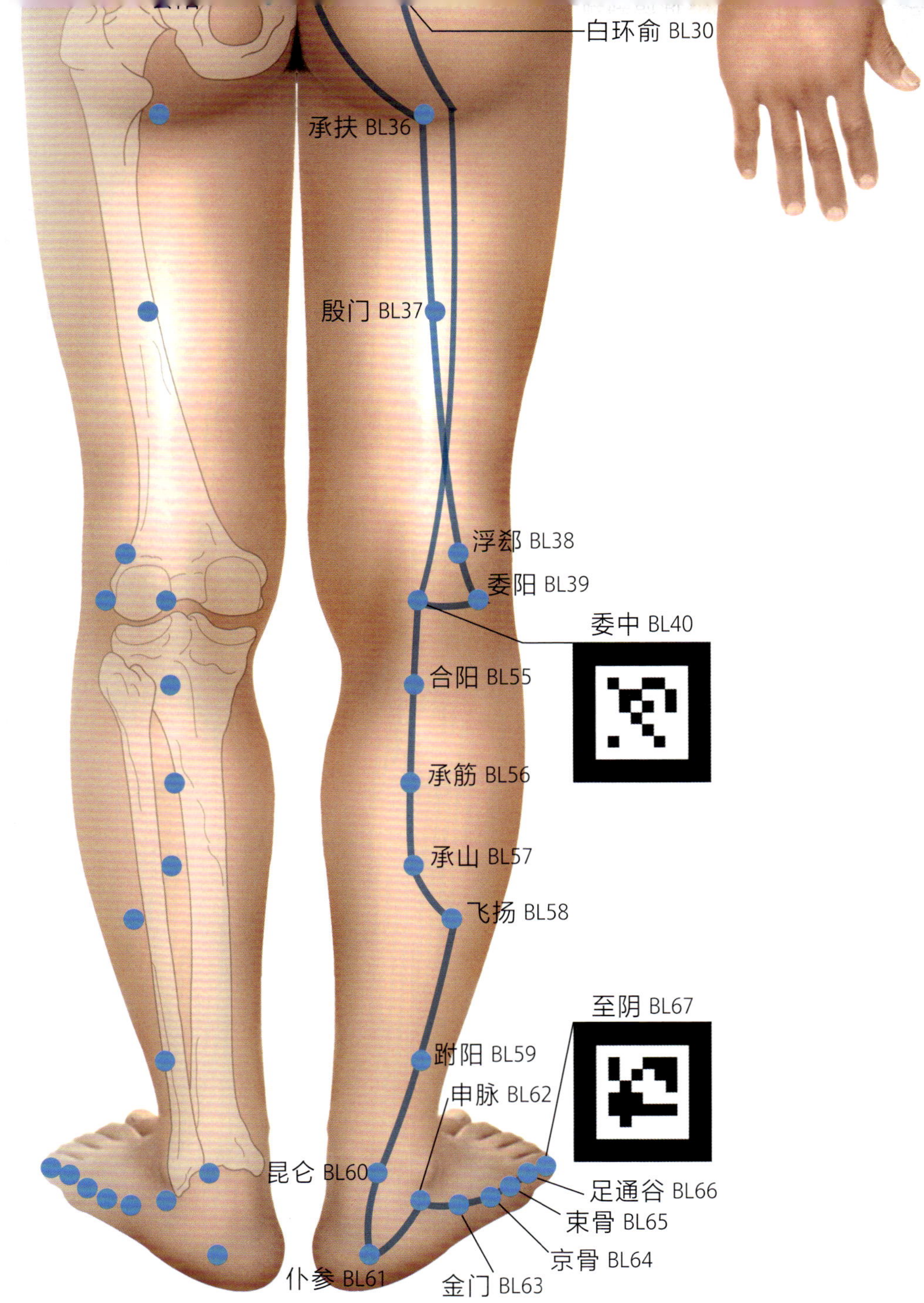

Shènshū(BL23)

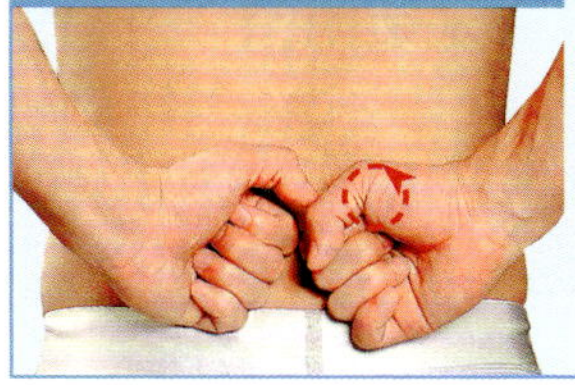

Put both clenched-fists on the waist, and use both metacarpophalangeal joints to knead Shenshu acupoint of both sides with a little heavy strength for 2 minutes.

Wěizhōng(BL40)

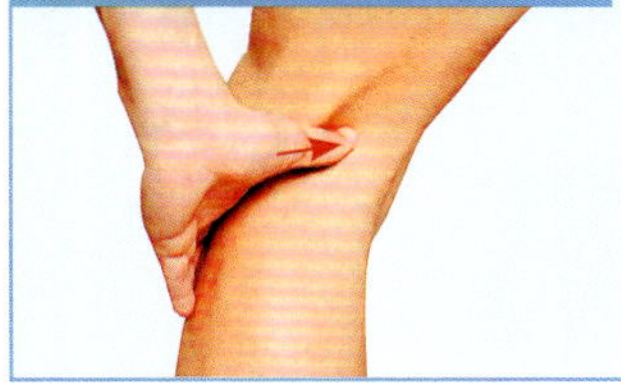

Use the thumb to press the Weizhong acupoint with a little heavy strength for a while, then relax. Repeat 5~6 times a day. Press the contralateral Weizhong acupoint with the same method.

Jīngmíng(BL1)

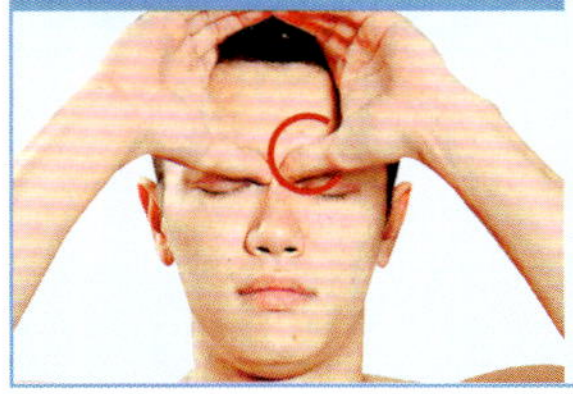

Use both thumbs to knead both Jingming acupoints with slight strength for 2 minutes.

Gānshū(BL18)

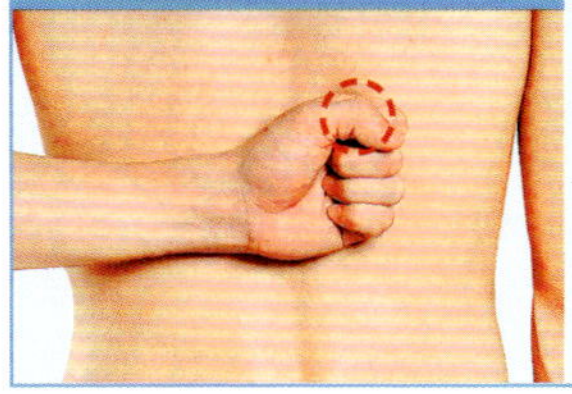

Put a clenched-fist on the back, and use the metacarpophalangeal joint to knead Ganshu acupoint with a little heavy strength for 2 minutes. Knead the contralateral Ganshu acupoint with the same method.

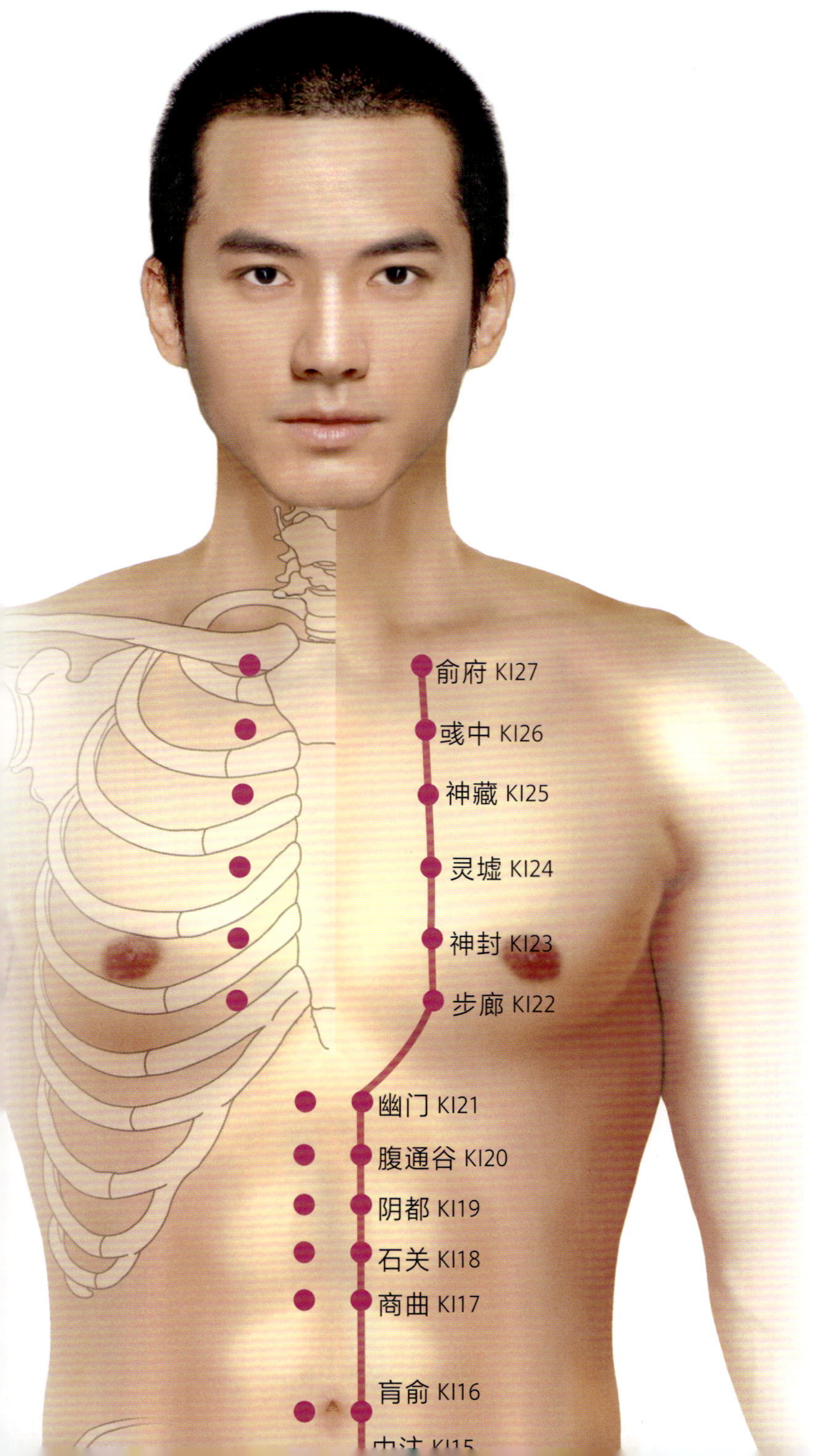

足少阴肾经

足少阴肾经起于脚掌心的涌泉穴，经腿部内侧上达胸前的俞府穴。本经一侧 27 穴，左右两侧共 54 穴。

肾经主治病症：①遗精、阳痿、小便不利、不育等泌尿生殖系统疾病。②癫狂、失眠、眩晕等神经精神系统疾病。③大腿内后侧痛、腰部痛、咽喉肿痛等经脉循行部位的疾患。④本经还可治疗月经不调、痛经、不孕等妇科疾病。

KI	穴名	主治
★ 1	涌泉	头顶痛、眩晕、昏厥、癫狂、失眠、便秘、小便不利、咽喉肿痛、失音、足心热
2	然谷	月经不调、遗精、小便不利、泄泻、咽喉肿痛、咯血、口噤
★ 3	太溪	月经不调、遗精、阳痿、小便频数、消渴、泄泻、腰痛、头痛、耳鸣、耳聋、咽喉肿痛、失眠、咳嗽、咯血
4	大钟	癃闭、遗尿、便秘、咯血、气喘、嗜睡、足跟痛
5	水泉	月经不调、痛经、小便不利
★ 6	照海	月经不调、痛经、带下、小便不利、咽喉痛、目赤肿痛、失眠
7	复溜	水肿、腹胀、泄泻、盗汗、热病无汗或汗出不止
8	交信	月经不调、崩漏、泄泻、便秘
9	筑宾	癫狂、呕吐、疝气、小腿疼痛

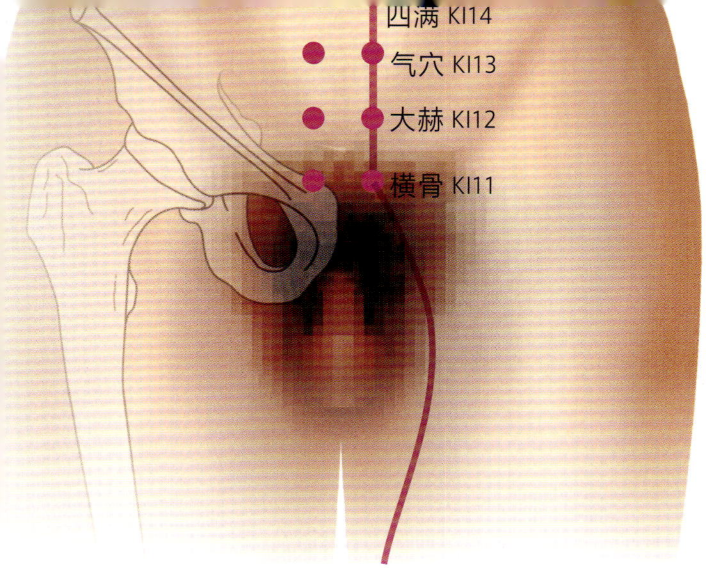

Kidney Meridian of Foot-Shaoyin,KI.

Kidney Meridian of Foot-Shaoyin starts from the center of the sole (Yongquan acupoint), it runs along the medial side of the legs upwardly to the chest (Shufu acupoint). There are 27 acupoints in each side of the meridian and 54 acupoints in total.

The Kidney Meridian indications: ① Urinary system and reproductive system diseases including spermatorrhea,erectile dysfunction,dysuria and infertility. ② Nervous system diseases including manic-depressive psychosis,insomnia and dizziness. ③ Diseases on the pathway of the meridian including pain in the medial posterior side of the thigh,abdominal pain, swelling and pain in the throat. ④ Gynecological diseases including irregular menstruation,dysmenorrhea and sterility.

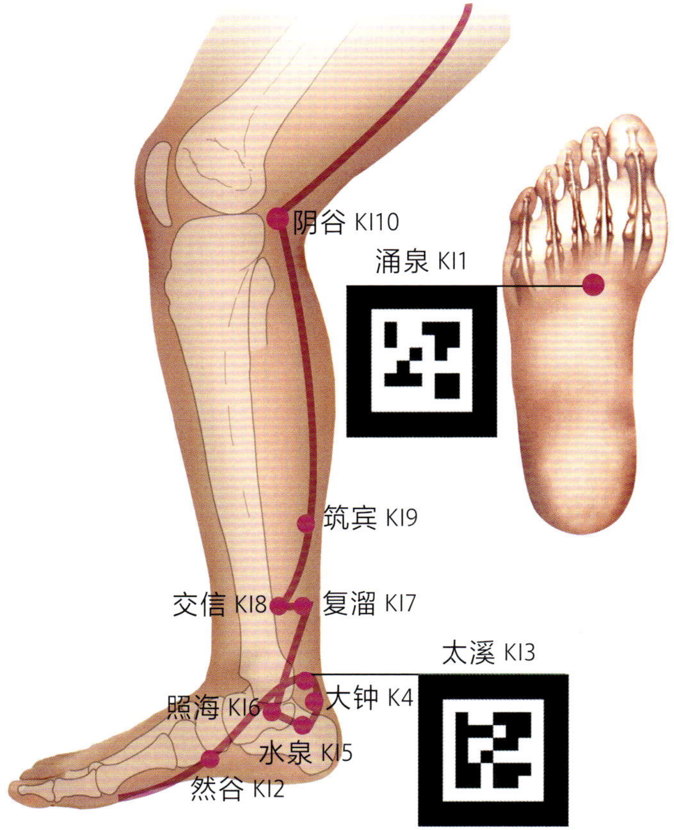

KI	Acupoints	Indications
★ 1	Yǒngquán	Pain in the top of head; dizziness; syncope; manic-depressive psychosis; insomnia; constipation; dysuria; swelling and pain in the throat; aphonia; heat in the center of the sole
2	Rángǔ	Irregular menstruation; spermatorrhea; dysuria; diarrhea; swelling and pain in the throat; hemoptysis; lockjaw
★ 3	Tàixī	Irregular menstruation; spermatorrhea; erectile dysfunction; frequent urination; diabetes mellitus; diarrhea; waist pain; headache; tinnitus; deafness; swelling and pain in the throat; insomnia; cough; hemoptysis
4	Dàzhōng	Retention of urine; enuresis; constipation; hemoptysis; asthma; somnolence; heel pain
5	Shuǐquán	Irregular menstruation; dysmenorrhea; dysuria
★ 6	Zhàohǎi	Irregular menstruation; leukorrheal diseases; dysmenorrhea; dysuria; throat pain; redness, swelling and pain in eyes; insomnia
7	Fùliū	Edema; abdominal distension; diarrhea; night sweating; heat disease with anhidrosis; heat disease with profuse sweating
8	Jiāoxìn	Irregular menstruation; metrorrhagia and metrostaxis; diarrhea; constipation
9	Zhùbīn	Manic-depressive psychosis; vomiting; hernia; pain in the lower leg

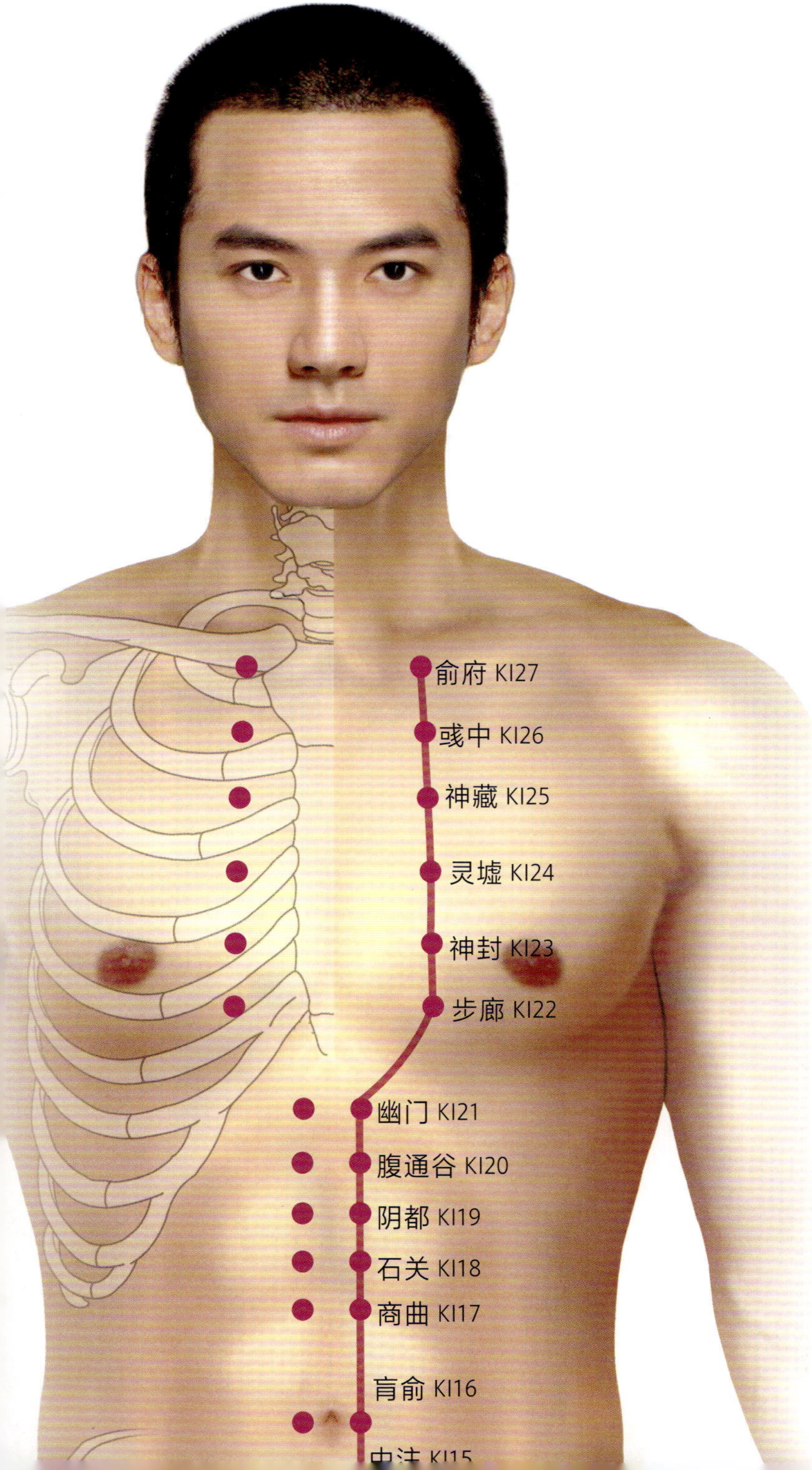

续表

KI	穴名	主治
10	阴谷	阳痿、疝气、崩漏、膝股痛、癫狂
11	横骨	少腹胀痛、小便不利、遗尿、遗精、阳痿、疝气
12	大赫	遗精、阳痿、带下
13	气穴	月经不调、带下、闭经、崩漏、小便不利、泄泻
14	四满	月经不调、带下、遗精、阳痿、便秘、腹痛、水肿
15	中注	腹痛、便秘、泄泻、月经不调、痛经
16	肓俞	腹痛、腹胀、呕吐、泄泻、便秘、月经不调、疝气、腰脊痛
17	商曲	腹痛、泄泻、便秘
18	石关	呕吐、腹痛、便秘、不孕
19	阴都	呕吐、腹痛、便秘、不孕
20	腹通谷	腹痛、腹胀、呕吐、心痛、心悸
21	幽门	腹痛、腹胀、呕吐、泄泻
22	步廊	咳嗽、气喘、胸胁胀满、呕吐
23	神封	咳嗽、气喘、胸胁胀满、呕吐、乳腺炎
24	灵墟	咳嗽、气喘、胸胁胀满、呕吐、乳腺炎
25	神藏	咳嗽、气喘、胸痛、呕吐
26	彧中	咳嗽、气喘、胸胁胀满
27	俞府	咳嗽、气喘、胸痛、呕吐

★为本经常用穴

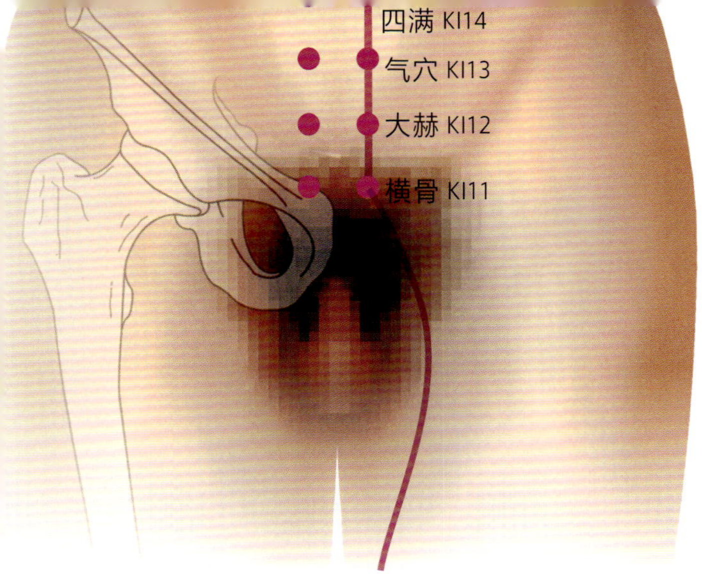

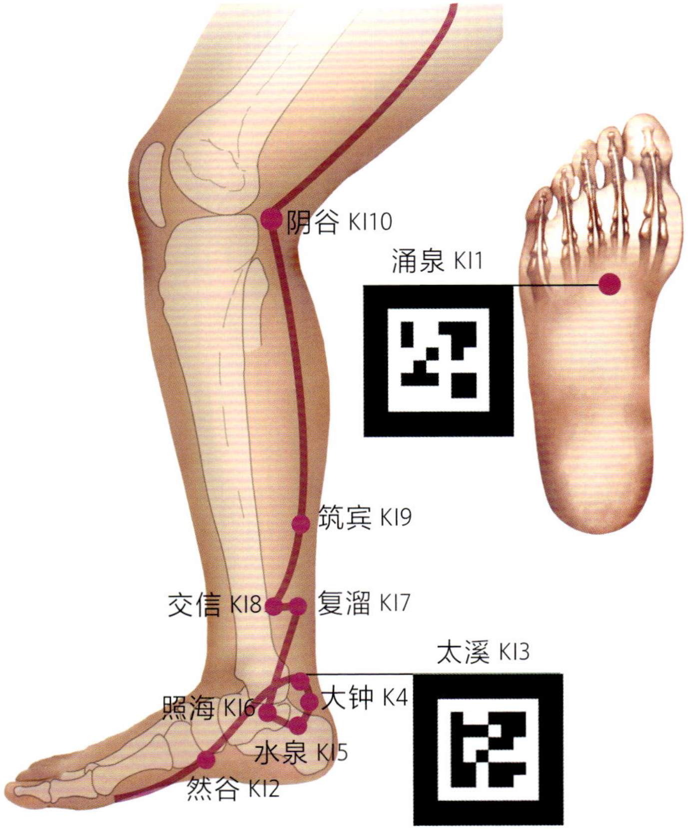

Continued

KI	Acupoints	Indications
10	Yīngǔ	Erectile dysfunction; hernia; metrorrhagia and metrostaxis; knee and thigh pain; manic-depressive psychosis
11	Hénggǔ	Distension and pain in the lateral abdomen; dysuria; enuresis; spermatorrhea; erectile dysfunction; hernia
12	Dàhè	Spermatorrhea; erectile dysfunction; leukorrheal diseases
13	Qìxué	Irregular menstruation; leukorrheal diseases; metrorrhagia and metrostaxis; amenorrhea; dysuria; diarrhea
14	Sìmǎn	Irregular menstruation; leukorrheal diseases; spermatorrhea; erectile dysfunction; constipation; abdominal pain; edema
15	Zhōngzhù	Abdominal pain; constipation; diarrhea; irregular menstruation; dysmenorrhea
16	Huāngshū	Abdominal pain; abdominal distension; vomiting; diarrhea; constipation; hernia; irregular menstruation; waist and spine pain
17	Shāngqū	Abdominal pain; diarrhea; constipation
18	Shíguān	Vomiting; abdominal pain; constipation; sterility
19	Yīndū	Vomiting; abdominal pain; constipation; sterility
20	Fùtōnggǔ	Abdominal pain; abdominal distension; vomiting; cardiac pain; palpitation
21	Yōumén	Abdominal pain; abdominal distension; diarrhea; vomiting
22	Bùláng	Cough; asthma; vomiting; distension in the chest and the hypochondrium
23	Shénfēng	Cough; asthma; vomiting; distension in the chest and the hypochondrium; mastitis
24	Língxū	Cough; asthma; vomiting; distension in the chest and the hypochondrium; mastitis
25	Shéncáng	Cough; asthma; chest pain; vomiting
26	Yùzhōng	Cough; asthma; distension in the chest and the hypochondrium
27	Shūfǔ	Cough; asthma; chest pain; vomiting

★ Common acupoint used in treatment

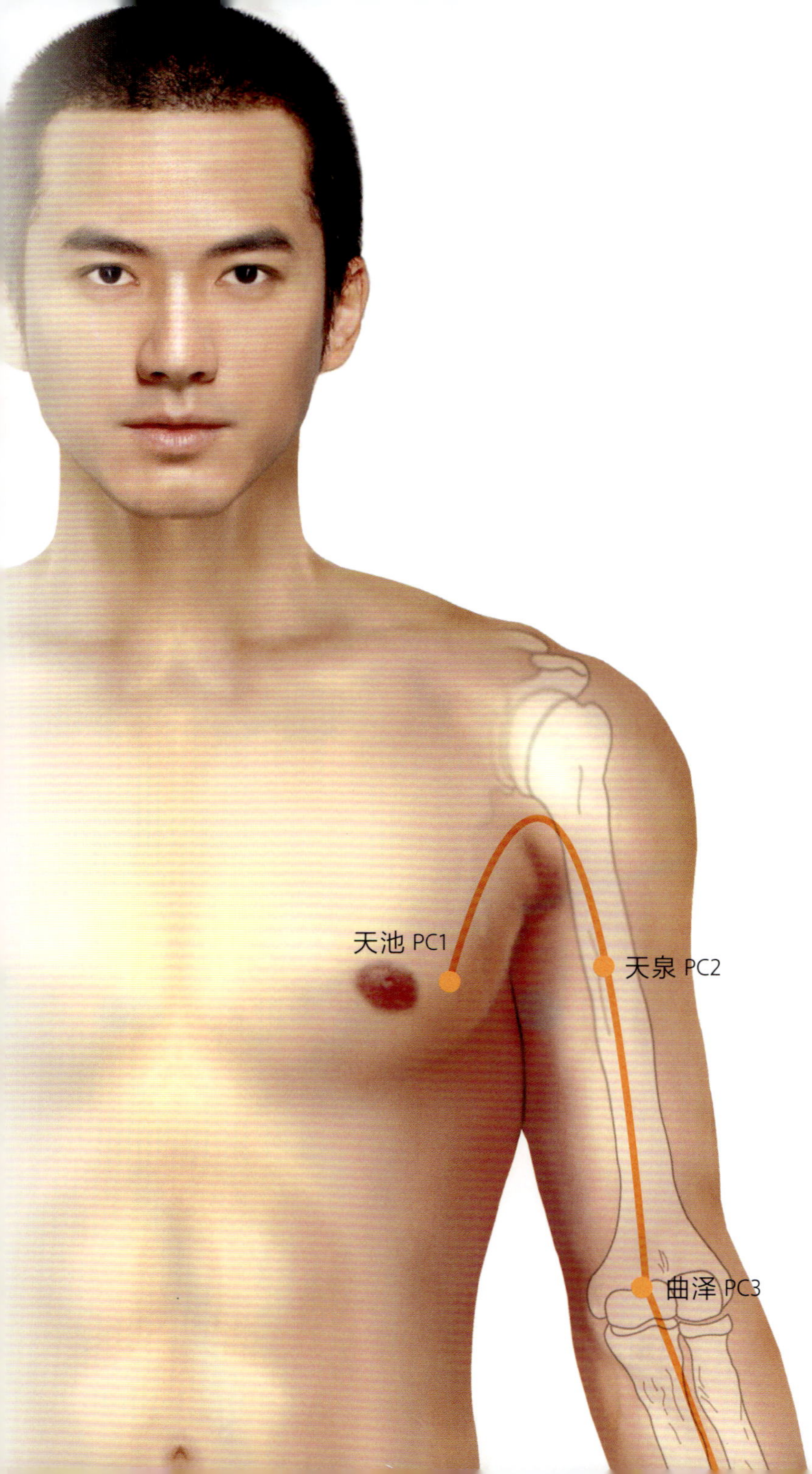

手厥阴心包经

手厥阴心包经起于乳房外侧的天池穴，经手臂内侧，止于手中指的中冲穴。本经一侧9 个穴，左右两侧共 18 个穴，8 个穴分布在上肢内侧中间，1 个穴在前胸部。

心包经主治病症：①心烦、胸闷、心悸、心痛等心胸疾病。②前臂痛、肘部痛等经脉循行部位的疾患。

PC	穴名	主治
1	天池	咳嗽、气喘、乳腺炎、乳少、胸闷、胸胁胀满
2	天泉	心痛、咳嗽、胸胁胀满、臂痛
★ 3	曲泽	心痛、心悸、热病、中暑、胃痛、呕吐、泄泻、肘臂疼痛
4	郄门	心痛、心悸、呕血、咯血
5	间使	心痛、心悸、癫狂、热病、胃痛、呕吐、肘臂痛
★ 6	内关	心痛、心悸、胸闷、眩晕、癫痫、失眠、偏头痛、胃痛、呕吐、泄泻、肘臂痛
★ 7	大陵	心痛、心悸、癫狂、胃痛、呕吐、手腕麻痛、胸胁胀痛

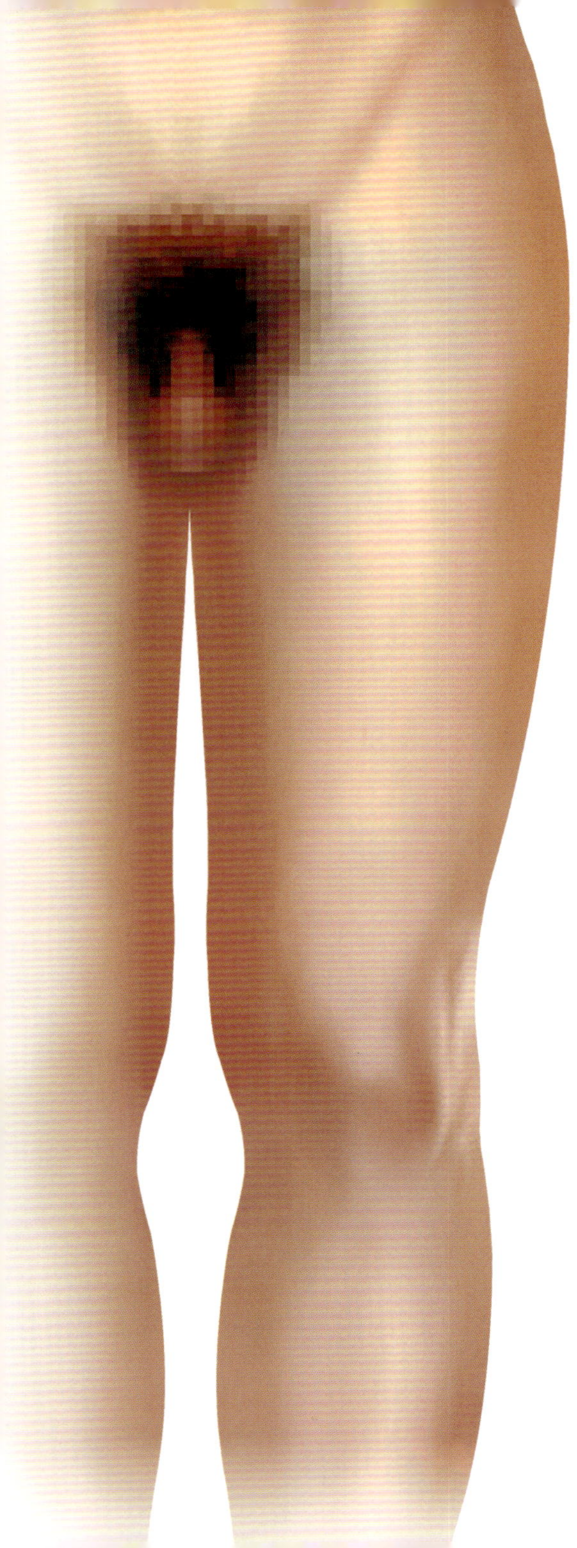

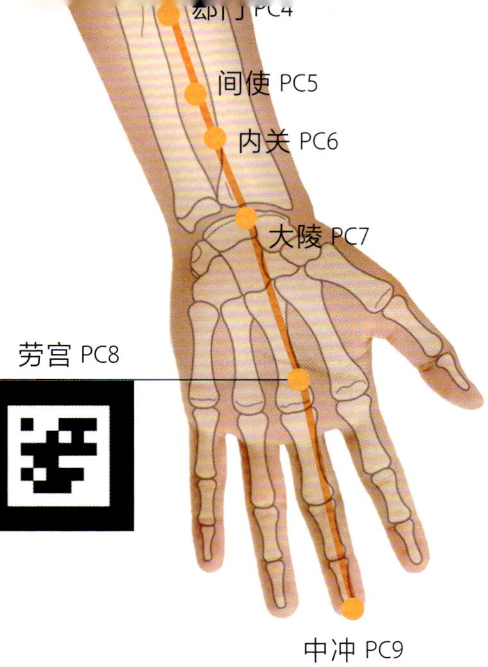

Pericardium Meridian of Hand-Jueyin,PC.

Pericardium Meridian of Hand-Jueyin originates from the lateral side of the breast (Tianchi acupoint). It runs along the medial aspect of the arm and ends at the middle finger (Zhongchong acupoint). There are 9 acupoints in each side of the meridian and 18 acupoints in total. There is an acupoint in the anterior chest, the other 8 acupoints are located in the interior medial aspect of the upper limb.

The Pericardium Meridian indications: ① Cardiothoracic diseases including vexation, chest tightness, palpitation, cardiac pain. ② Diseases on the pathway of the meridian including forearm pain, elbow pain.

PC	Acupoints	Indications
1	Tiānchí	Cough; asthma; mastitis; hypogalactia; chest tightness; chest tightness; distension in the chest and the hypochondrium
2	Tiānquán	Cardiac pain; cough; distension in the chest and the hypochondrium; arm pain
★ 3	Qūzé	Cardiac pain; palpitation; heat disease; heat stroke; stomachache; vomiting; diarrhea; pain in the arm and the elbow
4	Xìmén	Cardiac pain; palpitation; hematemesis; hemoptysis
5	Jiānshǐ	Cardiac pain; palpitation; manic-depressive psychosis; heat disease; stomachache; vomiting; pain in the arm and the elbow
★ 6	Nèiguān	Cardiac pain; palpitation; chest tightness; dizziness; manic-depressive psychosis; insomnia; migraine; stomachache; vomiting; diarrhea; pain in the arm and the elbow
★ 7	Dàlíng	Cardiac pain; palpitation; manic-depressive psychosis; stomachache; vomiting; numbness and pain in the wrist and the hand; distension and pain in the chest and the hypochondrium

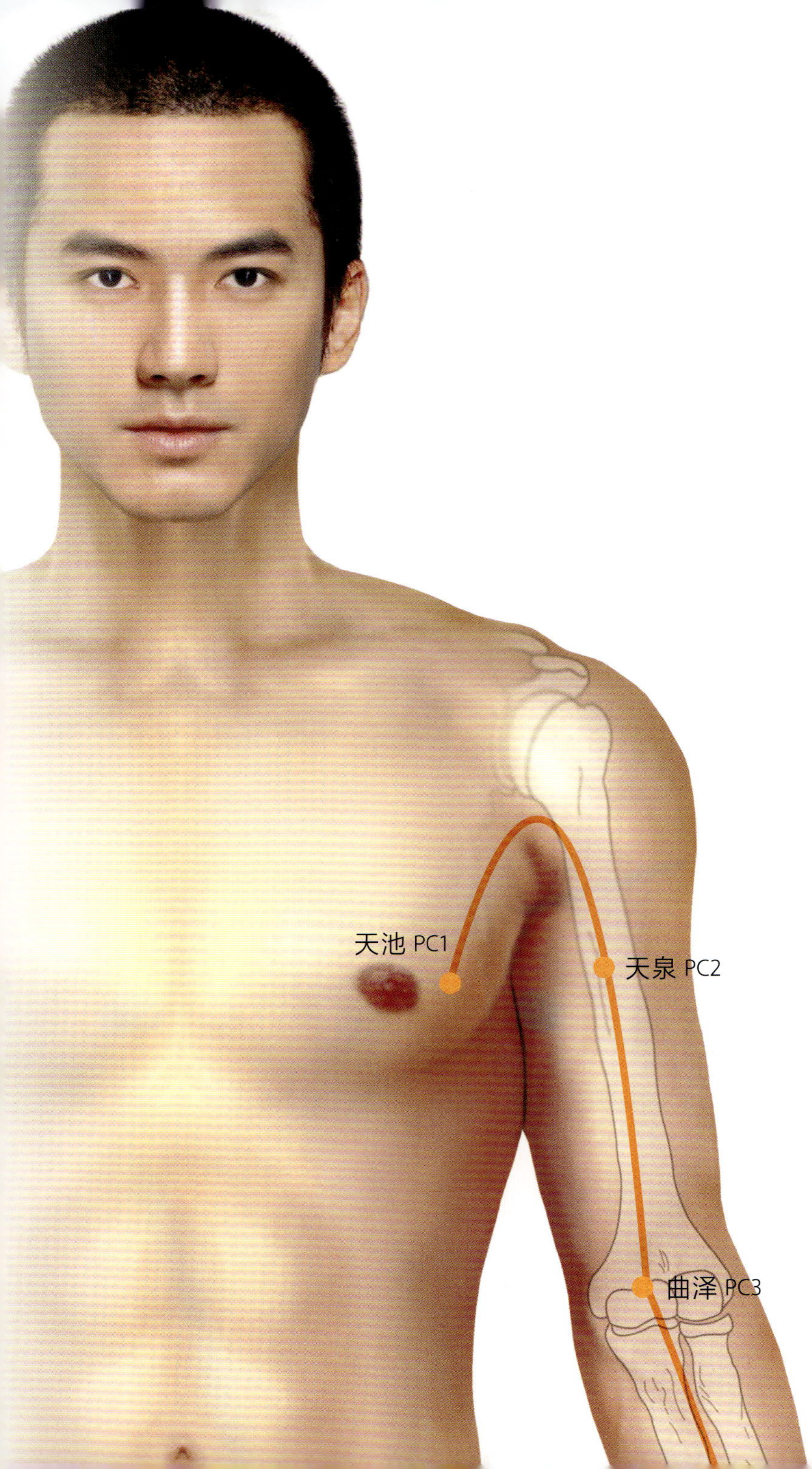

续表

PC	穴名	主治
★ 8	劳宫	癫狂、中风昏迷、中暑、心痛、口疮口臭
★ 9	中冲	中风昏迷、中暑、小儿惊风、热病、心烦、心痛、舌强（僵硬）肿痛

★为本经常用穴

内关

用拇指按揉内关穴 2 分钟，力度稍重。同法按揉对侧内关穴。

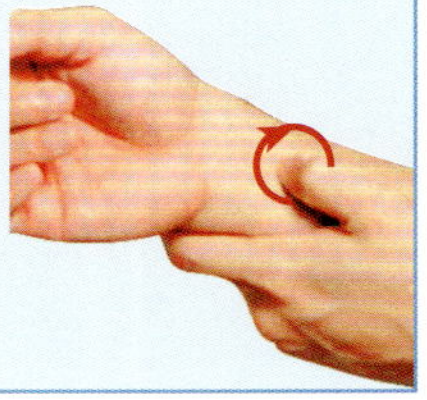

劳宫

用拇指按揉劳宫穴 2 分钟，力度稍重。同法按揉对侧劳宫穴。每日 2 次。

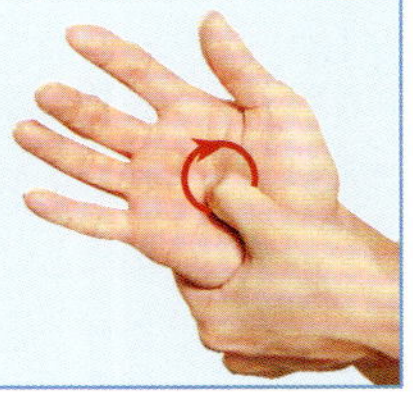

曲泽

用拇指按揉曲泽穴 2 分钟，力度稍重。同法按揉对侧曲泽穴。每日 2 次。

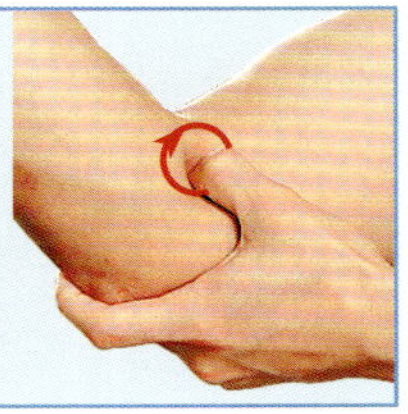

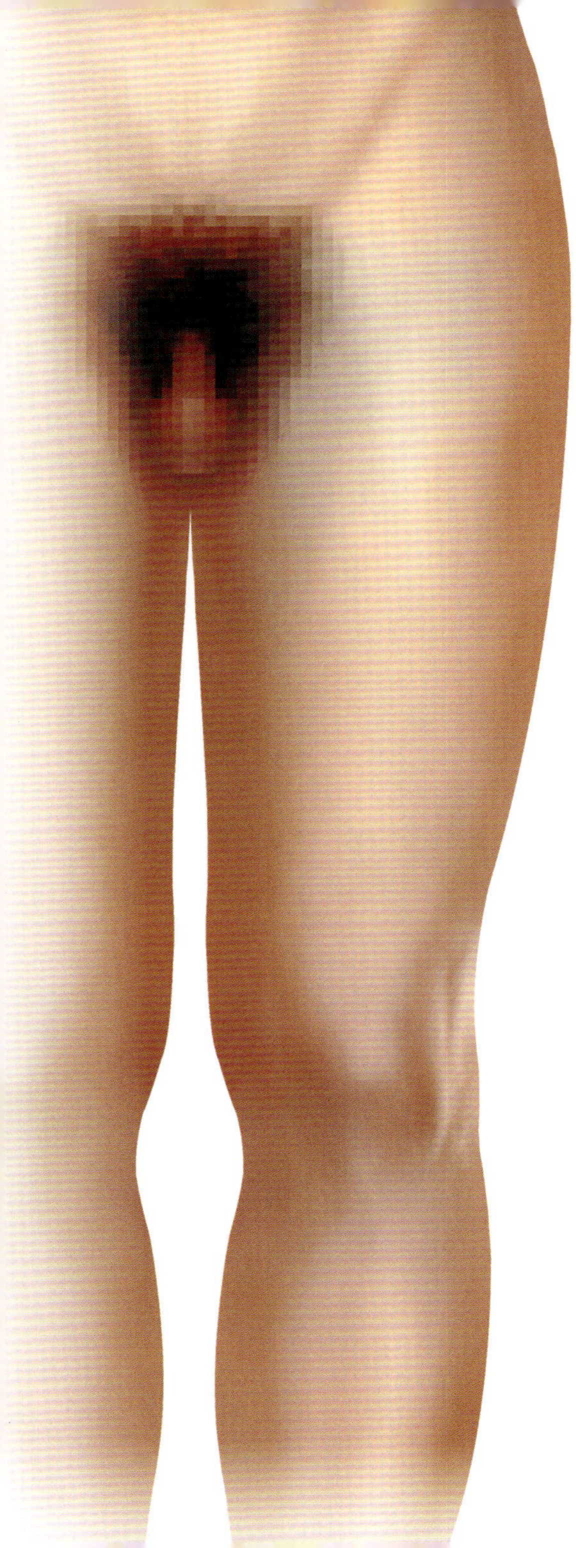

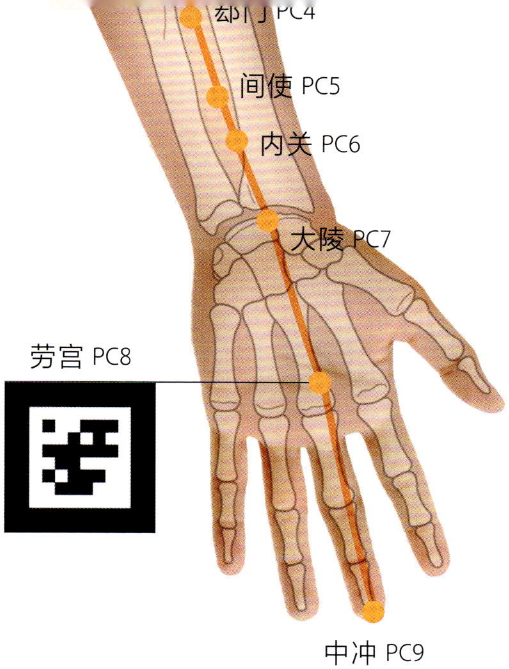

Continued

PC	Acupoints	Indications
★ 8	Láogōng	Manic-depressive psychosis; apoplectic coma; heat stroke; cardiac pain; aphtha; halitosis
★ 9	Zhōngchōng	Apoplectic coma; heat stroke; infantile convulsion; heat disease; vexation; cardiac pain; stiffness; swelling and pain in the tongue

★ Common acupoint used in treatment

Nèiguān(PC6)

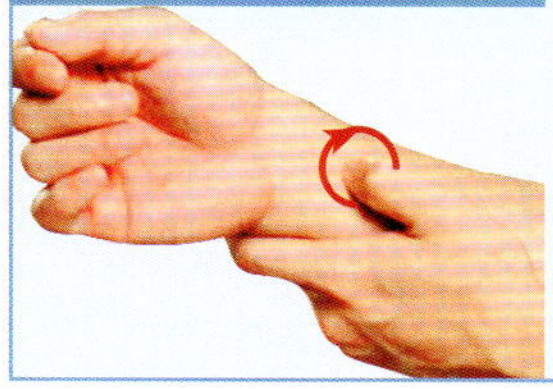

Use the thumb to knead the Neiguan acupoint with a little heavy strength for 2 minutes.Knead the contralateral Neiguan acupoint with the same method.

Láogōng(PC8)

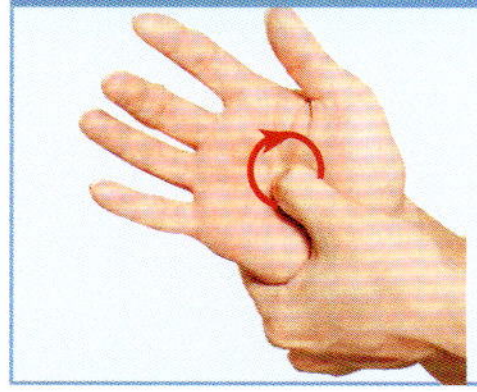

Use the thumb to knead the Laogong acupoint with a little heavy strength for 2 minutes. Knead the contralateral Laogong acupoint with the same method. Twice a day.

Qūzé(PC3)

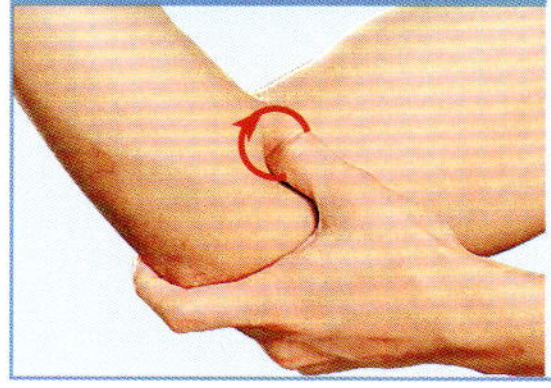

Use the thumb to knead the Quze acupoint with a little heavy strength for 2 minutes. Knead the contralateral Quze acupoint with the same method. Twice a day.

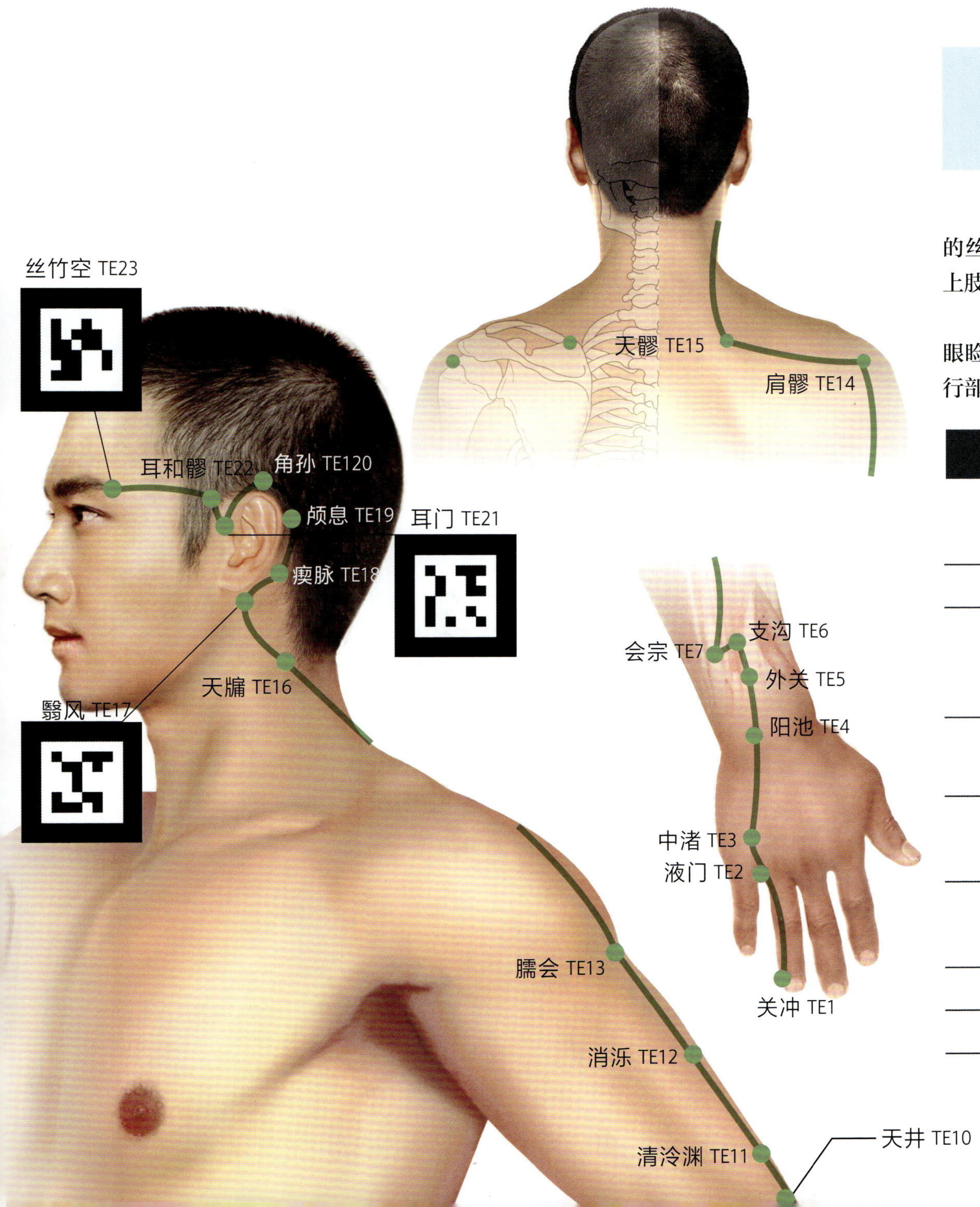

手少阳三焦经

手少阳三焦经从无名指关冲穴，经手臂外侧、耳后，止于眉梢的丝竹空穴。本经一侧 23 穴，左右两侧共 46 穴。13 个穴分布在上肢背面，10 个穴分布在颈部、侧头部。

三焦经主治病症：①头痛、耳鸣、耳聋、咽喉肿痛、面颊肿、眼睑瞤动等头面五官系统疾病。②手指屈伸不利、肘臂痛等经脉循行部位的疾患。

TE	穴名	主治
1	关冲	热病、昏厥、中暑、头痛、目赤、耳聋、咽喉肿痛
2	液门	头痛、目赤、耳聋、咽喉肿痛
3	中渚	头痛、目赤、耳鸣、耳聋、咽喉肿痛、热病、消渴、手指屈伸不利、肘臂肩背疼痛
4	阳池	耳聋、目赤肿痛、咽喉肿痛、消渴、腕痛
★ 5	外关	热病、头痛、目赤肿痛、耳鸣、耳聋、胸胁痛、上肢痿痹
★ 6	支沟	便秘、热病、胁肋痛、落枕、耳鸣、耳聋
7	会宗	耳鸣、耳聋、癫痫、上肢痹痛
8	三阳络	耳聋、暴喑（失音）、上肢痹痛

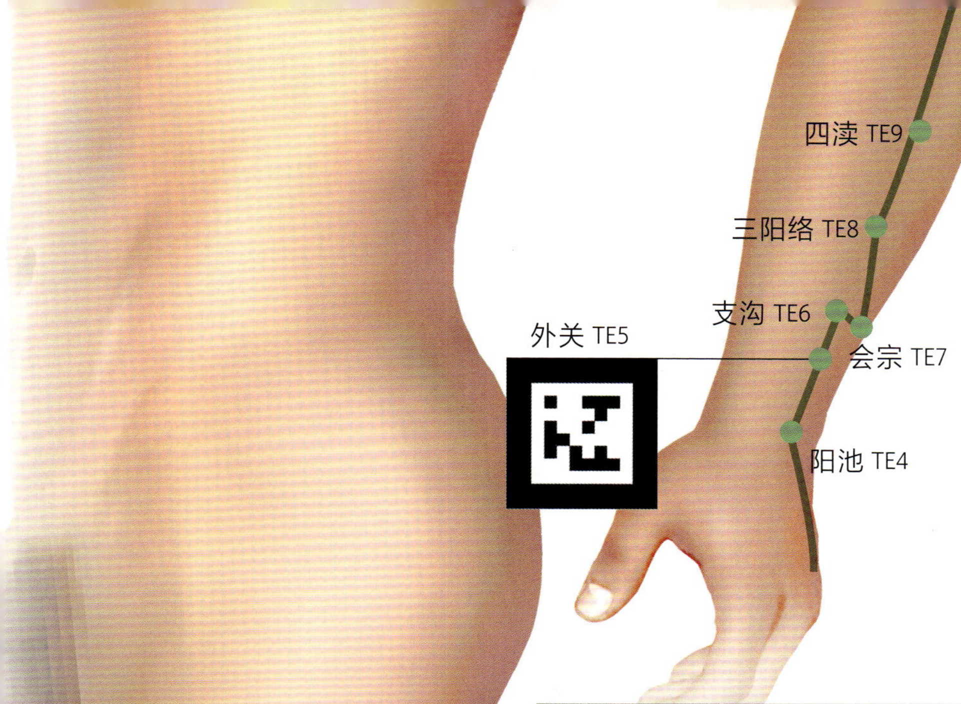

Triple Energizer Meridian of Hand-Shaoyang, TE.

Triple Energizer Meridian of Hand-Shaoyang originates from the ring finger (Guanchong acupoint). It passes through the lateral side of the arm and under the ear, it ends at the tip of the brow(Sizhukong acupoint). There are 23 acupoints in each side of the meridian and 46 acupoints in total. There are 13 acupoints on the dorsum of the upper limb, the other 10 acupoints are scattered in the lateral head and the neck.

The Triple Energizer Meridian indications: ① HEENT diseases including headache, tinnitus, deafness, swelling and pain in the throat, swollen cheek and eyelid twitching. ② Diseases on the pathway of the meridian including inhibited bending and stretching of the finger as well as pain in the elbow and the arm.

TE	Acupoints	Indications
1	Guānchōng	Heat disease; syncope; heat stroke; headache; red eyes; deafness; swelling and pain in the throat
2	Yèmén	Headache; red eyes; deafness; swelling and pain in the throat
3	Zhōngzhǔ	Headache; red eyes; tinnitus; deafness; swelling and pain in the throat; heat disease; diabetes mellitus; inhibited bending and stretching of the finger; pain in the elbow, arm, shoulder and back
4	Yángchí	Deafness; redness, swelling and pain of eyes; swelling and pain in throat; diabetes mellitus; wrist pain
★ 5	Wàiguān	Heat disease; headache; redness, swelling and pain of eyes; tinnitus; deafness; pain in the chest and the hypochondrium; flaccidity and motor impairment in the upper limb
★ 6	Zhīgōu	Constipation; heat disease; pain in the hypochondrium; stiff neck; tinnitus; deafness
7	Huìzōng	Tinnitus; deafness; epilepsy; pain and motor impairment of the upper limb
8	Sānyángluò	Deafness; aphonia; pain and motor impairment of the upper limb

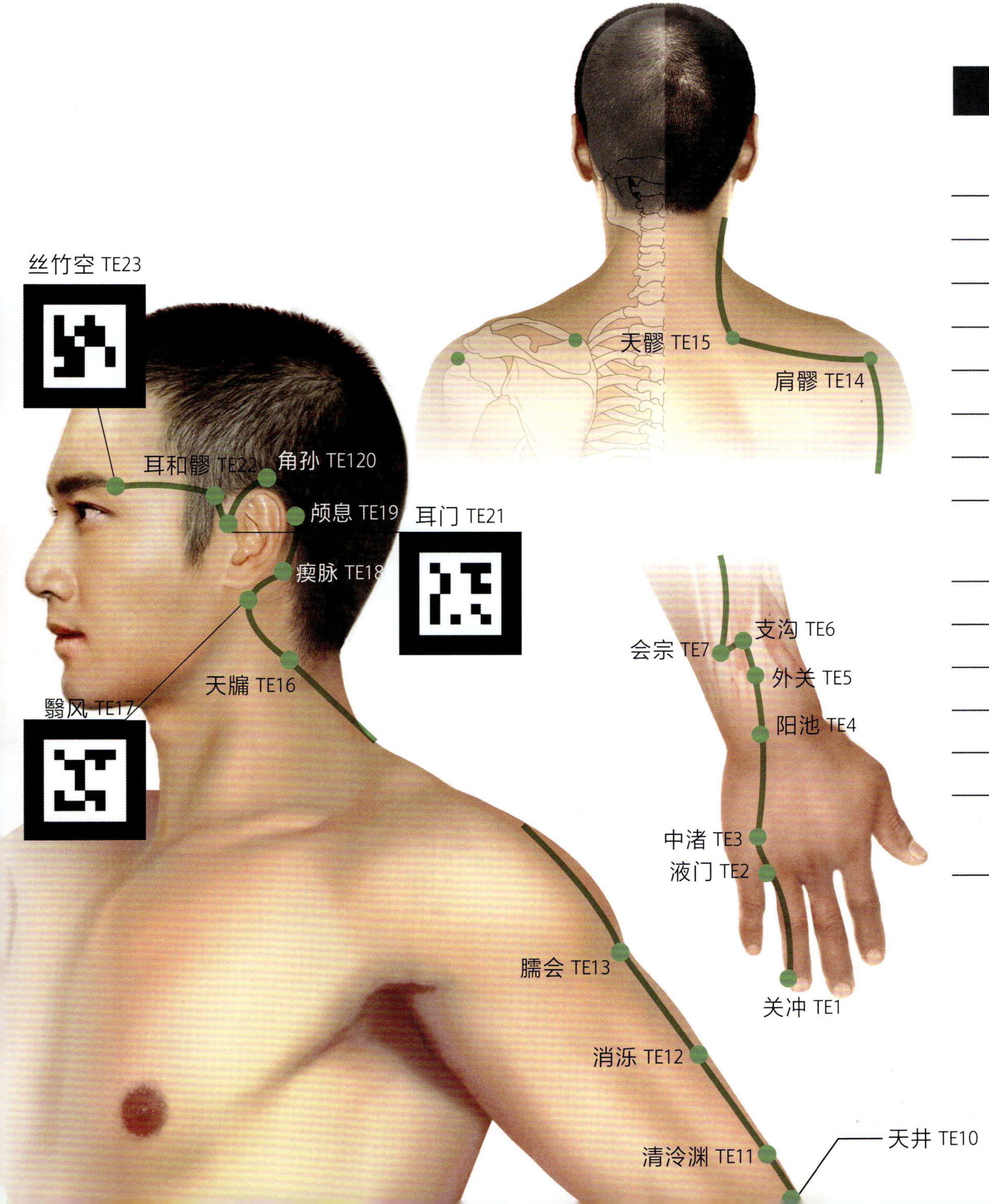

续表

TE	穴名	主治
9	四渎	耳聋、暴喑、齿痛、咽喉痛、偏头痛、上肢痹痛
10	天井	耳聋、偏头痛、癫痫、肘臂痛
11	清泠渊	头痛、目痛、胁痛、肩臂痛
12	消泺	头痛、项强、肩臂痛
13	臑会	上肢痿痹
14	肩髎	肩臂挛痛不遂
15	天髎	肩臂痛、颈项强痛
16	天牖	头痛、项强、目痛、耳聋、面肿
★ 17	翳风	耳鸣、耳聋、口㖞、牙关紧闭、齿痛、呃逆、颊肿
18	瘈脉	耳鸣、耳聋、小儿惊风、头痛
19	颅息	小儿惊风、头痛
20	角孙	目翳、齿痛、偏头痛、项强
★ 21	耳门	耳鸣、耳聋、齿痛
22	耳和髎	头痛、耳鸣、牙关紧闭、口㖞
23	丝竹空	目赤肿痛、眼睑瞤动、目眩、头痛、癫狂

★为本经常用穴

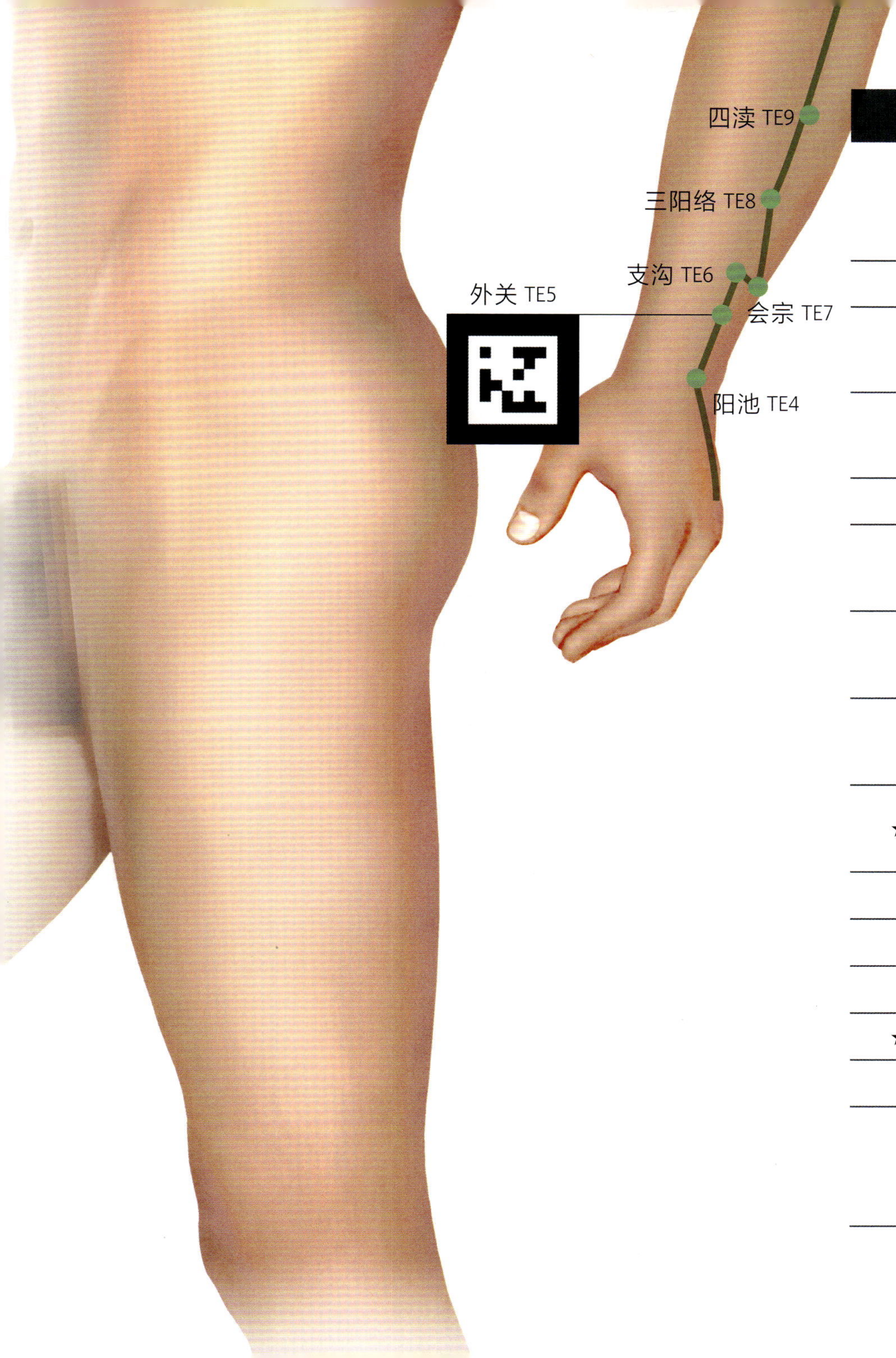

Continued

TE	Acupoints	Indications
9	Sìdú	Deafness; aphonia; toothache; throat pain; migraine; pain and motor impairment of the upper limb
10	Tiānjǐng	Deafness; migraine; epilepsy; elbow and arm pain
11	Qīnglíngyuān	Headache; eyes pain; pain in the hypochondrium; pain in the arm and the shoulder
12	Xiāoluò	Headache; stiffness in the neck; pain in the shoulder and the arm
13	Nàohuì	Flaccidity and motor impairment of the upper limb
14	Jiānliáo	Spasm, pain and motor impairment in the shoulder and the arm
15	Tiānliáo	Pain in the shoulder and the arm; stiffness and pain in the neck
16	Tiānyǒu	Headache; stiff neck; eyes pain; deafness; swollen face
★ 17	Yìfēng	Tinnitus; deafness; deviation of the mouth; lockjaw; toothache; hiccup; swollen face
18	Chìmài	Tinnitus; deafness; infantile convulsion; headache
19	Lúxī	Infantile convulsion; headache
20	Jiǎosūn	Nephelium; toothache; migraine; stiff neck
★ 21	Ěrmén	Tinnitus; deafness; toothache
22	Ěrhéliáo	Headache; tinnitus; lockjaw; deviation of the mouth
23	Sīzhúkōng	Redness, swelling and pain in the eye; eyelid twitching; dizziness; headache; manic-depressive psychosis

★ Common acupoint used in treatment

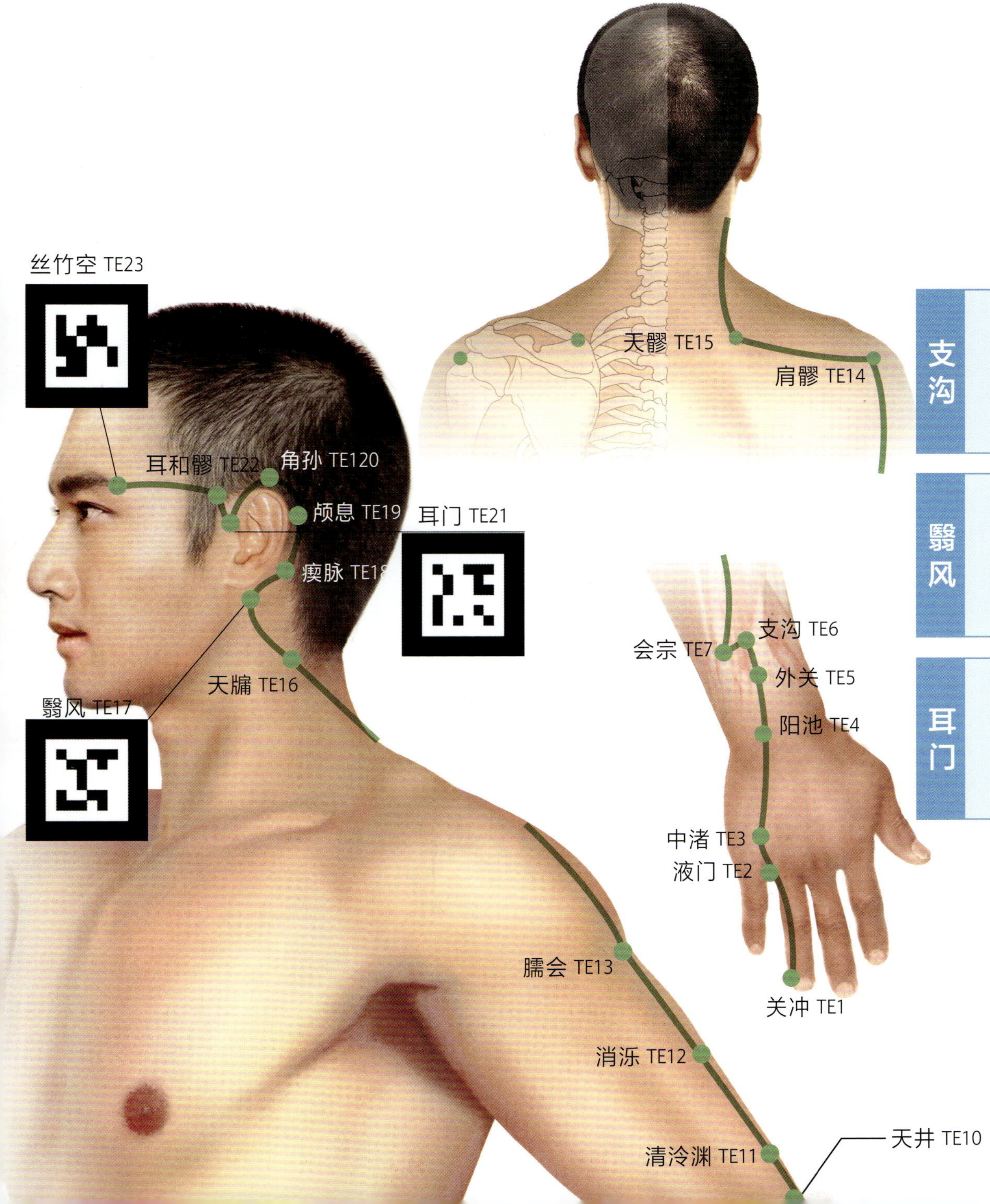

支沟

用拇指按揉支沟穴 2 分钟，力度稍重。同法按揉对侧支沟穴。

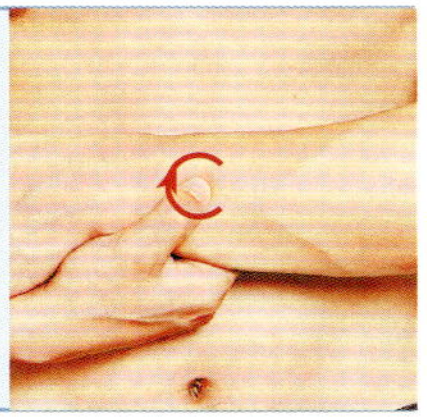

翳风

食、中二指并拢稍用力按压翳风穴，停留片刻后放松，反复 5~6 下。同法按压对侧翳风穴。

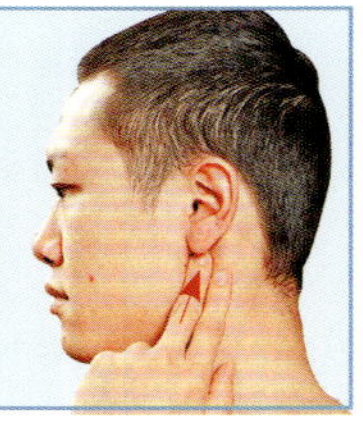

耳门

用中指按揉耳门穴 2 分钟，力度适中。同法按揉对侧耳门穴。每日 2 次。

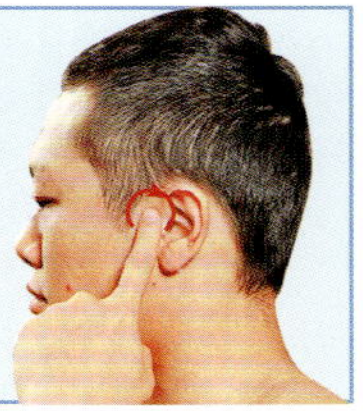

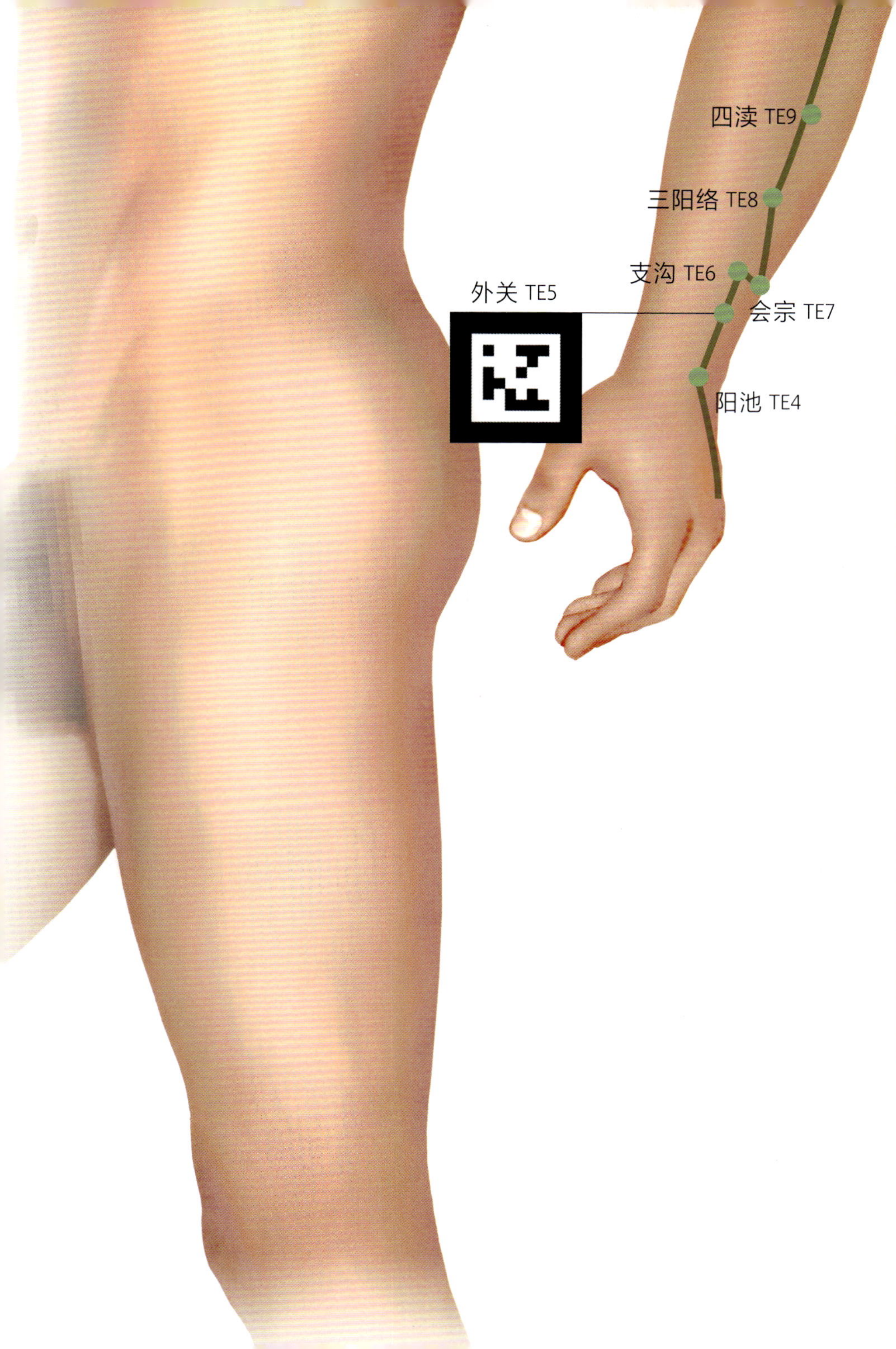

Zhīgōu(TE6)

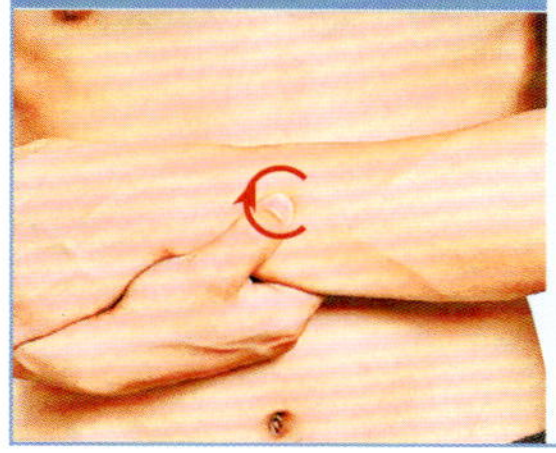

Use the thumb to knead the Zhigou acupoint with a little heavy strength for 2 minutes. Knead the contralateral Zhigou acupoint with the same method.

Yìfēng(TE17)

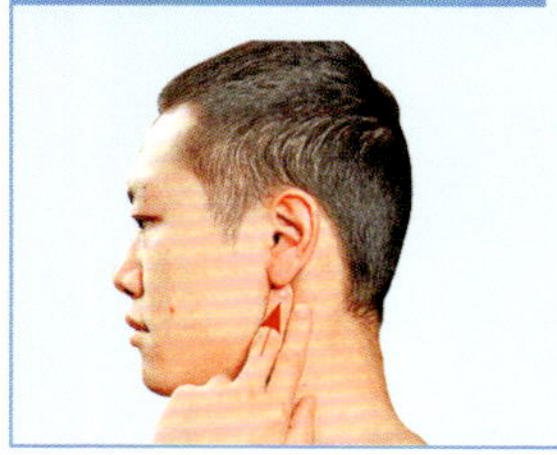

Use the index finger and middle finger to knead the Yifeng acupoint with a little heavy strength for a while, then relax, repeat 5~6 times. Knead the contralateral Yifeng acupoint with the same method.

Ěrmén(TE21)

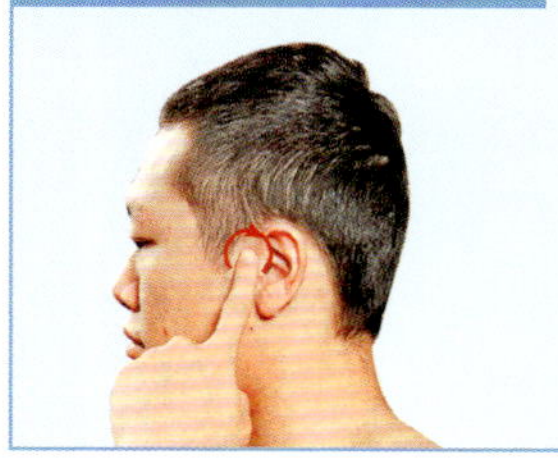

Use the middle finger to knead the Ermen acupoint with appropriate strength for 2 minutes. Knead the contralateral Ermen acupoint with the same method. Twice a day.

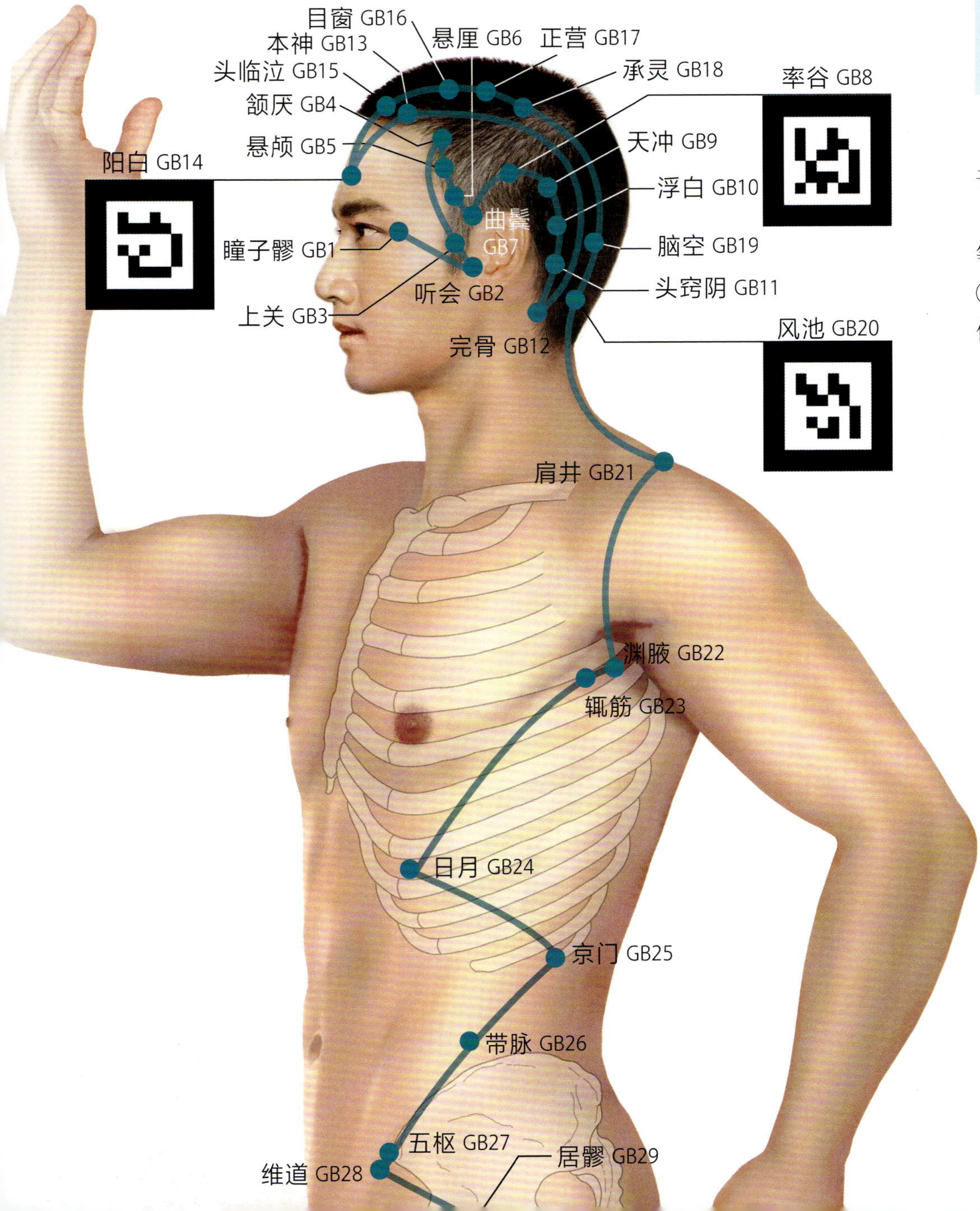

足少阳胆经

足少阳胆经起于眼睛外侧的瞳子髎穴，经耳后、颈、腿部外侧，止于第四趾外侧的足窍阴穴。本经一侧 44 穴，左右两侧共 88 穴。

胆经主治病症：①头痛、耳鸣、耳聋、咽喉肿痛、眼睑瞤动、鼻塞等头面五官疾病。②眩晕、小儿惊痫、中风昏迷等神经精神系统疾病。③疝气、黄疸等肝胆病。④颈项强痛、胸胁痛、下肢痿痹等经脉循行部位的疾患。

GB	穴名	主治
1	瞳子髎	目赤肿痛、目翳、头痛
2	听会	耳鸣、耳聋、颞颌关节炎
3	上关	耳鸣、耳聋、偏头痛、面痛
4	颔厌	偏头痛、眩晕、癫痫、中风后遗症
5	悬颅	偏头痛、目赤肿痛、中风后遗症
6	悬厘	偏头痛、目赤肿痛、中风后遗症
7	曲鬓	偏头痛、目赤肿痛、中风后遗症
8	率谷	头痛、眩晕、耳鸣、耳聋
9	天冲	头痛、耳鸣、耳聋、癫痫
10	浮白	头痛、耳鸣、耳聋、目痛
11	头窍阴	耳鸣、耳聋、头痛、眩晕
12	完骨	头痛、颈项强痛、失眠、吞咽障碍
13	本神	头痛、眩晕、目赤肿痛、癫痫
14	阳白	头痛、眩晕、视物模糊、目痛、眼睑下垂、面瘫、眼睑瞤动

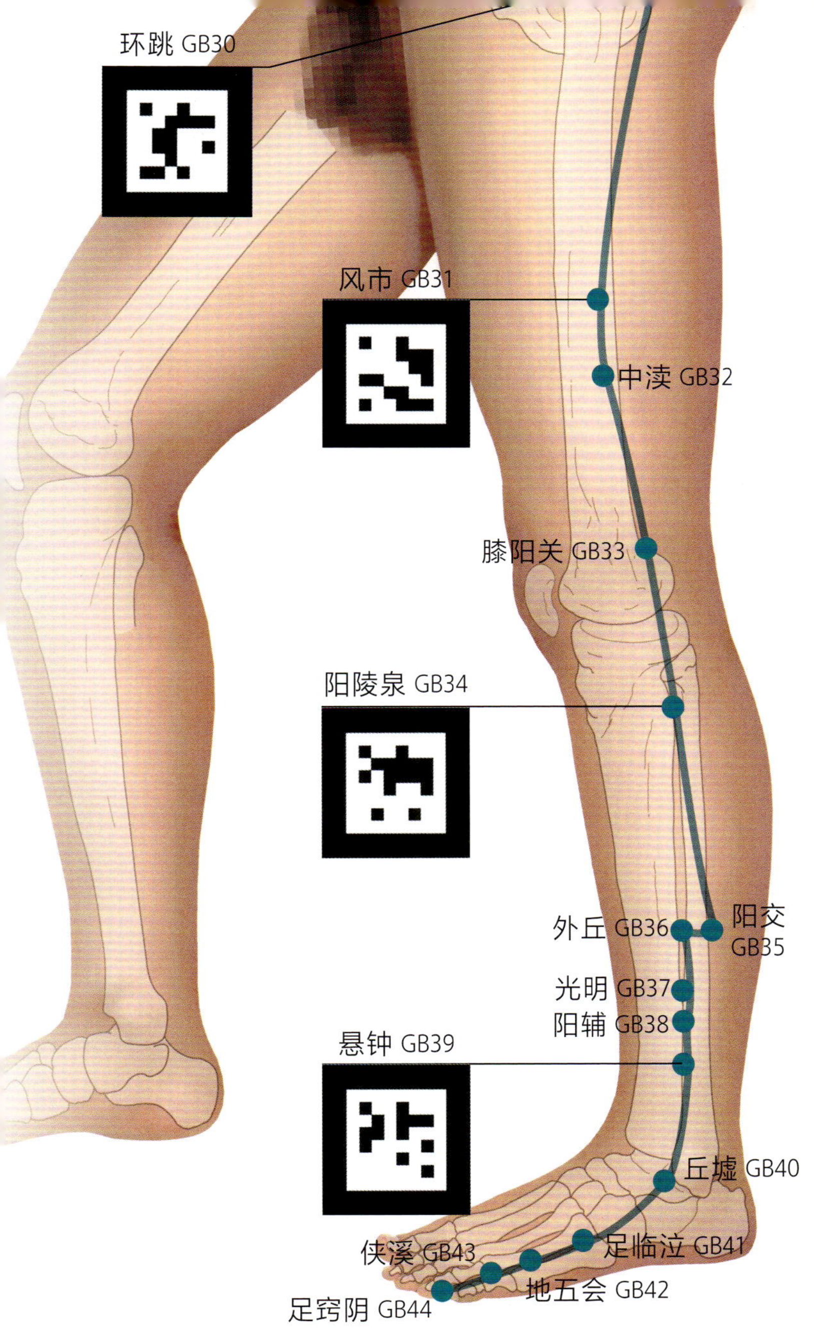

Gallbladder Meridian of Foot-Shaoyang, GB.

Gallbladder Meridian of Foot-Shaoyang starts in the lateral side of the eye (Tongziliao acupoint), it runs behind the ear and along the neck and the lateral side of the leg. It ends in the lateral side of the fourth toe(Zuqiaoyin acupoint). There are 44 acupoints in each side of the meridian,and 88 acupoints in total.

The Gallbladder Meridian indications: ① HEENT diseases including headache, tinnitus, deafness, swelling and pain in the throat, eyelid twitching, rhinobyon. ② Nervous system diseases including dizziness, infantile convulsion and apoplectic coma. ③ Hepatobiliary diseases including jaundice and hernia. ④ Diseases on the pathway of the meridian including stiffness in the neck, pain in the chest and the hypochondrium and flaccidity and motor impairment of the lower limb, etc.

GB	Acupoints	Indications
1	Tóngzǐliáo	Redness, swelling and pain in the eye; nephelium; headache
2	Tīnghuì	Tinnitus; deafness; temporomandibular arthritis
3	Shàngguān	Tinnitus; deafness; migraine; facial pain
4	Hànyàn	Migraine; dizziness; epilepsy; sequela of stroke
5	Xuánlú	Migraine; redness, swelling and pain in the eye; sequela of stroke
6	Xuánlí	Migraine; redness, swelling and pain in the eye; sequela of stroke
7	Qūbìn	Migraine; redness, swelling and pain in the eye; sequela of stroke
8	Shuàigǔ	Headache; dizziness; tinnitus; deafness
9	Tiānchōng	Headache; tinnitus; deafness; epilepsy
10	Fúbái	Headache; tinnitus; deafness; eyes pain
11	Tóuqiàoyīn	Headache; dizziness; tinnitus; deafness
12	Wángǔ	Headache; stiffness in the neck; insomnia; dysphagia
13	Běnshén	Headache; dizziness; redness, swelling and pain in the eye; epilepsy
14	Yángbái	Headache; dizziness; blurry vision; eyes pain; blepharoptosis; facial paralysis; eyelid twitching

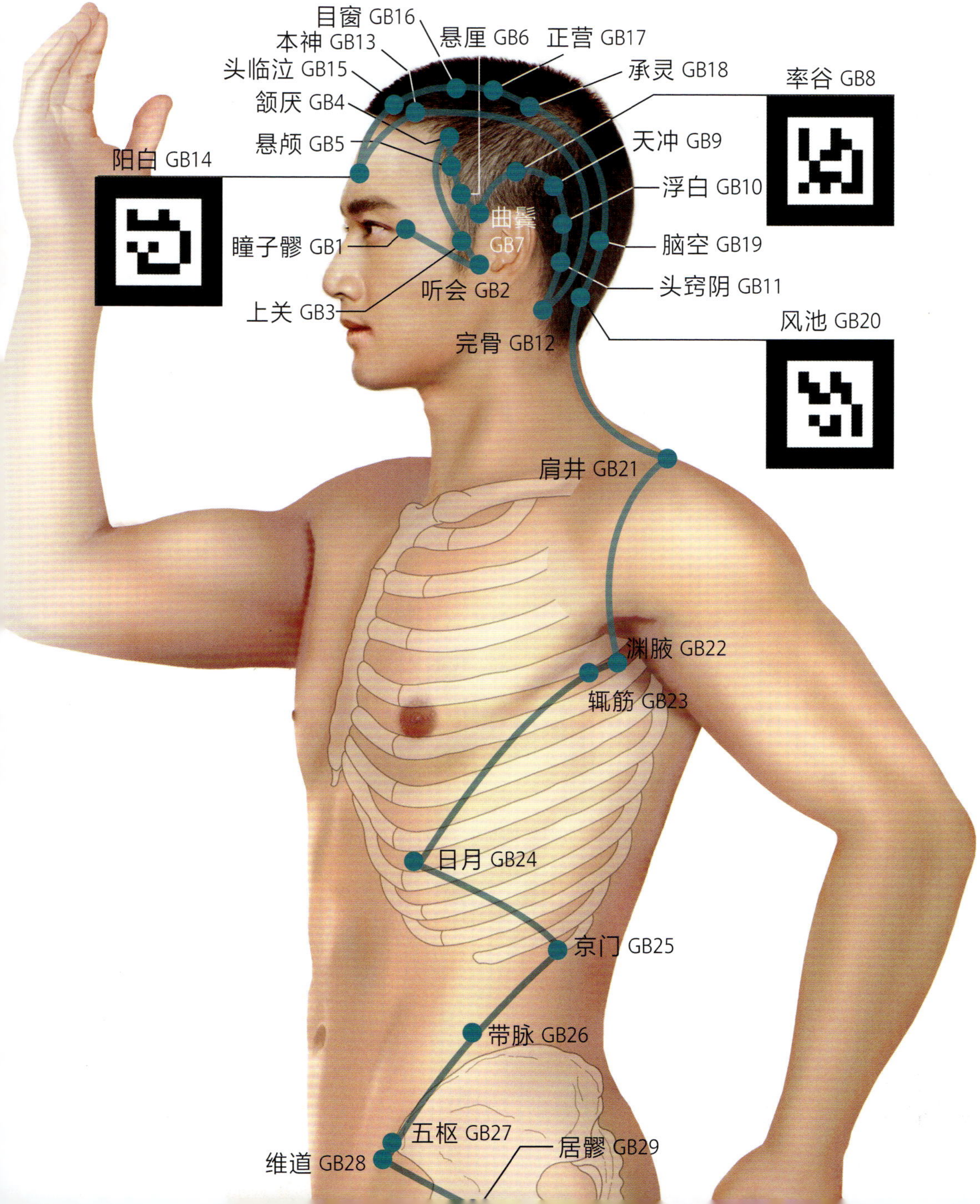

续表

GB	穴名	主治
15	头临泣	头痛、眩晕、癫痫
16	目窗	目赤肿痛、视物模糊、头痛、眩晕
17	正营	头痛、眩晕
18	承灵	头痛、眩晕、目痛
19	脑空	头痛、目眩、颈项强痛、癫狂、癫痫
★ 20	风池	头痛、眩晕、失眠、癫痫、中风、感冒、颈项强痛
★ 21	肩井	颈项强痛、肩背疼痛、上肢不遂
22	渊腋	胸痛、胁痛、上肢痹痛
23	辄筋	胸满、胁痛、呕吐、吞酸、气喘
24	日月	黄疸、呕吐、吞酸、呃逆、胃脘痛、胁肋胀痛
25	京门	小便不利、水肿、腹胀、泄泻、肠鸣、腰痛、胁痛
26	带脉	带下、月经不调、疝气、小腹痛、胁痛、腰痛
27	五枢	腹痛、便秘、带下、月经不调、疝气
28	维道	少腹痛、便秘、肠痈（阑尾炎）、月经不调、疝气
29	居髎	腰痛、下肢痿痹、疝气
★ 30	环跳	下肢痿痹、半身不遂、腰腿痛

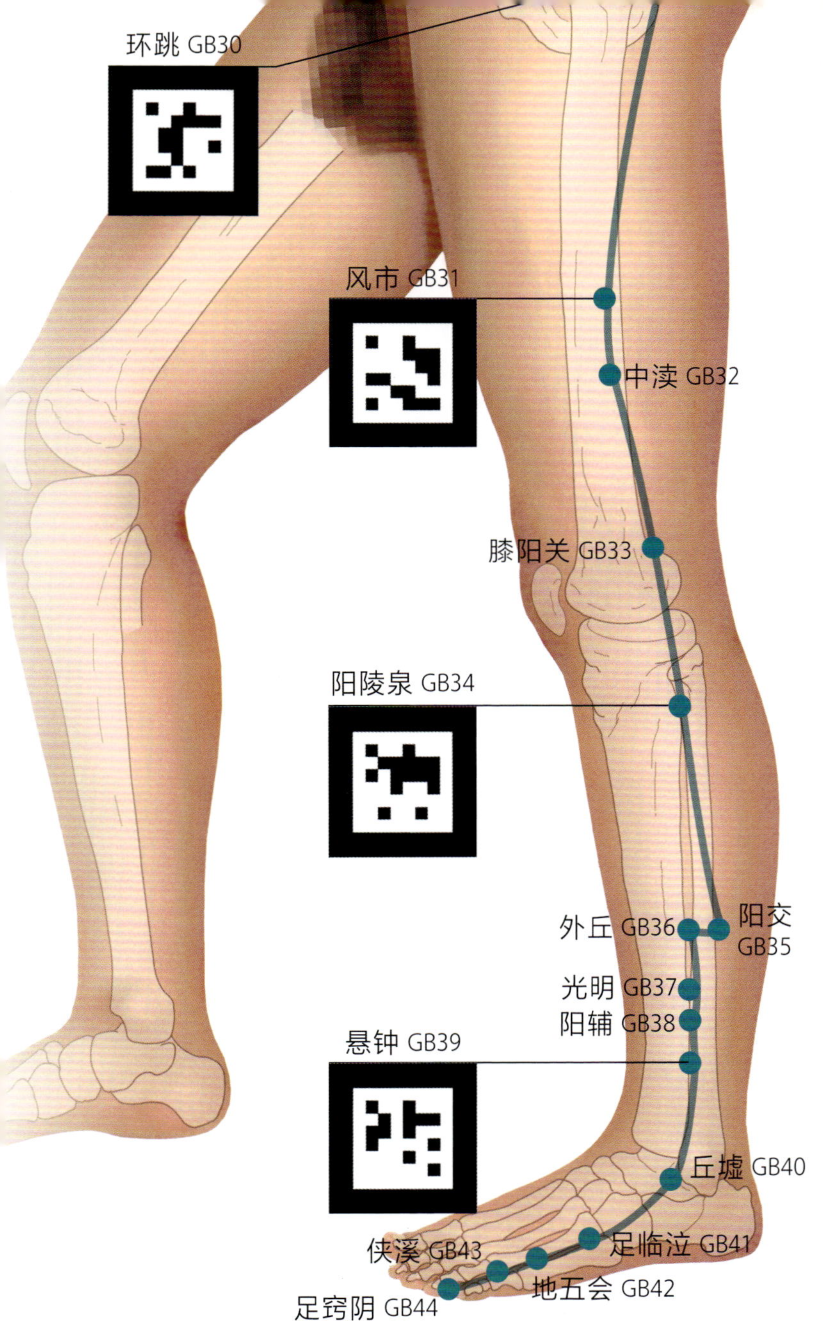

Continued

GB	Acupoints	Indications
15	Tóulínqì	Headache; dizziness; epilepsy
16	Mùchuāng	Redness, swelling and pain in the eye; blurry vision; headache; dizziness
17	Zhèngyíng	Headache; dizziness
18	Chénglíng	Headache; dizziness; eyes pain
19	Nǎokōng	Headache; dizziness; stiffness and pain in the neck; epilepsy; manic-depressive psychosis
★ 20	Fēngchí	Headache; dizziness; insomnia; epilepsy; wind stroke; cold; stiffness and pain in the neck
★ 21	Jiānjǐng	Stiffness and pain in the neck; pain in the shoulder and the back; motor impairment of the upper limb
22	Yuānyè	Chest pain; hypochondrium pain; motor impairment and pain of the upper limb
23	Zhéjīn	Chest tightness; pain in the hypochondrium; vomiting; acid swallowing; asthma
24	Rìyuè	Jaundice; vomiting; acid swallowing; hiccup; stomachache; pain and distension in the chest and the hypochondrium
25	Jīngmén	Dysuria; edema; abdominal distension; diarrhea; borborygmus; waist pain; pain in the hypochondrium
26	Dàimài	Leukorrheal diseases; irregular menstruation; hernia; pain in the lower abdomen; pain in the hypochondrium; waist pain
27	Wǔshū	Abdominal pain; constipation; leukorrheal diseases; irregular menstruation; hernia
28	Wéidào	Pain in the lateral abdomen; constipation; appendicitis; irregular menstruation; hernia
29	Jūliáo	Waist pain; flaccidity and motor impairment of the lower limb; hernia
★ 30	Huántiào	Flaccidity and motor impairment of the lower limb; hemiplegia; waist and leg pain

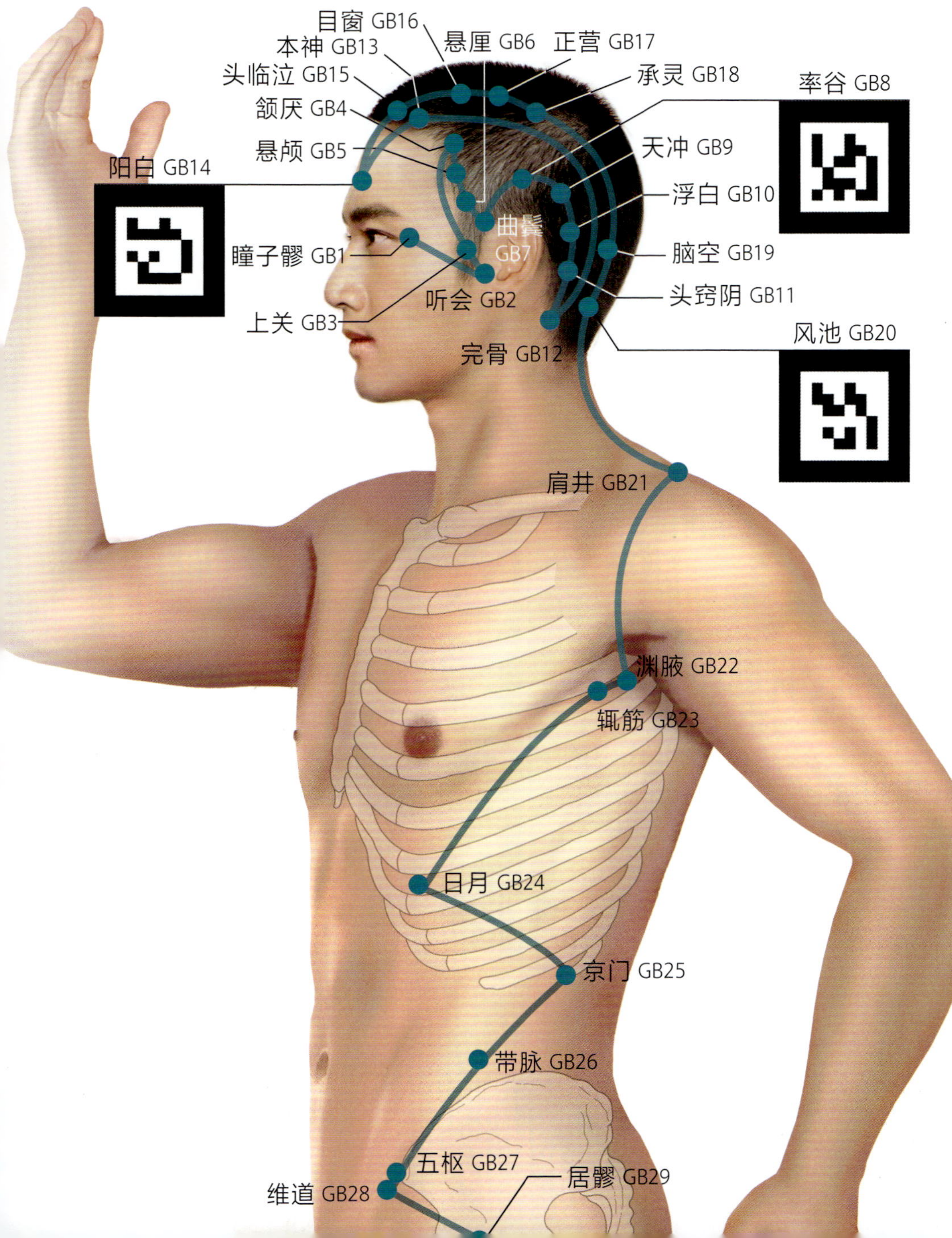

续表

GB	穴名	主治
31	风市	下肢痿痹、全身瘙痒、腰腿痛
32	中渎	下肢痿痹、半身不遂、股外侧皮神经炎
33	膝阳关	半身不遂、膝髌肿痛挛急、小腿麻木
★ 34	阳陵泉	下肢痿痹、膝髌肿痛、胆囊炎、偏头痛
35	阳交	下肢痿痹
36	外丘	下肢痿痹
37	光明	目痛、夜盲、目视不明、近视、干眼症
38	阳辅	下肢痿痹、胸胁胀痛
★ 39	悬钟	下肢痿痹、胸胁胀痛、颈项强痛、偏头痛、膝髌肿痛
40	丘墟	下肢痿痹、外踝肿痛、脚气（中医指足胫麻木、酸痛、软弱无力）、胸胁胀痛
41	足临泣	足跗肿痛、胁肋疼痛、偏头痛、目赤肿痛
42	地五会	足跗肿痛、胁肋疼痛、头痛、目赤、耳鸣、耳聋
43	侠溪	头痛、眩晕、目赤肿痛、耳鸣、耳聋、胸胁疼痛、乳腺炎
44	足窍阴	足肿痛、胁痛、目赤肿痛、耳鸣、耳聋、头痛、失眠

★为本经常用穴

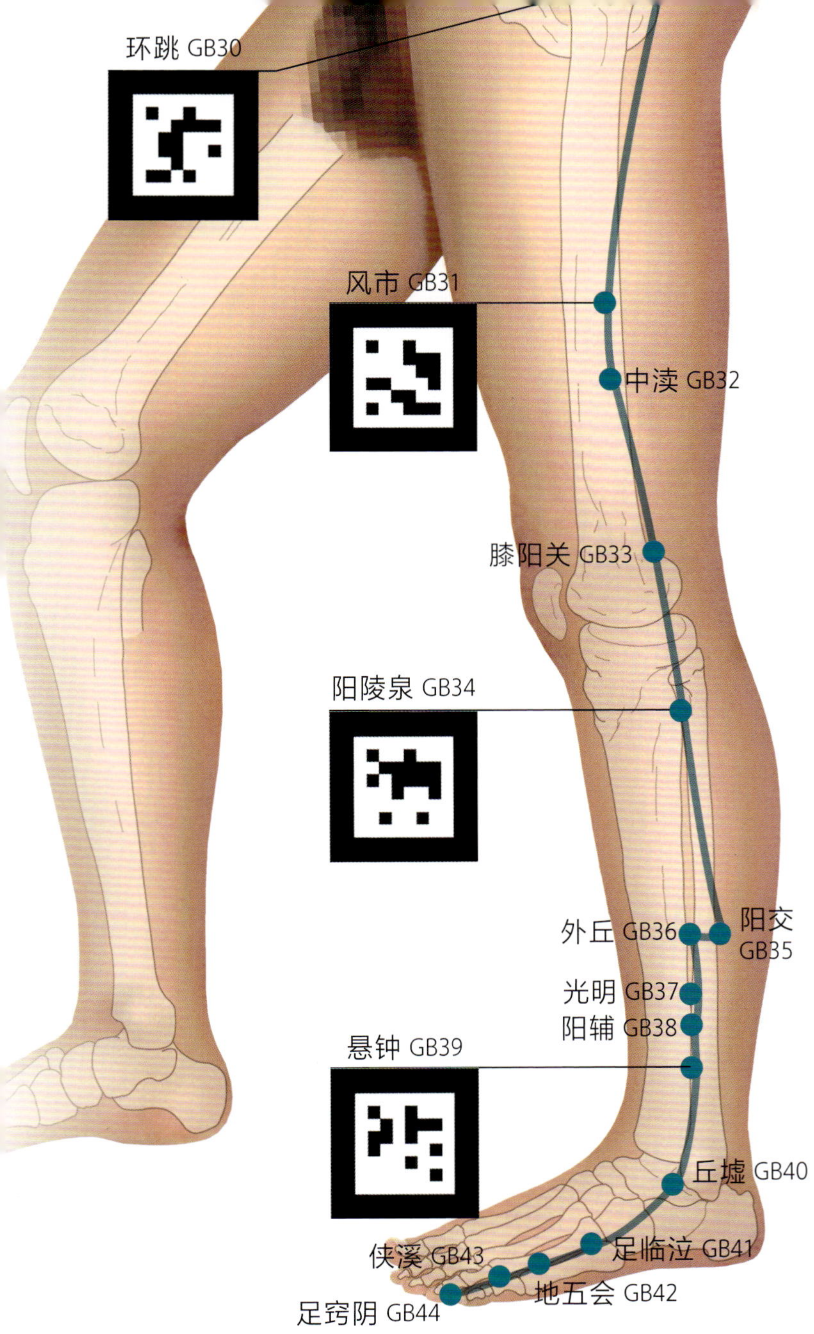

Continued

GB	Acupoints	Indications
31	Fēngshì	Flaccidity and motor impairment of the lower limb; skin itching; waist and leg pain
32	Zhōngdú	Flaccidity and motor impairment of the lower limb; hemiplegia; lateral femoral cutaneous neuritis
33	Xīyángguān	hemiplegia; spasm, swelling and pain in the knee; numbness in the crus
★ 34	Yánglíngquán	Flaccidity and motor impairment of the lower limb; swelling and pain of the knee; cholecystitis; migraine
35	Yángjiāo	Flaccidity and motor impairment of the lower limb
36	Wàiqiū	Flaccidity and motor impairment of the lower limb
37	Guāngmíng	Eyes pain; nyctalopia; blurry vision; myopia; xerophthalmia
38	Yángfǔ	Flaccidity and motor impairment of the lower limb; pain and distension in the chest and the hypochondrium
★ 39	Xuánzhōng	Flaccidity and motor impairment of the lower limb; distension and pain in the chest and the hypochondrium; stiffness and pain in the neck; migraine; swelling and pain in the knee
40	Qiūxū	Flaccidity and motor impairment of the lower limb; swelling and pain in the ankle; soreness, numbness, pain and flaccidity in the foot; distension and pain in the chest and the hypochondrium
41	Zúlínqì	Swelling and pain in the back of the foot; pain in the hypochondrium; migraine; redness, swelling and pain of the eye
42	Dìwǔhuì	Swelling and pain in the back of the foot; pain in the hypochondrium; headache; red eyes; tinnitus; deaf ness
43	Xiáxī	Headache; dizziness; redness, swelling and pain in the eye; tinnitus; deafness; pain in the hypochondrium; mastitis
44	Zúqiàoyīn	Foot swelling and pain; pain in the hypochondrium; redness, swelling and pain in the eye; tinnitus; deafness; headache; insomnia

★ Common acupoint used in treatment

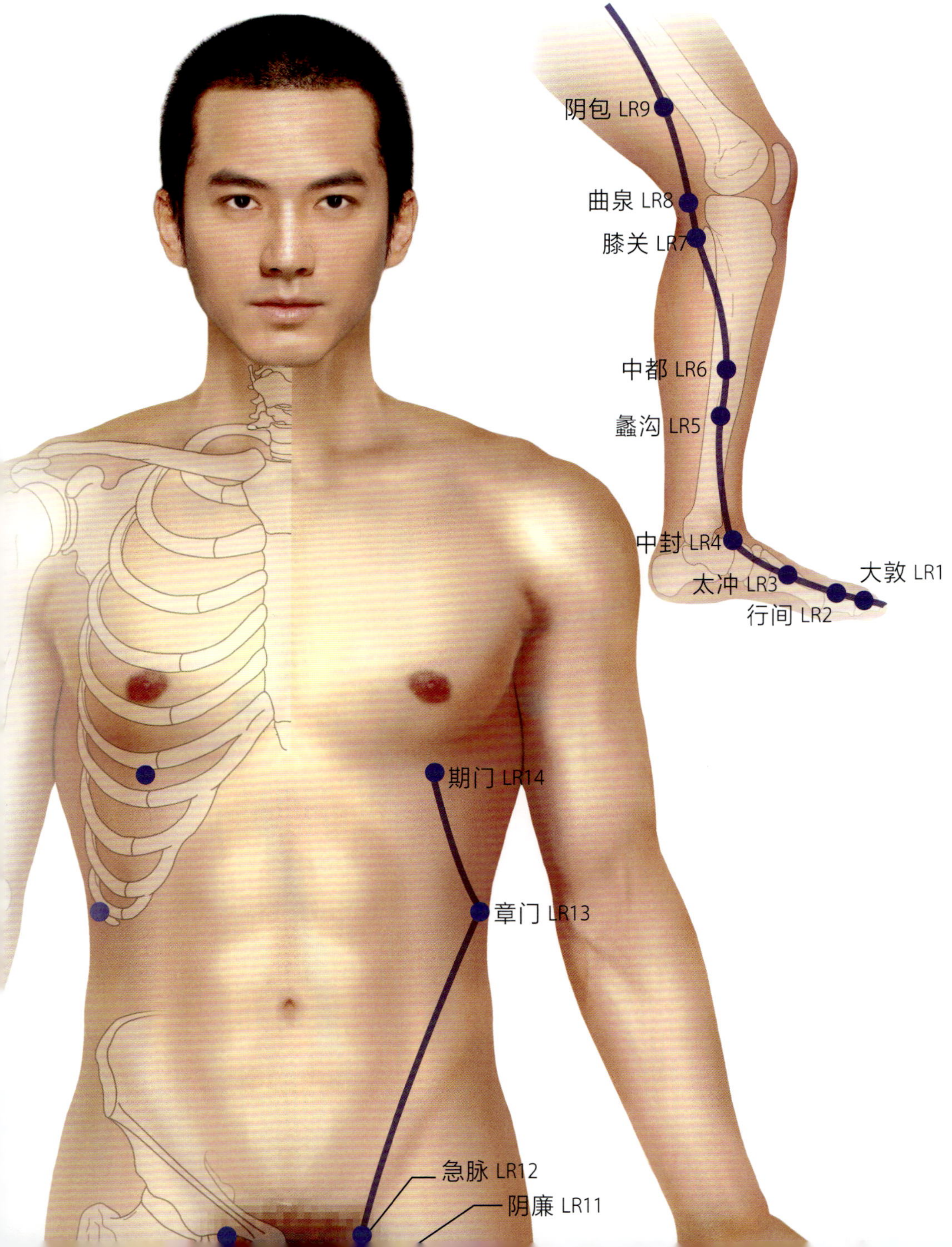

足厥阴肝经

足厥阴肝经起于脚拇趾外侧的大敦穴，沿腿部内侧往上，经腹部，止于乳房下方的期门穴。本经一侧 14 穴，左右两侧共 28 穴。

肝经主治病症：①偏头痛、咽喉肿痛、面颊肿、眼睑瞤动等头面五官疾病。②郁闷、急躁易怒等不良情绪。③中风、癫痫等神经系统疾病。④少腹、前阴疼痛等经脉循行部位的疾患。⑤本经还可治疗月经不调、崩漏、带下等妇科疾病。

LR	穴名	主治
1	大敦	遗尿、癃闭、经闭、月经不调、疝气、癫痫
★ 2	行间	头痛、目眩、目赤肿痛、月经不调、痛经、小便不利、中风、癫痫、胁肋疼痛、急躁易怒、黄疸
★ 3	太冲	头痛、目眩、目赤肿痛、耳鸣、耳聋、呃逆、月经不调、崩漏、痛经、小便不利、中风、癫痫、胁肋疼痛、急躁易怒、黄疸、下肢痿痹、失眠
4	中封	腹痛、小便不利、疝气、下肢痿痹、足踝肿痛
5	蠡沟	睾丸肿痛、外阴瘙痒、小便不利、遗尿、月经不调、足胫肿痛
6	中都	疝气、崩漏、腹痛、腹泻、胁痛、下肢痿痹
7	膝关	膝股疼痛、下肢痿痹

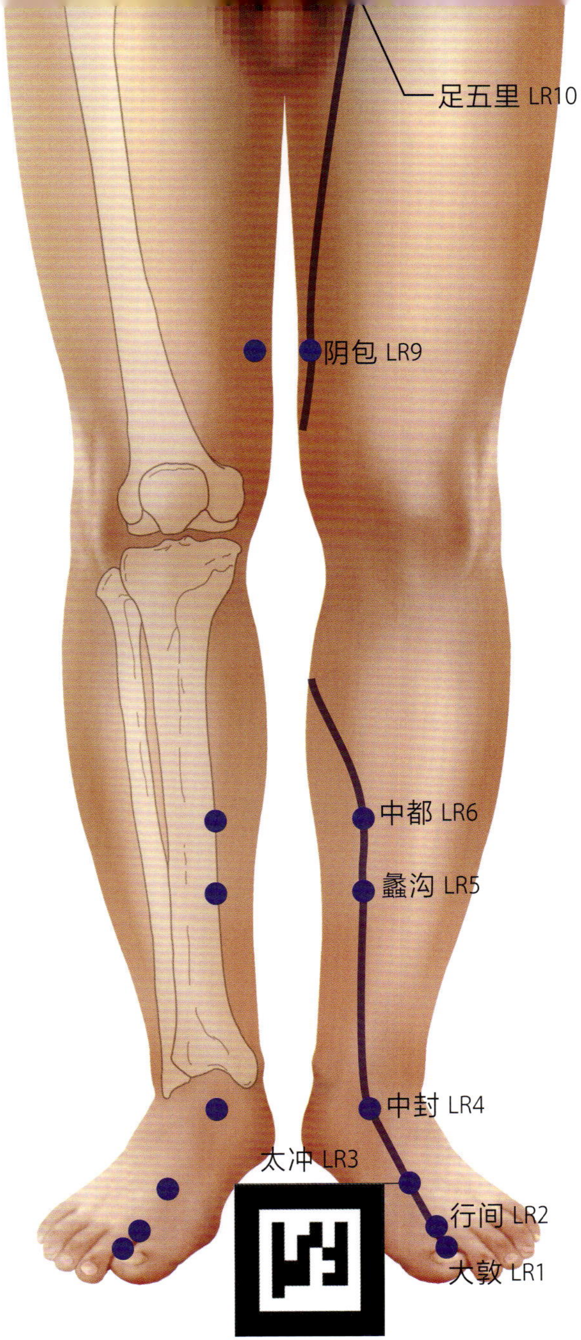

Liver Meridian of Foot-Jueyin, LR.

Liver Meridian of Foot-Jueyin originates from the lateral side of the great toe (Dadun acupoint). It ascends along the medial side of the leg, passes through the abdomen and ends under the breast (Qimen acupoint). There are 14 acupoints in each side of the meridian and 28 acupoints in total.

The Liver Meridian indications: ① HEENT diseases including: migraine, swelling and pain in the throat, swollen face, eyelid twitching. ② Uncomfortable emotions including depression and short temper, etc. ③ Nervous system diseases including wind stroke and epilepsy. ④ Diseases on the pathway of the meridian including pain in the lateral abdomen and external genitalia pain. ⑤ Gynecological diseases including irregular menstruation, leukorrheal diseases and metrorrhagia and metrostaxis.

LR	Acupoints	Indications
1	Dàdūn	Enuresis; retention of urine; amenorrhea; irregular menstruation; hernia; epilepsy
★ 2	Xíngjiān	Headache; dizziness; redness, swelling and pain in eyes; irregular menstruation; dysmenorrhea; dysuria; stroke; epilepsy; pain in the hypochondrium; short temper; jaundice
★ 3	Tàichōng	Headache; dizziness; redness, swelling and pain in the eye; tinnitus; deafness; hiccup; irregular menstruation; metrorrhagia and metrostaxis; dysmenorrhea; dysuria; wind stroke; epilepsy; pain in the hypochondrium; short temper; jaundice; flaccidity and motor impairment of the lower limb; insomnia
4	Zhōngfēng	Abdominal pain; dysuria; hernia; flaccidity and motor impairment of the lower limb; malleolus
5	Lígōu	Swelling and pain in the testicle; genitalia itching; dysuria; enuresis; irregular menstruation; swelling and pain in the shin
6	Zhōngdū	hernia; metrorrhagia and metrostaxis; abdominal pain; diarrhea; pain in the hypochondrium; flaccidity and motor impairment of the lower limb
7	Xīguān	Knee and thigh pain; flaccidity and motor impairment of the lower limb

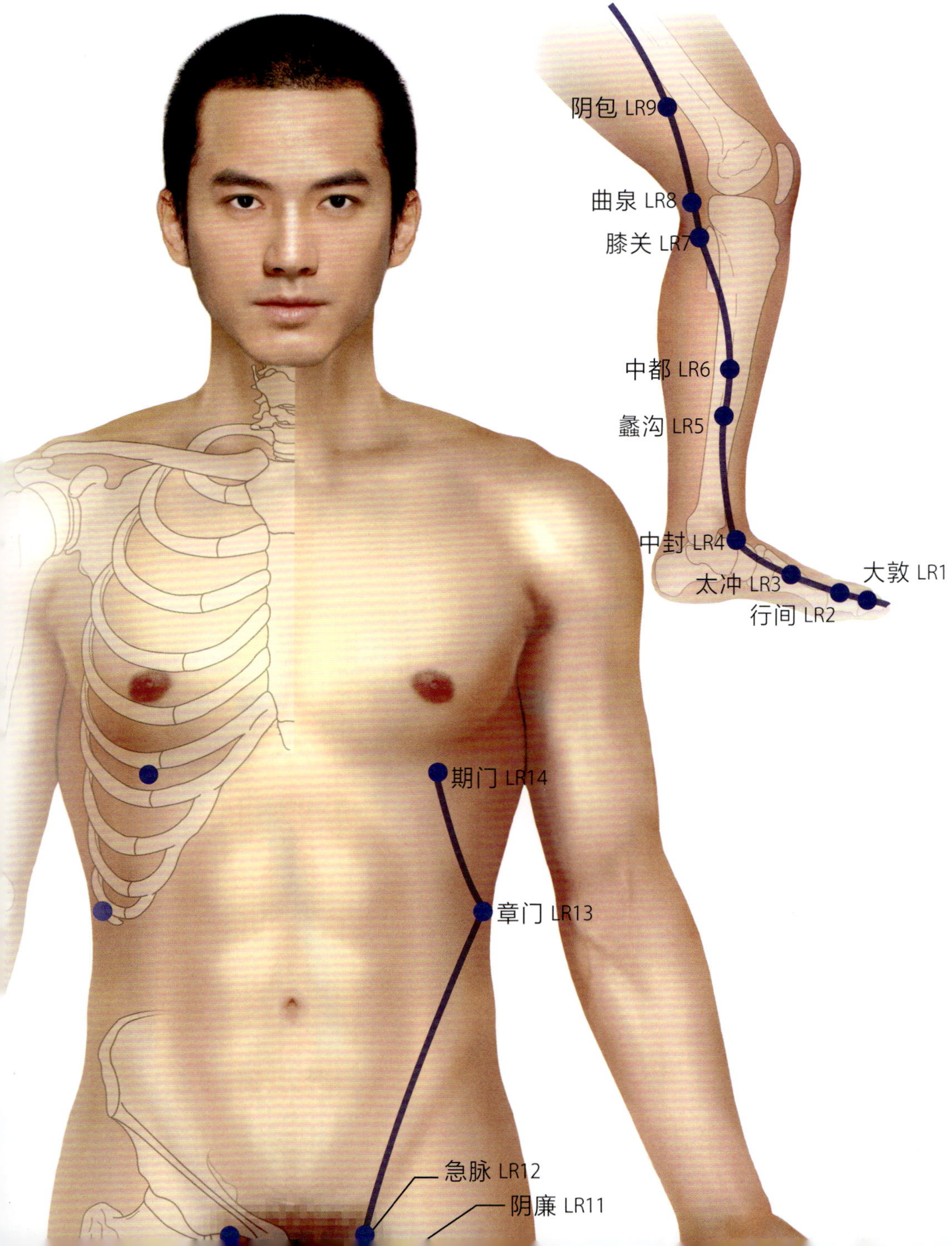

续表

LR	穴名	主治
8	曲泉	小腹痛、小便不利、淋证、癃闭、月经不调、痛经、阴痒、遗精、阳痿、膝股疼痛
9	阴包	月经不调、遗尿、小便不利、腰骶痛
10	足五里	小便不利、小腹胀痛、遗尿、阴囊湿痒、睾丸肿痛
11	阴廉	月经不调、带下、少腹胀痛
12	急脉	疝气、少腹痛、外阴肿痛
★ 13	章门	腹胀、泄泻、胁痛、黄疸
★ 14	期门	胸胁胀痛、腹胀、呃逆、乳腺炎、郁闷

★为本经常用穴

太冲

用拇指掐按太冲穴，停留片刻后放松，反复 5~6 下。同法掐按对侧太冲穴。

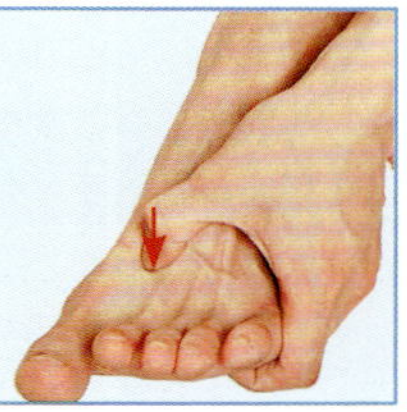

期门

食、中二指并拢按揉期门穴 2 分钟，力度稍重。同法按揉对侧期门穴。每日 2 次。

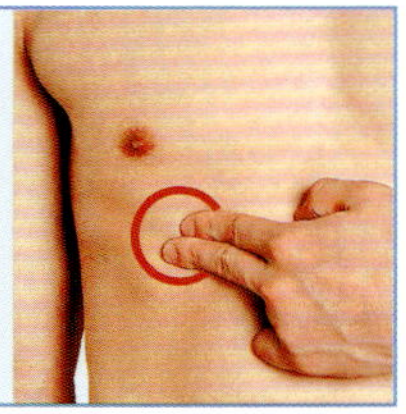

章门

用拇指按揉章门穴 2 分钟，力度稍重。同法按压对侧章门穴。每日 2 次。

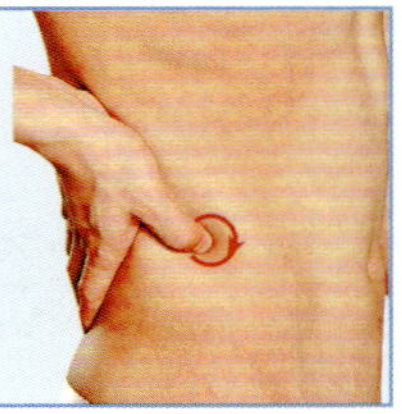

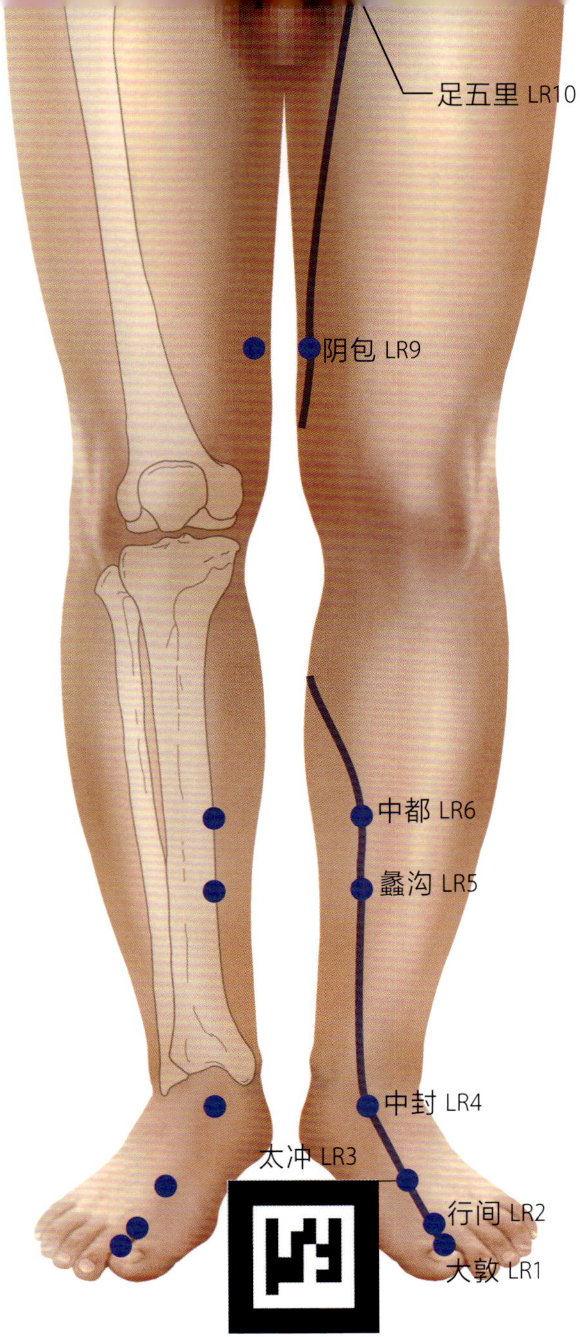

Continued

LR	Acupoints	Indications
8	Qūquán	lower abdominal pain; dysuria; gonorrhoea; retention of urine; irregular menstruation, dysmenorrhea; genitalia itching; spermatorrhea; erectile dysfunction; knee and thigh
9	Yīnbāo	Irregular menstruation; enuresis; dysuria; lumbosacral pain
10	Zúwǔlǐ	Dysuria; lower abdominal distension; enuresis; scrotum itching and dampness; swelling and pain of the testicle
11	Yīnlián	Irregular menstruation; leukorrheal diseases; lateral abdominal pain and distension
12	Jímài	Hernia; lateral abdominal pain; swelling and pain of the genitalia
★ 13	Zhāngmén	Abdominal distension; diarrhea; pain in the hypochondrium; jaundice
★ 14	Qīmén	Distension in the chest and the hypochondrium; abdominal distension; hiccup; mastitis; depression

★ Common acupoint used in treatment

Tàichōng(LR3)

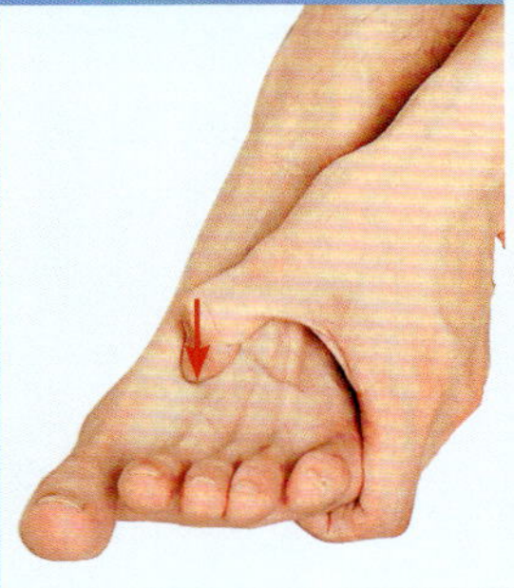

Use the thumb to press the Taichong acupoint for a while, then relax, repeat 5~6 times. Press the contralateral Taichong acupoint with the same method.

Qīmén(LR 14)

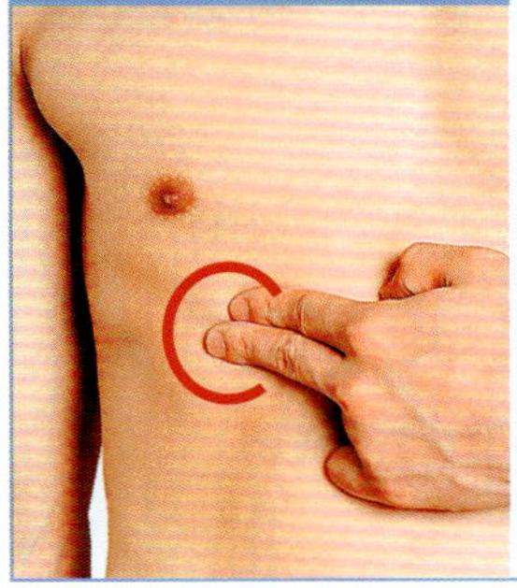

Use the index finger and middle finger to knead the Qimen acupoint with a little heavy strength for 2 minutes. Knead the contralateral Qimen acupoint with the same method. Twice a day.

Zhāngmén(LR13)

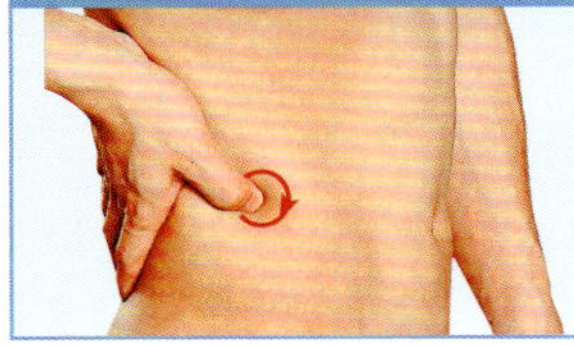

Use the thumb to press the Zhangmen acupoint with a little heavy strength for 2 minutes. Press the contralateral Zhangmen acupoint. Twice a day.

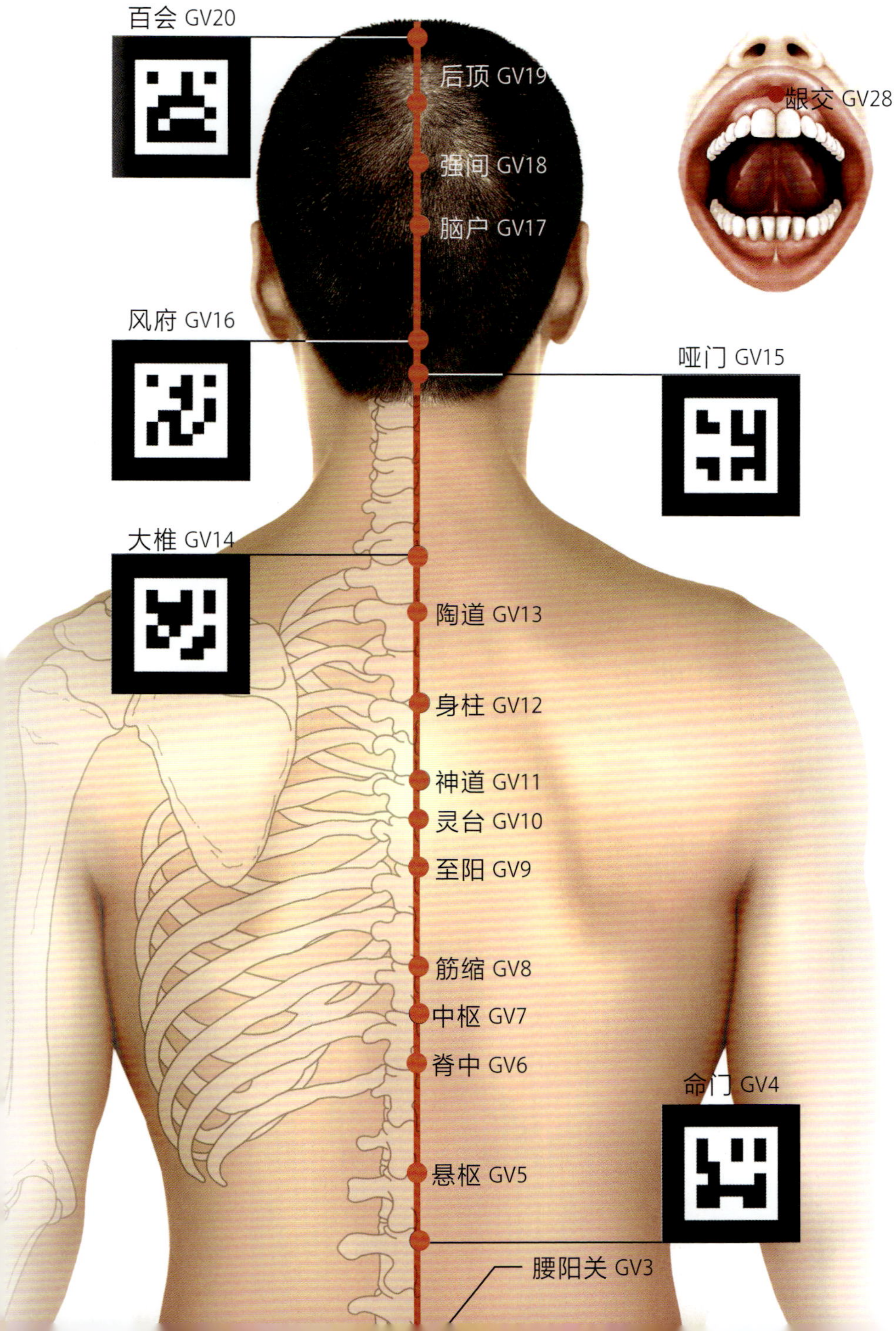

督脉

督脉起于腹部内，下出于会阴部，向后行于脊柱内部，上至头顶，沿前额下行鼻柱。起止穴分别为长强穴和龈交穴，本经共 29 穴。

督脉主治病症：①眩晕、耳鸣、失眠、癫痫、痴呆等神经精神系统疾病。②头项、背、腰骶等局部疾患及经脉循行部位的内脏疾病。③发热、中暑、流行性感冒等热病。④部分腧穴有强身健体作用 ，可用于日常保健。

GV	穴名	主治
1	长强	脱肛、泄泻、便秘、癫狂、腰骶痛、小儿痴呆
2	腰俞	腰脊疼痛、下肢痿痹、月经不调、脱肛、便秘、癫痫
★ 3	腰阳关	腰脊疼痛、下肢痿痹、月经不调、带下、遗精、阳痿
★ 4	命门	腰痛、下肢痿痹、遗精、阳痿、月经不调、带下、遗尿、尿频、泄泻
5	悬枢	腹痛、泄泻、肠鸣、腰脊强痛
6	脊中	泄泻、脱肛、黄疸、小儿疳积、癫痫、腰脊强痛

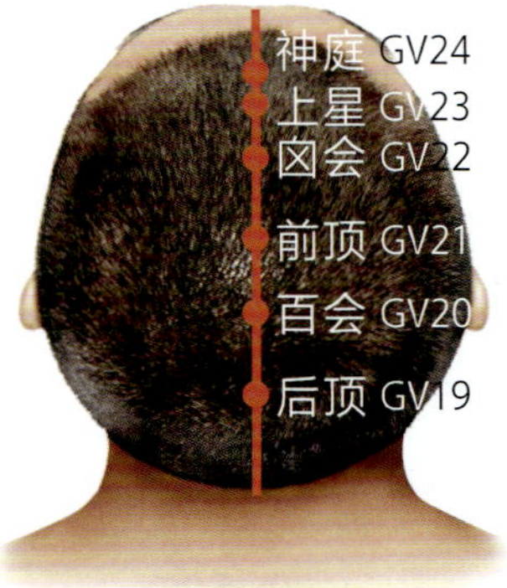

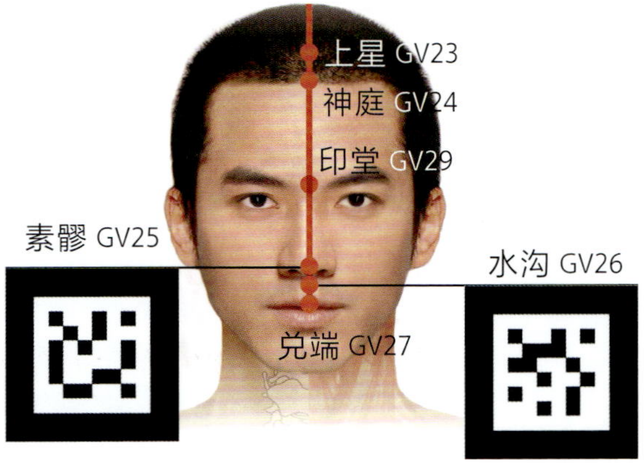

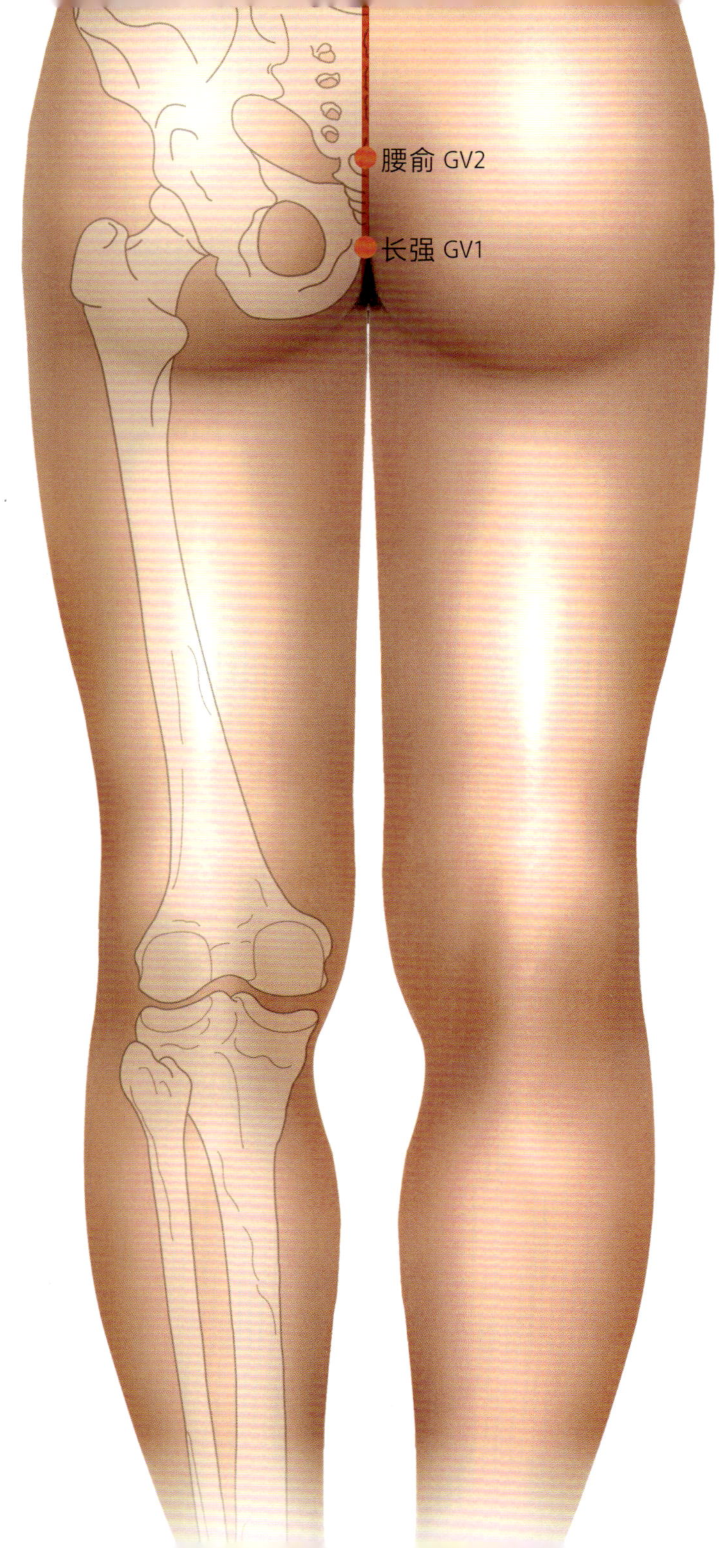

Governor Vessel Meridian, GV.

Governor Vessel Meridian starts from the abdomen. It upwardly comes out of the perineum, backwardly running along the spine upward to the top of the head the descends to the nasal septum along the forehead. The meridian starts from the Changqiang acupoint to the Yinjiao acupoint and there are 29 acupoints in total.

The Governor Vessel Meridian indications: ① Nervous system diseases including dizziness, tinnitus, insomnia, epilepsy and dementia. ② Diseases on the pathway of the meridian including head, neck, lumbosacral diseases and viscera diseases. ③ Heat diseases including fever, heat stroke and influenza. ④ Some acupoints have the function of health keeping which can be used in daily life.

GV	Acupoints	Indications
1	Chángqiáng	Prolapse of the rectum; diarrhea; constipation; manic-depressive psychosis; lumbosacral pain; infantile dementia
2	Yāoshū	Waist and spine pain; flaccidity and motor impairment of the lower limb; irregular menstruation; prolapse of the rectum; constipation; epilepsy
★ 3	Yāoyángguān	Waist and spine pain; flaccidity and motor impairment of the lower limb; irregular menstruation; leukorrheal diseases; spermatorrhea; erectile dysfunction
★ 4	Mìngmén	Waist pain; flaccidity and motor impairment of the lower limb; spermatorrhea; erectile dysfunction; irregular menstruation; leukorrheal diseases; enuresis; frequent urination; diarrhea
5	Xuánshū	Abdominal pain; diarrhea; borborygmus; stiffness and pain in the waist and the spine
6	Jǐzhōng	Diarrhea; prolapse of the rectum; jaundice; infantile malnutrition; epilepsy; stiffness and pain in the waist and the spine

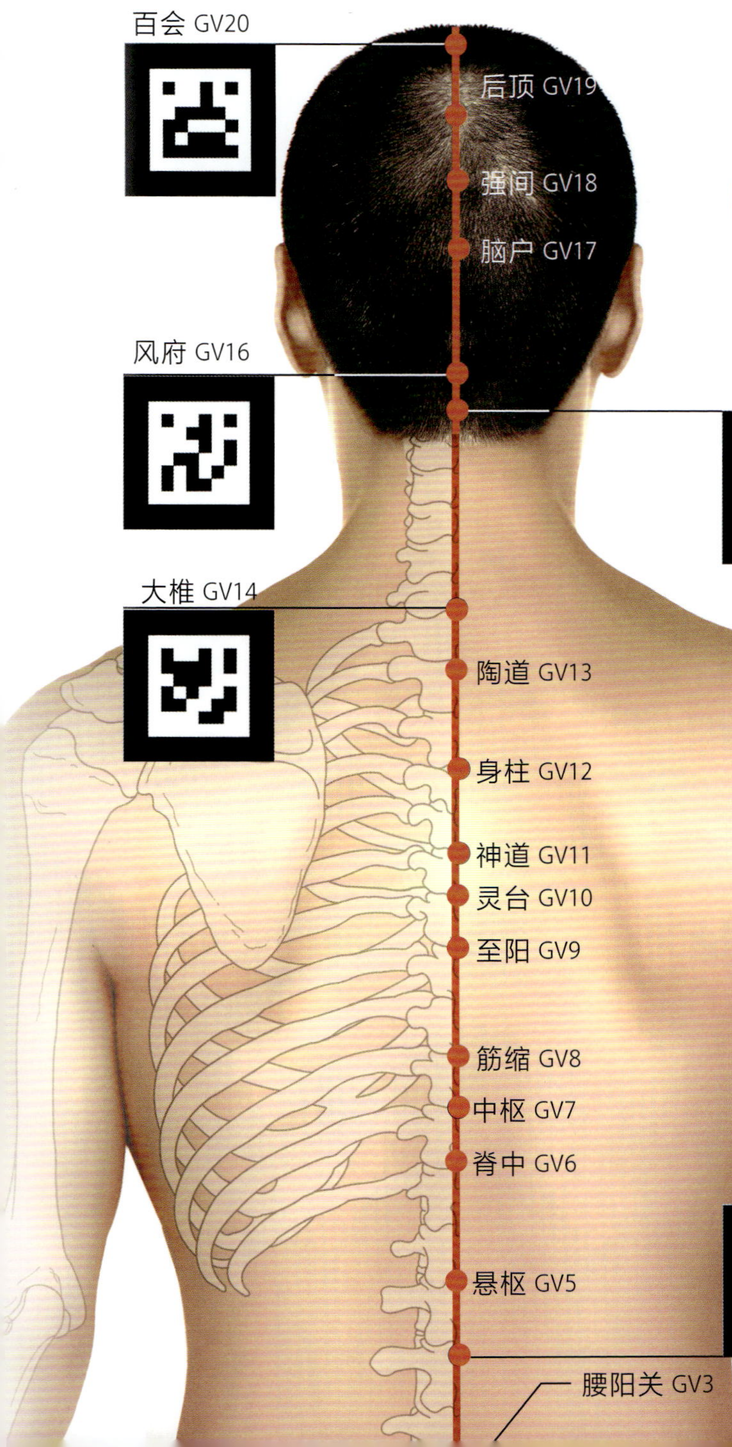

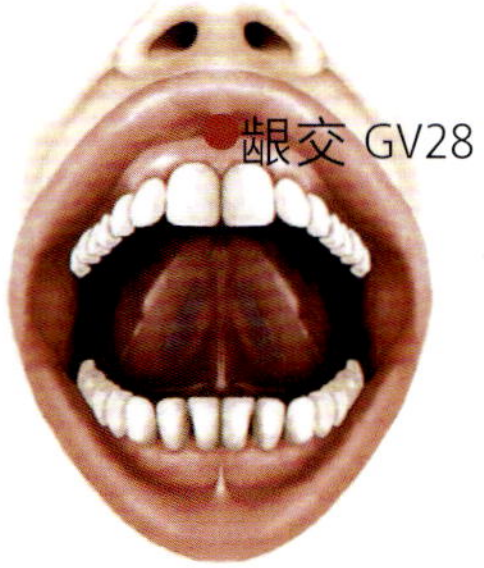

续表

GV	穴名	主治
7	中枢	呕吐、腹满、黄疸、腰背疼痛
8	筋缩	脊强、癫痫、抽搐、胃痛
9	至阳	黄疸、胸胁胀痛、身热、咳嗽、气喘、脊背强痛
10	灵台	咳嗽、气喘、胃痛、脊背强痛
11	神道	心悸、健忘、小儿惊痫、咳喘、脊背强痛
12	身柱	咳嗽、气喘、身热、癫痫、脊背强痛
13	陶道	热病、骨蒸潮热（形容发热自骨髓透发而出）、头痛、脊强、癫狂
★ 14	大椎	热病、骨蒸盗汗、咳嗽、气喘、癫痫、小儿惊风、感冒、胃寒、风疹、头项强痛、体虚怕冷
15	哑门	暴喑、舌强不语、癫狂、头痛、项强、中风
16	风府	头痛、眩晕、项强、中风不语、半身不遂、癫狂、目痛、咽喉肿痛
17	脑户	头痛、项强、目眩、癫狂
18	强间	头痛、项强、目眩、癫狂、失眠
19	后顶	头痛、项强、眩晕、癫狂

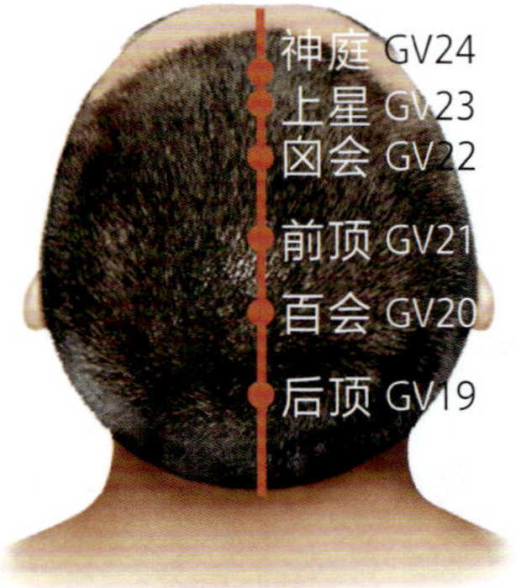

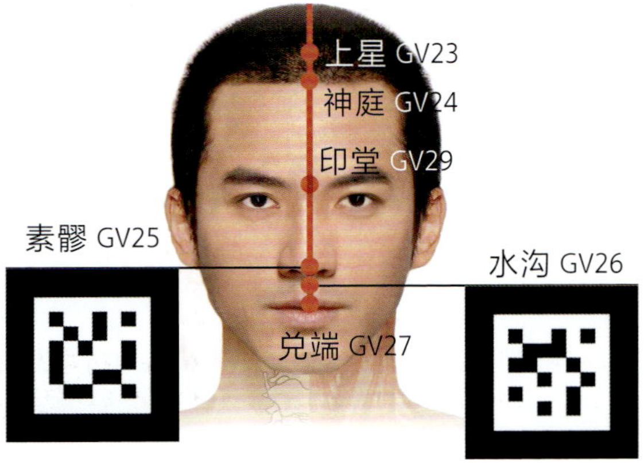

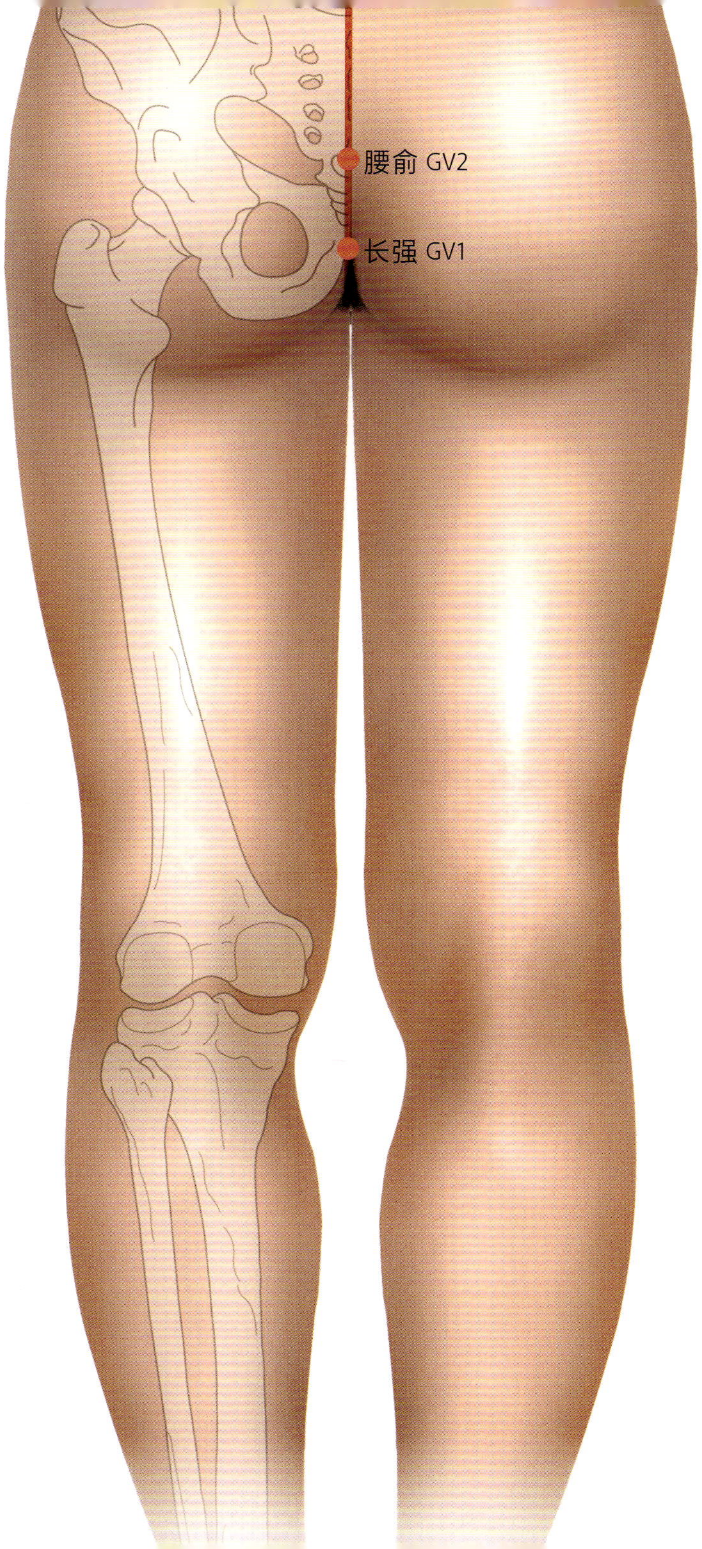

Continued

GV	Acupoints	Indications
7	Zhōngshū	Vomiting; abdominal distension; jaundice; waist and back pain
8	Jīnsuō	Spinal stiffness; epilepsy; convulsion; stomachache
9	Zhìyáng	Jaundice; distension in the chest and the hypochondrium; fever; cough; asthma; stiffness and pain in the spine and the back
10	Língtái	Cough; asthma; stomachache; stiffness and pain in the back and spine
11	Shéndào	Palpitation; amnesia; cough and asthma; stiffness and pain in the back and spine; infantile fright epilepsy
12	Shēnzhù	Cough; asthma; fever; epilepsy; stiffness and pain in the back and spine
13	Táodào	Heat disease; tidal fever due to steaming bone; headache; spine stiffness; manic-depressive psychosis
★ 14	Dàzhuī	Heat disease; night sweat due to steaming bone; cough; asthma; epilepsy; infantile convulsion; cold; stomach cold; rubella; stiffness in the head and the neck; weakness and fear of cold
15	Yǎmén	Aphonia; voice loss due to tongue stiffness; manic-depressive psychosis; headache; stiffness in the neck; wind stroke
16	Fēngfǔ	Headache; dizziness; stiffness in the neck; aphasia from wind stroke; hemiplegia; manic-depressive psychosis; eyes pain; swelling and pain in the throat
17	Nǎohù	Headache; stiffness in the neck; manic-depressive psychosis; dizziness
18	Qiángjiān	Headache; stiffness in the neck; manic-depressive psychosis; dizziness; insomnia
19	Hòudǐng	Headache; stiffness in the neck; manic-depressive psychosis; dizziness

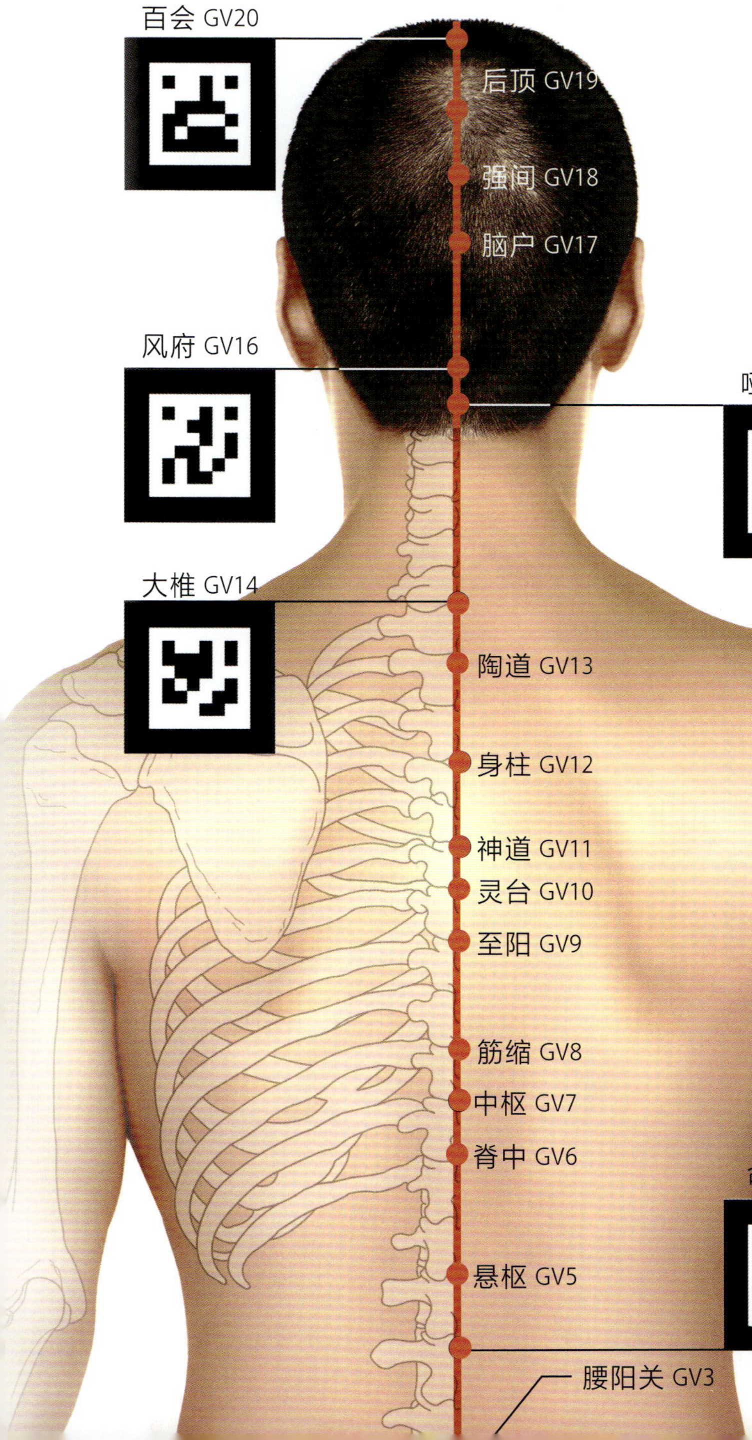

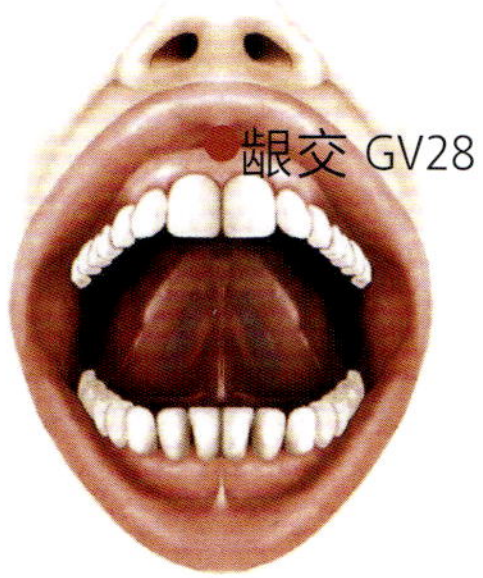

续表

GV	穴名	主治
★ 20	百会	头痛、眩晕、中风不语、癫狂、失眠、健忘、脱肛、久泻、胃下垂
21	前顶	头痛、眩晕、中风偏瘫、癫痫、目赤肿痛、鼻炎
22	囟会	头痛、眩晕、鼻炎、癫痫
23	上星	鼻炎、鼻出血、目痛、头痛、眩晕、癫狂、热病
★ 24	神庭	头痛、眩晕、失眠、癫痫、鼻炎、目痛
25	素髎	鼻塞、鼻炎、鼻出血、目痛、惊厥、昏迷、窒息
★ 26	水沟	昏迷、晕厥、中风、癫狂、抽搐、面瘫、齿痛、鼻塞、牙关紧闭、急性腰扭伤、消渴、黄疸、全身水肿
27	兑端	齿龈肿痛、鼻塞、鼻出血、昏厥
28	龈交	齿龈肿痛、鼻塞、鼻出血、癫狂、腰痛、项强
29	印堂	头痛、眩晕、失眠、小儿惊风、鼻塞、鼻炎、眉棱骨痛、目痛

★为本经常用穴

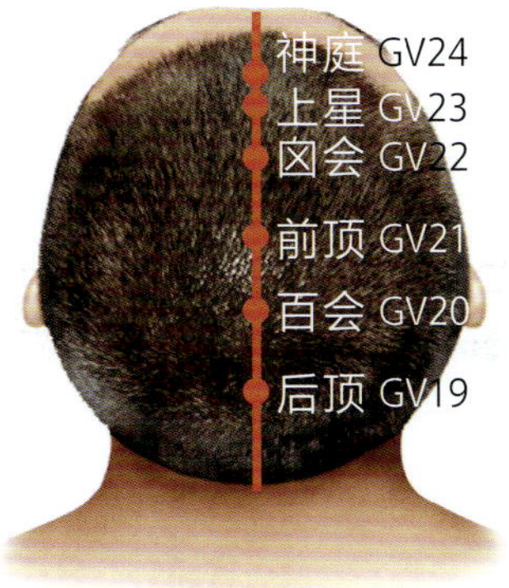

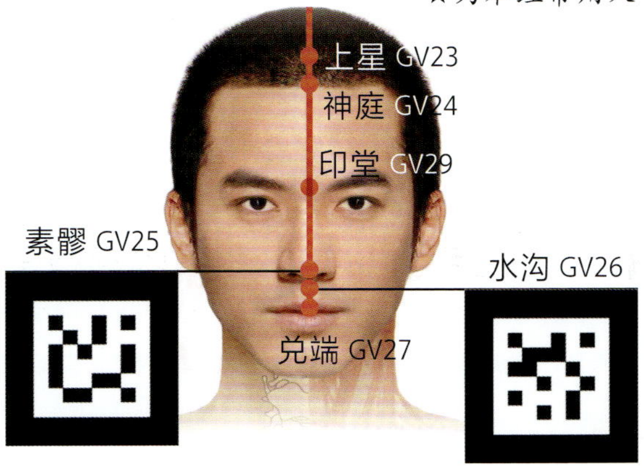

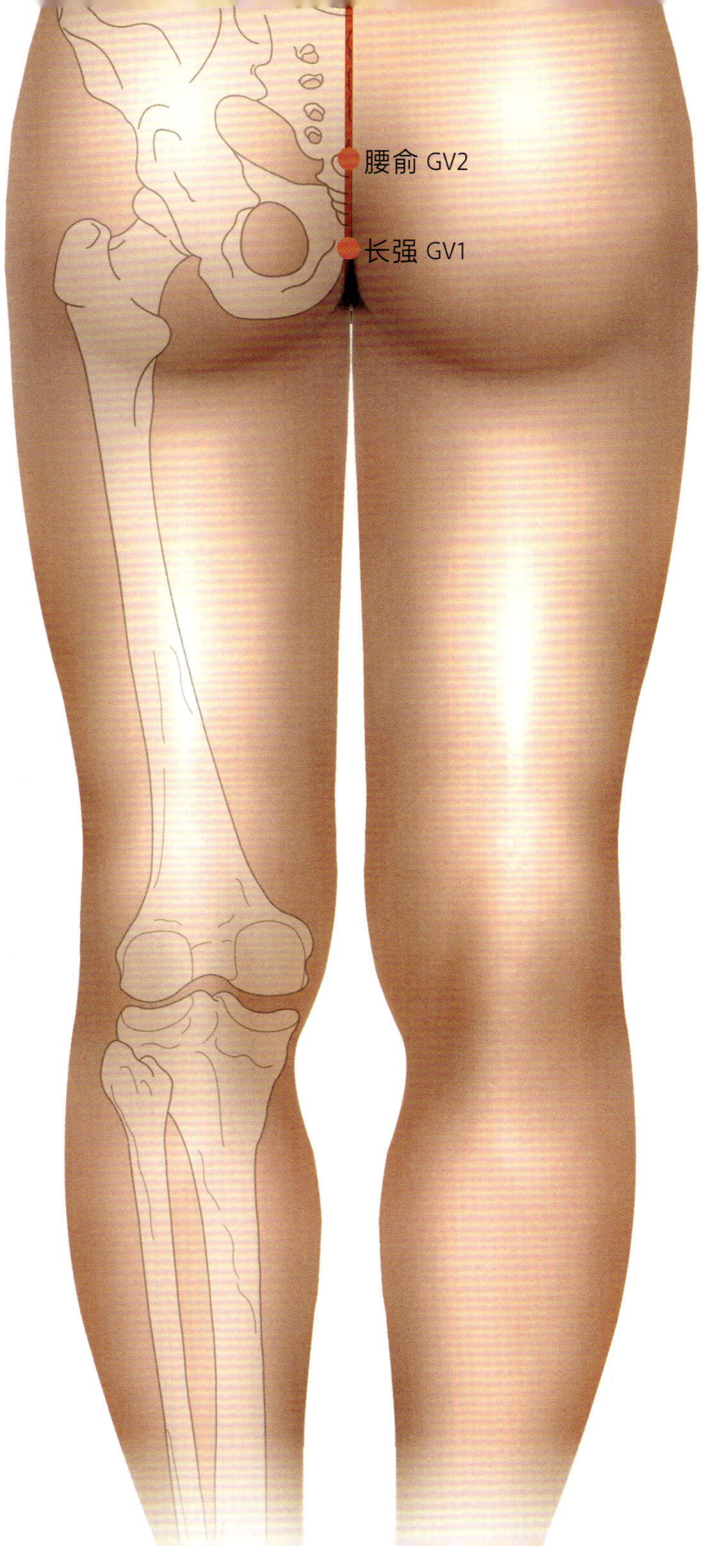

Continued

GV	Acupoints	Indications
★ 20	Bǎihuì	Headache; aphasia from wind stroke; dizziness; manic-depressive psychosis; insomnia; prolapse of rectum; chronic diarrhea; amnesia; gastroptosis
21	Qiándǐng	Headache; dizziness; hemiplegia due to wind stroke; epilepsy; redness,swelling and pain in eyes; rhinitis
22	Xìnhuì	Headache; dizziness; rhinitis; epilepsy
23	Shàngxīng	Rhinitis; nose bleeding; eyes pain; headache; dizziness; manic-depressive psychosis; heat disease
★ 24	Shéntíng	Headache; dizziness; insomnia; epilepsy; rhinitis; eyes pain
25	Sùliáo	Rhinitis; rhinobyon; nose bleeding; eyes pain; convulsion; coma; apnea
★ 26	Shuǐgōu	Coma; syncope; wind stroke; manic-depressive psychosis; convulsion; facial paralysis; toothache; rhinobyon; lockjaw; acute waist sprain; diabetes mellitus; jaundice; edema all over the body
27	Duìduān	Swelling and pain of the teeth and gum; rhinobyon; nose bleeding; syncope
28	Yínjiāo	Swelling and pain of the teeth and gum; rhinobyon; nose bleeding; manic-depressive psychosis; waist pain; stiffness in the neck
29	Yìntáng	Headache; dizziness; insomnia; infantile convulsion; rhinitis; rhinobyon; pain in the supraorbital ridge; eyes pain

★ Common acupoint used in treatment

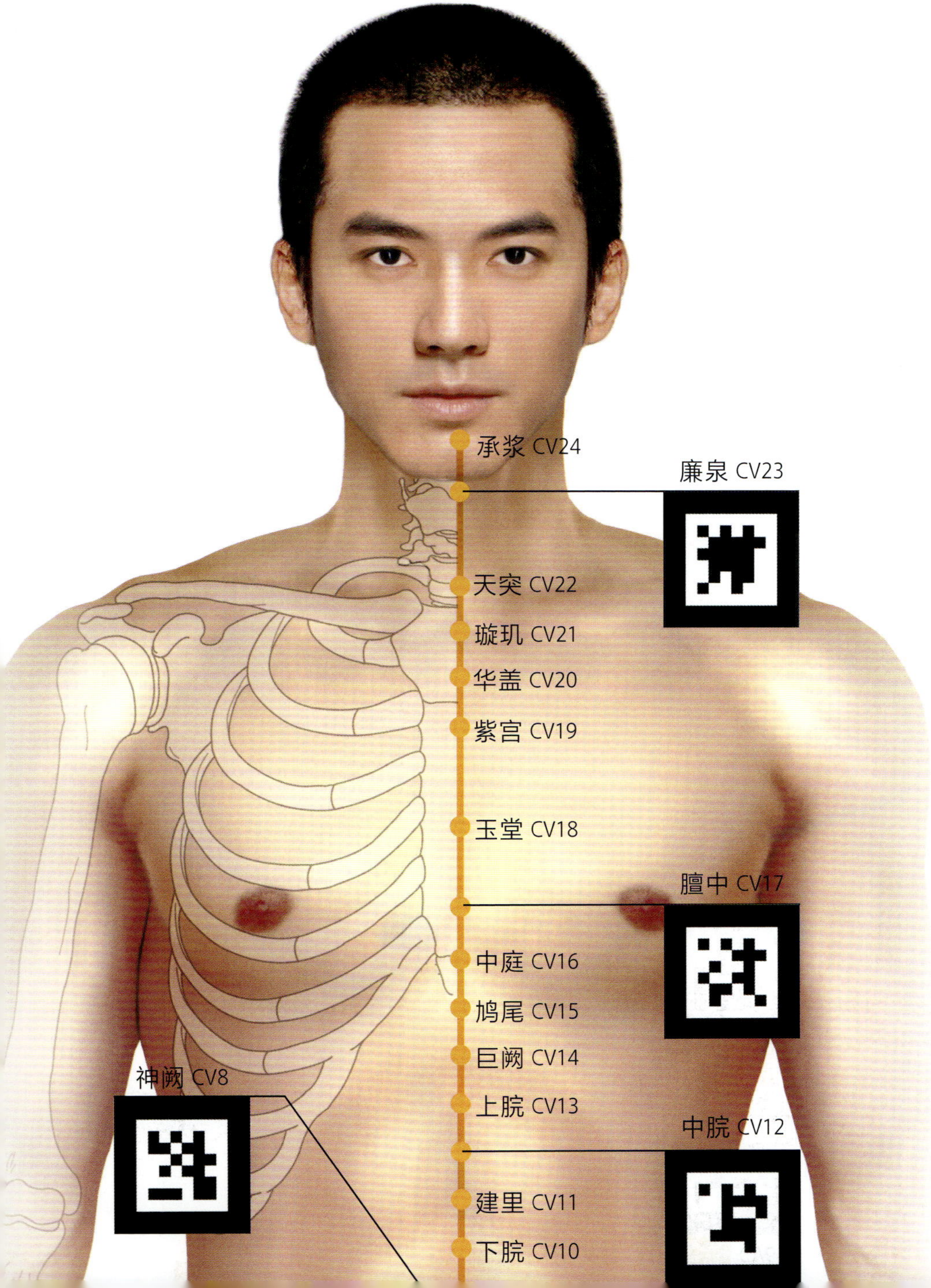

任脉

任脉起于小腹内，下出会阴，沿着腹部正中线到达咽喉部，再上行环绕口唇，经过面部，进入眼眶下，起止穴分别为会阴穴和承浆穴，本经共24穴。

任脉主治病症：①遗精、阳痿、早泄、遗尿等泌尿生殖系统疾病。②头面、咽喉、颈、胸、胃脘等局部疾患和经脉循行部位的内脏疾病。③部分腧穴有强身健体作用，可用于日常保健。④本经还可治疗月经不调、带下、不孕等妇科疾病。

CV	穴名	主治
1	会阴	昏迷、癫狂、小便不利、遗精、阴痒、脱肛、月经不调
2	曲骨	月经不调、痛经、带下、小便不利、遗尿、遗精、阳痿、阴囊湿疹
★3	中极	癃闭、遗尿、尿频、月经不调、带下、痛经、崩漏、遗精、阳痿、疝气
★4	关元	体虚、中风昏迷、眩晕、阳痿、遗精、月经不调、痛经、闭经、不孕、遗尿、小便频数、癃闭、疝气、腹痛、泄泻

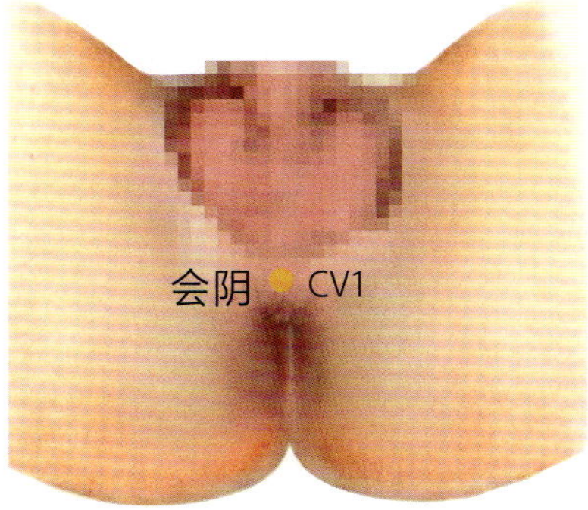

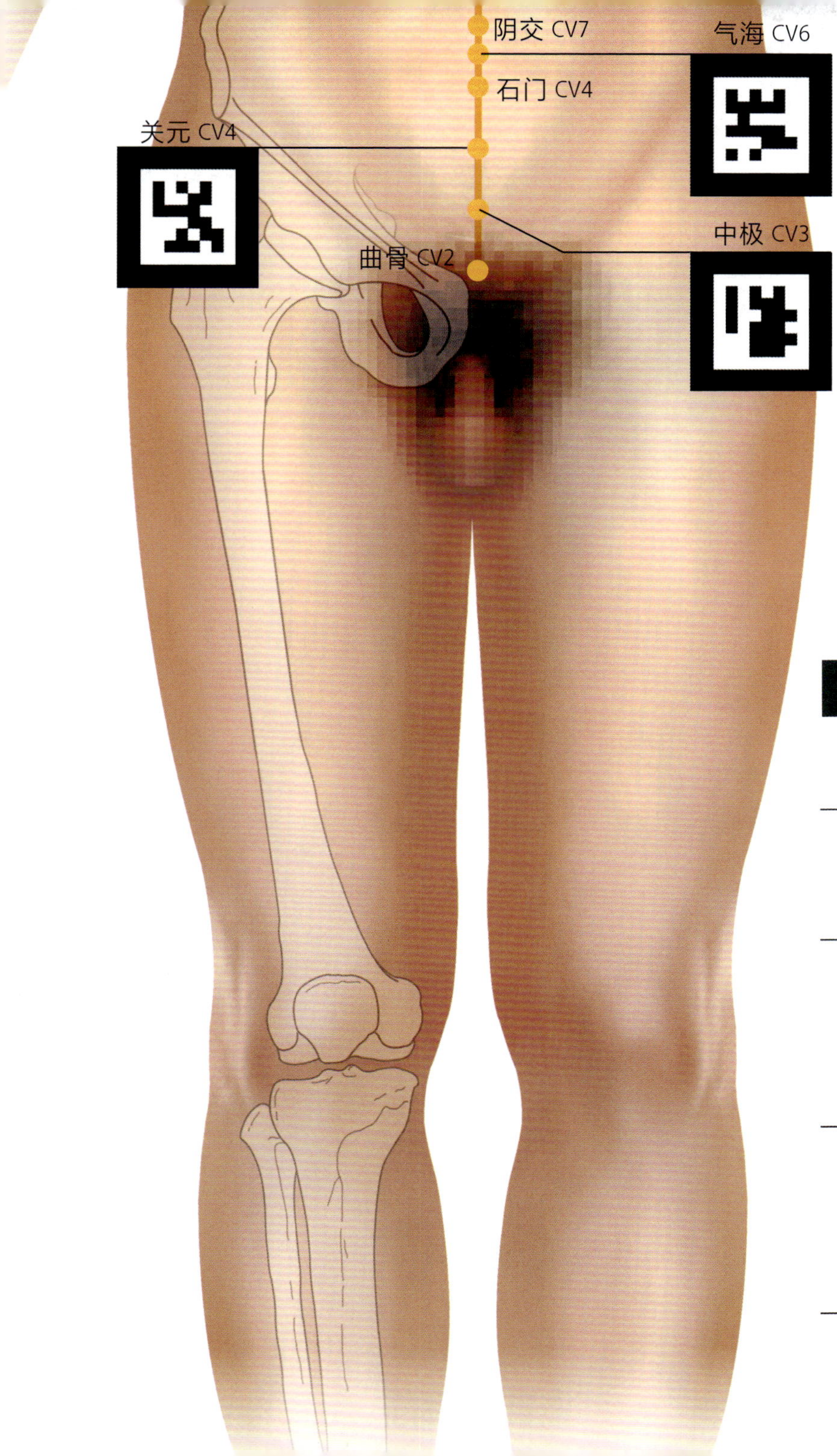

Conception Vessel Meridian, CV.

Conception Vessel Meridian starts from the lower abdomen. It comes out of the perineum and goes along the middle line of the abdomen to the throat, then it runs upwards around the mouth and lips through face entering the region under the orbit. The meridian starts from the Huiyin acupoint to the Chengjiang acupoint, there are 24 acupoints in total.

The Conception Vessel Meridian indications: ① Urogenital system diseases including spermatorrhea, erectile dysfunction, enuresis and prospermia. ② Regional diseases on the pathway of the meridian including head, face, neck, chest, abdominal diseases and viscera diseases. ③ Some acupoints have the function of keeping health which can be used in daily life. ④ Gynecological diseases including irregular menstruation, leukorrheal diseases and sterility.

CV	Acupoints	Indications
1	Huìyīn	Coma; manic-depressive psychosis; dysuria; spermatorrhea; genitalia itching; prolapse of rectum; irregular menstruation
2	Qūgǔ	Irregular menstruation; leukorrheal diseases; dysmenorrhea; dysuria; enuresis; spermatorrhea; erectile dysfunction; scrotal eczema
★ 3	Zhōngjí	Retention of urine; enuresis; frequent urination; irregular menstruation; leukorrheal diseases; dysmenorrhea; spermatorrhea; erectile dysfunction; metrorrhagia and metrostaxis; hernia
★ 4	Guānyuán	Weakness; coma due to wind stroke; dizziness; spermatorrhea; erectile dysfunction; irregular menstruation; dysmenorrhea; amenorrhea;sterility; enuresis; frequent urination; retention of urine; hernia; abdominal pain; diarrhea

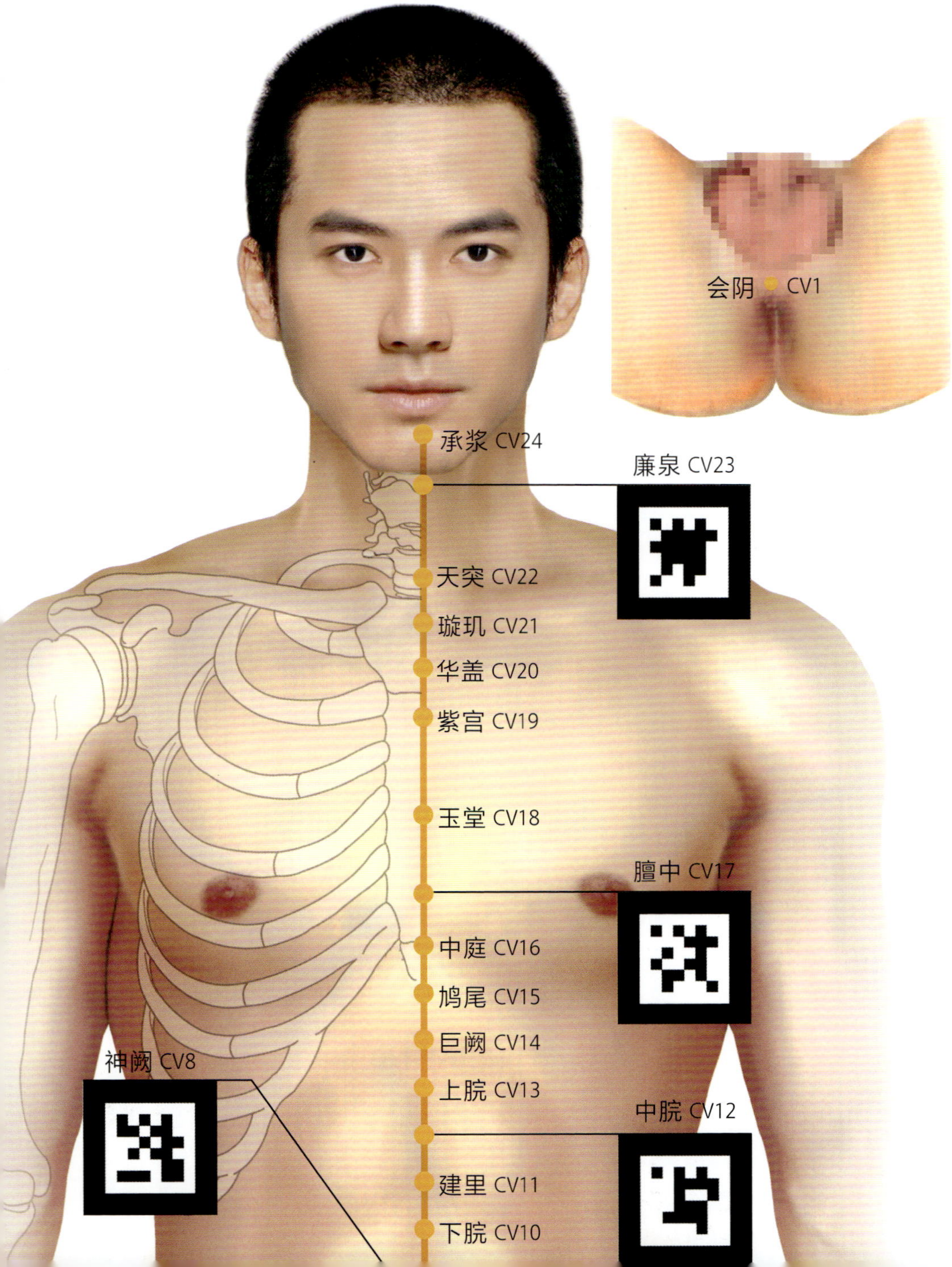

续表

CV	穴名	主治
5	石门	小便不利、遗精、阳痿、带下、崩漏、产后恶露不净、腹痛、腹胀、水肿、泄泻
★ 6	气海	腹痛、泄泻、便秘、遗尿、遗精、阳痿、月经不调、带下、闭经、崩漏、体虚、中风脱证
7	阴交	腹痛、水肿、泄泻、月经不调、带下、疝气
★ 8	神阙	腹痛、久泻、脱肛、水肿、虚脱
9	水分	腹痛、泄泻、反胃吐食、水肿、腹胀、小便不利
10	下脘	腹痛、腹胀、消化不良、呕吐、泄泻、虚肿、消瘦
11	建里	胃痛、腹胀、肠鸣、呕吐、水肿
★ 12	中脘	胃痛、呕吐、腹胀、消化不良、泄泻、黄疸、咳喘痰多、失眠
13	上脘	胃痛、呕吐、腹胀、消化不良、泄泻、黄疸、癫痫
14	巨阙	胃痛、吐酸、呕吐、心悸、癫狂
15	鸠尾	胸闷、心悸、心痛、呃逆、呕吐、腹胀、癫狂

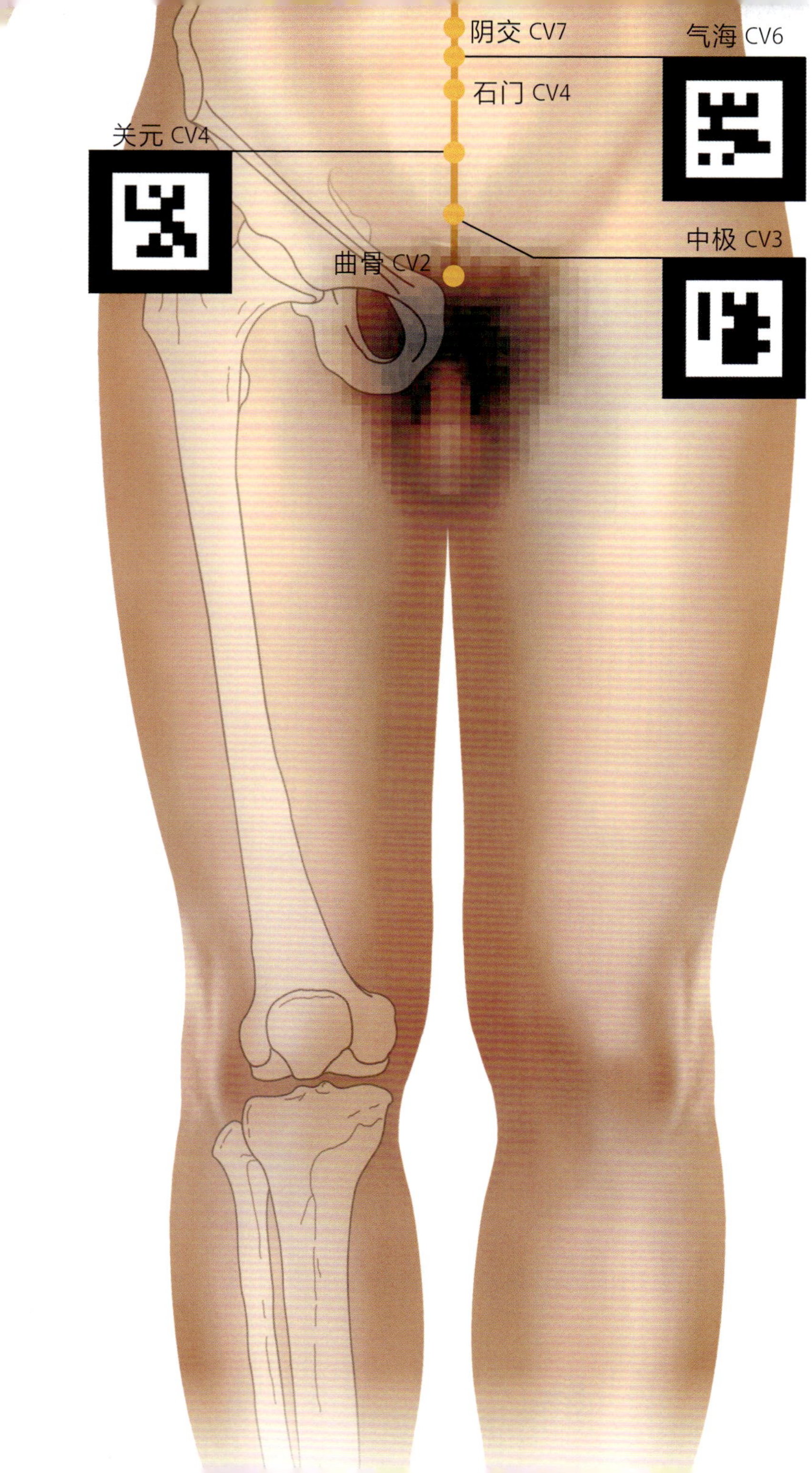

Continued

CV	Acupoints	Indications
5	Shímén	Dysuria; spermatorrhea; erectile dysfunction; leukorrheal diseases; metrorrhagia and metrostaxis; postpartum lochiorrhea; abdominal pain; abdominal distension; edema; diarrhea
★ 6	Qìhǎi	Abdominal pain; diarrhea; constipation; enuresis; spermatorrhea; erectile dysfunction; irregular menstruation; leukorrheal diseases; amenorrhea; metrorrhagia and metrostaxis; weakness; collapse syndrome due to wind stroke
7	Yīnjiāo	Abdominal pain; edema; diarrhea; irregular menstruation; leukorrheal diseases; hernia
★ 8	Shénquè	Abdominal pain; chronic diarrhea; prolapse of rectum; edema; collapse
9	Shuǐfēn	Abdominal pain; diarrhea; nausea and vomiting; edema; abdominal distension; dysuria
10	Xiàwǎn	Abdominal pain; abdominal distension; dyspepsia; vomiting; diarrhea; puffiness; emaciation
11	Jiànlǐ	Stomachache; abdominal distension; borborygmus; vomiting; edema
★ 12	Zhōngwǎn	Stomachache; vomiting; abdominal distension; dyspepsia; diarrhea; jaundice; cough with profuse phlegm; insomnia
13	Shàngwǎn	Stomachache; vomiting; abdominal distension; dyspepsia; diarrhea; jaundice; epilepsy
14	Jùquè	Stomachache; acid regurgitation; vomiting; palpitation; manic-depressive psychosis
15	Jiūwěi	Chest tightness; palpitation; cardiac pain; hiccup; vomiting; abdominal distension; manic-depressive psychosis

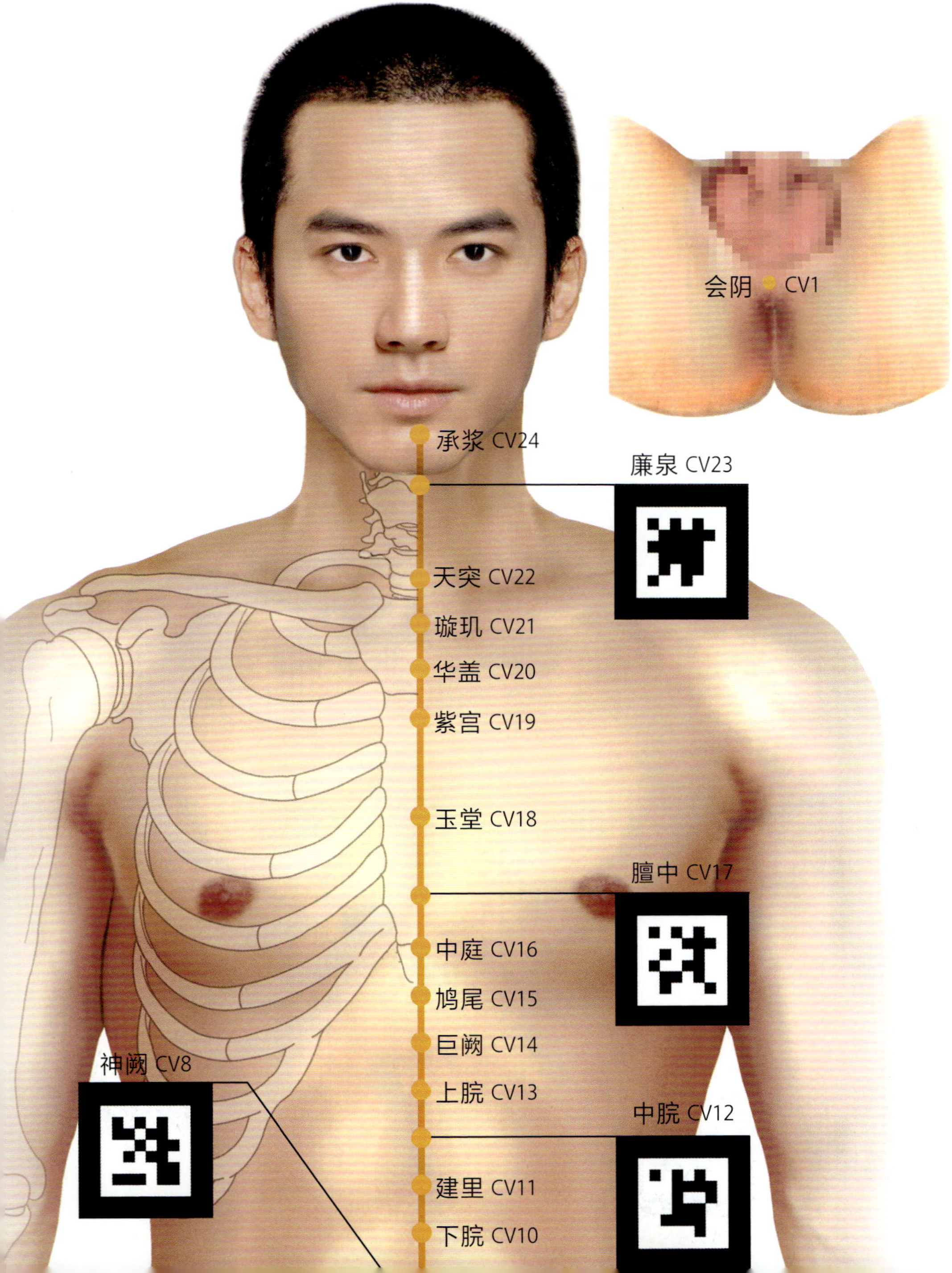

续表

CV	穴名	主治
16	中庭	胸胁胀满、心痛、呕吐、小儿吐乳
★ 17	膻中	胸闷、气短、胸痛、心悸、咳嗽、气喘、乳少、乳腺炎、呕吐、呃逆
18	玉堂	胸痛、胸闷、咳嗽、气喘、呕吐
19	紫宫	咳嗽、气喘、胸痛、胸闷
20	华盖	咳嗽、气喘、胸痛、咽喉痛
21	璇玑	咳嗽、气喘、胸痛、咽喉痛、胃中积滞
22	天突	咳嗽、气喘、胸痛、咽喉痛、暴喑及梅核气（喉中异物感，吞之不下，吐之不出）和噎膈（吞咽哽噎不顺，食入即吐）
23	廉泉	舌强不语、舌下肿痛、暴喑、吞咽困难、口舌生疮、咽喉肿痛
24	承浆	面瘫、齿龈肿痛、暴喑、消渴、癫痫

★为本经常用穴

神阙

用食指按揉神阙穴 2 分钟，力度宜深透，以感觉局部微热为佳。

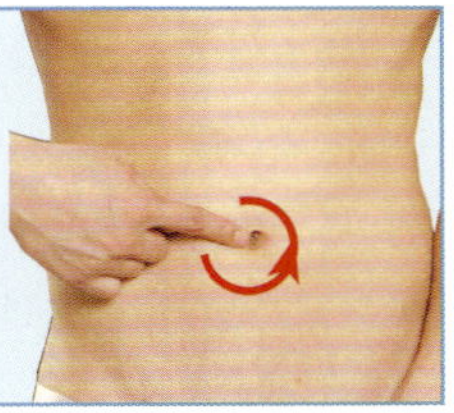

关元

用拇指按揉关元穴 2 分钟，力度适中。

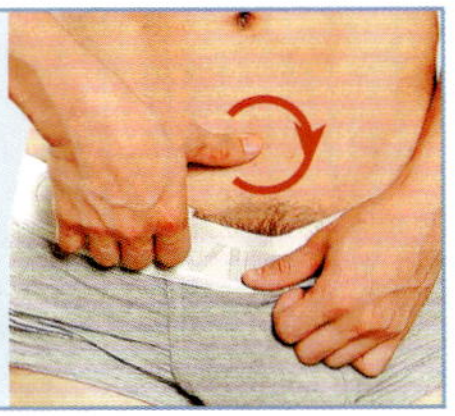

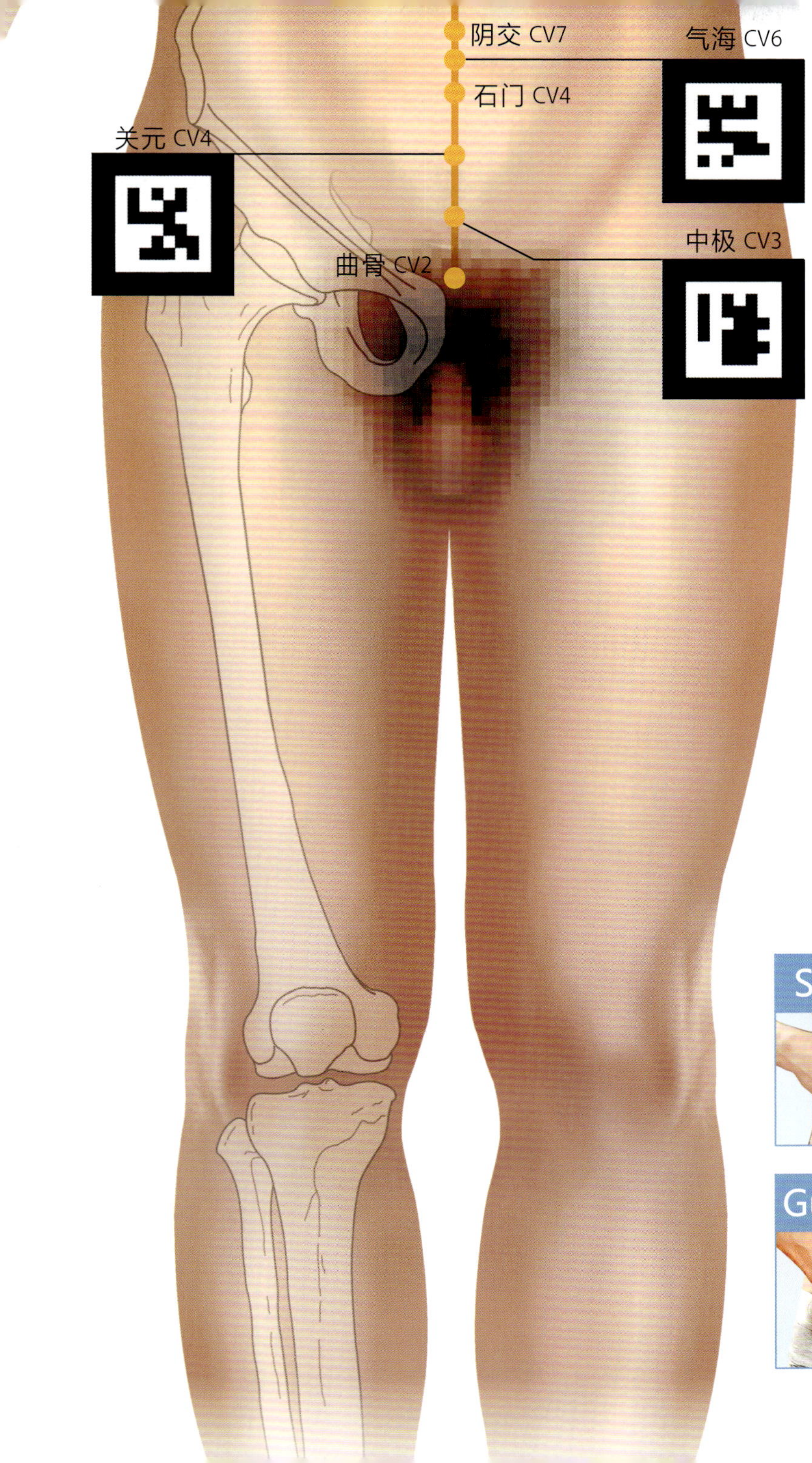

Continued

CV	Acupoints	Indications
16	Zhōngtíng	Distension and pain in the chest and the hypochondrium; cardiac pain; vomiting; vomiting of milk in children
★ 17	Dànzhōng	Chest tightness; shortness of breath; chest pain; palpitation; cough; asthma; hypogalactia; mastitis; vomiting; hiccup
18	Yùtáng	Chest pain; chest tightness; cough; asthma; vomiting
19	Zǐgōng	Cough; asthma; chest pain; chest distress
20	Huágài	Cough; asthma; chest pain; swelling and pain in the throat
21	Xuánjī	Cough; asthma; chest pain; throat pain; dyspepsia
22	Tiāntū	Cough; asthma; chest pain; swelling and pain in the throat; aphonia; globus hystericus (discomfort feeling in the throat which can neither be swallowed nor spat); dysphagia (difficulty in swallowing; vomiting after eating)
23	Liánquán	Voice loss due to stiff tongue; swelling and pain under the tongue; aphonia; dysphagia; aphtha; swelling and pain in the throat
24	Chéngjiāng	Facial paralysis; swelling and pain of the teeth and gum; aphonia; diabetes mellitus; epilepsy

★ Common acupoint used in treatment

Shénquè(CV8)

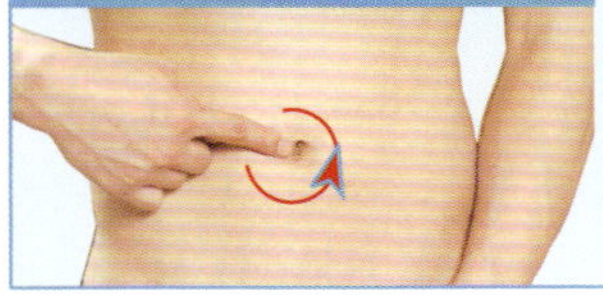

Use the thumb to knead the Shenque acupoint with heavy strength for 2 minutes. It will be better if you can feel the slight local heat.

Guānyuán(CV4)

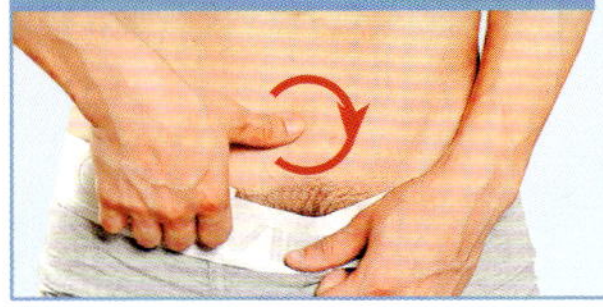

Use the thumb to knead the Guanyuan acupoint with appropriate strength for 2 minutes.

第二章　穴位分部图解

Chapter 2: Diagrams of Acupoints in Different Divisions

头颈肩部穴位

Acupoints of Head, Neck and Shoulder

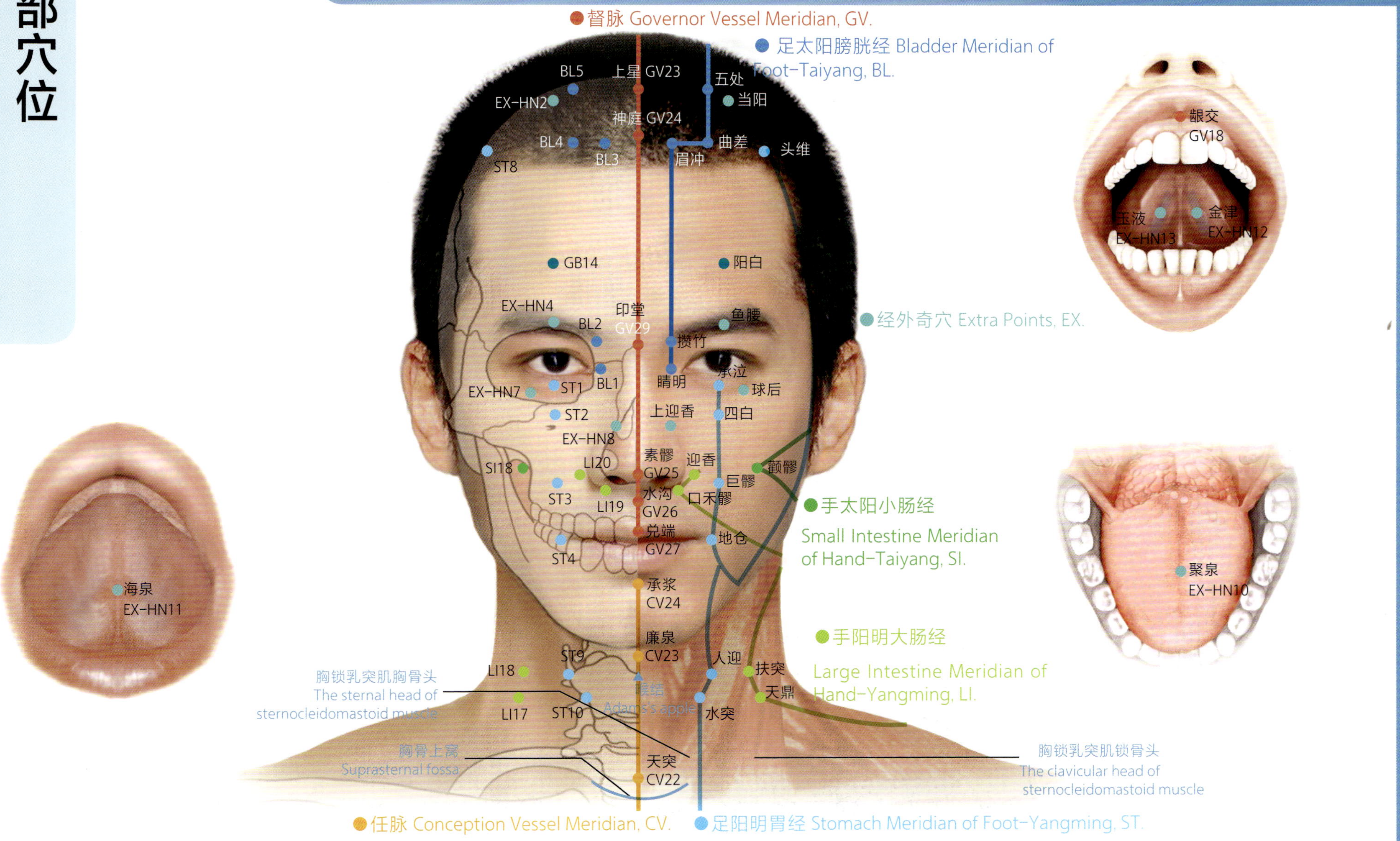

穴位	定位
肩髃	在三角肌区，肩峰外侧缘前端与肱骨大结节两骨间凹陷中
巨骨	在肩胛区，锁骨肩峰端与肩胛冈之间凹陷中
天鼎	在颈部，横平环状软骨，胸锁乳突肌后缘
扶突	在胸锁乳突肌区，横平喉结，胸锁乳突肌前、后缘中间
口禾髎	在面部，横平人中沟上 1/3 与下 2/3 交点，鼻孔外缘直下
迎香	在面部，鼻翼外缘中点旁，鼻唇沟中
承泣	在面部，眼球与眶下缘之间，瞳孔直下

穴位	定位
四白	在面部，眶下孔处
巨髎	在面部，横平鼻翼下缘，瞳孔直下
地仓	在面部，口角旁开 0.4 寸（指寸）
大迎	在面部，下颌角前方，咬肌附着部的前缘凹陷中，面动脉搏动处
颊车	在面部，下颌角前上方约一横指（中指）
下关	在面部，颧弓下缘中央与下颌切迹之间凹陷中
头维	在头部，额角发际直上 0.5 寸，头正中线旁开 4.5 寸

Acupoints	Location
Jiānyú(LI15)	In the region of the deltoid muscle, In the depression of anterior lateral margin of acromion and humerus greater tuberosity
Jùgǔ(LI16)	In the region of the scapula, in the depression of the acromion tip of clavicle and the spine of scapula
Tiāndǐng(LI17)	On the neck, level with the cricoid cartilage,on the posterior margin of the sternocleidomastoid muscle
Fútū(LI18)	In the region of the sternocleidomastoid muscle, level with the tip of Adam's apple, at the midpoint between the posterior and the anterior border of sternocleidomastoid muscle
Kǒuhéliáo(LI19)	On the face, level with the junction of upper 1/3 and lower 2/3 of the philtrum, directly below the lateral margin of the nostril
Yíngxiāng(LI20)	On the face, beside the midpoint of the lateral side of the ala nasi, in the nasolabial groove
Chéngqì(ST1)	On the face, directly below the pupil, between the eyeball and the infraorbital ridge
Sìbái(ST2)	On the face, at the infraorbital foramen
Jùliáo(ST3)	On the face, level with the lower border of the ala nasi, directly below the pupil
Dìcāng(ST4)	On the face, 0.4 cun lateral to the corner of the mouth
Dàyíng(ST5)	On the face, on the anterior aspect of the angle of the mandible and in the depression of the anterior border of the attached portion of the masseter muscle, on the pulsation place of facial artery
Jiáchē(ST6)	On the face,one finger breadth (middle finger) anterior and superior to the lower angle of the mandible
Xiàguān(ST7)	On the face, in the depression of the mandibular notch and the midpoint of lower margin of the zygomatic arch
Tóuwéi(ST8)	on the head, 0.5 cun above the hairline at the corner of the forehead, 4.5 cun lateral to the midline of the head

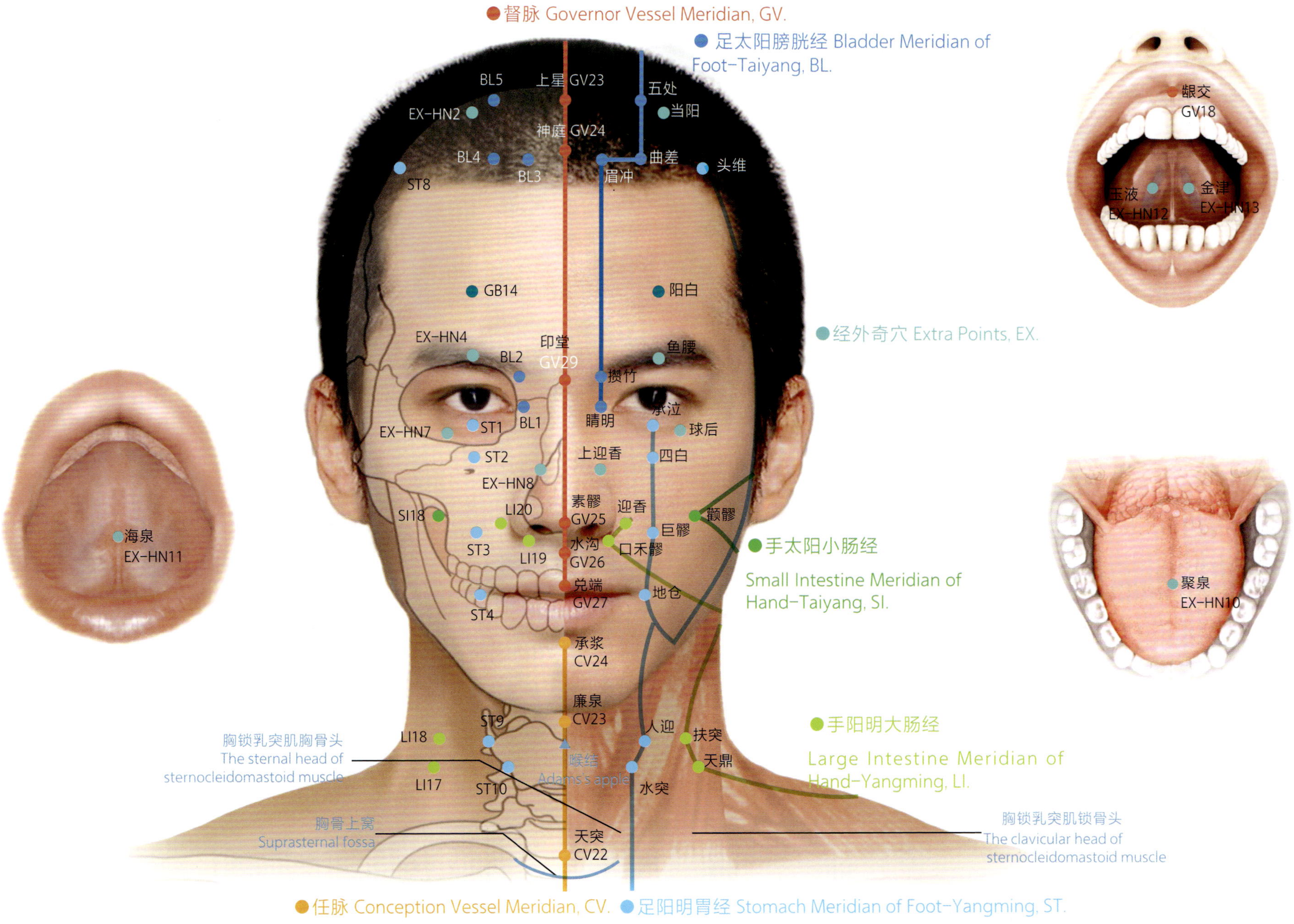
督脉 Governor Vessel Meridian, GV.
足太阳膀胱经 Bladder Meridian of Foot-Taiyang, BL.
经外奇穴 Extra Points, EX.
手太阳小肠经 Small Intestine Meridian of Hand-Taiyang, SI.
手阳明大肠经 Large Intestine Meridian of Hand-Yangming, LI.
任脉 Conception Vessel Meridian, CV.
足阳明胃经 Stomach Meridian of Foot-Yangming, ST.
BL5
上星 GV23
五处
EX-HN2
当阳
神庭 GV24
BL4
BL3
曲差
头维
ST8
眉冲
GB14
阳白
EX-HN4
印堂 GV29
鱼腰
BL2
攒竹
BL1
睛明
承泣
EX-HN7
ST1
球后
ST2
上迎香
四白
EX-HN8
素髎 GV25
迎香
颧髎
SI18
LI20
巨髎
ST3
LI19
水沟 GV26
口禾髎
兑端 GV27
地仓
ST4
承浆 CV24
廉泉 CV23
ST9
LI18
人迎
扶突
天鼎
胸锁乳突肌胸骨头
The sternal head of sternocleidomastoid muscle
喉结
Adams's apple
LI17
ST10
水突
胸骨上窝
Suprasternal fossa
天突 CV22
胸锁乳突肌锁骨头
The clavicular head of sternocleidomastoid muscle
龈交 GV18
玉液 EX-HN12
金津 EX-HN13
海泉 EX-HN11
聚泉 EX-HN10

续表

穴位	定位	穴位	定位
人迎	在颈部，横平喉结，胸锁乳突肌前缘，颈总动脉搏动处	睛明	在面部，目内眦内上方眶内侧壁凹陷中
水突	在颈部，横平环状软骨，胸锁乳突肌前缘	攒竹	在面部，眉头凹陷中，额切迹处
气舍	在胸锁乳突肌区，锁骨上小窝，锁骨胸骨端上缘，胸锁乳突肌胸骨头与锁骨头中间的凹陷中	眉冲	在头部，额切迹直上入发际 0.5 寸
天窗	在颈部，横平喉结，胸锁乳突肌的后缘	曲差	在头部，前发际正中直上 0.5 寸，旁开 1.5 寸
天容	在颈部，下颌角后方，胸锁乳突肌的前缘凹陷中	五处	在头部，前发际正中直上 1 寸，旁开 1.5 寸
颧髎	在面部，颧骨下缘，目外眦直下凹陷中	承光	在头部，前发际正中直上 2.5 寸，旁开 1.5 寸
听宫	在面部，耳屏正中与下颌骨髁突之间的凹陷中	通天	在头部，前发际正中直上 4 寸，旁开 1.5 寸

Continued

Acupoints	Location
Rényíng(ST9)	On the neck, level with the tip of the Adam's apple, in the anterior border of sternocleidomastoid muscle, on the pulsation place of arteria carotis communis
Shuǐtū(ST10)	On the neck, level with the cricoid cartilage, in the anterior margin of sternocleidomastoid muscle
Qìshè(ST11)	On the sternocleidomastoid muscle, in the superior border of the sternal extremity of the clavicle, in the depression of the sternal head and clavicular head of sternocleidomastoid muscle
Tiānchuāng(SI16)	On the neck, level with the Adam's apple, in the posterior margin of the sternocleidomastoid muscle
Tiānróng(SI17)	On the neck, in the posterior aspect of the angle of mandible, in the depression of the anterior margin of sternocleidomastoid muscle
Quánliáo(SI18)	On the face, in the lower margin of the zygoma and the depression directly below the outer canthus
Tīnggōng(SI19)	On the face, in the depression between the condyloid process of the mandible and the midpoint of the tragus
Jīngmíng(BL1)	On the face, in the depression of orbital wall, in the interior and superior border of inner canthus
Cuánzhú(BL2)	On the face, in the depression of interior extermity of the eyebrow, on the supraorbital notch
Méichōng(BL3)	On the head, 0.5 cun within the hairline that is directly above supraorbital notch
Qūchā(BL4)	On the head, 0.5 cun directly within the midpoint of the anterior hairline, 1.5 cun lateral to the midline
Wǔchù(BL5)	On the head, 1 cun directly within the midpoint of the anterior hairline, 1.5 cun lateral to the midline
Chéngguāng(BL6)	On the head, 2.5 cun directly within the midpoint of the anterior hairlint, 1.5 cun lateral to the midline
Tōngtiān(BL7)	On the head, 4 cun directly within the midpoint of the anterior hairline, 1.5 cun lateral to the midline

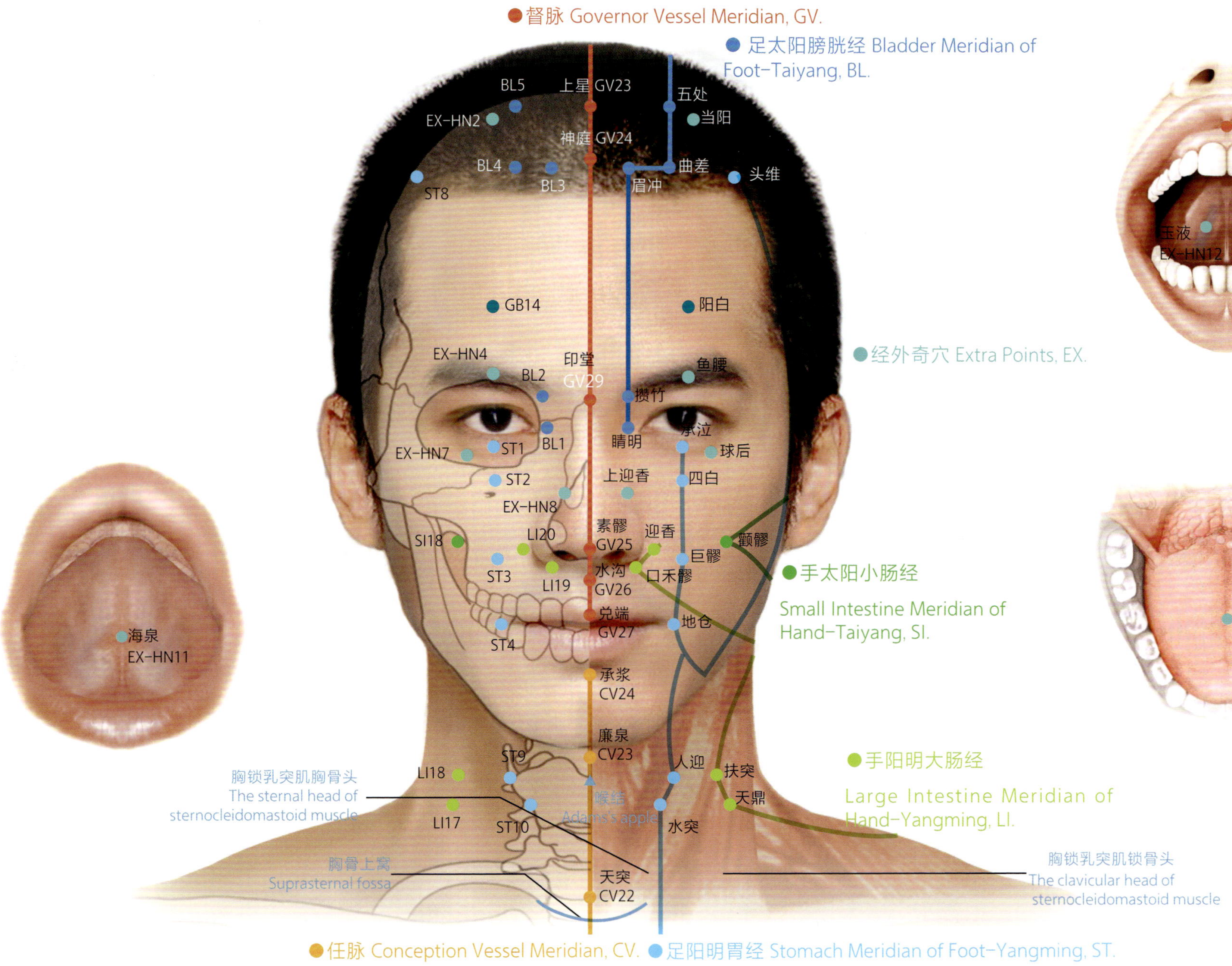
督脉 Governor Vessel Meridian, GV.
足太阳膀胱经 Bladder Meridian of Foot-Taiyang, BL.
经外奇穴 Extra Points, EX.
手太阳小肠经 Small Intestine Meridian of Hand-Taiyang, SI.
手阳明大肠经 Large Intestine Meridian of Hand-Yangming, LI.
任脉 Conception Vessel Meridian, CV.
足阳明胃经 Stomach Meridian of Foot-Yangming, ST.
BL5
上星 GV23
五处
当阳
EX-HN2
神庭 GV24
BL4
BL3
曲差
眉冲
头维
ST8
GB14
阳白
EX-HN4
印堂 GV29
BL2
鱼腰
攒竹
BL1
睛明
承泣
EX-HN7
ST1
球后
ST2
上迎香
四白
EX-HN8
素髎 GV25
迎香
颧髎
SI18
LI20
巨髎
ST3
LI19
水沟 GV26
口禾髎
兑端 GV27
地仓
ST4
承浆 CV24
廉泉 CV23
ST9
LI18
人迎
扶突
天鼎
LI17
ST10
水突
喉结 Adam's apple
天突 CV22
胸锁乳突肌胸骨头 The sternal head of sternocleidomastoid muscle
胸骨上窝 Suprasternal fossa
胸锁乳突肌锁骨头 The clavicular head of sternocleidomastoid muscle
龈交 GV18
玉液 EX-HN12
金津 EX-HN13
海泉 EX-HN11
聚泉 EX-HN10

续表

穴位	定位
络却	在头部，前发际正中直上 5.5 寸，旁开 1.5 寸
玉枕	在头部，横平枕外隆凸上缘，后发际正中线旁开 1.3 寸
天柱	在颈后区，横平第 2 颈椎棘突上际，斜方肌外缘凹陷中
天牖	在颈部，横平下颌角，胸锁乳突肌的后缘凹陷中
翳风	在颈部，耳垂后方，乳突下端前方凹陷中
瘈脉	在头部，乳突中央，角孙与翳风沿耳轮弧形连线的上 2/3 与下 1/3 的交点处
颅息	在头部，角孙与翳风沿耳轮弧形连线的上 1/3 与下 2/3 的交点处
角孙	在头部，耳尖正对发际处
耳门	在耳区，耳屏上切迹与下颌骨髁突之间的凹陷中
耳和髎	在头部，鬓发后缘，耳郭根的前方，颞浅动脉的后缘
丝竹空	在面部，眉梢凹陷中
瞳子髎	在面部，目外眦外侧 0.5 寸凹陷中
听会	在面部，耳屏间切迹与下颌骨髁突之间的凹陷中
上关	在面部，颧弓上缘中央凹陷中

Continued

Acupoints	Location
Luòquè(BL8)	On the head, 5.5 cun directly within the midpoint of the anterior hairline, 1.5 cun lateral to the midline
Yùzhěn(BL9)	On the head, level with the superior margin of the external occipital protuberance, 1.3 cun lateral to the midpoint of posterior hairline
Tiānzhù(BL10)	In the posterior neck region, level with the superior border of the spinous process of the 2nd cervical vertebra，in the depression of the lateral border of the trapezius muscle
Tiānyǒu(TE16)	On the neck, level with the lower angle of mandible, in the depression of the posterior border of the sternocleidomastoid muscle
Yìfēng(TE17)	On the neck, in the posterior aspect of the earlobe, in the depression anterior to the lower aspect of the mastoid process
Chìmài(TE18)	On the head, at the midpoint of the mastoid process, at the junction of upper 2/3 and lower 1/3 on the curved line along the helix from the Jiaosun acupoint to the Yifeng acupoint
Lúxī(TE19)	On the head, at the junction of the upper 1/3 and lower 2/3 on the curved line from the Jiaosun acupoint to the Yifeng acupoint
Jiǎosūn(TE20)	On the head, within the hairline and level with the ear apex
Ěrmén(TE21)	In the ear region, in the depression between the supratragic notch of the tragus and the condyloid process of the mandible
Ěrhéliáo(TE22)	On the head, on the posterior border of the hairline, anterior to the root of the auricle, on the posterior border of the superficial temporal artery
Sīzhúkōng(TE23)	On the face, in the depression of the lateral end of the eyebrow
Tóngzǐliáo(GB1)	On the face, in the depression 0.5 cun lateral to the outer canthus
Tīnghuì(GB2)	On the face, in the depression between the intertragic notch and the condyloid process of the mandible
Shàngguān(GB3)	On the face, in the middle depression superior to the upper margin of the zygomatic arch

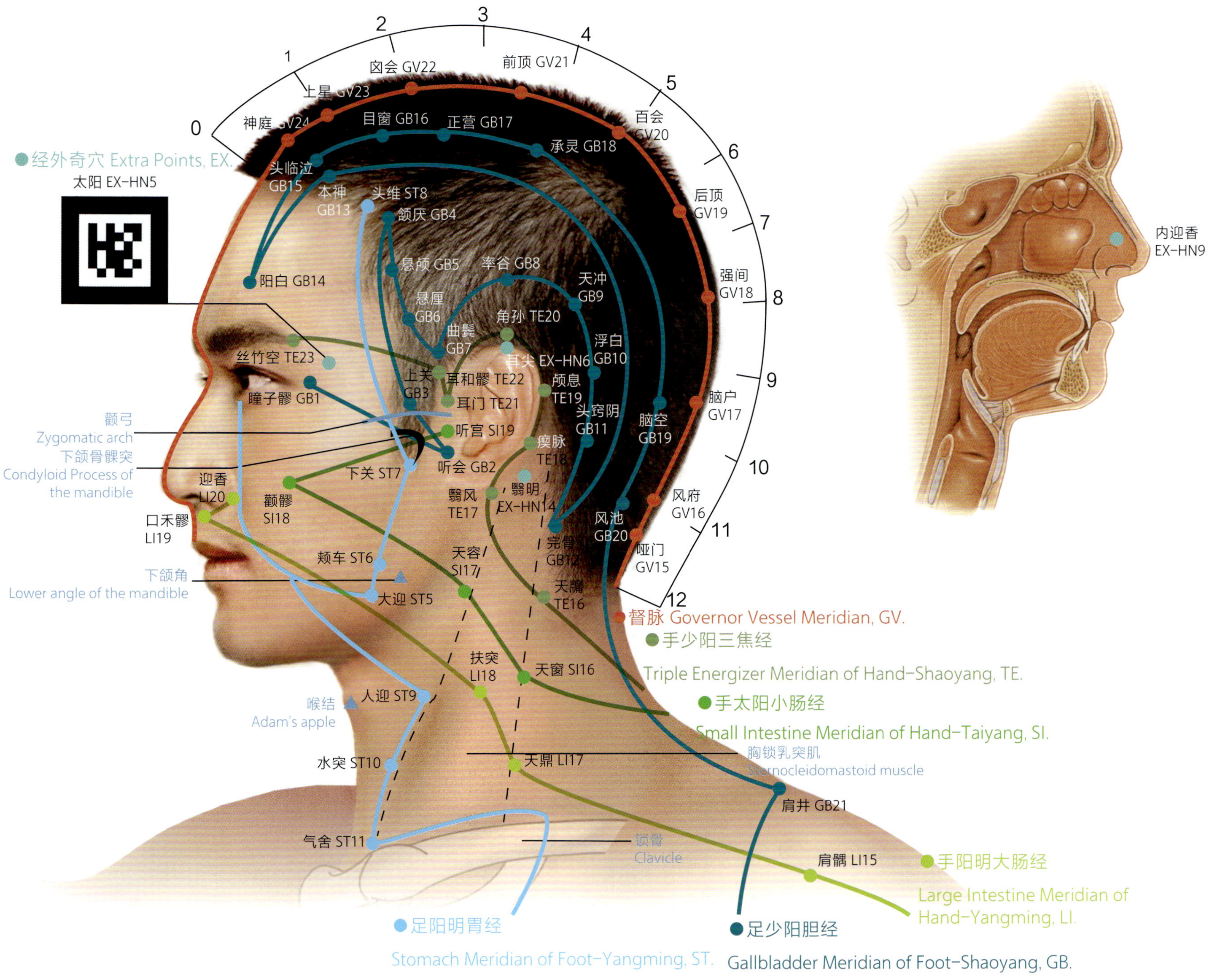
0
1
2
3
4
5
6
7
8
9
10
11
12
神庭 GV24
上星 GV23
囟会 GV22
前顶 GV21
百会 GV20
后顶 GV19
强间 GV18
脑户 GV17
风府 GV16
哑门 GV15
目窗 GB16
正营 GB17
承灵 GB18
头临泣 GB15
本神 GB13
头维 ST8
颔厌 GB4
悬颅 GB5
率谷 GB8
天冲 GB9
悬厘 GB6
角孙 TE20
曲鬓 GB7
浮白 GB10
耳尖 EX-HN6
上关 GB3
耳和髎 TE22
颅息 TE19
耳门 TE21
头窍阴 GB11
脑空 GB19
听宫 SI19
瘈脉 TE18
听会 GB2
翳明 EX-HN14
翳风 TE17
风池 GB20
完骨 GB12
天容 SI17
天牖 TE16
阳白 GB14
经外奇穴 Extra Points, EX.
太阳 EX-HN5
丝竹空 TE23
瞳子髎 GB1
颧弓 Zygomatic arch
下颌骨髁突 Condyloid Process of the mandible
下关 ST7
迎香 LI20
颧髎 SI18
口禾髎 LI19
颊车 ST6
下颌角 Lower angle of the mandible
大迎 ST5
扶突 LI18
天窗 SI16
喉结 Adam's apple
人迎 ST9
水突 ST10
天鼎 LI17
胸锁乳突肌 Sternocleidomastoid muscle
肩井 GB21
气舍 ST11
锁骨 Clavicle
肩髃 LI15
督脉 Governor Vessel Meridian, GV.
手少阳三焦经
Triple Energizer Meridian of Hand-Shaoyang, TE.
手太阳小肠经
Small Intestine Meridian of Hand-Taiyang, SI.
手阳明大肠经
Large Intestine Meridian of Hand-Yangming, LI.
足阳明胃经
Stomach Meridian of Foot-Yangming, ST.
足少阳胆经
Gallbladder Meridian of Foot-Shaoyang, GB.
内迎香 EX-HN9

续表

穴位	定位	穴位	定位
颔厌	在头部，从头维至曲鬓的弧形连线（其弧度与鬓发弧度相应）的上 1/4 与下 3/4 交点处	浮白	在头部，耳后乳突的后上方，从天冲至完骨的弧形连线（其弧度与耳郭弧度相应）的上 1/3 与下 2/3 交点处
悬颅	在头部，从头维至曲鬓的弧形连线（其弧度与鬓发弧度相应）的中点处	头窍阴	在头部，耳后乳突的后上方，从天冲至完骨的弧形连线（其弧度与耳郭弧度相应）的上 2/3 与下 1/3 交点处
悬厘	在头部，从头维至曲鬓的弧形连线（其弧度与鬓发弧度相应）的上 3/4 与下 1/4 交点处	完骨	在头部，耳后乳突的后下方凹陷中
曲鬓	在头部，耳前鬓角发际后缘与耳尖水平线的交点处	本神	在头部，前发际上 0.5 寸，头正中线旁开 3 寸
率谷	在头部，耳尖直上入发际 1.5 寸	阳白	在头部，眉上 1 寸，瞳孔直上
天冲	在头部，耳根后缘直上，入发际 2 寸	头临泣	在头部，前发际上 0.5 寸，瞳孔直上

Continued

Acupoints	Location
Hànyàn(GB4)	On the head, at the junction of the upper 1/4 and lower 3/4 of the curved line from the Touwei acupoint to the Qubin acupoint
Xuánlú(GB5)	On the head, at the midpoint of the curved line from the Touwei acupoint to the Qubin acupoint
Xuánlí(GB6)	On the head, at the junction of the upper 3/4 and lower 1/4 of the curved line from the Touwei acupoint to the Qubin acupoint
Qūbìn(GB7)	On the head, at the junction between the posterior margin of the temple hairline and the horizontal line of the ear apex
Shuàigǔ(GB8)	On the head, 1.5 cun directly within the hairline above the apex of the ear
Tiānchōng(GB9)	On the head, 2 cun directly within the hairline above the posterior border of the ear
Fúbái(GB10)	On the head, posterior and superior to the mastoid process, at the junction of the upper 1/3 and lower 2/3 of the curved line from Tianchong acupoint to Wangu acupoint
Tóuqiàoyīn(GB11)	On the head, posterior and superior to the mastoid process, at the junction of the upper 2/3 and lower 1/3 of the curved line from Tianchong acupoint to Wangu acupoint
Wángǔ(GB12)	On the head, in the depression posterior and inferior to the mastoid process
Běnshén(GB13)	On the head, 0.5 cun above the front hairline, 3 cun lateral to the midline of the head
Yángbái(GB14)	On the head, 1 cun above the eyebrow, directly above the pupil
Tóulínqì(GB15)	On the head, 0.5 cun above the front hairline, directly above the pupil

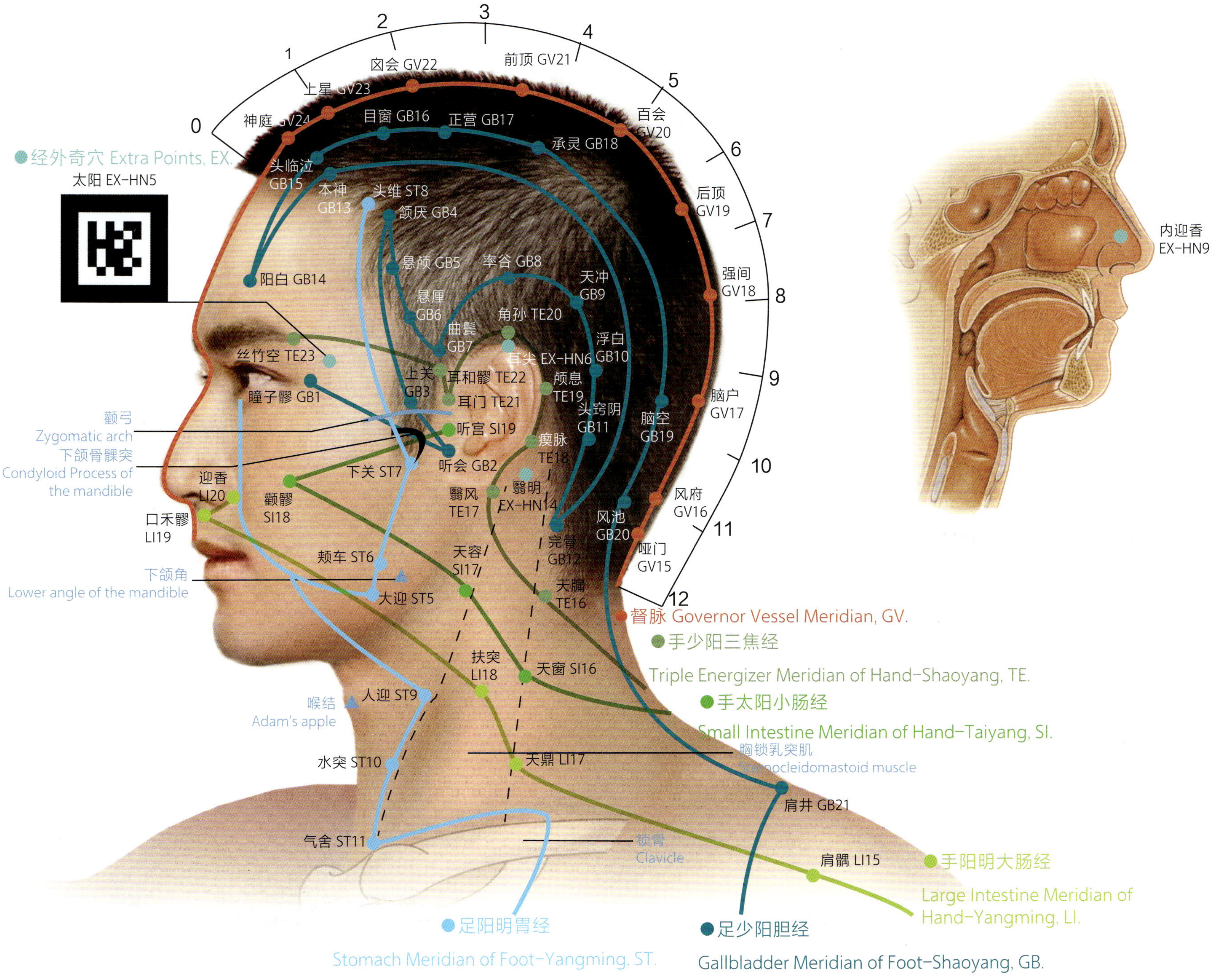
0
1
2
3
4
5
6
7
8
9
10
11
12
神庭 GV24
上星 GV23
囟会 GV22
前顶 GV21
百会 GV20
后顶 GV19
强间 GV18
脑户 GV17
风府 GV16
哑门 GV15
头临泣 GB15
目窗 GB16
正营 GB17
承灵 GB18
本神 GB13
头维 ST8
颔厌 GB4
阳白 GB14
悬颅 GB5
率谷 GB8
天冲 GB9
悬厘 GB6
角孙 TE20
曲鬓 GB7
浮白 GB10
耳尖 EX-HN6
丝竹空 TE23
上关 GB3
耳和髎 TE22
颅息 TE19
瞳子髎 GB1
耳门 TE21
头窍阴 GB11
脑空 GB19
听宫 SI19
瘈脉 TE18
听会 GB2
下关 ST7
翳明 EX-HN14
翳风 TE17
风池 GB20
完骨 GB12
迎香 LI20
颧髎 SI18
口禾髎 LI19
颊车 ST6
天容 SI17
天牖 TE16
大迎 ST5
扶突 LI18
天窗 SI16
人迎 ST9
水突 ST10
天鼎 LI17
肩井 GB21
气舍 ST11
肩髃 LI15
经外奇穴 Extra Points, EX.
太阳 EX-HN5
颧弓
Zygomatic arch
下颌骨髁突
Condyloid Process of the mandible
下颌角
Lower angle of the mandible
喉结
Adam's apple
胸锁乳突肌
Sternocleidomastoid muscle
锁骨
Clavicle
督脉 Governor Vessel Meridian, GV.
手少阳三焦经
Triple Energizer Meridian of Hand-Shaoyang, TE.
手太阳小肠经
Small Intestine Meridian of Hand-Taiyang, SI.
手阳明大肠经
Large Intestine Meridian of Hand-Yangming, LI.
足阳明胃经
Stomach Meridian of Foot-Yangming, ST.
足少阳胆经
Gallbladder Meridian of Foot-Shaoyang, GB.
内迎香
EX-HN9

续表

穴位	定位	穴位	定位
目窗	在头部，前发际上 1.5 寸，瞳孔直上	大椎	在脊柱区，第 7 颈椎棘突下凹陷中，后正中线上
正营	在头部，前发际上 2.5 寸，瞳孔直上	哑门	在颈后区，第 2 颈椎棘突上际凹陷中，后正中线上
承灵	在头部，前发际上 4 寸，瞳孔直上	风府	在颈后区，枕外隆凸直下，两侧斜方肌之间凹陷中
脑空	在头部，横平枕外隆凸的上缘，风池直上	脑户	在头部，枕外隆凸的上缘凹陷中
风池	在颈后区，枕骨之下，胸锁乳突肌上端与斜方肌上端之间的凹陷中	强间	在头部，后发际正中直上 4 寸
肩井	在肩胛区，第 7 颈椎棘突与肩峰最外侧点连线的中点	后顶	在头部，后发际正中直上 5.5 寸

Continued

Acupoints	Location
Mùchuāng(GB16)	On the head, 1.5 cun above the front hairline, directly above the pupil
Zhèngyíng(GB17)	On the head, 2.5 cun above the front hairline, directly above the pupil
Chénglíng(GB18)	On the head, 4 cun above the front hairline, directly above the pupil
Nǎokōng(GB19)	On the head, level with the upper margin of the external occipital protuberance, directly above Fengchi acupoint
Fēngchí(GB20)	In the posterior region of the neck, below the occipital bone, in the depression between the superior margin of the sternocleidomastoid muscle and the superior margin of the trapezius
Jiānjǐng(GB21)	In the region of the scapular, at the midpoint of the joining line from the spinous process of the 7th cervical vertebra and the outmost point of the acromion
Dàzhuī(GV14)	In the spinal region, in the depression below the spinous process of the 7th cervical vertebra, on the posterior midline
Yǎmén(GV15)	In the posterior neck region, in the depression of the superior borcler of the spinous process of the 2nd cervical vertebra, on the posterior midline
Fēngfǔ(GV16)	In the posterior neck region, directly below the external occipital protuberance, in the depression between two trapezius muscles
Nǎohù(GV17)	On the head, in the depression of the superior margin of the external occipital protuberance
Qiángjiān(GV18)	On the head, 4 cun directly above the middle of the posterior hairline
Hòudǐng(GV19)	On the head, 5.5 cun directly above the middle of the posterior hairline

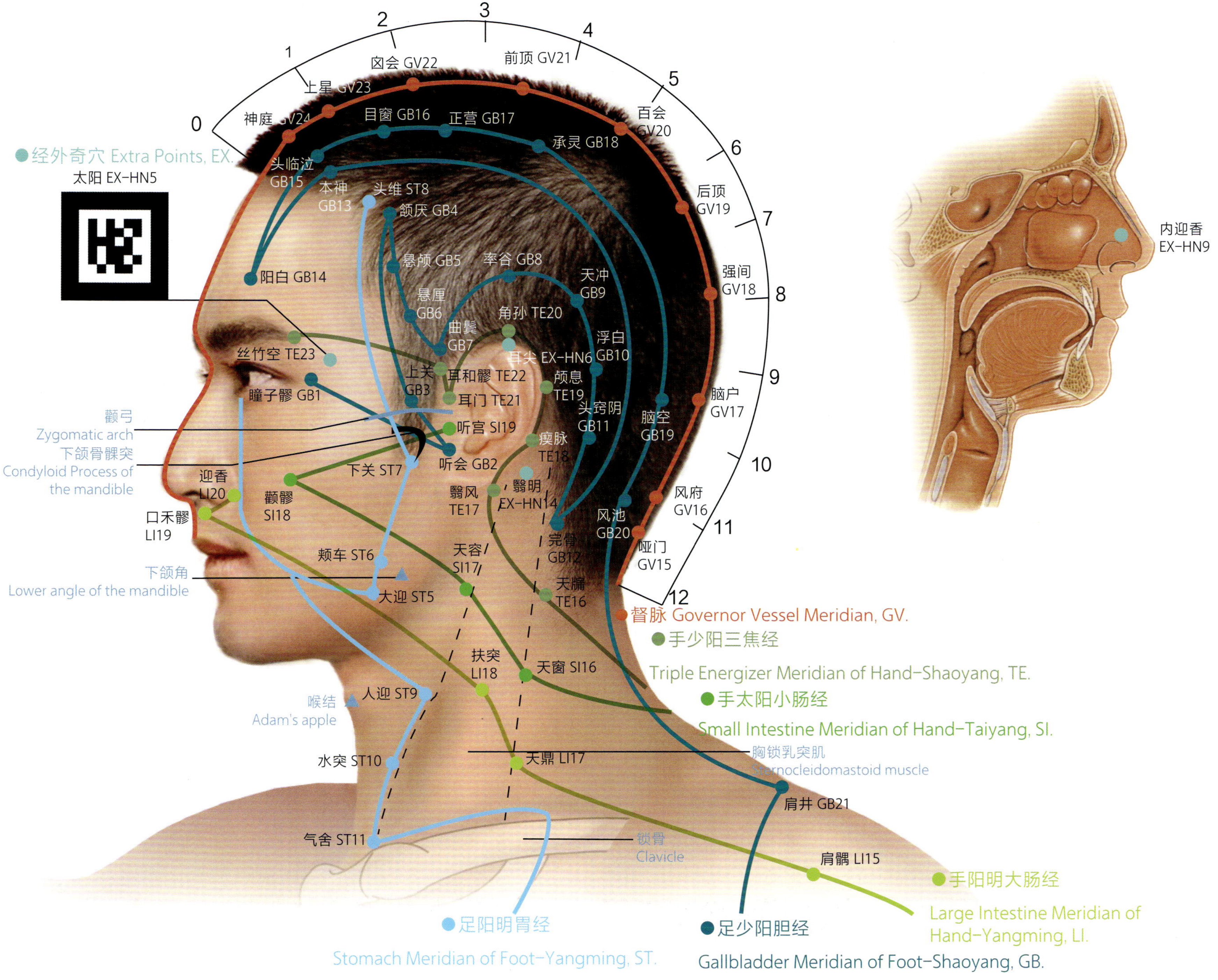
0
1
2
3
4
5
6
7
8
9
10
11
12
上星 GV23
神庭
囟会 GV22
前顶 GV21
百会 GV20
后顶 GV19
强间 GV18
脑户 GV17
风府 GV16
哑门 GV15
目窗 GB16
正营 GB17
承灵 GB18
头临泣 GB15
本神 GB13
头维 ST8
颔厌 GB4
阳白 GB14
悬颅 GB5
率谷 GB8
天冲 GB9
悬厘 GB6
角孙 TE20
曲鬓 GB7
浮白 GB10
耳尖 EX-HN6
上关 GB3
耳和髎 TE22
颅息 TE19
耳门 TE21
头窍阴 GB11
脑空 GB19
听宫 SI19
瘈脉 TE18
听会 GB2
下关 ST7
翳风 TE17
翳明 EX-HN14
风池 GB20
完骨 GB12
经外奇穴 Extra Points, EX.
太阳 EX-HN5
丝竹空 TE23
瞳子髎 GB1
颧弓 Zygomatic arch
下颌骨髁突 Condyloid Process of the mandible
迎香 LI20
颧髎 SI18
口禾髎 LI19
颊车 ST6
天容 SI17
下颌角 Lower angle of the mandible
大迎 ST5
天牖 TE16
督脉 Governor Vessel Meridian, GV.
手少阳三焦经
Triple Energizer Meridian of Hand-Shaoyang, TE.
扶突 LI18
天窗 SI16
人迎 ST9
喉结 Adam's apple
手太阳小肠经
Small Intestine Meridian of Hand-Taiyang, SI.
胸锁乳突肌
Sternocleidomastoid muscle
水突 ST10
天鼎 LI17
肩井 GB21
气舍 ST11
锁骨 Clavicle
肩髃 LI15
手阳明大肠经
Large Intestine Meridian of Hand-Yangming, LI.
足阳明胃经
Stomach Meridian of Foot-Yangming, ST.
足少阳胆经
Gallbladder Meridian of Foot-Shaoyang, GB.
内迎香 EX-HN9

续表

穴位	定位
百会	在头部，前发际正中直上 5 寸
前顶	在头部，前发际正中直上 3.5 寸
囟会	在头部，前发际正中直上 2 寸
上星	在头部，前发际正中直上 1 寸
神庭	在头部，前发际正中直上 0.5 寸
素髎	在面部，鼻尖的正中央
水沟	在面部，人中沟的上 1/3 与中 1/3 交点处
兑端	在面部，上唇结节的中点
龈交	在上唇内，上唇系带与上齿龈的交点
印堂	在头部，两眉毛内侧端中间的凹陷中
天突	在颈前区，胸骨上窝中央，前正中线上
廉泉	在颈前区，喉结上方，舌骨上缘凹陷中，前正中线上
承浆	在面部，颏唇沟的正中凹陷处

Continued

Acupoints	Location
Bǎihuì(GV20)	On the head, 5 cun directly above the middle of the front hairline
Qiándǐng(GV21)	On the head, 3.5 cun directly above the middle of the front hairline
Xìnhuì(GV22)	On the head, 2 cun directly above the middle of the front hairline
Shàngxīng(GV23)	On the head, 1 cun directly above the middle of the front hairline
Shéntíng(GV24)	On the head, 0.5 cun directly above the middle of the front hairline
Sùliáo(GV25)	On the face, in the middle of the tip of the nose
Shuǐgōu(GV26)	On the face, at the junction of upper 1/3 and lower 2/3 of the philtrum
Duìduān(GV27)	On the face, in the middle of upper lip tubercle
Yínjiāo(GV28)	Within the upper lip, at the junction of the frenulum of the upper lip and the upper gum
Yìntáng(GV29)	On the head, in the depression of midpoint of interior margin of two eyebrows
Tiāntū(CV22)	In the anterior region of the neck, in the center of the sterna fossa, on the anterior midline
Liánquán(CV23)	In the anterior region of the neck, above the Adam's apple, in the depression of the superior hyoid bone, on the anterior midline
Chéngjiāng(CV24)	On the face, in the depression of the midpoint of the mentolabial groove

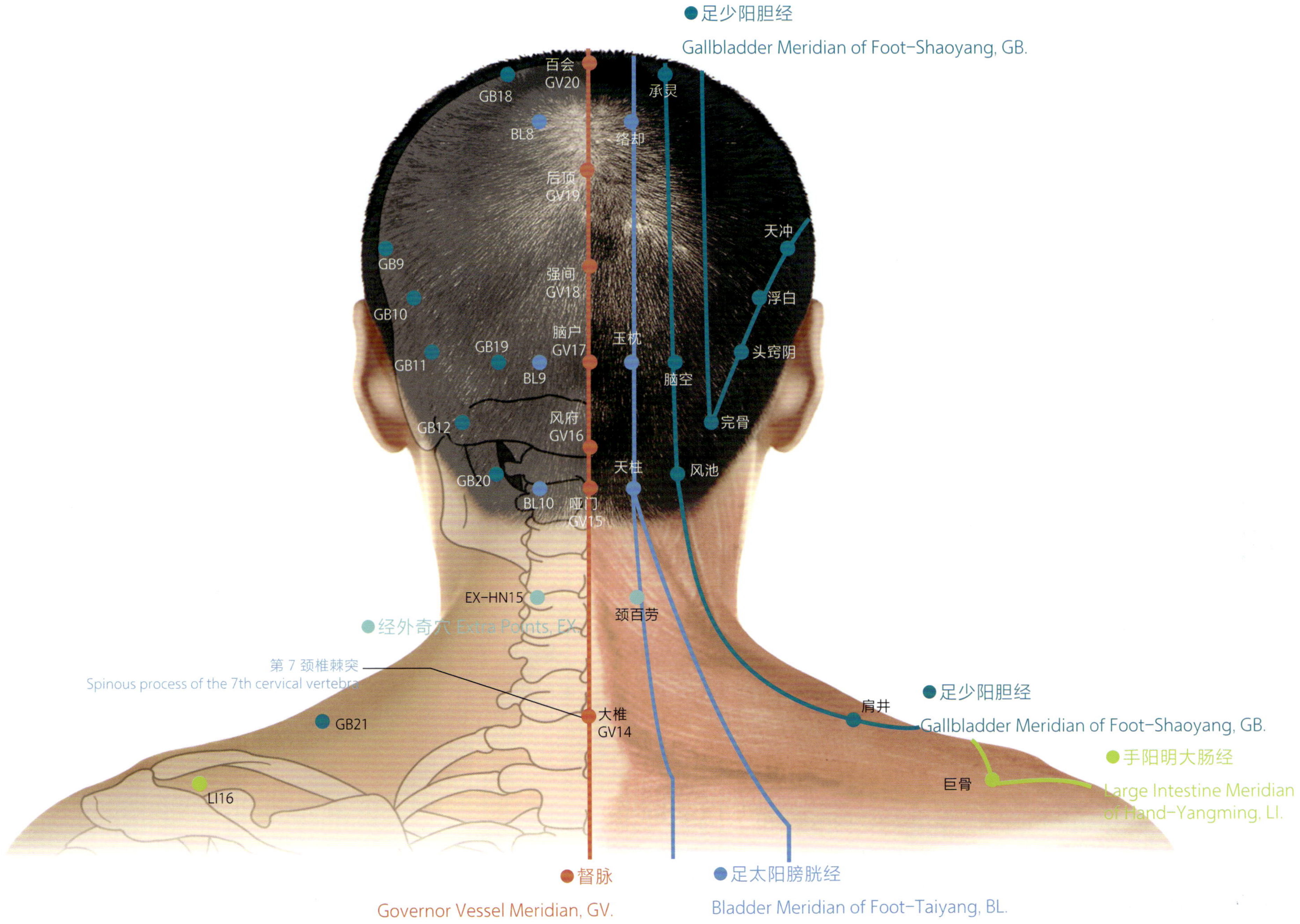
足少阳胆经
Gallbladder Meridian of Foot-Shaoyang, GB.
百会
GV20
GB18
承灵
BL8
络却
后顶
GV19
GB9
强间
GV18
天冲
浮白
GB10
脑户
GV17
玉枕
头窍阴
GB19
GB11
BL9
脑空
完骨
风府
GV16
GB12
天柱
风池
GB20
BL10
哑门
GV15
EX-HN15
颈百劳
经外奇穴 Extra Points, EX.
第 7 颈椎棘突
Spinous process of the 7th cervical vertebra
肩井
足少阳胆经
大椎
GV14
GB21
Gallbladder Meridian of Foot-Shaoyang, GB.
手阳明大肠经
巨骨
Large Intestine Meridian
of Hand-Yangming, LI.
LI16
督脉
Governor Vessel Meridian, GV.
足太阳膀胱经
Bladder Meridian of Foot-Taiyang, BL.

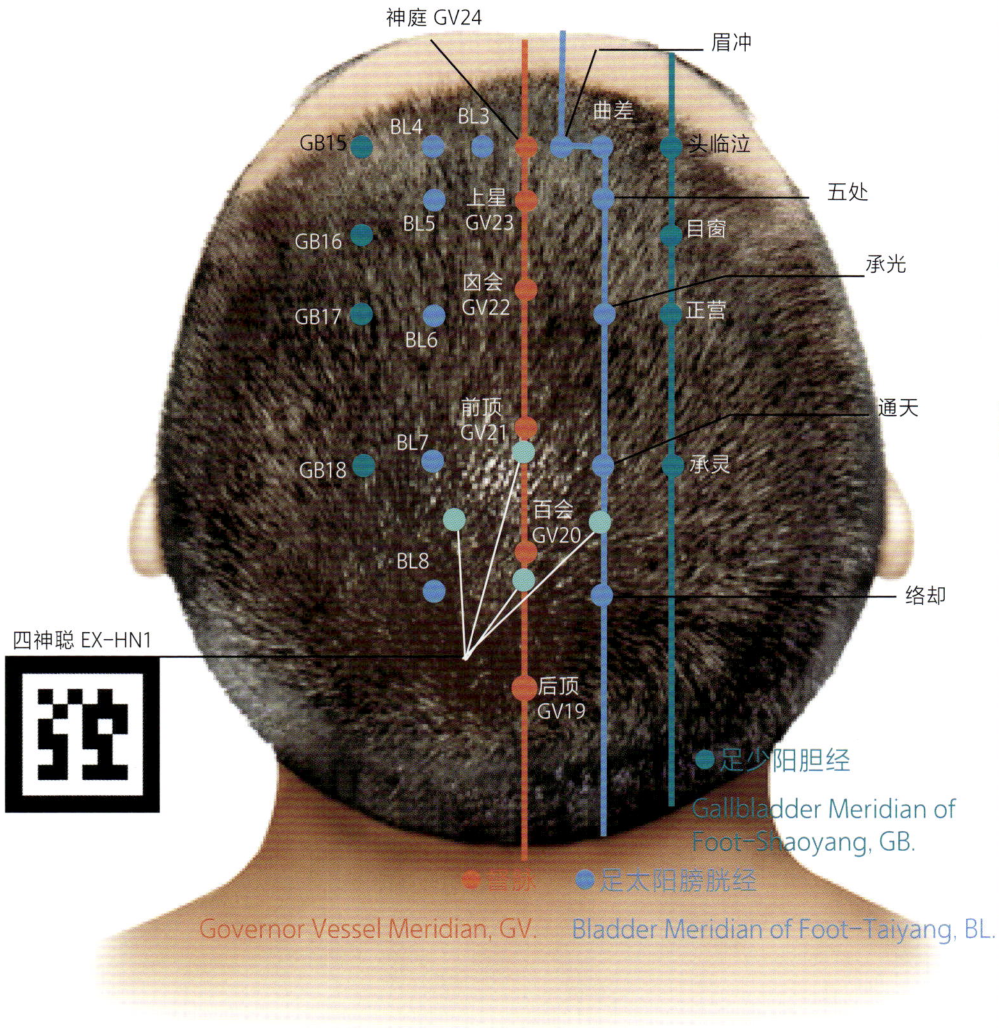

续表

穴位	定位
四神聪	在头部，百会前后左右各旁开 1 寸，共 4 穴
当阳	在头部，瞳孔直上，前发际上 1 寸
鱼腰	在头部，瞳孔直上，眉毛中
太阳	在头部，眉梢与目外眦之间，向后约一横指的凹陷中
耳尖	在耳区，在外耳轮的最高点
球后	在面部，眶下缘外 1/4 与内 3/4 交界处
上迎香	在面部，鼻翼软骨与鼻甲的交界处，近鼻唇沟上端处

Continued

Acupoints	Location
Sìshéncōng(EX-HN1)	On the head, 1 cun respectively posterior, anterior and lateral to the Baihui acupoint, altogether 4 acupoints
Dāngyáng(EX-HN2)	On the head, 1 cun within the anterior hairline, directly above the pupil
Yúyāo(EX-HN4)	On the head, inside the eyebrow, directly above the pupil
Tàiyáng(EX-HN5)	On the head, in the depression about 1 finger breadth posterior to the midpoint of the eyebrow and the outer canthus
Ěrjiān(EX-HN6)	In the region of the ear, at the apex of the auricle
Qiúhòu(EX-HN7)	On the face, at the junction of outer 1/4 and inner 3/4 of the infraorbital margin
Shàngyíngxiāng (EX-HN8)	On the face, at the junction of ala nasi cartilage and the turbinate, near the superior border of the nasolabial groove

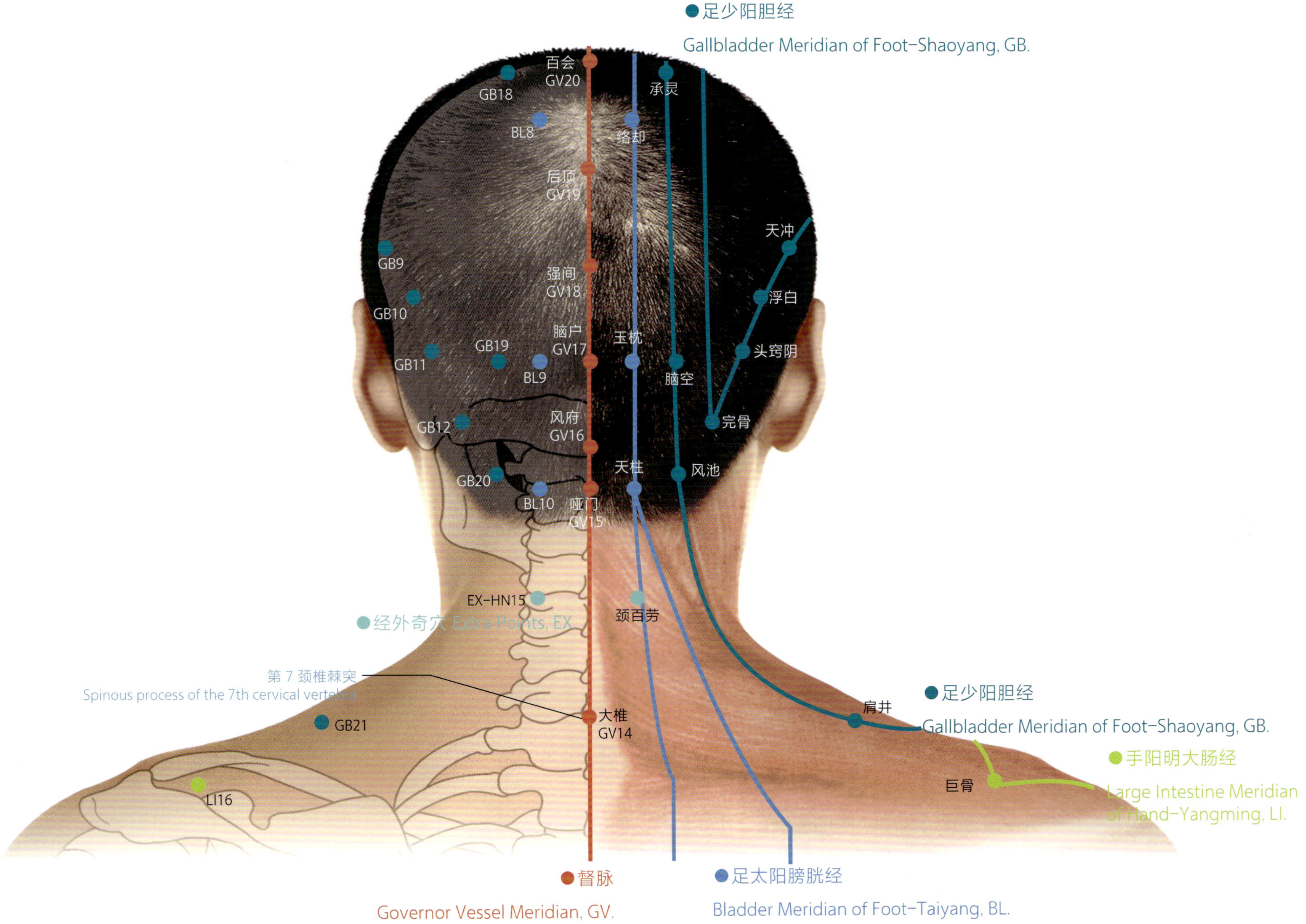
足少阳胆经
Gallbladder Meridian of Foot-Shaoyang, GB.
百会
GV20
GB18
承灵
BL8
络却
后顶
GV19
天冲
GB9
强间
GV18
浮白
GB10
脑户
GV17
玉枕
头窍阴
GB19
GB11
BL9
脑空
风府
GV16
完骨
GB12
天柱
风池
GB20
BL10
哑门
GV15
EX-HN15
颈百劳
经外奇穴 Extra Points, EX
第 7 颈椎棘突
Spinous process of the 7th cervical vertebra
肩井
足少阳胆经
大椎
GV14
Gallbladder Meridian of Foot-Shaoyang, GB.
GB21
手阳明大肠经
巨骨
Large Intestine Meridian
of Hand-Yangming, LI.
LI16
督脉
Governor Vessel Meridian, GV.
足太阳膀胱经
Bladder Meridian of Foot-Taiyang, BL.

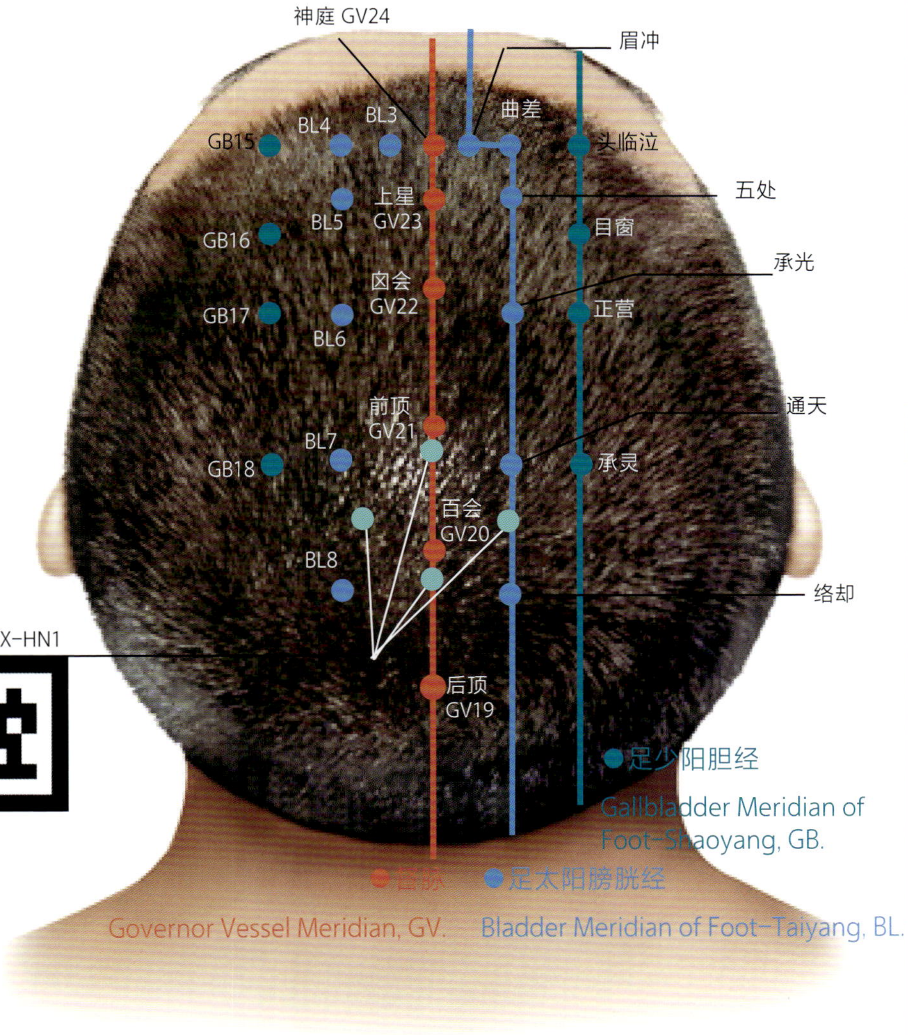

续表

穴位	定位
内迎香	在鼻孔处，鼻翼软骨与鼻甲交界的黏膜处
聚泉	在口腔内，舌背正中缝的中点处
海泉	在口腔内，舌下系带中点处
金津	在口腔内，舌下系带左侧的静脉上
玉液	在口腔内，舌下系带右侧的静脉上
翳明	在颈部，翳风后 1 寸
颈百劳	在颈部，第 7 颈椎棘突直上 2 寸，后正中线旁开 1 寸

Continued

Acupoints	Location
Nèiyíngxiāng (EX-HN9)	Inside nostril, at the conjunctive mucosa of ala nasi cartilage and the turbinate
Jùquán(EX-HN10)	In the mouth, at the midpoint of median raphe of back of the tongue
Hǎiquán(EX-HN11)	In the mouth, at the midpoint of the frenulum of the tongue
Jīnjīn(EX-HN12)	In the mouth, on the left vein of the frenulum of the tongue
Yùyè(EX-HN13)	In the mouth, on the right vein of the frenulum of the tongue
Yìmíng(EX-HN14)	On the neck, 1 cun posterior to the Yifeng acupoint
Jìngbǎiláo(EX-HN15)	On the neck, 2 cun directly above the 7th cervical vertebra, 1 cun lateral to the posterior midline

胸腹部穴位

Acupoints of Chest and Abdomen

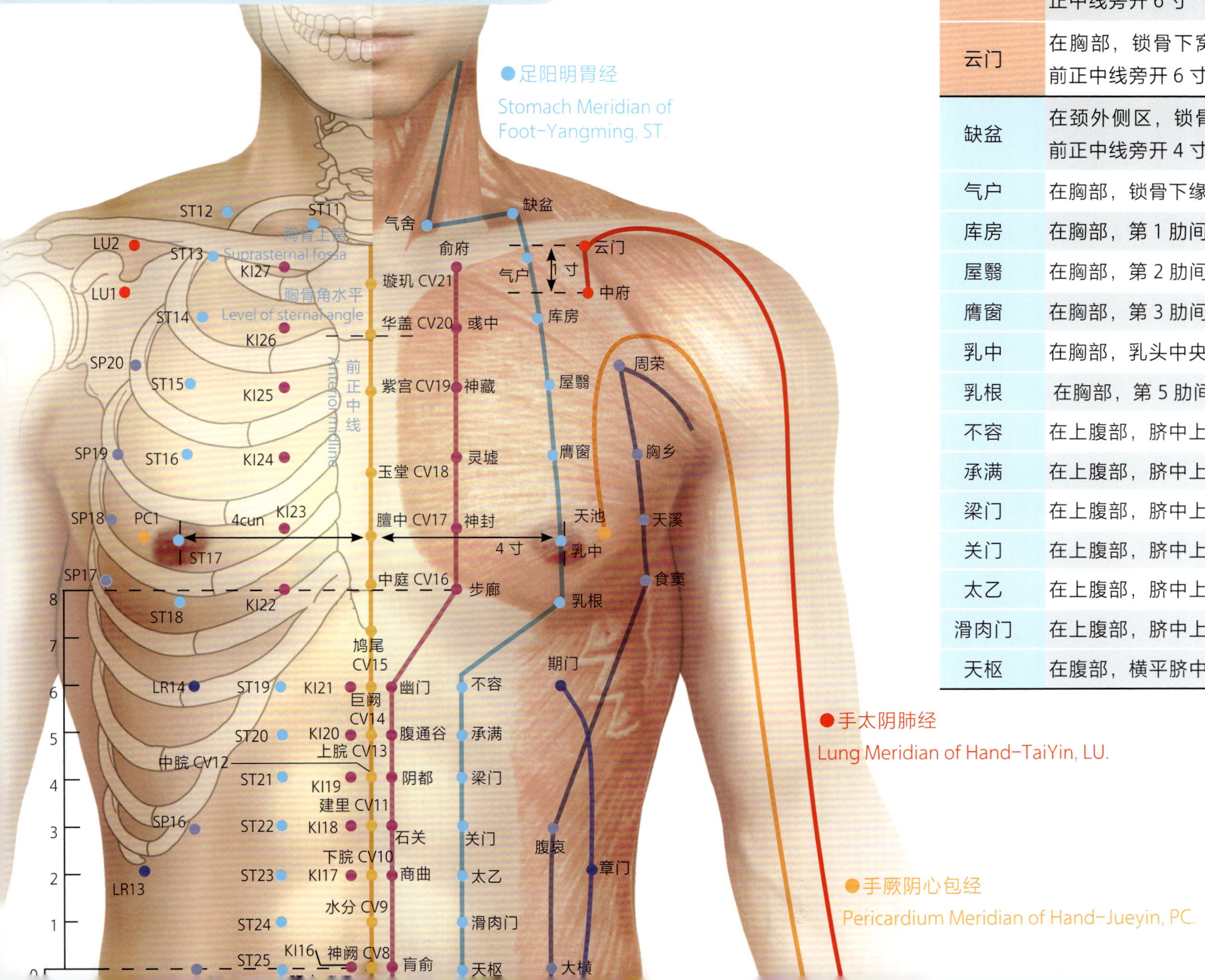

穴位	定位
中府	在胸部，横平第 1 肋间隙，锁骨下窝外侧，前正中线旁开 6 寸
云门	在胸部，锁骨下窝凹陷中，肩胛骨喙突内缘，前正中线旁开 6 寸
缺盆	在颈外侧区，锁骨上大窝，锁骨上缘凹陷中，前正中线旁开 4 寸
气户	在胸部，锁骨下缘，前正中线旁开 4 寸
库房	在胸部，第 1 肋间隙，前正中线旁开 4 寸
屋翳	在胸部，第 2 肋间隙，前正中线旁开 4 寸
膺窗	在胸部，第 3 肋间隙，前正中线旁开 4 寸
乳中	在胸部，乳头中央
乳根	在胸部，第 5 肋间隙，前正中线旁开 4 寸
不容	在上腹部，脐中上 6 寸，前正中线旁开 2 寸
承满	在上腹部，脐中上 5 寸，前正中线旁开 2 寸
梁门	在上腹部，脐中上 4 寸，前正中线旁开 2 寸
关门	在上腹部，脐中上 3 寸，前正中线旁开 2 寸
太乙	在上腹部，脐中上 2 寸，前正中线旁开 2 寸
滑肉门	在上腹部，脐中上 1 寸，前正中线旁开 2 寸
天枢	在腹部，横平脐中，前正中线旁开 2 寸

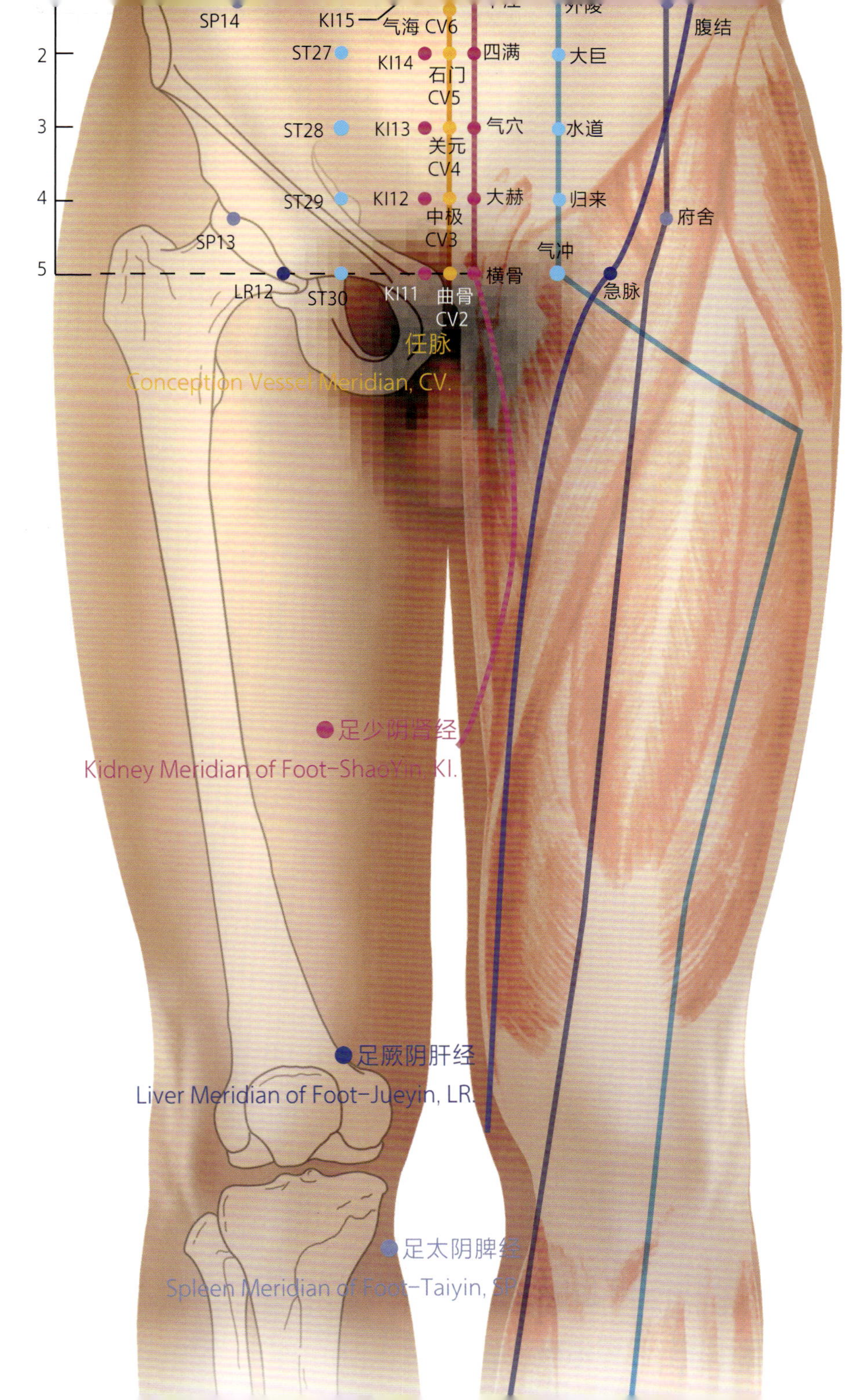

Acupoints	Location
Zhōngfǔ(LU1)	On the chest, level with the 1st intercostal space, in lateral side of the infraclavicular fossa, 6 cun lateral to the anterior midline
Yúnmén(LU2)	On the chest, in the depression of the infraclavicular fossa, in the interior margin of the coracoid process, 6 cun lateral to the anterior midline
Quēpén(ST12)	In the lateral region of the neck, in the great supraclavicular fossa, 4 cun lateral to the anterior midline
Qìhù(ST13)	On the chest, in the inferior margin of the clavicle, 4 cun lateral to the anterior midline
Kùfáng(ST14)	On the chest, in the 1st intercostal space, 4 cun lateral to the anterior midline
Wūyì(ST15)	On the chest, in the 2nd intercostal space, 4 cun lateral to the anterior midline
Yīngchuāng(ST16)	On the chest, in the 3rd intercostal space, 4 cun lateral to the anterior midline
Rǔzhōng(ST17)	On the chest, in the center of the nipple
Rǔgēn(ST18)	On the chest, in the 5th intercostal space, 4 cun lateral to the anterior midline
Bùróng(ST19)	On the upper abdomen, 6 cun above the navel, 2 cun lateral to the anterior midline
Chéngmǎn(ST20)	On the upper abdomen, 5 cun above the navel, 2 cun lateral to the anterior midline
Liángmén(ST21)	On the upper abdomen, 4 cun above the navel, 2 cun lateral to the anterior midline
Guānmén(ST22)	On the upper abdomen, 3 cun above the navel, 2 cun lateral to the anterior midline
Tàiyǐ(ST23)	On the upper abdomen, 2 cun above the navel, 2 cun lateral to the anterior midline
Huáròumén(ST24)	On the upper abdomen, 1 cun above the navel, 2 cun lateral to the anterior midline
Tiānshū(ST25)	On the abdomen, level with the navel, 2 cun lateral to the anterior midline

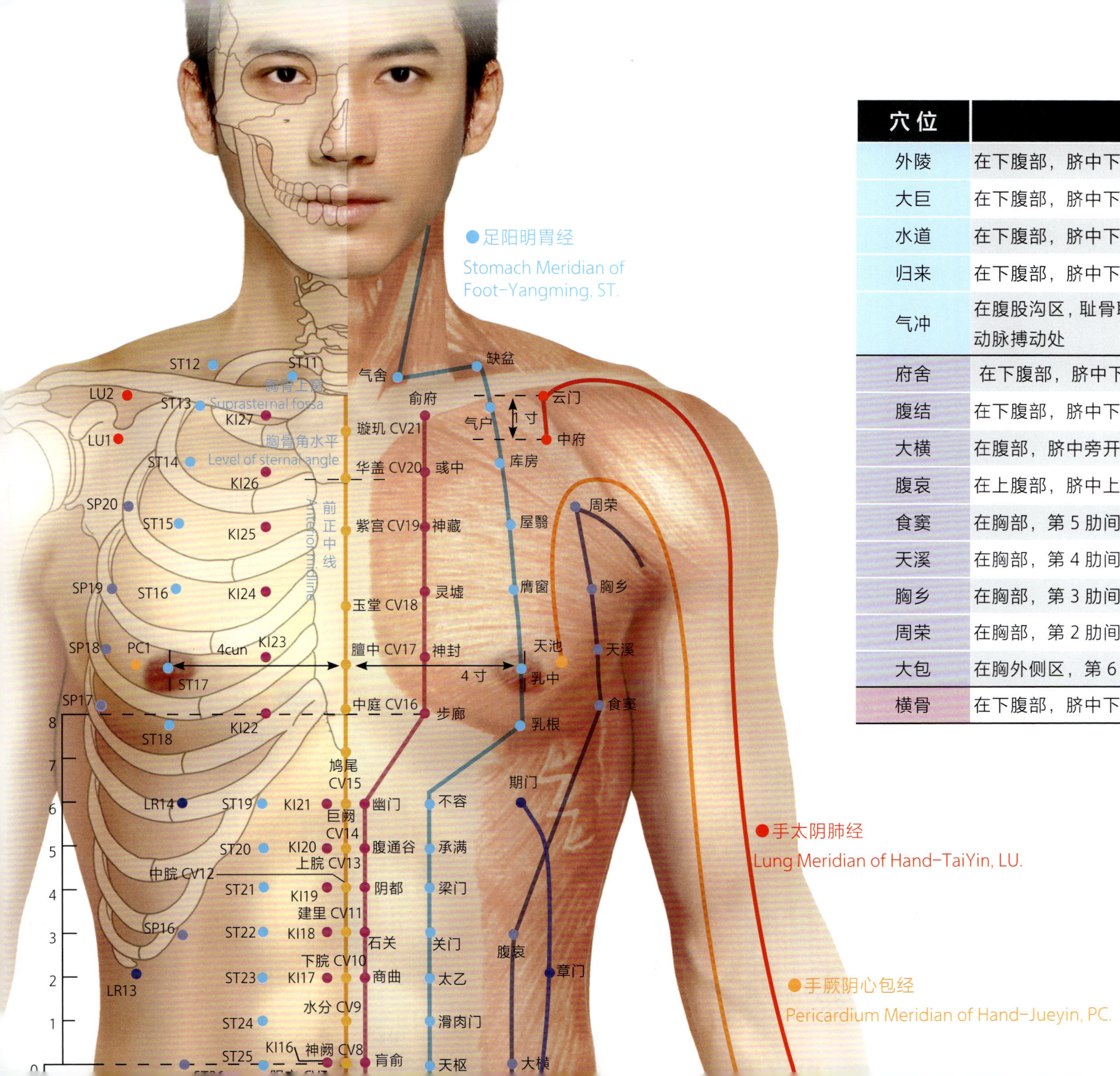

续表

穴位	定位
外陵	在下腹部，脐中下 1 寸，前正中线旁开 2 寸
大巨	在下腹部，脐中下 2 寸，前正中线旁开 2 寸
水道	在下腹部，脐中下 3 寸，前正中线旁开 2 寸
归来	在下腹部，脐中下 4 寸，前正中线旁开 2 寸
气冲	在腹股沟区，耻骨联合上缘，前正中线旁开 2 寸，动脉搏动处
府舍	在下腹部，脐中下 4.3 寸，前正中线旁开 4 寸
腹结	在下腹部，脐中下 1.3 寸，前正中线旁开 4 寸
大横	在腹部，脐中旁开 4 寸
腹哀	在上腹部，脐中上 3 寸，前正中线旁开 4 寸
食窦	在胸部，第 5 肋间隙，前正中线旁开 6 寸
天溪	在胸部，第 4 肋间隙，前正中线旁开 6 寸
胸乡	在胸部，第 3 肋间隙，前正中线旁开 6 寸
周荣	在胸部，第 2 肋间隙，前正中线旁开 6 寸
大包	在胸外侧区，第 6 肋间隙，在腋中线上
横骨	在下腹部，脐中下 5 寸，前正中线旁开 0.5 寸

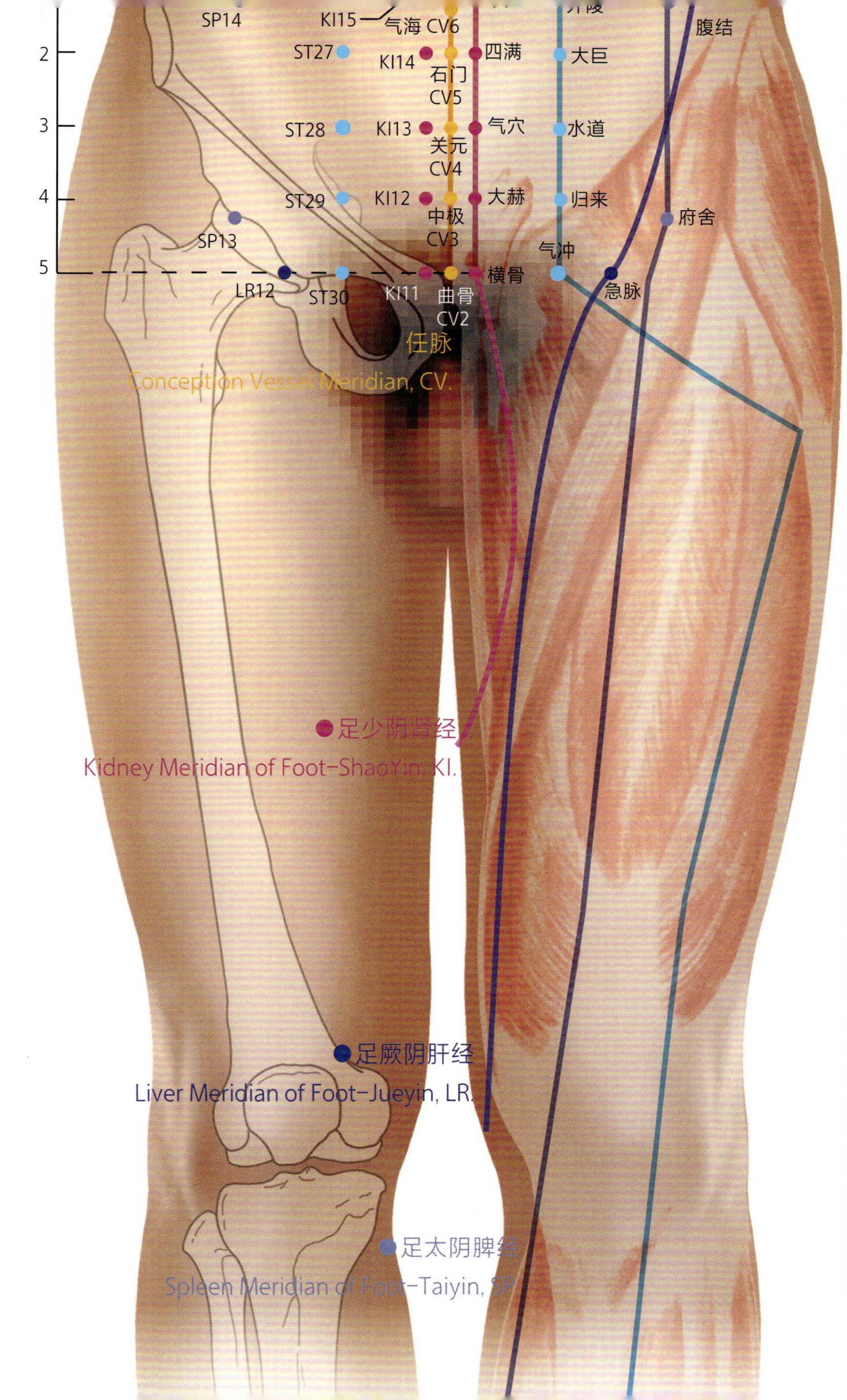

Continued

Acupoints	Location
Wàilíng(ST26)	On the lower abdomen, 1 cun below the navel, 2 cun lateral to the anterior midline
Dàjù(ST27)	On the lower abdomen, 2 cun below the navel, 2 cun lateral to the anterior midline
Shuǐdào(ST28)	On the lower abdomen, 3 cun below the navel, 2 cun lateral to the anterior midline
Guīlái(ST29)	On the lower abdomen, 4 cun below the navel, 2 cun lateral to the anterior midline
Qìchōng(ST30)	In the region of the groin, in the superior margin of the symphysis pubis, 2 cun lateral to the anterior midline, on the pulsation place of artery
Fǔshè(SP13)	On the lower abdomen, 4.3 cun below the navel, 4 cun lateral to the anterior midline
Fùjié(SP14)	On the lower abdomen, 1.3 cun below the navel, 4 cun lateral to the anterior midline
Dàhéng(SP15)	On the abdomen, 4 cun lateral to the navel
Fù'āi(SP16)	On the upper abdomen, 3 cun above the navel, 4 cun lateral to the anterior midline
Shídòu(SP17)	On the chest, in the 5th intercostal space, 6 cun lateral to the anterior midline
Tiānxī(SP18)	On the chest, in the 4th intercostal space, 6 cun lateral to the anterior midline
Xiōngxiāng (SP19)	On the chest, in the 3rd intercostal space, 6 cun lateral to the anterior midline
Zhōuróng(SP20)	On the chest, in the 2nd intercostal space, 6 cun lateral to the anterior midline
Dàbāo(SP21)	In the lateral region of the chest, in the 6th intercostal space, on the midaxillary line
Hénggǔ(KI11)	On the lower abdomen, 5 cun below the navel, 0.5 cun lateral to the anterior midline

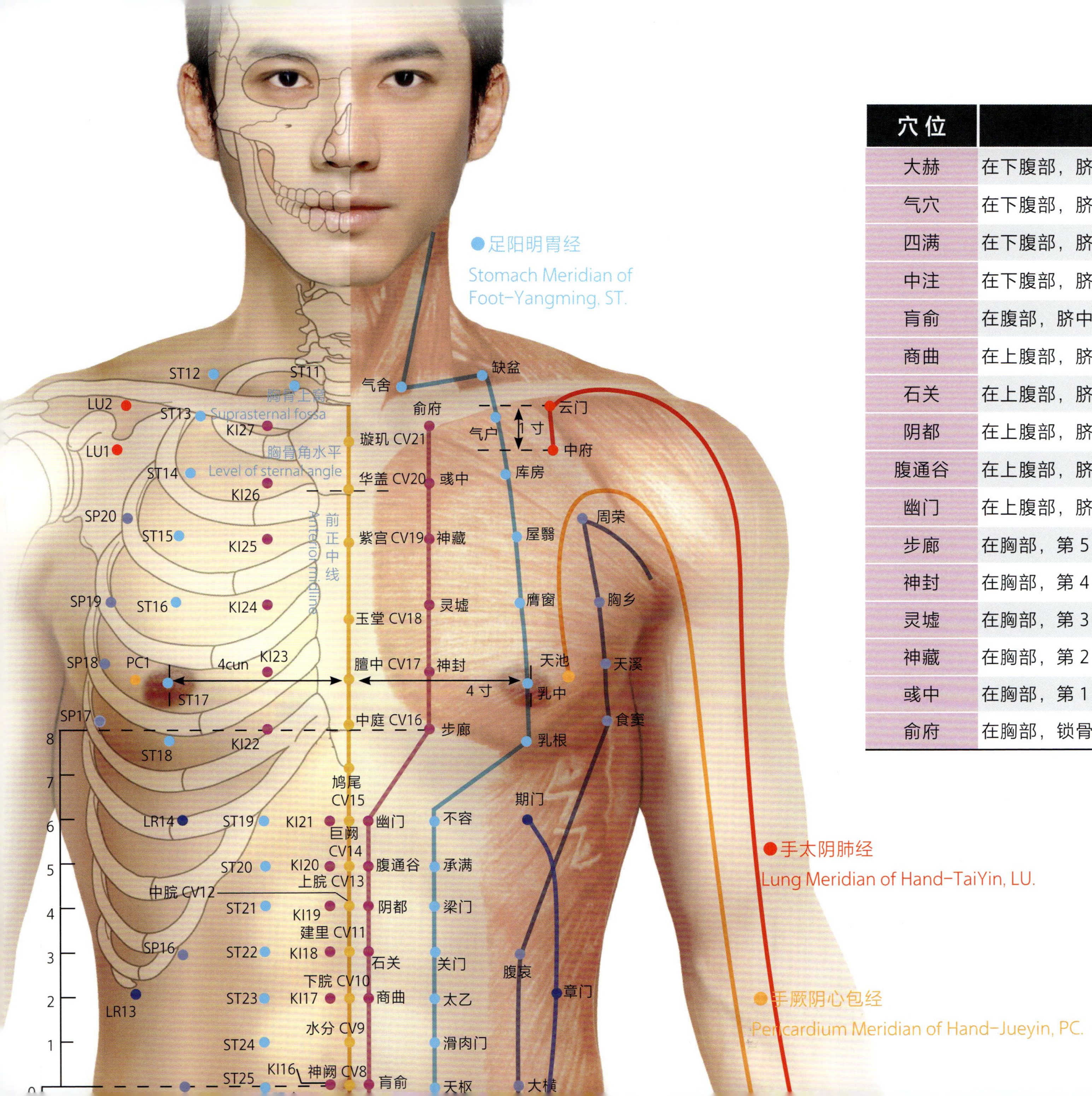

续表

穴位	定位
大赫	在下腹部，脐中下 4 寸，前正中线旁开 0.5 寸
气穴	在下腹部，脐中下 3 寸，前正中线旁开 0.5 寸
四满	在下腹部，脐中下 2 寸，前正中线旁开 0.5 寸
中注	在下腹部，脐中下 1 寸，前正中线旁开 0.5 寸
肓俞	在腹部，脐中旁开 0.5 寸
商曲	在上腹部，脐中上 2 寸，前正中线旁开 0.5 寸
石关	在上腹部，脐中上 3 寸，前正中线旁开 0.5 寸
阴都	在上腹部，脐中上 4 寸，前正中线旁开 0.5 寸
腹通谷	在上腹部，脐中上 5 寸，前正中线旁开 0.5 寸
幽门	在上腹部，脐中上 6 寸，前正中线旁开 0.5 寸
步廊	在胸部，第 5 肋间隙，前正中线旁开 2 寸
神封	在胸部，第 4 肋间隙，前正中线旁开 2 寸
灵墟	在胸部，第 3 肋间隙，前正中线旁开 2 寸
神藏	在胸部，第 2 肋间隙，前正中线旁开 2 寸
彧中	在胸部，第 1 肋间隙，前正中线旁开 2 寸
俞府	在胸部，锁骨下缘，前正中线旁开 2 寸

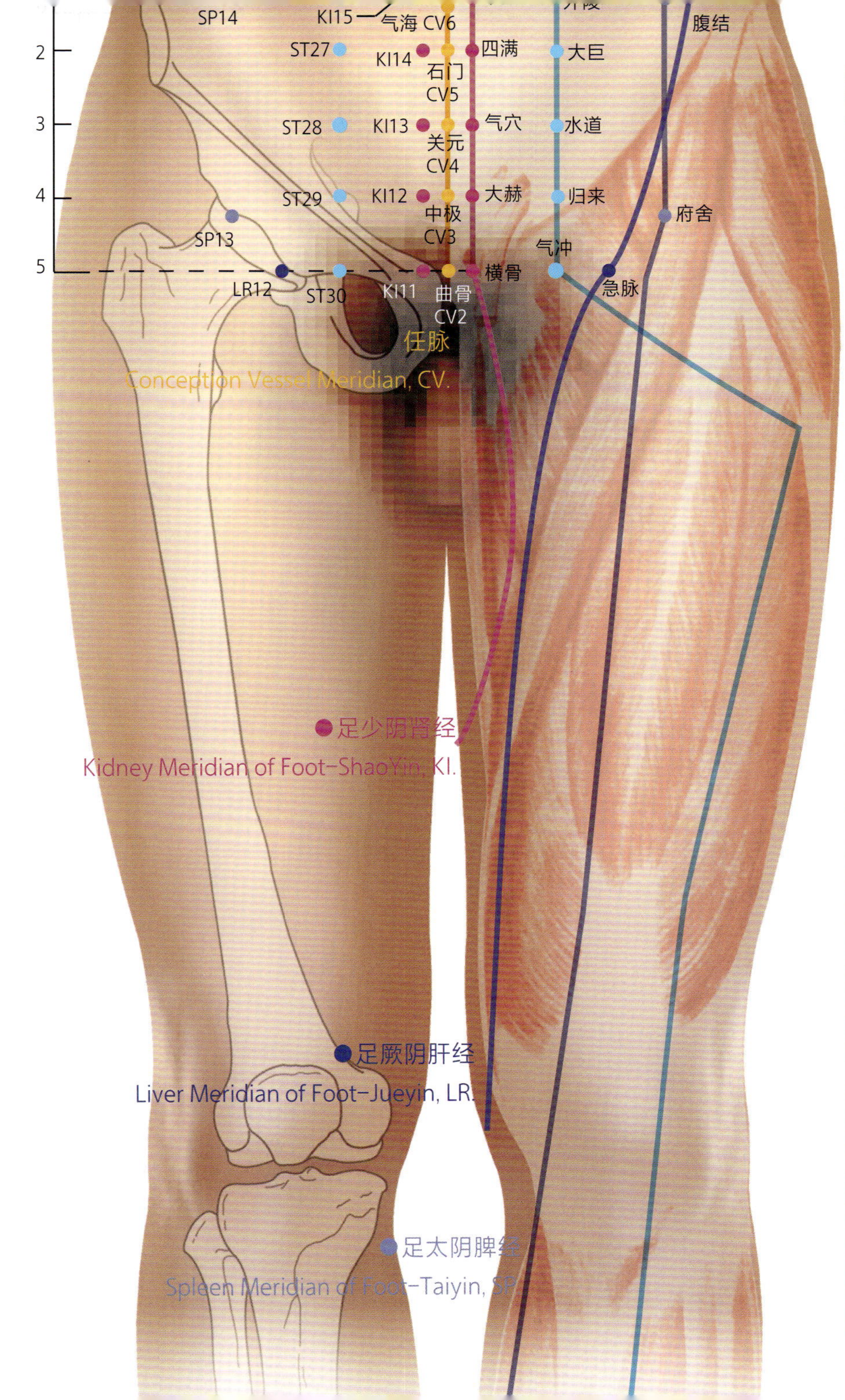

Continued

Acupoints	Location
Dàhè(KI12)	On the lower abdomen, 4 cun below the navel, 0.5 cun lateral to the anterior midline
Qìxué(KI13)	On the lower abdomen, 3 cun below the navel, 0.5 cun lateral to the anterior midline
Sìmǎn(KI14)	On the lower abdomen, 2 cun below the navel, 0.5 cun lateral to the anterior midline
Zhōngzhù(KI15)	On the lower abdomen, 1 cun below the navel, 0.5 cun lateral to the anterior midline
Huāngshū(KI16)	On the abdomen, 0.5 cun lateral to the navel
Shāngqū(KI17)	On the upper abdomen, 2 cun above the navel, 0.5 cun lateral to the anterior midline
Shíguān(KI18)	On the upper abdomen, 3 cun above the navel, 0.5 cun lateral to the anterior midline
Yīndū(KI19)	On the upper abdomen, 4 cun above the navel, 0.5 cun lateral to the anterior midline
Fùtōnggǔ(KI20)	On the upper abdomen, 5 cun above the navel, 0.5 cun lateral to the anterior midline
Yōumén(KI21)	On the upper abdomen, 6 cun above the navel, 0.5 cun lateral to the anterior midline
Bùláng(KI22)	On the chest, in the 5th intercostal space, 2 cun lateral to the anterior midline
Shénfēng(KI23)	On the chest, in the 4th intercostal space, 2 cun lateral to the anterior midline
Língxū(KI24)	On the chest, in the 3rd intercostal space, 2 cun lateral to the anterior midline
Shéncáng(KI25)	On the chest, in the 2nd intercostal space, 2 cun lateral to the anterior midline
Yùzhōng(KI26)	On the chest, in the 1st intercostal space, 2 cun lateral to the anterior midline
Shūfǔ(KI27)	On the chest, in the inferior margin of the clavicle, 2 cun lateral to the anterior midline

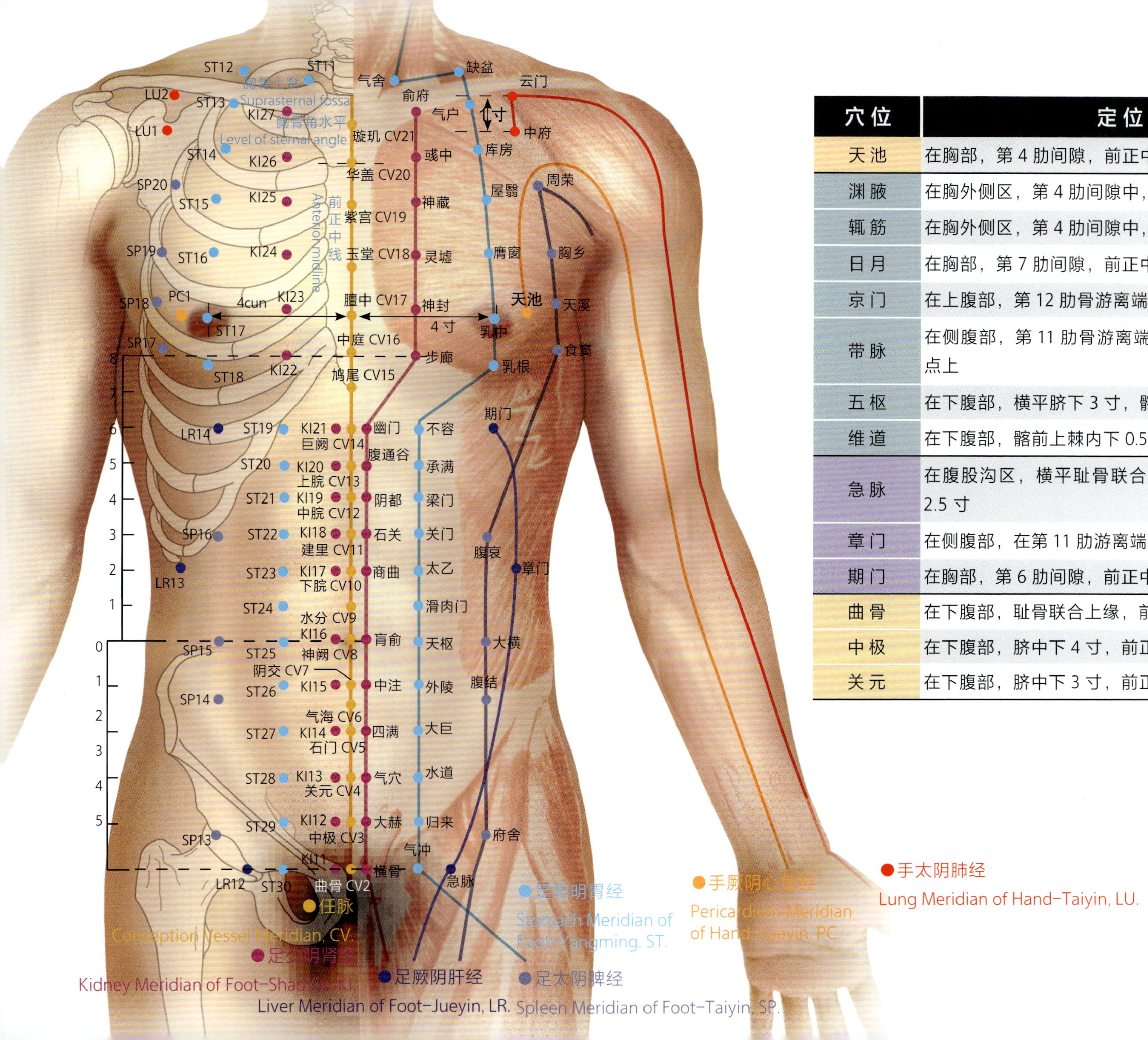

续表

穴位	定位
天池	在胸部，第 4 肋间隙，前正中线旁开 5 寸
渊腋	在胸外侧区，第 4 肋间隙中，在腋中线上
辄筋	在胸外侧区，第 4 肋间隙中，在腋中线前 1 寸
日月	在胸部，第 7 肋间隙，前正中线旁开 4 寸
京门	在上腹部，第 12 肋骨游离端的下际
带脉	在侧腹部，第 11 肋骨游离端垂线与脐水平线的交点上
五枢	在下腹部，横平脐下 3 寸，髂前上棘内侧
维道	在下腹部，髂前上棘内下 0.5 寸
急脉	在腹股沟区，横平耻骨联合上缘，前正中线旁开 2.5 寸
章门	在侧腹部，在第 11 肋游离端的下际
期门	在胸部，第 6 肋间隙，前正中线旁开 4 寸
曲骨	在下腹部，耻骨联合上缘，前正中线上
中极	在下腹部，脐中下 4 寸，前正中线上
关元	在下腹部，脐中下 3 寸，前正中线上

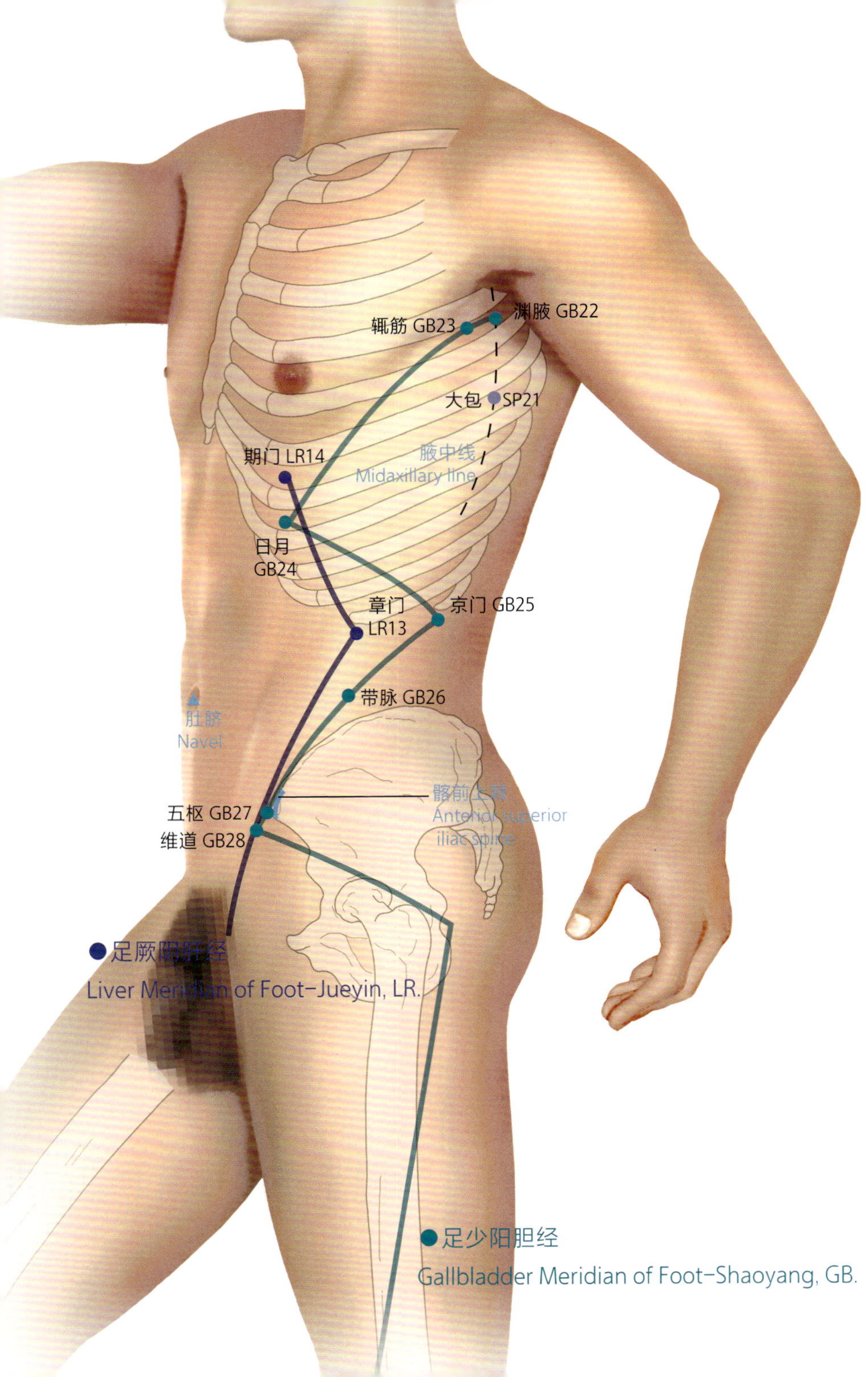

Continued

Acupoints	Location
Tiānchí(PC1)	On the chest, in the 4th intercostal space, 5 cun lateral to the anterior midline
Yuānyè(GB22)	In the exterior region of the chest, in the 4th intercostal space, on the midaxillary line
Zhéjīn(GB23)	In the exterior region of the chest, in the 4th intercostal space, 1 cun anterior to the midaxillary line
Rìyuè(GB24)	On the chest, in the 7th intercostal space, 4 cun lateral to the anterior midline
Jīngmén(GB25)	On the upper abdomen, in the inferior border of the free end of the 12th rib
Dàimài(GB26)	On the lateral abdomen, at the junction of the vertical line of the free end of the 11th rib and the horizontal line of the umbilicus
Wǔshū(GB27)	On the lower abdomen, in the interior side of the anterior superior iliac spine, 3 cun below the umbilicus
Wéidào(GB28)	On the lower abdomen, 0.5 cun interior and inferior to the anterior superior iliac spine
Jímài(LR12)	In the region of groin, level with the superior margin of the symphysis pubis, 2.5 cun lateral to the anterior midline
Zhāngmén(LR13)	On the lateral abdomen, in the inferior border of the free end of the 11th rib
Qīmén(LR14)	On the chest, in the 6th intercostal space, 4 cun lateral to the anterior midline
Qūgǔ(CV2)	On the lower abdomen, in the superior margin of the symphysis pubis, on the anterior midline
Zhōngjí(CV3)	On the lower abdomen, 4 cun below the navel, on the anterior midline
Guānyuán(CV4)	On the lower abdomen, 3 cun below the navel, on the anterior midline

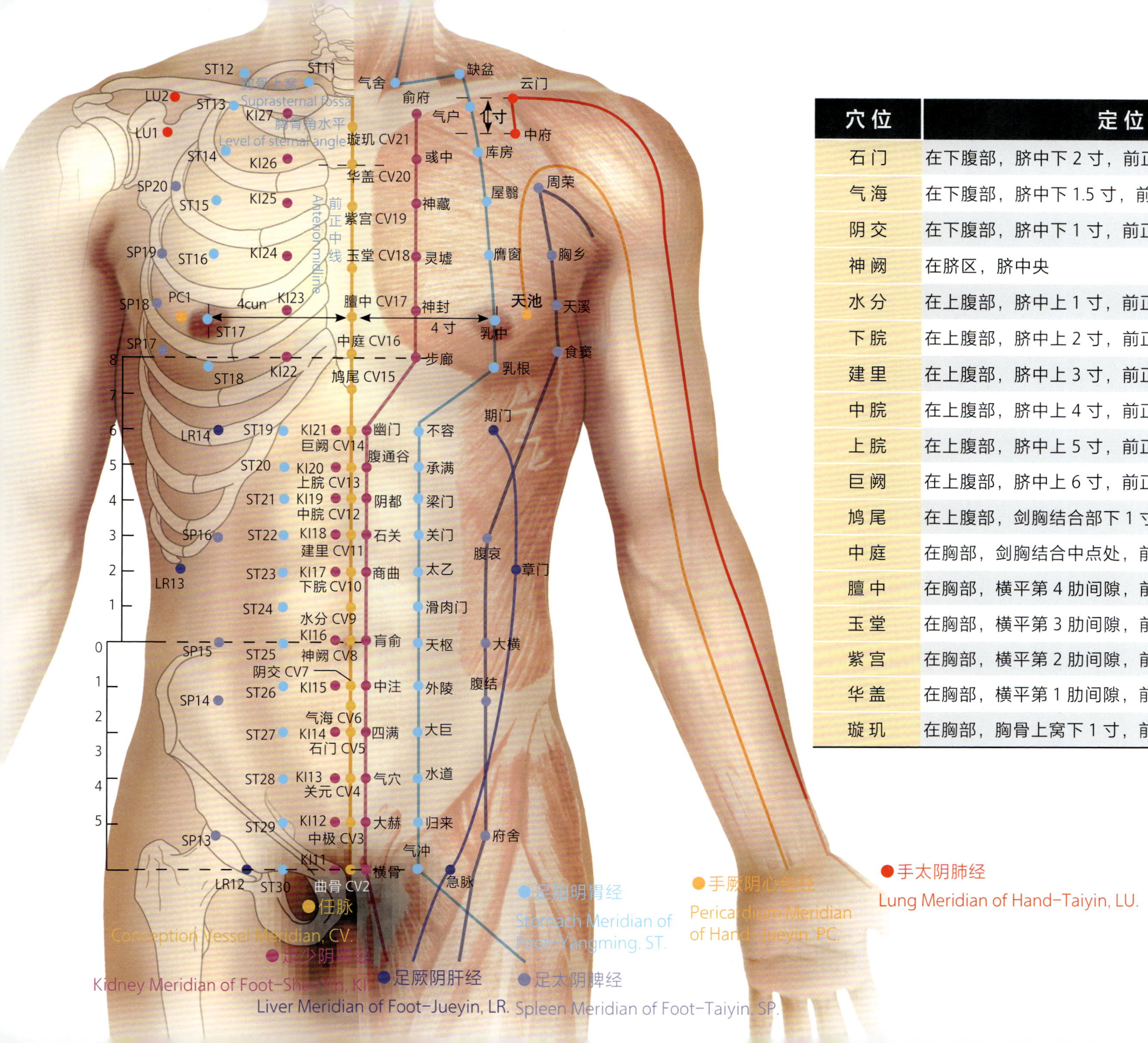

续表

穴 位	定 位
石 门	在下腹部，脐中下 2 寸，前正中线上
气 海	在下腹部，脐中下 1.5 寸，前正中线上
阴 交	在下腹部，脐中下 1 寸，前正中线上
神 阙	在脐区，脐中央
水 分	在上腹部，脐中上 1 寸，前正中线上
下 脘	在上腹部，脐中上 2 寸，前正中线上
建 里	在上腹部，脐中上 3 寸，前正中线上
中 脘	在上腹部，脐中上 4 寸，前正中线上
上 脘	在上腹部，脐中上 5 寸，前正中线上
巨 阙	在上腹部，脐中上 6 寸，前正中线上
鸠 尾	在上腹部，剑胸结合部下 1 寸，前正中线上
中 庭	在胸部，剑胸结合中点处，前正中线上
膻 中	在胸部，横平第 4 肋间隙，前正中线上
玉 堂	在胸部，横平第 3 肋间隙，前正中线上
紫 宫	在胸部，横平第 2 肋间隙，前正中线上
华 盖	在胸部，横平第 1 肋间隙，前正中线上
璇 玑	在胸部，胸骨上窝下 1 寸，前正中线上

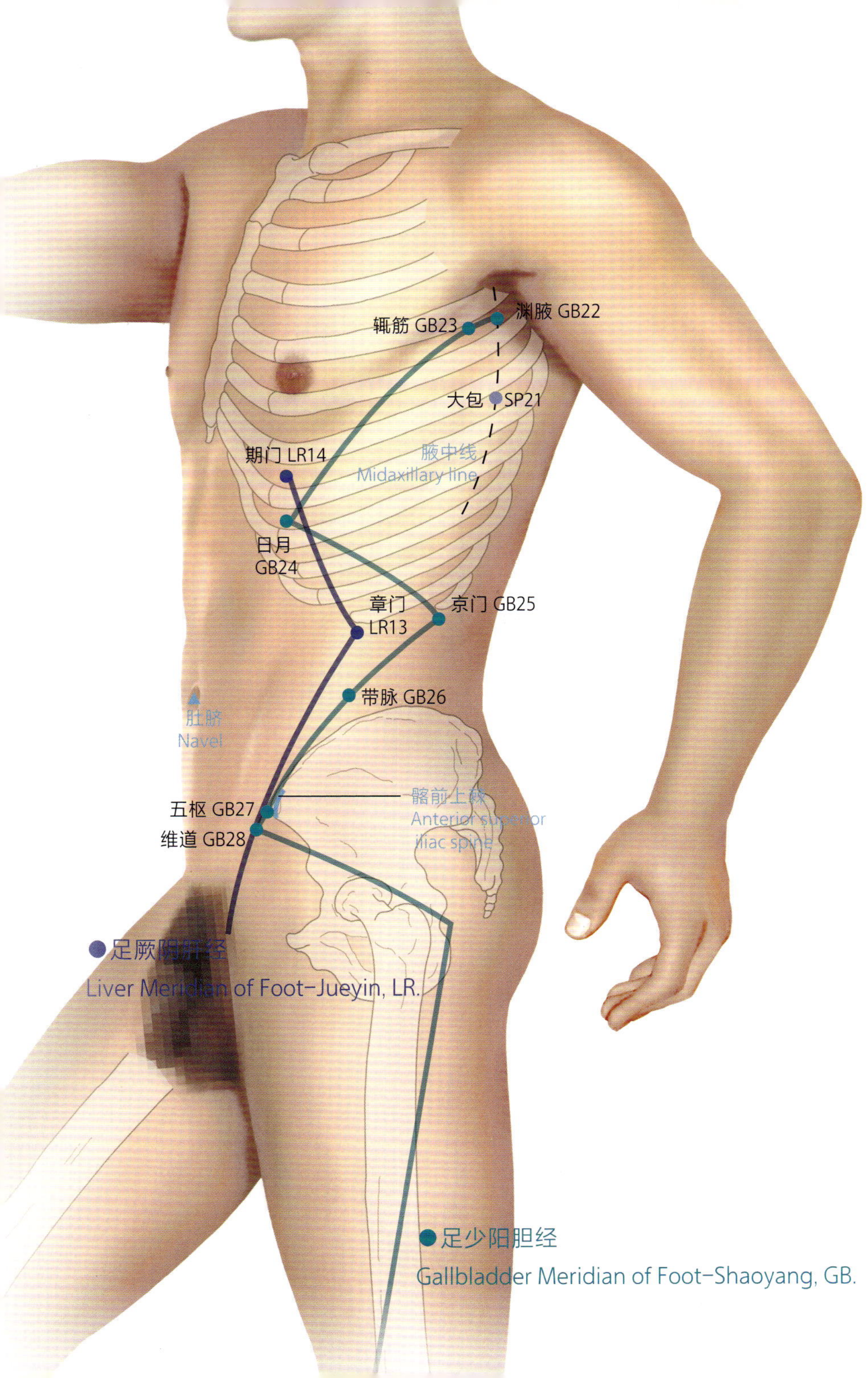

Continued

Acupoints	Location
Shímén(CV5)	On the lower abdomen, 5 cun below the navel, on the anterior midline
Qìhǎi(CV6)	On the lower abdomen, 1.5 cun below the navel, on the anterior midline
Yīnjiāo(CV7)	On the lower abdomen, 1 cun below the navel, on the anterior midline
Shénquè(CV8)	In the region of umbilicus in the center of the navel
Shuǐfēn(CV9)	On the upper abdomen, 1 cun above the navel, on the anterior midline
Xiàwǎn(CV10)	On the upper abdomen, 2 cun above the navel, on the anterior midline
Jiànlǐ(CV11)	On the upper abdomen, 3 cun above the navel, on the anterior midline
Zhōngwǎn(CV12)	On the upper abdomen, 4 cun above the navel, on the anterior midline
Shàngwǎn(CV13)	On the upper abdomen, 5 cun above the navel, on the anterior midline
Jùquè(CV14)	On the upper abdomen, 6 cun above the navel, on the anterior midline
Jiūwěi(CV15)	On the upper abdomen, 1 cun below the xiphosternal synchondrosis, on the anterior midline
Zhōngtíng(CV16)	On the chest, at the midpoint of the xiphosternal synchondrosis, on the anterior midline
Dànzhōng(CV17)	On the chest, level with the 4th intercostal space, on the anterior midline
Yùtáng(CV18)	On the chest, level with the 3rd intercostal space, on the anterior midline
Zǐgōng(CV19)	On the chest, level with the 2nd intercostal space, on the anterior midline
Huágài(CV20)	On the chest, level with the 1st intercostal space, on the anterior midline
Xuánjī(CV21)	On the chest, 1 cun below the suprasternal fossa, on the anterior midline

腰背臀部穴位

Acupoints of Waist, Back and Buttock

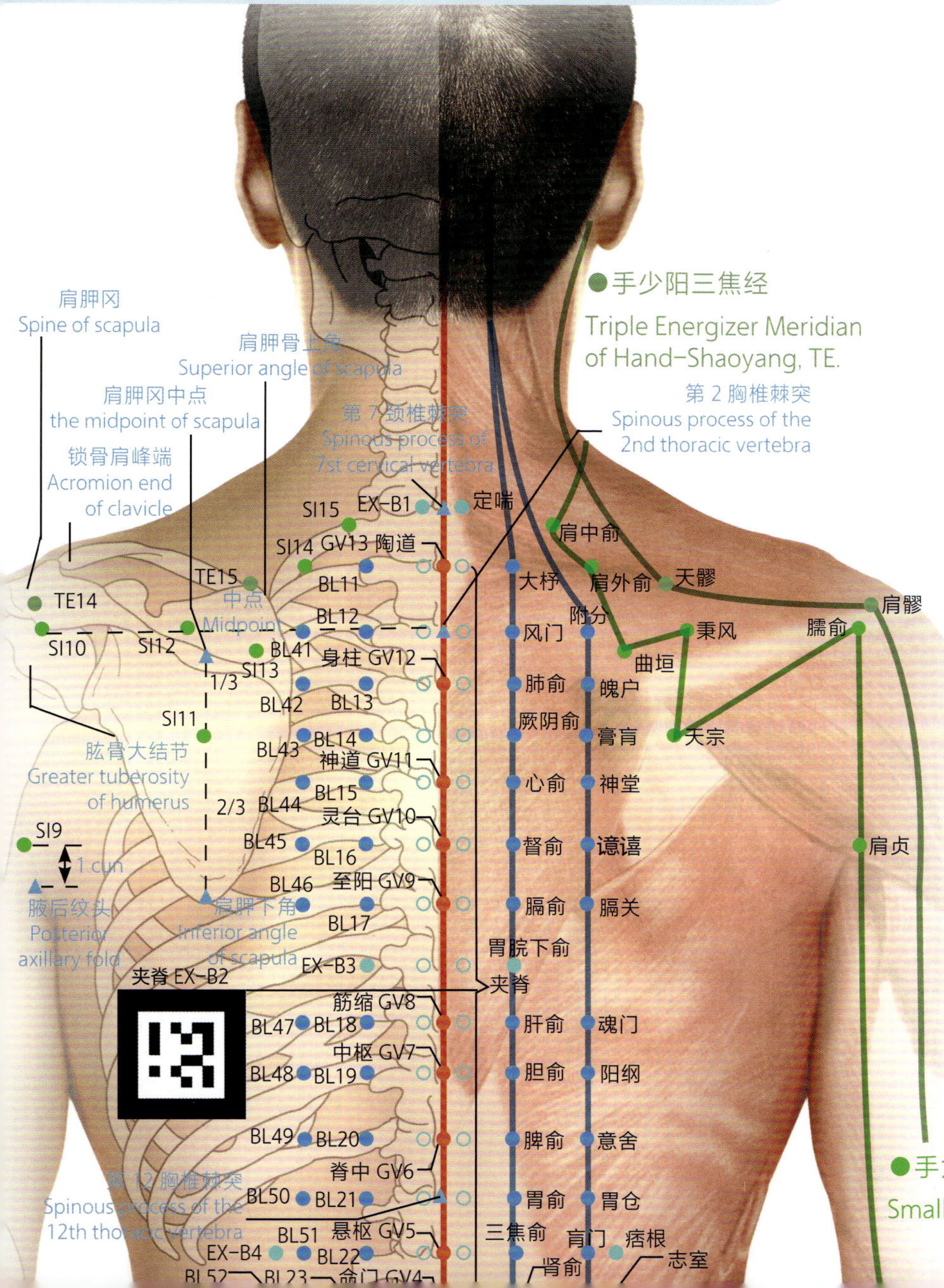

穴位	定位
肩贞	在肩胛区，肩关节后下方，腋后纹头直上 1 寸
臑俞	在肩胛区，腋后纹头直上，肩胛冈下缘凹陷中
天宗	在肩胛区，肩胛冈中点与肩胛下角连线上 1/3 与下 2/3 交点凹陷中
秉风	在肩胛区，肩胛冈中点上方冈上窝中
曲垣	在肩胛区，肩胛冈内侧端上缘凹陷中
肩外俞	在脊柱区，第 1 胸椎棘突下，后正中线旁开 3 寸
肩中俞	在脊柱区，第 7 颈椎棘突下，后正中线旁开 2 寸
大杼	在脊柱区，第 1 胸椎棘突下，后正中线旁开 1.5 寸
风门	在脊柱区，第 2 胸椎棘突下，后正中线旁开 1.5 寸
肺俞	在脊柱区，第 3 胸椎棘突下，后正中线旁开 1.5 寸
厥阴俞	在脊柱区，第 4 胸椎棘突下，后正中线旁开 1.5 寸
心俞	在脊柱区，第 5 胸椎棘突下，后正中线旁开 1.5 寸
督俞	在脊柱区，第 6 胸椎棘突下，后正中线旁开 1.5 寸
膈俞	在脊柱区，第 7 胸椎棘突下，后正中线旁开 1.5 寸
肝俞	在脊柱区，第 9 胸椎棘突下，后正中线旁开 1.5 寸

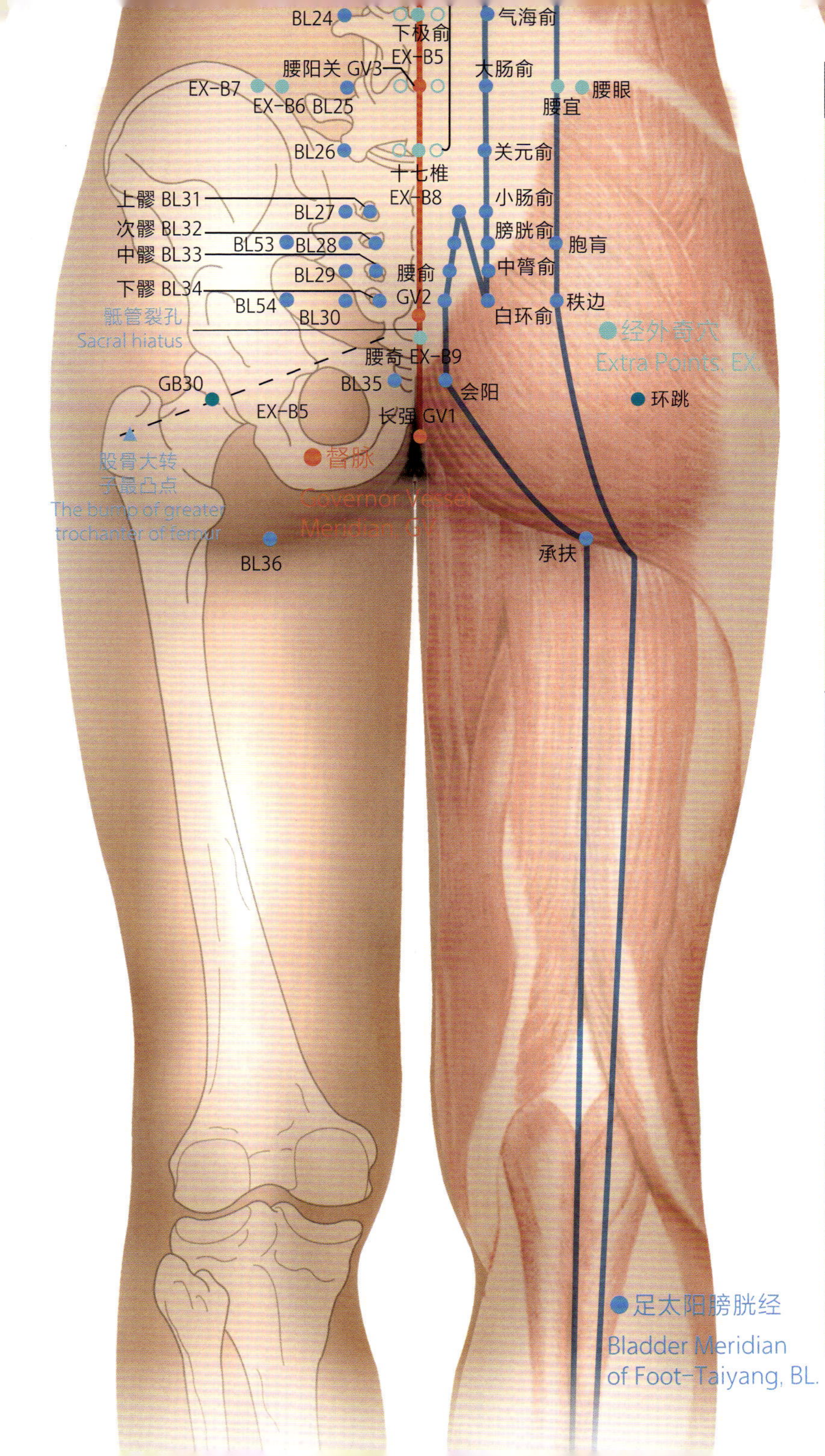

Acupoints	Location
Jiānzhēn(SI9)	In the scapular region, in the posterior and inferior aspect of the shoulder joint, 1 cun directly above the posterior axillary fold
Nàoshū(SI10)	In the scapular region, directly above the posterior axillary fold, in the depression of the inferior margin of the scapular spine
Tiānzōng(SI11)	In the scapular region, in the depression of the upper 1/3 and lower 2/3 of the line joining the midpoint of the scapular spine and the inferior angle of the scapula
Bǐngfēng(SI12)	In the scapular region, in the supraspinous fossa above the midpoint of the scapular spine
Qūyuán(SI13)	In the scapular region, in the depression of the superior margin of the interior scapular spine
Jiānwàishū(SI14)	In the spinal region, inferior to the spinous process of the 3rd thoracic vertebra, 3 cun lateral to the posterior midline
Jiānzhōngshū(SI15)	In the spinal region, inferior to the spinous process of the 7th cervical vertebra, 2 cun lateral to the posterior midline
Dàzhù(BL11)	In the spinal region, inferior to the spinous process of the 1st thoracic vertebra, 1.5 cun lateral to posterior midline
Fēngmén(BL12)	In the spinal region, inferior to the spinous process of the 2nd thoracic vertebra, 1.5 cun lateral to the posterior midline
Fèishū(BL13)	In the spinal region, inferior to the spinous process of the 3rd thoracic vertebra, 1.5 cun lateral to the posterior midline
Juéyīnshū(BL14)	In the spinal region, inferior to the spinous process of the 4th thoracic vertebra, 1.5 cun lateral to the posterior midline
Xīnshū(BL15)	In the spinal region, inferior to the spinous process of the 5th thoracic vertebra, 1.5 cun lateral to the posterior midline
Dūshū(BL16)	In the spinal region, inferior to the spinous process of the 6th thoracic vertebra, 1.5 cun lateral to the posterior midline
Géshū(BL17)	In the spinal region, inferior to the spinous process of the 7th thoracic vertebra, 1.5 cun lateral to the posterior midline
Gānshū(BL18)	In the spinal region, inferior to the spinous process of the 9th thoracic vertebra, 1.5 cun lateral to the posterior midline

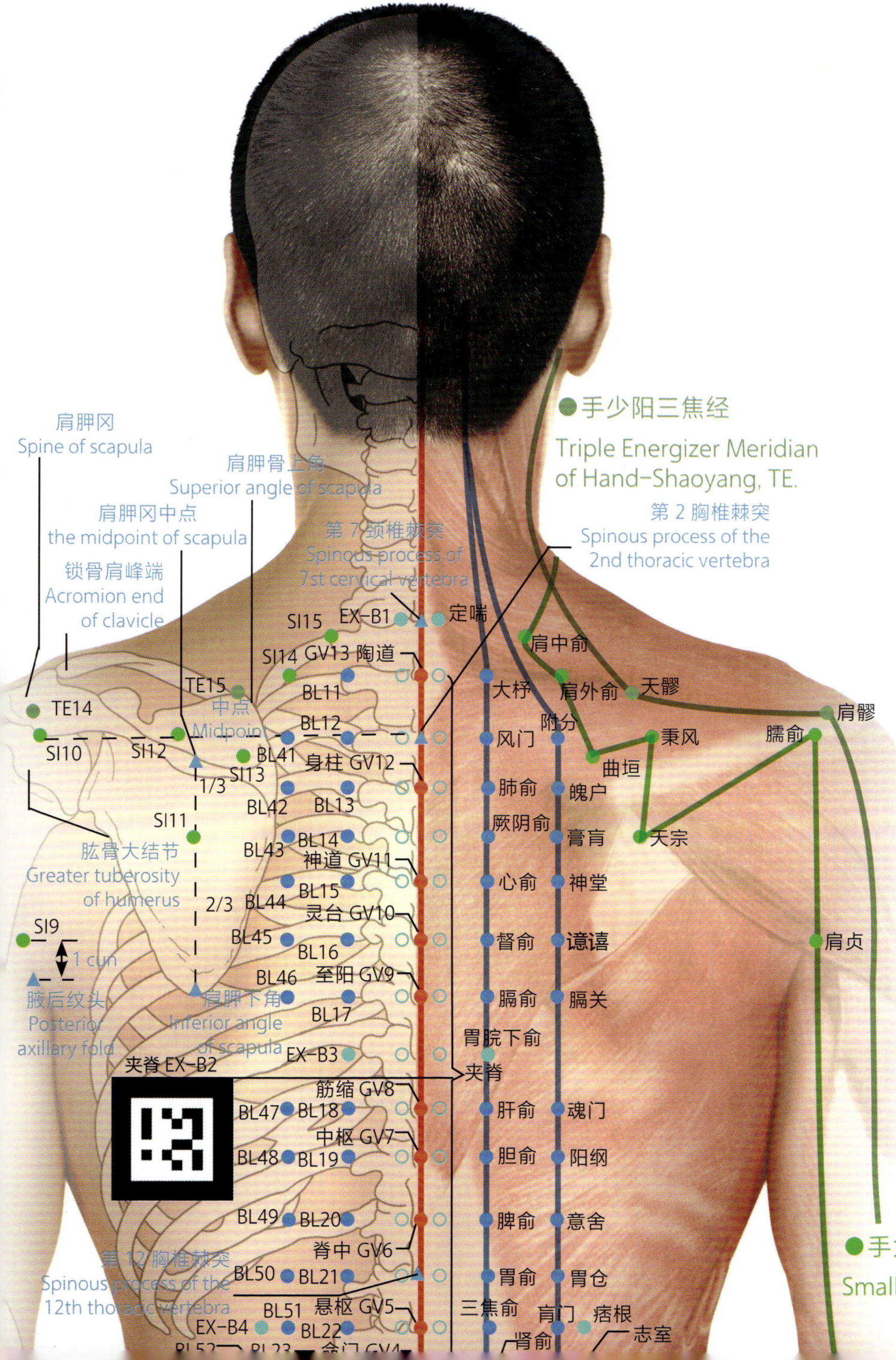

续表

穴位	定位
胆俞	在脊柱区，第 10 胸椎棘突下，后正中线旁开 1.5 寸
脾俞	在脊柱区，第 11 胸椎棘突下，后正中线旁开 1.5 寸
胃俞	在脊柱区，第 12 胸椎棘突下，后正中线旁开 1.5 寸
三焦俞	在脊柱区，第 1 腰椎棘突下，后正中线旁开 1.5 寸
肾俞	在脊柱区，第 2 腰椎棘突下，后正中线旁开 1.5 寸
气海俞	在脊柱区，第 3 腰椎棘突下，后正中线旁开 1.5 寸
大肠俞	在脊柱区，第 4 腰椎棘突下，后正中线旁开 1.5 寸
关元俞	在脊柱区，第 5 腰椎棘突下，后正中线旁开 1.5 寸
小肠俞	在骶区，横平第 1 骶后孔，骶正中嵴旁开 1.5 寸
膀胱俞	在骶区，横平第 2 骶后孔，骶正中嵴旁开 1.5 寸
中膂俞	在骶区，横平第 3 骶后孔，骶正中嵴旁开 1.5 寸
白环俞	在骶区，横平第 4 骶后孔，骶正中嵴旁开 1.5 寸
上髎	在骶区，正对第 1 骶后孔处
次髎	在骶部，正对第 2 骶后孔中
中髎	在骶部，正对第 3 骶后孔中
下髎	在骶部，正对第 4 骶后孔中
会阳	在骶区，尾骨端旁开 0.5 寸

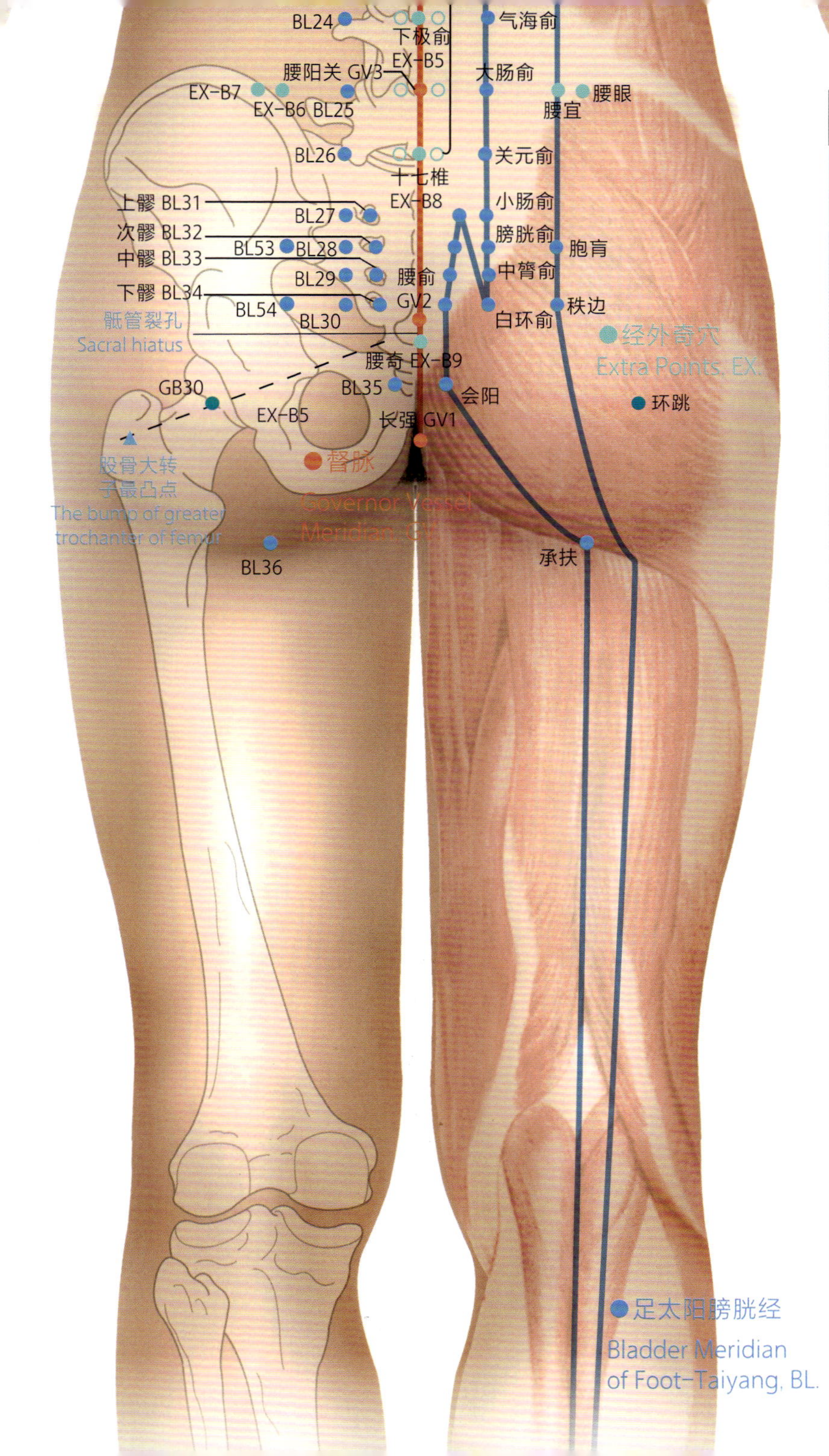

Continued

Acupoints	Location
Dǎnshū(BL19)	In the spinal region, inferior to the spinous process of the 10th thoracic vertebra, 1.5 cun lateral to the posterior midline
Píshū(BL20)	In the spinal region, inferior to the spinous process of the 11th thoracic vertebra, 1.5 cun lateral to the posterior midline
Wèishū(BL21)	In the spinal region, inferior to the spinous process of the 12th thoracic vertebra, 1.5 cun lateral to the posterior midline
Sānjiāoshū(BL22)	In the spinal region, inferior to the spinous process of the 1st lumbar vertebra, 1.5 cun lateral to the posterior midline
Shènshū(BL23)	In the spinal region, inferior to the spinous process of the 2nd lumbar vertebra, 1.5 cun lateral to the posterior midline
Qìhǎishū(BL24)	In the spinal region, inferior to the spinous process of the 3rd lumbar vertebra, 1.5 cun lateral to the posterior midline.
Dàchángshū(BL25)	In the spinal region, inferior to the spinous process of the 4th lumbar vertebra, 1.5 cun lateral to the posterior midline
Guānyuánshū(BL26)	In the spinal region, inferior to the spinous process of the 5th lumbar vertebra, 1.5 cun lateral to the posterior midline
Xiǎochángshū(BL27)	In the sacral region, level with the 1st posterior sacral foramen, 1.5 cun lateral to the median sacral crest
Pángguāngshū(BL28)	In the sacral region, level with the 2nd posterior sacral foramen, 1.5 cun lateral to the median sacral crest
Zhōnglǚshū(BL29)	In the sacral region, level with the 3rd posterior sacral foramen, 1.5 cun lateral to the median sacral crest
Báihuánshū(BL30)	In the sacral region, level with the 4th posterior sacral foramen, 1.5 cun lateral to the median sacral crest
Shàngliáo(BL31)	In the sacral region, directly faced with the 1st posterior sacral foramen
Cìliáo(BL32)	In the sacral region, directly faced with the 2nd posterior sacral foramen
Zhōngliáo(BL33)	In the sacral region, directly faced with the 3rd posterior sacral foramen
Xiàliáo(BL34)	In the sacral region, directly faced with the 4th posterior sacral foramen
Huìyáng(BL35)	In the sacral region, 0.5 cun lateral to the coccyx end

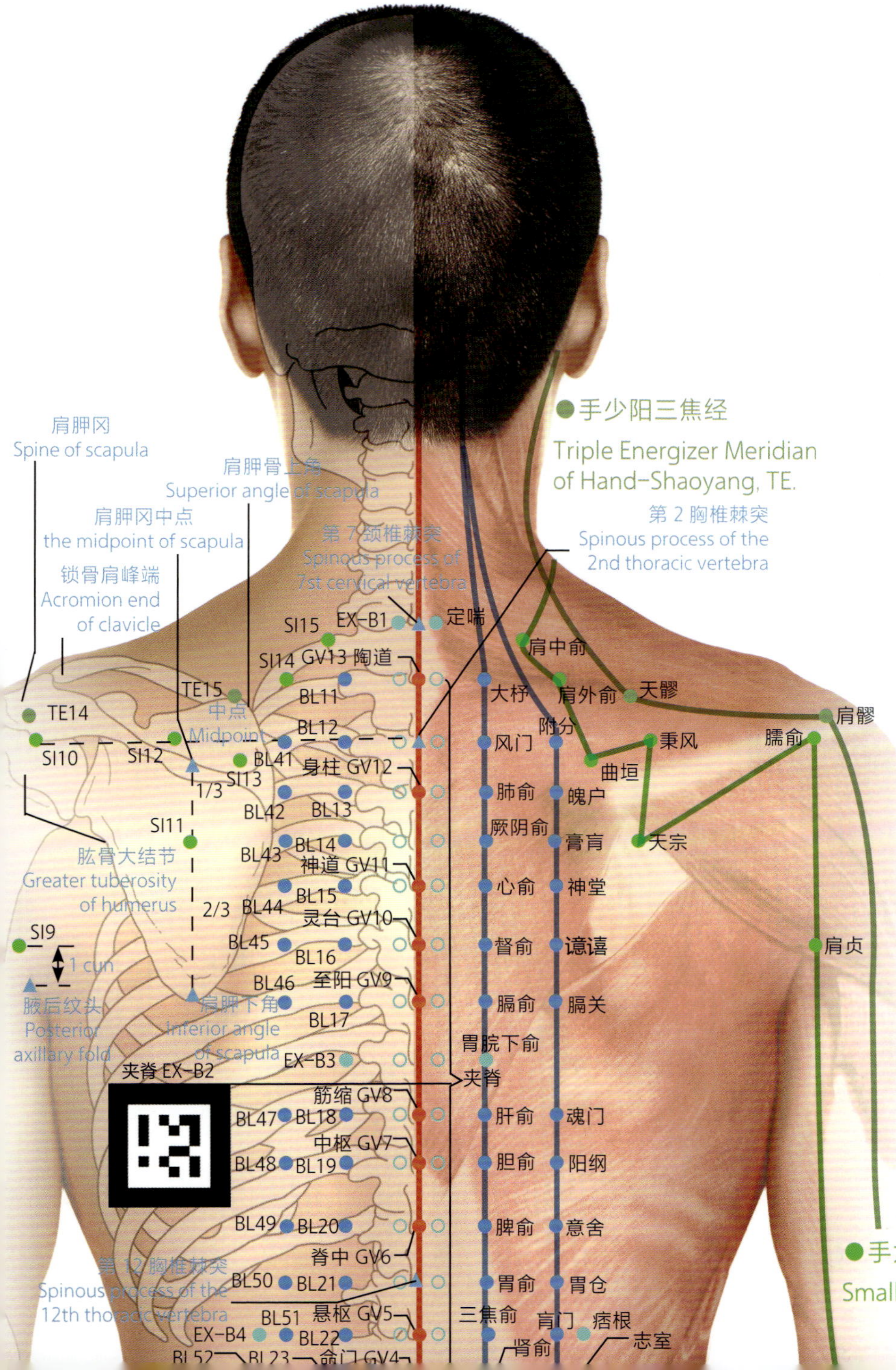

续表

穴位	定位
承扶	在股后区，臀沟的中点
附分	在脊柱区，第 2 胸椎棘突下，后正中线旁开 3 寸
魄户	在脊柱区，第 3 胸椎棘突下，后正中线旁开 3 寸
膏肓	在脊柱区，第 4 胸椎棘突下，后正中线旁开 3 寸
神堂	在脊柱区，第 5 胸椎棘突下，后正中线旁开 3 寸
譩譆	在脊柱区，第 6 胸椎棘突下，后正中线旁开 3 寸
膈关	在脊柱区，第 7 胸椎棘突下，后正中线旁开 3 寸
魂门	在脊柱区，第 9 胸椎棘突下，后正中线旁开 3 寸
阳纲	在脊柱区，第 10 胸椎棘突下，后正中线旁开 3 寸
意舍	在脊柱区，第 11 胸椎棘突下，后正中线旁开 3 寸
胃仓	在脊柱区，第 12 胸椎棘突下，后正中线旁开 3 寸
肓门	在腰区，第 1 腰椎棘突下，后正中线旁开 3 寸
志室	在腰区，第 2 腰椎棘突下，后正中线旁开 3 寸
胞肓	在骶区，横平第 2 骶后孔，骶正中嵴旁开 3 寸
秩边	在骶区，横平第 4 骶后孔，骶正中嵴旁开 3 寸

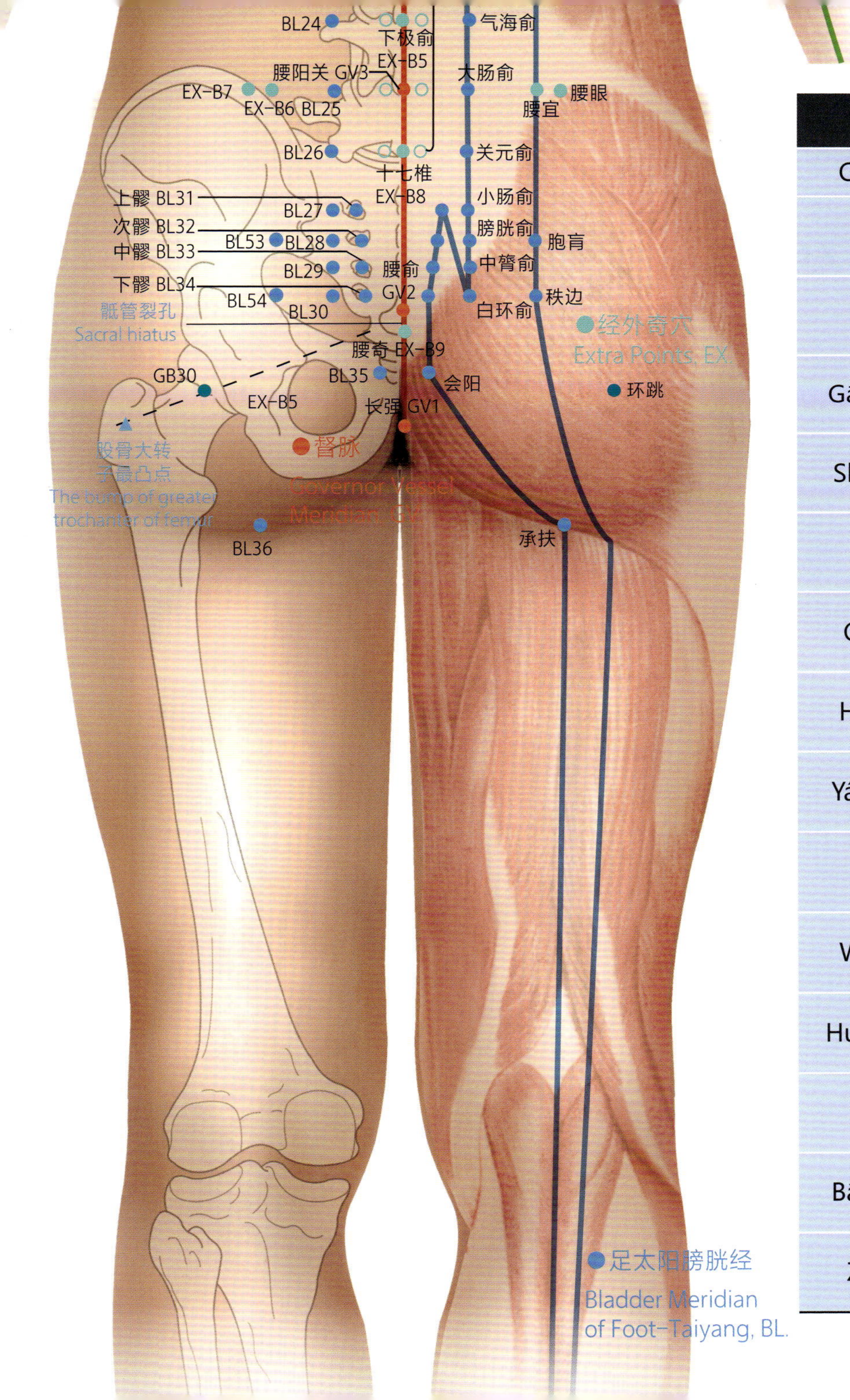

Continued

Acupoints	Location
Chéngfú(BL36)	In the posterior region of thigh, at the midpoint of the gluteal fold
Fùfēn(BL41)	In the spinal region, inferior to the spinous process of the 2nd thoracic vertebra, 3 cun lateral to the posterior midline
Pòhù(BL42)	In the spinal region, inferior to the spinous process of the 3rd thoracic vertebra, 3 cun lateral to the posterior midline
Gāohuāng(BL43)	In the spinal region, inferior to the spinous process of the 4th thoracic vertebra, 3 cun lateral to the posterior midline
Shéntáng(BL44)	In the spinal region, inferior to the spinous process of the 5th thoracic vertebra, 3 cun lateral to the posterior midline
Yìxǐ(BL45)	In the spinal region, inferior to the spinous process of the 6th thoracic vertebra, 3 cun lateral to the posterior midline
Géguān(BL46)	In the spinal region, inferior to the spinous process of the 7th thoracic vertebra, 3 cun lateral to the posterior midline
Húnmén(BL47)	In the spinal region, inferior to the spinous process of the 9th thoracic vertebra, 3 cun lateral to the posterior midline
Yánggāng(BL48)	In the spinal region, inferior to the spinous process of the 10th thoracic vertebra, 3 cun lateral to the posterior midline
Yìshè(BL49)	In the spinal region, inferior to the spinous process of the 11th thoracic vertebra, 3 cun lateral to the posterior midline
Wèicāng(BL50)	In the spinal region, inferior to the spinous process of the 12th thoracic vertebra, 3 cun lateral to the posterior midline
Huāngmén(BL51)	In the lumbar region, inferior to the spinous process of the 1st lumbar vertebra, 3 cun lateral to the posterior midline
Zhìshǐ(BL52)	In the lumbar region, inferior to the spinous process of the 2nd lumbar vertebra, 3 cun lateral to the posterior midline
Bāohuāng(BL53)	In the sacral region, level with the 2nd posterior sacral foramen, 3 cun lateral to the median sacral crest
Zhìbiān(BL54)	In the sacral region, level with the 4th posterior sacral foramen, 3 cun lateral to the median sacral crest

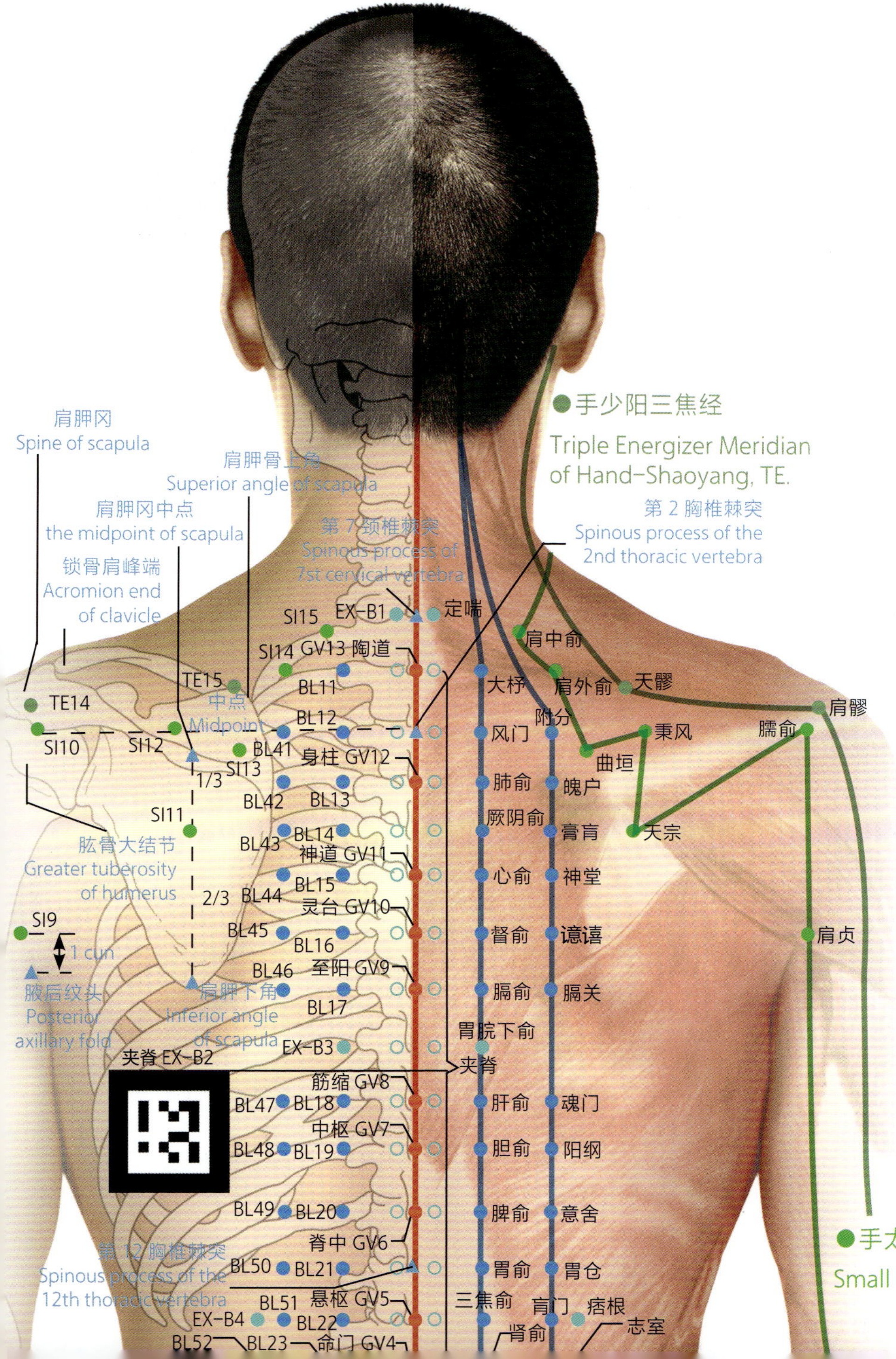

续表

穴位	定位
肩髎	在三角肌区，肩峰角与肱骨大结节两骨间凹陷中
天髎	在肩胛区，肩胛骨上角骨际凹陷中
居髎	在臀区，髂前上棘与股骨大转子最凸点连线的中点处
环跳	在臀区，股骨大转子最凸点与骶管裂孔连线的外 1/3 与内 2/3 交点处
长强	在会阴部，尾骨下方，尾骨端与肛门连线的中点处
腰俞	在骶区，正对骶管裂孔，后正中线上
腰阳关	在脊柱区，第 4 腰椎棘突下凹陷中，后正中线上
命门	在脊柱区，第 2 腰椎棘突下凹陷中，后正中线上
悬枢	在脊柱区，第 1 腰椎棘突下凹陷中，后正中线上
脊中	在脊柱区，第 11 胸椎棘突下凹陷中，后正中线上
中枢	在脊柱区，第 10 胸椎棘突下凹陷中，后正中线上
筋缩	在脊柱区，第 9 胸椎棘突下凹陷中，后正中线上
至阳	在脊柱区，第 7 胸椎棘突下凹陷中，后正中线上

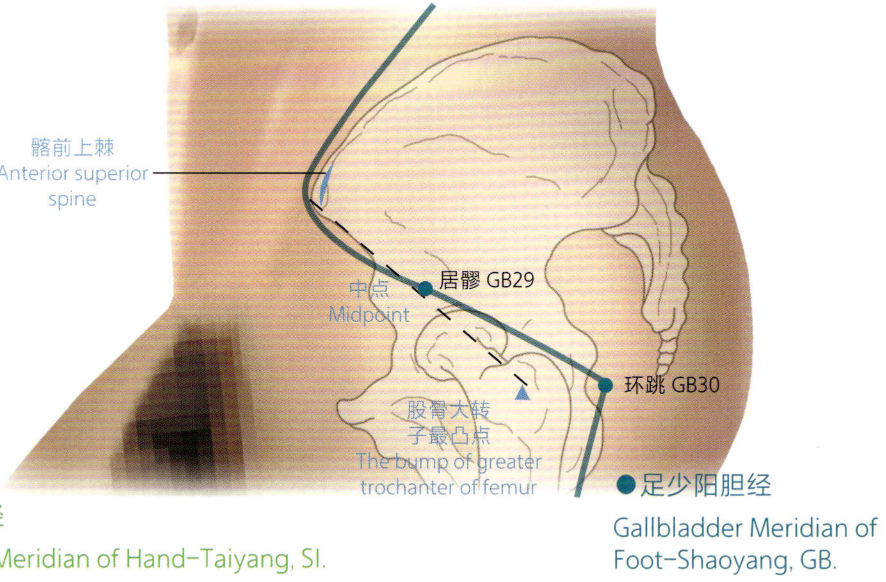

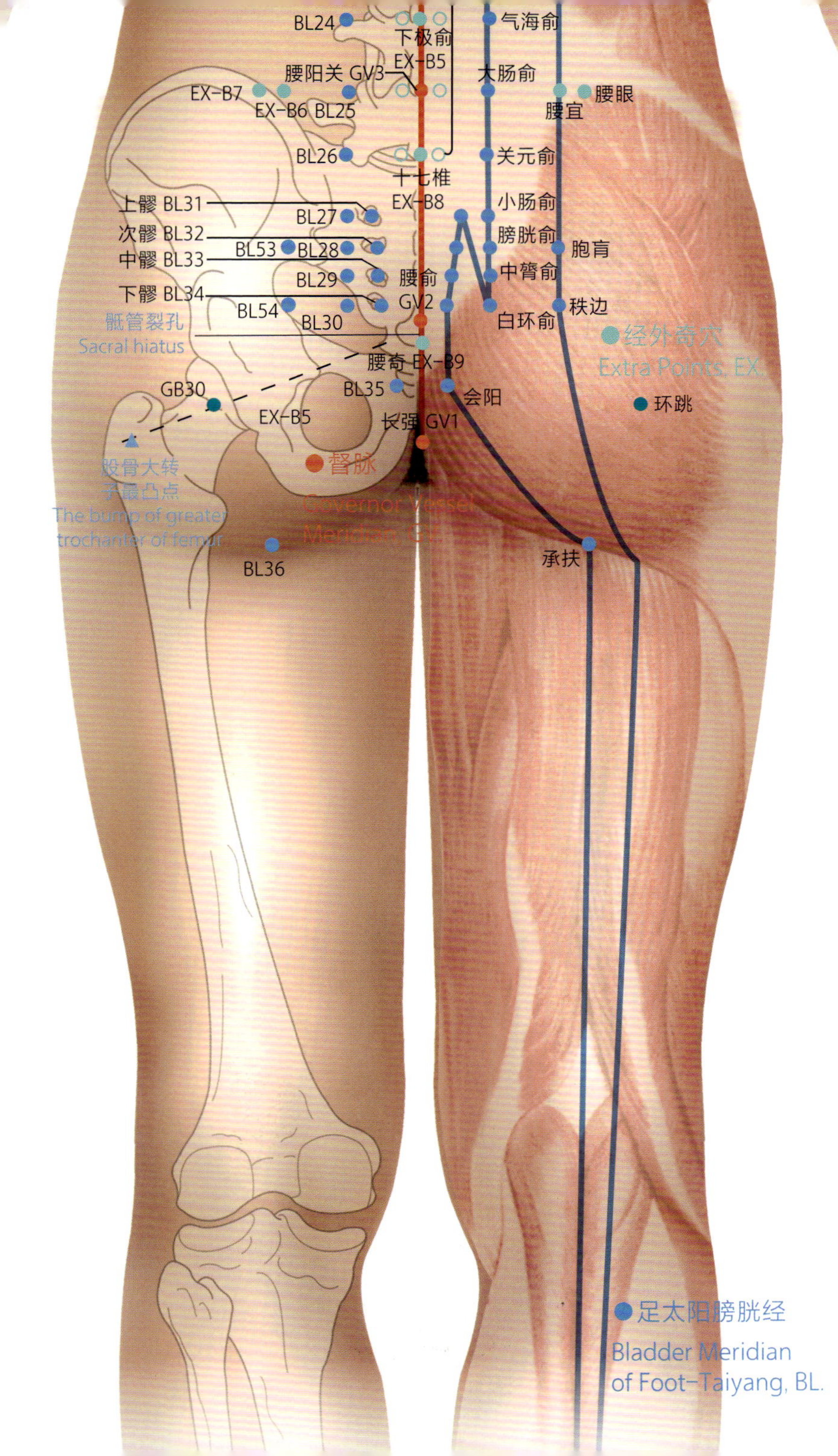

Continued

Acupoints	Location
Jiānliáo(TE14)	In the deltoid region, in the depression of the acromial angle and the greater tuberosity of the humerus
Tiānliáo(TE15)	In the scapular region, in the skeletal depression of the superior angle of the scapula
Jūliáo(GB29)	In the gluteal region, at the midpoint of the line joining the anterior superior iliac spine and the greater trochanter of the femur
Huántiào(GB30)	In the gluteal region, at the junction of the lateral 1/3 and interior 2/3 of the line joining the greater trochanter of the femur and the sacral hiatus
Chángqiáng (GV1)	In the perineum region, inferior to the coccyx, at the midpoint of the coccyx end and the anus
Yāoshū(GV2)	In the sacral region, directly faced with the sacral hiatus, on the posterior midline
Yāoyángguān (GV3)	In the spinal region, in the depression inferior to the spinous process of the 4th lumbar vertebra, on the dorsal midline
Mìngmén(GV4)	In the spinal region, in the depression inferior to the spinous process of the 2nd lumbar vertebra, on the posterior midline
Xuánshū(GV5)	In the spinal region, in the depression inferior to the spinous process of the 1st lumbar vertebra, on the posterior midline
Jǐzhōng(GV6)	In the spinal region, in the depression inferior to the spinous process of the 11th thoracic vertebra, on the posterior midline
Zhōngshū(GV7)	In the spinal region, in the depression inferior to the spinous process of the 10th thoracic vertebra, on the posterior midline
Jīnsuō(GV8)	In the spinal region, in the depression inferior to the spinous process of the 9th thoracic vertebra, on the posterior midline
Zhìyáng(GV9)	In the spinal region, in the depression inferior to the spinous process of the 7th thoracic vertebra, on the posterior midline

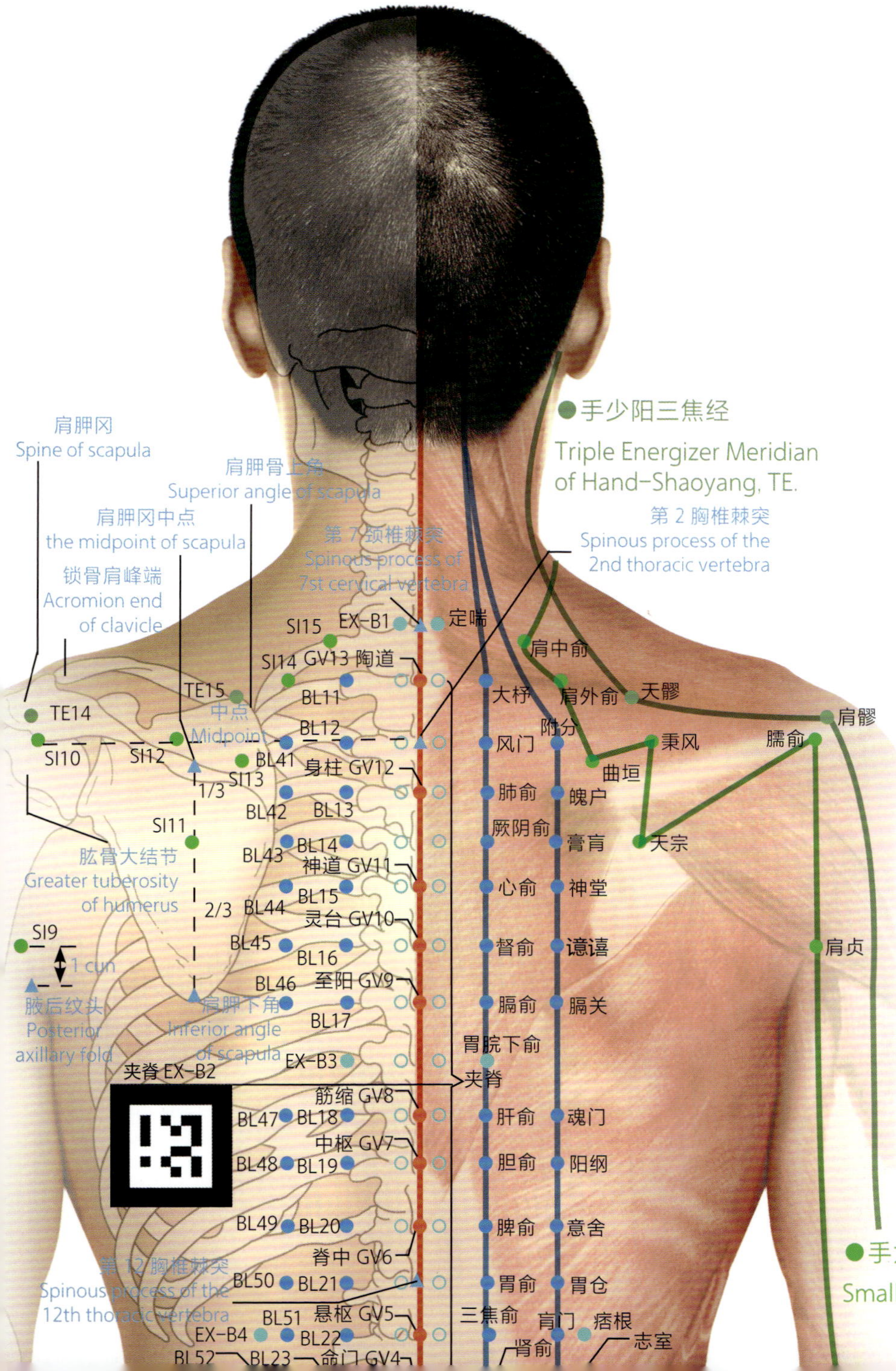

续表

穴位	定位
灵台	在脊柱区，第 6 胸椎棘突下凹陷中，后正中线上
神道	在脊柱区，第 5 胸椎棘突下凹陷中，后正中线上
身柱	在脊柱区，第 3 胸椎棘突下凹陷中，后正中线上
陶道	在脊柱区，第 1 胸椎棘突下凹陷中，后正中线上
定喘	在脊柱区，横平第 7 颈椎棘突下，后正中线旁开 0.5 寸
夹脊	在脊柱区，第 1 胸椎至第 5 腰椎棘突下两侧，后正中线旁开 0.5 寸，一侧 17 穴
胃脘下俞	在脊柱区，横平第 8 胸椎棘突下，后正中线旁开 1.5 寸
痞根	在腰区，横平第 1 腰椎棘突下，后正中线旁开 3.5 寸
下极俞	在腰区，第 3 腰椎棘突下
腰宜	在腰区，横平第 4 腰椎棘突下，后正中线旁开 3 寸
腰眼	在腰区，横平第 4 腰椎棘突下，后正中线旁开约 3.5 寸凹陷中
十七椎	在腰区，第 5 腰椎棘突下凹陷中
腰奇	在骶区，尾骨端直上 2 寸，骶角之间凹陷中

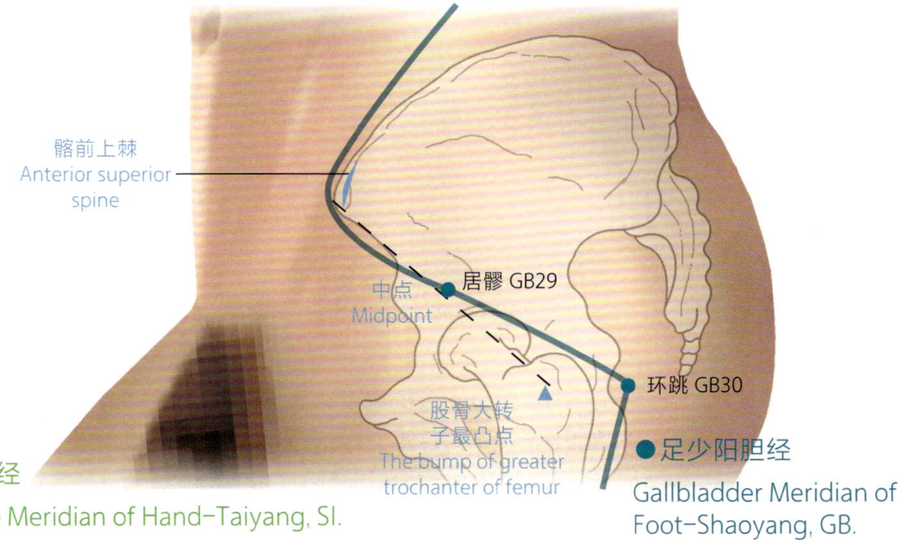

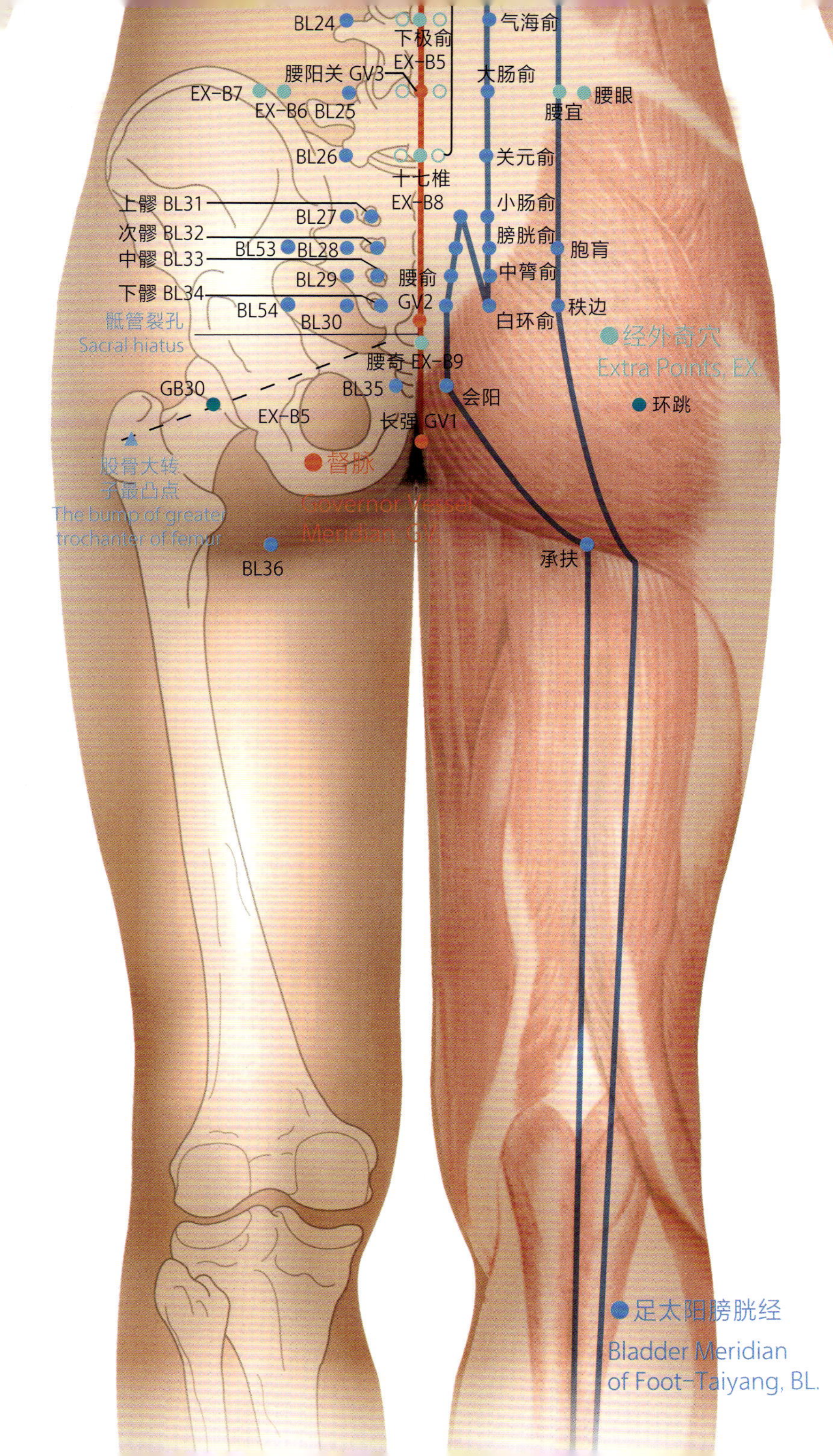

Continued

Acupoints	Location
Língtái(GV10)	In the spinal region, in the depression inferior to the spinous process of the 6th thoracic vertebra, on the posterior midline
Shéndào(GV11)	In the spinal region, in the depression inferior to the spinous process of the 5th thoracic vertebra, on the posterior midline
Shēnzhù(GV12)	In the spinal region, in the depression inferior to the spinous process of the 3rd thoracic vertebra, on the posterior midline
Táodào(GV13)	In the spinal region, in the depression inferior to the spinous process of the 1st thoracic vertebra, on the posterior midline
Dìngchuǎn (EX-B1)	In the spinal region, level with the inferior side of spinous process of the 7th cervical vertebra, 0.5 cun lateral to the dorsal midline
Jiájǐ(EX-B2)	In the spinal region, in two sides of the inferior aspect of the spinous process of the 1st thoracic vertebra to the 5th lumbar vertebra, 0.5 cun lateral to the posterior midline, with 17 acupoints of each side
Weìwǎnxiàshū (EX-B3)	In the spinal region, level with the inferior aspect of the spinous process of the 8th thoracic vertebra, 1.5 cun lateral to the posterior midline
Pǐgēn(EX-B4)	In the lumbar region, level with the inferior aspect of the spinous process of the 1st lumbar vertebra, 3.5 cun lateral to the posterior midline
Xiàjíshū(EX-B5)	In the lumbar region, inferior to the spinous process of the 3rd lumbar vertebra
Yāoyí(EX-B6)	In the lumbar region, level with the inferior aspect of the spinous process of the 4th lumbar vertebra, 3 cun lateral to the posterior midline
Yāoyǎn(EX-B7)	In the lumbar region, level with the inferior aspect of the spinous process of the 4th lumbar vertebra, in the depression about 3.5 cun lateral to the posterior midline
Shíqīzhuī(EX-B8)	In the lumbar region, in the depression of the inferior aspect of the spinous process of the 5th lumbar vertebra
Yāoqí(EX-B9)	In the sacral region, 2 cun directly above the coccyx end, in the depression between two sacral angles

上肢部穴位

Acupoints of Upper Limbs

穴位	定位
天府	在臂前区，腋前纹头下 3 寸，肱二头肌桡侧缘处
侠白	在臂前区，腋前纹头下 4 寸处，肱二头肌桡侧缘处
尺泽	在肘区，肘横纹上，肱二头肌腱桡侧缘凹陷中
孔最	在前臂前区，腕掌侧远端横纹上 7 寸，尺泽与太渊连线上
列缺	在前臂，腕掌侧远端横纹上 1.5 寸，拇短伸肌腱与拇长展肌腱之间，拇长展肌腱沟的凹陷中
经渠	在前臂前区，腕掌侧远端横纹上 1 寸，桡骨茎突与桡动脉之间
太渊	在腕前区，桡骨茎突与舟状骨之间，拇长展肌腱尺侧凹陷中
鱼际	在手外侧，第 1 掌骨桡侧中点赤白肉际处
少商	在手指，拇指末节桡侧，指甲根角侧上方 0.1 寸（指寸）
极泉	在腋区，腋窝中央，腋动脉搏动处
青灵	在臂前区，肘横纹上 3 寸，肱二头肌的内侧沟中

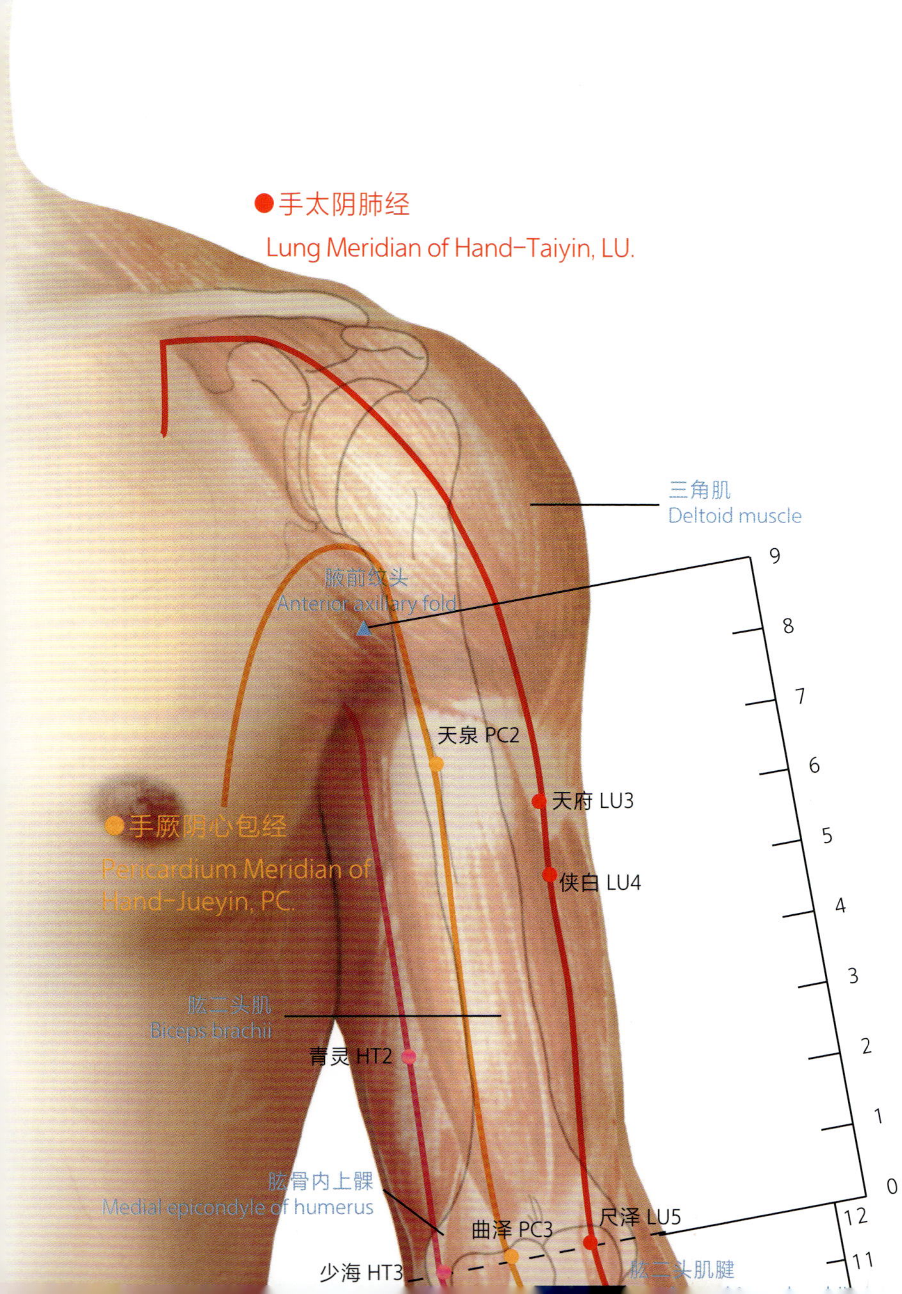

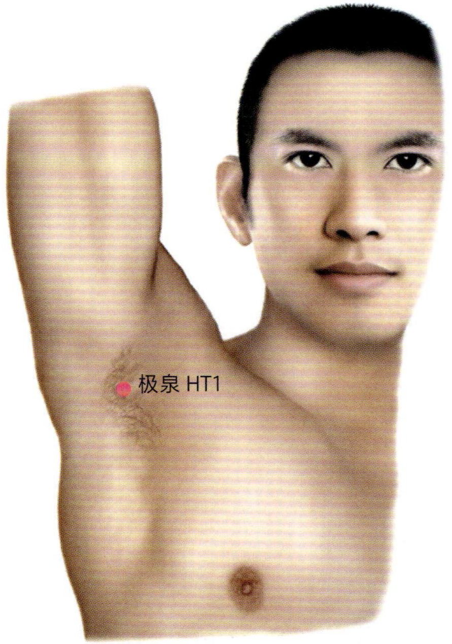

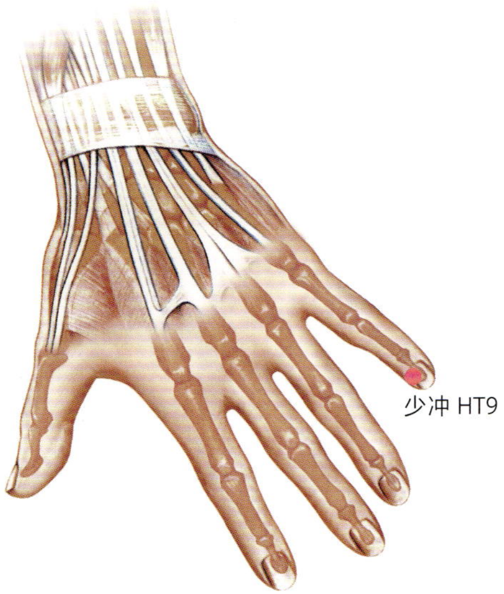

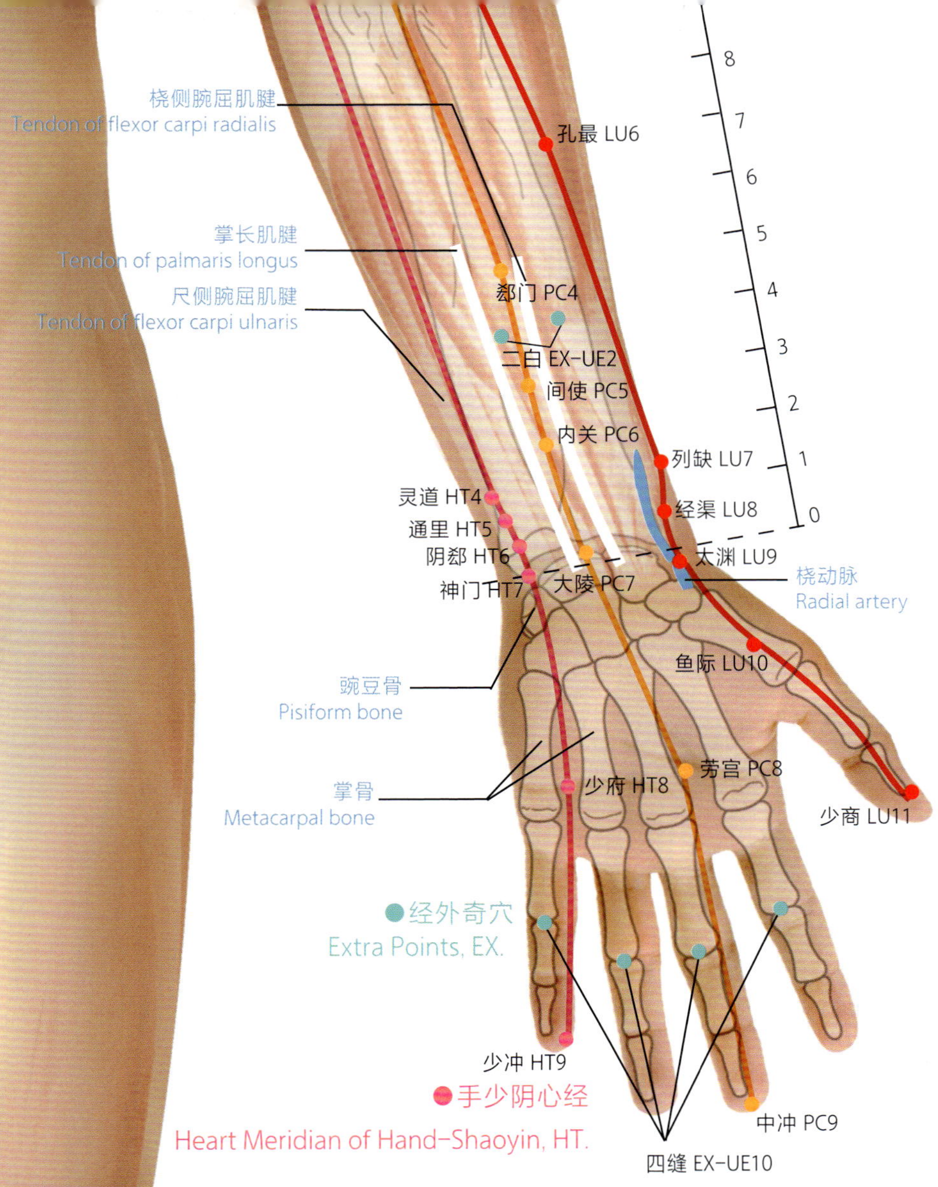

Acupoints	Location
Tiānfǔ(LU3)	In the anterior region of the arm, 3 cun below the anterior axillary fold, in the radial margin of the biceps brachii
Xiábái(LU4)	In the anterior region of the arm, 4 cun below the anterior axillary fold, in the radial margin of the biceps brachii
Chǐzé(LU5)	In the elbow region, on the cubital, in the depression of the radial margin of the biceps brachii
Kǒngzuì(LU6)	In the anterior region of the forearm, 7 cun above the distal transverse crease of the palmar wrist, on the line between the Chize acupoint and theTaiyuan acupoint
Lièquē(LU7)	In the forearm region, 1.5 cun above the distal transverse crease of the palmar wrist, in the middle between the tendon of extensor pollicis brevis and the tendon of abductor pollicis longus, in the depression of tendon groove of the extensor pollicis longus
Jīngqú(LU8)	In the anterior region of the forearm, 1 cun above the distal transverse crease of the palmar wrist, between the styloid process of the radius and the radial artery
Tàiyuān(LU9)	In the anterior region of the wrist, between the styloid process of the radius and the navicular bone, in the ulnar depression of the tendon of abductor pollicis longus
Yújì(LU10)	In the lateral region of the hand, at the midpoint of 1st metacarpal bone, at the junction of the red and white skin of the hand
Shàoshāng (LU11)	In the finger, 0.1 cun posterior and lateral to the thumb nail, on the radial side
Jíquán(HT1)	In the axilla region, in the center of the armpit where the axillary artery pulses
Qīnglíng(HT2)	In the anterior region of the arm, 3 cun above the transverse crease of elbow, in the interior sulcus of the biceps brachii

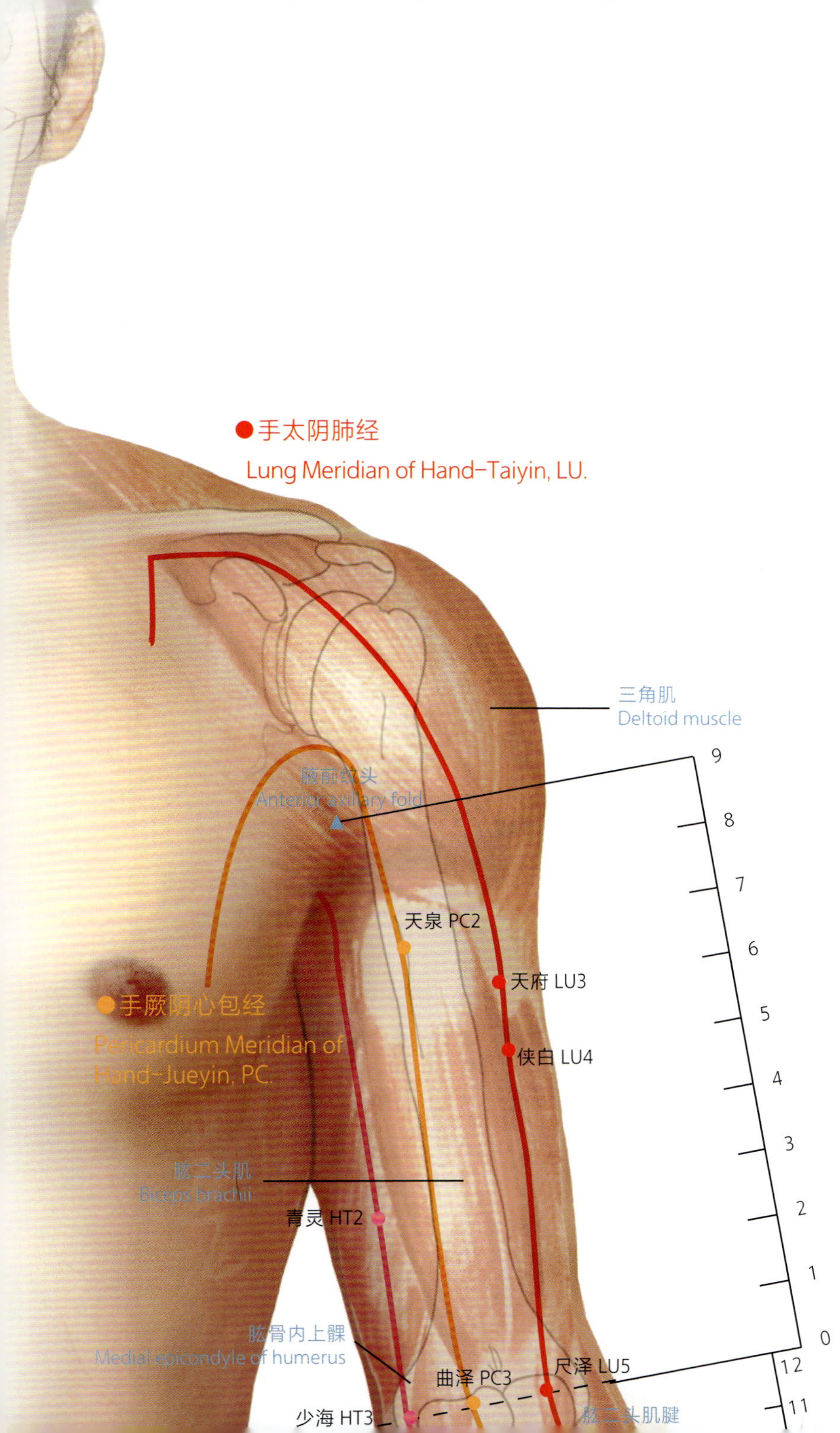

续表

穴位	定位
少海	在肘前区，横平肘横纹，肱骨内上髁前缘
灵道	在前臂前区，腕掌侧远端横纹上 1.5 寸，尺侧腕屈肌腱的桡侧缘
通里	在前臂前区，腕掌侧远端横纹上 1 寸，尺侧腕屈肌腱的桡侧缘
阴郄	在前臂前区，腕掌侧远端横纹上 0.5 寸，尺侧腕屈肌腱的桡侧缘
神门	在腕前区，腕掌侧远端横纹尺侧端，尺侧腕屈肌腱的桡侧缘
少府	在手掌，横平第 5 掌指关节近端，第 4、5 掌骨之间
少冲	小指末节桡侧，指甲根角侧上方 0.1 寸（指寸）
天泉	在臂前区，腋前纹头下 2 寸，肱二头肌的长、短头之间
曲泽	在肘前区，肘横纹上，肱二头肌腱的尺侧缘凹陷中

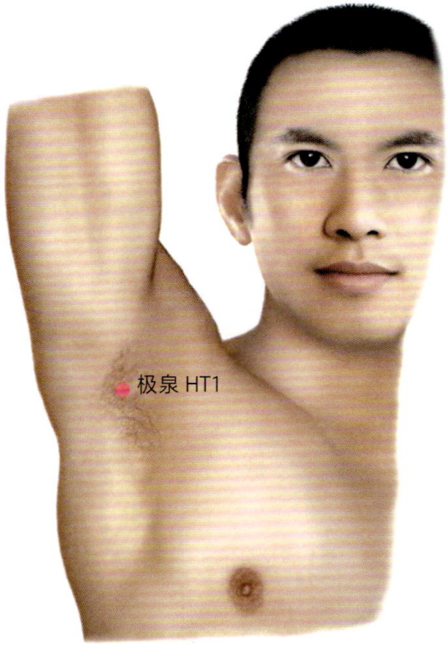

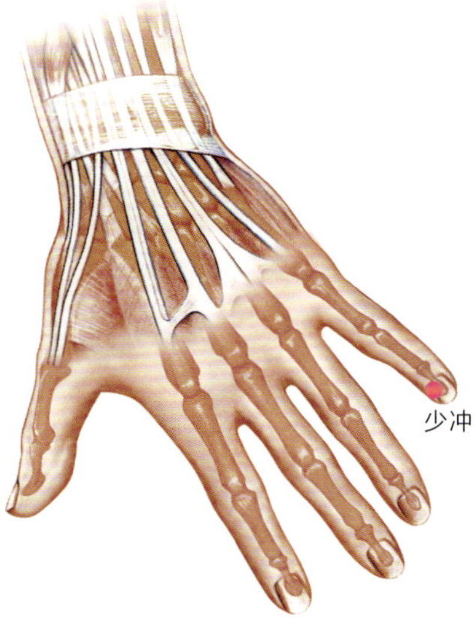

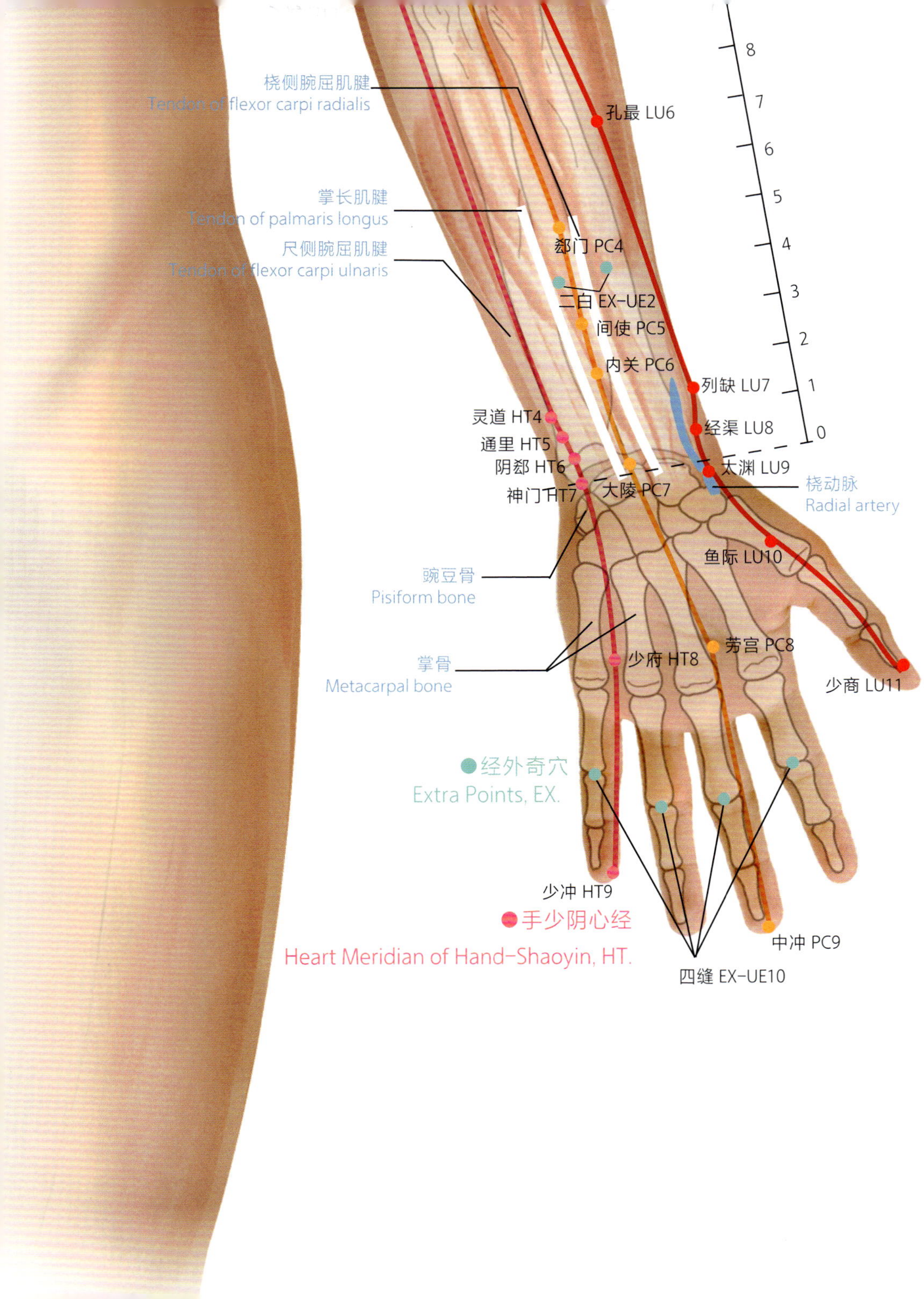

Continued

Acupoints	Location
Shàohǎi(HT3)	In the anterior region of the elbow, level with the transverse crease of elbow, in the anterior margin of the interior epicondyle of the humerus
Língdào(HT4)	In the anterior region of the forearm,1.5 cun above the distal transverse crease of the palmar wrist, in the radial margin of the tendor of flexor carpi ulnaris
Tōnglǐ(HT5)	In the anterior region of the forearm, 1 cun above the distal transverse crease of the palmar trist, in the radial margin of the tendor of flexor carpi ulnaris
Yīnxì(HT6)	In the anterior region of the forearm, 0.5 cun above the distal transverse crease of the palmar wrist, in the radial margin of the tendor of flexor carpi ulnaris
Shénmén(HT7)	In the anterior region of the wrist, in the distal transverse crease of the palmar wrist, in the radial margin of the tendor of flexor carpi ulnaris
Shàofǔ(HT8)	On the palm, level with the proximal end of the 5th metacarpophalangeal joint, between the 4th and 5th metacarpal bones
Shàochōng (HT9)	0.1 cun from the corner of the nail, in the radial side of the little finger
Tiānquán(PC2)	In the anterior region of the arm, 2 cun below the end of the anterior axillary fold, between the longus and the brevis of biceps brachii
Qūzé(PC3)	In the anterior region of the elbow, on the transverse crease of the elbow, in the depression of ulnar margin of the tendor of biceps brachii

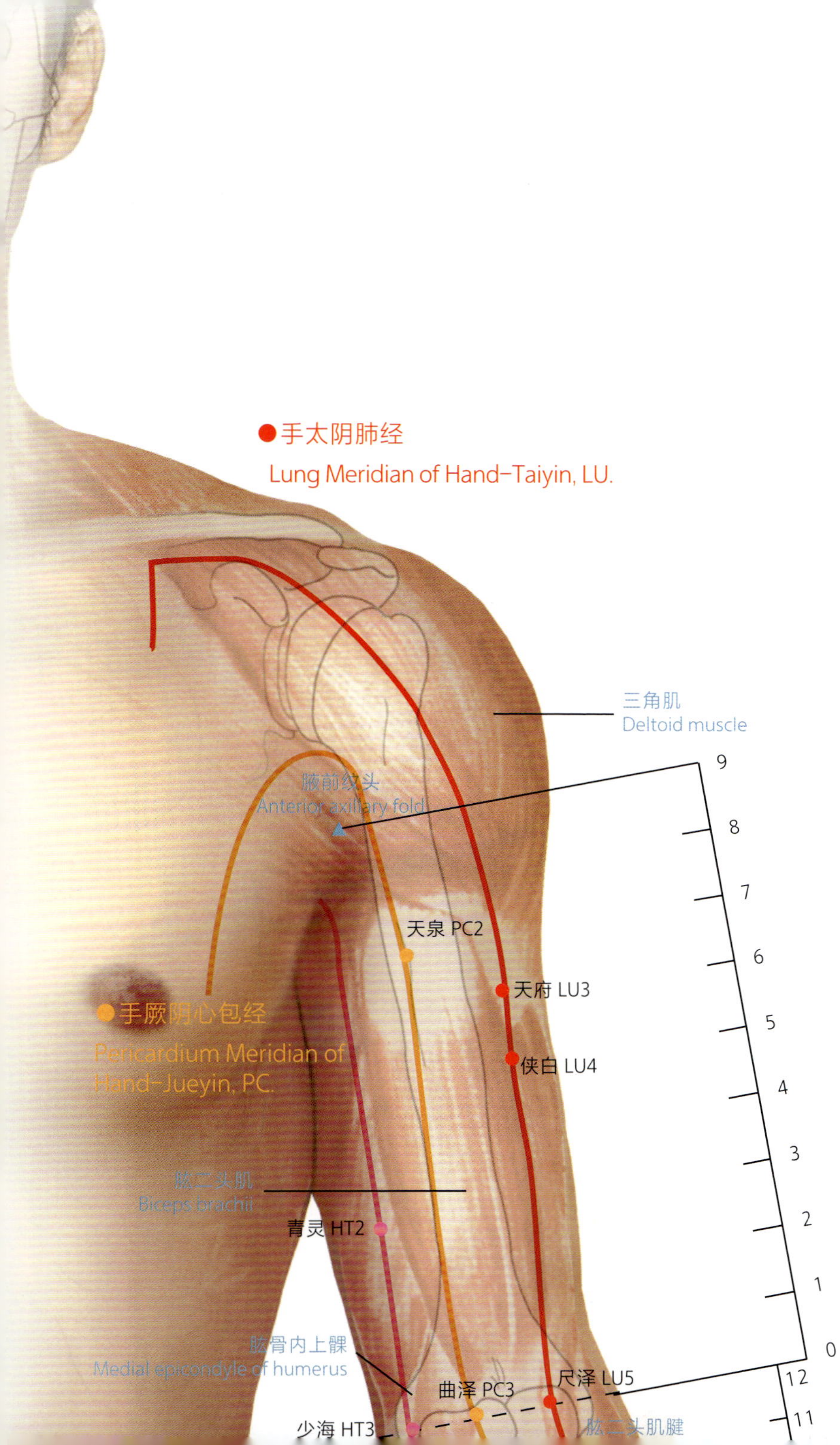

续表

穴位	定位
郄门	在前臂前区，腕掌侧远端横纹上 5 寸，掌长肌腱与桡侧腕屈肌腱之间
间使	在前臂前区，腕掌侧远端横纹上 3 寸，掌长肌腱与桡侧腕屈肌腱之间
内关	在前臂前区，腕掌侧远端横纹上 2 寸，掌长肌腱与桡侧腕屈肌腱之间
大陵	在腕前区，腕掌侧远端横纹中，掌长肌腱与桡侧腕屈肌腱之间
劳宫	在掌区，横平第 3 掌指关节近端，第 2、3 掌骨之间偏于第 3 掌骨
中冲	在手指，中指末节最高点
二白	在前臂前区，腕掌侧远端横纹上 4 寸，桡侧腕屈肌腱的两侧，左右上肢各 2 穴
四缝	在手指，第 2~5 指掌面的近侧指间关节横纹的中央，一手 4 穴

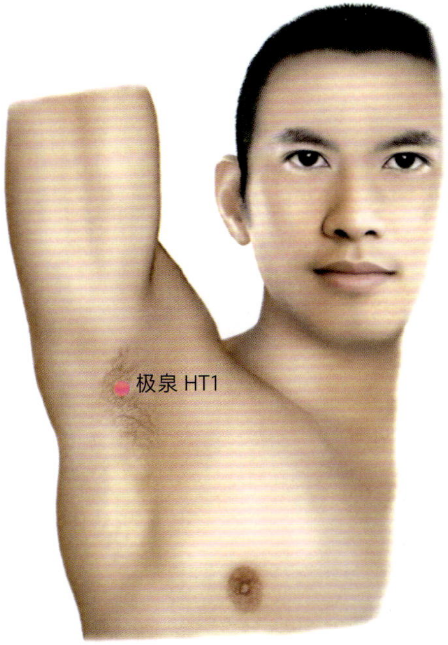

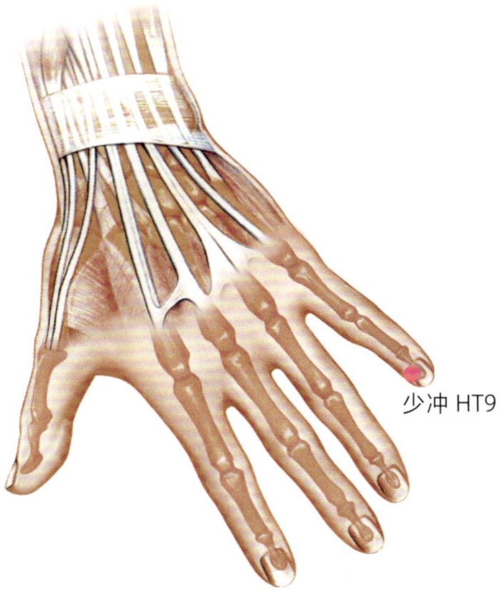

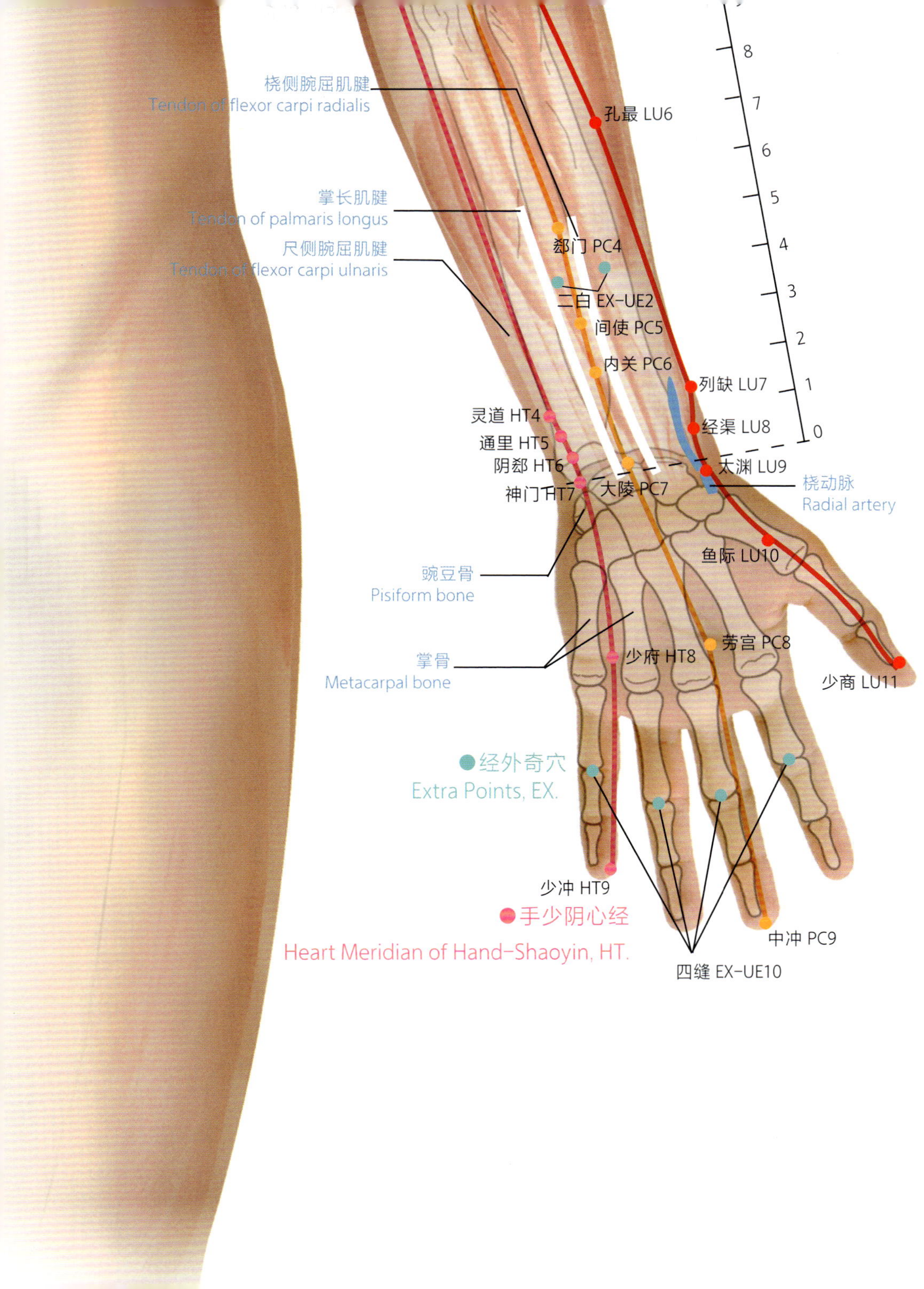

Continued

Acupoints	Location
Xìmén(PC4)	In the anterior region of the forearm, 5 cun above the distal transverse crease of palmar wrist, between the tendon of palmaris longus and radial flexor tendor of wrist
Jiānshǐ(PC5)	In the anterior region of the forearm, 3 cun above the distal transverse crease of palmar wrist, between the tendon of palmaris longus and radial flexor tendor of wrist
Nèiguān(PC6)	In the anterior region of the forearm, 2 cun above the distal transverse crease of palmar wrist, between the tendon of palmaris longus and radial flexor tendor of wrist
Dàlíng(PC7)	In the anterior region of the wrist, on the distal transverse crease of palmar wrist, between the tendon of palmaris longus and radial flexor tendor of wrist
Láogōng(PC8)	In the region of the palm, level with the near end of the 3th metacarpophalangeal joint, between the 2nd and 3rd metacarpal bones, closer to the 3rd metacarpal bone
Zhōngchōng (PC9)	On the finger, in the apex of the middle finger
Erbái(EX-UE2)	In the anterior region of the forearm, 4 cun above the distal transverse crease of palmar wrist, on both sides of the radial flexor tendor of the wrist, with 2 acupoints of each upper limb
Sìfèng(EX-UE10)	On the finger, in the center of the transverse crease of the proximal interphalangeal joints of the 2nd to the 5th finger on the palmar side, with 4 acupoints in each hand

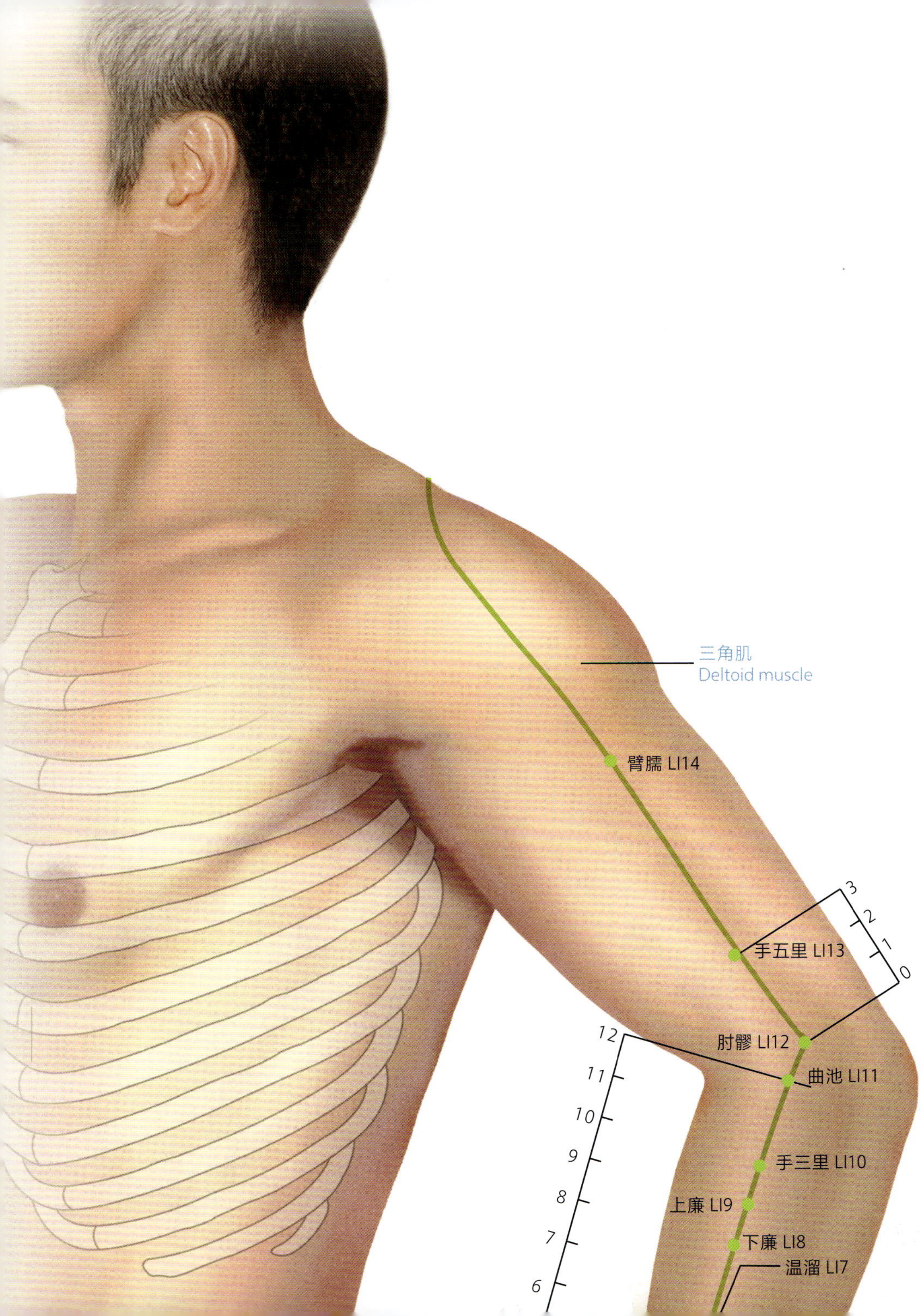

续表

穴位	定位
商阳	在手指，食指末节桡侧，指甲根角侧上方 0.1 寸（指寸）
二间	在手指，第 2 掌指关节桡侧远端赤白肉际处
三间	在手背，第 2 掌指关节桡侧近端凹陷处
合谷	在手背，第 2 掌骨桡侧的中点处
阳溪	在腕区，腕背侧远端横纹桡侧，桡骨茎突远端，解剖学“鼻烟窝”凹陷中
偏历	在前臂，腕背侧远端横纹上 3 寸，阳溪与曲池连线上
温溜	在前臂，腕背侧远端横纹上 5 寸，阳溪与曲池连线上
下廉	在前臂，肘横纹下 4 寸，阳溪与曲池连线上
上廉	在前臂，肘横纹下 3 寸，阳溪与曲池连线上
手三里	在前臂，肘横纹下 2 寸，阳溪与曲池连线上
曲池	在肘区，尺泽与肱骨外上髁连线的中点处
肘髎	在肘区，肱骨外上髁上缘，髁上嵴的前缘
手五里	在臂部，肘横纹上 3 寸处，曲池与肩髃连线上
臂臑	在臂部，曲池上 7 寸，三角肌前缘处

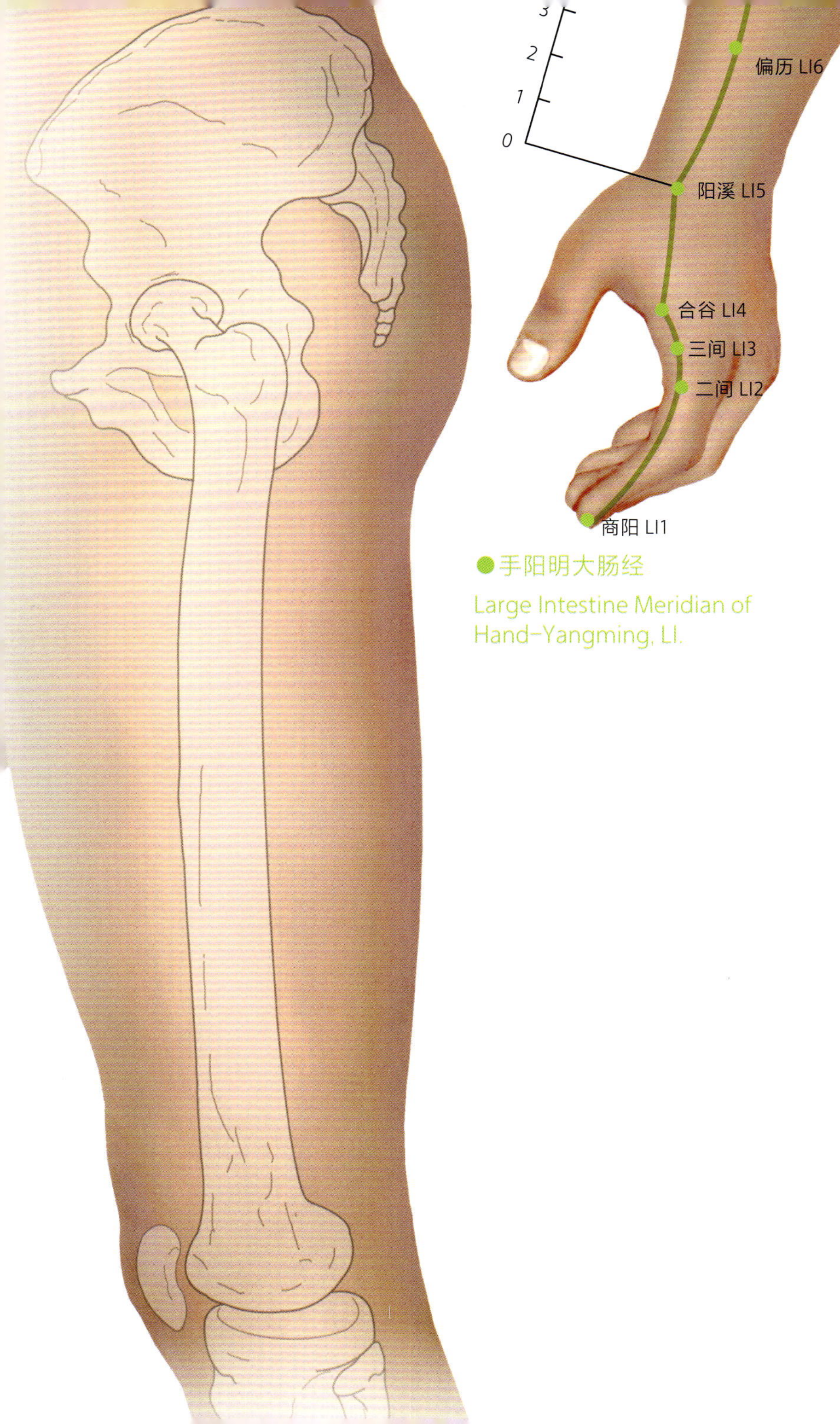

●手阳明大肠经

Large Intestine Meridian of Hand-Yangming, LI.

Continued

Acupoints	Location
Shāngyáng (LI1)	On the finger, 0.1 cun from the corner of the nail, in the radial side of the index finger
Èrjiān (LI2)	On the finger, in the distal radial side of the 2nd metacarpophalangeal joint, at the junction of the red and white skin
Sānjiān (LI3)	On the dorsum of the hand, in the proximal radial side of the 2nd metacarpophalangeal joint
Hégǔ (LI4)	On the dorsum of the hand , at the midpoint of the radial side of the 2nd metacarpal bone
Yángxī (LI5)	In the region of the wrist, in the radial side of the distal transverse crease of dorsal wrist, in the distal end of styloid process of radius, in the depression of anatomist's snuff-box
Piānlì (LI6)	In the region of the forearm, 3 cun above the distal transverse crease of dorsal wrist, on the line between the Yangxi acupoint and the Quchi acupoint
Wēnliū (LI7)	In the region of the forearm, 5 cun above the distal transverse crease of dorsal wrist, in the line between the Yangxi acupoint and the Quchi acupoint
Xiàlián (LI8)	In the region of the forearm, 4 cun below the transverse crease of the elbow, in the line between the Yangxi acupoint and the Quchi acupoint
Shànglián (LI9)	In the region of the forearm, 3 cun below the transverse crease of the elbow, in the line between the Yangxi acupoint and the Quchi acupoint
Shǒusānlǐ (LI10)	In the region of the forearm, 2 cun below the transverse crease of the elbow, in the line between the Yangxi acupoint and the Quchi acupoint
Qūchí (LI11)	In the region of the elbow, at the midpoint of the line between Chize acupoint and the external epicondyle of the humerus
Zhǒuliáo (LI12)	In the region of the elbow, in the superior margin of the external epicondyle of humerus, in the anterior margin of the supracondylar ridge
Shǒuwǔlǐ (LI13)	In the region of the arm, 3 cun above the transverse crease of the elbow, on the line between the Quchi acupoint and the Jianyu acupoint
Bìnào (LI14)	In the region of the arm, 7 cun above the Quchi acupoint, in the anterior margin of the deltoid

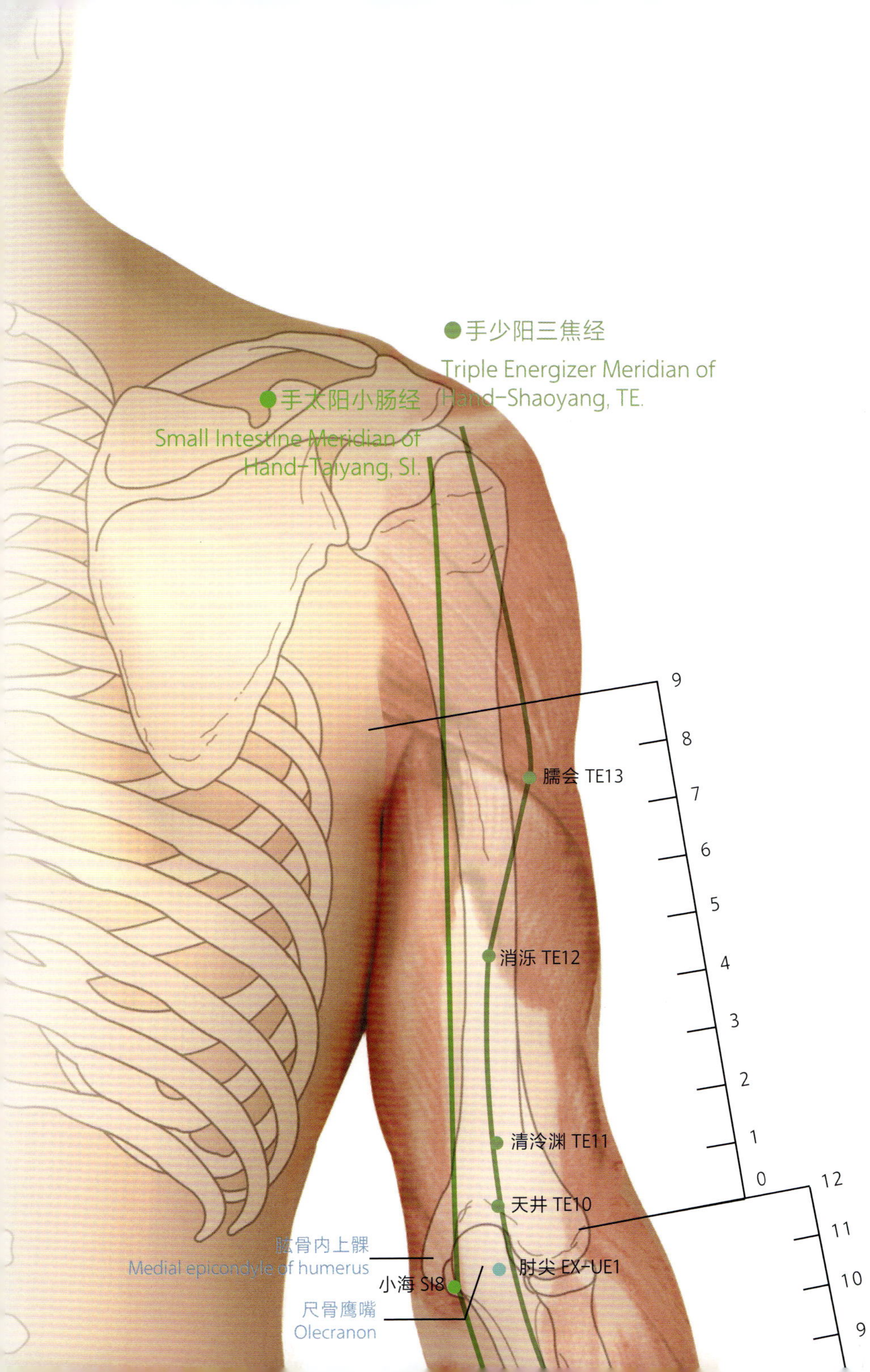

续表

穴位	定位
少泽	在手指，小指末节尺侧，指甲根角侧上方 0.1 寸（指寸）
前谷	在手指，第 5 掌指关节尺侧远端赤白肉际凹陷中
后溪	在手内侧，第 5 掌指关节尺侧近端赤白肉际凹陷中
腕骨	在腕区，第 5 掌骨底与三角骨之间的赤白肉际凹陷中
阳谷	在腕后区，尺骨茎突与三角骨之间的凹陷中
养老	在前臂后区，腕背横纹上 1 寸，尺骨头桡侧凹陷中
支正	在前臂后区，腕背侧远端横纹上 5 寸，尺骨尺侧与尺侧腕屈肌之间
小海	在肘后区，尺骨鹰嘴与肱骨内上髁之间凹陷中
肘尖	在肘后区，尺骨鹰嘴的尖端
中泉	在前臂后区，腕背侧远端横纹上，指总伸肌腱桡侧的凹陷中
中魁	在手指，中指背面，近侧指间关节的中点处

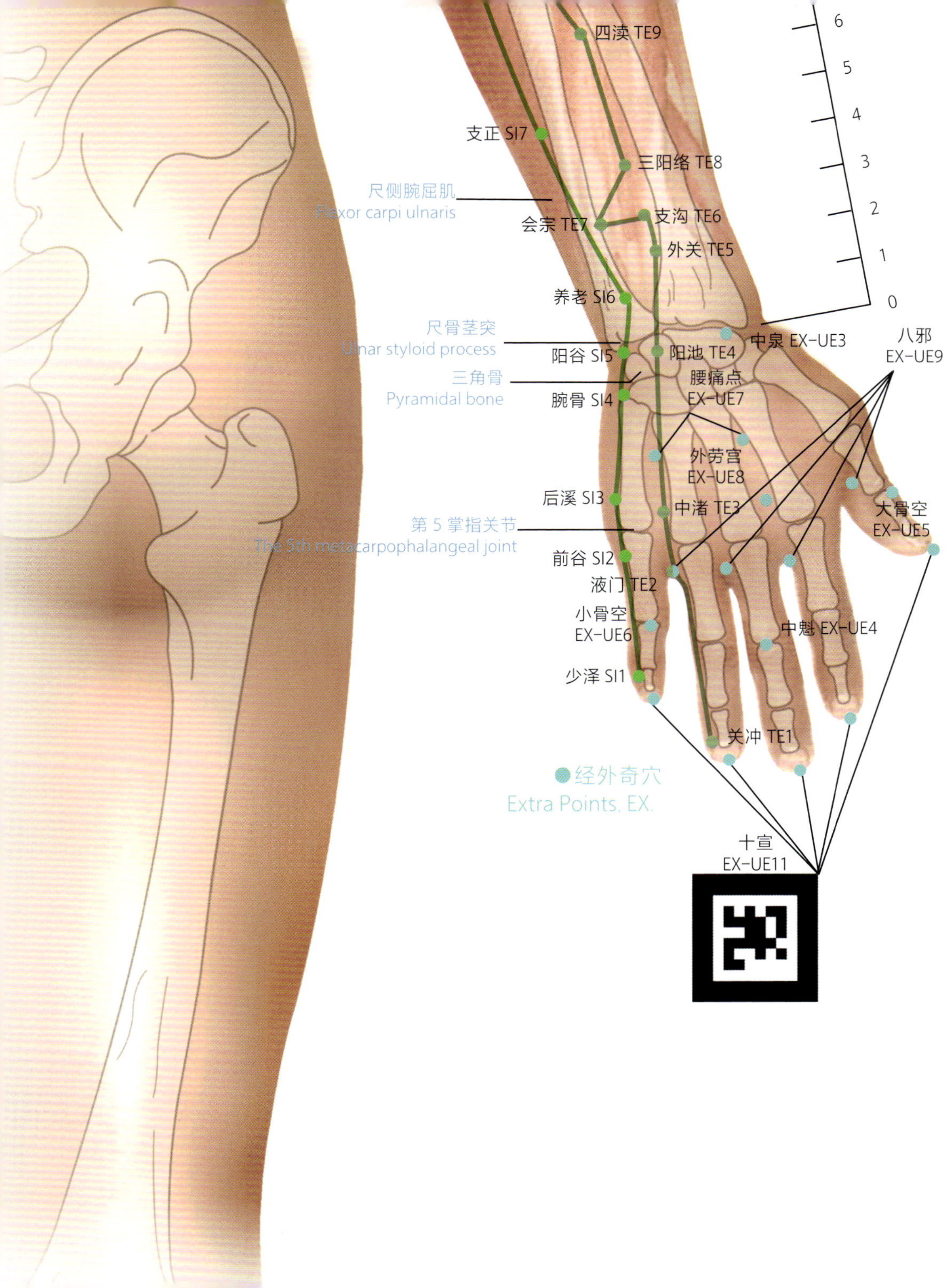

Continued

Acupoints	Location
Shàozé(SI1)	On the finger, 0.1 cun from the corner of the nail, in the ulnar side of the little finger
Qiángǔ(SI2)	On the finger, at the ulnar distal side of the 5th metacarpophalangeal joint, at the junction of the red and white skin
Hòuxī(SI3)	In the interior aspect of the hand, in the ulnar proximal side of the 5th metacarpophalangeal joint, at the junction of the red and white skin
Wàngǔ(SI4)	In the region of the wrist, in the depression of the junction of the red and white skin between the basis of the 5th metacarpal bone and the triangular bone
Yánggǔ(SI5)	In the posterior region of the wrist, in a fossa between the styloid process of the ulna and the triangular bone
Yǎnglǎo(SI6)	In the posterior region of the forearm, 1 cun above the transverse crease of the dorsal wrist, in the depression on the radial side of the ulna head
Zhīzhèng(SI7)	In the posterior region of the forearm, 5 cun above the distal transverse crease of the dorsal wrist, in the middle of the ulnar side of the ulna and ulnar flexor of the wrist
Xiǎohǎi(SI8)	In the posterior region of the elbow, in the depression between the ulna olecroanon and the medial epicondyle of the humerus
Zhǒujiān (EX-UE1)	In the posterior region of the elbow, in the tip of the ulna olecroanon
Zhōngquán (EX-UE3)	In the posterior region of the forearm, on the distal transverse crease of the dorsal wrist, in the depression of the radial side of the tendon of extensor digitorum communis
Zhōngkuí (EX-UE4)	On the finger, on the dorsum of middle finger, at the midpoint of the proximal interphalangeal joint

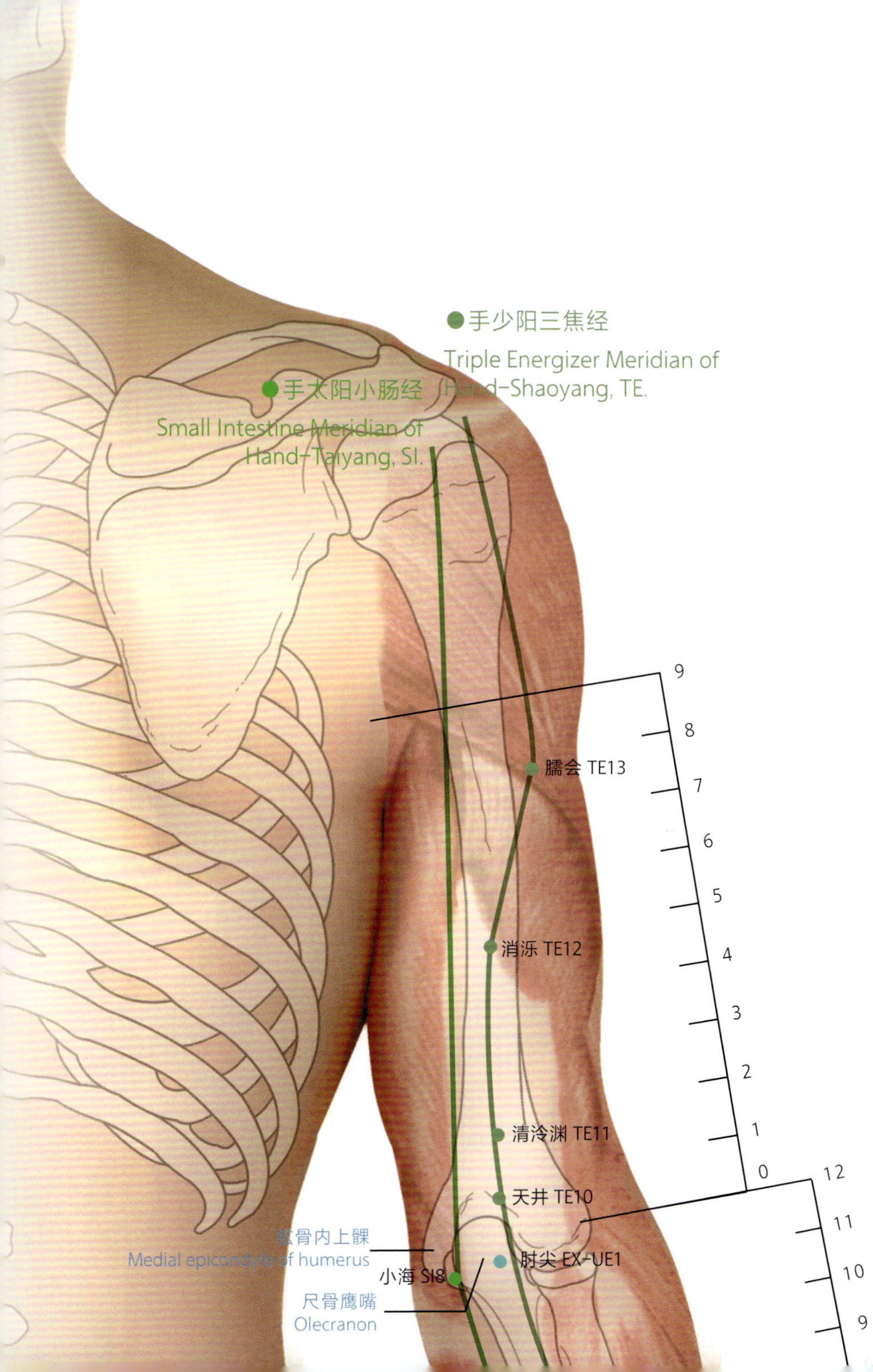

续表

穴位	定位
大骨空	在手指，拇指背面，指间关节的中点处
小骨空	在手指，小指背面，近侧指间关节的中点处
腰痛点	在手背，第 2、3 掌骨间及第 4、5 掌骨间，腕背侧远端横纹与掌指关节的中点处，一手 2 穴
外劳宫	在手背，第 2、3 掌骨间，掌指关节后 0.5 寸（指寸）凹陷中
八邪	在手背，第 1~5 指间，指蹼缘后方赤白肉际处，左右共 8 穴
十宣	在手指，十指尖端，距指甲游离缘 0.1 寸（指寸），左右共 10 穴
关冲	在手指，第 4 指末节尺侧，指甲根角侧上方 0.1 寸（指寸）
液门	在手背，第 4、5 指间，指蹼缘上方赤白肉际凹陷中
中渚	在手背，第 4、5 掌骨间，第 4 掌指关节近端凹陷中
阳池	在腕后区，腕背侧远端横纹上，指伸肌腱的尺侧缘凹陷中

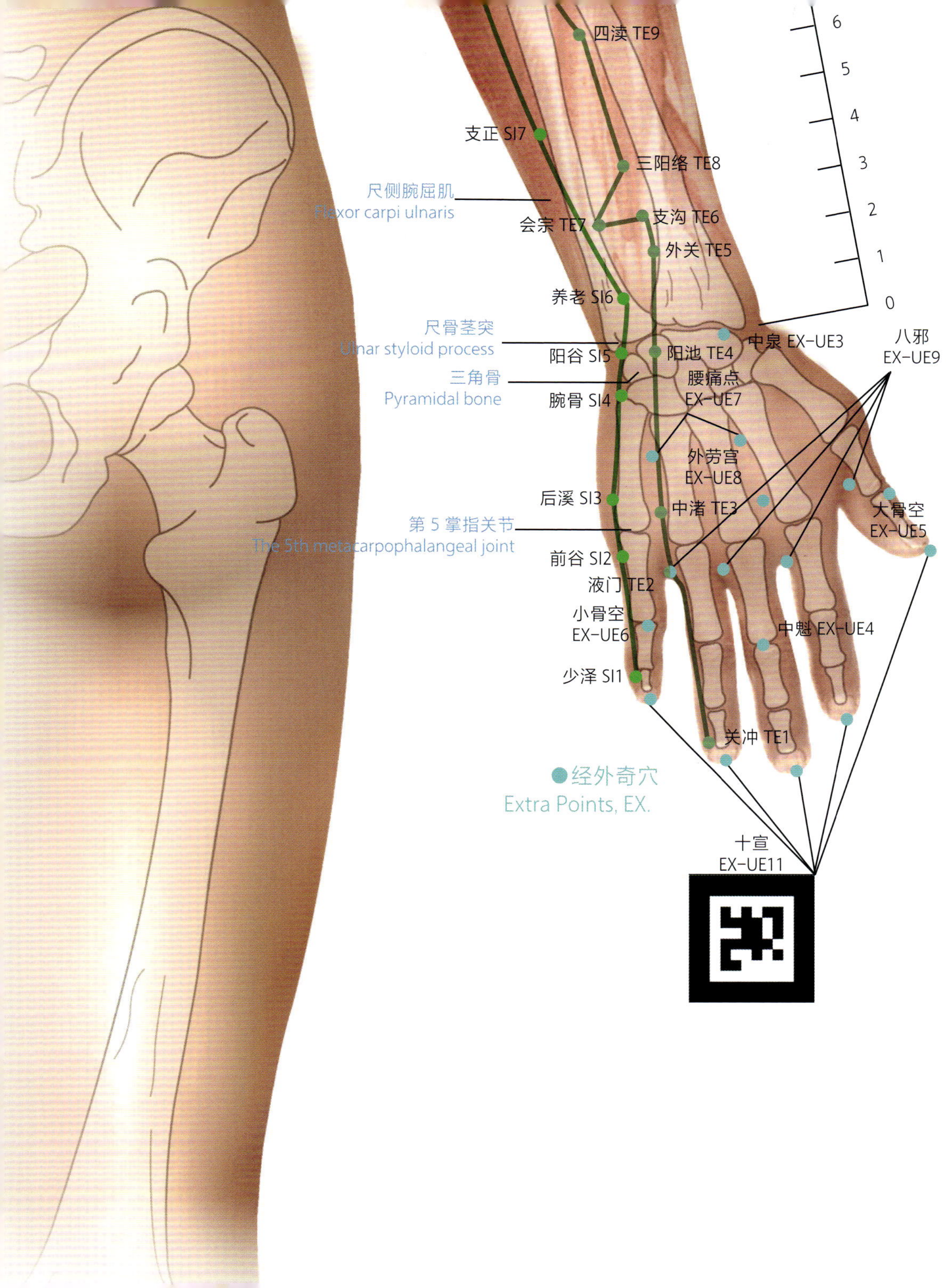

Continued

Acupoints	Location
Dàgǔkōng (EX-UE5)	On the finger, on the dorsum of the thumb, at the midpoint of the interphalangeal joint
Xiǎogǔkōng (EX-UE6)	On the finger, on the dorsum of the little finger, at the midpoint of the proximal interphalangeal joint
Yāotòngdiǎn (EX-UE7)	On the dorsum of the hand, between the 2nd and the 3rd metacarpal bone, and between the 4th and the 5th metacarpal bone at the midpoint of the distal transverse crease of dorsal wrist and the metacarpophalangeal joint, with 2 acupoints of each hand
Wàiláogōng (EX-UE8)	On the dorsum of the hand, between the 2nd and the 3rd metacarpal bone, in the depression 0.5 cun posterior to the metacarpophalangeal joint
Bāxié (EX-UE9)	On the dorsum of the hand, between all five fingers, at the junction of the red and white skin posterior to the natatory edge, with eight points in total
Shíxuān (EX-UE11)	On the finger, in the tip of ten fingers, 0.1 cun from the free edge of the nail, with ten points in total
Guānchōng (TE1)	On the finger, 0.1 cun from the corner of the nail, in the ulnar side of the ring finger
Yèmén (TE2)	On the dorsum of the hand, between the ring finger and the little finger, in the depression of the junction of the red and white skin above the natatory edge
Zhōngzhǔ (TE3)	On the dorsum of the hand, between the 4th and the 5th metacarpal bone, in the depression of the proximal 4th metacarpophalangeal joint
Yángchí (TE4)	In the posterior region of the wrist, on the distal transverse crease of the dorsal wrist, in the depression of the ulnar margin of the tendon of extensor digitorum

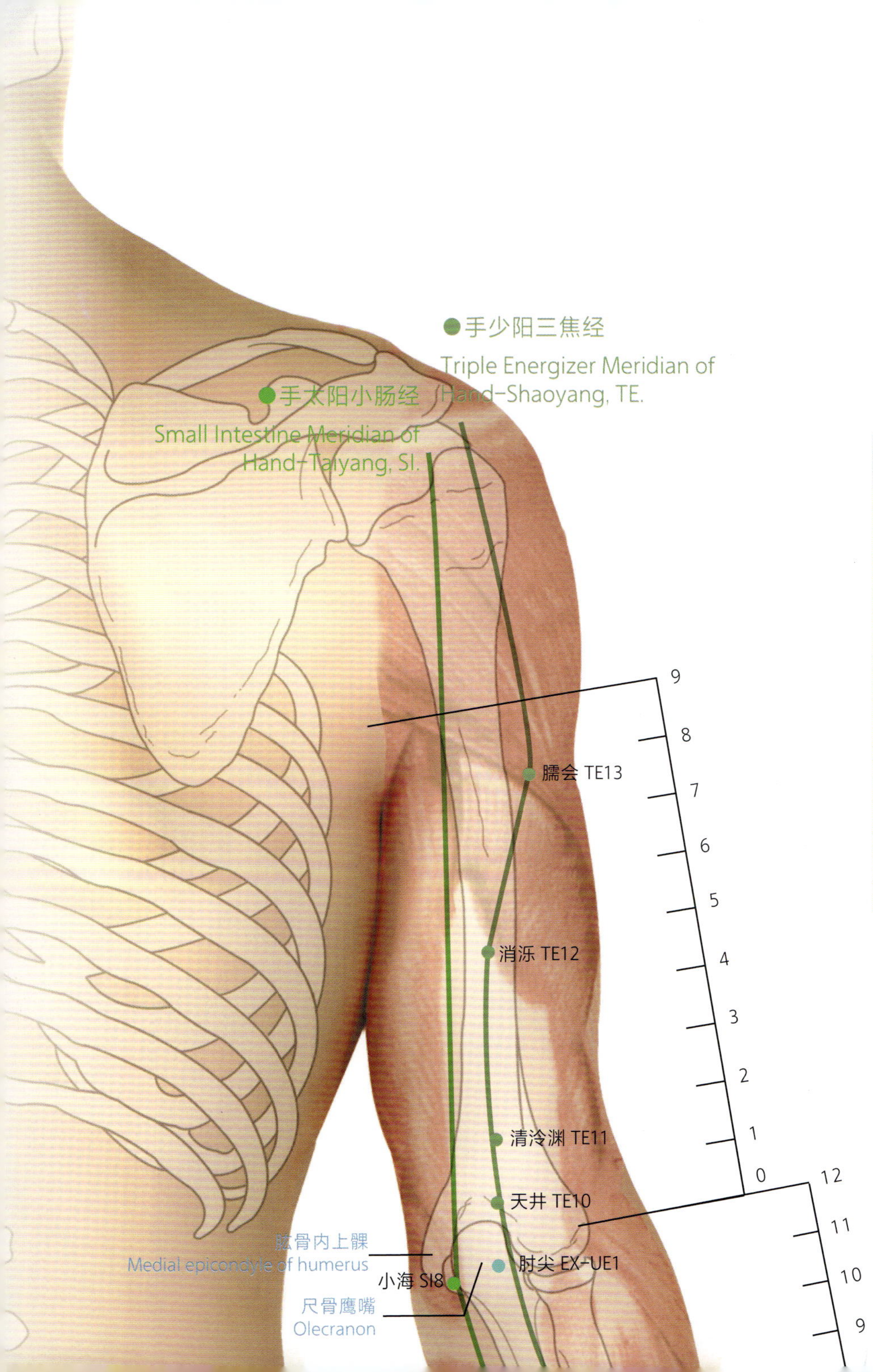

续表

穴位	定位
外关	在前臂后区，腕背侧远端横纹上 2 寸，尺骨与桡骨间隙中点
支沟	在前臂后区，腕背侧远端横纹上 3 寸，尺骨与桡骨间隙中点
会宗	在前臂后区，腕背侧远端横纹上 3 寸，尺骨的桡侧缘
三阳络	在前臂后区，腕背侧远端横纹上 4 寸，尺骨与桡骨间隙中点
四渎	前臂后区，肘尖下 5 寸，尺骨与桡骨间隙中点
天井	在肘后区，肘尖上 1 寸凹陷中
清泠渊	在臂后区，肘尖与肩峰角连线上，肘尖上 2 寸
消泺	在臂后区，肘尖与肩峰角连线上，肘尖上 5 寸
臑会	在臂后区，肩峰角下 3 寸，三角肌的后下缘

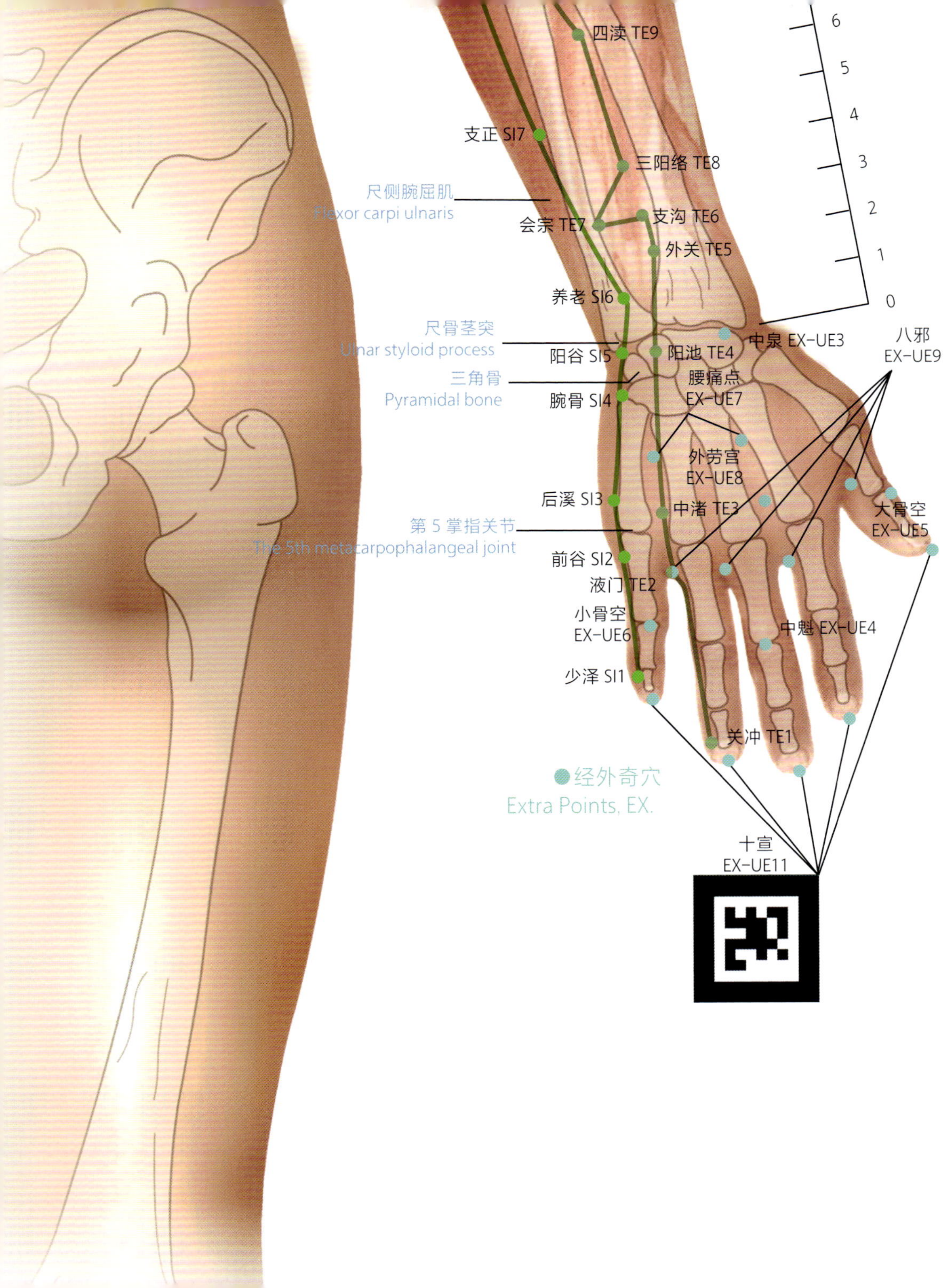

Continued

Acupoints	Location
Wàiguān (TE5)	In the posterior region of the forearm, 2 cun above the distal transverse crease of the dorsal wrist, at the midpoint of the ulna and the radius
Zhīgōu (TE6)	In the posterior region of the forearm, 3 cun above the distal transverse crease of the dorsal wrist, at the midpoint of the ulna and the radius
Huìzōng (TE7)	In the posterior region of the forearm, 3 cun above the distal transverse crease of the dorsal wrist, in the radial margin of the ulna
Sānyángluò (TE8)	In the posterior region of the forearm, 4 cun above the distal transverse crease of the dorsal wrist, at the midpoint of the ulna and the radius
Sìdú (TE9)	In the posterior region of the forearm, 5 cun below the tip of the elbow, at the midpoint of the ulna and the radius
Tiānjǐng (TE10)	In the posterior region of the elbow, in the depression 1 cun above the tip of the elbow
Qīnglíngyuān (TE11)	In the posterior region of the arm, on the line between the tip of the elbow and the acromial angle, 2 cun above the tip of the elbow
Xiāoluò (TE12)	In the posterior region of the upper arm, on the line between the tip of the elbow and the acromial angle, 5 cun above the tip of the elbow
Nàohuì (TE13)	In the posterior region of the arm, 3 cun below the acromial angle, in the posterior margin of the deltoid

下肢部穴位

Acupoints of Lower Limbs

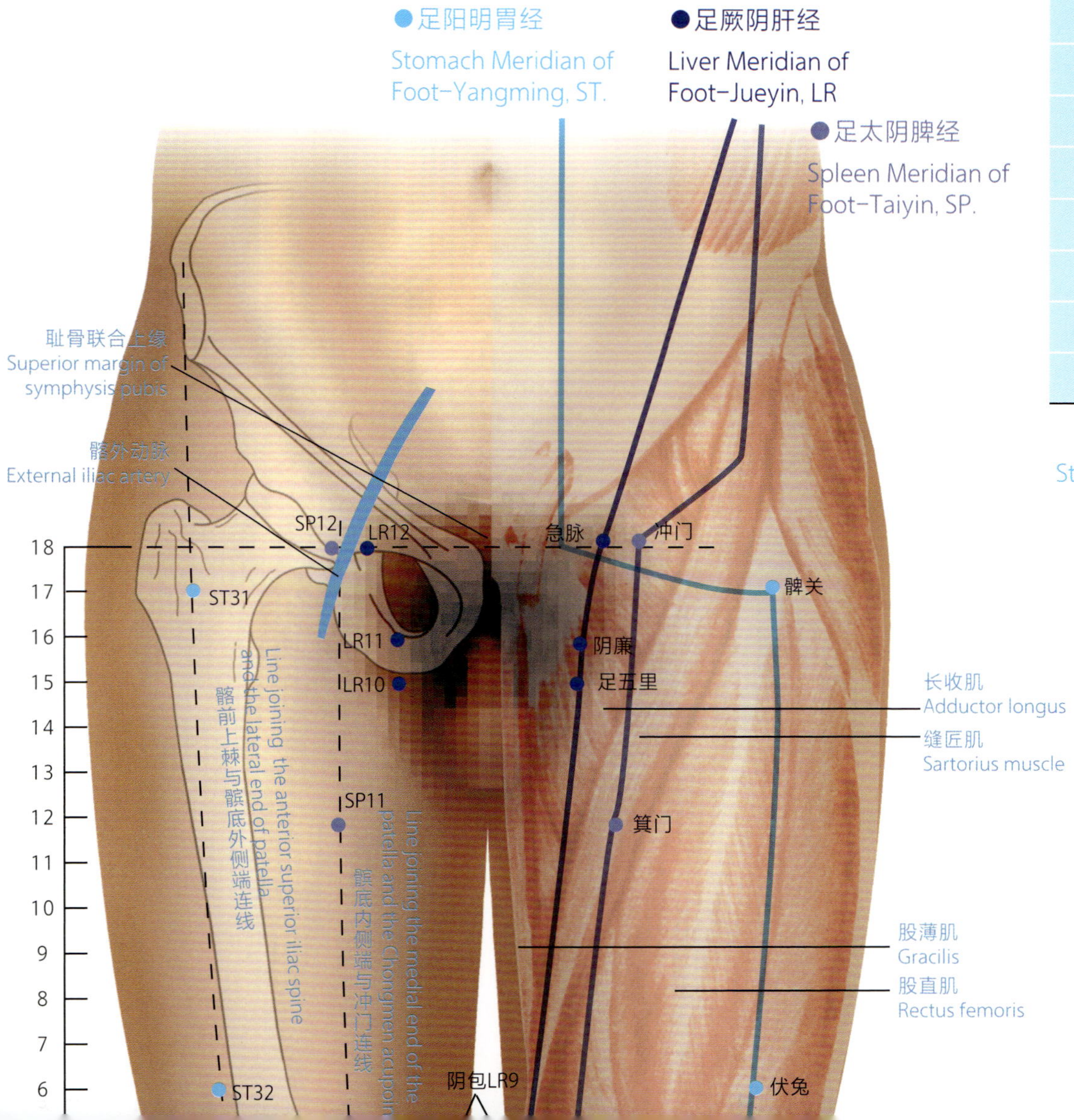

穴位	定位
髀关	在股前区，股直肌近端，缝匠肌与阔筋膜张肌 3 条肌肉之间凹陷中
伏兔	在股前区，髌底上 6 寸，髂前上棘与髌底外侧端的连线上
阴市	在股前区，髌底上 3 寸，股直肌肌腱外侧缘
梁丘	在股前区，髌底上 2 寸，股外侧肌与股直肌肌腱之间
犊鼻	在膝前区，髌韧带外侧凹陷中
足三里	在小腿前外侧，犊鼻下 3 寸，犊鼻与解溪连线上
上巨虚	在小腿外侧，犊鼻下 6 寸，犊鼻与解溪连线上
条口	在小腿外侧，犊鼻下 8 寸，犊鼻与解溪连线上
下巨虚	在小腿外侧，犊鼻下 9 寸，犊鼻与解溪连线上
丰隆	在小腿外侧，外踝尖上 8 寸，胫骨前缘的外侧

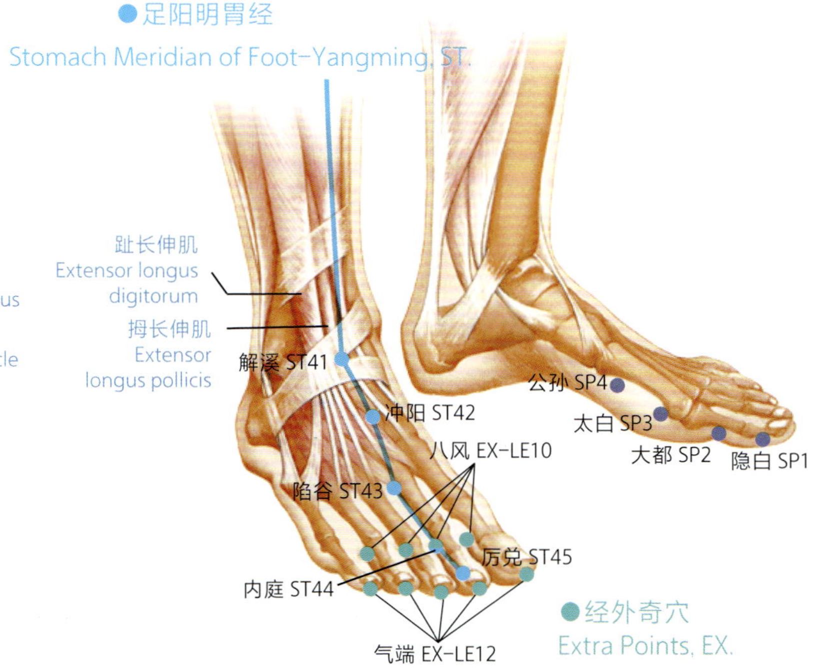

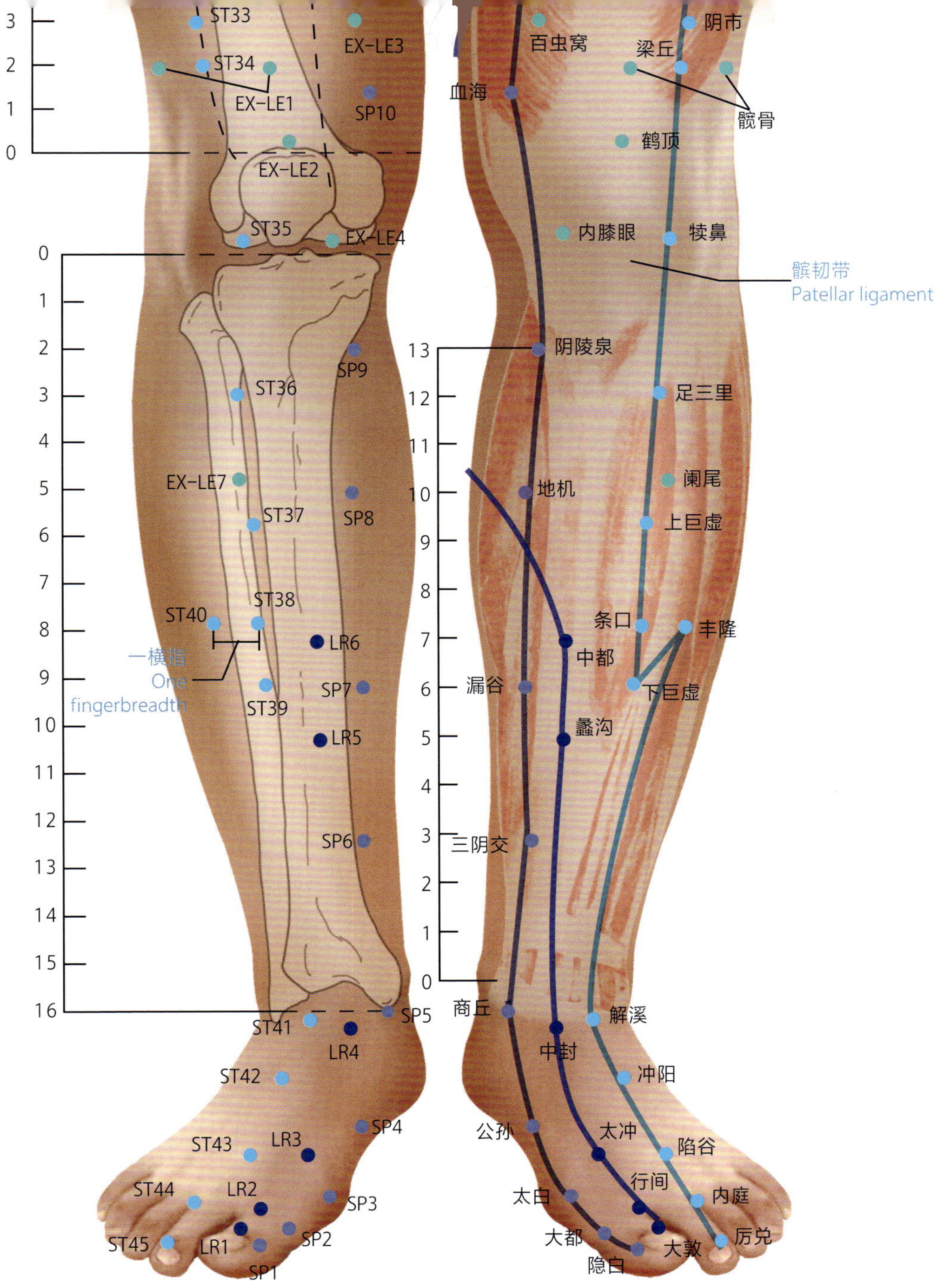

Acupoints	Location
Bìguān (ST31)	In the anterior region of the thigh, in the proximal rectus femoris, in the depression between the sartorius and three muscles of the tensor fasciae latae
Fútù (ST32)	In the anterior region of the thigh, 6 cun above the base of patella, on the line between the anterior superior iliac spine and the lateral end of the base of patella
Yīnshì (ST33)	In the anterior region of the thigh, 3 cun above the base of patella, in the lateral margin of the tendon of rectus femoris
Liángqiū (ST34)	In the anterior region of the thigh, 2 cun above the base of patella, in the middle of the vastus lateralis and the tendon of rectus femoris
Dúbí (ST35)	In the anterior region of the knee, in the lateral depression of the patellar tendon
Zúsānlǐ (ST36)	In the anterior-lateral side of crus, 3 cun below the Dubi acupoint, on the line between the Dubi acupoint and the Jiexi acupoint
Shàngjùxū (ST37)	In the lateral side of crus, 6 cun below the Dubi acupoint, on the line between the Dubi acupoint and the Jiexi acupoint
Tiáokǒu (ST38)	In the lateral side of crus, 8 cun below the Dubi acupoint, on the line between the Dubi acupoint and the Jiexi acupoint
Xiàjùxū (ST39)	In the lateral side of crus, 9 cun below the Dubi acupoint, on the line between the Dubi acupoint and the Jiexi acupoint
Fēnglóng (ST40)	In the lateral side of crus, 8 cun above the prominence of lateral malleolus, in the lateral side of the anterior margin of the tibia

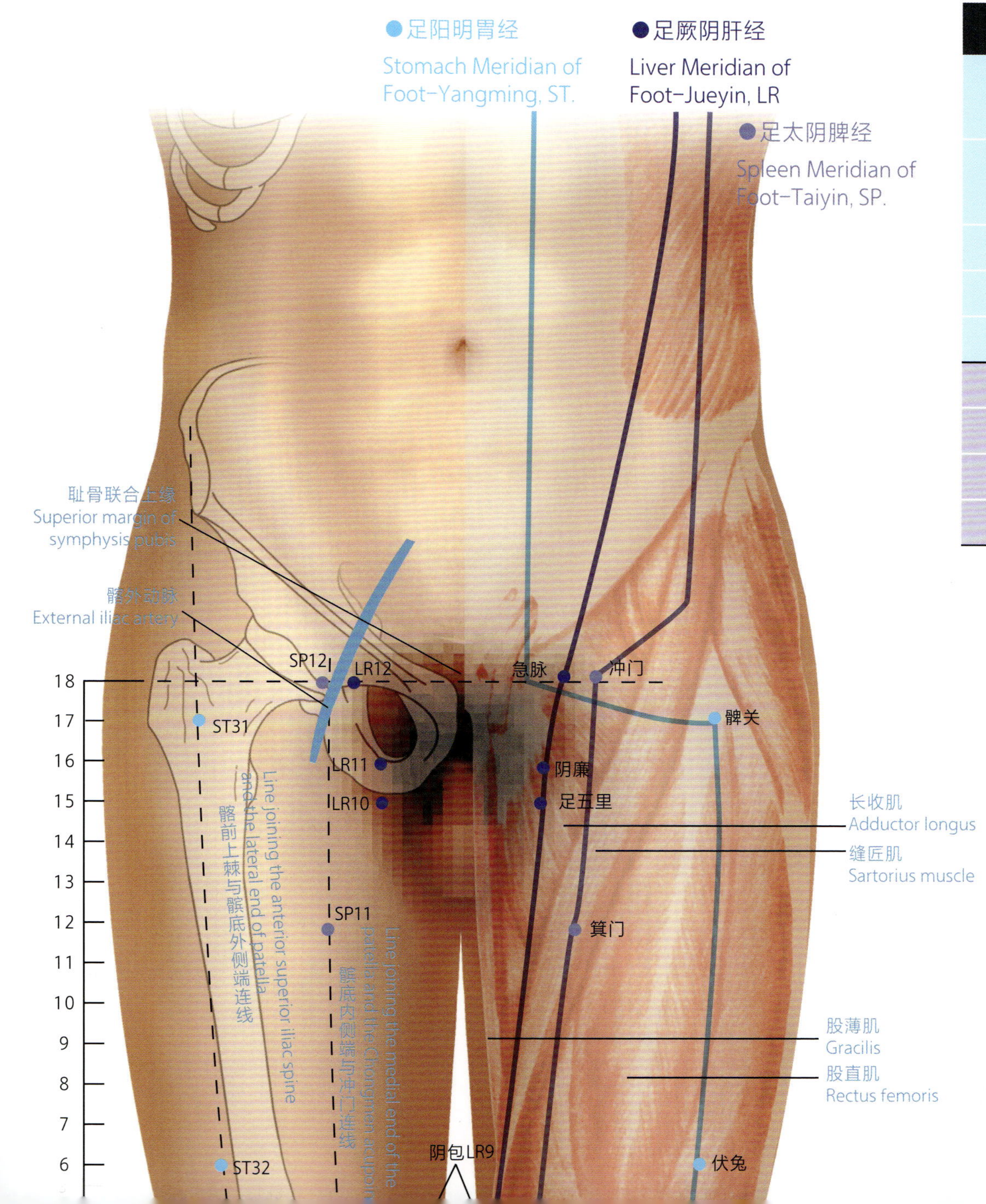

续表

穴位	定位
解溪	在踝部，踝关节前面中央凹陷中，当拇长伸肌腱与趾长伸肌腱之间
冲阳	在足背，第 2 跖骨基底部与中间楔状骨关节处，可触及足背动脉
陷谷	在足背，当第 2、3 跖骨间，第 2 跖趾关节近端凹陷中
内庭	在足背，第 2、3 趾间，趾蹼缘后方赤白肉际处
厉兑	在足趾，第 2 趾末节外侧，趾甲根角侧后方 0.1 寸（指寸）
隐白	在足趾，大趾末节内侧，趾甲根角侧后方 0.1 寸（指寸）
大都	在足趾，第 1 跖趾关节远端赤白肉际凹陷中
太白	在跖区，第 1 跖趾关节近端赤白肉际凹陷中
公孙	在跖区，第 1 跖骨底的前下缘赤白肉际处

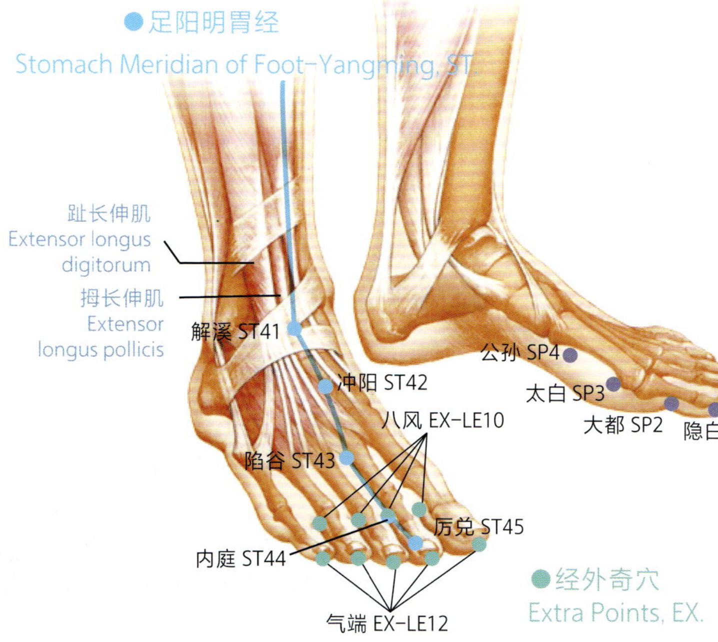

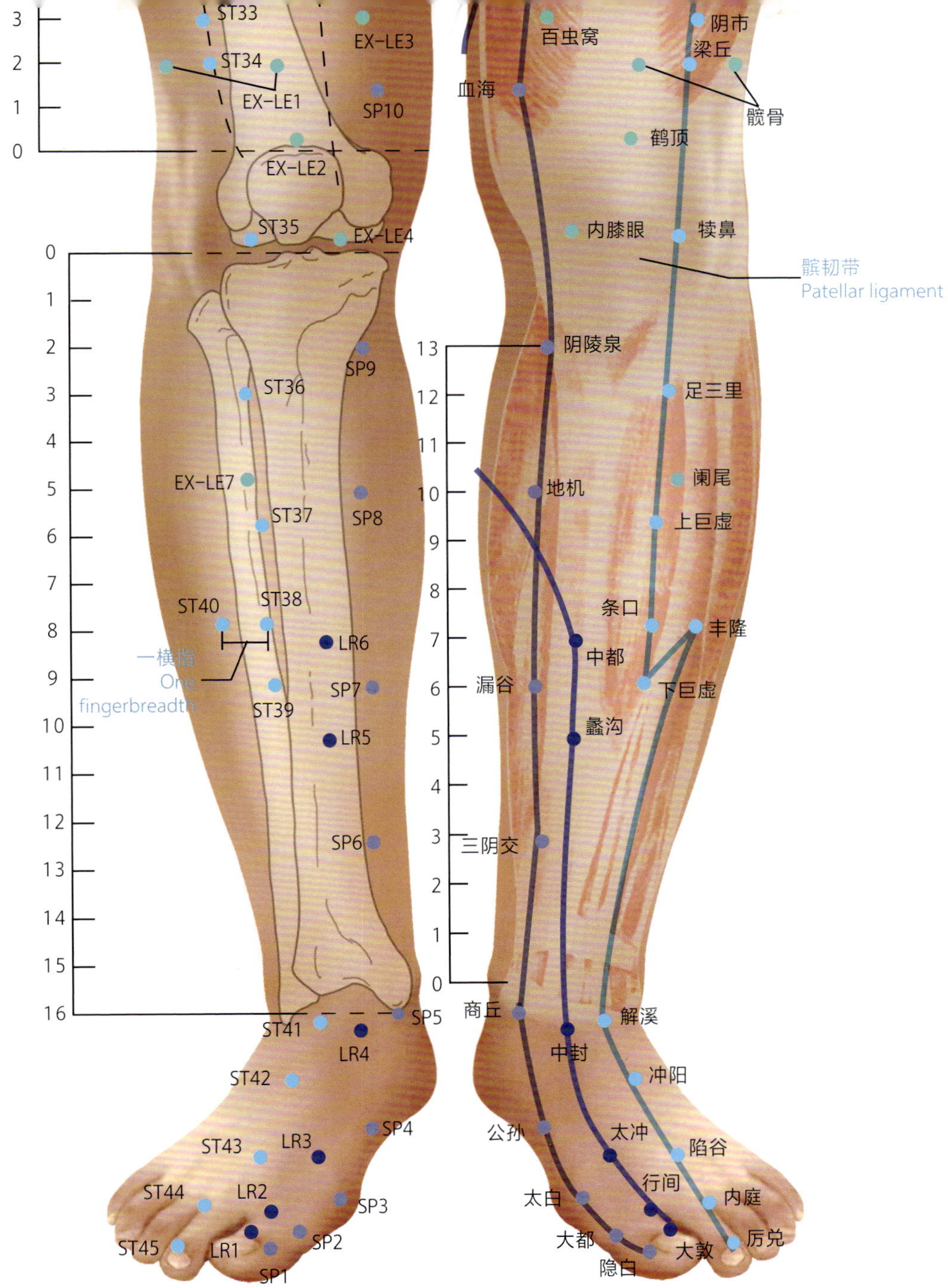

Continued

Acupoints	Location
Jiěxī (ST41)	In the region of the ankle, in the medial depression of the anterior side of ankle joint, between the tendon of extensor pollicis longus and the tendon of extensor digitorum longus
Chōngyáng (ST42)	On the dorsum of foot, between the 2nd metatarsal base and the joint of middle sphenoid bone where dorsal artery of foot can be palpated
Xiàngǔ (ST43)	On the dorsum of foot, between the 2nd and the 3rd metatarsal bone, in the proximal depression of the 2nd metatarsophalangeal joint
Nèitíng (ST44)	On the dorsum of foot, between the 2nd and the 3rd toe, at the junction of the red and white skin posterior to the border of web
Lìduì (ST45)	On the toe, in the lateral side of the end of the 2nd toe, 0.1 cun lateral and posterior to the corner of the nail
Yǐnbái (SP1)	On the toe, in the interior aspect of the end of the great toe, 0.1 cun lateral and posterior to the corner of the nail
Dàdū (SP2)	On the toe, in the depression at the junction of the red and white skin of the distal end of the 1st metatarsophalangeal joint
Tàibái (SP3)	On the sole of foot, in the depression at the junction of the red and white skin of the proximal end of the 1st metatarsophalangeal joint
Gōngsūn (SP4)	On the sole of foot, at the junction of the red and white skin anterior and inferior to the base of the 1st metatarsal bone

续表

穴位	定位
商丘	在踝区，内踝前下方，舟骨粗隆与内踝尖连线中点凹陷中
三阴交	在小腿内侧，内踝尖上 3 寸，胫骨内侧缘后际
漏谷	在小腿内侧，内踝尖上 6 寸，胫骨内侧缘后际
地机	在小腿内侧，阴陵泉下 3 寸，胫骨内侧缘后际
阴陵泉	在小腿内侧，胫骨内侧髁下缘与胫骨内侧缘之间的凹陷中
血海	在股前区，髌底内侧端上 2 寸，股内侧肌隆起处
箕门	在股前区，髌底内侧端与冲门的连线上 1/3 与下 2/3 交点，长收肌和缝匠肌交角的动脉搏动处
冲门	在腹股沟区，腹股沟斜纹中，髂外动脉搏动处的外侧

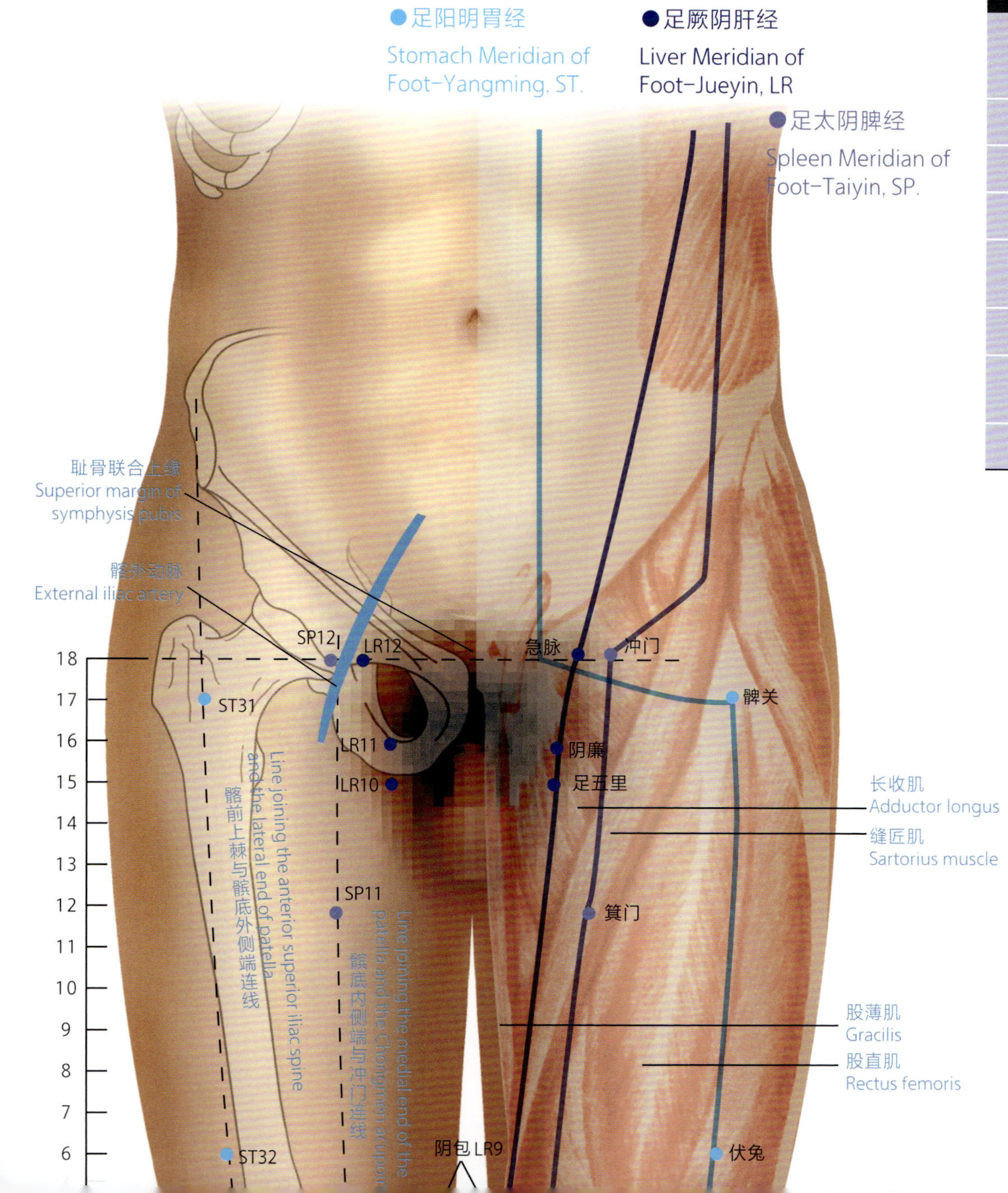

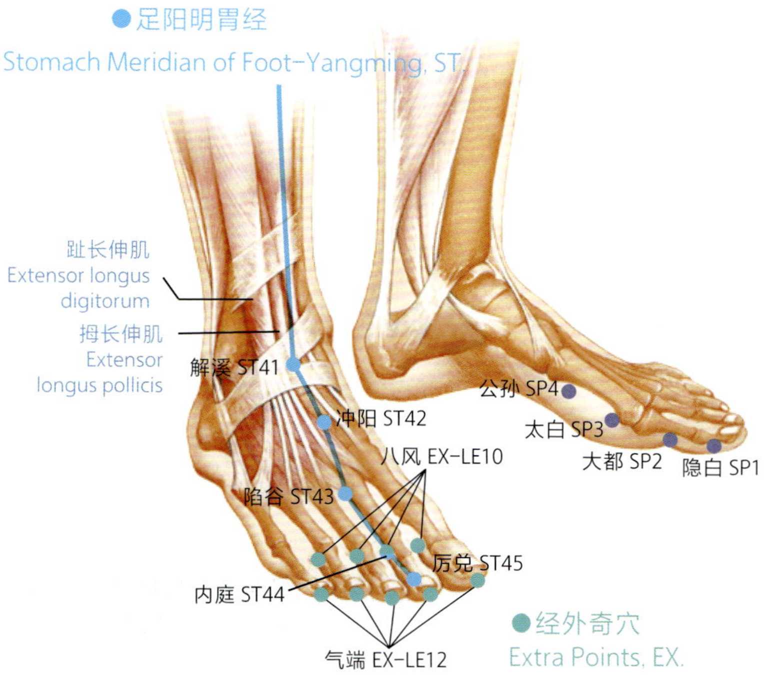

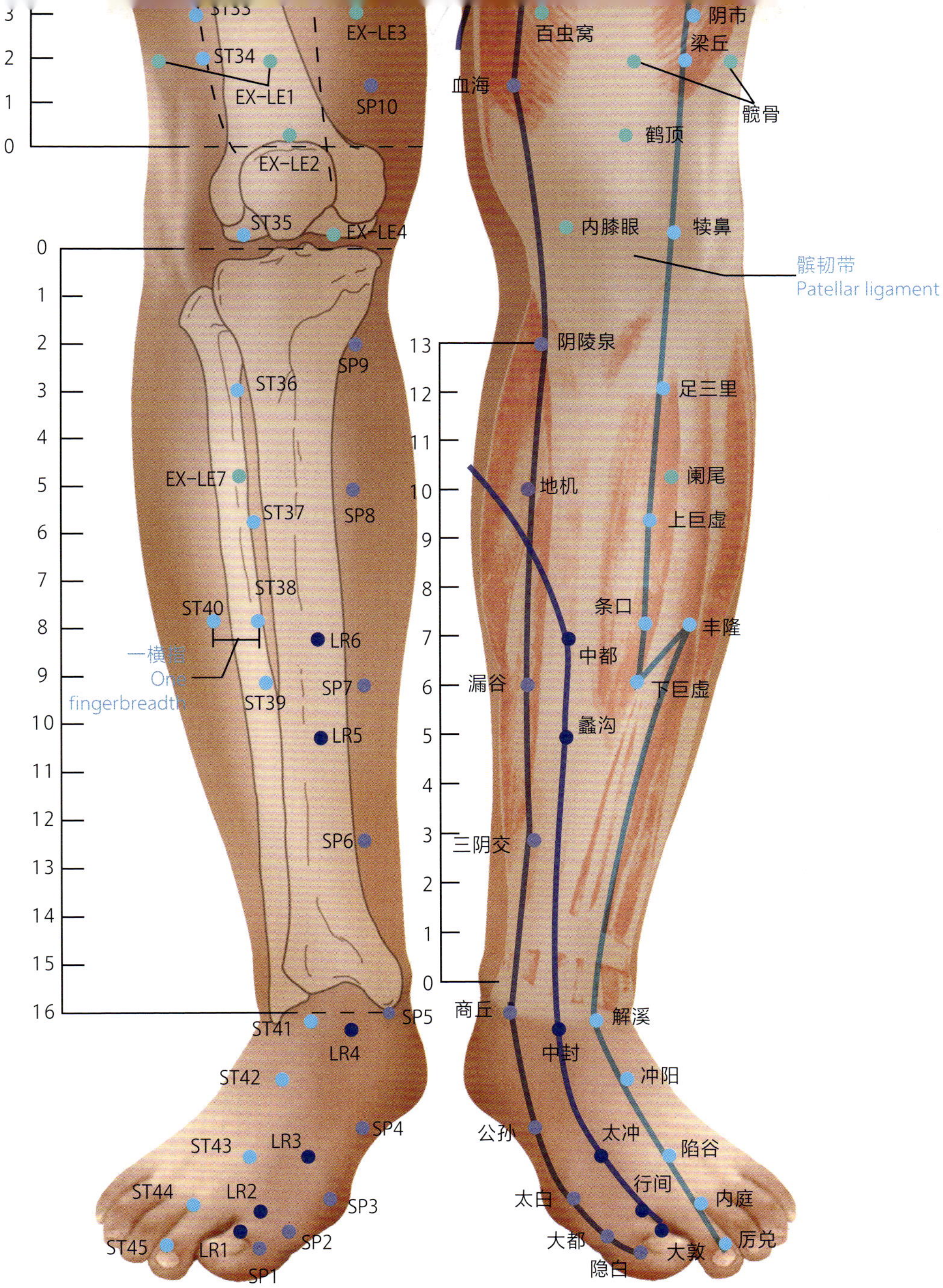

Continued

Acupoints	Location
Shāngqiū (SP5)	In the region of the ankle, anterior and inferior to the medial malleolus, in the depression at the midpoint of line between the tuberosity of navicular bone and the tip of the medial malleolus
Sānyīnjiāo (SP6)	In the interior side of the crus, 3 cun above the tip of the medial malleolus, in the posterior border of the interior margin of the tibia
Lòugǔ (SP7)	In the interior side of the crus, 6 cun above the tip of the medial malleolus, in the posterior border of the interior margin of the tibia
Dìjī (SP8)	In the interior side of the crus, 3 cun below the Yinlingquan acupoint, in the posterior border of the interior margin of the tibia
Yīnlíngquán (SP9)	In the interior side of the crus, in the depression between the inferior margin of the medial tibial condyle and the interior margin of the tibia
Xuèhǎi (SP10)	In the anterior region of the thigh, 2 cun above the interior side of the base of patella, at the bump of the medial vastus muscle
Jīmén (SP11)	In the anterior region of the thigh, at the junction of upper 1/3 and lower 2/3 on the line between Chongmen acupoint and interior side of the base of patella, on the angle of intersection of adductor longus and sartorius where the pulse can be palpated
Chōngmén (SP12)	In the region of the groin, in the inguinal twill, at the lateral side of the pulse of external iliac artery

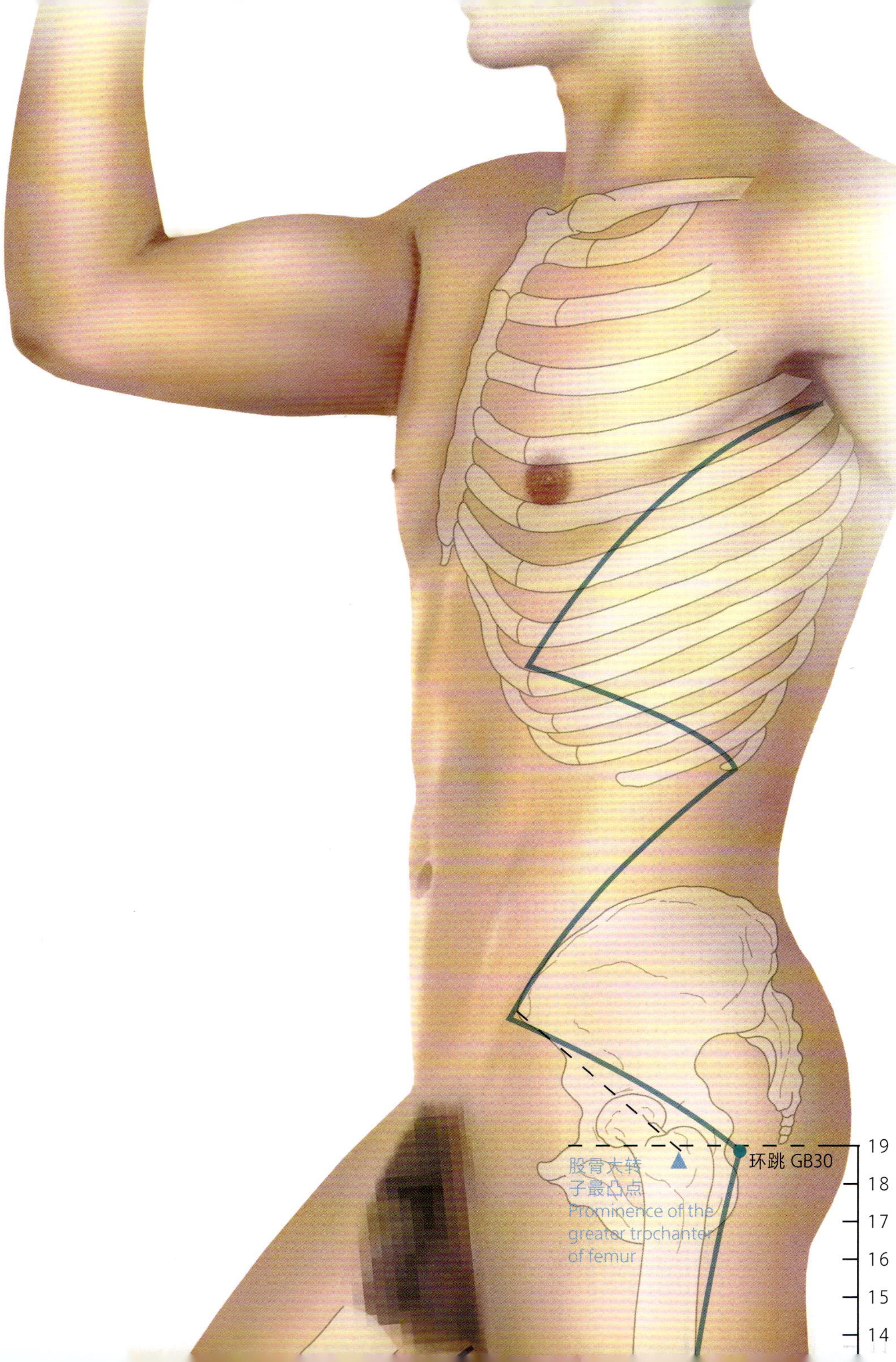

续表

穴位	定位
殷门	在股后区，臀沟下 6 寸，股二头肌与半腱肌之间
浮郄	在膝后区，腘横纹上 1 寸，股二头肌腱的内侧缘
委阳	在膝部，腘横纹上，股二头肌腱的内侧缘
委中	在膝后区，腘横纹中点
合阳	在小腿后区，腘横纹下 2 寸，腓肠肌内、外侧头之间
承筋	在小腿后区，腘横纹下 5 寸，腓肠肌两肌腹之间
承山	在小腿后区，腓肠肌两肌腹与肌腱交角处
飞扬	在小腿后区，昆仑直上 7 寸，腓肠肌外下缘与跟腱移行处
跗阳	在小腿后区，昆仑直上 3 寸，腓骨与跟腱之间

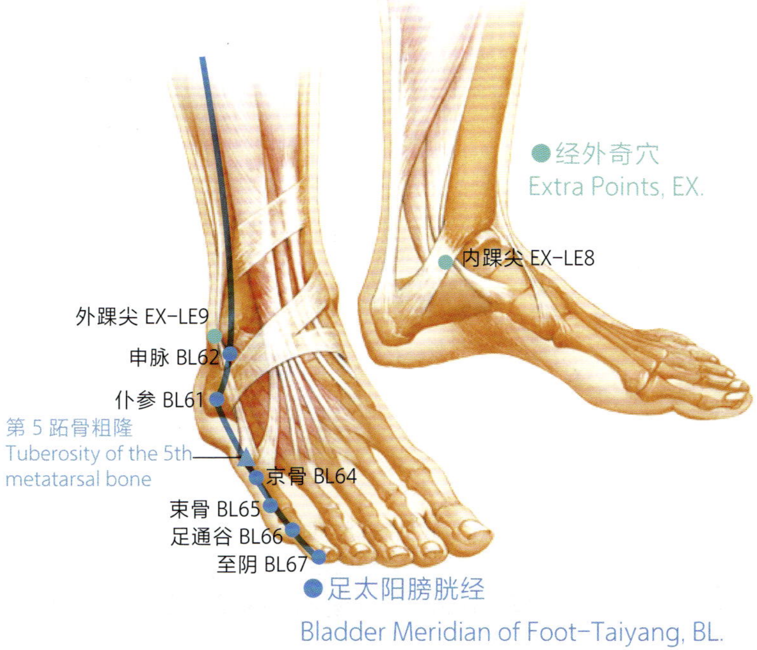

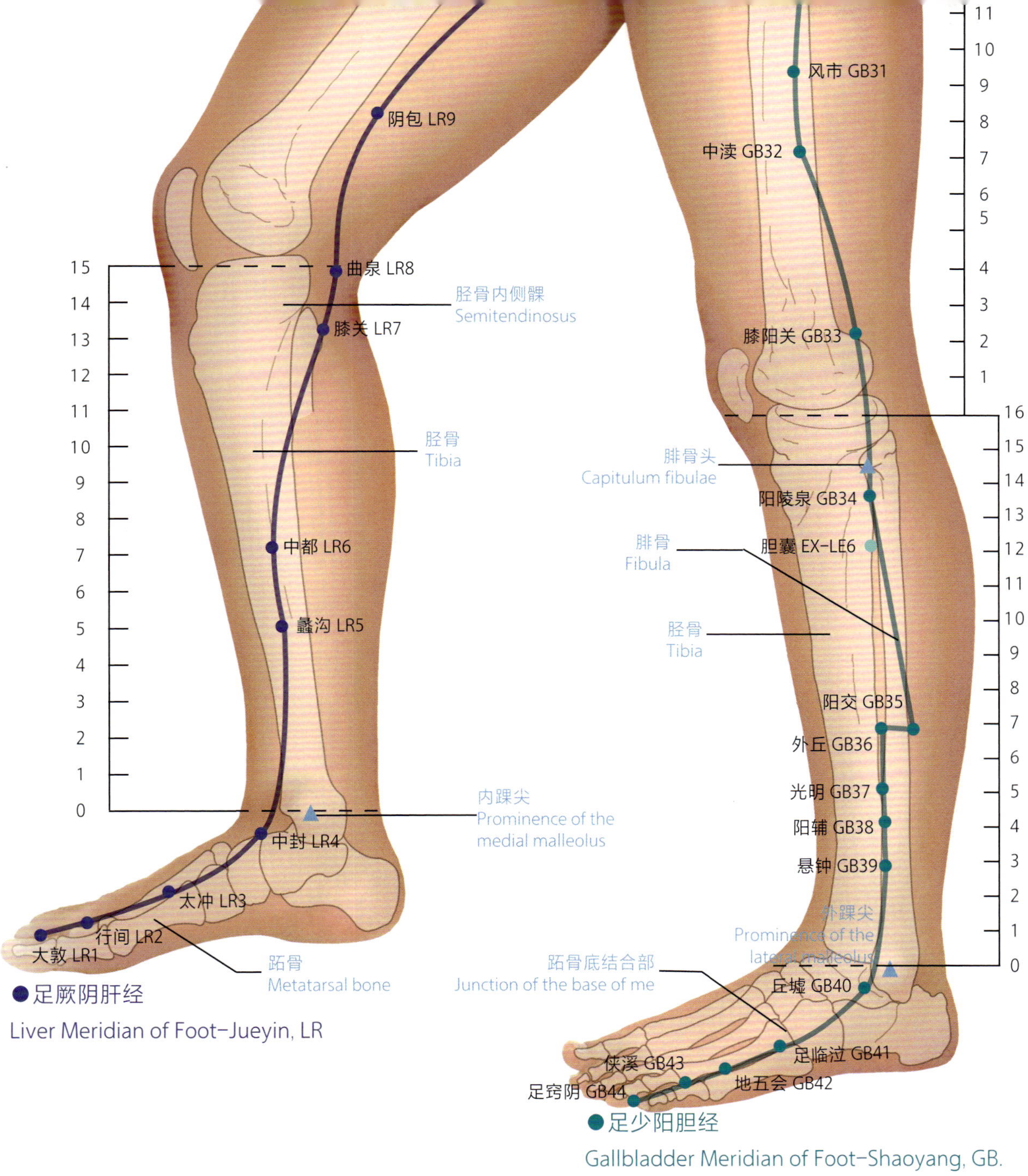

Continued

Acupoints	Location
Yīnmén (BL37)	In the posterior region of the thigh, 6 cun below the gluteal fold, between the biceps femoris muscle and the semitendinosus
Fúxì (BL38)	In the posterior region of the knee, 1 cun above the popliteal crease, in the medial margin of the biceps femoris tendon
Wěiyáng (BL39)	In the region of the knee, in the popliteal crease, in the medial margin of the biceps femoris tendon
Wěizhōng (BL40)	In the posterior region of the knee, at the midpoint of the popliteal crease
Héyáng (BL55)	In the posterior region of crus, 2 cun below the popliteal crease, between the lateral head and the medial head of gastrocnemius
Chéngjīn (BL56)	In the posterior region of crus, 5 cun below the popliteal crease, between the two gastrocnemius muscle bellies
Chéngshān (BL57)	In the posterior region of crus, at the junction between two gastrocnemius muscle bellies and the tendon
Fēiyáng (BL58)	In the posterior region of crus, 7 cun directly above the Kunlun acupoint, at the junction of the lateral and inferior margin of the gastrocnemius and the tendon
Fūyáng (BL59)	In the posterior region of crus, 3 cun directly above the Kunlun acupoint, between the fibula and the tendon

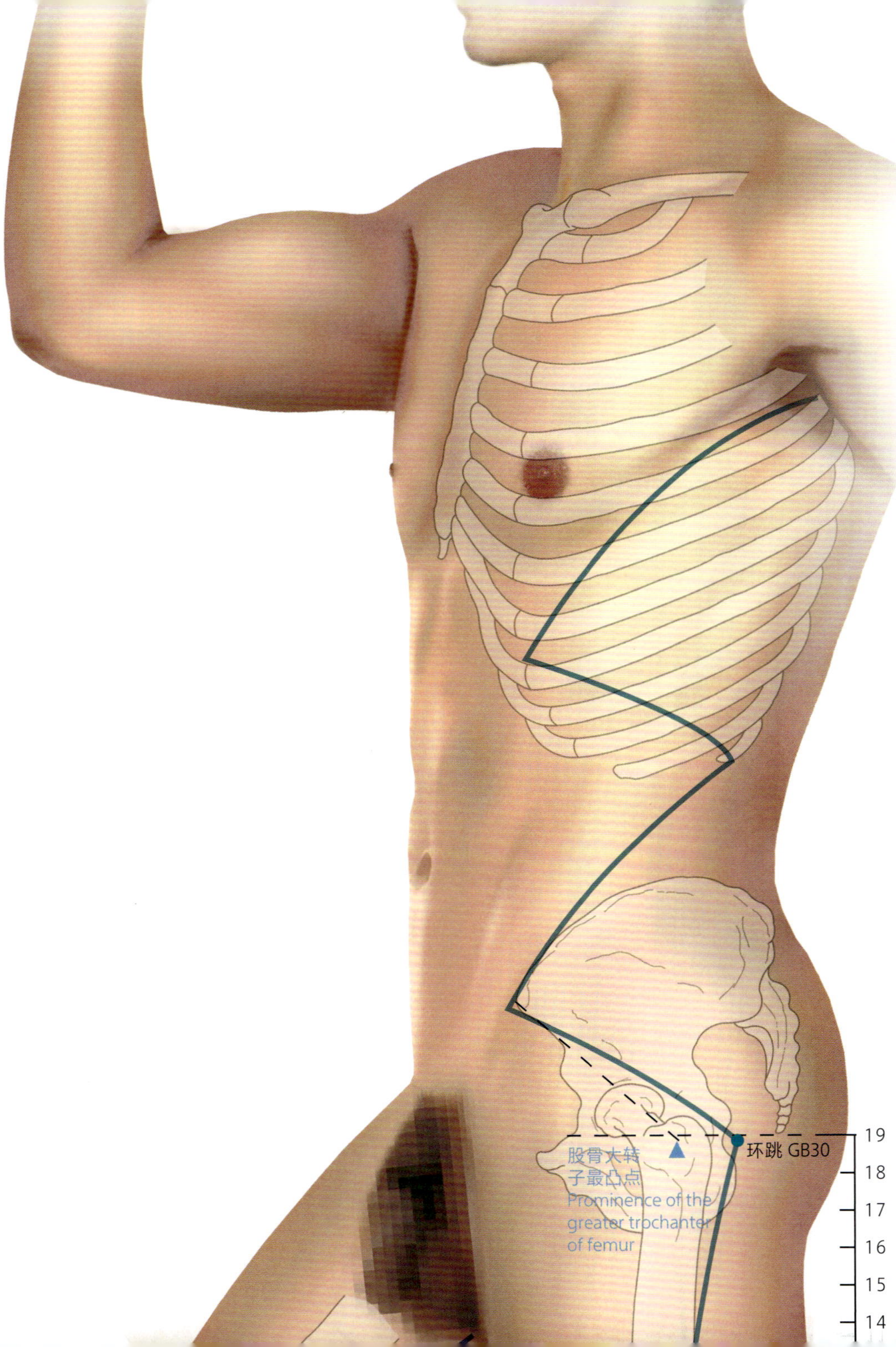

续表

穴位	定位
昆仑	在踝区，外踝尖与跟腱之间的凹陷中
仆参	在跟区，昆仑直下，跟骨外侧，赤白肉际处
申脉	在踝区，外踝尖直下，外踝下缘与跟骨之间凹陷中
金门	在足背，外踝前缘直下。第 5 跖骨粗隆后方，骰骨下缘凹陷中
京骨	在跖区，第 5 跖骨粗隆前下方，赤白肉际处
束骨	在跖区，第 5 跖趾关节的近端，赤白肉际处
足通谷	在跖区，第 5 跖趾关节的远端，赤白肉际处
至阴	在足趾，小趾末节外侧，趾甲根角侧后方 0.1 寸（指寸）

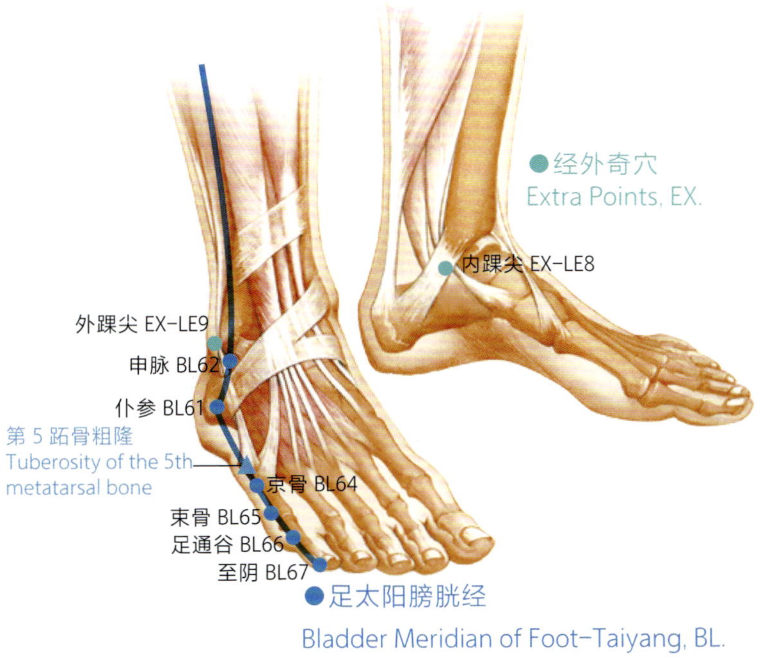

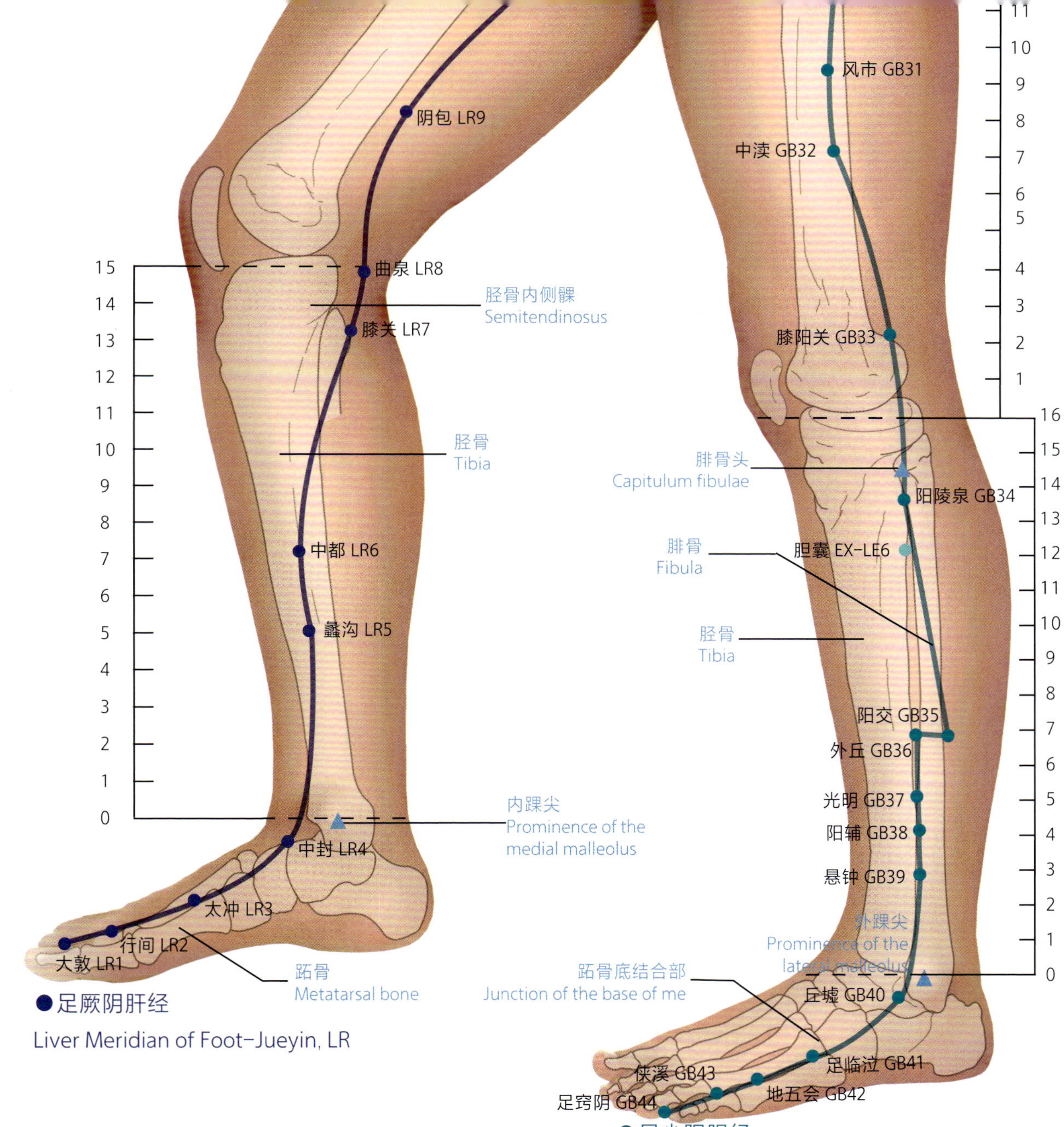

●足厥阴肝经

Liver Meridian of Foot-Jueyin, LR

●足少阳胆经

Gallbladder Meridian of Foot-Shaoyang, GB.

Continued

Acupoints	Location
Kūnlún (BL60)	In the region of the ankle, in the fossa between the tendon and the prominence of lateral malleolus
Púcān (BL61)	In the region of the heel, right below the Kunlun acupoint, in the side of the calcaneus, at the junction of the red and white skin
Shēnmài (BL62)	In the region of the ankle, directly below the tip of the lateral malleolus, in the depression between the inferior margin of the lateral malleolus and the calcaneus
Jīnmén (BL63)	On the dorsum of the foot, directly below the anterior prominence of lateral malleolus. In the posterior side of the tuberosity of the 5th metatarsal bone, in the depression of the inferior margin of the cuboid bone
Jīnggǔ (BL64)	On the sole of foot, in the anterior and inferior side of the tuberosity of the 5th metatarsal bone, at the junction of the red and white skin
Shùgǔ (BL65)	On the sole of foot, in the proximal side of the 5th metatarsophalangeal joint, at the junction of the red and white skin
Zútōnggǔ (BL66)	On the sole of foot, in the distal side of the 5th metatarsophalangeal joint, at the junction of the red and white skin
Zhìyīn (BL67)	On the toe, in the lateral side of the tip of little toe, 0.1 cun lateral and posterior to the corner of the nail

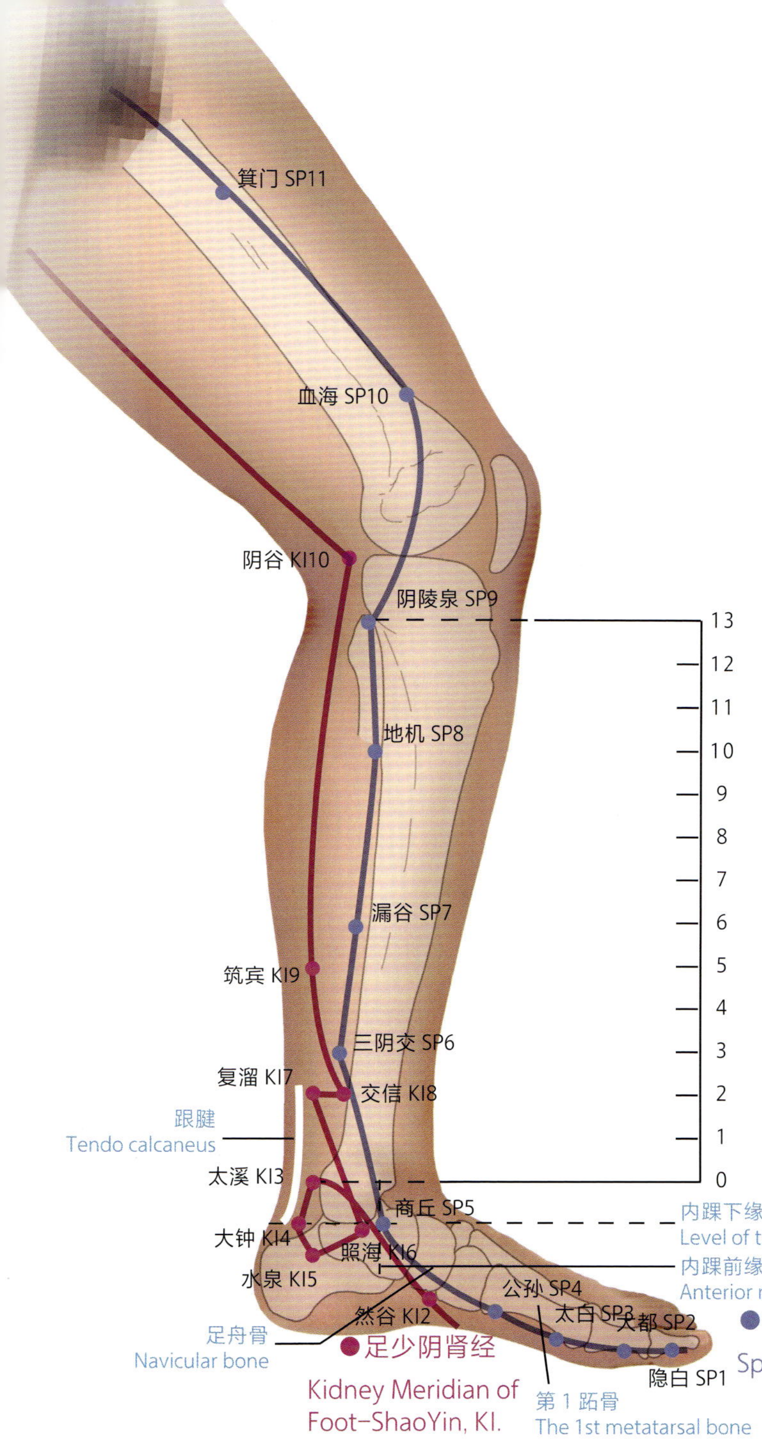

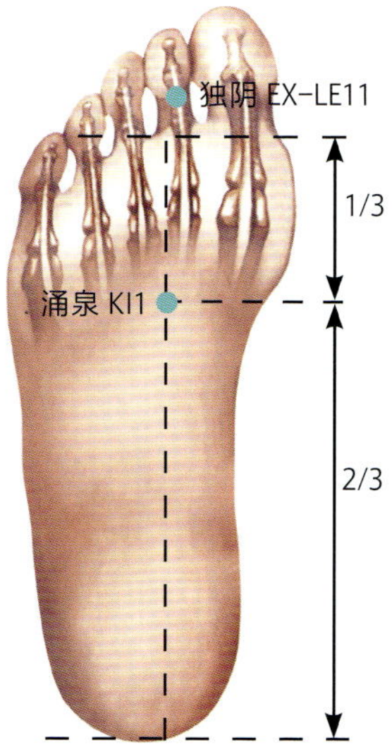

续表

穴位	定位
涌泉	在足底，屈足卷趾时足心最凹陷中
然谷	在足内侧，足舟骨粗隆下方，赤白肉际处
太溪	在踝区，内踝尖与跟腱之间的凹陷中
大钟	在跟区，内踝后下方，跟骨上缘，跟腱附着部前缘凹陷中
水泉	在跟区，太溪直下 1 寸，跟骨结节内侧凹陷中
照海	在踝区，内踝尖下 1 寸，内踝下缘边际凹陷中
复溜	在小腿内侧，内踝尖直上 2 寸，跟腱的前缘
交信	在小腿内侧，内踝尖上 2 寸，胫骨内侧缘后际凹陷中
筑宾	在小腿内侧，太溪直上 5 寸，比目鱼肌与跟腱之间
阴谷	在膝后区，腘横纹上，半腱肌肌腱外侧缘
风市	在股部，直立垂手，掌心贴于大腿时，中指尖所指凹陷中，髂胫束（大腿外侧的筋膜）后缘
中渎	在股部，腘横纹上 7 寸，髂胫束后缘

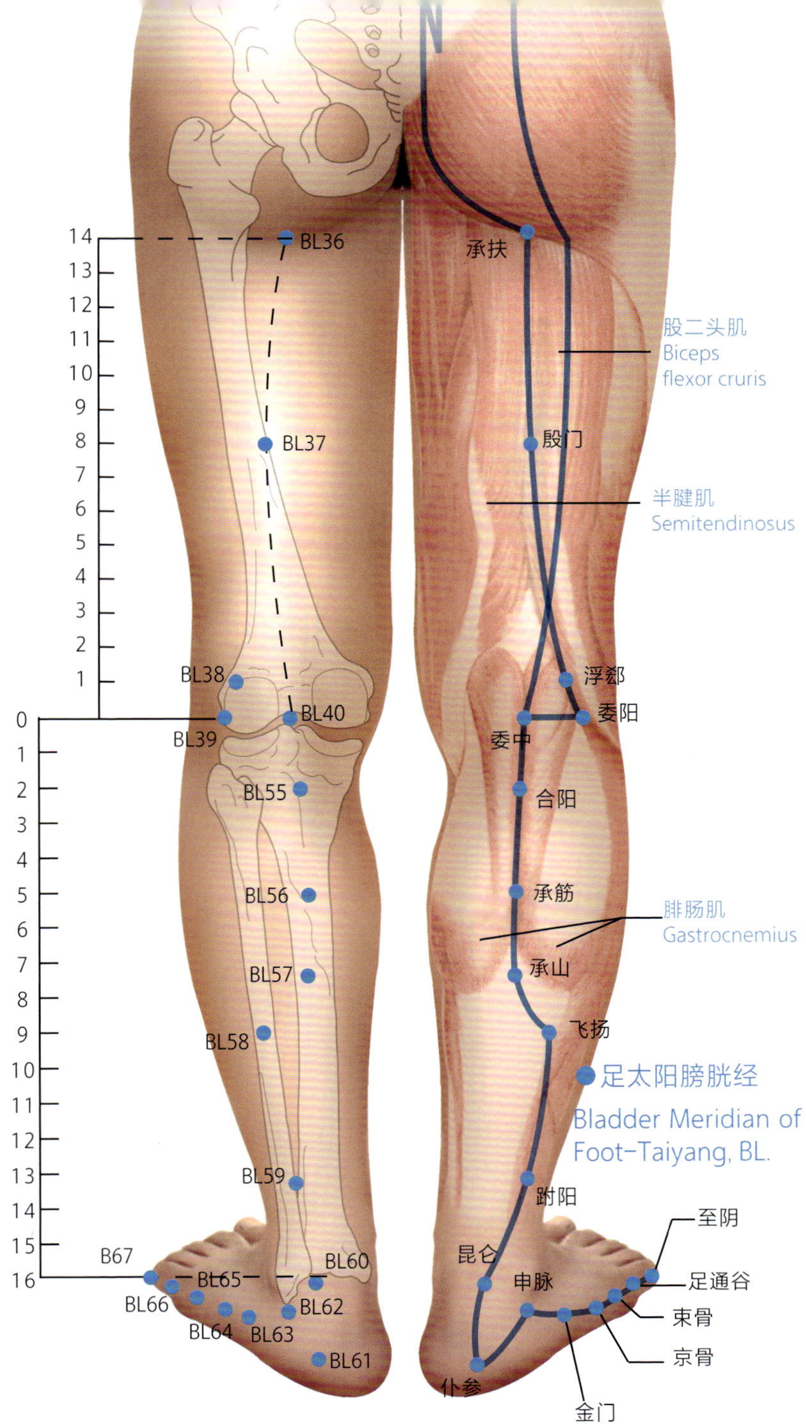

Continued

Acupoints	Location
Yǒngquán(KI1)	On the sole, in the depression occuring when you bend the leg and toes
Rángǔ(KI2)	In the medial region of the foot, below the tuberosity of the navicular bone, at the junction of the red and white skin
Tàixī(KI3)	In the region of the ankle, in the depression between the prominence of the medial malleolus and the tendon calcaneus
Dàzhōng(KI4)	In the region of the heel, posterior and inferior to the medial malleolus, in the superior margin of the calcaneus, in the depression of the anterior margin of the adhesion of the tendon calcaneus
Shuǐquán(KI5)	In the region of the heel, 1 cun directly below the Taixi acupoint, in the depression of the interior side of tubercle of the calcaneus
Zhàohǎi(KI6)	In the region of the ankle, 1 cun below the prominence of the medial malleolus, in the depression of the inferior margin of medial malleolus
Fùliū(KI7)	In the interior region of crus, 2 cun directly above the prominence of medial malleolus, in the anterior margin of tendon calcaneus
Jiāoxìn(KI8)	In the interior region of crus, 2 cun above the prominence of medial malleolus, in the lateral depression of the interior margin of the tibia
Zhùbīn(KI9)	In the interior region of crus, 5 cun directly above the Taixi acupoint, between the tendon calcaneus and the soleus
Yīngǔ(KI10)	In the posterior region of the knee, in the popliteal crease, in the lateral margin between of semitendinosus
Fēngshì(GB31)	In the region of the thigh, when the patient is standing with the hands down and palm affixed to the thigh, the acupoint is in the depression pointed by the middle finger, in the posterior side of iliotibial tract
Zhōngdú(GB32)	In the region of the thigh, 7 cun above the popliteal crease line, in the lateral margin of the iliotibial tract

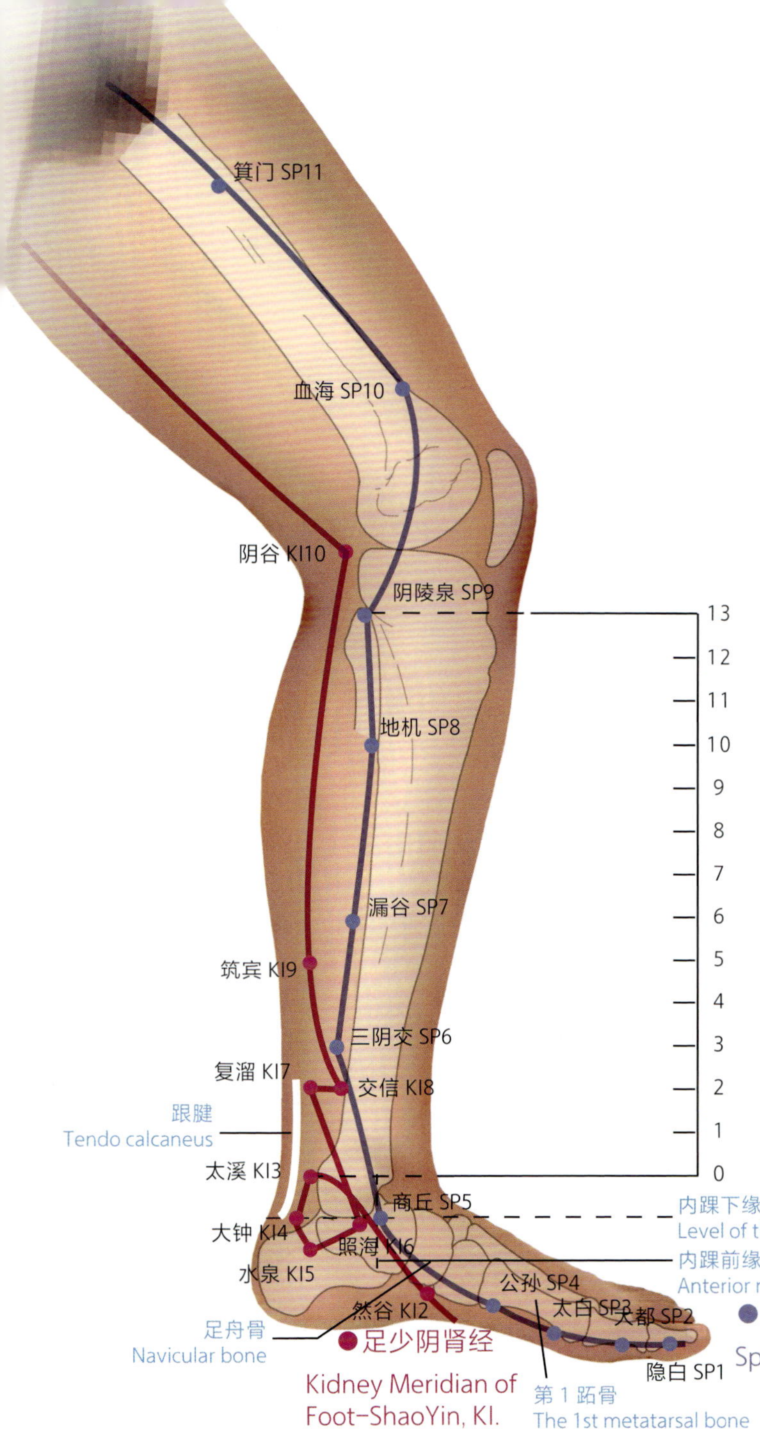

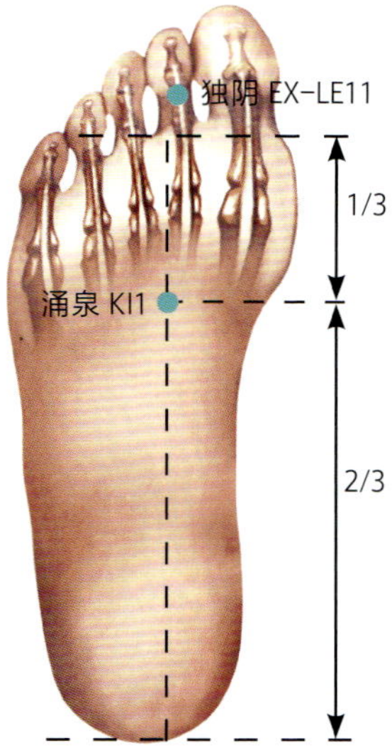

续表

穴位	定位
膝阳关	在膝部，股骨外上髁后上缘，股二头肌腱与髂胫束之间的凹陷中
阳陵泉	在小腿外侧，腓骨头前下方凹陷中
阳交	在小腿外侧，外踝尖上 7 寸，腓骨后缘
外丘	在小腿外侧，外踝尖上 7 寸，腓骨前缘
光明	在小腿外侧，外踝尖上 5 寸，腓骨前缘
阳辅	在小腿外侧，外踝尖上 4 寸，腓骨前缘
悬钟	在小腿外侧，外踝尖上 3 寸，腓骨前缘
丘墟	在踝区，外踝的前下方，趾长伸肌腱的外侧凹陷中
足临泣	在足背，第 4、5 跖骨底结合部的前方，第 5 趾长伸肌腱外侧凹陷中
地五会	在足背，第 4、5 跖骨间，第 4 跖趾关节近端凹陷中
侠溪	在足背，第 4、5 趾间，趾蹼缘后方赤白肉际处
足窍阴	在足趾，第 4 趾末节外侧，趾甲根角侧后方 0.1 寸（指寸）

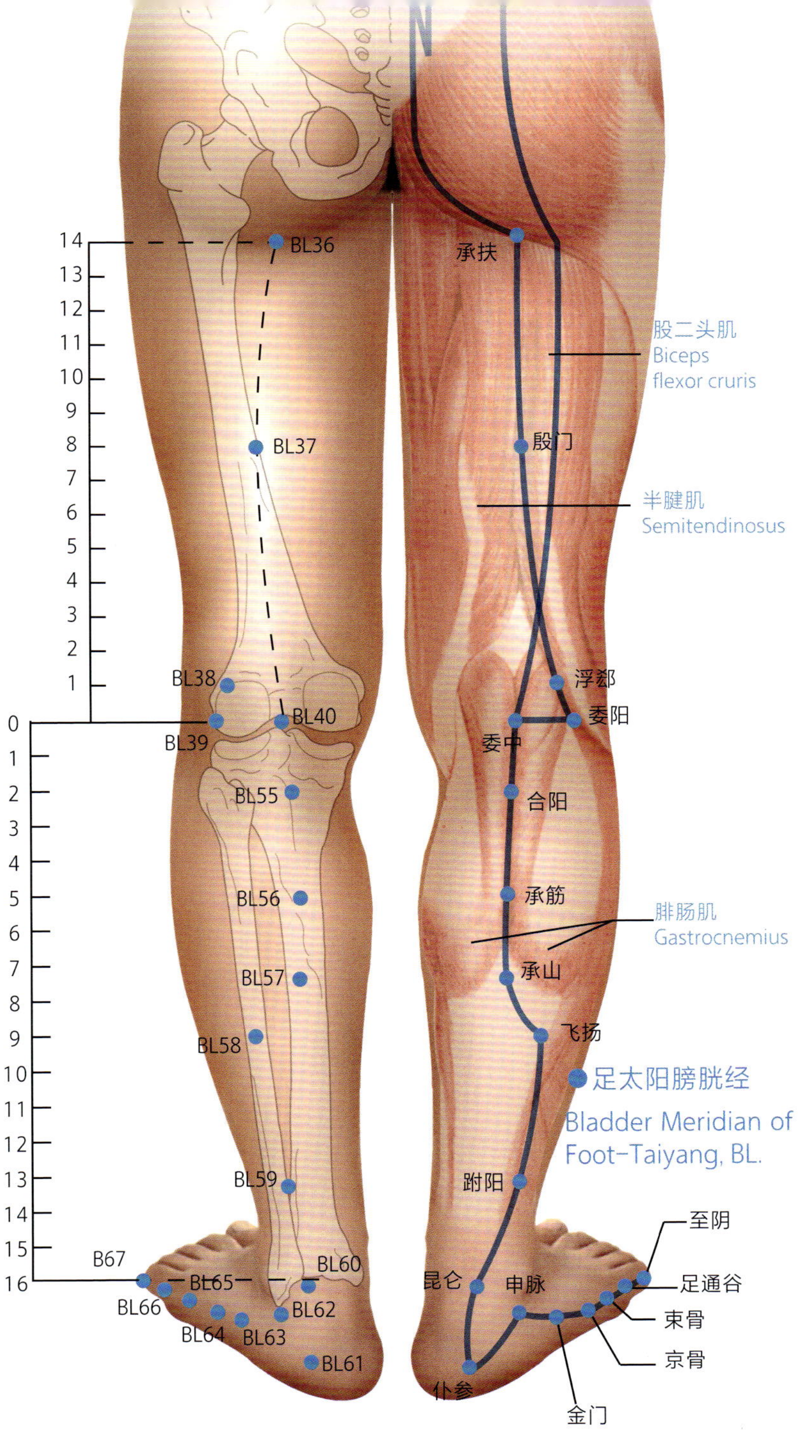

Continued

Acupoints	Location
Xīyángguān(GB33)	In the region of the knee, in the lateral and superior margin of the lateral femoral epicondyle, in the depression of the iliotibial tract and the tendon of biceps femoris
Yánglíngquán(GB34)	In the lateral region of crus, in the anterior and inferior depression of the fibula
Yángjiāo(GB35)	In the lateral region of crus, 7 cun above the prominence of lateral malleolus, in the lateral margin of the fibula
Wàiqiū(GB36)	In the lateral region of crus, 7 cun above the prominence of lateral malleolus, in the anterior margin of the fibula
Guāngmíng(GB37)	In the lateral region of crus, 5 cun above the prominence of lateral malleolus, in the anterior margin of the fibula
Yángfǔ(GB38)	In the lateral region of crus, 4 cun above the prominence of lateral malleolus, in the anterior margin of the fibula
Xuánzhōng(GB39)	In the lateral region of crus, 3 cun above the prominence of lateral malleolus and in the anterior margin of the fibula
Qiūxū(GB40)	In the region of the ankle, anterior and inferior to the lateral malleolus, in the lateral depression of the tendon of extensor digitorum longus
Zúlínqì(GB41)	On the dorsum of the foot, in the anterior side of the junction of the 4th and the 5th metatarsal base joint, in the lateral depression of the tendon of 5th extensor digitorum longus
Dìwǔhuì(GB42)	On the dorsum of the foot, between the 4th and the 5th metatarsal bone, in the depression of the proximal 4th metatarsophalangeal joint
Xiáxī(GB43)	On the dorsum of the foot, between the 4th and the 5th toe, at the junction of red and white skin posterior to the foot web
Zúqiàoyīn(GB44)	On the toe, in the lateral side of the 4th toe, 0.1 cun lateral and posterior to the corner of the nail

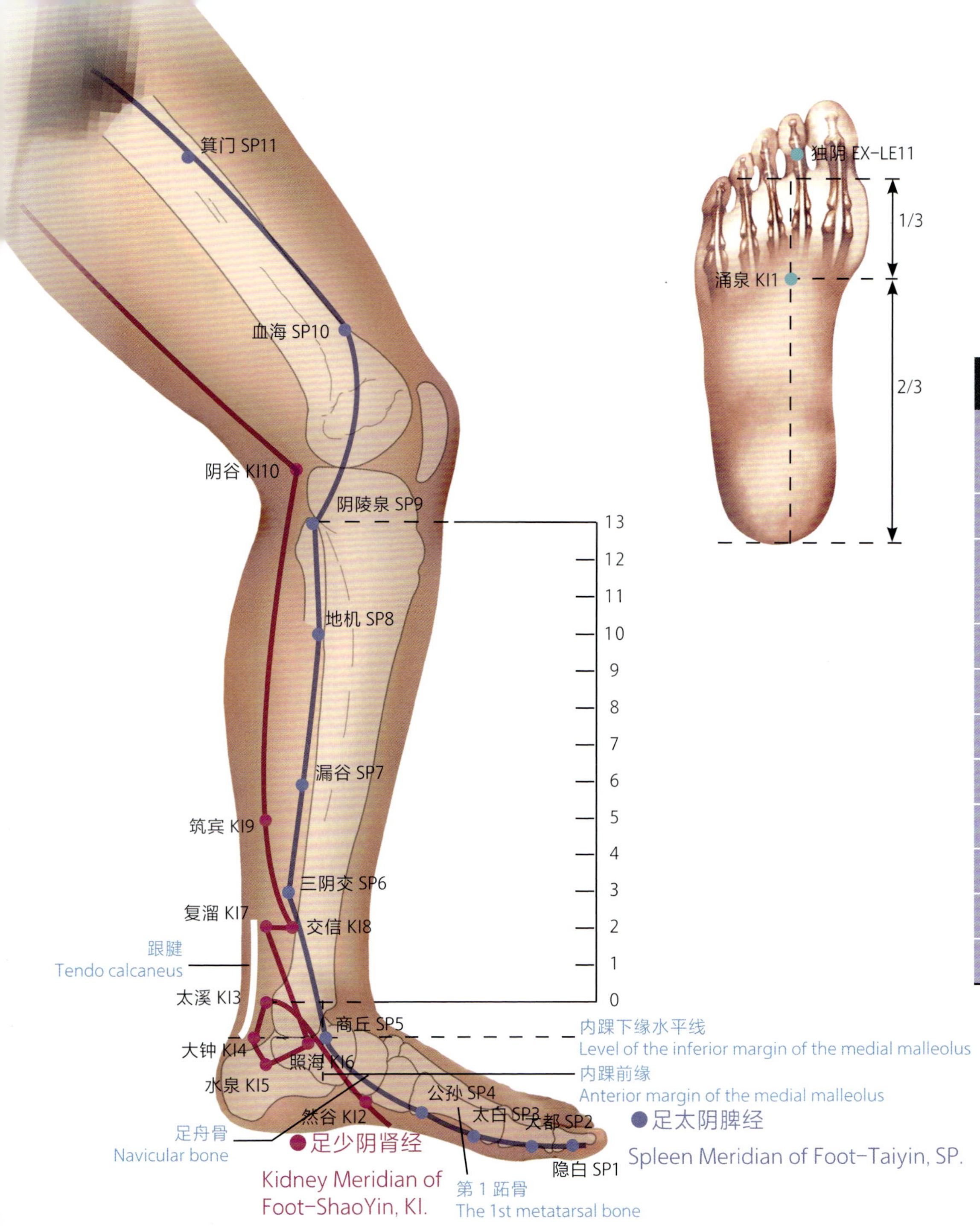

续表

穴位	定位
大敦	在足趾，大趾末节外侧，趾甲根角侧后方 0.1 寸（指寸）
行间	在足背，第 1、2 趾间，趾蹼缘后方赤白肉际处
太冲	在足背，第 1、2 跖骨间，跖骨底结合部前方凹陷中，或触及动脉搏动
中封	在踝区，内踝前，胫骨前肌肌腱的内侧凹陷中
蠡沟	在小腿内侧，内踝尖上 5 寸，胫骨内侧面的中央
中都	在小腿内侧，内踝尖上 7 寸，胫骨内侧面的中央
膝关	在膝部，胫骨内侧髁的下方，阴陵泉后 1 寸
曲泉	在膝部，腘横纹内侧端，半腱肌肌腱内缘凹陷中
阴包	在股前区，髌底上 4 寸，股薄肌与缝匠肌之间
足五里	在股前区，气冲直下 3 寸，动脉搏动处
阴廉	在股前区，气冲直下 2 寸

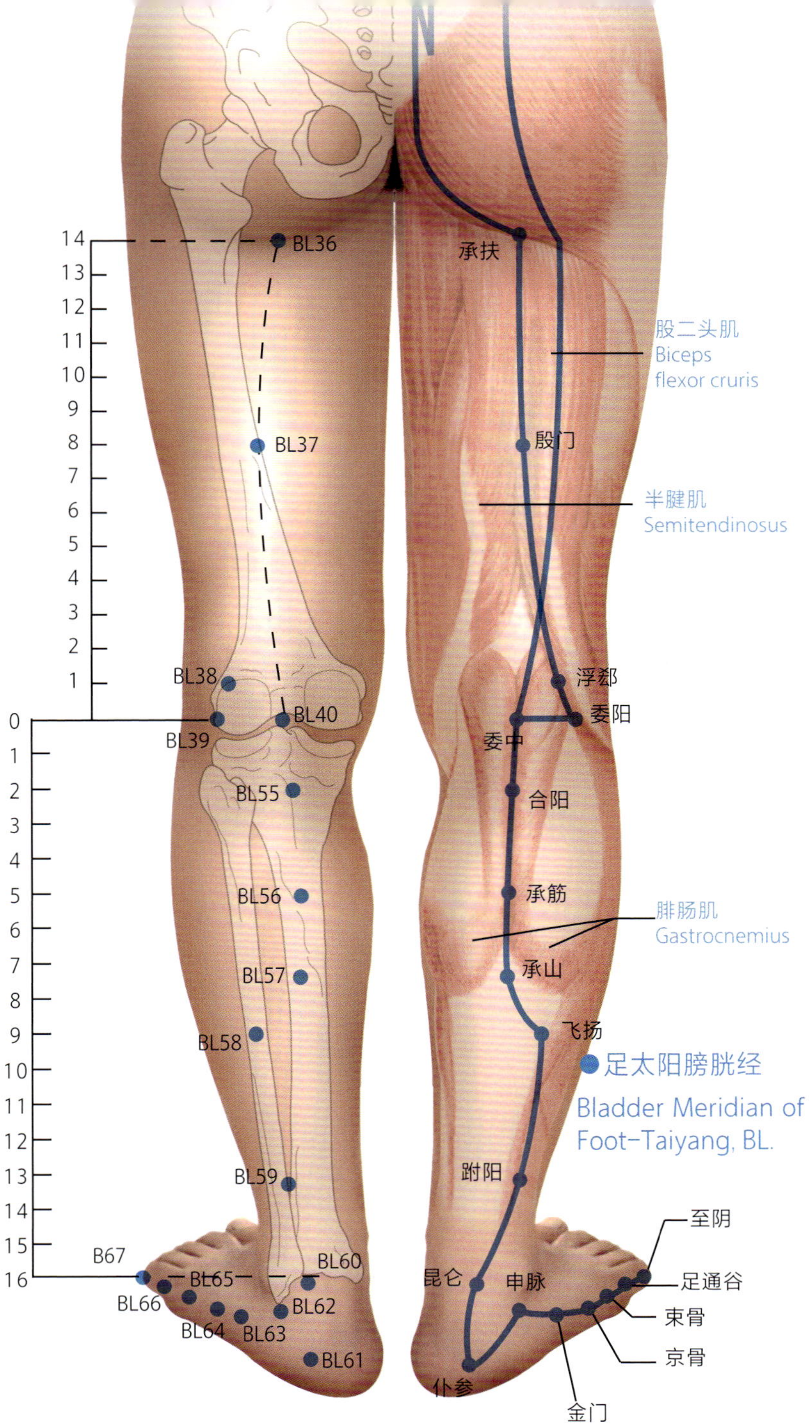

Continued

Acupoints	Location
Dàdūn(LR1)	On the toe, in the lateral side of the great toe, 0.1 cun lateral and posterior to the corner of the nail
Xíngjiān(LR2)	On the dorsum of foot, between the 1st and the 2nd toe, at the junction of the red and white skin posterior to the web
Tàichōng(LR3)	On the dorsum of foot, between the 1st and the 2nd metatarsal bone, in the depression anterior to the junction of the base of the metatarsal bone where the artery pulse can be palpated
Zhōngfēng(LR4)	In the region of the ankle, anterior to the medial malleolus, in the interior depression of the tendor of anterior tibial muscle
Lígōu(LR5)	In the interior region of crus, 5 cun above the prominence of medial malleolus, in the center of the interior aspect of the tibia
Zhōngdū(LR6)	In the interior region of crus, 7 cun above the prominence of medial malleolus, in the center of the interior aspect of the tibia
Xīguān(LR7)	In the region of the knee, below the medial tibial condyle, 1 cun posterior to the Yinlinquan acupoint
Qūquán(LR8)	In the region of the knee, in the interiol side of the popliteal crease, in the depression of the interior margin of the tendon of semitendinosus
Yīnbáo(LR9)	In the anterior region of the thigh, 4 cun above the base of patella, between the gracilis and the sartorius
Zúwǔlǐ(LR10)	In the anterior region of the thigh, 3 cun directly below the Qichong acupoint where arterial pulse can be palpated
Yīnlián(LR11)	In the anterior region of the thigh, 2 cun directly below the Qichong acupoint

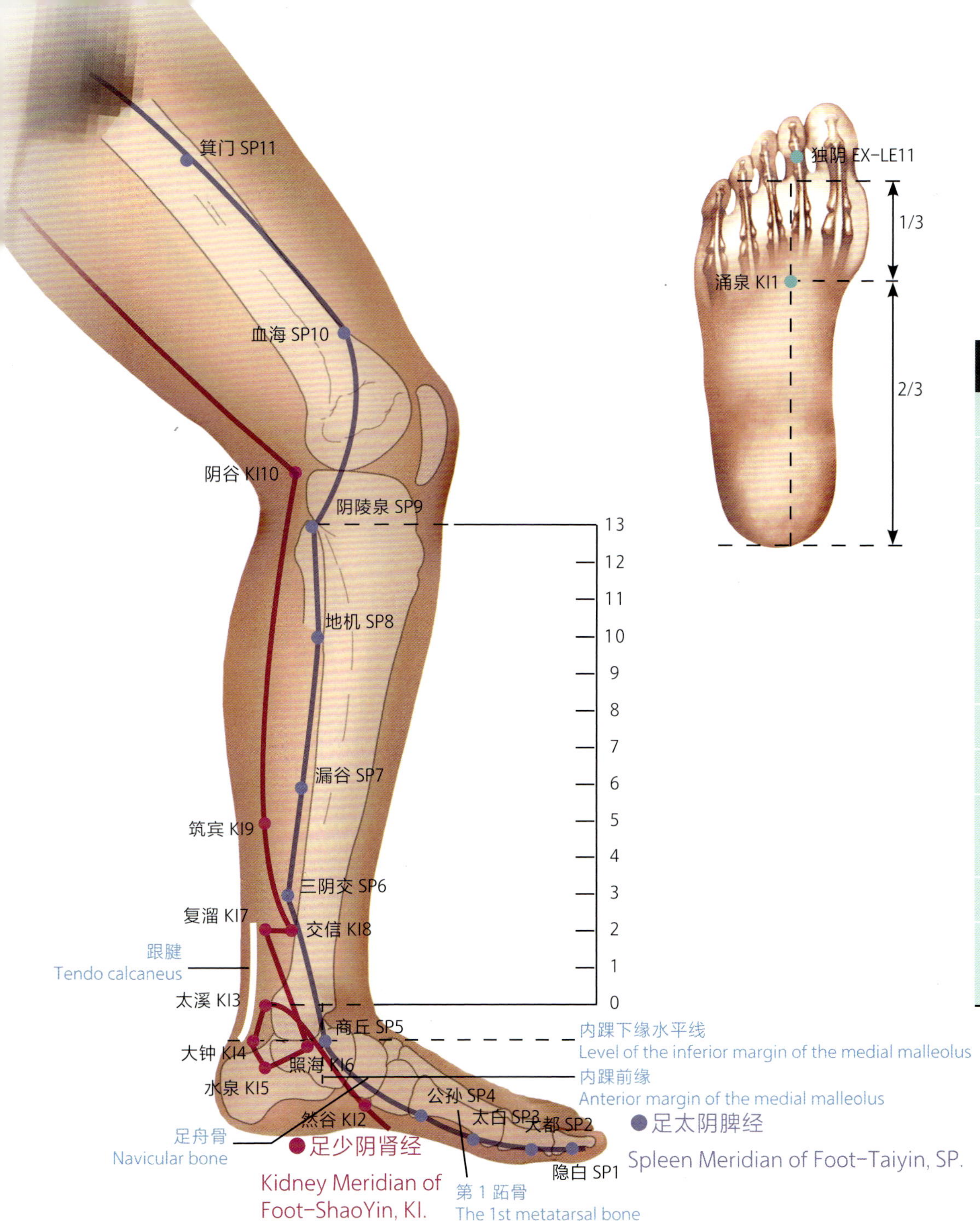

续表

穴位	定位
髋骨	在股前区，梁丘两旁各 1.5 寸，一肢 2 穴
鹤顶	在膝前区，髌底中点的上方凹陷中
百虫窝	在股前区，髌底内侧端上 3 寸
内膝眼	在膝部，髌韧带内侧凹陷处的中央
胆囊	在小腿外侧，腓骨小头直下 2 寸
阑尾	在小腿外侧，髌韧带外侧凹陷下 5 寸，胫骨前嵴外一横指（中指）
内踝尖	在踝区，内踝的最凸起处
外踝尖	在踝区，外踝的最凸起处
八风	在足背，第 1~5 趾间，趾蹼缘后方赤白肉际处，左右共 8 穴
独阴	在足底，第 2 趾的跖侧远端趾间关节的中点
气端	在足趾，十趾端的中央，距趾甲游离缘 0.1 寸（指寸），左右共 10 穴

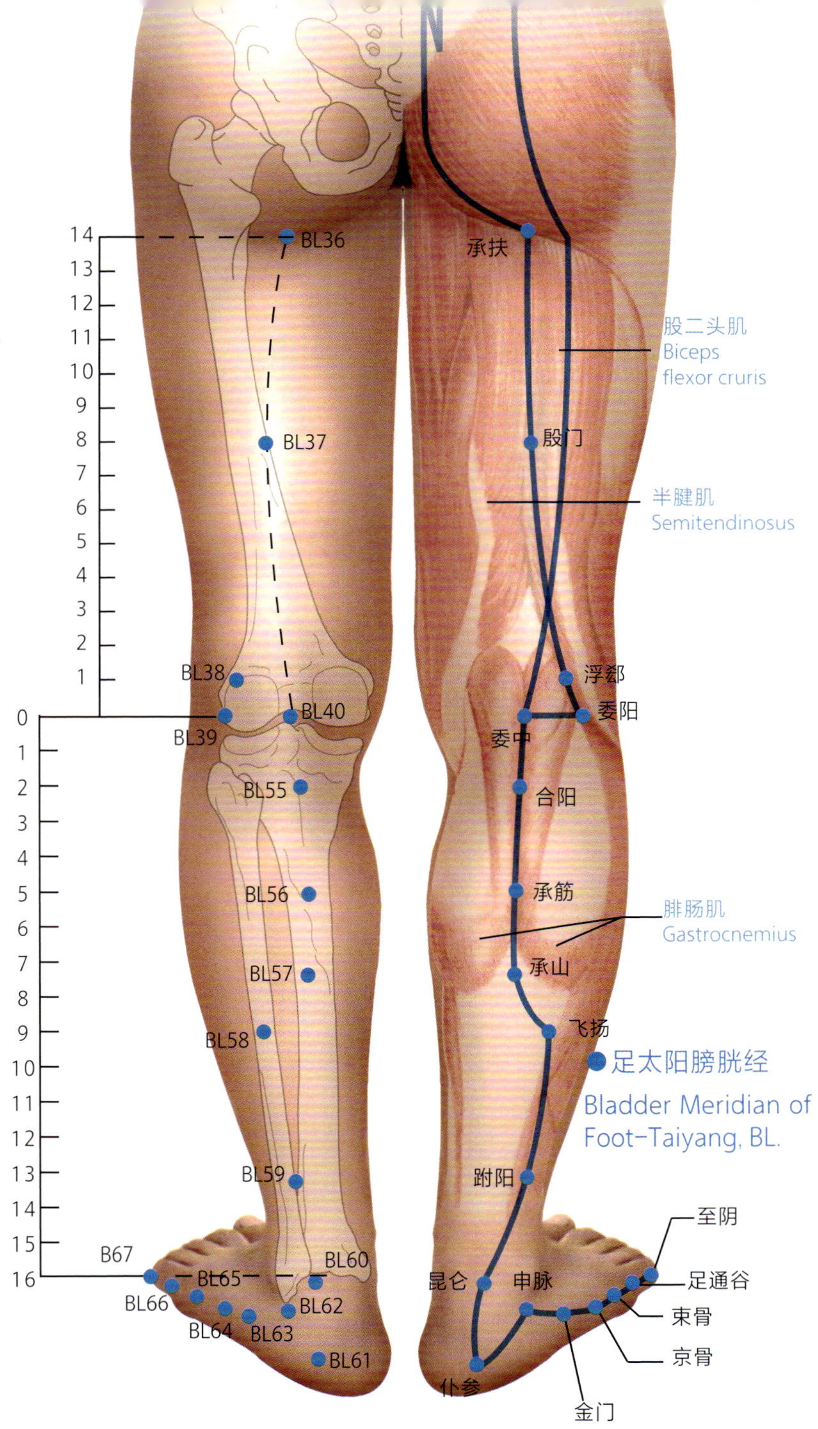

Continued

Acupoints	Location
Kuāngǔ (EX-LE1)	In the anterior region of the thigh, 1.5 cun lateral to the Liangqiu acupoint of both sides, with 2 acupoints of each lower limb
Hèdǐng (EX-LE2)	In the anterior region of the knee, in the superior depression of the midpoint of the base of patella
Bǎichóngwō (EX-LE3)	In the anterior region of the thigh, 3 cun above the medial base of patella
Nèixīyǎn (EX-LE4)	In the region of the knee, in the center of the interior depression of the patellar ligament
Dǎnnáng (EX-LE6)	In the posterior region of crus, 2 cun directly below the fibula head
Lánwěi (EX-LE7)	In the posterior region of crus, 5 cun below the depression of the lateral patellar ligament, one finger breadth lateral to the anterior tibia eminence
Nèihuáijiān (EX-LE8)	In the region of the ankle, at the most obvious embossment of the medial malleolus
Wàihuáijiān (EX-LE9)	In the region of the ankle, at the most obvious embossment of the lateral malleolus
Bāfēng (EX-LE10)	On the dorsum of foot, between all five toes, at the junction of the red and white skin, with 8 points in total
Dúyīn (EX-LE11)	On the sole, at the midpoint of the distal interphalangeal joint of the metatarsal side of the 2nd toe
Qìduān (EX-LE12)	On the toe, in the center of all toes, 0.1 cun from the free edge of the nail, with 10 acupoints in total

第三章　超速效三步对症按摩法

1 强腰壮肾

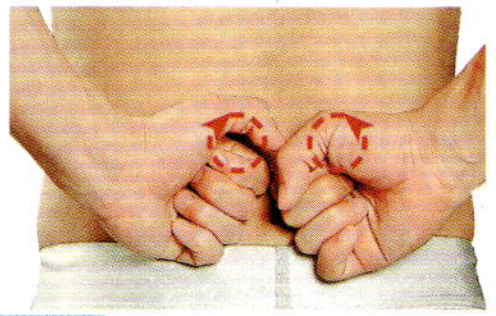

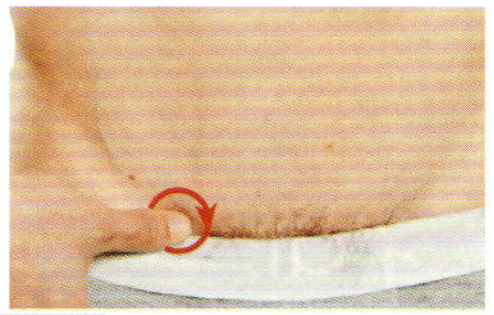

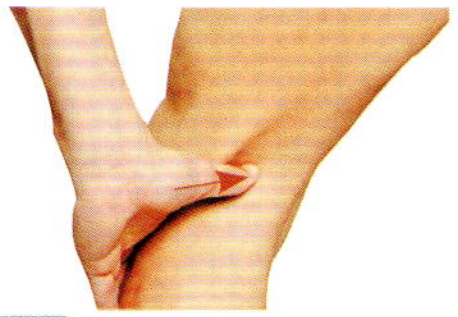

肾俞 两手握拳绕于背后腰部，用掌指关节稍用力按揉两侧肾俞穴 2 分钟。

气冲 用拇指按揉气冲穴 2 分钟，力度稍重。同法按揉对侧气冲穴。

委中 用拇指用力按压委中穴，停留片刻后放松，反复 5~6 下。同法按压对侧委中穴。

2 强筋健骨

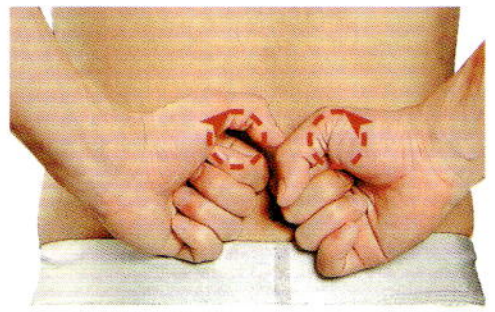

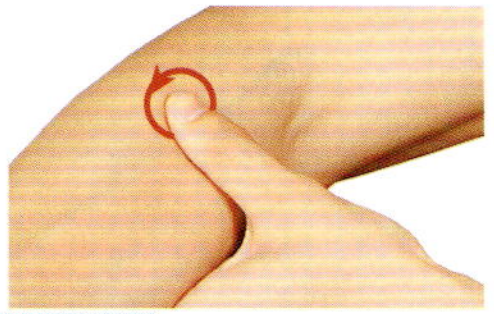

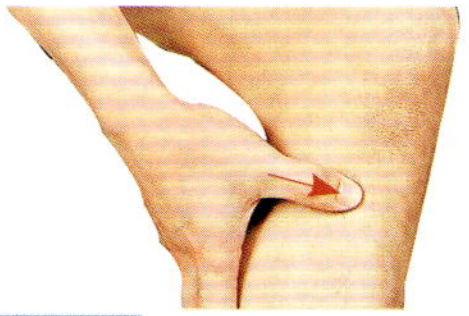

肾俞 两手握拳绕于背后腰部，用掌指关节稍用力按揉两侧肾俞穴 2 分钟。

手三里 用拇指按揉手三里穴 2 分钟，力度稍重。同法按揉对侧手三里穴。

足三里 用拇指稍用力按压足三里穴，停留片刻后放松，反复 5~6 下。同法按压对侧足三里穴。

3 明目养肝

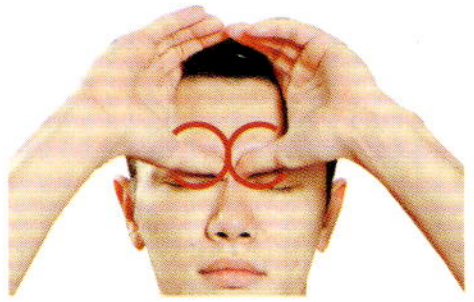

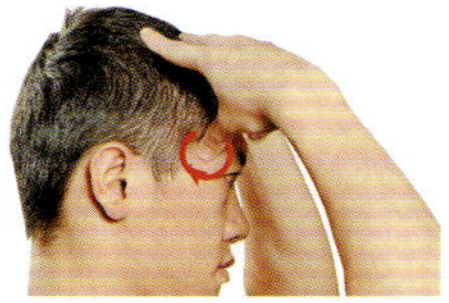

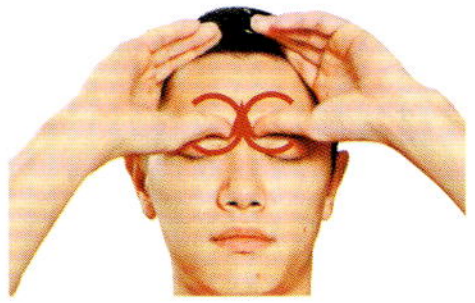

睛明 用双手拇指按揉两侧睛明穴 2 分钟，力度稍轻。

太阳 用双手拇指按揉两侧太阳穴 2 分钟，力度适中。

攒竹 将两手拇指按揉两侧攒竹穴 2 分钟，力度稍轻。

4 补心健脑

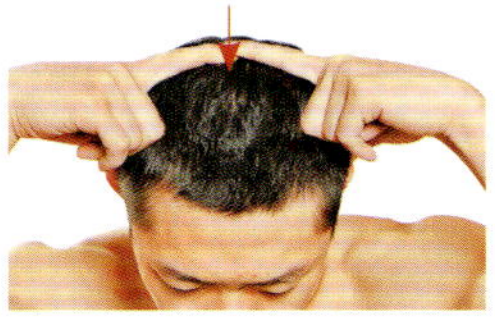

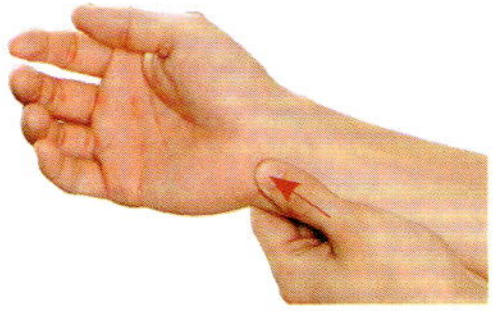

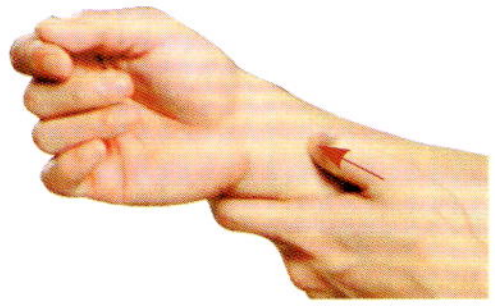

百会 两手食指重叠稍用力按压百会穴，停留片刻后放松，反复 5~6 下。

神门 用拇指稍用力按压神门穴，停留片刻后放松，反复 5~6 下。同法按压对侧神门穴。

内关 用拇指稍用力按压内关穴，停留片刻后放松，反复 5~6 下。同法按压对侧内关穴。

5 缓解压力

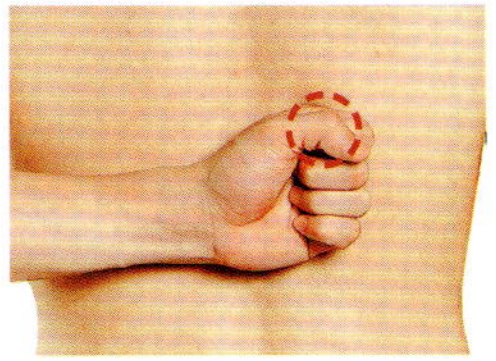

肝俞 一手握拳绕于背后，用掌指关节按揉肝俞穴 2 分钟，力度稍重。同法按揉对侧肝俞穴。

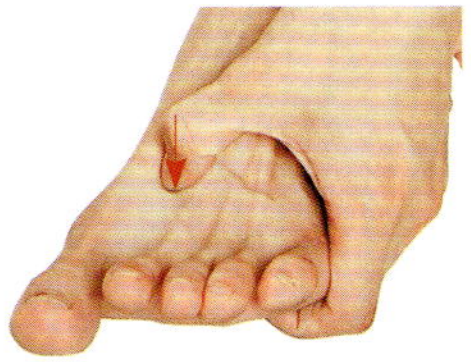

太冲 用拇指掐按太冲穴，停留片刻后放松，反复5~6下。同法掐按对侧太冲穴。

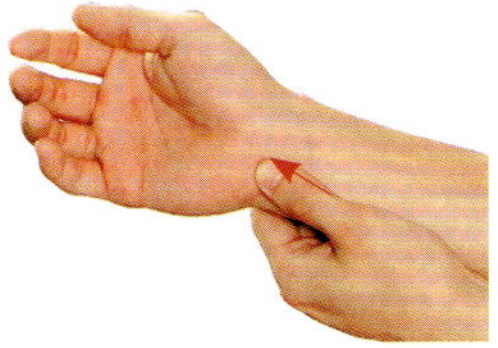

神门 用拇指稍用力按压神门穴，停留片刻后放松，反复 5~6 下。同法按压对侧神门穴。

Chapter 3: Super Quick-acting Three-step Symptomatic Massage Manipulations

1 Strengthening Waist and Kidney

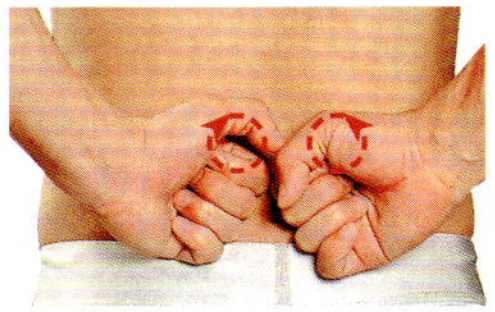

Shènshū(BL23): Put both clenched-fists on the waist and use both metacarpophalangeal joints to knead both Shenshu acupoints with a little heavy strength for 2 minutes.

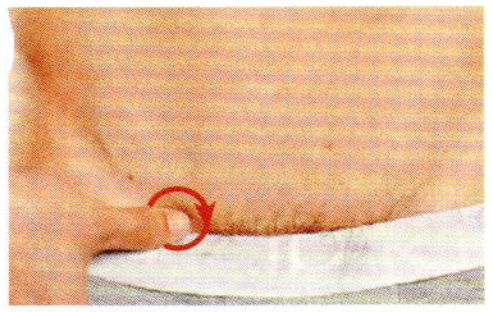

Qìchōng(ST30): Use the thumb to knead the Qichong acupoint for 2 minutes with a little heavy strength. Knead the contralateral Qichong acupoint with the same method.

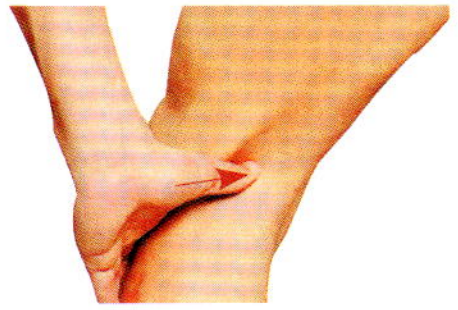

Wěizhōng(BL40): Use the thumb to press the Weizhong acupoint with a little heavy strength for a while, then relax, repeated 5~6 times a day. Press the contralateral Weizhong acupoint with the same method.

2 Strengthening Tendon and Bone

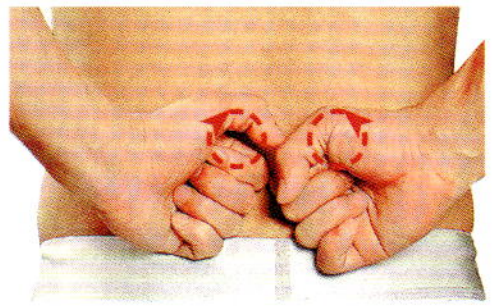

Shènshū(BL23): Put both clenched-fists on the waist and use both metacarpophalangeal joints to knead both Shenshu acupoints with a little heavy strength for 2 minutes.

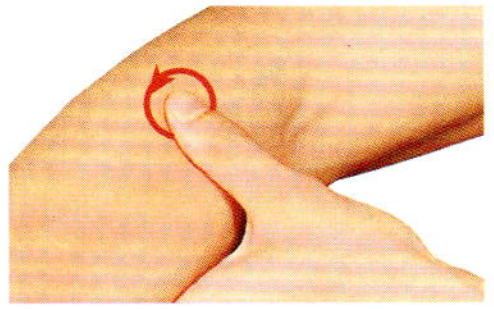

Shǒusānlǐ(LI10): Use the thumb to knead the Shousanli acupoint for 2 minutes with a little heavy strength. Knead the contralateral Shousanli acupoint with the same method.

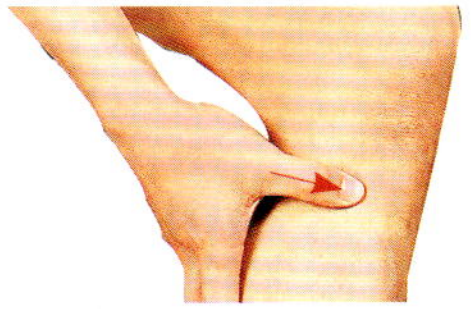

Zúsānlǐ(ST36): Use the thumb to press the Zusanli acupoint with a little heavy strength for a while then relax, repeat 5~6 times a day. Press the contralateral Zusanli acupoint with the same method.

3 Nourishing Liver and Improving Eyesight

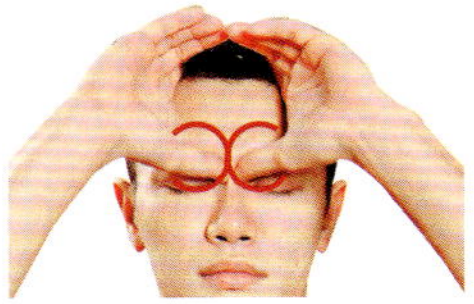

Jīngmíng(BL1): Use both thumbs to knead both Jingming acupoints with slight strength for 2 minutes.

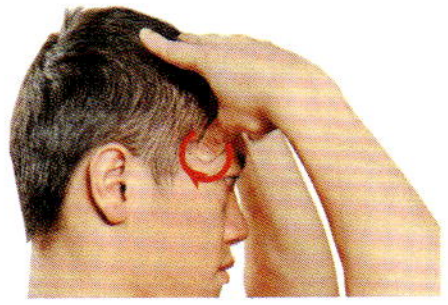

Tàiyáng(EX-HN5): Use both thumbs to knead both Taiyang acupoints with appropriate strength for 2 minutes.

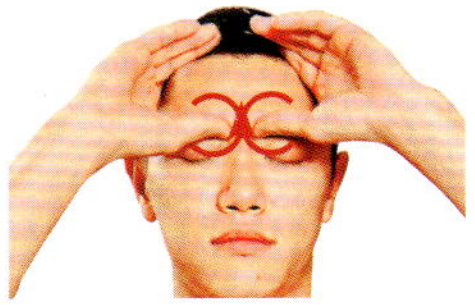

Cuánzhú(BL2): Use both thumbs to knead both Cuanzhu acupoints with slight strength for 2 minutes.

4 Nourishing Heart and Brain

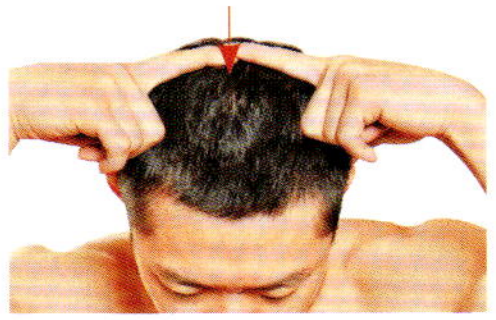

Bǎihuì(GV20): Overlap both index fingers together and press the Baihui acupoint with a little heavy strength for 2 minutes then relax, repeat 5~6 times a day.

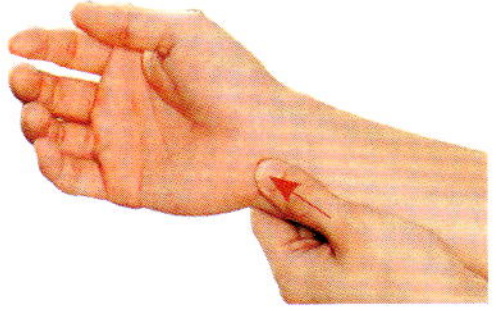

Shénmén(HT7): Use the thumb to press the Shenmen acupoint for a while then relax, repeat 5~6 times with slight strength. Press the contralateral Shenmen acupoint with the same method.

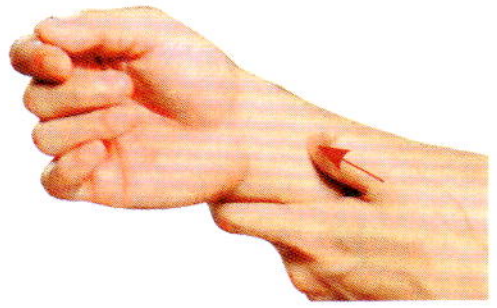

Nèiguān(PC6): Use the thumb to press the Neiguan acupoint for a while then relax,repeat 5~6 times with slight strength. Press the contralateral Neiguan acupoint with the same method.

5 Relieving Pressure

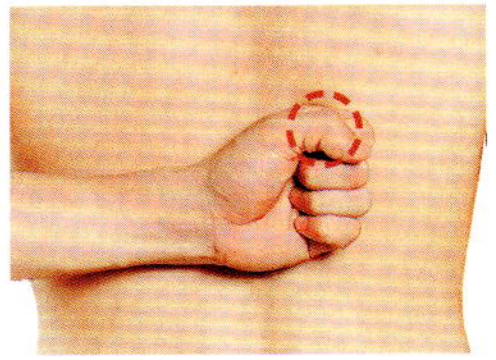

Gānshū(BL18): Put a clenched-fist on the waist and use the metacarpophalangeal joint to knead Ganshu acupoint with a little heavy strength for 2 minutes. Knead the contralateral Ganshu acupoint with the same method.

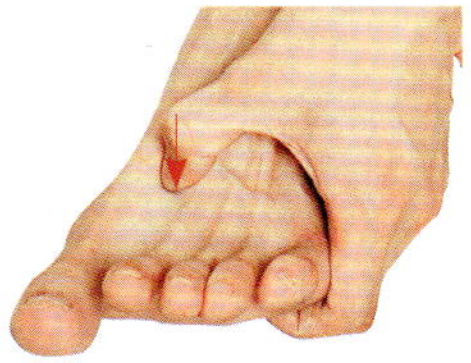

Tàichōng(LR3): Use the thumb to press the Taichong acupoint for a while then relax, repeat 5~6 times. Press the contralateral Taichong acupoint with the same method.

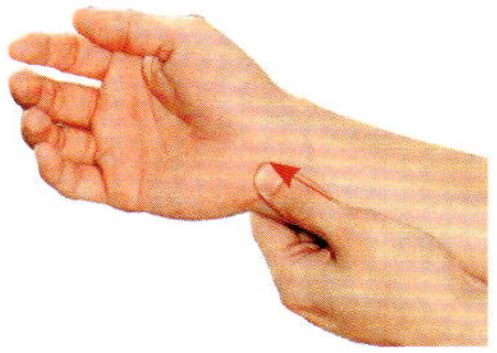

Shénmén(HT7): Use the thumb to press the Shenmen acupoint for a while then relax, repeat 5~6 times with slight strength. Press the contralateral Shenmen acupoint with the same method.

6 延年益寿

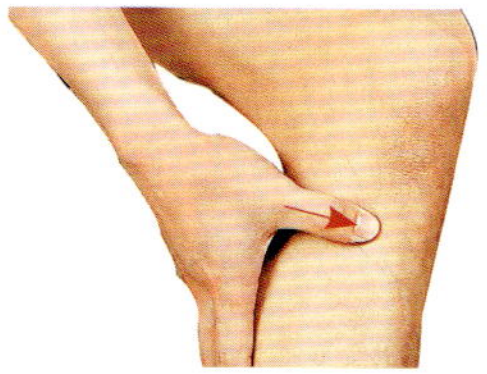

足三里 用拇指稍用力按压足三里穴，停留片刻后放松，反复5~6下。同法按压对侧足三里穴。

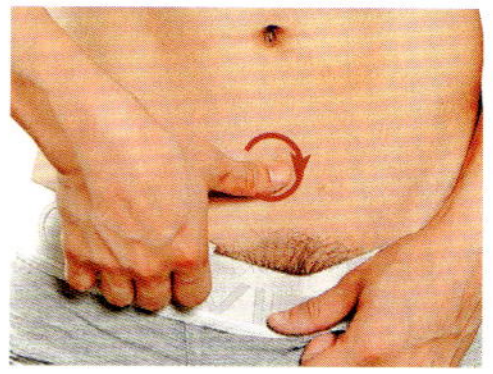

关元 用拇指按揉关元穴2分钟，力度适中。

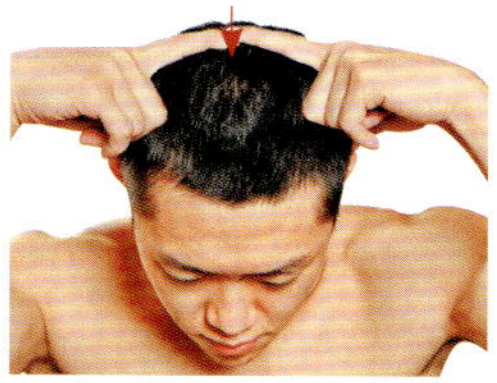

百会 两手食指重叠稍用力按压百会穴，停留片刻后放松，反复5~6下。

7 阳痿

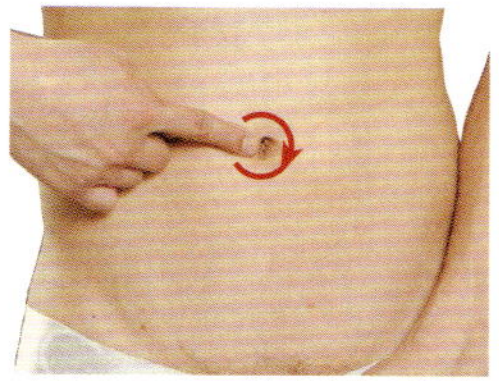

神阙 用拇指按揉神阙穴2分钟，力度适中。

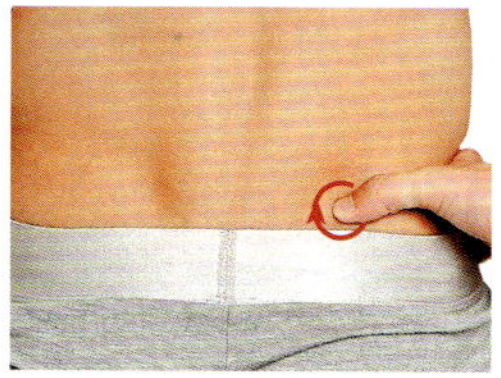

腰眼 用拇指稍用力按揉腰眼穴2分钟。同法按揉对侧腰眼穴。

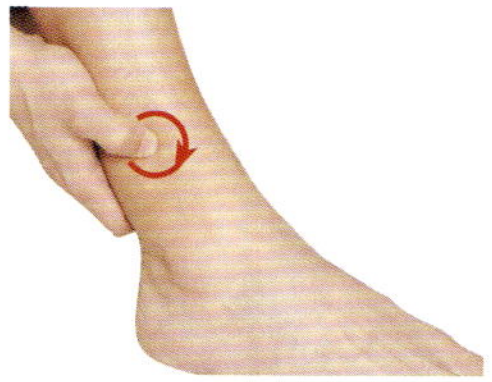

悬钟 用拇指按揉悬钟穴2分钟，力度稍重。同法按揉对侧悬钟穴。

8 早泄

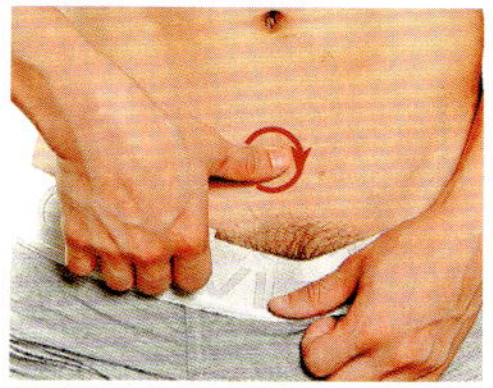

关元 用拇指按揉关元穴2分钟，力度适中。

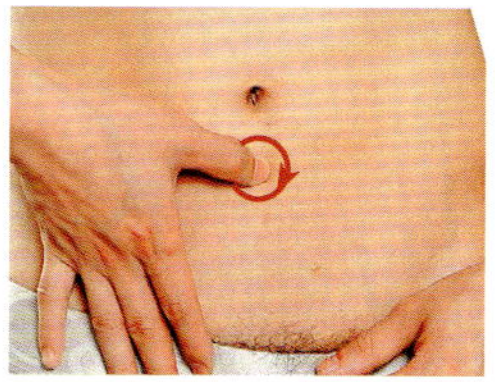

气海 用拇指按揉气海穴2分钟，力度适中。

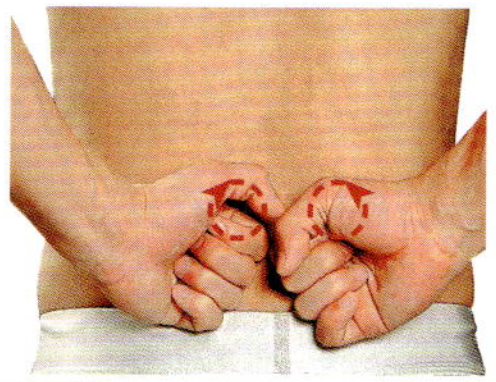

肾俞 两手握拳绕于背后腰部，用掌指关节稍用力按揉两侧肾俞穴2分钟。

9 遗精

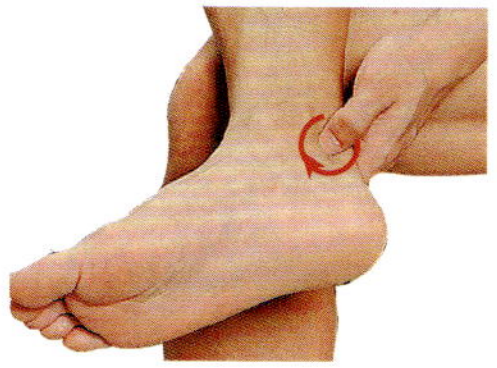

太溪 用拇指按揉太溪穴2分钟，力度稍重。同法按揉对侧太溪穴。

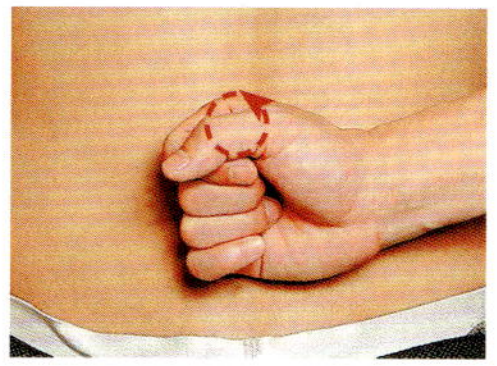

命门 一手握拳绕于背后，用掌指关节稍用力按揉命门穴2分钟。

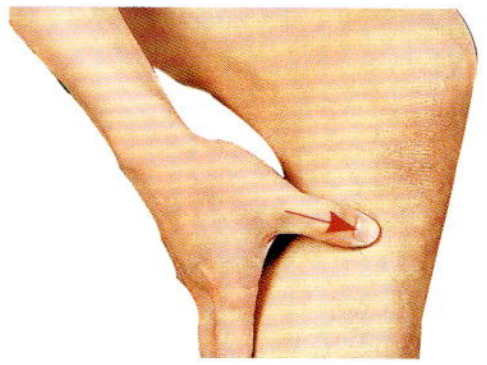

足三里 用拇指稍用力按压足三里穴，停留片刻后放松，反复5~6下。同法按压对侧足三里穴。

10 睾丸炎

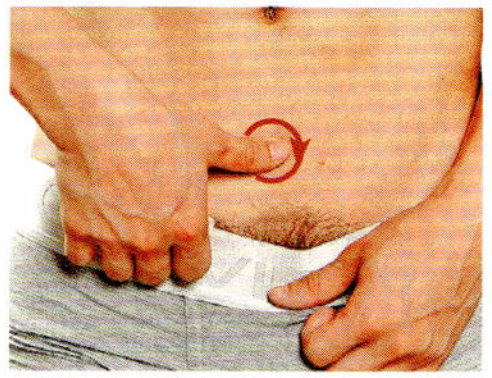

关元 用拇指按揉关元穴2分钟，力度适中。

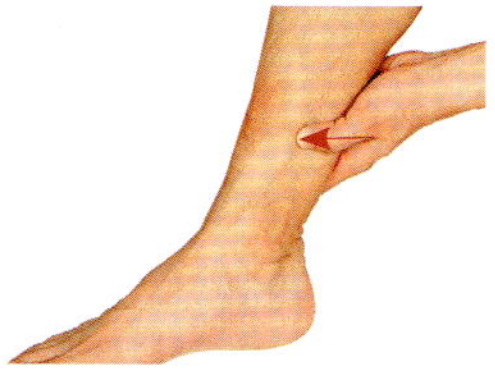

三阴交 用拇指稍用力按压三阴交穴，停留片刻后放松，反复5~6下。同法按压对侧三阴交穴。

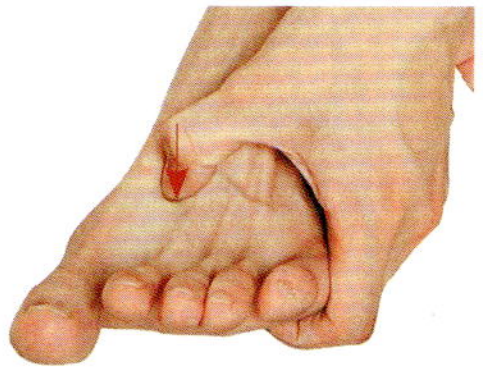

太冲 用拇指掐按太冲穴，停留片刻后放松，反复5~6下。同法掐按对侧太冲穴。

11 前列腺炎

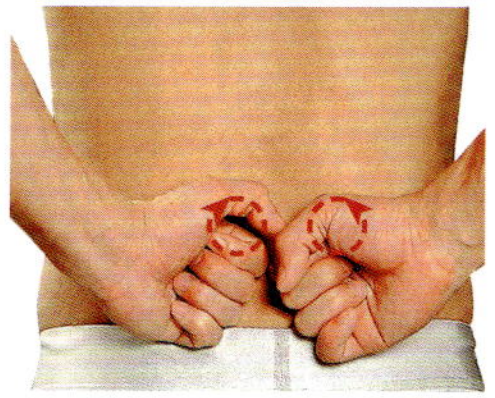

肾俞 两手握拳绕于背后腰部，用掌指关节稍用力按揉两侧肾俞穴2分钟。

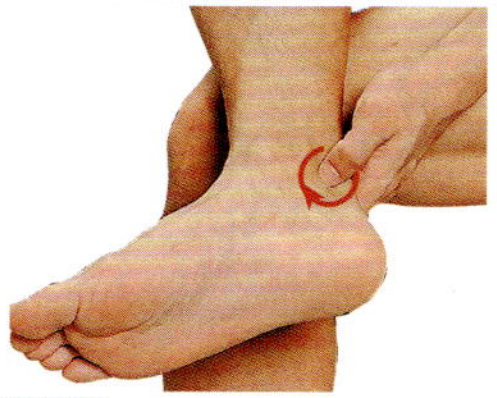

太溪 用拇指按揉太溪穴2分钟，力度稍重。同法按揉对侧太溪穴。

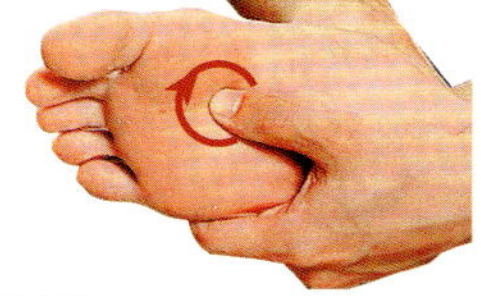

涌泉 用拇指按揉涌泉穴2分钟，力度稍重。同法按揉对侧涌泉穴。

6 Prolonging Life

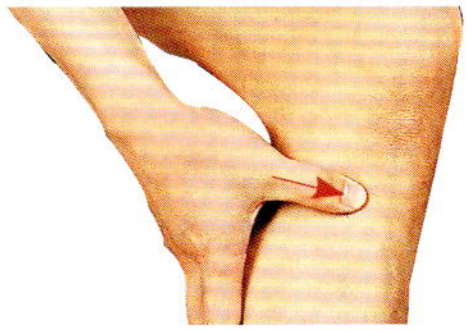

Zúsānlǐ(ST36): Use the thumb to press the Zusanli acupoint with a little heavy strength for a while, then relax, repeat 5~6 times a day. The contralateral Zusanli acupoint with the same method.

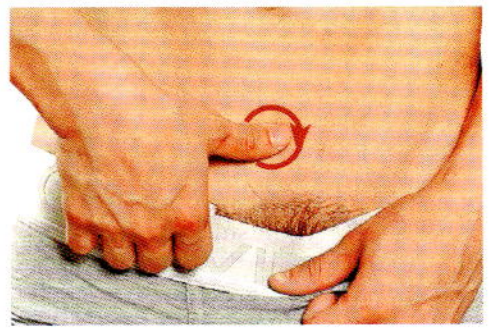

Guānyuán(CV4): Use the thumb to knead the Guanyuan acupoint with appropriate strength for 2 minutes.

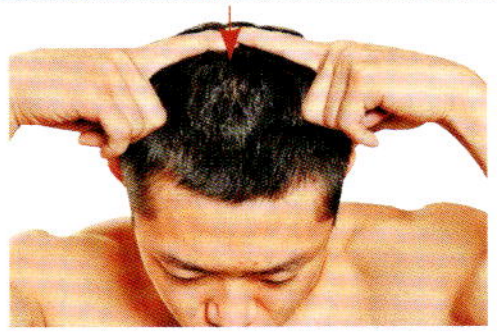

Bǎihuì(GV20): Overlap both index fingers and knead the Baihui acupoint with a little heavy strength for 2 minutes, then relax, repeat 5~6 times a day.

7 Erectile Dysfunction

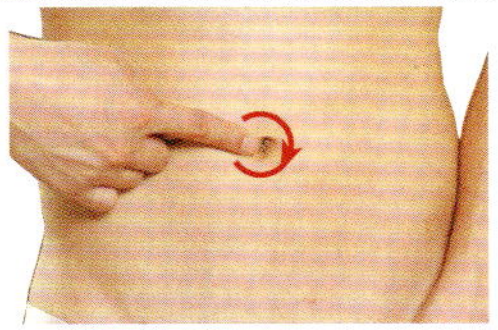

Shénquè(CV8): Use the thumb to knead the Shenque acupoint with appropriate strength for 2 minutes.

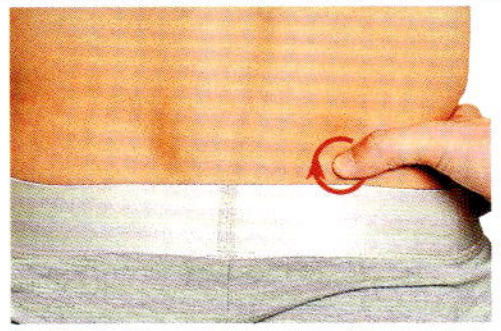

Yāoyǎn(EX-B7): Use the thumb to knead the Yaoyan acupoint with appropriate strength for 2 minutes.

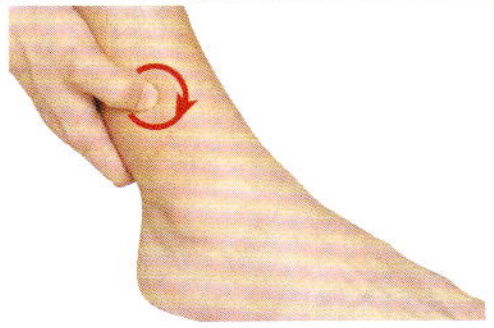

Xuánzhōng(GB39): Use the thumb to knead the Xuanzhong acupoint with a little heavy strength for 2 minutes. Knead the contralateral Xuanzhong acupoint with the same method.

8 Prospermia

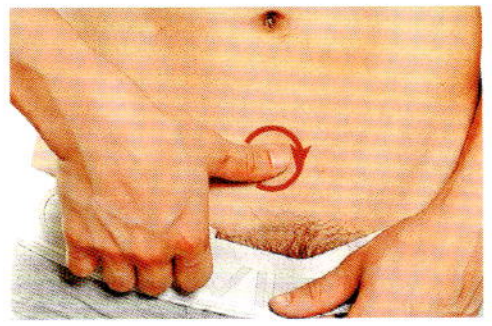

Guānyuán(CV4): Use the thumb to knead the Guanyuan acupoint with appropriate strength for 2 minutes.

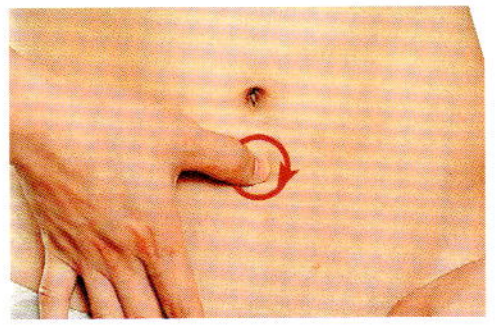

Qìhǎi(CV6): Use the thumb to knead the Qihai acupoint with appropriate strength for 2 minutes.

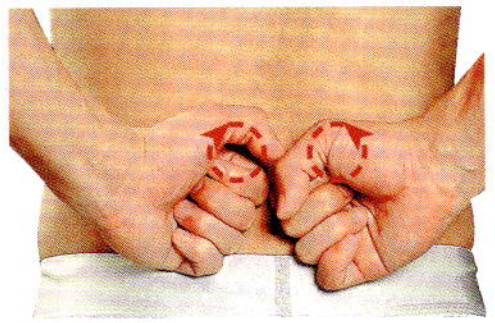

Shènshū(BL23): Put both clenched-fists on the waist and use both metacarpophalangeal joints to knead both Shenshu acupoints with a little heavy strength for 2 minutes.

9 Spermatorrhea

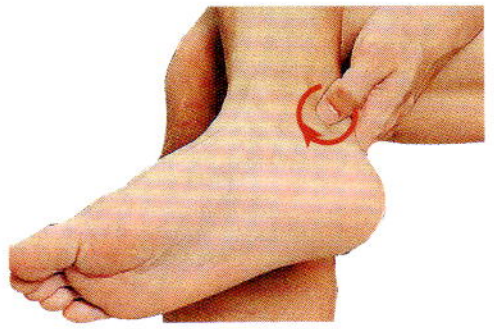

Tàixī(KI3): Use the thumb to knead the Taixi acupoint with a little heavy strength for 2 minutes. Knead the contralateral Taixi acupoint with the same method.

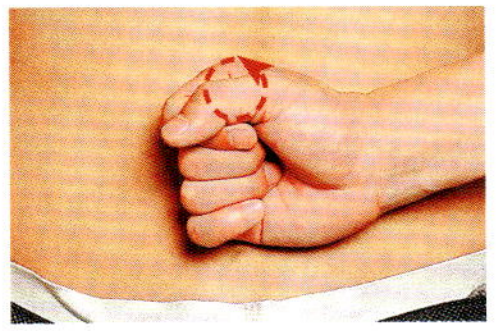

M ìngmén(GV4): Put a clenched-fist on the waist, use the metacarpophalangeal joint to knead Mingmen acupoint with a little heavy strength for 2 minutes.

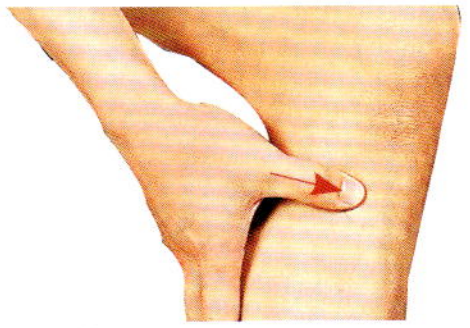

Zúsānlǐ(ST36): Use the thumb to press the Zusanli acupoint with a little heavy strength for a while, then relax, repeat 5~6 times a day. Press the contralateral Zusanli acupoint with the same method.

10 Testitis

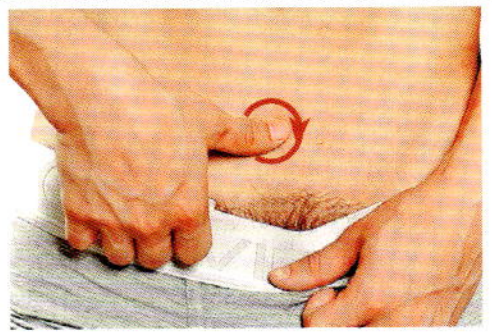

Guānyuán(CV4): Use the thumb to knead the Guanyuan acupoint with appropriate strength for 2 minutes.

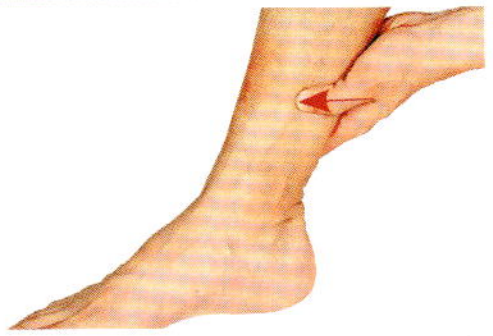

Sānyīnjiāo(SP6): Use the thumb to press the Sanyinjiao acupoint with a little heavy strength for a while,then relax. repeat 5~6 times a day. Press the contralateral Sanyinjiao acupoint with the same method.

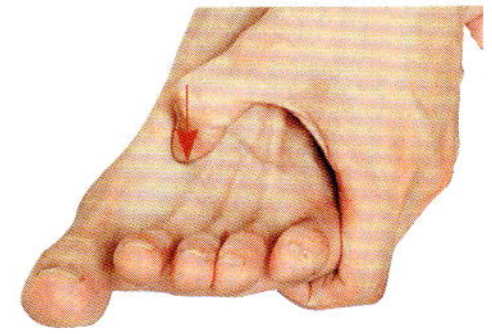

Tàichōng(LR3): Use the thumb to press the Taichong acupoint for a while, then relax,repeat 5~6 times. Press the contralateral Taichong acupoint with the same method.

11 Prostatitis

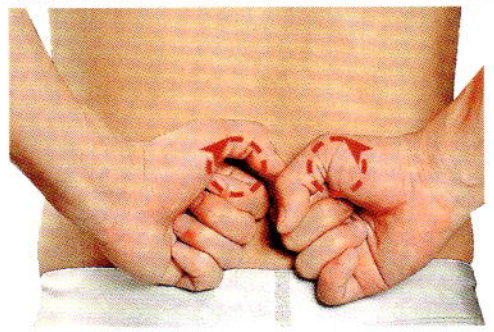

Shènshū(BL23): Put both clenched-fists on the waist and use both metacarpophalangeal joints to knead both Shenshu acupoints with a little heavy strength for 2 minutes.

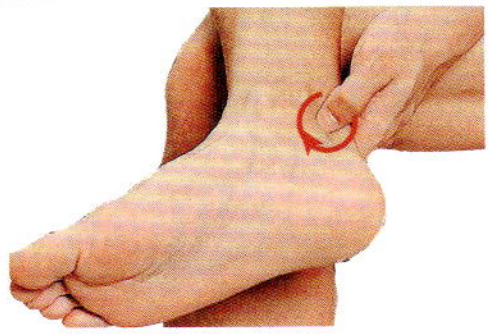

Tàixī(KI3): Use the thumb to knead the Taixi acupoint with a little heavy strength for 2 minutes. Knead the contralateral Taixi acupoint.

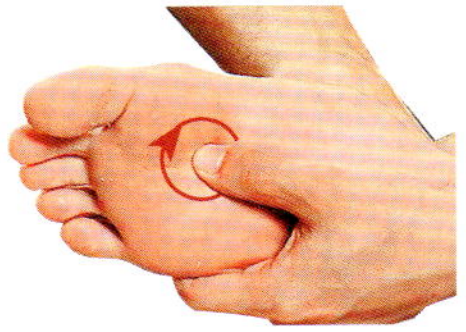

Yǒngquán(KI1): Use the thumb to knead the Yongquan acupoint with a little heavy strength for 2 minutes. Knead the contralateral Yongquan acupoint with the same method.

12 男性不育症

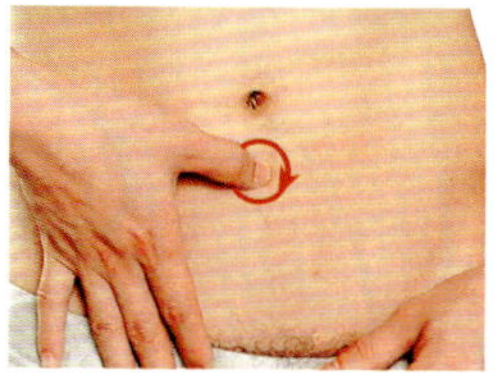

气海 用拇指按揉气海穴2分钟，力度适中。

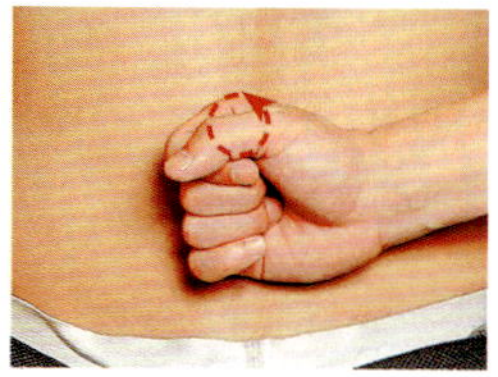

命门 一手握拳绕于背后，用掌指关节稍用力按揉命门穴2分钟。

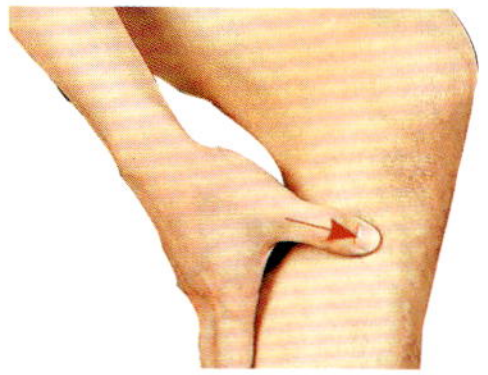

足三里 用拇指稍用力按压足三里穴，停留片刻后放松，反复5~6下。同法按压对侧足三里穴。

13 不射精症

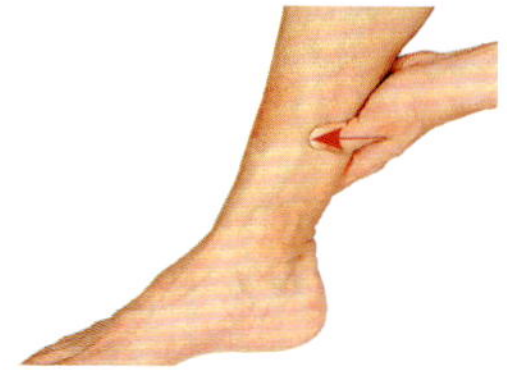

三阴交 用拇指稍用力按压三阴交穴，停留片刻后放松，反复5~6下。同法按压对侧三阴交穴。

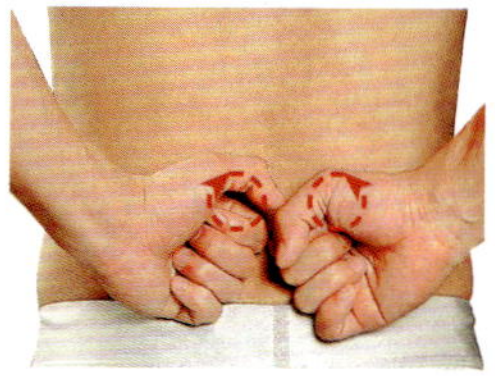

肾俞 两手握拳绕于背后腰部，用掌指关节稍用力按揉两侧肾俞穴2分钟。

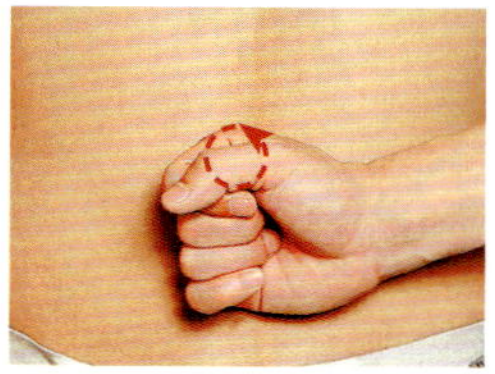

命门 一手握拳绕于背后，用掌指关节稍用力按揉命门穴2分钟。

14 前列腺囊肿

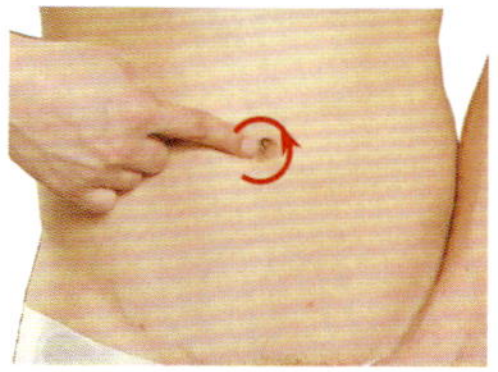

神阙 用食指按揉神阙穴2分钟，力度宜深透，以感觉局部微热为佳。

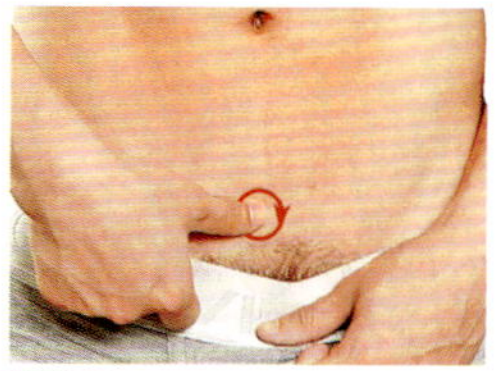

中极 用拇指按揉中极穴2分钟，力度适中。

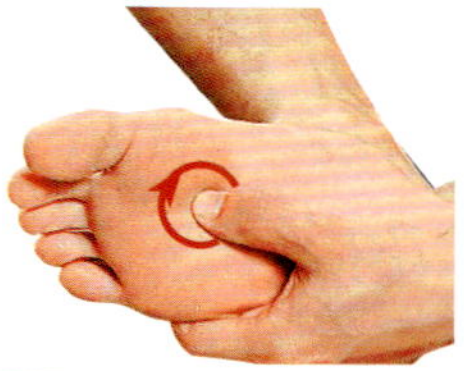

涌泉 用拇指按揉涌泉穴2分钟，力度稍重。同法按揉对侧涌泉穴。

15 少精子症

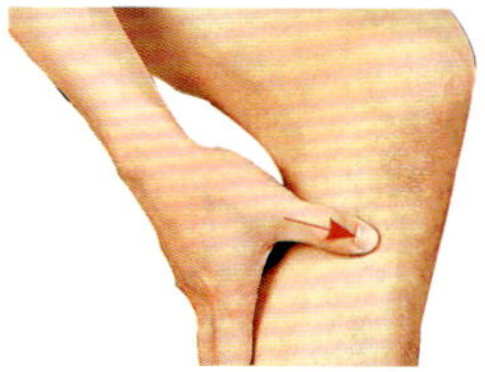

足三里 用拇指稍用力按压足三里穴，停留片刻后放松，反复5~6下。同法按压对侧足三里穴。

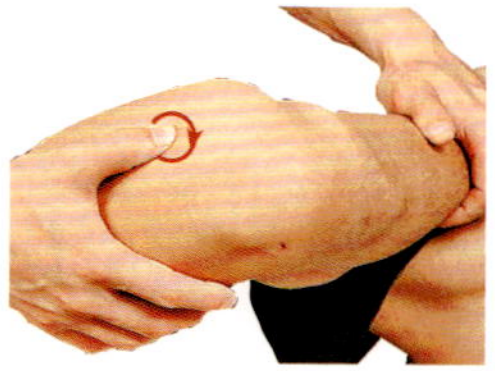

血海 用拇指按揉血海穴2分钟，力度稍重。同法按揉对侧血海穴。

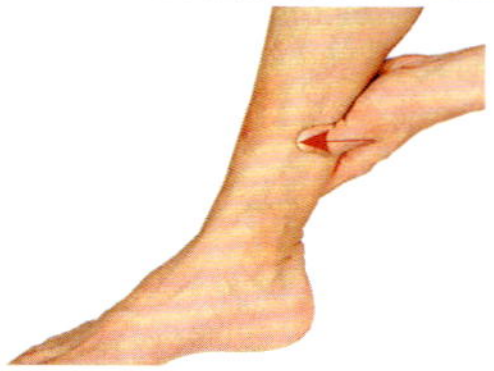

三阴交 用拇指用力按压三阴交穴，停留片刻后放松，反复5~6下。同法按压对侧三阴交穴。

16 男性更年期综合征

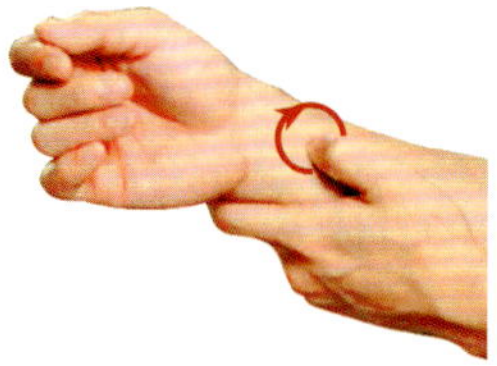

内关 用拇指按揉内关穴2分钟，力度稍重。同法按揉对侧内关穴。

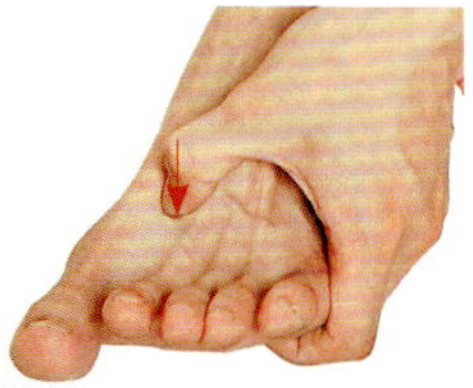

太冲 用拇指稍用力按压太冲穴，停留片刻后放松，反复5~6下。同法按压对侧太冲穴。

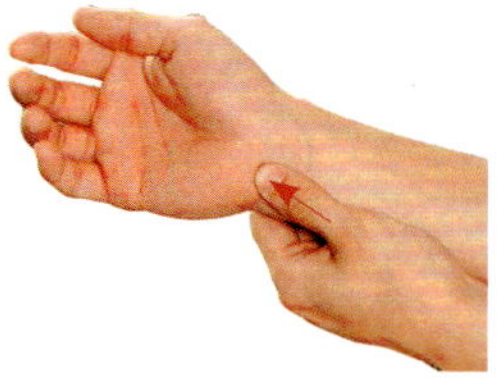

神门 用拇指稍用力按压神门穴，停留片刻后放松，反复5~6下。同法按压对侧神门穴。

17 感冒

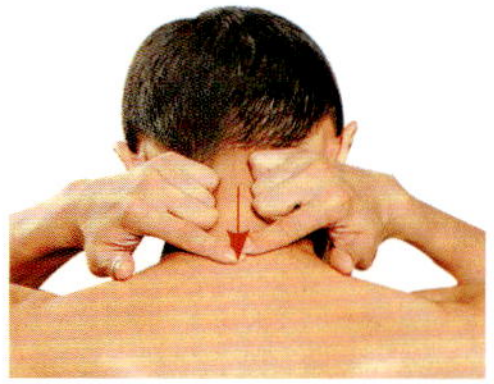

大椎 两手食指重叠稍用力按压大椎穴，停留片刻后放松，反复5~6下。

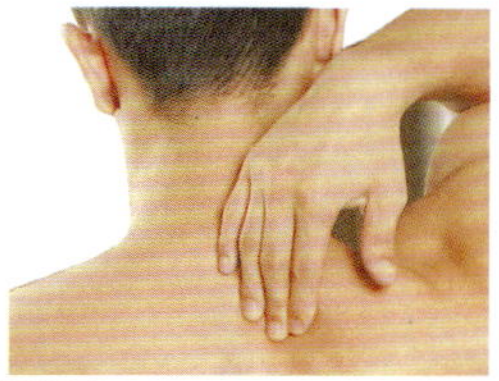

风门 用手的中指按揉穴位2分钟，力度宜稍重，也可用手按揉对侧穴位。

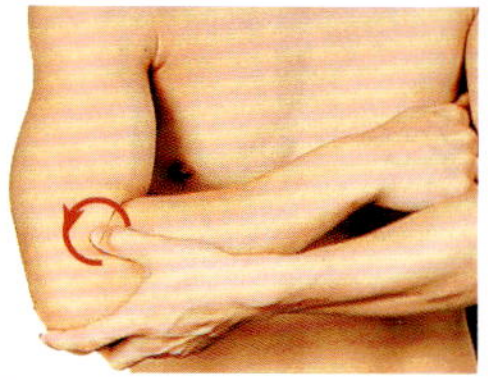

曲池 用拇指按揉曲池穴2分钟，力度稍重。同法按揉对侧曲池穴。

12 Male Infertility

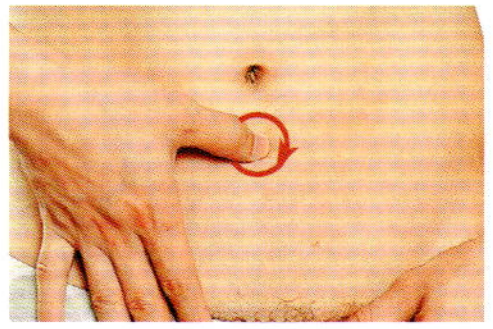

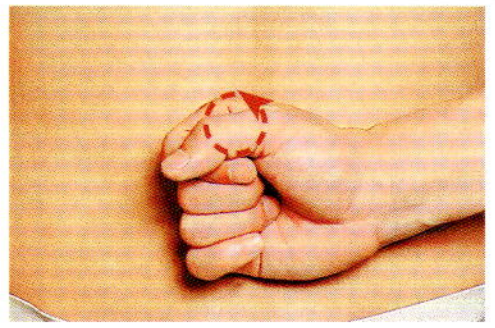

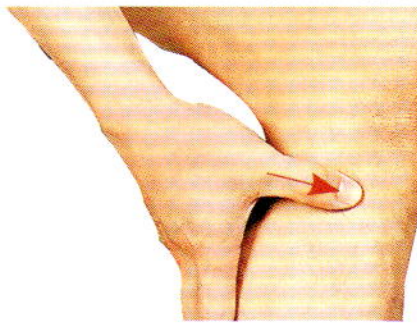

Qìhǎi(CV6) : Use the thumb to knead the Qihai acupoint with appropriate strength for 2 minutes.

Mìngmén(GV4) : Put a clenched-fist on the waist, use the metacarpophalangeal joint to knead Mingmen acupoint with a little heavy strength for 2 minutes. Knead the contralateral Mingmen acupoint with the same method.

Zúsānlǐ(ST36) : Use the thumb to press the Zusanli acupoint with a little heavy strength for a while, then relax, repeat 5~6 times a day. Press the contralateral Zusanli acupoint.

13 Anejaculation

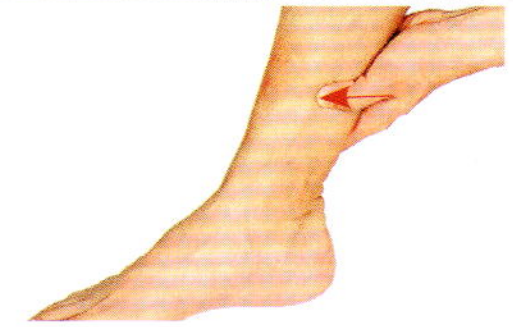

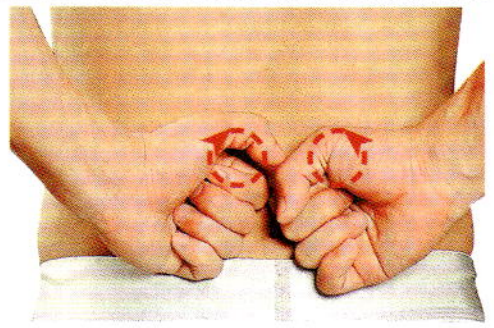

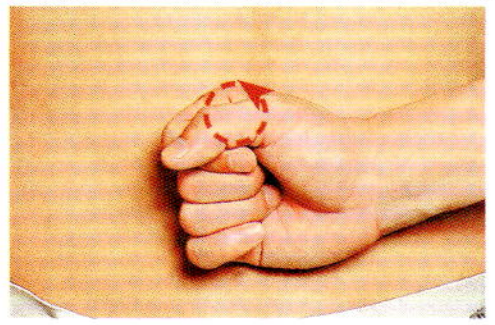

Sānyīnjiāo(SP6) : Use the thumb to press the Sanyinjiao acupoint with a little heavy strength for a while, then relax, repeat 5~6 times a day. Press the contralateral Sanyinjiao acupoint.

Shènshū(BL23) : Put both clenched-fists on the waist and use both metacarpophalangeal joints to knead both Shenshu acupoints with a little heavy strength for 2 minutes.

M ìngmén(GV4) : Put a clenched-fist on the waist, use the metacarpophalangeal joint to knead Mingmen acupoint with a little heavy strength for 2 minutes. Knead the contralateral Mingmen acupoint.

14 Cyst of Prostate

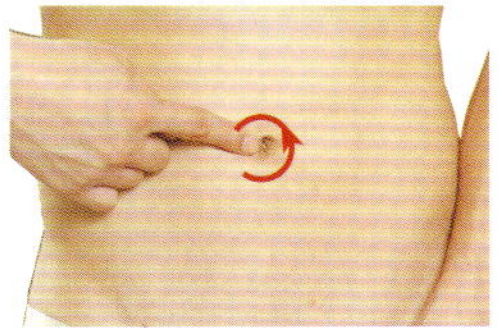

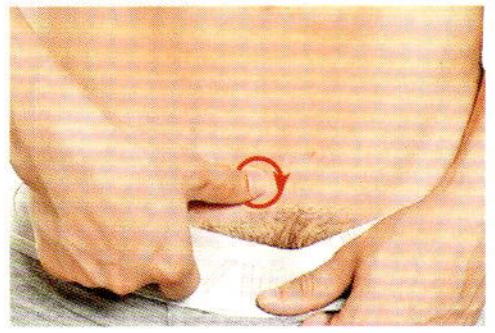

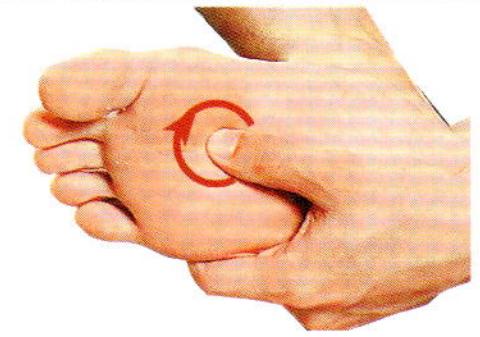

Shénquè(CV8) : Use the thumb to knead the Shenque acupoint with appropriate strength for 2 minutes, it will be better if slight local heat can be felt.

Zhōngjí(CV3) : Use the thumb to knead the Zhongji acupoint with appropriate strength for 2 minutes.

Yǒngquán(KI1) : Use the thumb to knead the Yongquan acupoint with a little heavy strength for 2 minutes. Knead the contralateral Yongquan acupoint.

15 Oligospermia

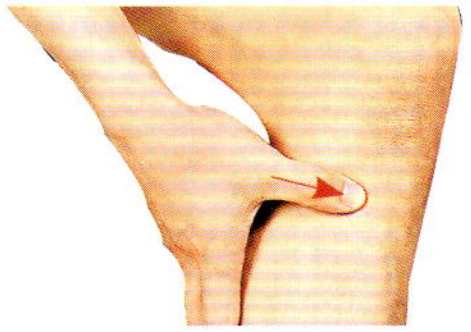

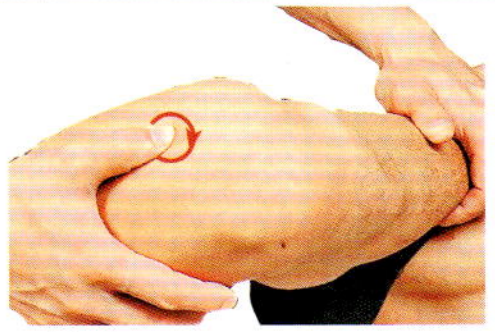

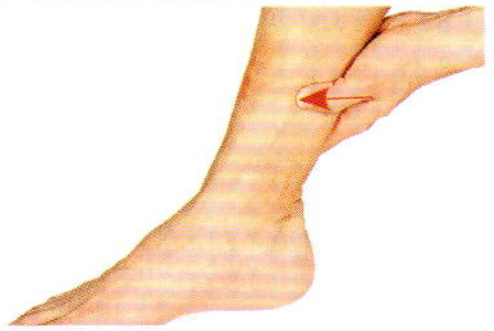

Zúsānlǐ(ST36) : Use the thumb to press the Zusanli acupoint with a little heavy strength for a while, then relax, repeat 5~6 times a day. Press the contralateral Zusanli acupoint.

Xuèhǎi(SP10): Use the thumb to knead the Xiehai acupoint with a little heavy strength for 2 minutes.Knead the contralateral Xiehai acupoint with the same method.

Sānyīnjiāo(SP6): Use the thumb to press the Sanyinjiao acupoint with a little heavy strength for a while,then relax, repeat 5~6 times a day. Press the contralateral Sanyinjiao acupoint with the same method.

16 Male Climacteric Syndrome

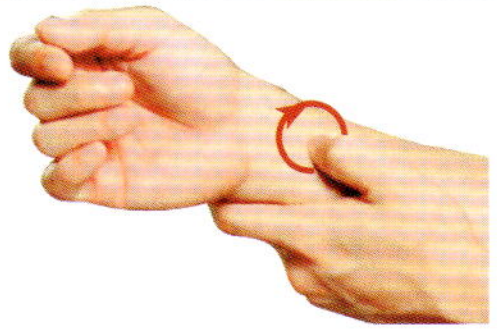

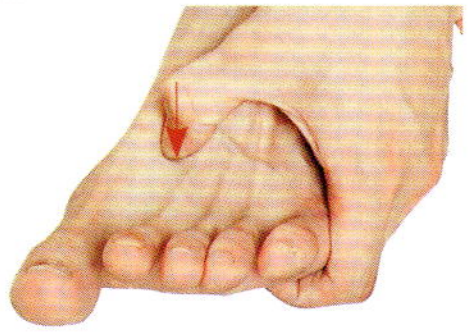

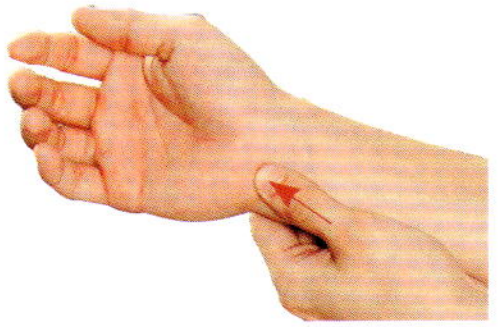

Nèiguān(PC6) : Use the thumb to knead the Neiguan acupoint with a little heavy strength for 2 minutes. Knead the contralateral Neiguan acupoint with the same method.

Tàichōng(LR3) : Use the thumb to press the Taichong acupoint for a while,then relax, repeat 5~6 times. Press the contralateral Taichong acupoint with the same method.

Shénmén(HT7) : Use the thumb to press the Shenmen acupoint with a little heavy strength for a moment, then relax, repeat 5~6 times. Press the contralateral Shenmen acupoint with the same metnod.

17 Cold

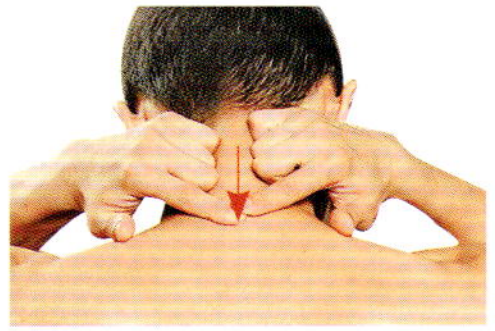

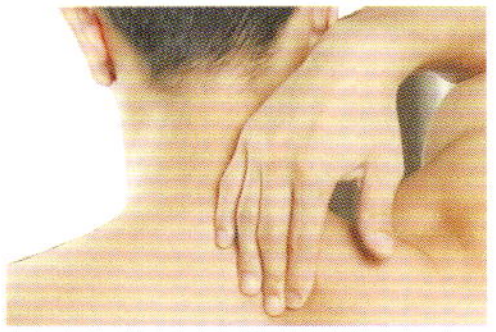

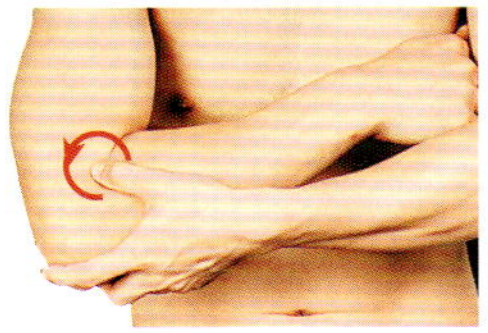

Dàzhuī(GV14):Overlap both index fingers and press the Dazhui acupoint with a little heavy strength for a moment, then relax, repeat 5~6 times a day.

Fēngmén(BL12) : Use the middle finger to knead the Fengmen acupoint with a little heavy strength for 2 minutes, or use the contralateral Fengmen acupoint.

Qūchí(LI11) : Use the thumb to knead Quchi acupoint for 2 minutes with a little heavy strength. Knead the contralateral acupoint with the same method.

18 发热

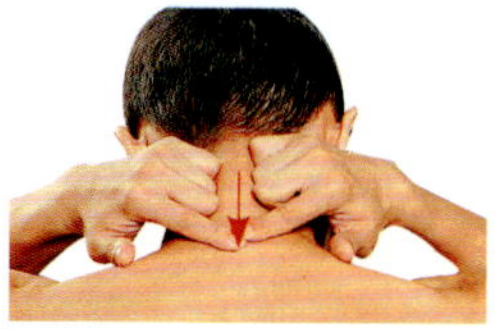
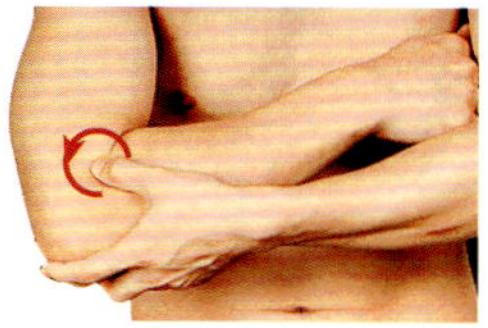
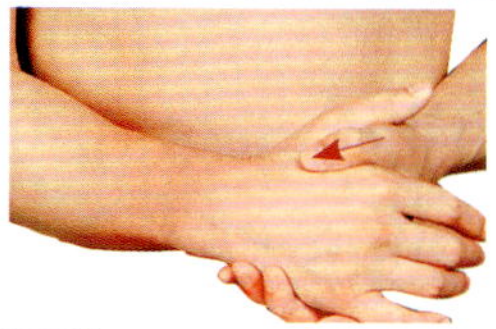

大椎 两手食指重叠，稍用力按压大椎穴，停留片刻后放松，反复 5~6 下。

曲池 用拇指按揉曲池穴 2 分钟，力度稍重。同法按揉对侧曲池穴。

合谷 用拇指用力按压合谷穴，停留片刻后放松，反复 5~6 下。同法按压对侧合谷穴。

19 咳嗽

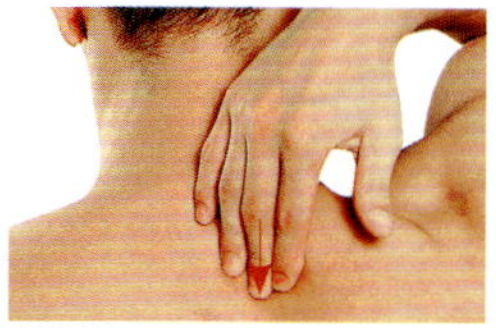
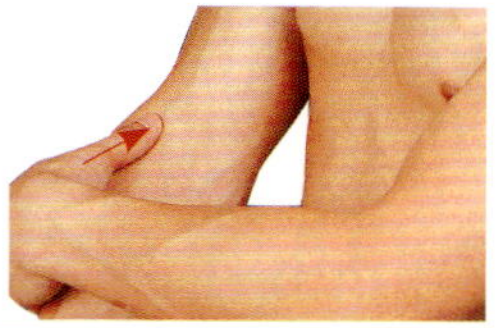
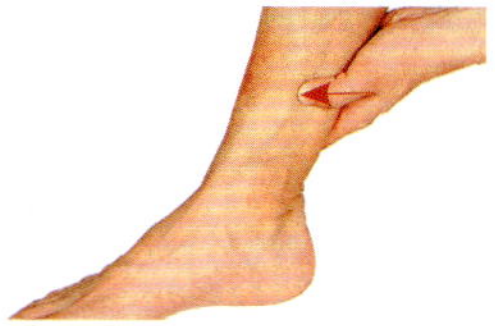

肺俞 将手抬起放于背后，用手指稍用力按压肺俞穴，停留片刻后放松，反复 5~6 下。同法按压对侧肺俞穴。

尺泽 用拇指点按尺泽穴，可配按揉法，操作 2 分钟，力度适中。

三阴交 用拇指用力按压三阴交穴，停留片刻后放松，反复 5~6 下。同法按压对侧三阴交穴。

20 哮喘

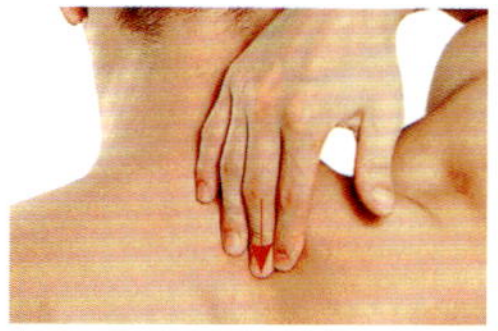
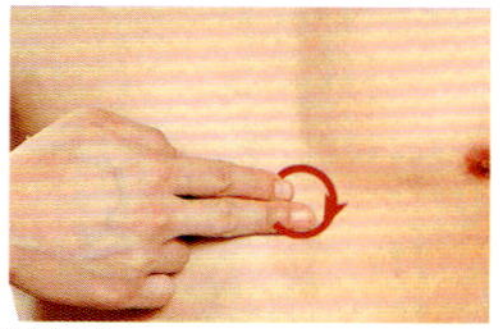
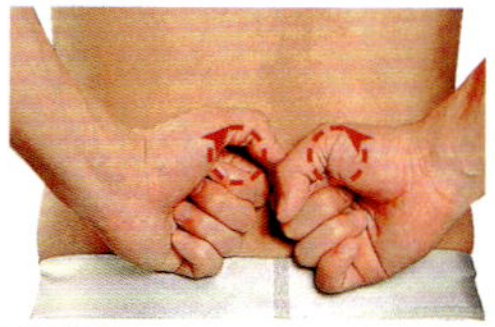

肺俞 将手抬起放于背后，用手指稍用力按压肺俞穴，停留片刻后放松，反复 5~6 下。同法按压对侧肺俞穴。

膻中 先用食、中二指按揉膻中穴 1 分钟，力度稍轻；再用拇指从胸骨上窝向下直推到胸骨下角 5~6 下。

肾俞 两手握拳绕于背后腰部，用掌指关节稍用力按揉两侧肾俞穴 2 分钟。

21 高血压

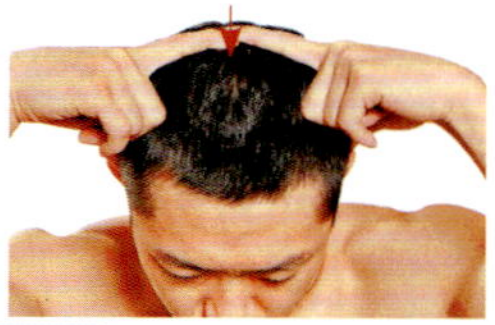
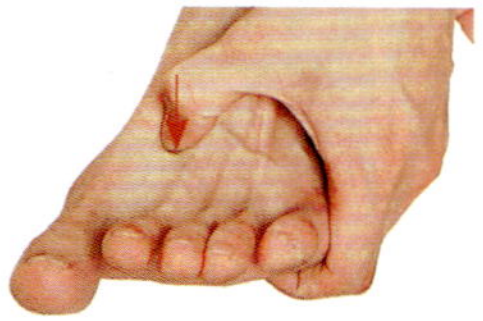
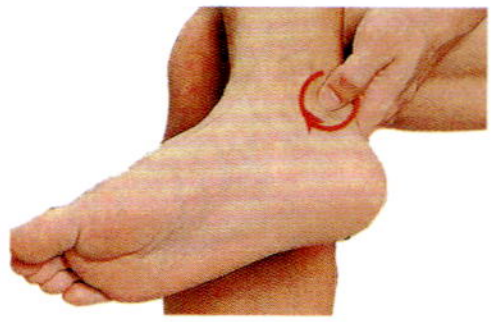

百会 两手食指重叠稍用力按压百会穴，停留片刻后放松，反复 5~6 下。

太冲 用拇指掐揉太冲穴，力度稍重。同法掐揉对侧太冲穴。

太溪 用拇指按揉太溪穴 2 分钟，力度稍重。同法按揉对侧太溪穴。

22 冠心病

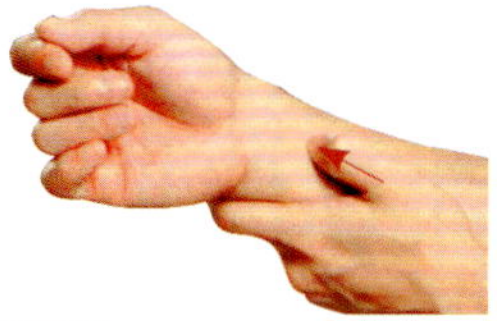
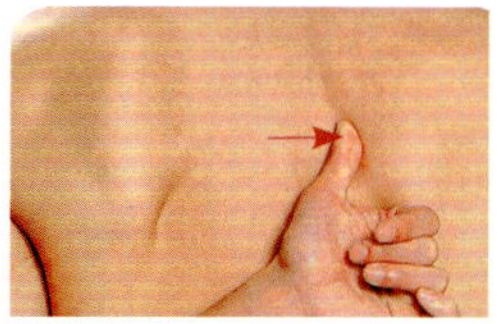
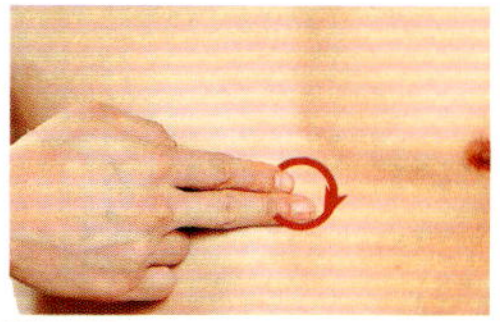

内关 用拇指稍用力按压内关穴，停留片刻后放松，反复 5~6 下。同法按压对侧内关穴。

心俞 一手绕于背后，用拇指稍用力推按心俞穴，停留片刻后放松，反复 5~6 下。同法按压对侧心俞穴。

膻中 先用食、中二指按揉膻中穴 1 分钟，力度稍轻；再用拇指从胸骨上窝向下直推到胸骨下角 5~6 下。

23 胃痛

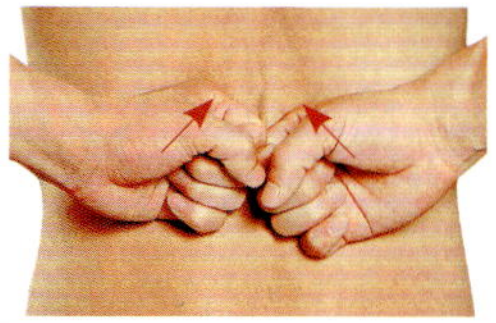
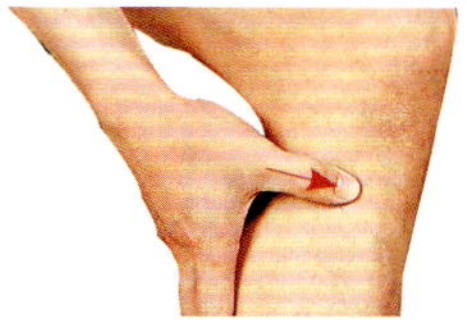
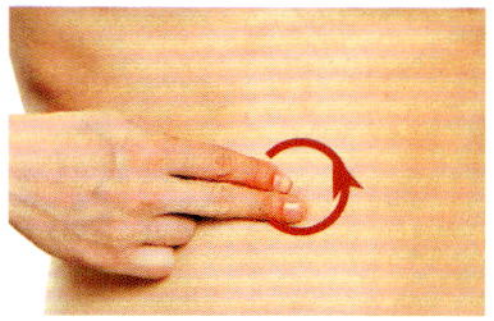

脾俞 双手握拳绕于背后，用掌指关节稍用力按压两侧脾俞穴，停留片刻后放松，反复 5~6 下。

足三里 用拇指稍用力按压足三里穴，停留片刻后放松，反复 5~6 下。同法按压对侧足三里穴。

中脘 用手指按揉中脘穴，逆时针方向揉转 2 分钟，力度稍重。

18 Fever

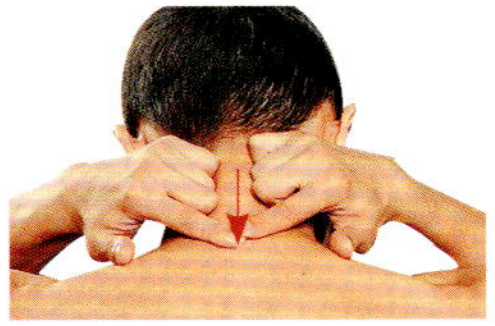

Dàzhuī(GV14) : Overlap both index fingers and press the Dazhui acupoint with a little heavy strength for 2 minutes, then relax, repeat 5~6 times a day.

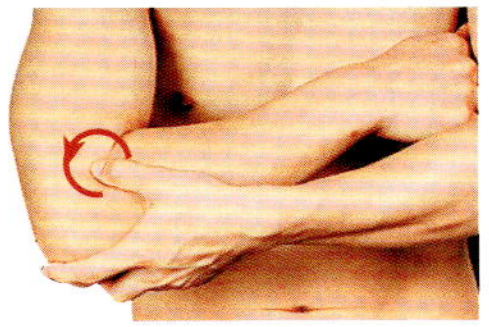

Qūchí(LI11) : Use the thumb to knead the Quchi acupoint with a little heavy strength for 2 minutes. Knead the contralateral Quchi acupoint with the same method.

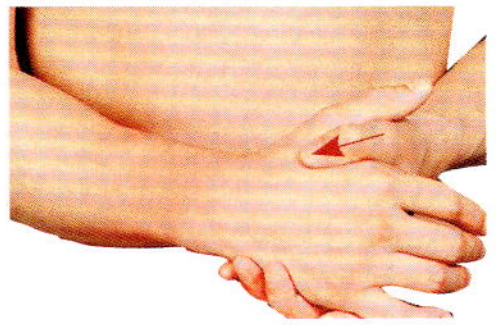

Hégǔ(LI 4) : Use the thumb to press the Hegu acupoint for a while, then relax, repeat 5~6 times. Press the contralateral Hegu acupoint with the same method.

19 Cough

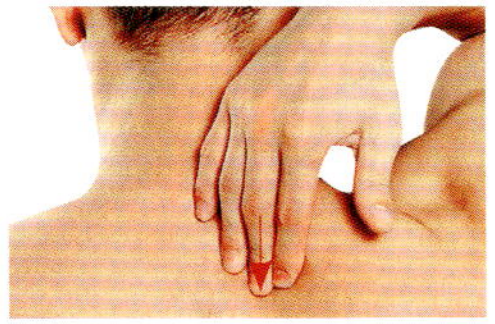

Fèishū(BL13):Put the hand on the back and use the finger to press the Feishu acupoint with a little heavy strength for a while, then relax, repeat 5~6 times a day. Press the contralateral Feishu acupoint.

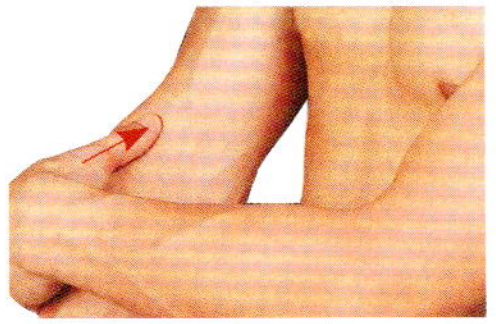

Chǐzé(LU5) : Use the thumb to press or knead Chize acupoint with appropriate strength for 2 minutes.

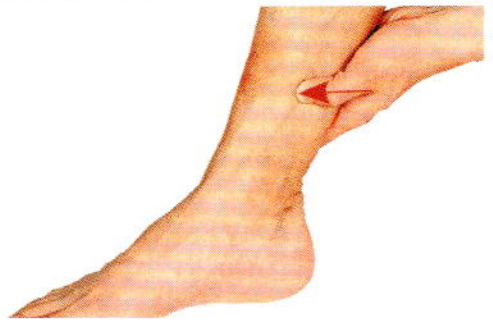

Sānyīnjiāo(SP6): Use the thumb to press the Sanyinjiao acupoint with a little heavy strength for a while, then relax, repeat 5~6 times a day. Press the contralateral Sanyinjiao acupoint with the same method.

20 Asthma

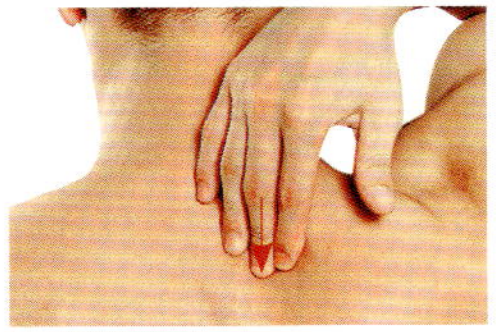

Fèishū(BL13): Put the hand on the back and use the finger to press the Feishu acupoint with a little heavy strength for a while, then relax, repeat 5~6 times a day. Press the contralateral Feishu acupoint with the same method.

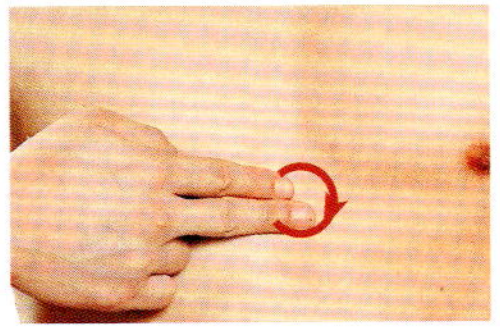

Dànzhōng(CV17):Use the index finger and middle finger to knead the Danzhong acupoint with slight strength for a minute, then use the thumb to push downward from the fossa suprasternalis to the infrasternal angle,repeat 5~6 times.

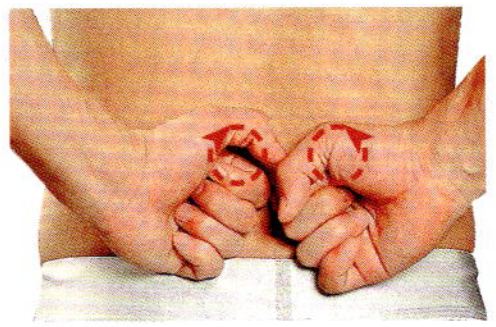

Shènshū(BL23) : Put both clenched-fists on the waist and use both metacarpophalangeal joints to knead both Shenshu acupoints with a little heavy strength for 2 minutes.

21 Hypertension

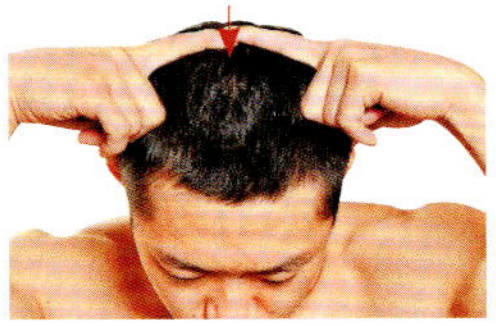

Bǎihuì(GV20): Overlap both index fingers to knead the Baihui acupoint with a little heavy strength for a moment, then relax, repeat 5~6 times a day.

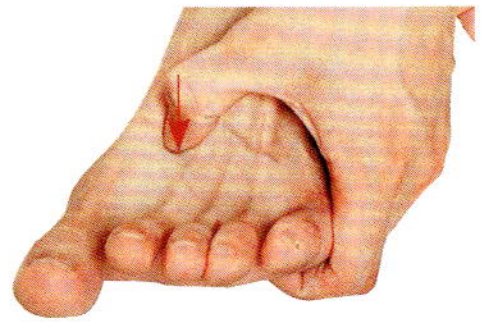

Tàichōng(LR3) : Use the thumb to press the Taichong acupoint for a while, then relax,repeat 5~6 times. Knead the contralateral Taichong acupoint.

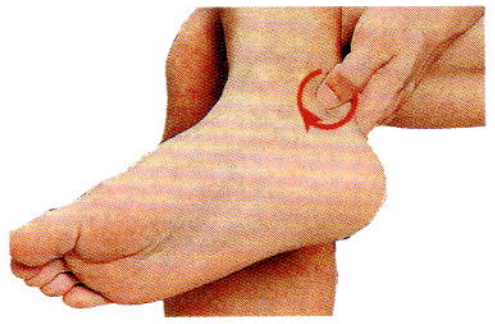

Tàixī(KI3): Use the thumb to knead the Taixi acupoint with a little heavy strength for 2 minutes. Knead the contralateral Taixi acupoint.

22 Coronary Heart Disease

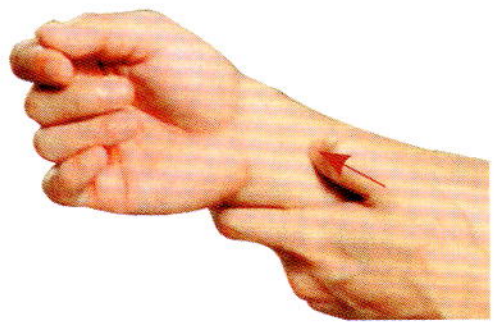

Nèiguān(PC6) : Use the thumb to press the Neiguan acupoint for a while, then relax,repeat 5~6 times with slight strength. Press the contralateral Neiguan acupoint.

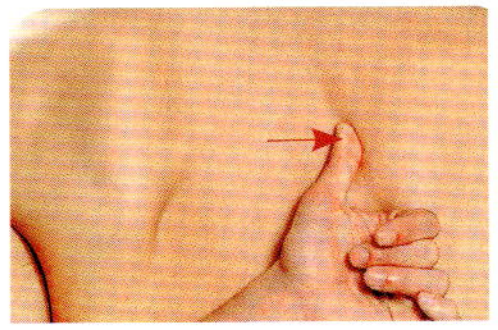

Xīnshū(BL15) : Put the hand on the back and use the thumb to press the Xinshu acupoint with a little heavy strength for a while, then relax, repeat 5~6 times a day. Press the contralateral Xinshu acupoint with the same method.

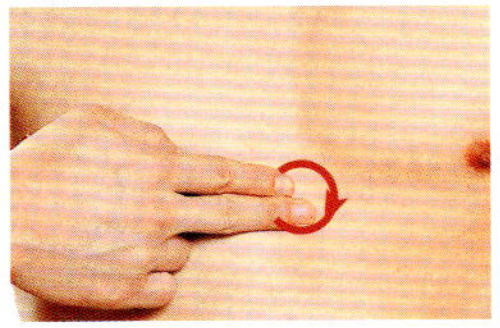

Dànzhōng(CV17) : Use the index finger and middle finger to knead the Danzhong acupoint with slight strength for a minute, use the thumb to push downward from the fossa suprasternalis to the infrasternal angle, repeat 5~6 times.

23 Stomachache

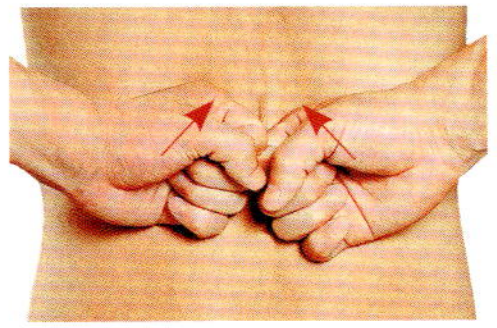

Píshū(BL20): Put both clenched-fists on the waist, use both metacarpophalangeal joints to knead both Pishu acupoints with a little heavy strength for a moment, repeat 5~6 times.

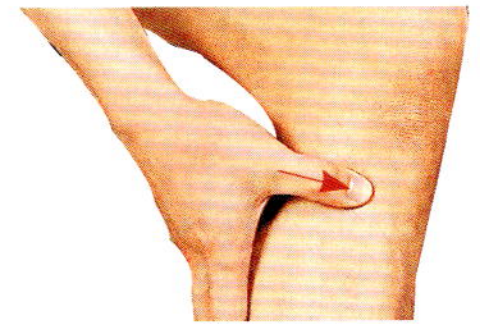

Zúsānlǐ(ST36): Use the thumb to press the Zusanli acupoint with a little heavy strength for a while, then relax, repeat 5~6 times a day. Press the contralateral Zusanli acupoint with the same method.

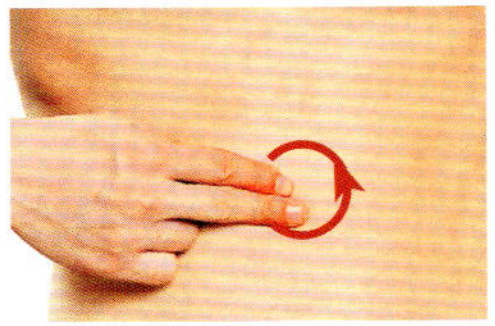

Zhōngwǎn(CV12) : Use the finger to knead the Zhongwan acupoint in counterclockwise direction with a little heavy strength for 2 minutes.

24 腹泻

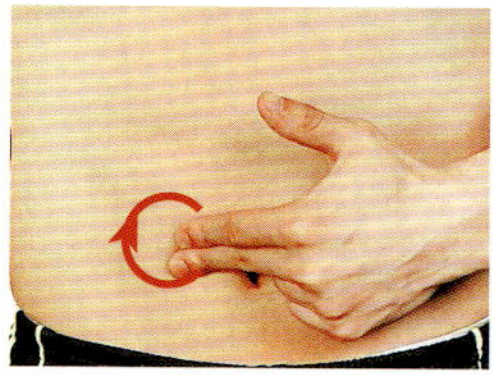

天枢 食、中二指并拢按揉天枢穴，顺时针方向揉转2分钟，力度稍重。同法按揉对侧天枢穴。

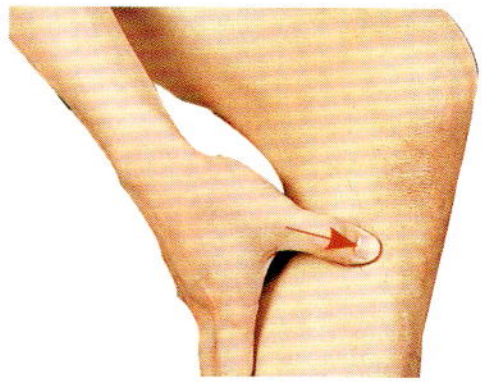

足三里 用拇指稍用力按压足三里穴，停留片刻后放松，反复5~6下。同法按压对侧足三里穴。

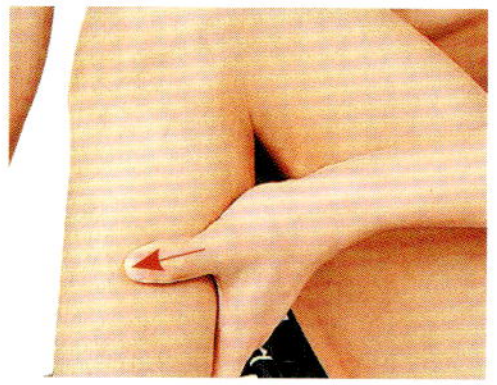

上巨虚 用拇指稍用力按压上巨虚穴，停留片刻后放松，反复5~6下。同法按压对侧上巨虚穴。

25 便秘

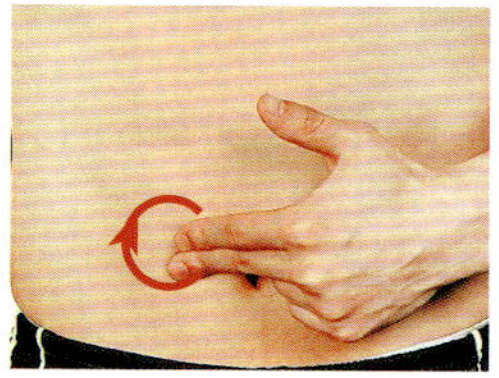

天枢 食、中二指并拢按揉天枢穴，顺时针方向揉转2分钟，力度稍重。同法按揉对侧天枢穴。

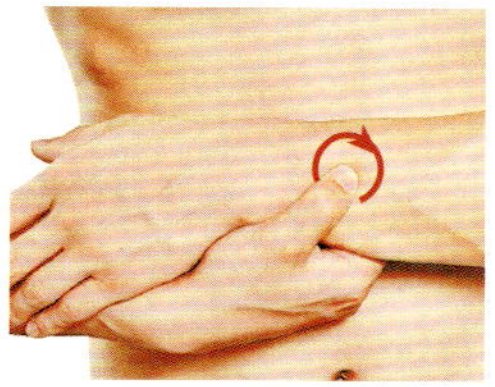

支沟 用拇指按揉支沟穴2分钟，力度稍重。同法按揉对侧支沟穴。

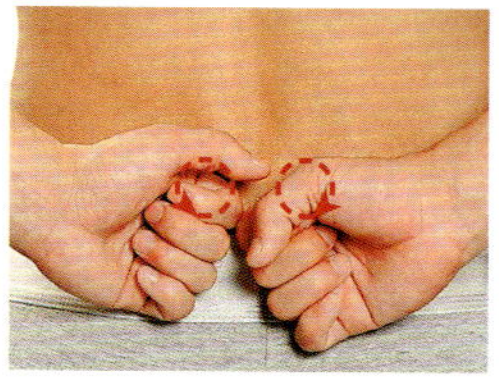

大肠俞 两手握拳绕于背后，用掌指关节稍用力按压两侧大肠俞穴，停留片刻后放松，反复5~6下。

26 糖尿病

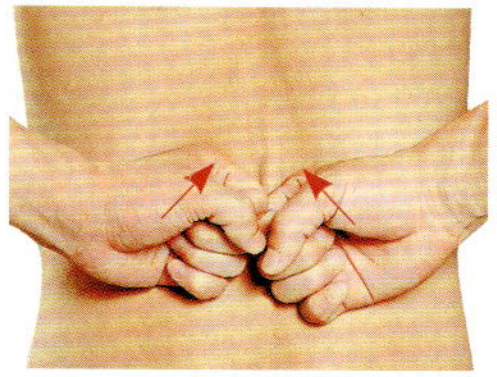

脾俞 双手握拳绕于背后，用掌指关节稍用力按压两侧脾俞穴，停留片刻后放松，反复5~6下。

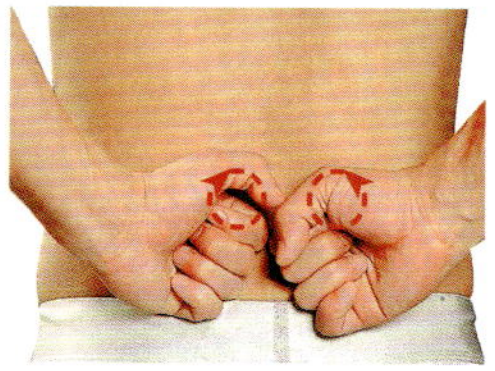

肾俞 双手握拳绕于背后，用掌指关节按揉两侧肾俞穴，力度稍重。

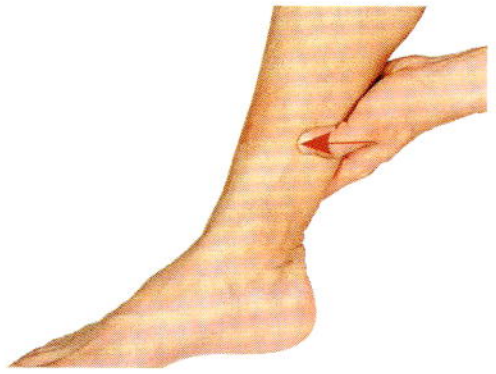

三阴交 用拇指用力按压三阴交穴，停留片刻后放松，反复5~6下。同法按压对侧三阴交穴。

27 高脂血症

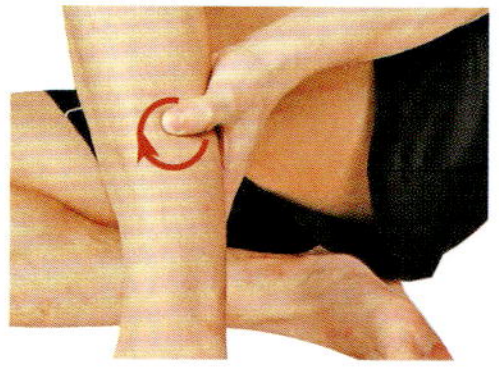

丰隆 用拇指按揉丰隆穴2分钟，力度稍重。同法按揉对侧丰隆穴。

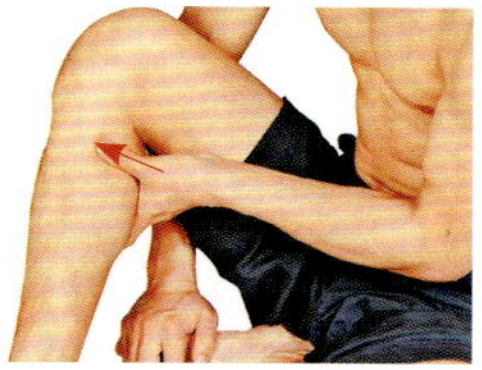

阴陵泉 用拇指按压阴陵泉穴，停留片刻后放松，反复5~6下。同法按压对侧阴陵泉穴，每次2分钟。

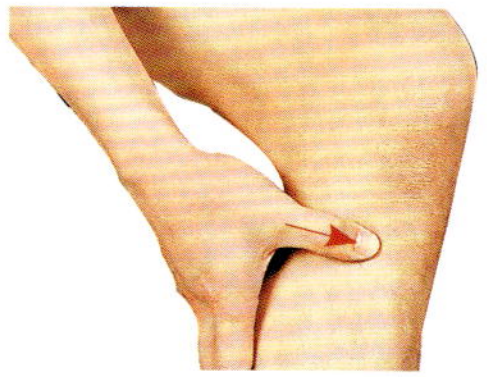

足三里 用拇指稍用力按压足三里穴，停留片刻后放松，反复5~6下。同法按压对侧足三里穴。

28 头痛

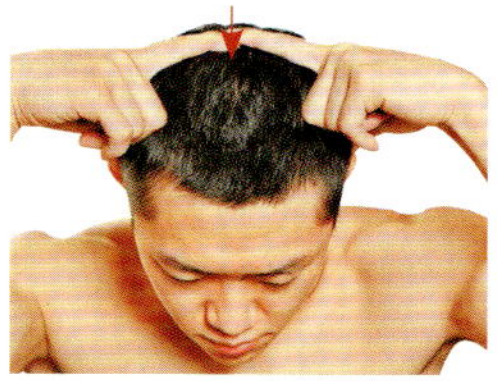

百会 两手食指重叠稍用力按压百会穴，停留片刻后放松，反复5~6下。

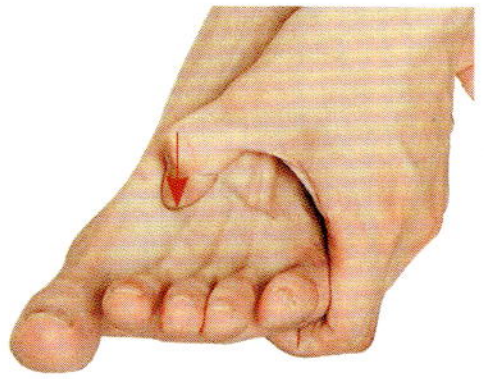

太冲 用拇指掐揉太冲穴，力度稍重。同法掐揉对侧太冲穴。

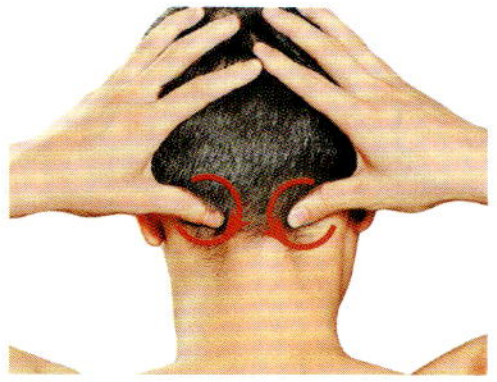

风池 用两手拇指勾揉两侧风池穴2分钟，力度稍重。

29 失眠

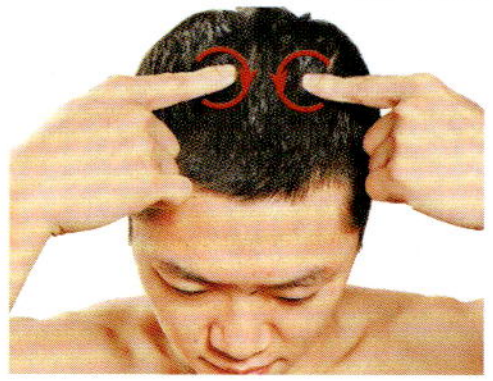

四神聪 用两手食指按揉四神聪穴，每个穴位1分钟，力度稍重。

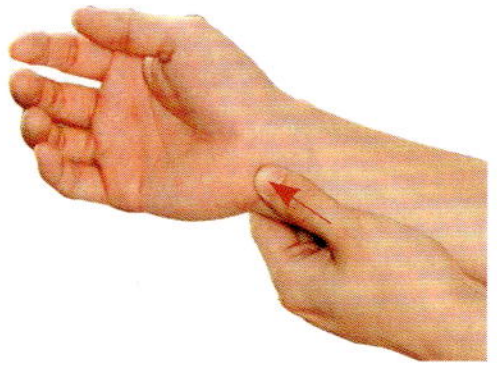

神门 用拇指稍用力按压神门穴，停留片刻后放松，反复5~6下。同法按压对侧神门穴。

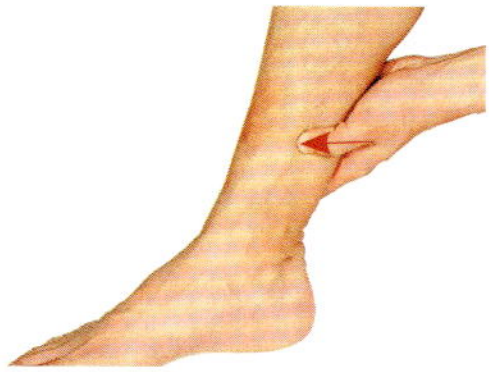

三阴交 用拇指用力按压三阴交穴，停留片刻后放松，反复5~6下。同法按压对侧三阴交穴。

24 Diarrhea

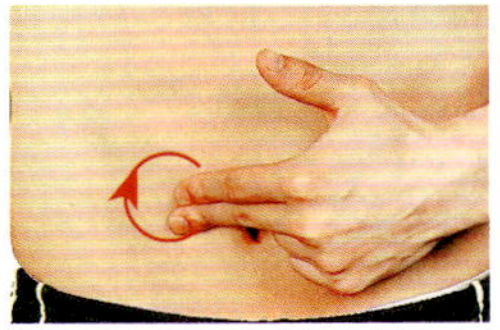

Tiānshū(ST25) : Use the index finger and middle finger to knead the Tianshu acupoint in clockwise direction with a little heavy strength for 2 minutes.

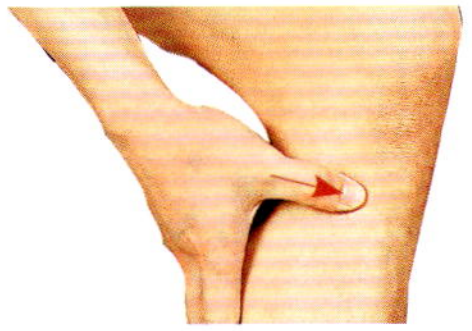

Zúsānlǐ(ST36) : Use the thumb to press the Zusanli acupoint with a little heavy strength for a while, then relax, repeat 5~6 times a day. Knead the contralateral Zusanli acupoint with the same method.

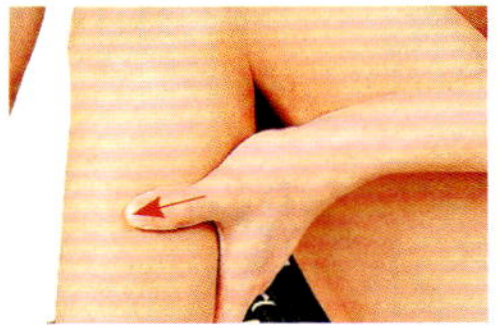

Shàngjùxū(ST37) : Use the thumb to press the Shangjuxu acupoint for a while, then relax, repeat 5~6 times with slight strength. Press the contralateral Shangjuxu acupoint with the same method.

25 Constipation

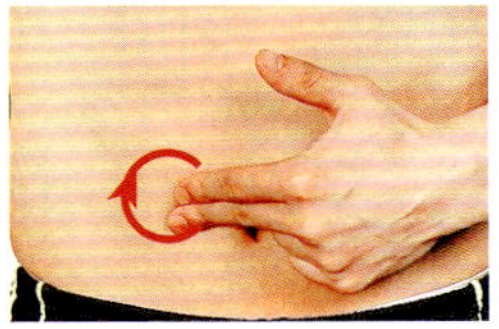

Tiānshū(ST25): Use the index finger and middle finger to knead the Tianshu acupoint in clockwise direction with a little heavy strength for 2 minutes.

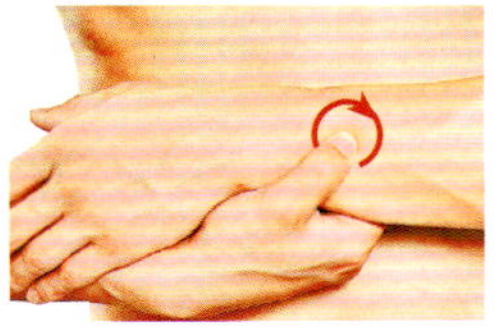

Zhīgōu(TE6) : Use the thumb to knead the Zhigou acupoint with a little heavy strength for 2 minutes. Knead the contralateral Zhigou acupoint.

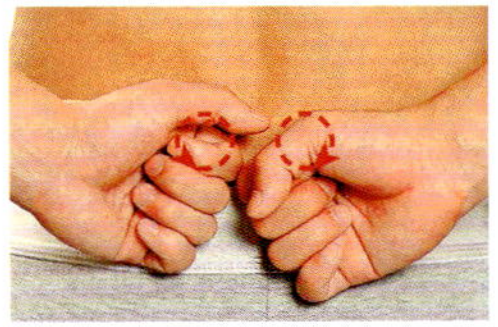

Dàchángshū(BL 25) : Put both clenched-fists on the waist and use both metacarpophalangeal joints to knead both Dachangshu acupoints with a little heavy strength for a moment, repeat 5~6 times.

26 Diabetes Mellitus

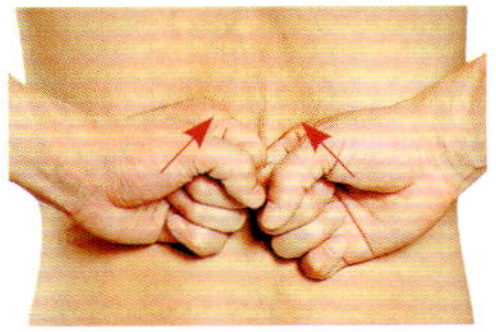

Píshū(BL26) : Put both clenched-fists on the back and use both metacarpophalangeal joints to press both Pishu acupoints with a little heavy strength for a moment, then relax, repeat 5~6 times.

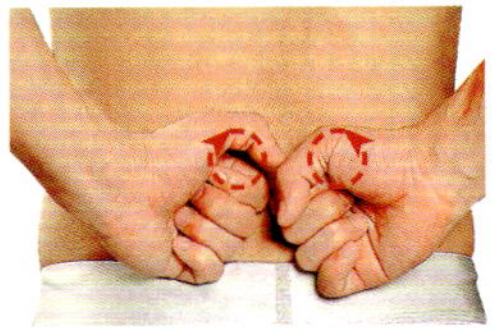

Shènshū(BL23) : Put both clenched-fists on the back and use both metacarpophalangeal joints to knead both Shenshu acupoints with a little heavy strength.

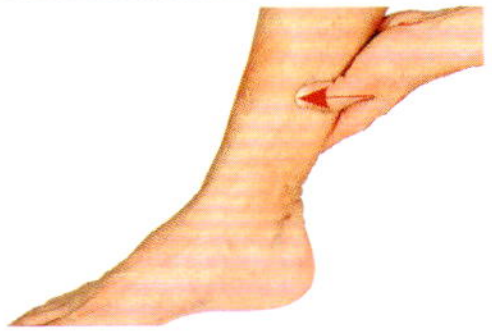

Sānyīnjiāo(SP6) : Use the thumb to press the Sanyinjiao acupoint with a little heavy strength for a while,then relax, repeat 5~6 times a day. Press the contralateral Sanyinjiao acupoint with the same method.

27 Hyperlipemia

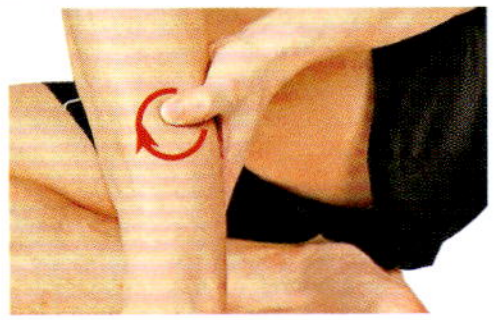

Fēnglóng(ST40) : Use the thumb to knead the Fenglong acupoint with a little heavy strength for 2 minutes. Knead the contralateral Fenglong acupoint with the same method.

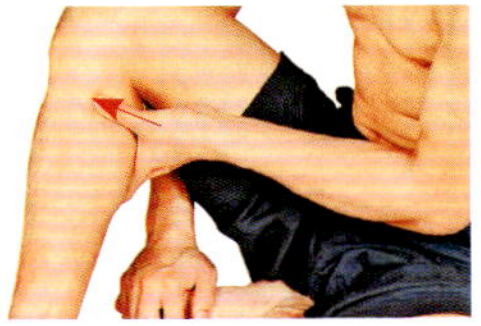

Yīnlíngquán(SP9) : Use the thumb to press the Yinlingquan acupoint with a little heavy strength for a while, then relax, repeat 5~6 times a day. Press the contralateral Yinlingquan acupoint with the same method for 2 minutes.

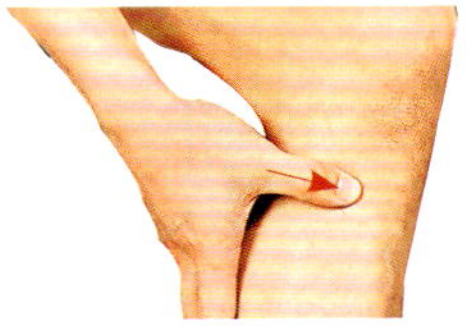

Zúsānlǐ(ST36) : Use the thumb to press the Zusanli acupoint with a little heavy strength for a while,then relax, repeat 5~6 times a day. Press the contralateral Zusanli acupoint.

28 Headache

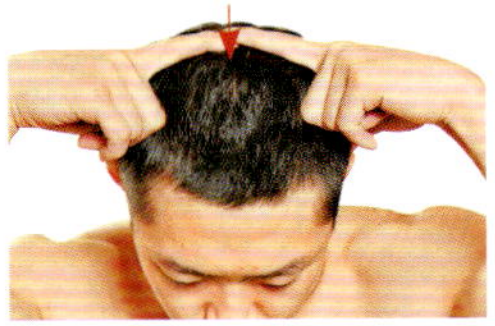

Bǎihuì(GV20) : Overlap both index fingers and press the Baihui acupoint with a little heavy strength for a moment, then relax, repeat 5~6 times a day.

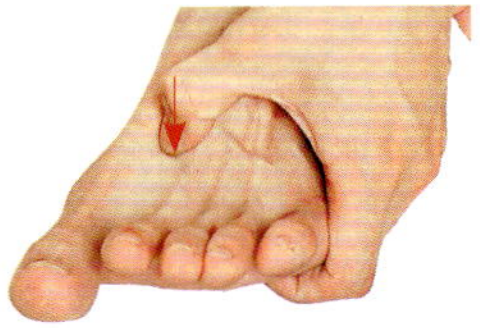

Tàichōng(LR3) : Use the thumb to press the Taichong acupoint with a little heavy strength, press the contralateral Taichong acupoint with the same method.

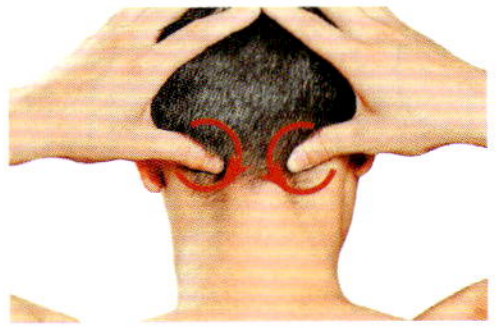

Fēngchí(GB20) : Use both thumbs to knead Fengchi acupoints with a little heavy strength for 2 minutes.

29 Insomnia

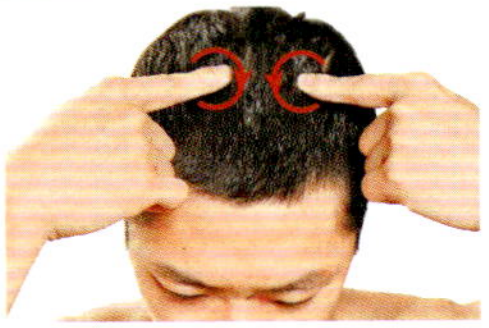

Sìshéncōng(EX-HN1) : Use both index fingers to knead Sishencong acupoints with a little heavy strength for a minute.

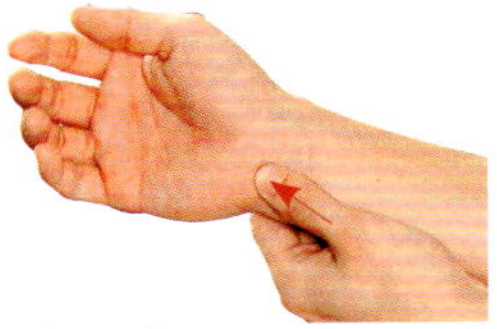

Shénmén(HT7) : Use the thumb to press the Shenmen acupoint for a while, then relax, repeat 5~6 times with slight strength. Press the contralateral ShenMen acupoint.

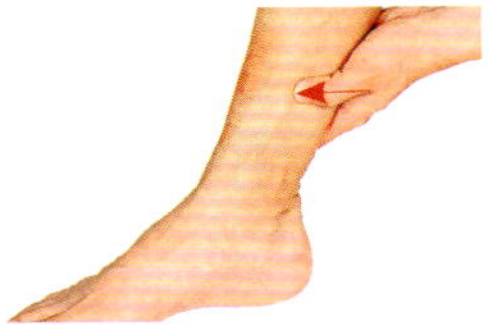

Sānyīnjiāo(SP6) : Use the Thumb to press the Sanyinjiao acupoint with a little heavy strength for a while, then relax, repeat 5~6 times. Press the contralateral Sanyinjiao acupoint with the same method.

30 健忘

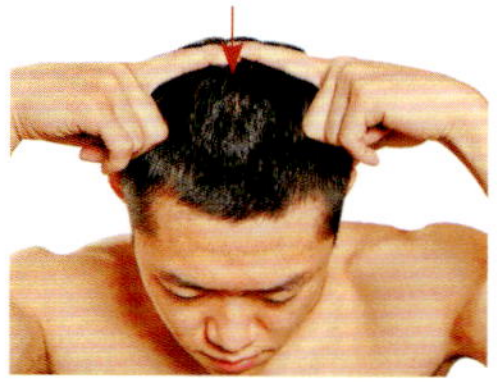

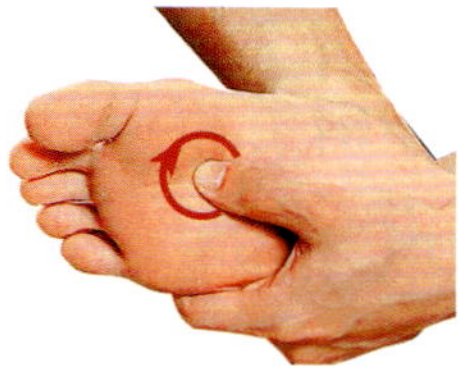

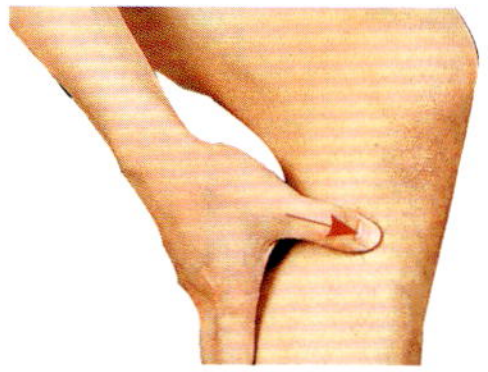

百会 两手食指重叠稍用力按压百会穴，停留片刻后放松，反复5~6下。

涌泉 用拇指按揉涌泉穴2分钟，力度稍重。同法按揉对侧涌泉穴。

足三里 用拇指稍用力按压足三里穴，停留片刻后放松，反复5~6下。同法按压对侧足三里穴。

31 慢性咽炎

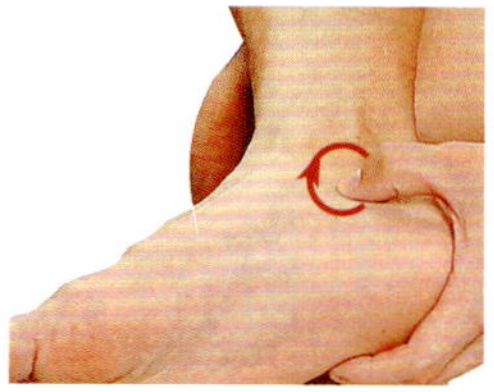

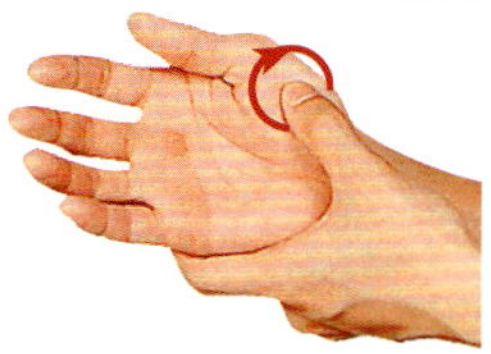

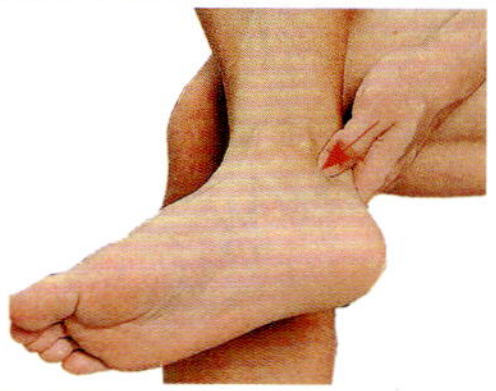

照海 用拇指按揉照海穴2分钟，力度稍重。同法按揉对侧照海穴。

鱼际 用拇指按揉鱼际穴2分钟，力度稍重。同法按揉对侧鱼际穴。

太溪 用拇指稍用力按压太溪穴，停留片刻后放松，反复5~6下。同法按压对侧太溪穴。

32 慢性鼻炎

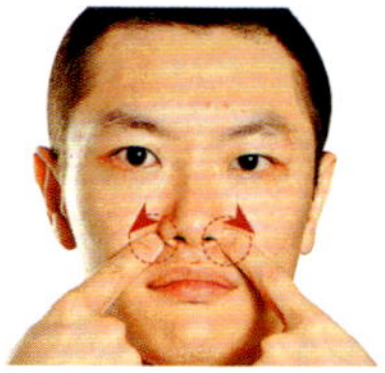

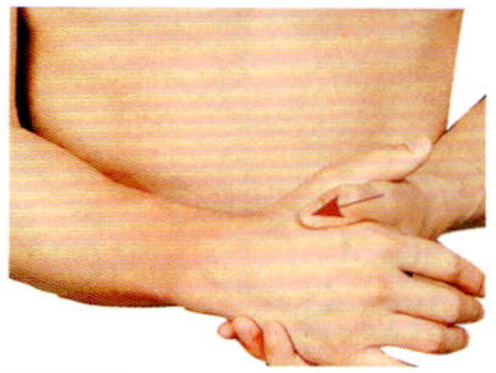

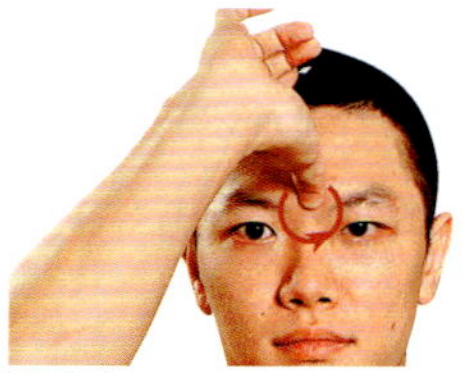

迎香 用两手食指按揉两侧迎香穴2分钟，力度稍重。

合谷 用拇指用力按压合谷穴，停留片刻后放松，反复5~6下。同法按压对侧合谷穴。

印堂 用拇指掐揉印堂穴2分钟，力度稍重。

33 落枕

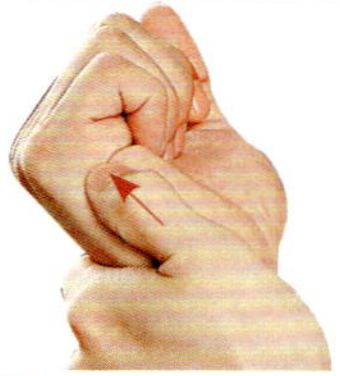

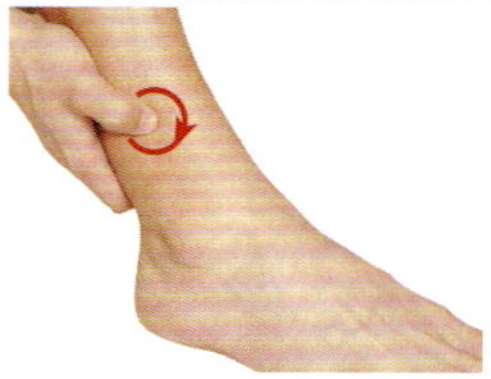

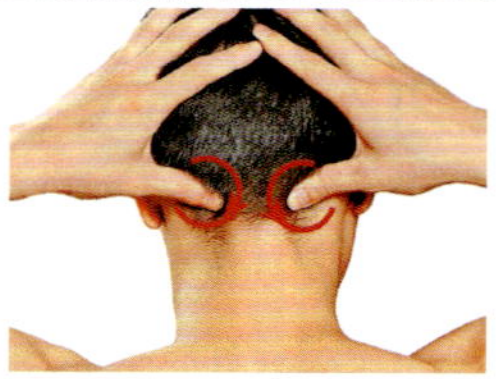

后溪 用拇指稍用力按压后溪穴，停留片刻后放松，反复5~6下。同法按压对侧后溪穴。

悬钟 用拇指按揉悬钟穴2分钟，力度稍重。同法按揉对侧悬钟穴。

风池 两手拇指勾揉两侧风池穴2分钟，力度稍重。

34 颈椎病

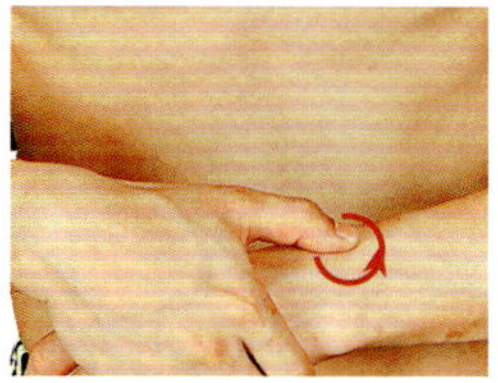

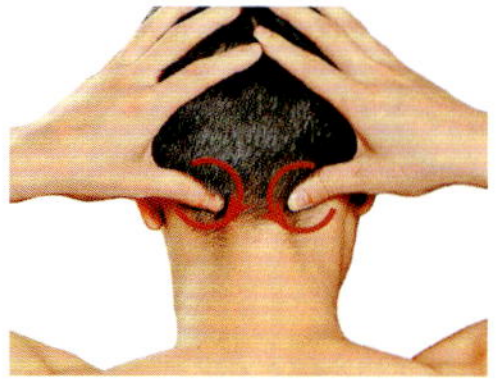

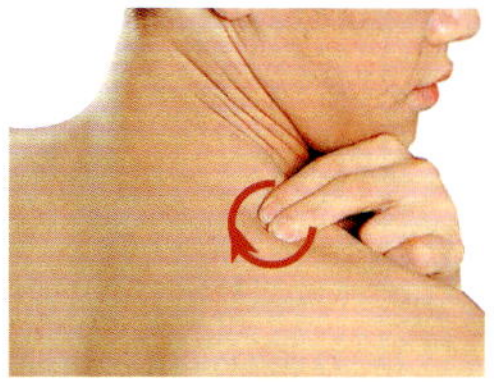

列缺 用拇指按揉列缺穴2分钟，力度稍重。同法按揉对侧列缺穴。

风池 两手拇指勾揉两侧风池穴2分钟，力度稍重。

肩井 食、中二指并拢按揉肩井穴2分钟，力度稍重。同法按揉对侧肩井穴。

35 肩周炎

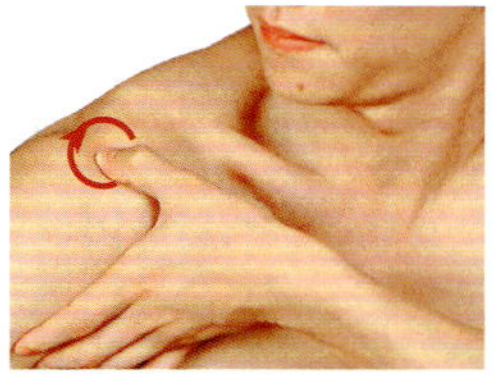

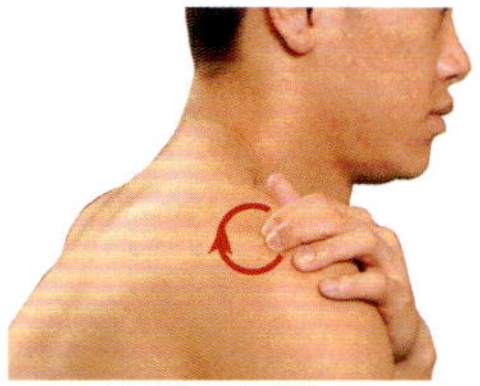

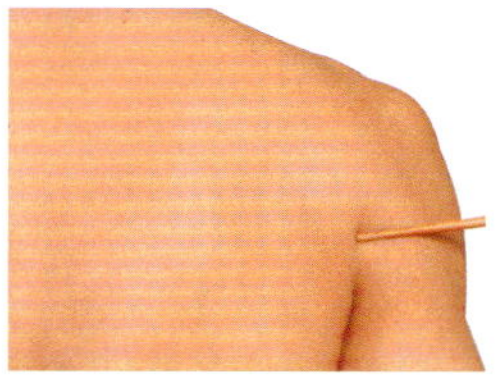

肩髃 用拇指按揉肩髃穴2分钟，力度稍重。同法按揉对侧肩髃穴。

肩髎 用食指、中指按揉对侧肩髎穴2分钟，力度适宜。

肩贞 此穴在腋后纹头直上1寸，三角肌后缘。可请他人帮忙按摩，用拇指点按本穴2分钟。

30 Amnesia

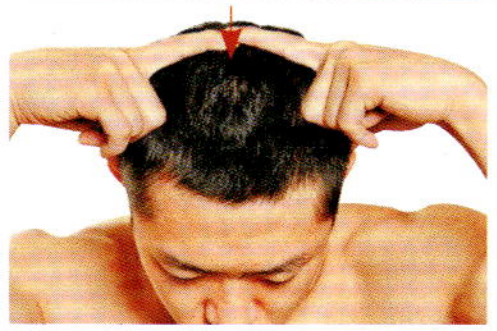

Bǎihuì(GV20) : Overlap both index fingers to press the Baihui acupoint with a little heavy strength for a moment, then relax, repeat 5~6 times.

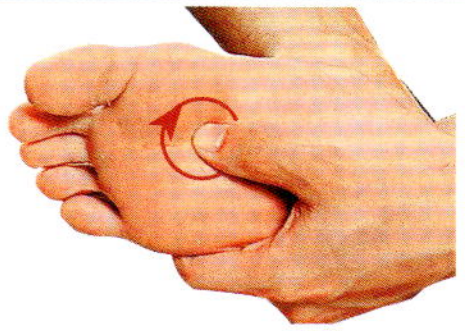

Yǒngquán(KI1) : Use the thumb to knead the Yongquan acupoint with a little heavy strength for 2 minutes. Knead the contralateral Yongquan acupoint.

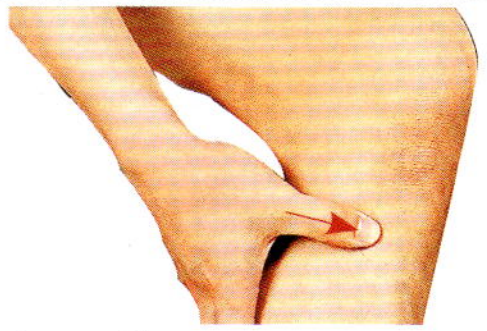

Zúsānlǐ(ST36) : Use the thumb to press the Zusanli acupoint with a little heavy strength for a while,then relax, repeat 5~6 times. Press the contralateral Zusanli acupoint with the same method.

31 Chronic Pharyngitis

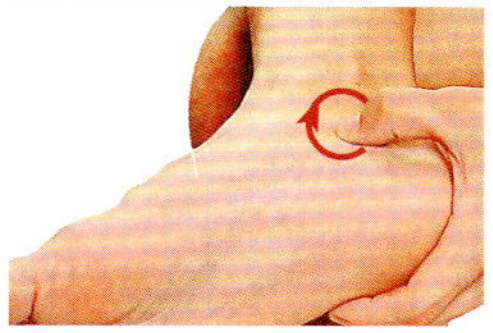

Zhàohǎi(KI6) : Use the thumb to knead the Zhaohai acupoint with a little heavy strength for 2 minutes. Knead the contralateral Zhaohai acupoint with the same method.

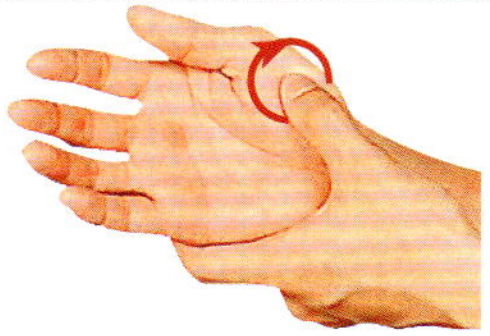

Yújì(LU10) : Use the thumb to knead the Yuji acupoint with a little heavy strength for 2 minutes. Knead the contralateral Yuji acupoint.

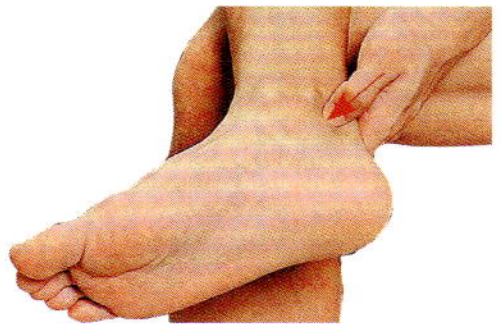

Tàixī(KI3) : Use the thumb to knead the Taixi acupoint with a little heavy strength for 2 minutes, then relax, repeat 5~6 times. Knead the contralateral Taixi acupoint with the same method.

32 Chronic Rhinitis

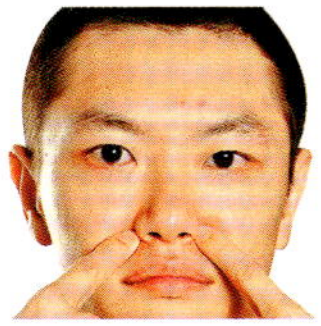

Yíngxiāng(LI20) : Use both index fingers to knead both side Yingxiang acupoints with a little heavy strength for 2 minutes.

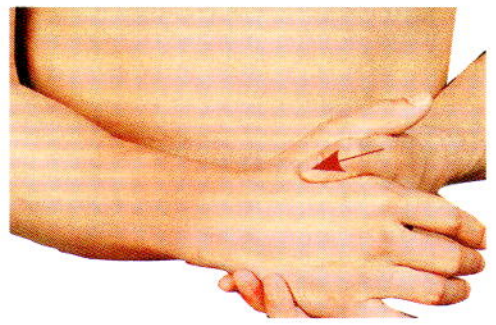

Hégǔ(LI 4) : Use the thumb to press the Hegu acupoint for a while,then relax, repeat 5~6 times. Press the contralateral Hegu acupoint with the same method.

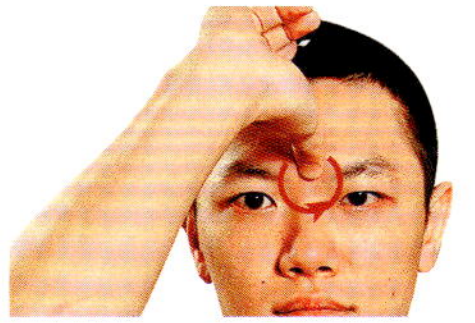

Yìntáng(GV29) : Use the thumb to knead the Yintang acupoint with a little heavy strength for 2 minutes.

33 Stiff Neck

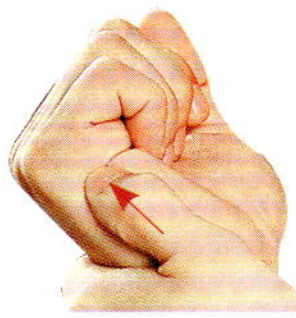

Hòuxī(SI3) : Use the thumb to press the Houxi acupoint for a while, then relax, repeat 5~6 times. Press the contralateral Houxi acupoint with the same method.

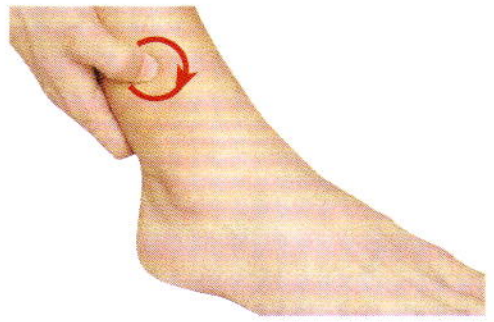

Xuánzhōng(GB39) : Use the thumb to knead the acupoint with a little heavy strength for 2 minutes. Knead the contralateral acupoint with the same method.

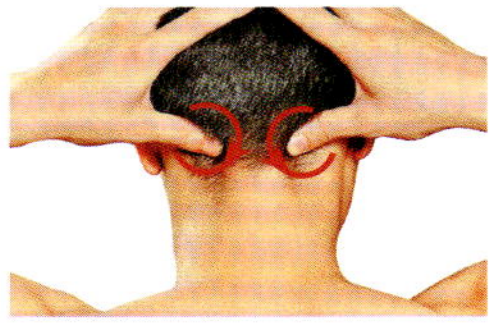

Fēngchí(GB20) : Use both thumbs to knead Fengchi acupoints with a little heavy strength for 2 minutes.

34 Cervical Spondylosis

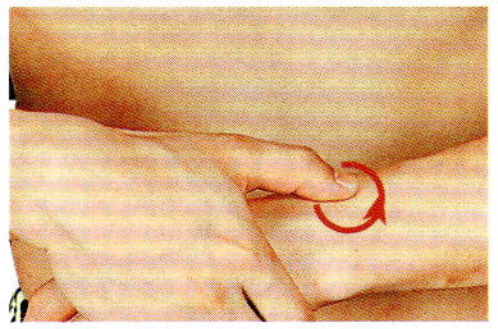

Lièquē(LU7) : Use the thumb to knead the Lieque acupoint for 2 minutes with a little heavy strength, knead the contralateral Lieque acupoint with the same method.

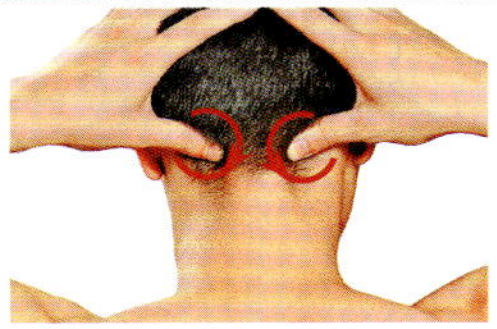

Fēngchí(GB20) : Use both thumbs to knead Fengchi acupoint with a little heavy strength for 2 minutes.

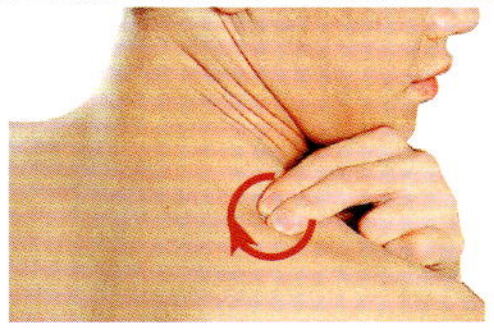

Jiānjǐng(GB21) : Use the index finger and middle finger to knead the Jianjing acupoint with a little heavy strength for 2 minutes. Knead the contralateral Jianjing acupoint with the same method.

35 Shoulder Periarthritis

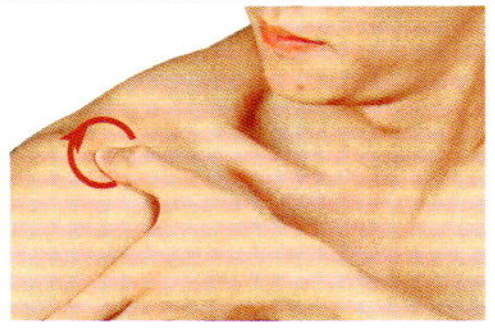

Jiānyú(LI15) : Use the thumb to knead Jianyu acupoint with a little heavy strength for 2 minutes. Knead the contralateral Jianyu acupoint with the same method.

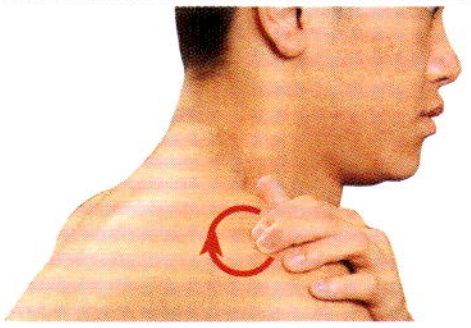

Jiānliáo(TE14) : Use the index finger and middle finger to knead contralateral Jianliao acupoint with a little heavy strength for 2 minutes.

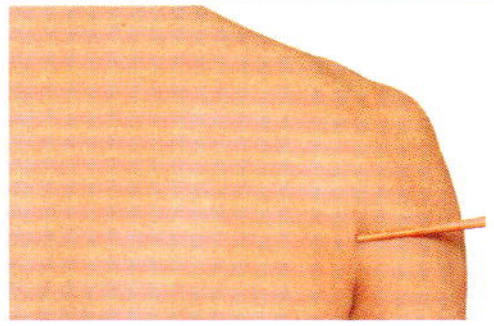

Jiānzhēn(SI9): This acupoint is located 1 cun above the posterior end of the axillary, in the posterior margin of the deltoid. Let others to help you knead Jianzhen acupoint with thumb for 2 minutes.

36 网球肘（肱骨外上髁炎）

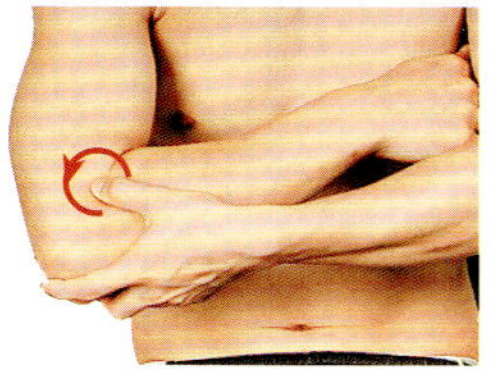

曲池 用拇指按揉曲池穴2分钟，力度稍重。同法按揉对侧曲池穴。

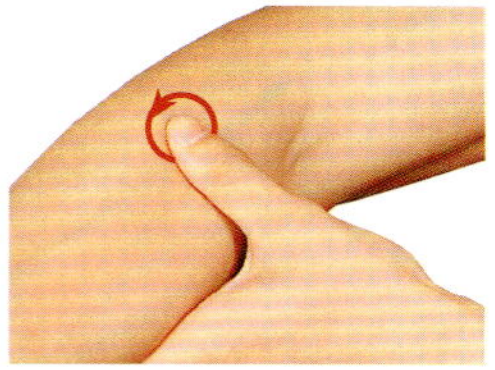

手三里 用拇指按揉手三里穴2分钟，力度稍重。同法按揉对侧手三里穴。

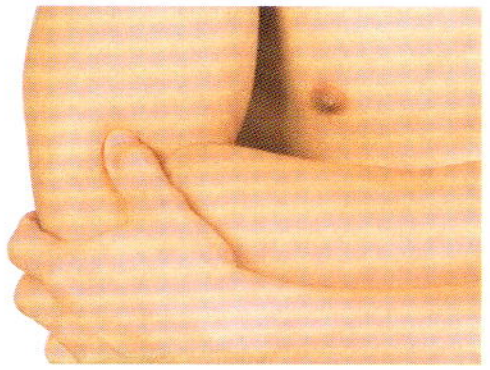

肘髎 用拇指按揉肘髎穴2分钟，力度适宜。同法按揉对侧肘髎穴。

37 急性腰扭伤

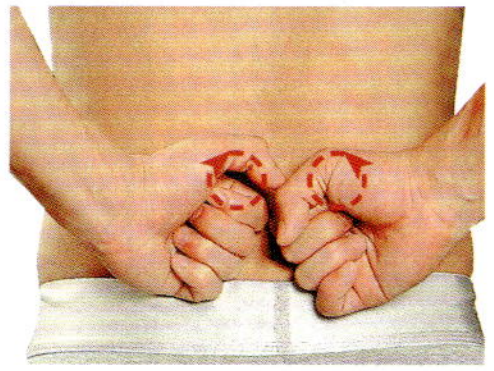

肾俞 两手握拳绕于背后腰部，用掌指关节稍用力按揉两侧肾俞穴2分钟。

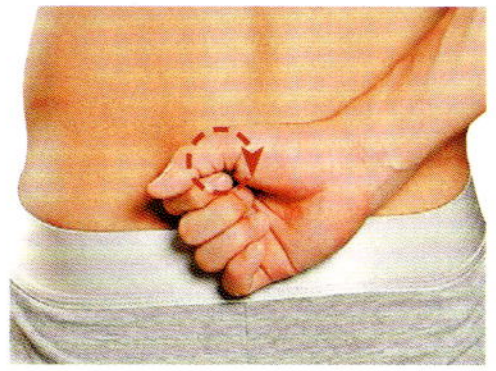

腰阳关 一手握拳绕于背后，用掌指关节稍用力按揉腰阳关穴2分钟。

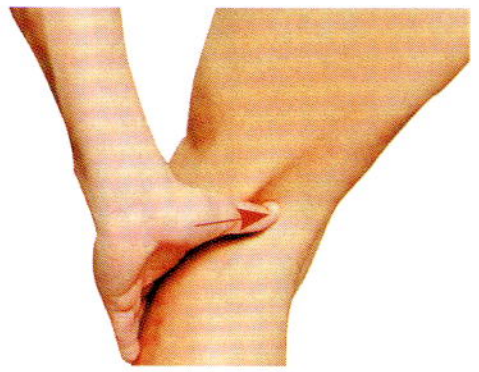

委中 用拇指用力按压委中穴，停留片刻后放松，反复5~6下。同法按压对侧委中穴。

38 腰痛

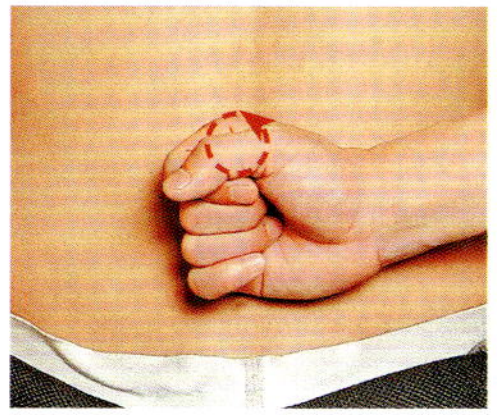

命门 一手握拳绕于背后，用掌指关节稍用力按揉命门穴2分钟。

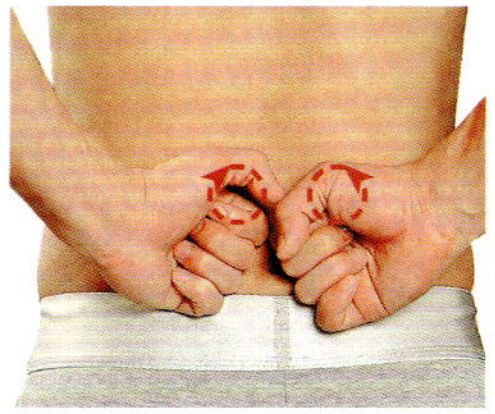

肾俞 两手握拳绕于背后腰部，用掌指关节稍用力按揉两侧肾俞穴2分钟。

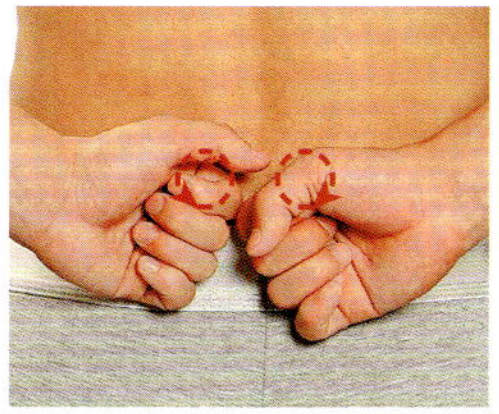

大肠俞 两手握拳绕于腰部，用掌指关节稍用力按揉两侧大肠俞穴2分钟。

39 坐骨神经痛

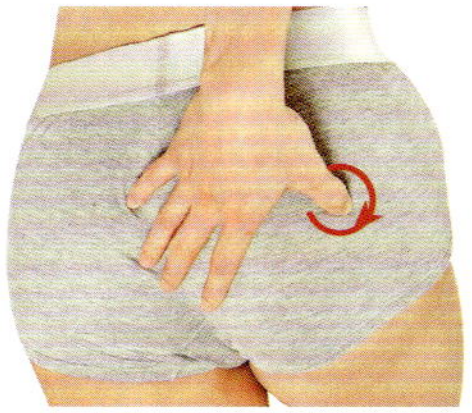

环跳 用拇指按揉环跳穴2分钟，力度稍重。同法按揉对侧环跳穴。

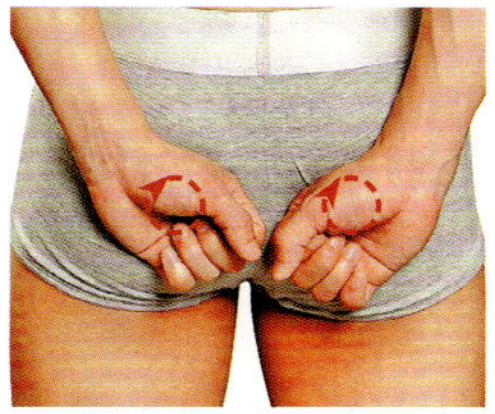

秩边 两手握拳绕于背后腰骶部，用掌指关节稍用力按揉两侧秩边穴2分钟。

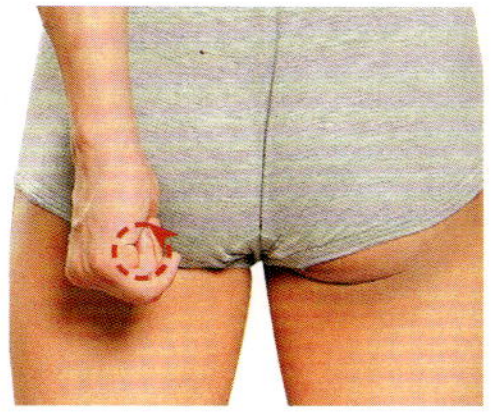

承扶 用拇指按揉承扶穴2分钟，力度稍重。同法按揉对侧承扶穴。

40 膝关节炎

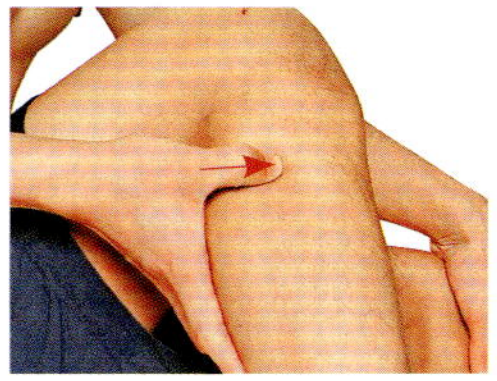

阳陵泉 用拇指稍用力按压阳陵泉穴，停留片刻后放松，反复5~6下。同法按压对侧阳陵泉穴。

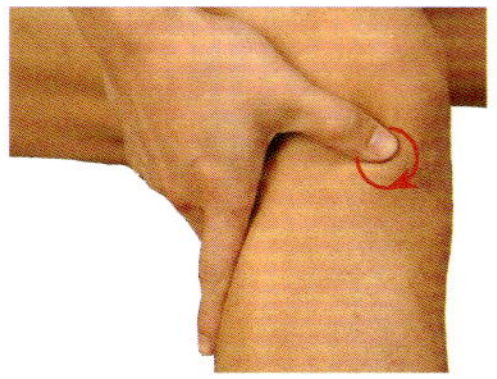

犊鼻 用拇指按揉犊鼻穴2分钟，力度适宜。同法按揉对侧犊鼻穴。

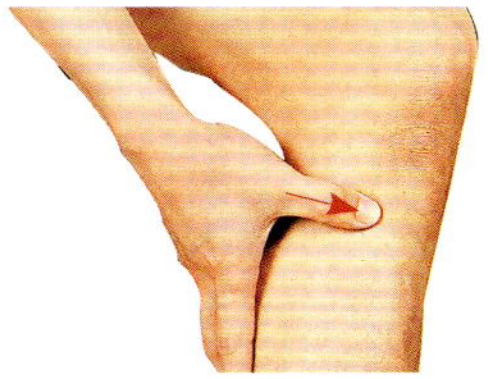

足三里 用拇指稍用力按压足三里穴，停留片刻后放松，反复5~6下。同法按压对侧足三里穴。

41 斑秃

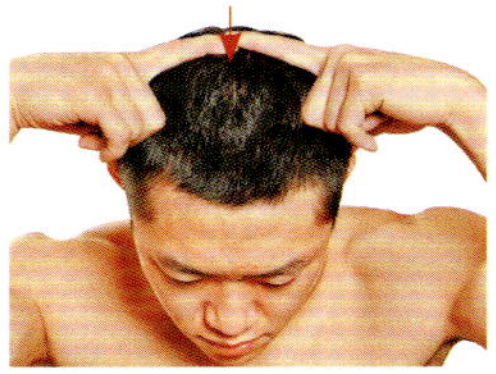

百会 两手食指重叠，稍用力按压百会穴，停留片刻后放松，反复5~6下。

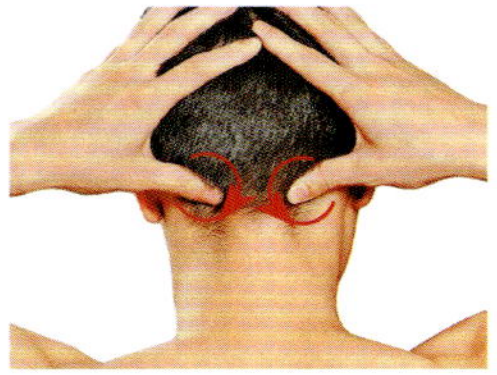

风池 用两手拇指勾揉两侧风池穴2分钟，力度稍重。

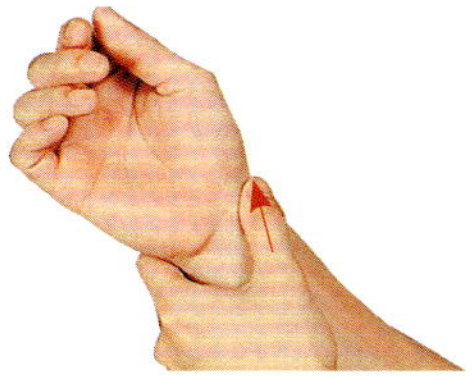

太渊 用拇指按压太渊穴，停留片刻后放松，反复5~6下，力度稍重。同法按压对侧太渊穴。

36 Tennis Elbow (Lateral Epicondylitis)

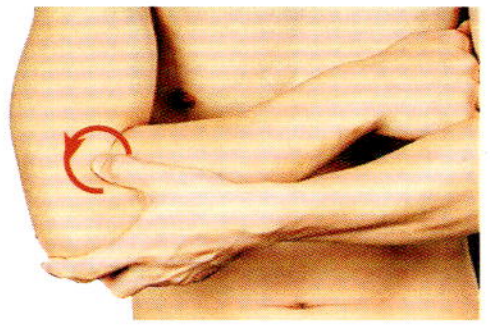

Qūchí(LI 11): Use the thumb to knead the Quchi acupoint with a little heavy strength for 2 minutes. Knead the contralateral Quchi acupoint with the same method.

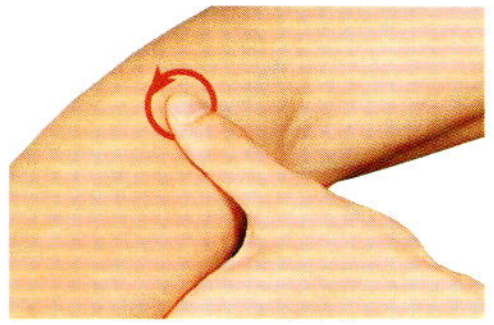

Shǒusānlǐ(LI10):Use the thumb to knead the Shousanli acupoint for 2 minutes with a little heavy strength. Knead the contralateral Shousanli acupoint with the same method.

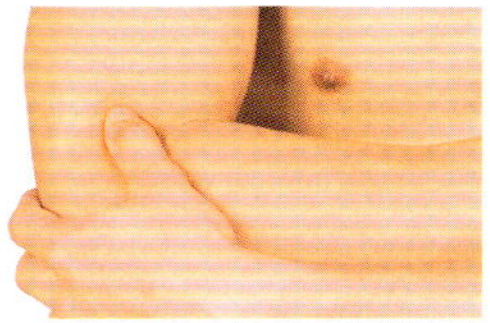

Zhǒuliáo(LI12) : Use the thumb to knead the Zhouliao acupoint for 2 minutes with appropriate strength. Use the same method to the contralateral Zhouliao acupoint.

37 Acute Waist Sprain

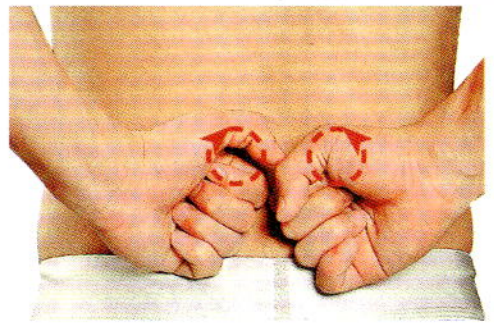

Shènshū(BL23) : Put both clenched-fists on the waist and use both metacarpophalangeal joints to knead both Shenshu acupoints with a little heavy strength for 2 minutes.

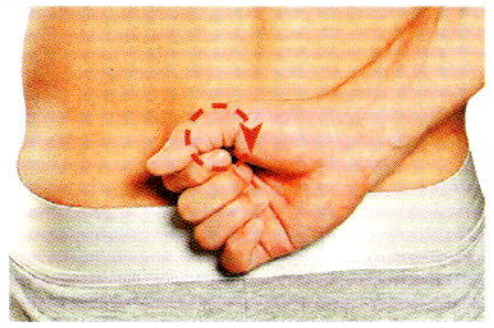

Yāoyángguān(GV3) : Put the clenched-fists on the back, use the metacarpophalangeal joint to knead the acupoint with a little heavy strength for 2 minutes.

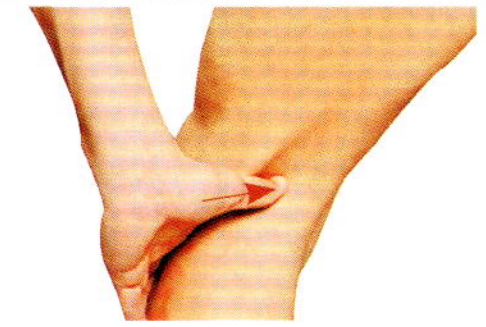

Wěizhōng(BL 40) : Use the thumb to press the Weizhong acupoint with a little heavy strength for a while,then relax, repeat 5~6 times. Press the contralateral Weizhong acupoint with the same method.

38 Waist Pain

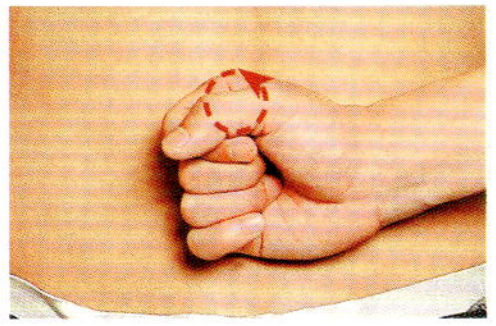

Mìngmén(GV4) : Put a clenched-fists on the back, use the metacarpophalangeal joint to knead Mingmen acupoint with a little heavy strength for 2 minutes.

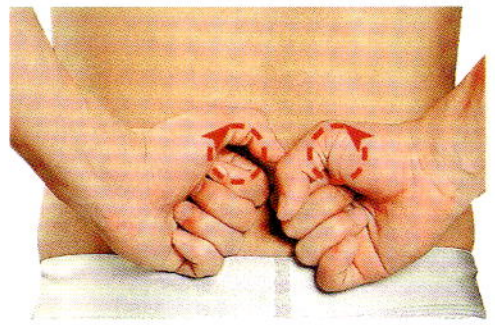

Shènshū(BL23) : Put both clenched-fists on the waist and use both metacarpophalangeal joints to knead both Shenshu acupoints with a little heavy strength for 2 minutes.

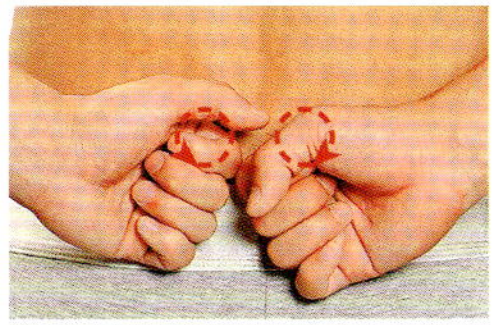

Dàchángshū(BL25) : Put both clenched-fists on the waist and use both metacarpophalangeal joints to knead both Dachangshu acupoints with a little heavy strength for 2 minutes.

39 Sciatica

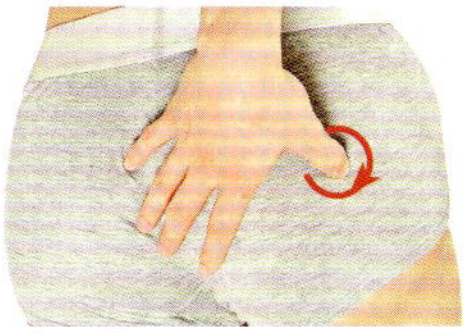

Huántiào(GB30) : Use the thumb to knead Huantiao acupoint with a little heavy strength for 2 minutes. Knead the contralateral Huantiao acupoint with the same method.

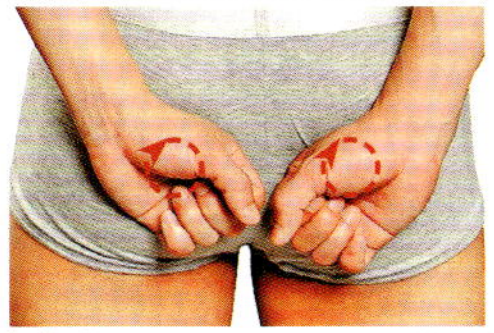

Zhìbiān(BL54): Put both clenched-fists on the lumbosacral region, use both metacarpophalangeal joints to knead both Zhibian acupoints with a little heavy strength for 2 minutes.

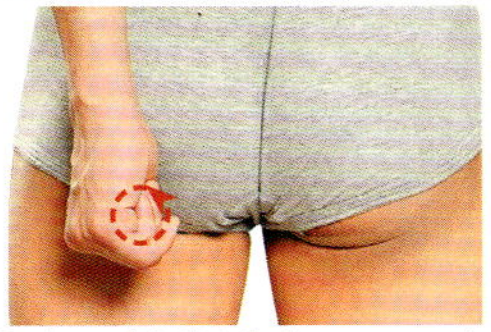

Chéngfú(BL36) : Use the thumb to knead Chengfu acupoint with a little heavy strength for 2 minutes. Knead the contralateral Chengfu acupoint with the same method.

40 Gonitis

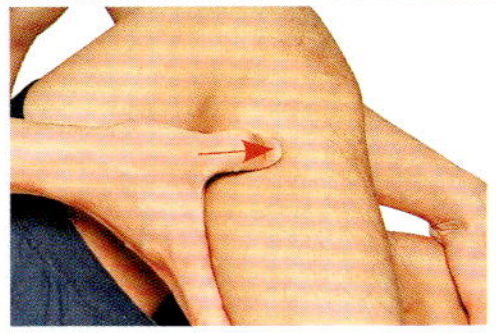

Yánglíngquán(GB34) : Use the thumb to press the Yanglingquan acupoint for a while, then relax, repeat 5~6 times.Press the contralateral Yanglingquan acupoint with the same method.

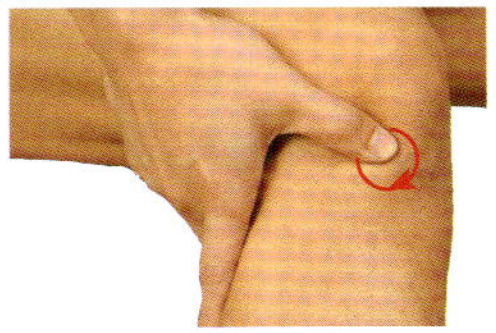

Dúbí(ST35) : Use the thumb to knead the Dubi acupoint with appropriate strength for 2 minutes. Knead the contralateral Dubi acupoint with the same method.

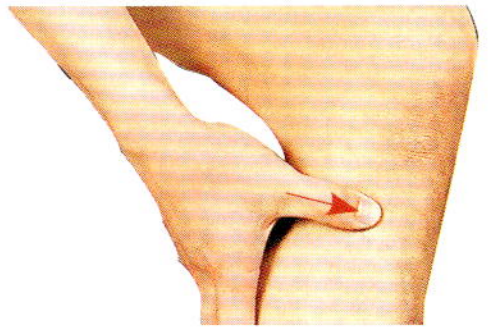

Zúsānlǐ(ST36) : Use the thumb to press the Zusanli acupoint with a little heavy strength for a while, then relax, repeat 5~6 times. Press the contralateral Zusanli acupoint with the same method.

41 Alopecia Areata

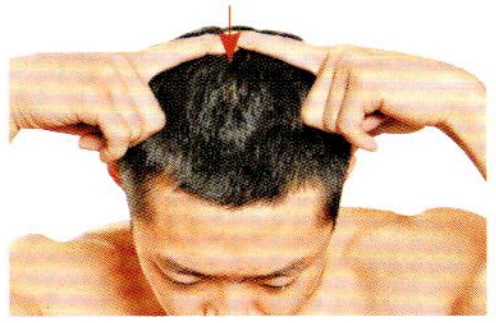

Bǎihuì(GV20) : Overlap both index fingers and press the Baihui acupoint with a little heavy strength for a moment, then relax, repeat 5~6 times.

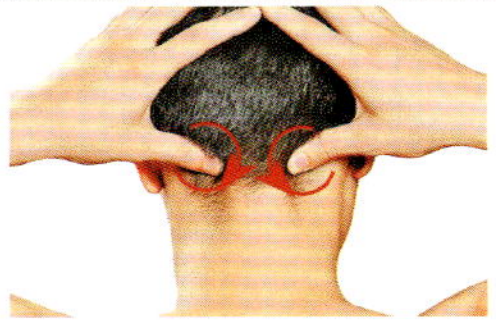

Fēngchí(GB20) : Use both thumbs to knead both Fengchi acupoints with a little heavy strength for 2 minutes.

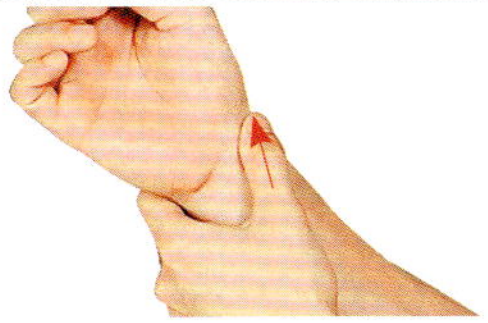

Tàiyuān(LU9) : Use the thumb to press the Taiyuan acupoint for a while,then relax, repeat 5~6 times. Press the contralateral Taiyuan acupoint with the same method.

42 痤疮

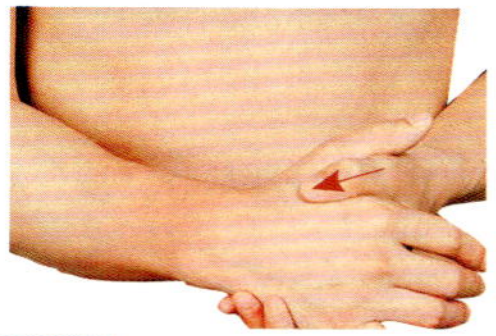

合谷 用拇指用力按压合谷穴，停留片刻后放松，反复 5~6 下。同法按压对侧合谷穴。

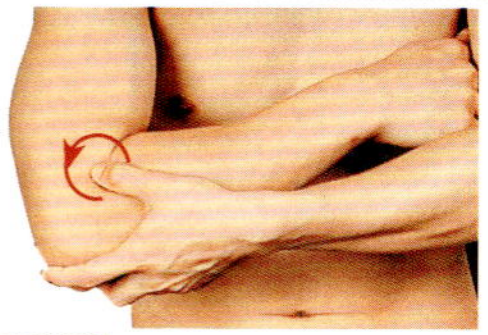

曲池 用拇指按揉曲池穴 2 分钟，力度稍重。同法按揉对侧曲池穴。

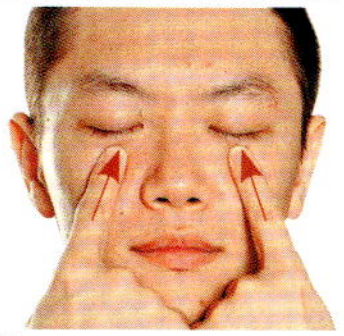

四白 用双手食指按压两侧四白穴，停留片刻后放松，反复 5~6 下，力度稍轻。

43 戒烟

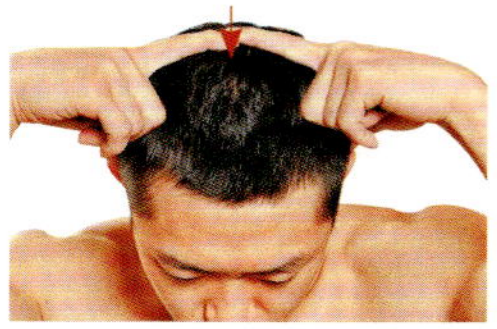

百会 两手食指重叠，稍用力按压百会穴，停留片刻后放松，反复 5~6 下。

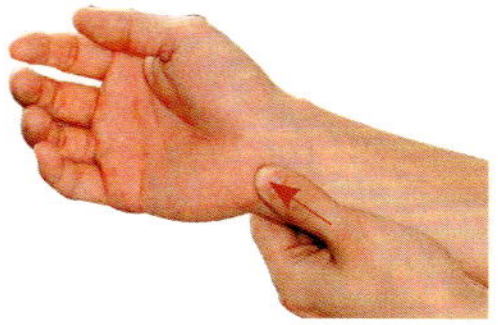

神门 用拇指稍用力按压神门穴，停留片刻后放松，反复 5~6 下。同法按压对侧神门穴。

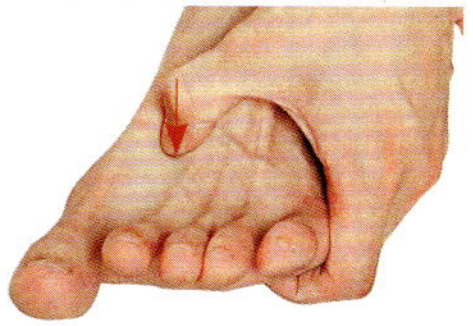

太冲 用拇指掐按太冲穴，停留片刻后放松，反复 5~6 下。同法掐按对侧太冲穴。

44 减肥

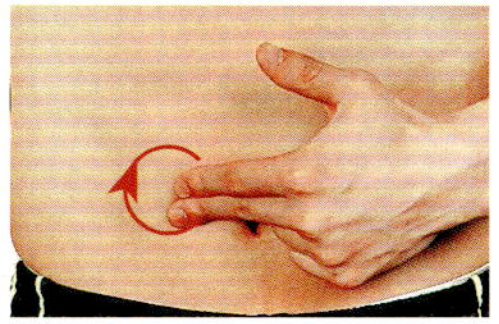

天枢 食、中二指并拢按揉天枢穴 2 分钟，力度适中。同法按揉对侧天枢穴。

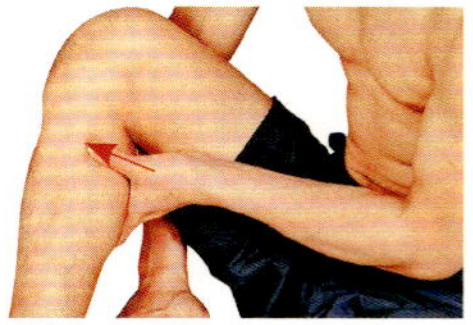

阴陵泉 用拇指稍用力按压阴陵泉穴，停留片刻后放松，反复 5~6 下。同法按压对侧阴陵泉穴。

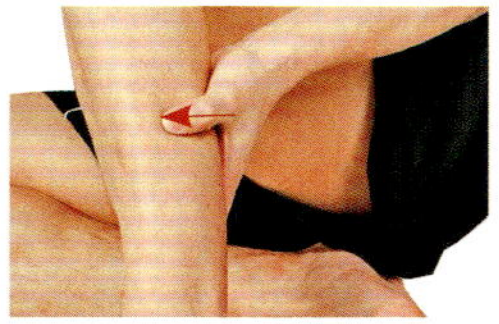

丰隆 用拇指用力按压丰隆穴，停留片刻后放松，反复 5~6 下。

42 Acne

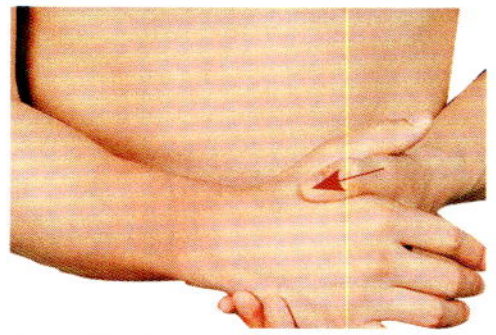

Hégǔ(LI4) : Use the thumb to press the Hegu acupoint for a while,then relax,repeat 5–6 times. Press the contralateral Hegu acupoint with the same method.

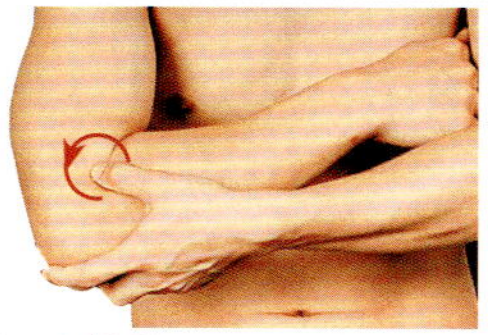

Qūchí(LI11) : Use the thumb to knead the Quchi acupoint with a little heavy strength for 2 minutes.Knead the contralateral Quchi acupoint with the same method.

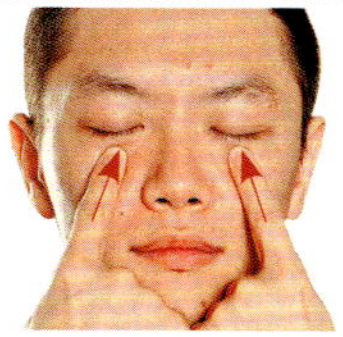

Sìbái(ST2) : Use both index fingers to press both Sibai acupoints for a while, then relax, repeat 5~6 times.

43 Smoking Cessation

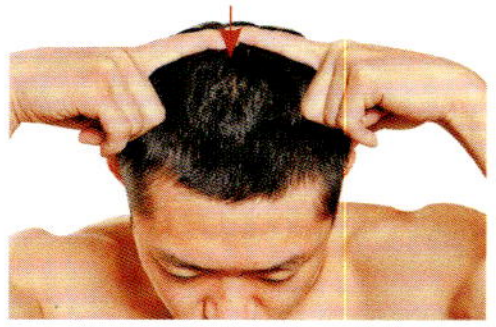

Bǎihuì(GV20) : Overlap both index fingers to press the Baihui acupoints with a little heavy strength for a while, then relax, repeat 5~6 times.

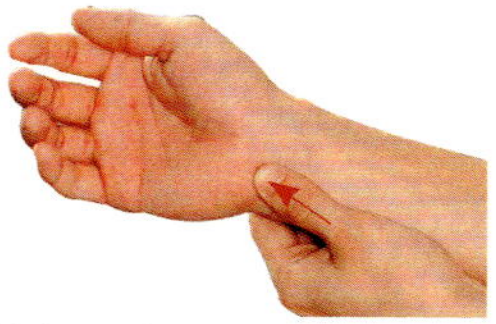

Shénmén(HT7) : Use the thumb to press the Shenmen acupoint for a while,then relax, repeat 5~6 times with a little heavy strength. Press the contralateral Shenmen acupoint with the same method.

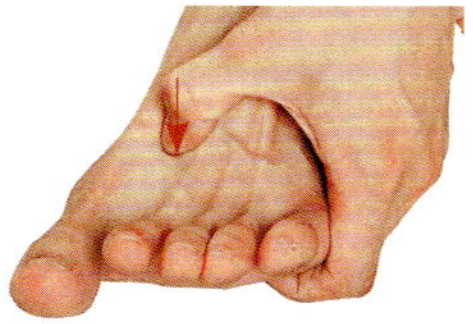

Tàichōng(LR3) : Use the thumb to press the Taichong acupoint for a while,then relax, repeat 5~6 times. Press the contralateral Taichong acupoint with the same method.

44 Weight Reduction

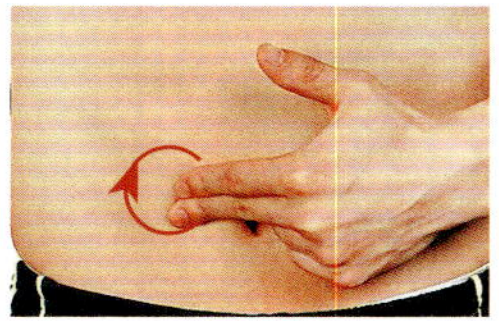

Tiānshū(ST25) : Use the index finger and middle finger to knead the Tianshu acupoint with appropriate strength. Knead the contralateral acupoint with the same method.

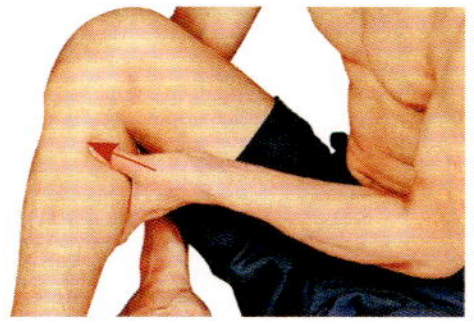

Yīnlíngquán(SP9) : Use the thumb to press the Yinlingquan acupoint with a little heavy strength for a while, then relax. Repeat 5~6 times. Press the contralateral Yinlingquan acupoint with the same method.

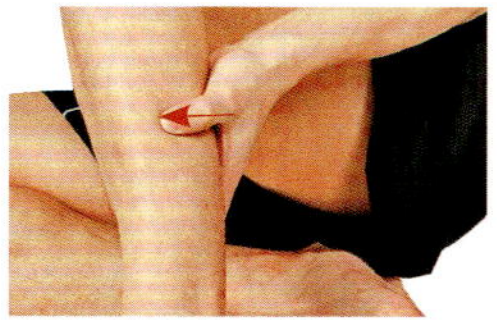

Fēnglóng(ST40) : Use the thumb to knead the Fenglong acupoint with heavy strength for a while, then relax, repeat 5~6 times.

Three-Dimension

Colored Diagrams for

Meridians and Acupoints

(Chinese-English Edition)

三维经络穴位全彩图集

（中英对照版）

编　著　（按姓氏笔画排序）

老中医养生堂　刘嘉瑶
许博捷　杨丽雯
余骏腾　张金金
张晓雯　张淑巧
陈谷超　林　芳
段牡薇　贾荣曼
高玉伟　郭修兵
曹柏川　曹琳琰

Female Meridians and Acupoints

女性经络穴位

编　著　（按姓氏笔画排序）

老中医养生堂　杨丽雯
张金金　曹柏川
曹琳琰

海峡出版发行集团 | 福建科学技术出版社
THE STRAITS PUBLISHING & DISTRIBUTING GROUP | FUJIAN SCIENCE & TECHNOLOGY PUBLISHING HOUSE

目录 CONTENTS

第二章　穴位分部图解 —— 90
Chapter 2: Diagrams of Acupoints in Different Divisions

第三章　超速效三步对症按摩法 —— 188
Chapter 3: Super Quick-acting Three-step Symptomatic Massage Manipulations

附录　经外奇穴图解 —— 200
Appendix: Diagrams of Extra Points

本书特色与使用说明

1. 本书以最新国家标准《腧穴名称与定位》为依据，穴位英文名由拼音与代码组成，图中的穴位中文名旁仅上代码。除在句子中出现的穴名拼音不标声调外，其余穴名拼音均标声调。

2. 本书结合 AR 技术展示十四经脉循行和部分穴位的取穴，形象直观。读者扫描封底二维码并关注“健康乐读汇”微信公众号，按提示下载客户端，扫描识别码即可观看。

3. 经络腧穴内容全面，查找方便：先以十四经脉为纲，按经脉展示穴位，随图附穴位主治病症，并以“★”标出本经常用穴；接着再分部位解析各个穴位定位。从整体到局部帮您梳理相关知识。

4. 穴位应用不求人：收录 35 种常见病症的超速效对症按摩，简单实用疗效佳。

5. 另附“经外奇穴图解”供使用参考。

Features and Instructions

1. This book is based on the newest national standard proclaimed by *Nomenclature and Location of Acupuncture Points*. Each international acupuncture nomenclature consists of spelling and code, whereas only code is added to the acupoints of the picture beside the Chinese name considering limited space. Each spelling is marked with tone except for those occurring in sentences.

2. Circulations of the fourteen meridians and locations of some acupoints are displayed vividly and straightforwardly combined with AR technology. Readers may scan the QR code in back cover and focus on WeChat public account of *Happy Reading on Health*. Download the application under the instructions, then you can easily watch the video after scanning the identification code.

3. Overall contents of meridians and acupoints are contained, convenient for search: The contents first takes the fourteen meridians as main thread, displays acupoints respectively according to meridians, encloses indications of points and marks the common-used acupoints of the meridians with " ★ ", and then analyzes the location of every point according to different divisions. Acupoints knowledge is arranged from the whole to the parts for better understanding.

4. Acupoints massage self-application: Super quick-acting symptomatic massage manipulations for 35 common diseases are included. It is simple and practical with well curative effect.

5.The extra acupoints diagram is also enclosed for reference.

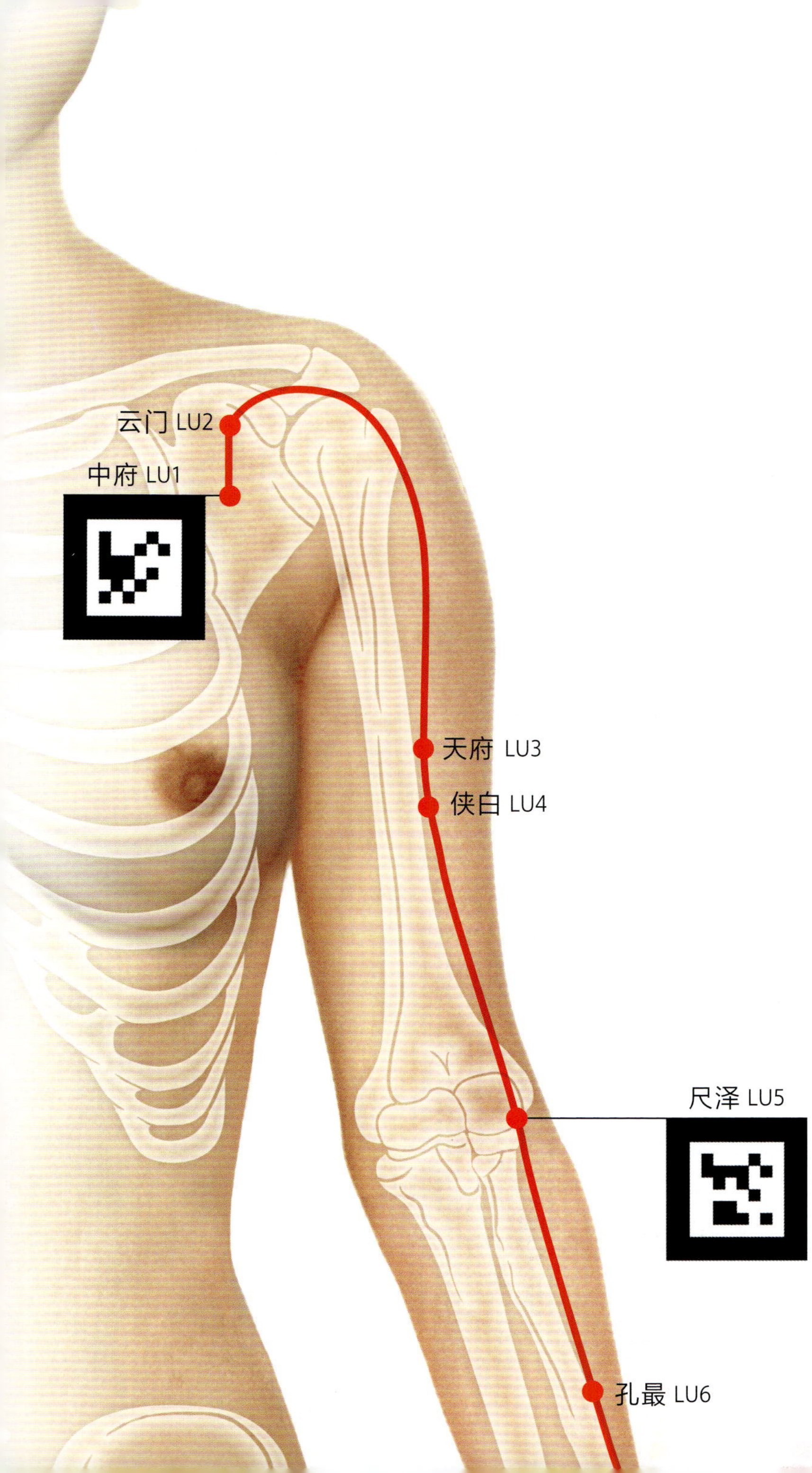

第一章　十四经穴图解

手太阴肺经

手太阴肺经从胸部走向手指，起于胸部的中府，经手臂内侧，止于手拇指的少商。

肺经主治病症：咳嗽、气急、喘息等呼吸系统疾患；上臂及前臂内侧疼痛不适等经脉循行部位的疾患。

LU	穴 名	主 治
★ 1	中府	咳嗽、气喘、胸痛、肩背痛
2	云门	咳嗽、气喘、胸痛、肩背痛
3	天府	咳嗽、气喘、鼻出血、上臂痛
4	侠白	咳嗽、气喘、干呕、上臂痛
★ 5	尺泽	咳嗽、气喘、咯血、咽喉肿痛、肘臂挛痛、急性吐泻、中暑、小儿惊风
6	孔最	咳嗽、咯血、气喘、咽喉肿痛、肘臂挛痛
★ 7	列缺	咳嗽、气喘、咽喉肿痛、头痛、齿痛、项强、口眼歪斜
8	经渠	咳嗽、气喘、胸痛、咽喉肿痛、手腕痛
9	太渊	咳嗽、气喘、无脉症、腕臂痛
10	鱼际	咳嗽、咯血、咽干、咽喉肿痛、失音、小儿疳积
★ 11	少商	咽喉肿痛、鼻出血、高热、昏迷、癫狂

★为本经常用穴

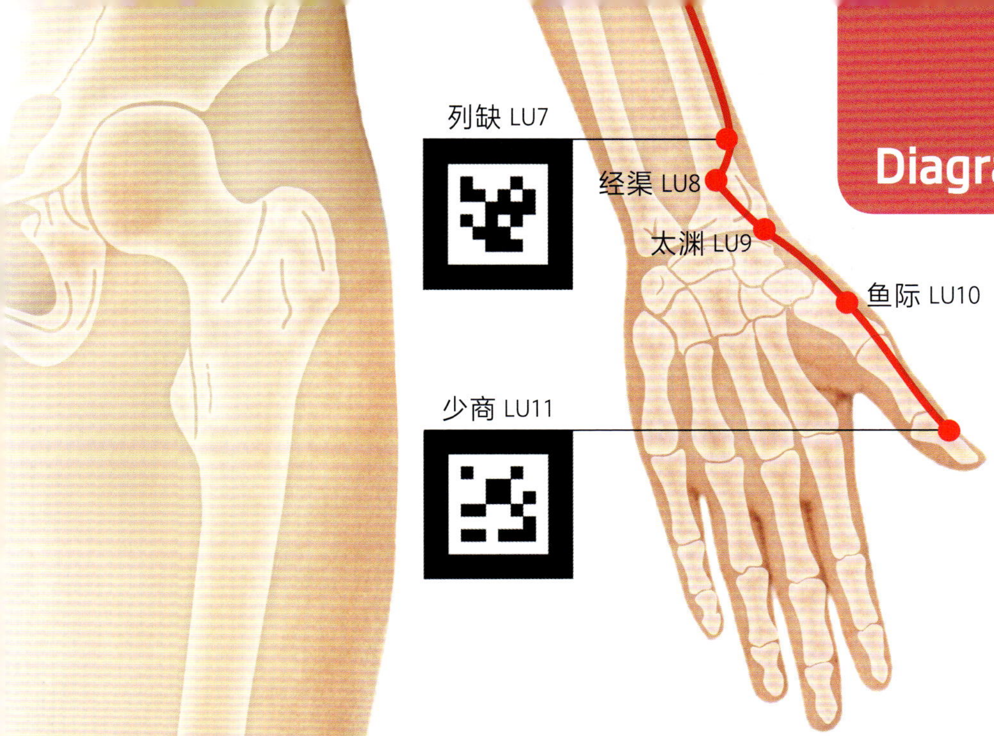

Chapter 1: Diagrams of Acupoints in the Fourteen Meridians

Lung Meridian of Hand-Taiyin, LU.

Lung Meridian of Hand-Taiyin originates from the chest to fingers, emerges from Zhongfu (LU1) in the chest, runs along the medial side of the arm and ends at Shaoshang (LU11) in the thumb of the hand.

Lung Meridian mainly treats the diseases of respiratory system including cough, short breath and asthma and diseases of running courses of the meridian including pain in medial side of upper arm and forearm.

LU	Acupoints	Indications
★ 1	Zhōngfǔ	Cough; asthma; chest pain; shoulder and back pain
2	Yúnmén	Cough; asthma; chest pain; shoulder and back pain
3	Tiānfǔ	Cough; asthma; nose bleeding; pain in upper arm
4	Xiábái	Cough; asthma; retch; pain in upper arm
★ 5	Chǐzé	Cough; asthma; hemoptysis; swelling and pain in throat; spasm and pain of elbow and arm; acute vomiting and diarrhea; heat stroke; infantile convulsion
6	Kǒngzuì	Cough; hemoptysis; asthma; swelling and pain in throat; spasm and pain in elbow and arm
★ 7	Lièquē	Cough; asthma; swelling and pain in throat; headache; toothache; stiff neck; deviation of mouth and eye
8	Jīngqú	Cough; asthma; chest pain; swelling and pain in throat; hand and wrist pain
9	Tàiyuān	Cough; asthma; pulseless disease; wrist and arm pain
10	Yújì	Cough; hemoptysis; dry throat; swelling and pain in throat; aphonia; infantile malnutrition
★ 11	Shàoshāng	Swelling and pain in throat ; nose bleeding; high fever; coma; manic and depressive psychosis

★ Common acupoint used in treatment

手阳明大肠经

手阳明大肠经起于食指末端的商阳，沿手臂外侧经过肩头，止于脸部鼻旁的迎香。

大肠经主治病症：目赤、咽喉肿痛、齿痛、口歪、耳鸣耳聋等头面五官疾患；中暑、发热等热病；腹痛、腹泻、便秘等肠胃疾患；上臂部疼痛等经脉循行部位的疾患。

LI	穴 名	主 治
1	商阳	齿痛、咽喉肿痛、昏迷、热病、急症
2	二间	鼻出血、齿痛、热病
3	三间	齿痛、咽喉肿痛、腹胀、肠鸣、嗜睡
★ 4	合谷	头痛、目赤肿痛、齿痛、鼻出血、口眼歪斜、耳聋、发热、恶寒、经闭、滞产
5	阳溪	头痛、目赤肿痛、耳聋、手腕痛

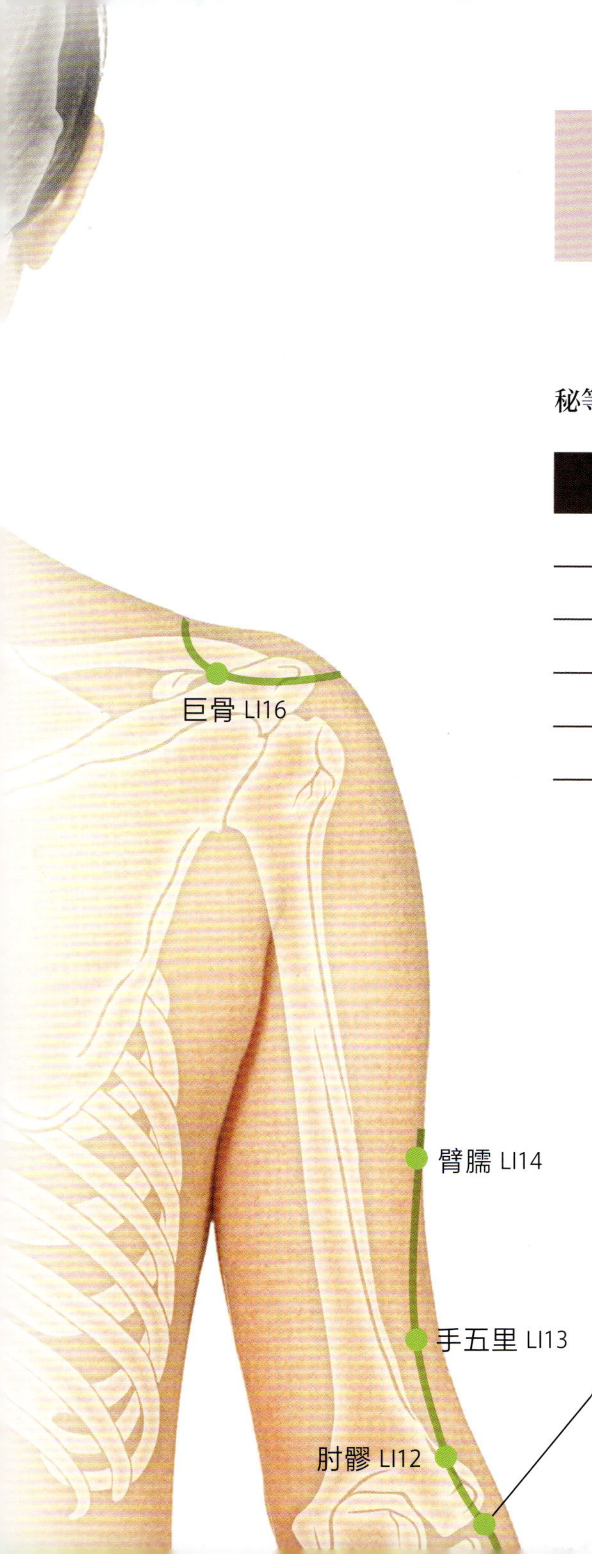

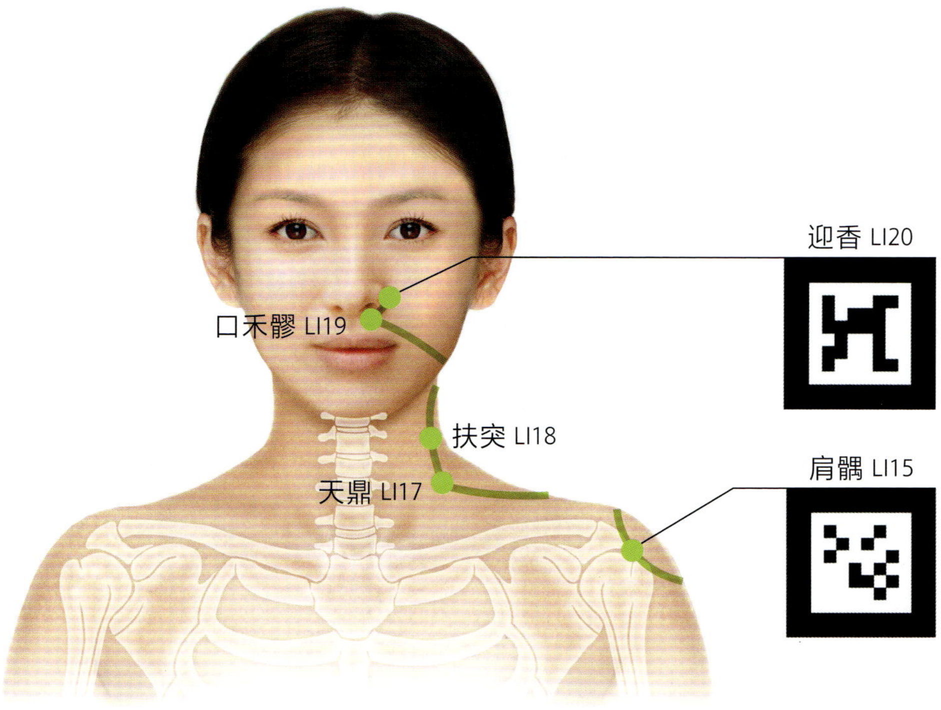

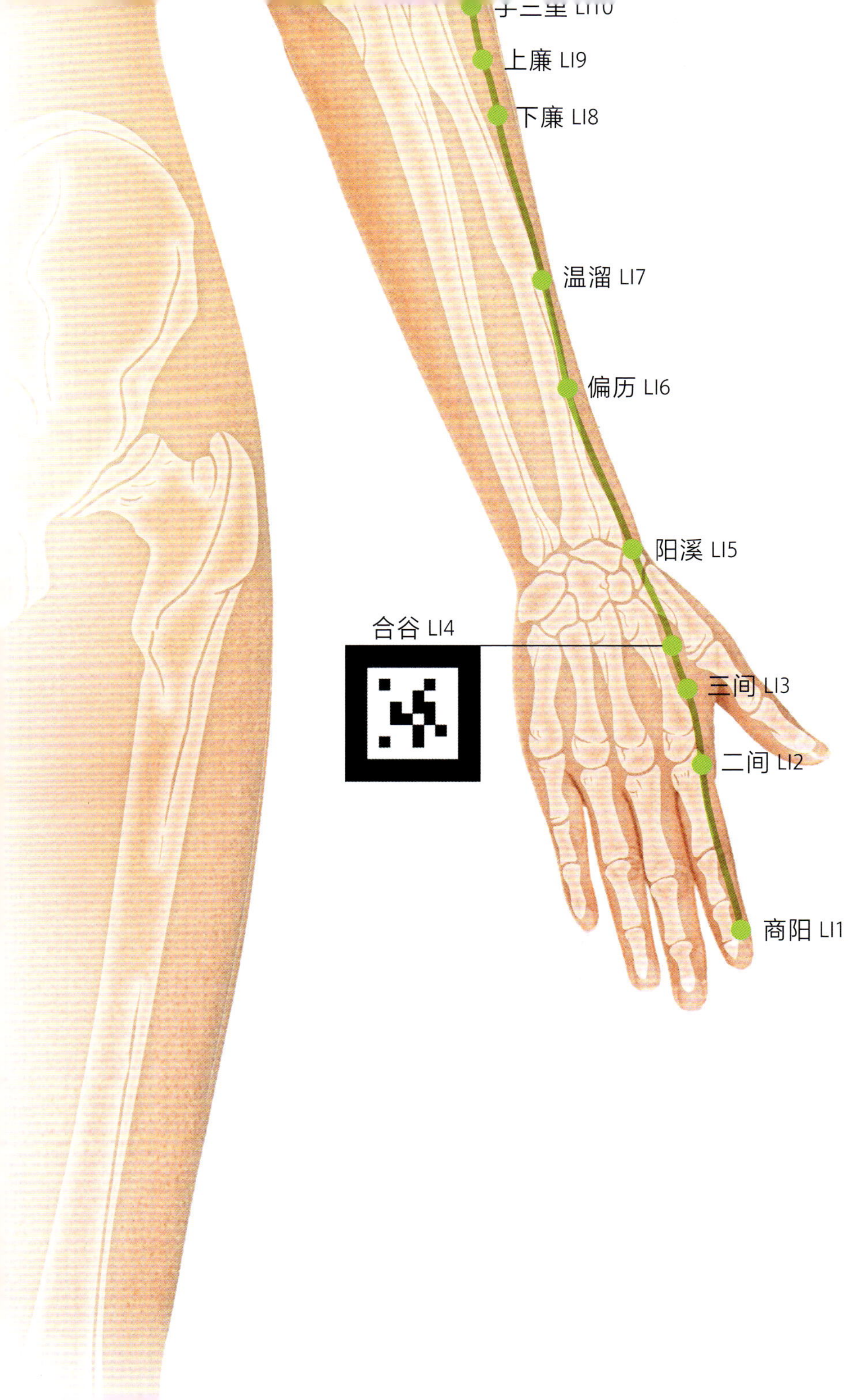

Large Intestine Meridian of Hand-Yangming, LI.

Large Intestine Meridian of Hand-Yangming emerges from Shangyang (LI1) at the end of the index finger, runs along the lateral part of the arm and through the shoulder, then terminates at Yingxiang (LI20) near the nose ala in the face.

Large Intestine Meridian mainly treats diseases of head, face and five sensory organs including red eyes, swelling and pain in throat, toothache, deviation of mouth, tinnitus and deafness; febrile diseases including heatstroke and fever; diseases of intestine and stomach including abdominal pain, diarrhea and constipation; diseases of running courses of meridian including upper arm pain.

LI	Acupoints	Indications
1	Shāngyáng	Toothache; swelling and pain in throat; coma; febrile diseases; emergency syndromes
2	Èrjiān	Nose bleeding; toothache; febrile diseases
3	Sānjiān	Toothache; swelling and pain in throat; distention of abdomen; borborygmus; somnolence
★ 4	Hégǔ	Headache; redness, swelling and pain of eyes; toothache; nose bleeding; deviation of mouth and eye; deafness; fever; aversion to cold; amenorrhea; prolonged delivery
5	Yángxī	Headache; redness, swelling and pain of eyes; deafness; hand and wrist pain

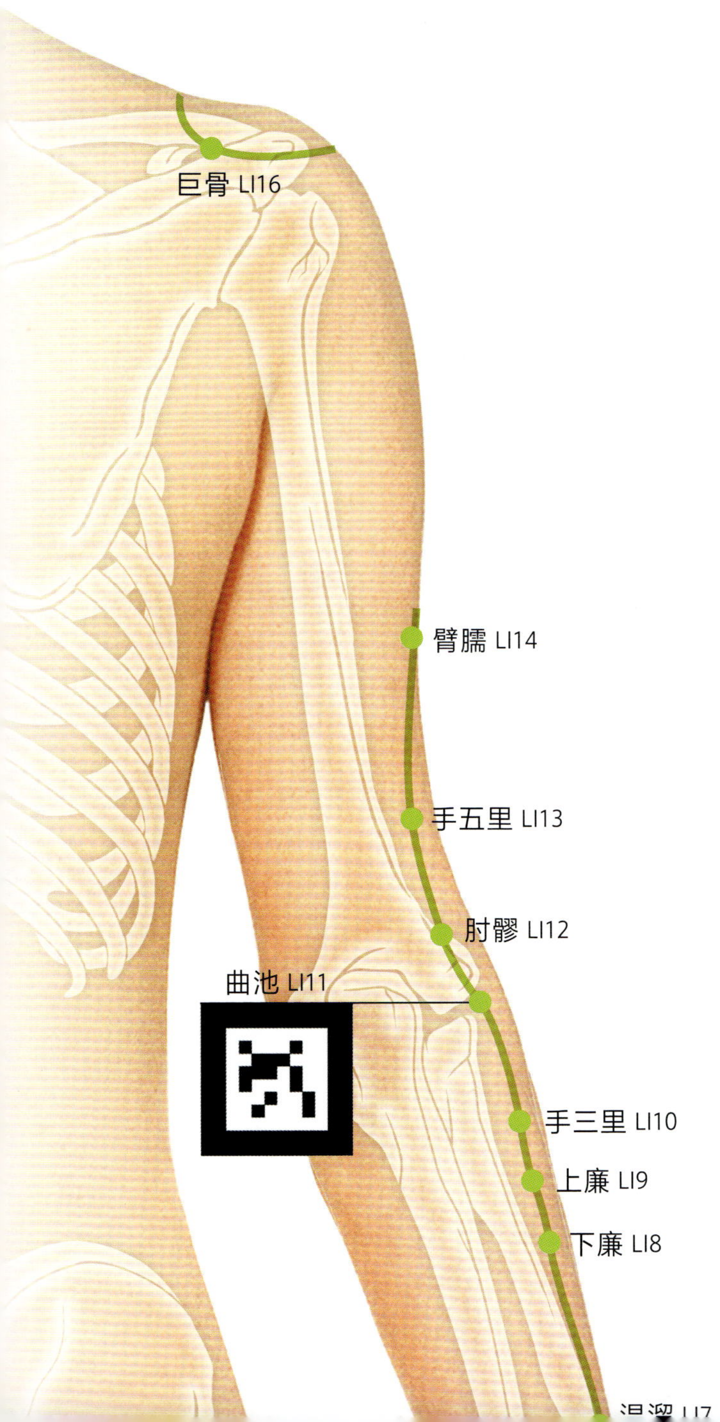

续表

LI	穴 名	主 治
6	偏历	耳鸣、耳聋、目赤、鼻出血、喉痛、手臂酸痛、水肿
7	温溜	肠鸣、腹痛、头痛、面肿、咽喉肿痛、肩周炎、背酸痛
8	下廉	肘臂痛、头痛、眩晕、目痛、腹胀、腹痛
9	上廉	肘臂痛、半身不遂、手臂麻木、头痛、肠鸣、腹痛
10	手三里	手臂无力、上肢不遂、腹痛、腹泻、齿痛、颊肿
★ 11	曲池	手臂痹痛、上肢不遂、热病、高血压、癫狂、腹痛、吐泻、咽喉肿痛、齿痛、目赤肿痛、荨麻疹、湿疹、颈淋巴结结核
12	肘髎	肘臂部疼痛、麻木、挛急
13	手五里	肘臂部疼痛或挛急，颈淋巴结结核
14	臂臑	肩周炎、颈项拘挛、颈淋巴结结核、目疾
★ 15	肩髃	肩周炎、上肢不遂、荨麻疹
16	巨骨	肩周炎、颈淋巴结结核、甲状腺肿大
17	天鼎	急性咽喉炎、气哽、咽喉肿痛、颈淋巴结结核、甲状腺肿大
18	扶突	咽喉肿痛、急性咽喉炎、颈淋巴结结核、甲状腺肿大、咳嗽、气喘，是颈部手术针麻用穴
19	口禾髎	口歪、鼻塞不通、鼻出血
★ 20	迎香	鼻塞、鼻出血、口歪、胆道蛔虫症

Continued

LI	Acupoints	Indications
6	Piānlì	Tinnitus; deafness; red eyes; nose bleeding; sore throat; sourness and pain in hand and arm; edema
7	Wēnliū	Borborygmus; abdominal pain; headache; facial edema; swelling and pain in throat; periarthritis of the shoulder; sourness and pain of back
8	Xiàlián	Elbow and arm pain; headache; dizziness; eyes pain; distention of abdomen; abdominal pain

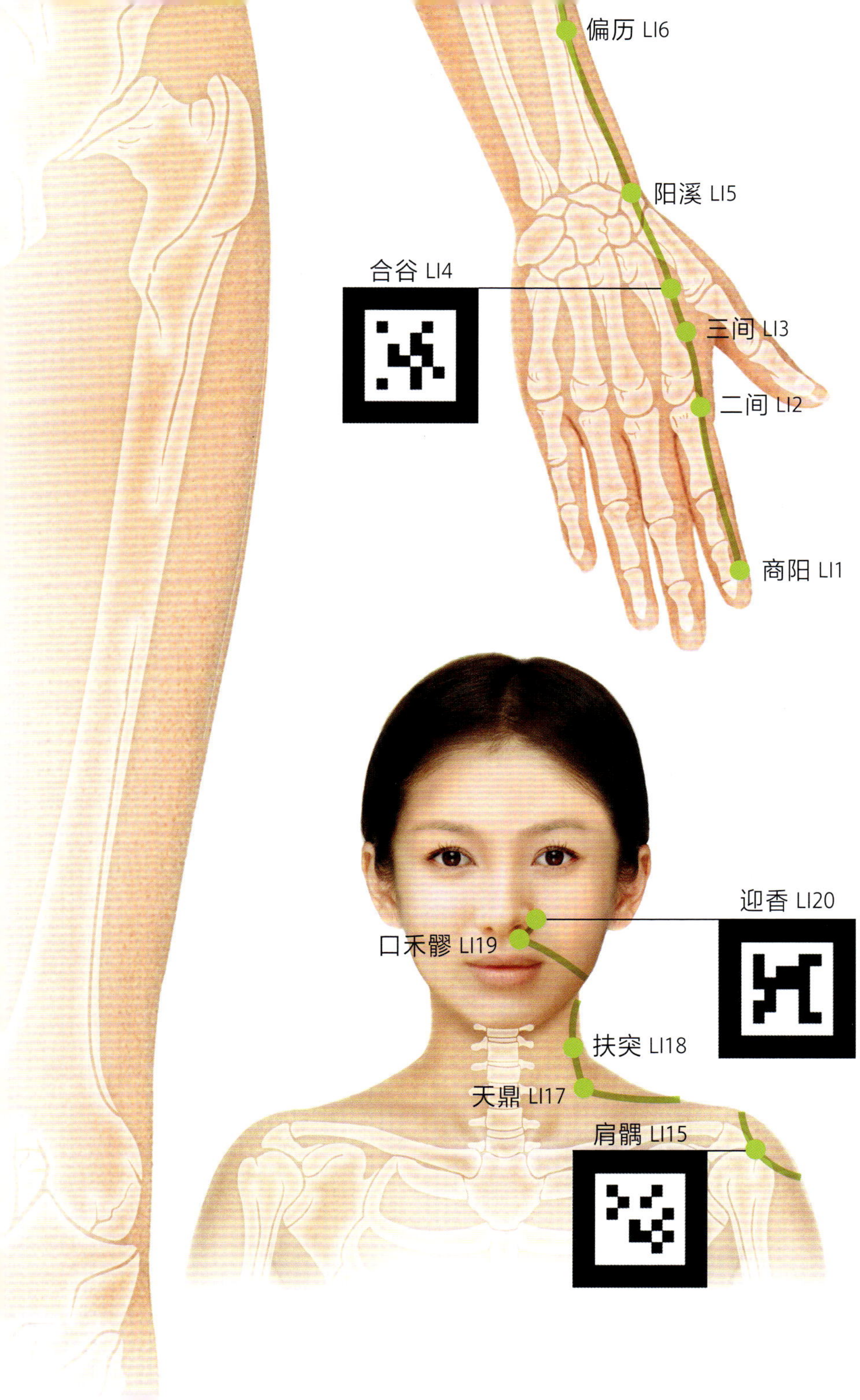

LI	Acupoints	Indications
9	Shànglián	Elbow and arm pain; hemiplegia; numbness of hand and arm; headache; borborygmus; abdominal pain
10	Shǒusānlǐ	Flaccidity of hand and arm; motor impairment of upper limbs; abdominal pain; diarrhea; toothache; swollen cheek
★ 11	Qūchí	Arthralgia of hand and arm; motor impairment of upper limbs; febrile diseases; hypertension; manic and depressive psychosis; abdominal pain; vomiting and diarrhea; swelling and pain in throat; toothache; redness, swelling and pain of eyes; measles; eczema; cervical lymph node tuberculosis
12	Zhǒuliáo	Pain, numbness and spasm of elbow and arm
13	Shǒuwǔlǐ	Pain and spasm of elbow and arm; cervical lymph node tuberculosis
14	Bìnào	Periarthritis of shoulder; neck spasm; cervical lymph node tuberculosis; eyes disease
★ 15	jiānyú	Periarthritis of shoulder; motor impairment of upper limbs; measles
16	Jùgǔ	Periarthritis of shoulder; cervical lymph node tuberculosis; goiter
17	Tiāndǐng	Acute sphagitis; choke; swelling and pain in throat; cervical lymph node tuberculosis; goiter
18	Fútū	Swelling and pain in throat; acute sphagitis; cervical lymph node tuberculosis; goiter; cough; short breath; acupuncture anaesthesia point for neck surgery
19	Kǒuhéliáo	Deviation of mouth; nasal obstruction; nose bleeding
★ 20	Yíngxiāng	Nasal obstruction; nose bleeding; deviation of mouth; biliary tract ascariasis

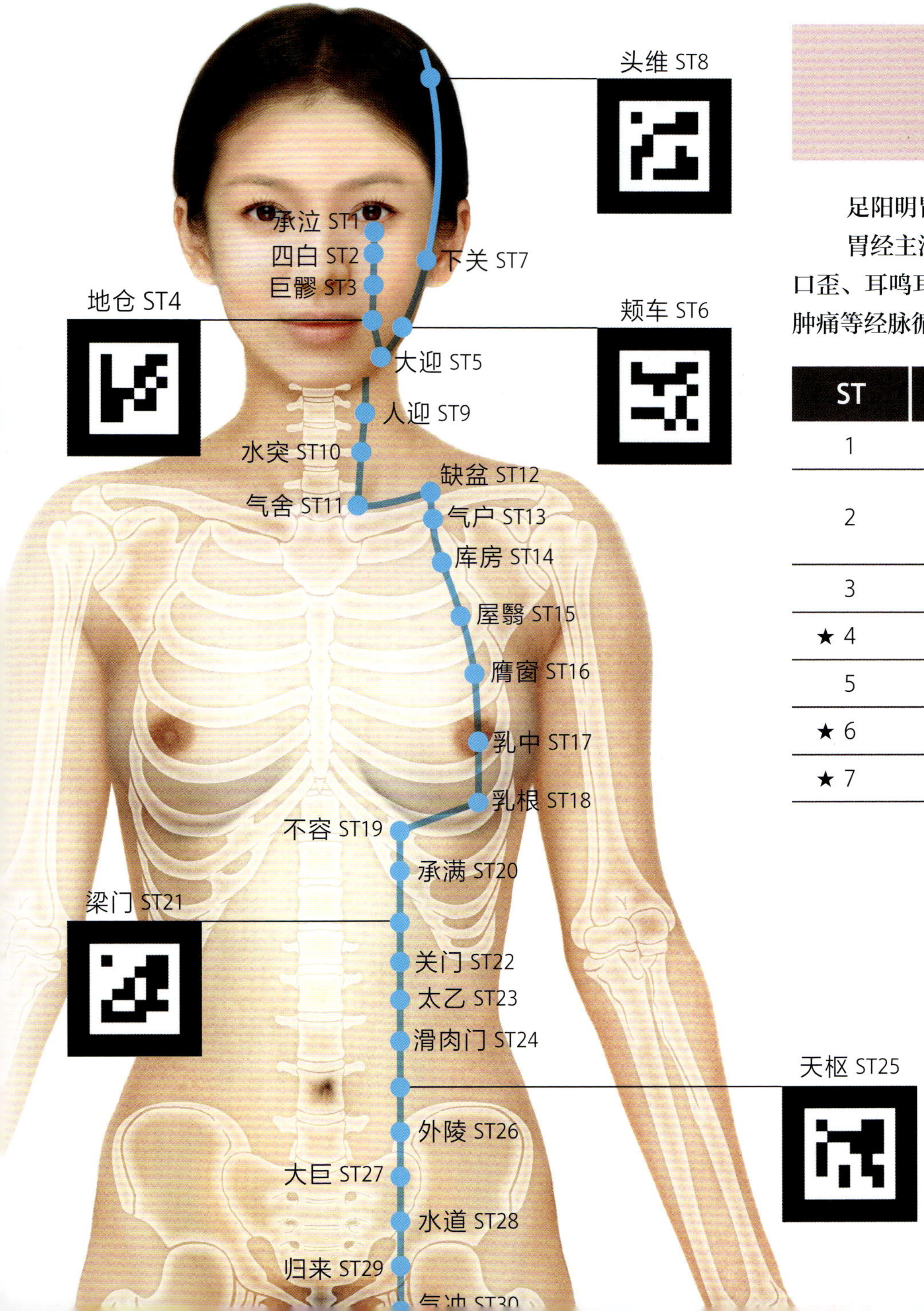

足阳明胃经

足阳明胃经起于头部，往下经过胸部、腹部、下肢外侧前缘达到足背。

胃经主治病症：呕吐、腹胀、腹痛、水肿、食欲不振等肠胃疾患；目赤、咽喉肿痛、齿痛、口歪、耳鸣耳聋等头面五官疾患；昏迷、癫狂、中风等神经精神疾病；咳嗽、气喘、膝关节肿痛等经脉循行部位的疾患。另外，本经的部分腧穴有强身健体的作用，常用于日常保健。

ST	穴 名	主 治
1	承泣	眼睑瞤动、迎风流泪、夜盲、近视、口眼歪斜、面肌痉挛
2	四白	目赤痛痒、眼睑瞤动、口眼歪斜、三叉神经痛、面肌痉挛、头痛、眩晕
3	巨髎	口眼歪斜、鼻出血、齿痛、唇颊肿
★ 4	地仓	口眼歪斜、流涎、三叉神经痛
5	大迎	口眼歪斜、唇颊肿、齿痛
★ 6	颊车	口眼歪斜、齿痛、牙关不利、唇颊肿
★ 7	下关	牙关不利、三叉神经痛、齿痛、口眼歪斜、耳聋、耳鸣

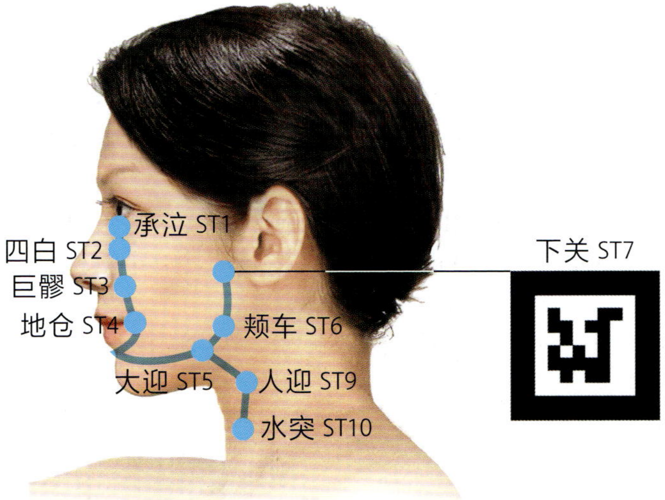

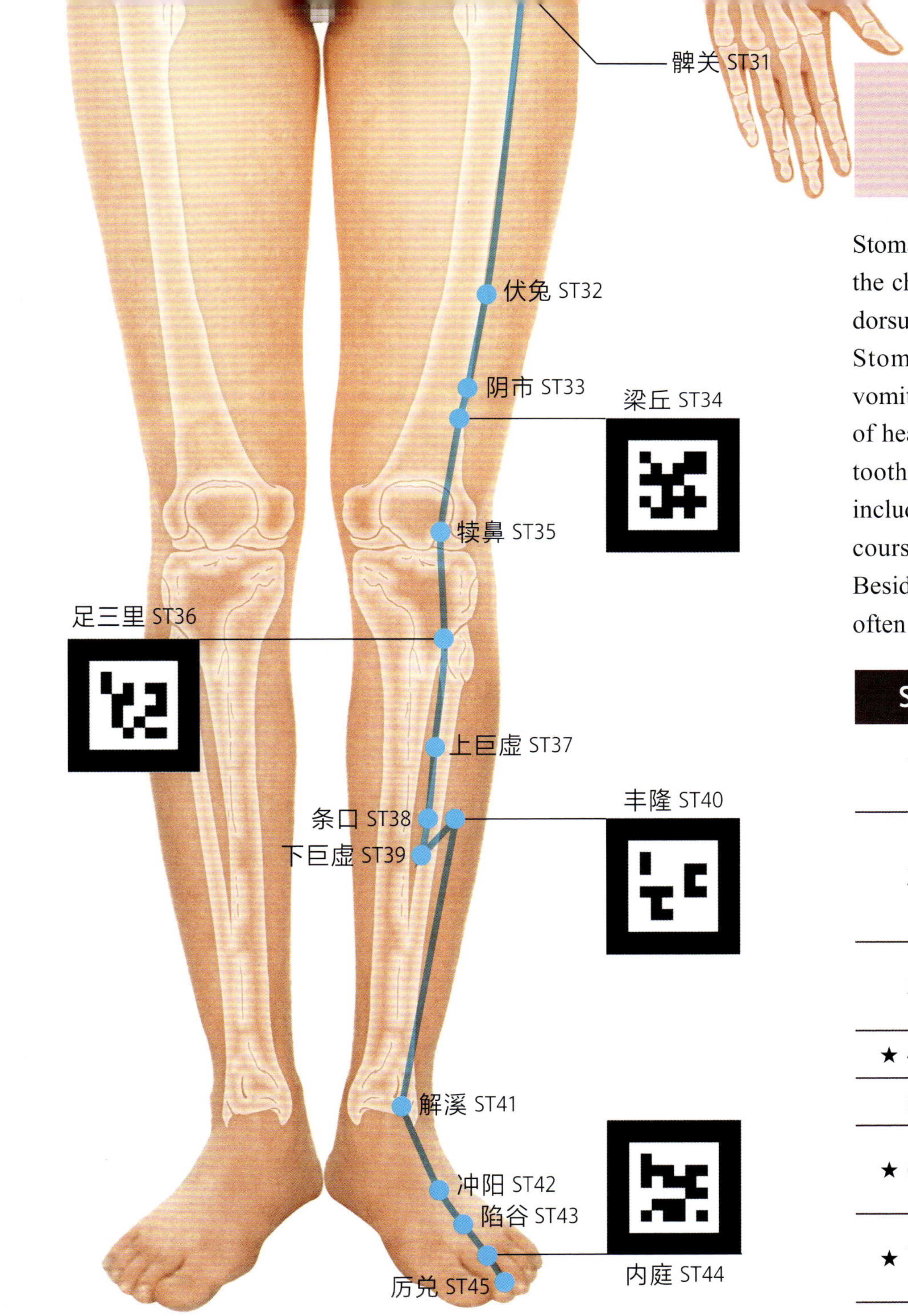

Stomach Meridian of Foot-Yangming, ST.

Stomach Meridian of Foot-Yangming emerges from the head, runs downward through the chest and abdomen and lateral frontal side of lower limbs, then terminates on the dorsum of foot.

Stomach Meridian mainly treats diseases of intestine and stomach including vomiting, distention of abdomen, abdominal pain, edema and poor appetite; diseases of head, face and five sensory organs including red eyes, swelling and pain in throat, toothache, deviation of mouth, tinnitus and deafness; diseases of nervous system including coma, manic and depressive psychosis and wind stroke; diseases of running courses of meridian including cough, asthma and swelling and pain of the knees. Besides, some points of Stomach Meridian has the effect of physical fitness, which is often used for daily health care.

ST	Acupoints	Indications
1	Chéngqì	Eyelid twitching; tearing induced by the wind; nyctalopia; myopia; deviation of mouth and eye; spasm of facial muscle
2	Sìbái	Redness; pain and itch of the eyes; eyelid twitching; deviation of mouth and eye; prosopalgia; spasm of facial muscle; headache; dizziness
3	Jùliáo	Deviation of mouth and eye; nose bleeding; toothache; swollen lip and cheek
★ 4	Dìcāng	Deviation of mouth and eye; salivation; prosopalgia
5	Dàyíng	Deviation of mouth and eye; swollen lip and cheek; toothache
★ 6	Jiáchē	Deviation of mouth and eye; toothache; difficulty in opening and closing tooth; swollen lip and cheek
★ 7	Xiàguān	Difficulty in opening and closing tooth; prosopalgia; toothache; deviation of mouth and eye; deafness; tinnitus

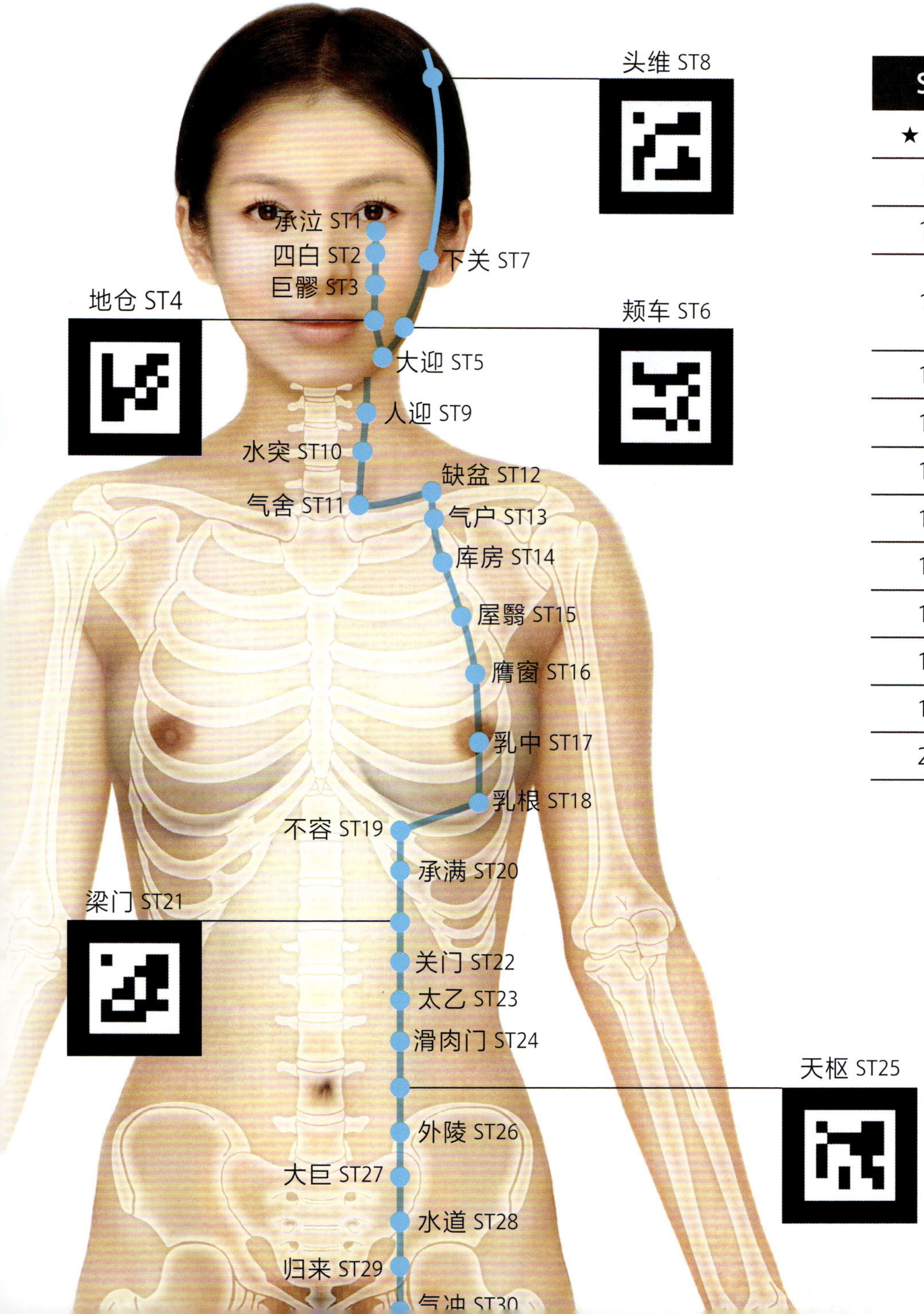

续表

ST	穴名	主治
★ 8	头维	头痛、目眩、目痛
9	人迎	甲状腺肿大、颈淋巴结结核、咽喉肿痛、气喘、高血压
10	水突	咽喉肿痛、咳嗽、气喘、偏头痛
11	气舍	咽喉肿痛、甲状腺肿瘤、颈淋巴结结核、气喘、呃逆、颈项强
12	缺盆	咳嗽、气喘、咽喉肿痛、颈淋巴结结核
13	气户	咳嗽、气喘、呃逆、肺气肿、胸痛
14	库房	咳嗽、气喘、咳唾脓血、胸胁胀痛
15	屋翳	咳嗽、气喘、咳唾脓血、胸胁胀痛、乳腺炎、乳腺纤维瘤
16	膺窗	咳嗽、气喘、胸胁胀痛、乳腺炎
17	乳中	本穴不针不灸，只作胸腹部腧穴的定位标志
18	乳根	乳部疾患、咳嗽、气喘、呃逆、胸痛
19	不容	呕吐、胃痛、纳少、腹胀
20	承满	胃痛、吐血、纳少

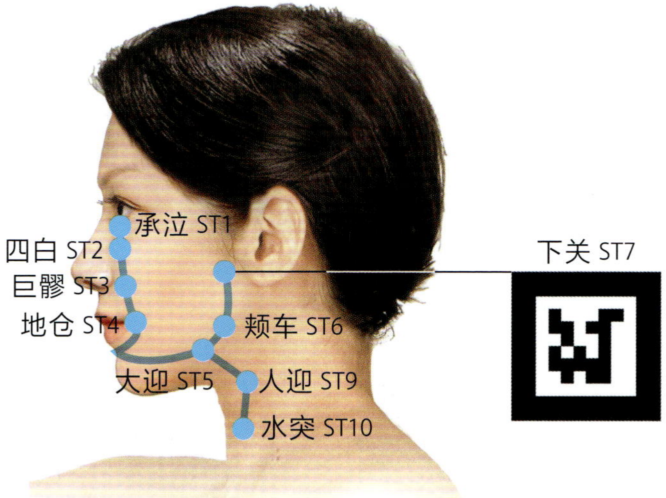

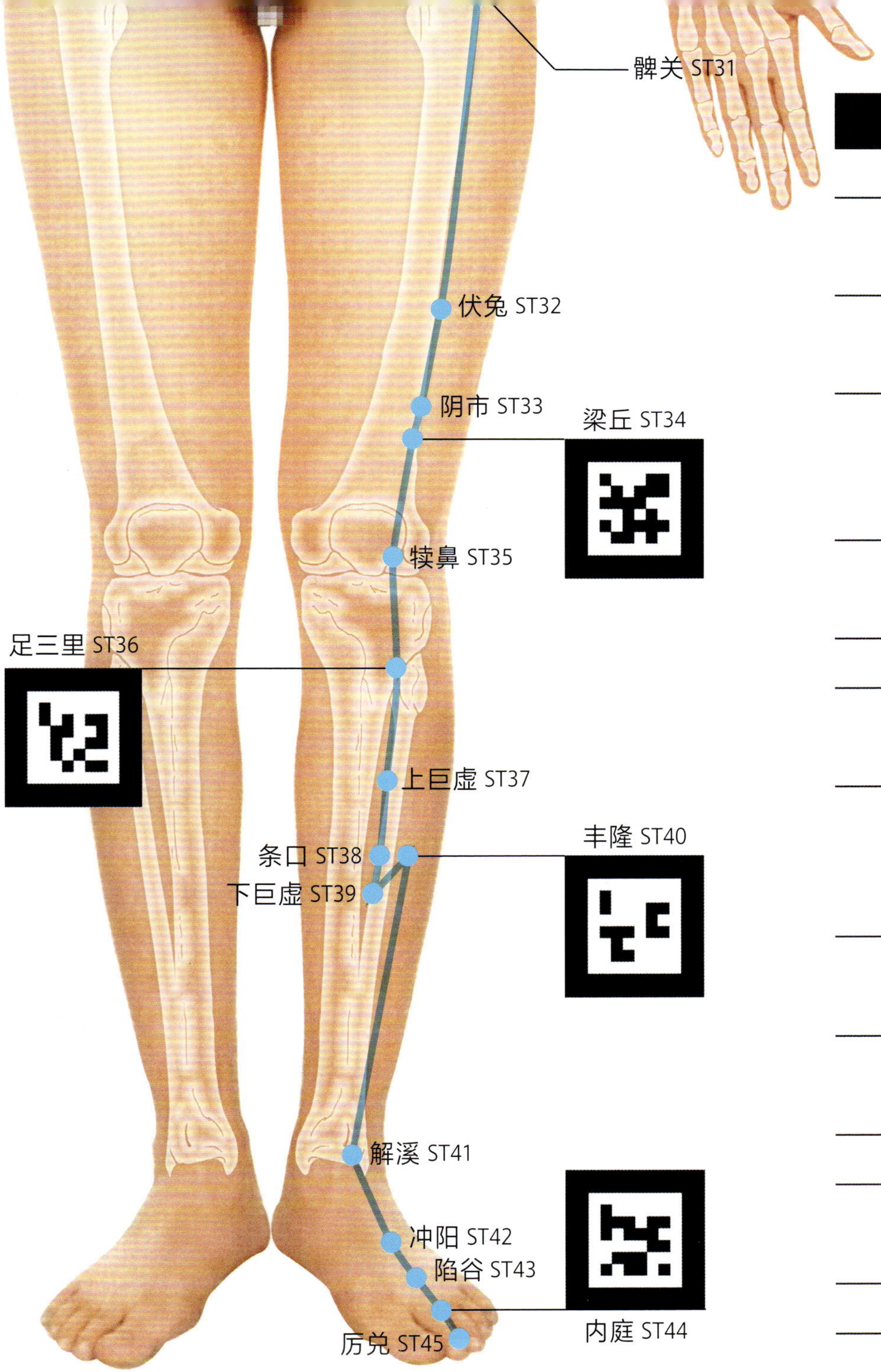

Continued

ST	Acupoints	Indications
★ 8	Tóuwéi	Headache; dizziness; eyes pain
9	Rényíng	Goiter; cervical lymph node tuberculosis; swelling and pain in throat; asthma; hypertension
10	Shuǐtū	Swelling and pain in throat; cough; asthma; migraine
11	Qìshè	Swelling and pain in throat; thyroid tumor; cervical lymph node tuberculosis; asthma; hiccup; neck stiffness
12	Quēpén	Cough; asthma; swelling and pain in throat; cervical lymph node tuberculosis
13	Qìhù	Cough; asthma; hiccup; emphysema; chest pain
14	Kùfáng	Cough; asthma; coughing up saliva and purulent blood; distending pain of chest and hypochondrium
15	Wūyì	Cough; asthma; coughing up saliva and purulent blood; distending pain of chest and hypochondrium; mastitis; fibroadenoma of breast
16	Yīngchuāng	Cough; asthma; distending pain of chest and hypochondrium; mastitis
17	Rǔzhōng	Not for acupuncture or moxa, just as the landmark for locating acupoints in the chest and abdomen
18	Rǔgēn	Breast diseases; cough; asthma; hiccup; chest pain
19	Bùróng	Vomiting; stomachache; poor appetite; distention of abdomen
20	Chéngmǎn	Stomachache; hematemesis; poor appetite

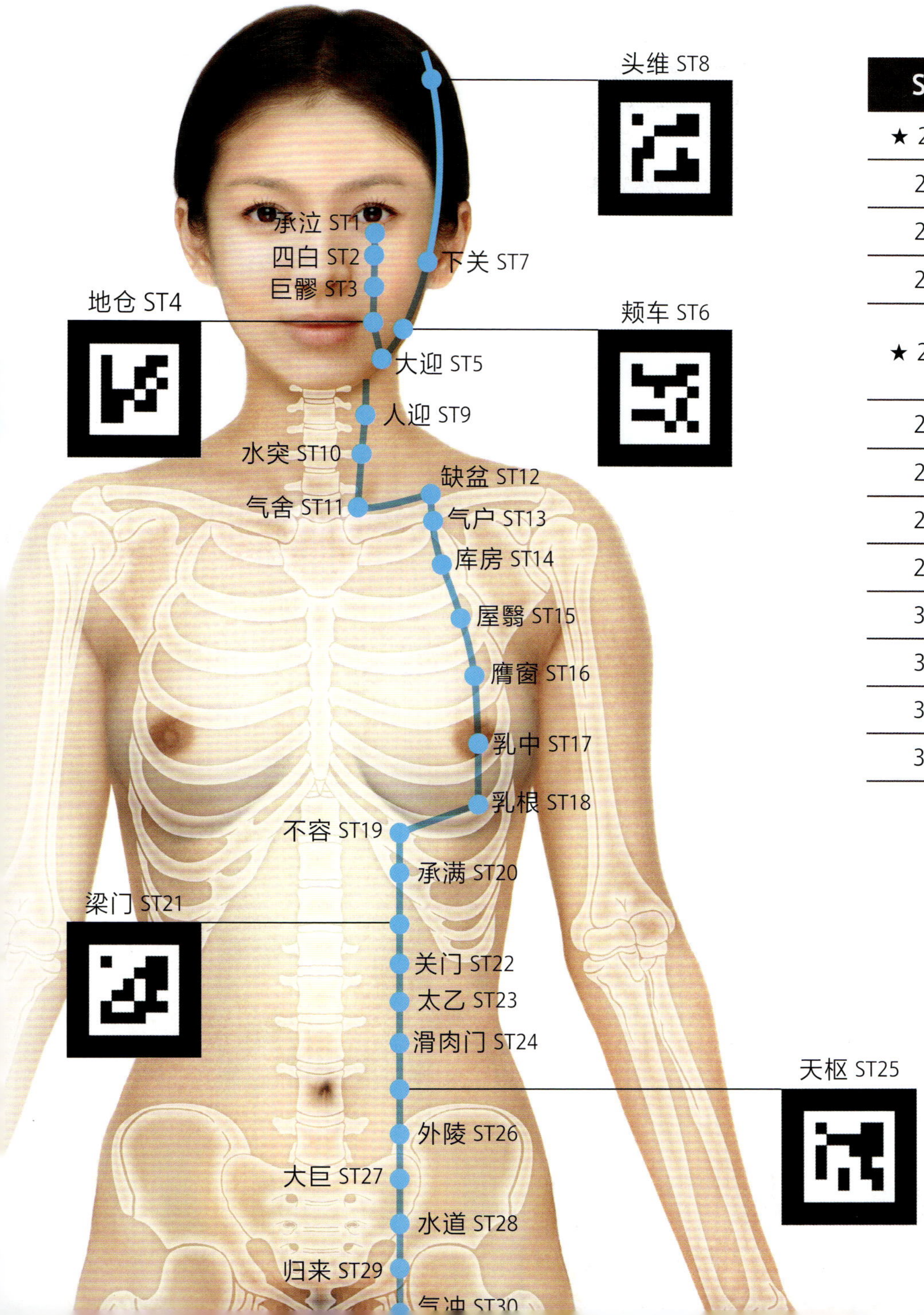

续表

ST	穴 名	主 治
★ 21	梁门	纳少、胃痛、呕吐
22	关门	腹胀、腹痛、肠鸣、腹泻
23	太乙	胃病、心烦、癫狂
24	滑肉门	胃痛、呕吐、癫狂
★ 25	天枢	腹痛、腹胀、肠鸣、泄泻、便秘、阑尾炎、月经不调、痛经
26	外陵	腹痛、疝气、痛经
27	大巨	小腹胀满、小便不利、疝气、遗精、早泄
28	水道	小腹胀满、小便不利、疝气、痛经、不孕
29	归来	小腹痛、疝气、月经不调、带下、子宫或阴道脱垂
30	气冲	肠鸣腹痛、疝气、月经不调、不孕、阳痿
31	髀关	下肢痿痹、腰痛、膝冷
32	伏兔	下肢痿痹、腰痛、膝冷、疝气
33	阴市	膝关节痛、下肢痿痹、腰痛、疝气

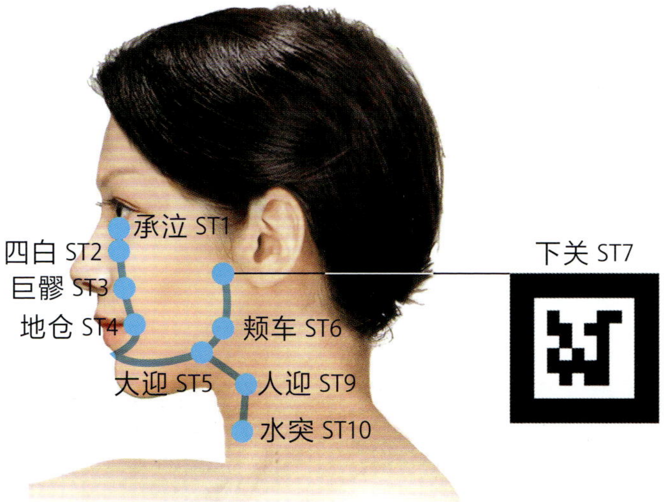

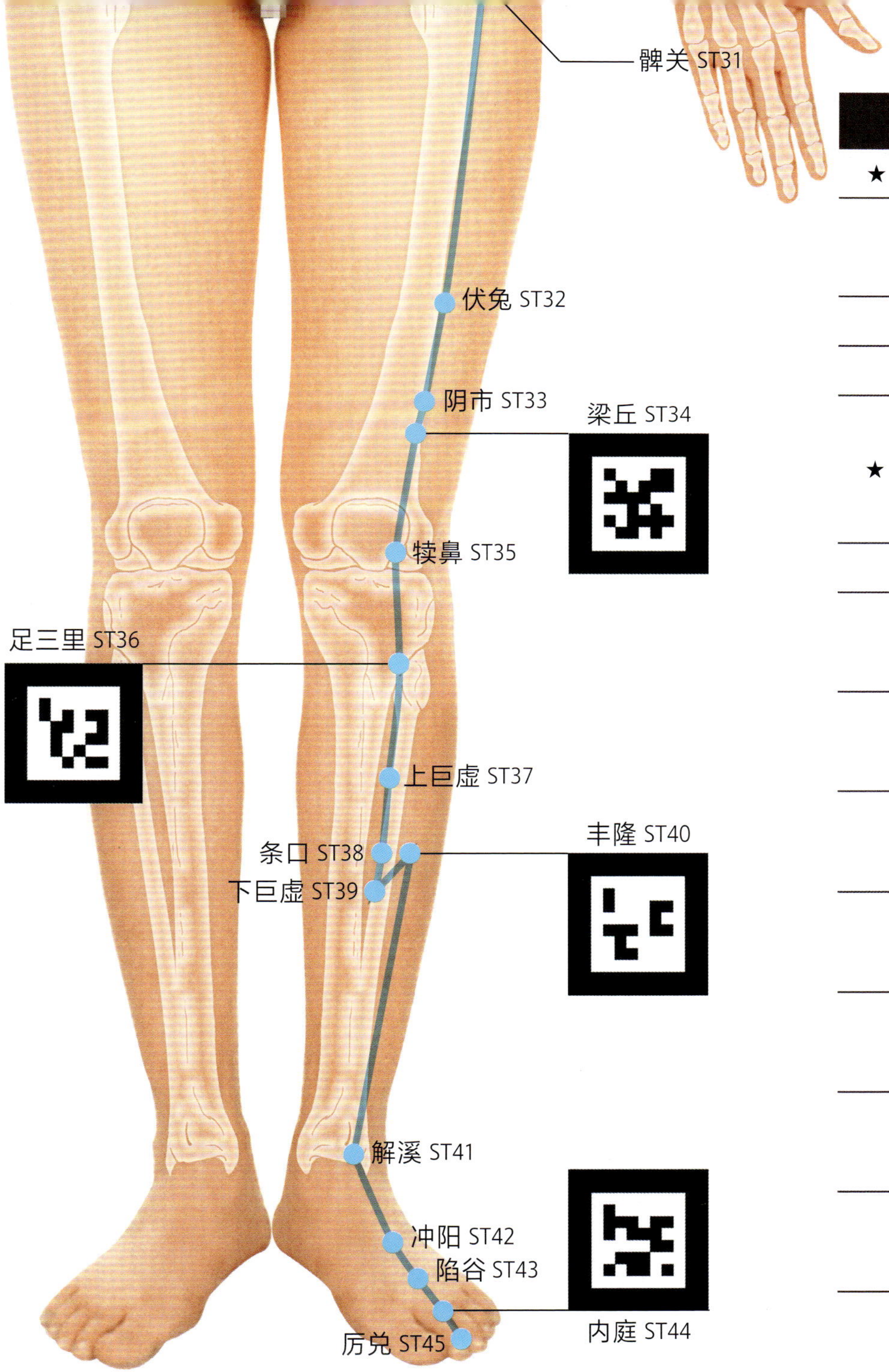

Continued

ST	Acupoints	Indications
★ 21	Liángmén	Poor appetite; stomachache; vomiting
22	Guānmén	Distention of abdomen; abdominal pain; borborygmus; diarrhea
23	Tàiyǐ	Stomach diseases; upset; manic and depressive psychosis
24	Huáròumén	Stomachache; vomiting; manic and depressive psychosis
★ 25	Tiānshū	Abdominal pain; distention of abdomen; borborygmus; diarrhea; constipation; appendicitis; irregular menstruation; dysmenorrhea
26	Wàilíng	Distention of abdomen; hernia; dysmenorrhea
27	Dàjù	Distention and fullness of lower abdomen; dysuria; hernia; seminal emission; premature ejaculation
28	Shuǐdào	Distention and fullness of lower abdomen; dysuria; hernia; dysmenorrhea; sterility
29	Guīlái	Pain in lower abdomen; hernia; irregular menstruation; leukorrheal diseases; uterus prolapse and vagina prolapse
30	Qìchōng	Borborygmus and abdominal pain; hernia; irregular menstruation; sterility; impotence
31	Bìguān	flaccidity and motor impairment of lower limbs; lower back pain; coldness in knees
32	Fútù	flaccidity and motor impairment of lower limbs; lower back pain; coldness in knees; hernia
33	Yīnshì	Knees pain; flaccidity and motor impairment of lower limbs; lower back pain; hernia

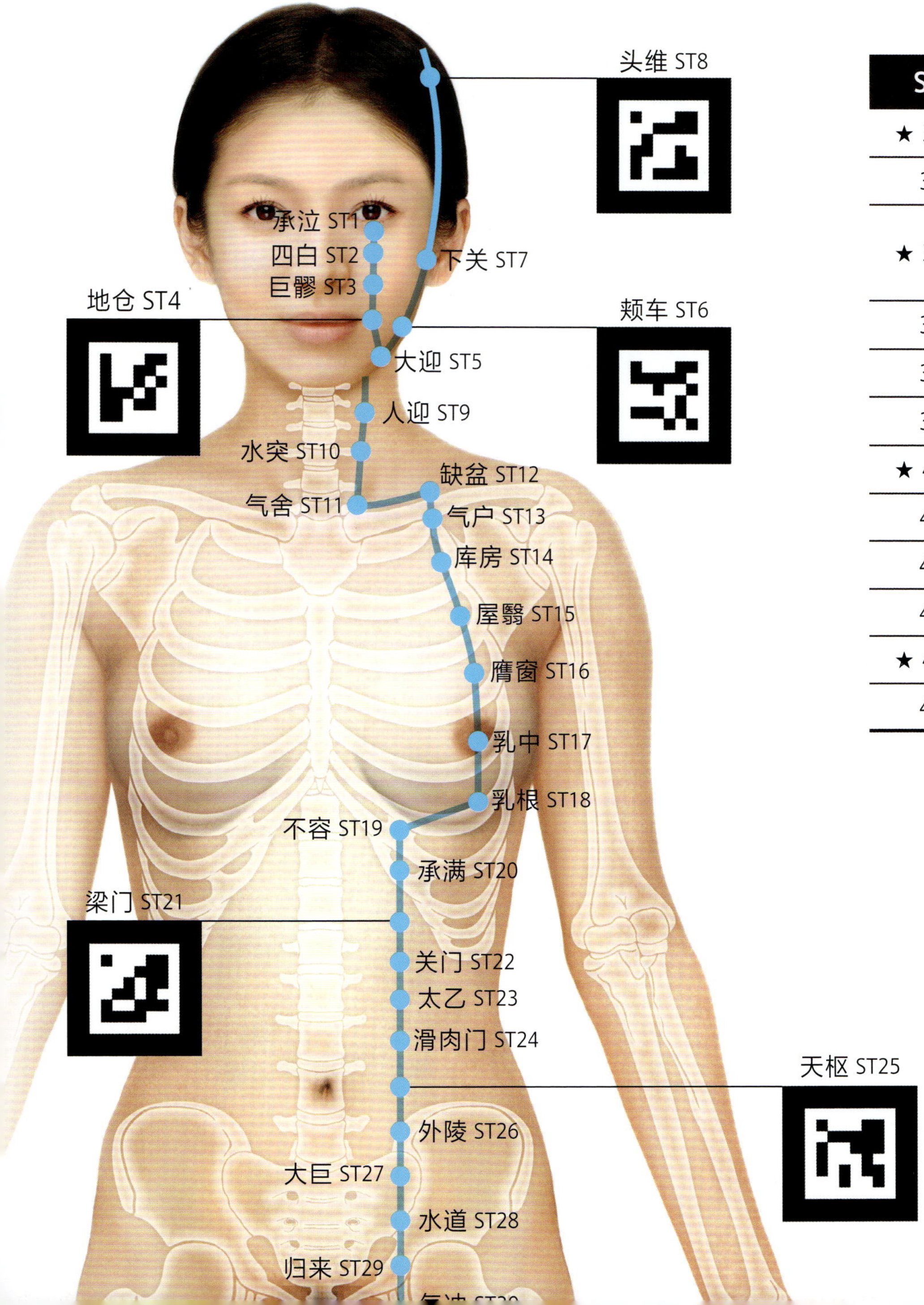

续表

ST	穴 名	主 治
★ 34	梁丘	急性胃病、膝肿痛、下肢不遂、乳部疾患
35	犊鼻	膝痛、屈伸不利、下肢麻痹
★ 36	足三里	胃痛、呕吐、吞咽困难、腹泻、腹胀、痢疾、便秘、下肢痿痹、癫狂、乳房肿痛、阑尾炎、虚劳
37	上巨虚	肠鸣、腹痛、腹泻、便秘、阑尾炎、下肢痿痹
38	条口	下肢痿痹、肌肉痉挛、肩周炎、臂痛、脘腹疼痛
39	下巨虚	腹泻、痢疾、小腹痛、下肢痿痹、乳房肿痛
★ 40	丰隆	头痛、眩晕、癫狂、咳嗽痰多、下肢痿痹、腹胀、便秘
41	解溪	下肢痿痹、足下垂、头痛、眩晕、癫狂、腹胀、便秘
42	冲阳	胃痛、口眼歪斜、癫狂、足痿无力
43	陷谷	面肿、水肿、足背肿痛、肠鸣腹痛
★ 44	内庭	齿痛、咽喉肿痛、鼻出血、热病、腹泻、便秘、足背肿痛
45	厉兑	鼻出血、齿痛、咽喉肿痛、热病、多梦、癫狂

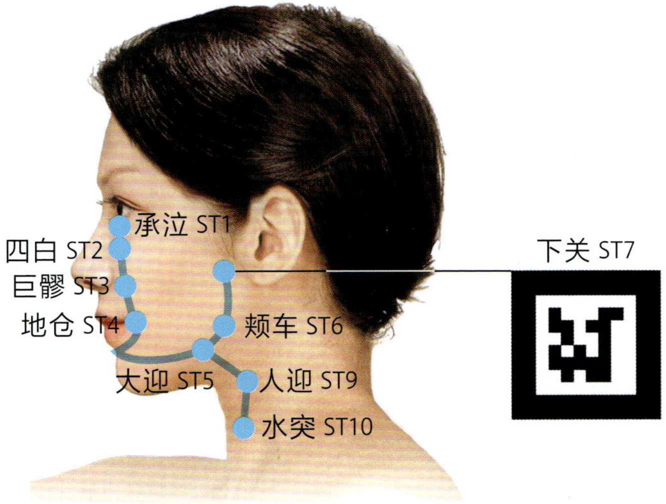

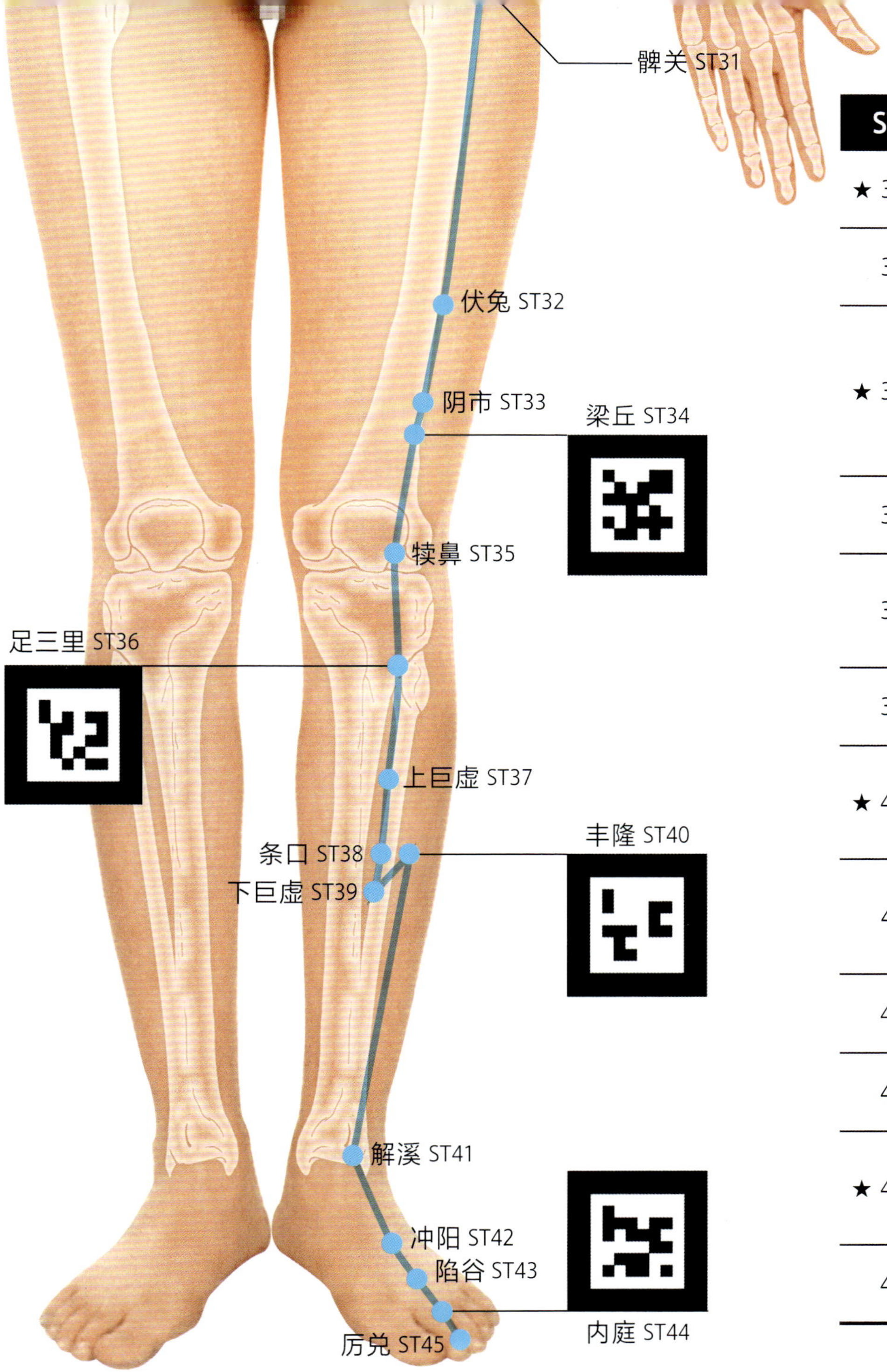

Continued

ST	Acupoints	Indications
★ 34	Liángqiū	Acute stomach diseases; swelling and pain in knees; motor impairment of lower limbs; breast diseases
35	Dúbí	Knees pain; difficulty in bending and stretching; numbness and motor impairment of lower limbs
★ 36	Zúsānlǐ	Stomachache; vomiting; difficulty in swallowing; diarrhea; distention of abdomen; dysentery; constipation; flaccidity and motor impairment of lower limbs; manic and depressive psychosis; swelling and pain of breast; appendicitis; consumptive diseases
37	Shàngjùxū	Borborygmus; abdominal pain; diarrhea; constipation; appendicitis; flaccidity and motor impairment of lower limbs
38	Tiáokǒu	flaccidity and motor impairment of lower limbs; muscle spasm; shoulder periarthritis; arm pain; pain in epigastrium and abdomen
39	Xiàjùxū	Diarrhea; dysentery; lower abdominal pain; flaccidity and motor impairment of lower limbs; swelling and pain of breast
★ 40	Fēnglóng	Headache; dizziness; manic and depressive psychosis; cough with profuse phlegm; flaccidity and motor impairment of lower limbs; distention of abdomen; constipation
41	Jiěxī	Flaccidity and motor impairment of lower limbs; drooping foot; headache; dizziness; manic and depressive psychosis; distention of abdomen; constipation
42	Chōngyáng	Stomachache; deviation of mouth and eye; manic and depressive psychosis; flaccidity of the foot
43	Xiàngǔ	Swollen face; edema; swelling and pain on the dorsum of foot; borborygmus and abdominal pain
★ 44	Nèitíng	Toothache; swelling and pain in throat; nose bleeding; febrile diseases; diarrhea; constipation; swelling and pain on the dorsum of foot
45	Lìduì	Nose bleeding; toothache; swelling and pain in throat; febrile diseases; dreaminess; manic and depressive psychosis

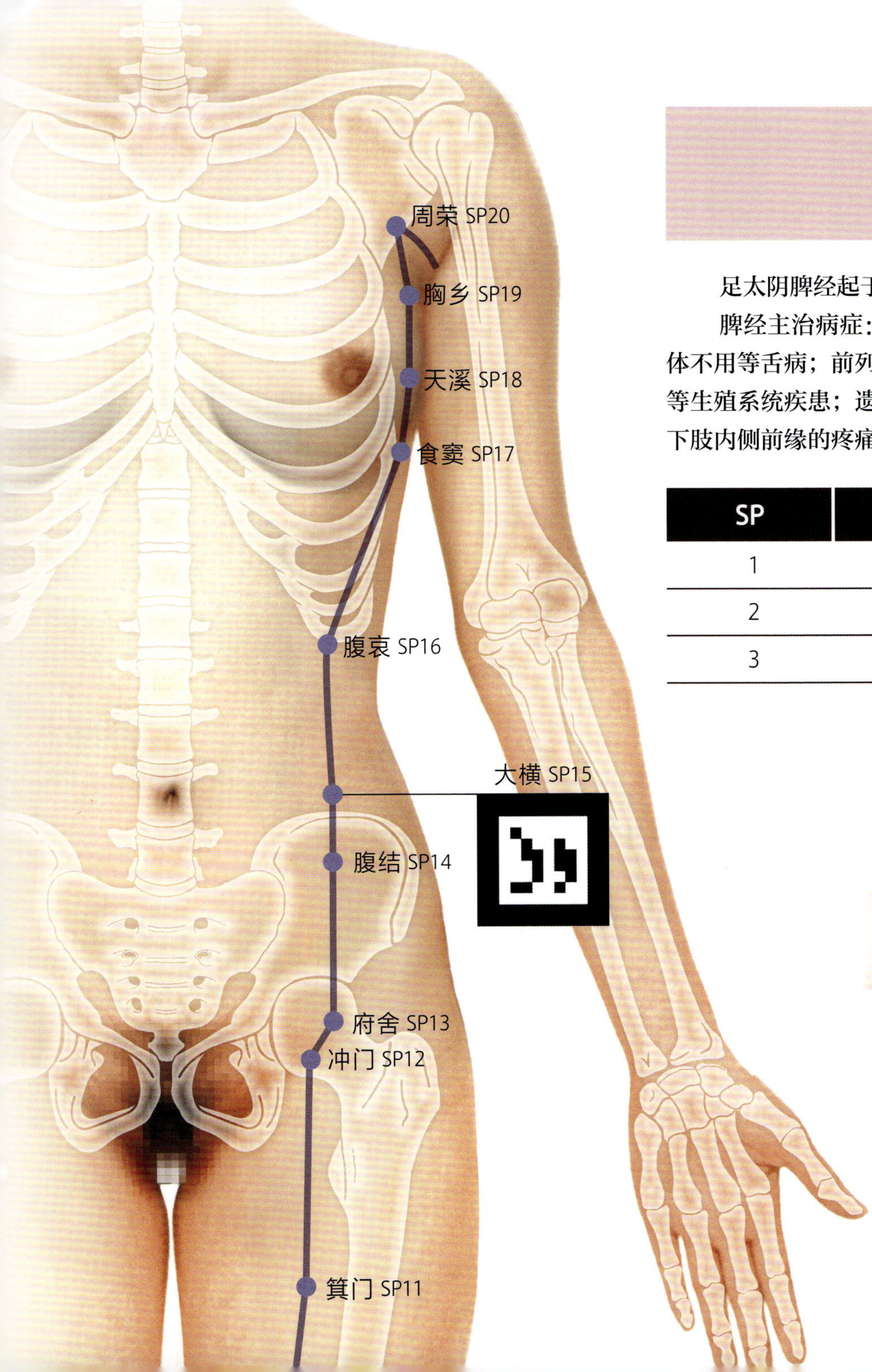

足太阴脾经

足太阴脾经起于足踇趾内侧隐白，经过腿部内侧，止于胸部的大包。

脾经主治病症：呕吐、胃痛、腹胀、便稀、泄泻、水肿、黄疸等脾胃疾患；中风后言语謇涩、舌体不用等舌病；前列腺炎、遗精、阳痿、痛经、月经不调、阴道炎、妊娠呕吐、难产、恶露不尽、不孕等生殖系统疾患；遗尿、尿频、尿急、尿潴留等泌尿系统疾患；皮肤瘙痒、湿疹、荨麻疹等皮肤疾患；下肢内侧前缘的疼痛、麻木、瘫痪等经脉循行部位的疾患。

SP	穴 名	主 治
1	隐白	月经过多、崩漏、便血、尿血、癫狂、多梦、惊风、腹满、暴泻
2	大都	腹胀、胃痛、呕吐、腹泻、便秘、热病、无汗
3	太白	肠鸣、腹胀、腹泻、便秘、体重肢痛

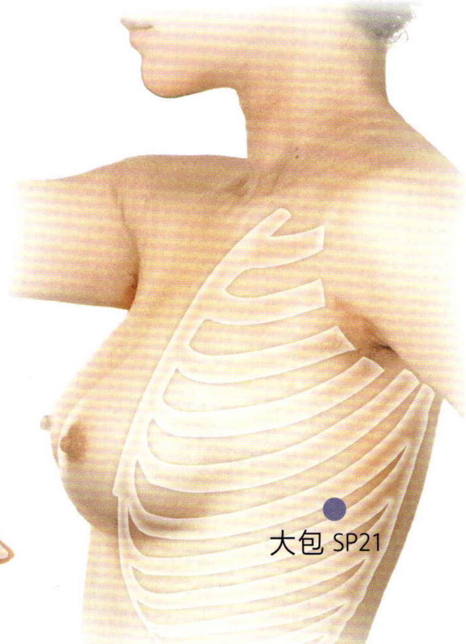

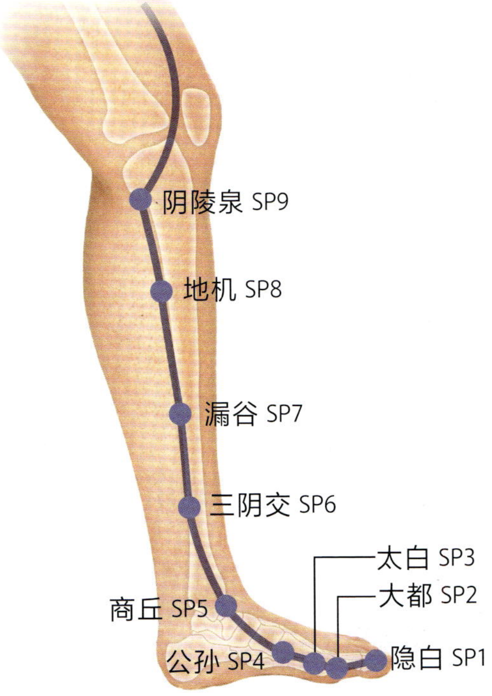

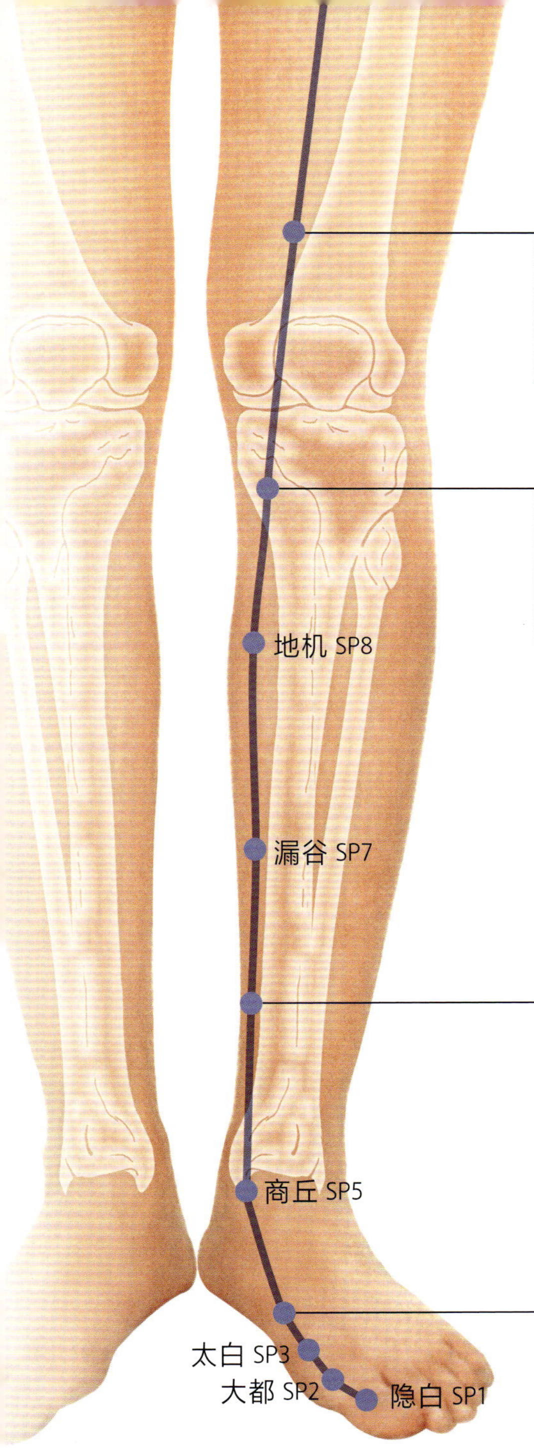

Spleen Meridian of Foot-Taiyin, SP.

Spleen Meridian of Foot-Taiyin emerges from Yinbai (SP1) at medial side of foot great toe, runs along the medial side of thigh and terminates at Dabao (SP21) in the chest.

Spleen Meridian mainly treats diseases of intestine and stomach including vomiting, stomachache, abdominal distention, loose stool, diarrhea, edema and jaundice; tongue diseases including retraction of the tongue and stiffness of tongue body after wind stroke; diseases of reproductive system including prostatitis, seminal emission, impotence, dysmenorrhea, irregular menstruation, vaginitis, vomiting of pregnancy, dystocia, prolonged lochia and sterility; diseases of urogenital system including enuresis, frequent urine, urgent urine and uroschesis; and skin diseases including skin itch, eczema and measles; diseases of running courses of meridian including numbness and motor impairment of frontal medial side of lower limbs.

SP	Acupoints	Indications
1	Yǐnbái	Hypermenorrhea; metrorrhalgia and metrostaxis; hematochezia; hematuria; manic and depressive psychosis; dreaminess; convulsion; fullness of abdomen; fulminant diarrhea
2	Dàdū	Distention of abdomen; stomachache; vomiting; diarrhea; constipation; febrile diseases; anidrosis
3	Tàibái	Borborygmus; distention of abdomen; diarrhea; constipation; body heaviness and extremities pain

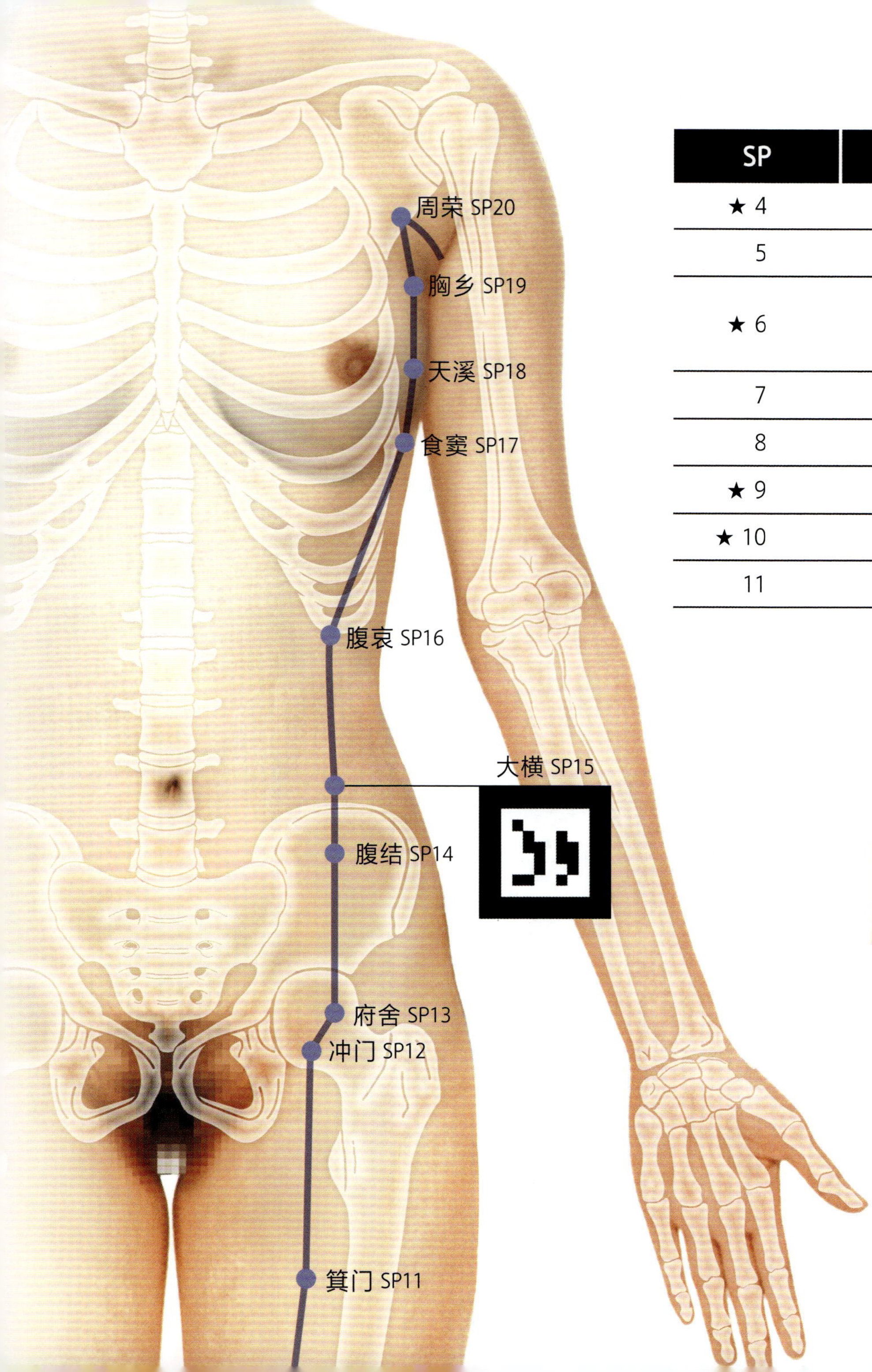

续表

SP	穴 名	主 治
★ 4	公孙	胃痛、呕吐、腹痛、腹泻、痢疾、心烦失眠、狂证、气上冲心
5	商丘	腹胀、腹泻、便秘、黄疸、足踝痛
★ 6	三阴交	肠鸣腹胀、腹泻、月经不调、带下、子宫或阴道脱垂、不孕、滞产、遗精、阳痿、遗尿、心悸、失眠、高血压、下肢痿痹、阴虚诸证
7	漏谷	腹胀、肠鸣、小便不利、遗精、下肢痿痹
8	地机	痛经、崩漏、月经不调、腹痛、腹泻、小便不利、水肿
★ 9	阴陵泉	腹胀、腹泻、水肿、黄疸、小便不利、膝痛
★ 10	血海	月经不调、痛经、经闭、荨麻疹、湿疹、丹毒
11	箕门	小便不利、遗尿、腹股沟肿痛

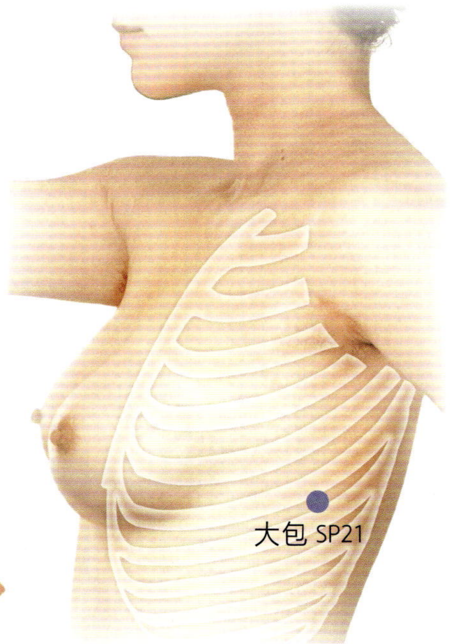

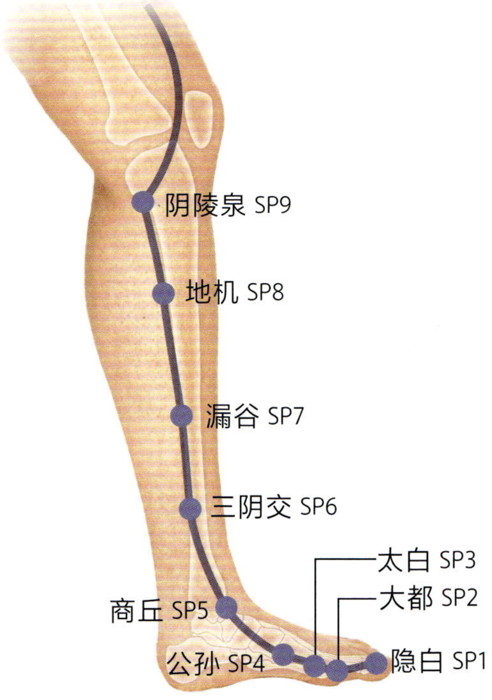

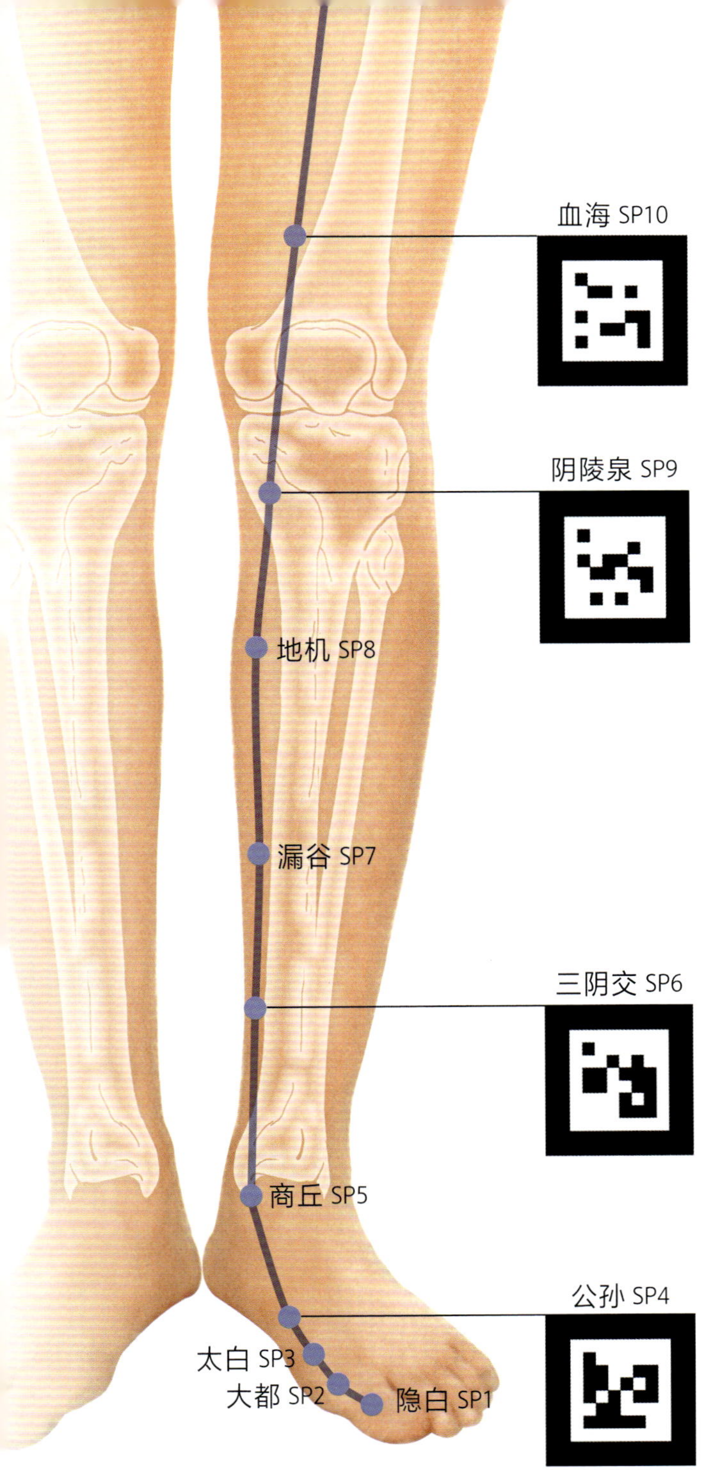

Continued

SP	Acupoints	Indications
★ 4	Gōngsūn	Stomachache; vomiting; abdominal pain, diarrhea; dysentery; upset and insomnia; manic psychosis; Qi rushing upward to heart
5	Shāngqiū	Distention of abdomen; diarrhea; constipation; jaundice; foot and malleolus pain
★ 6	Sānyīnjiāo	Borborygmus and abdominal pain; diarrhea; irregular menstruation; leukorrheal diseases; uterus prolapse and vagina prolapse; sterility; prolonged delivery; seminal emission; impotence; enuresis; palpitation; insomnia; hypertension; flaccidity and motor impairment of lower limbs; Yin deficiency syndromes
7	Lòugǔ	Distention of abdomen; borborygmus; dysuria; seminal emission; flaccidity and motor impairment of lower limbs
8	Dìjī	Dysmenorrhea; metrorrhalgia and metrostaxis; irregular menstruation; abdominal pain; diarrhea; dysuria; edema
★ 9	Yīnlíngquán	Distention of abdomen; diarrhea; edema; jaundice; dysuria; knees pain
★ 10	Xuèhǎi	Irregular menstruation; dysmenorrhea; amenorrhea; measles; eczema; erysipelas
11	Jīmén	Dysuria; enuresis; swelling and pain of groin

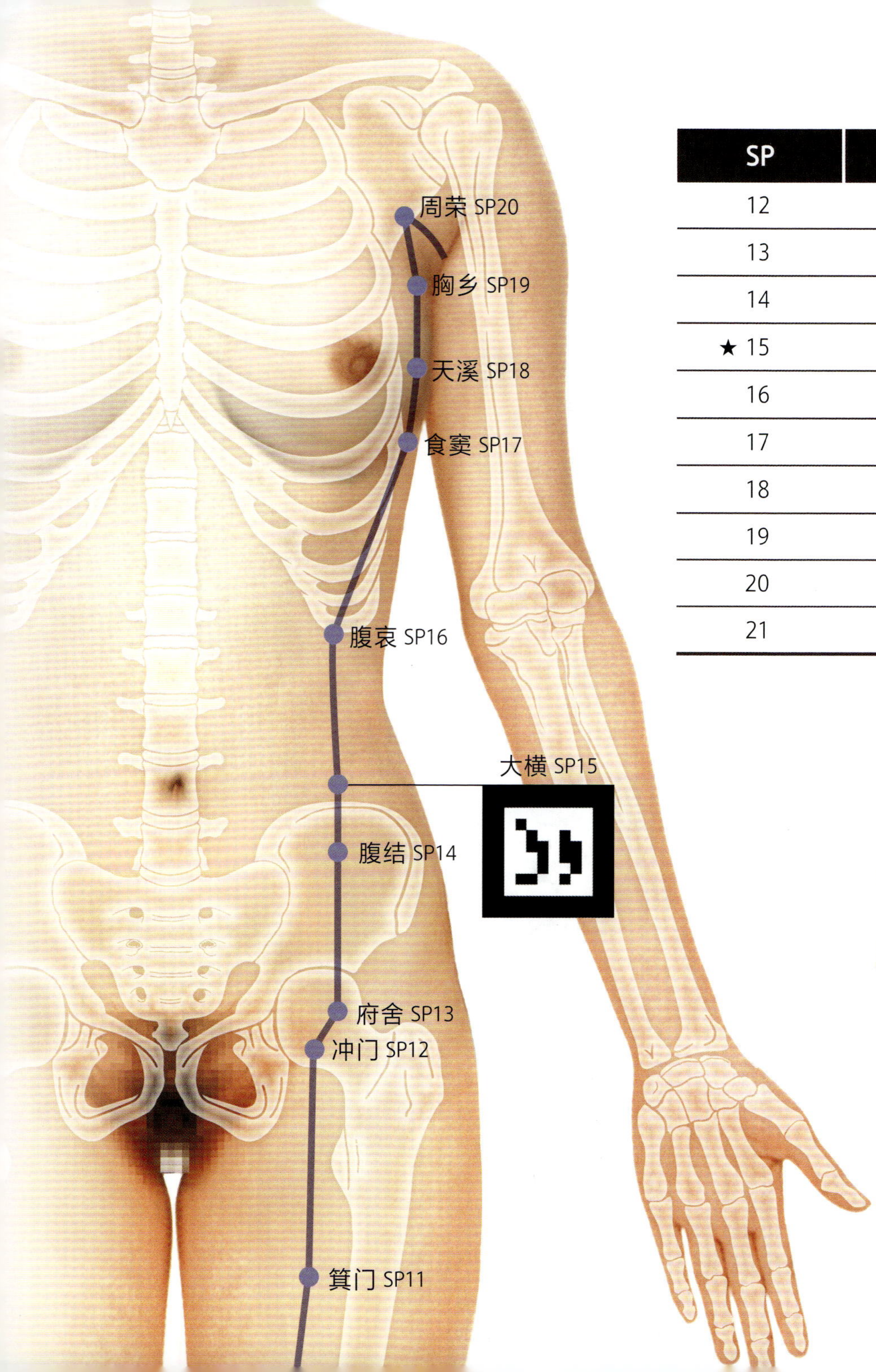

续表

SP	穴 名	主 治
12	冲门	腹痛、疝气、崩漏、带下、胎气上冲
13	府舍	腹痛、积聚、疝气
14	腹结	腹痛、腹泻、疝气
★ 15	大横	腹痛、腹泻、便秘
16	腹哀	消化不良、腹痛、便秘、痢疾
17	食窦	胸胁胀痛、嗳气、反胃、腹胀、水肿
18	天溪	胸痛、咳嗽、乳房肿痛、乳汁少
19	胸乡	胸胁胀痛
20	周荣	胸胁胀满、咳嗽、气喘
21	大包	气喘、胸胁痛、全身疼痛、岔气、四肢无力

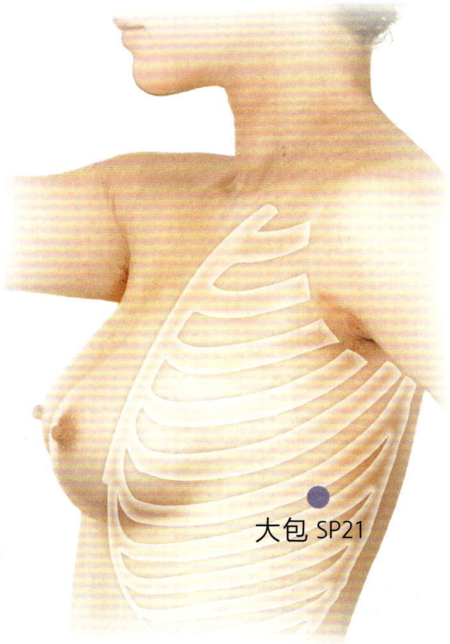

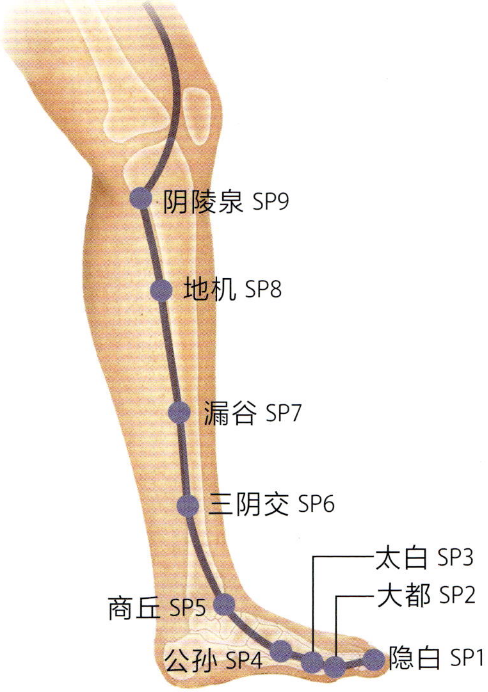

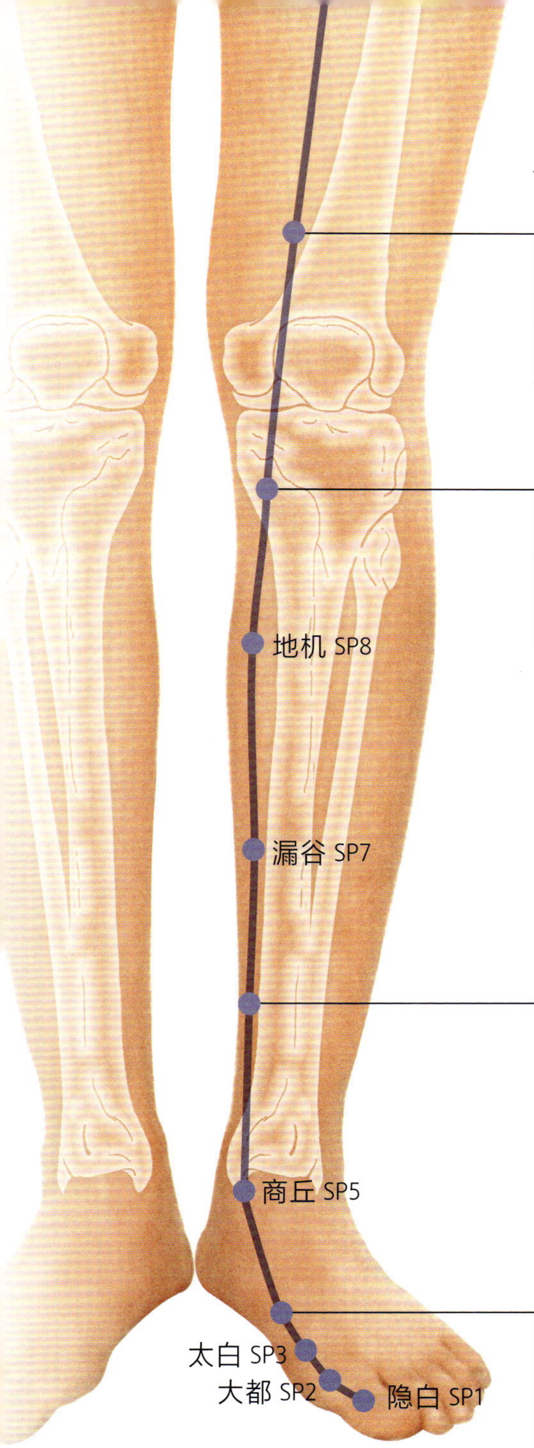

Continued

SP	Acupoints	Indications
12	Chōngmén	Abdominal pain; hernia; metrorrhalgia and metrostaxis; leukorrheal diseases; upward flow of fetus Qi
13	Fŭshè	Abdominal pain; abdominal mass; hernia
14	Fùjié	Abdominal pain; diarrhea; hernia
★ 15	Dàhéng	Abdominal pain; diarrhea; constipation
16	Fù'āi	Poor indigestion; abdominal pain; constipation; dysentery
17	Shídòu	Distending pain of chest and hypochondrium; belching; regurgitation; distention of abdomen; edema
18	Tiānxī	Chest pain; cough; swelling and pain of breast; lack of breast milk
19	Xiōngxiāng	Distending pain of chest and hypochondrium
20	Zhōuróng	Distending pain of chest and hypochondrium; cough; asthma
21	Dàbāo	Asthma; pain in the chest and hypochondrium; pain all over the body; feeling of pain in the chest when breath; flaccidity of four extremities

手少阴心经

手少阴心经起于腋窝中央的极泉，沿手臂内侧走到手小指内侧的少冲。

心经主治病症：舌强、失语等舌病；心绞痛、心律不齐、自主神经功能紊乱、失眠、神经分裂症等心神疾患；上肢内侧前缘的疼痛、麻木等经脉循行部位的疾患。

HT	穴 名	主 治
1	极泉	心痛、心悸、肩周炎、臂痛、胁肋疼痛、臂丛神经损伤、颈淋巴结结核、狐臭，还可作为上肢针麻用穴
2	青灵	头痛、胁痛、肩周炎、臂痛
★ 3	少海	心痛、癔症、肘臂挛痛、臂麻手颤、头项痛、腋胁部痛、颈淋巴结结核
4	灵道	心痛、精神异常、急性咽喉炎、肘臂挛痛
5	通里	心悸、怔忡、舌强不语、急性咽喉炎、腕臂痛
6	阴郄	心痛、惊悸、骨蒸盗汗、吐血、黏膜出血
★ 7	神门	心痛、心烦、惊悸、怔忡、健忘、失眠、痴呆、癫狂、高血压、胸胁痛
8	少府	心悸、胸痛、外阴瘙痒、阴痛、痈疡、小指挛痛
9	少冲	心悸、心痛、癫狂、昏迷、热病、胸胁痛

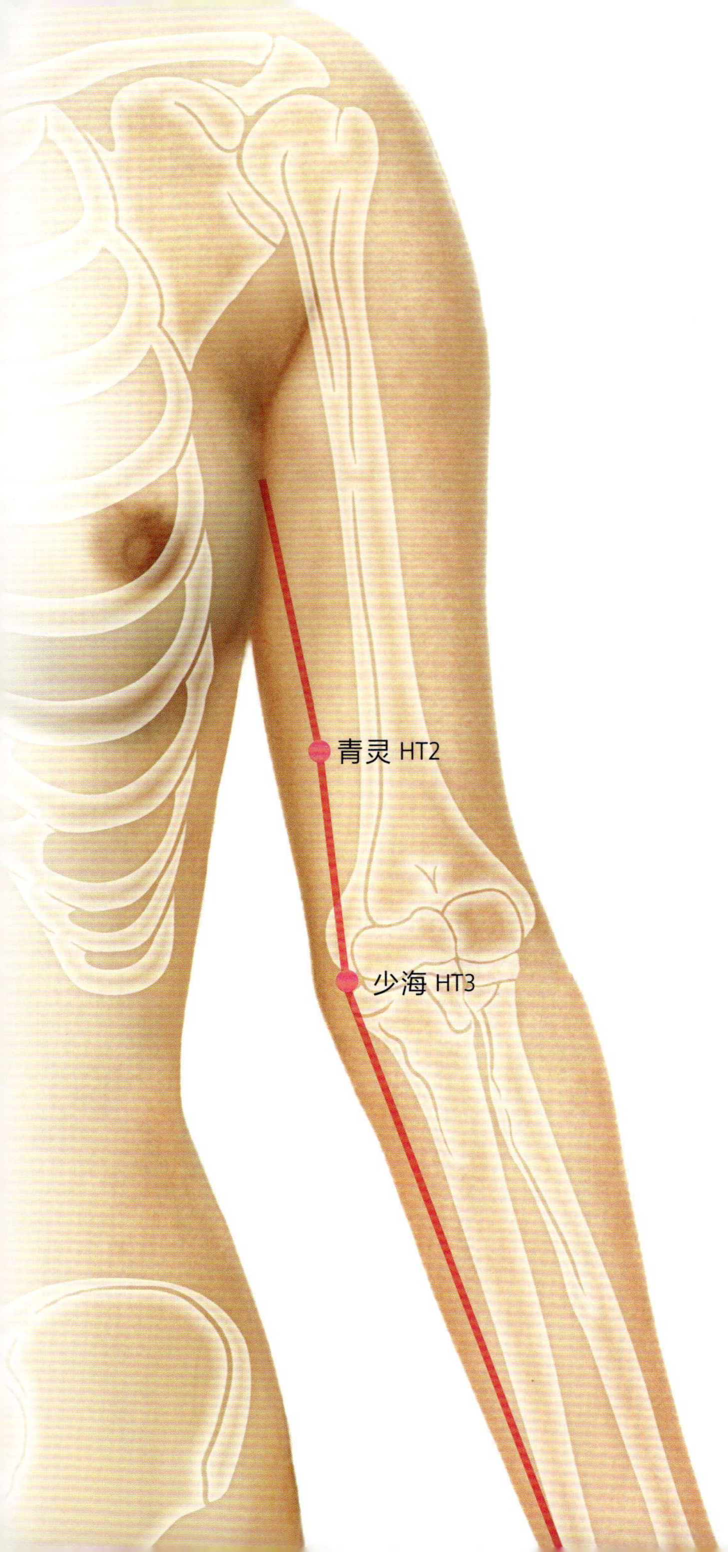

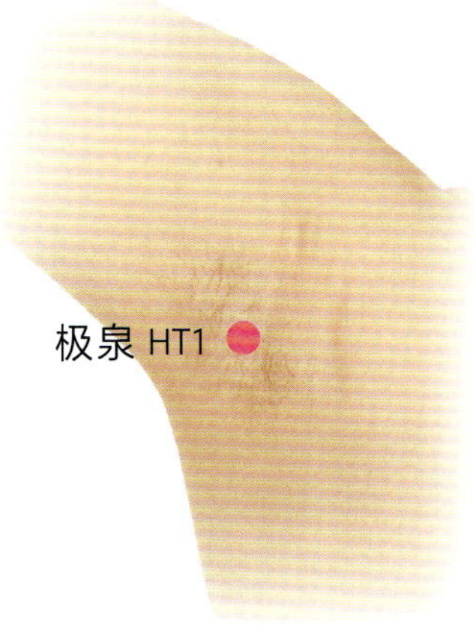

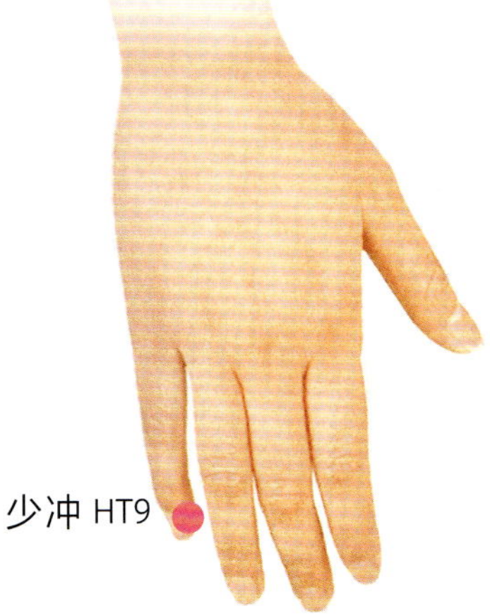

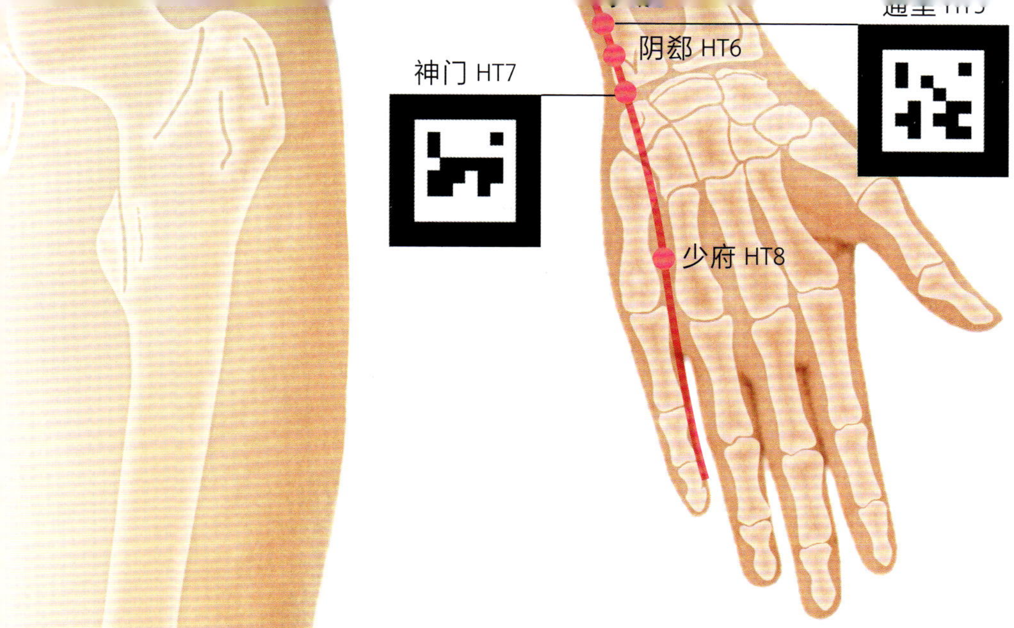

Heart Meridian of Hand-Shaoyin, HT.

Heart Meridian of Hand-Shaoyin emerges from Jiquan (HT1) in the middle of armpit, runs along medial side of arm and terminates at Shaochong (HT9) in medial side of little finger.

Heart Meridian mainly treats the tongue diseases including tongue stiffness and voice loss; diseases of heart and mind including angina, arrhythmia, dysfunction of autonomic nerves, insomnia and schizophrenia; diseases of running courses of meridian including pain and numbness in frontal medial side of upper limbs.

HT	Acupoints	Indications
1	Jíquán	Cardiac pain; palpitation; shoulder periarthritis; chest and hypochondrium pain; damage of brachial plexus; cervical lymph node tuberculosis; hircus; also used as acupuncture anesthesia common point for upper limbs
2	Qīnglíng	Headache; hypochondrium pain; shoulder periarthritis; arm pain
★ 3	Shàohǎi	Cardiac pain; hysteria; spasm and pain of elbow and arm; numbness of arm and hand tremor; pain in head and neck; pain in armpit and hypochondrium; cervical lymph node tuberculosis
4	Língdào	Cardiac pain; mental disorder; acute sphagitis; spasm and pain in elbow and arm
5	Tōnglǐ	Palpitation; severe palpitation; voice loss due to tongue stiffness; acute sphagitis; wrist and arm pain
6	Yīnxì	Cardiac pain; palpitation due to fright; night sweat and steaming bone; hematemesis; mucosa bleeding
★ 7	Shénmén	Cardiac pain; upset; palpitation due to fright; severe palpitation; amnesia; insomnia; dementia; manic and depressive psychosis; hypertension; chest and hypochondrium pain
8	Shàofǔ	Palpitation; chest pain; itch of vulva; genitalia pain; carbuncles; spasm and pain of the little finger
9	Shàochōng	Palpitation; cardiac pain; manic and depressive psychosis; coma; febrile disease; chest and hypochondrium pain

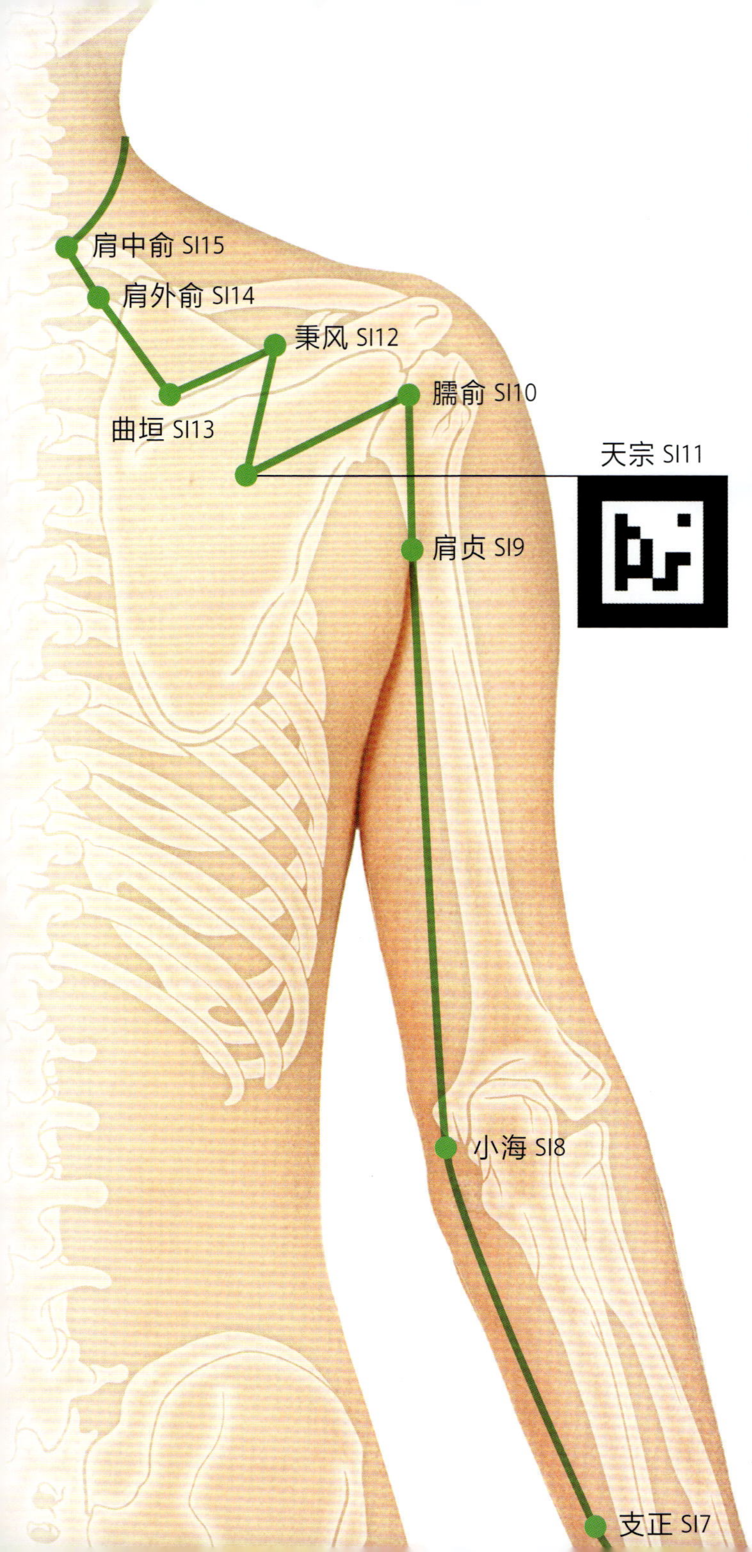

手太阳小肠经

手太阳小肠经起于手小指少泽，从手臂外侧到颈部，止于耳部的听宫。

小肠经主治病症：耳聋、耳鸣、中耳炎等耳部疾患；脑血管意外后遗症、面痛、面瘫、落枕、颈椎病、肩周炎、背痛、腰痛等经脉循行部位的疾患。

SI	穴 名	主 治
1	少泽	乳房肿痛、乳汁少、昏迷、热病、头痛、白内障、咽喉肿痛
2	前谷	热病、乳房肿痛、乳汁少、头痛、目痛、耳鸣、咽喉肿痛
★ 3	后溪	头项强痛、腰背痛、手指及肘臂挛痛、耳聋、目赤、癫狂、寒战发热
4	腕骨	指挛腕痛、头项强痛、白内障、黄疸、热病、寒战发热
5	阳谷	颈或颔部肿大、臂外侧痛、腕痛、头痛、目眩、耳鸣、耳聋、热病、癫狂
6	养老	目视不明，肩、背、肘、臂酸痛

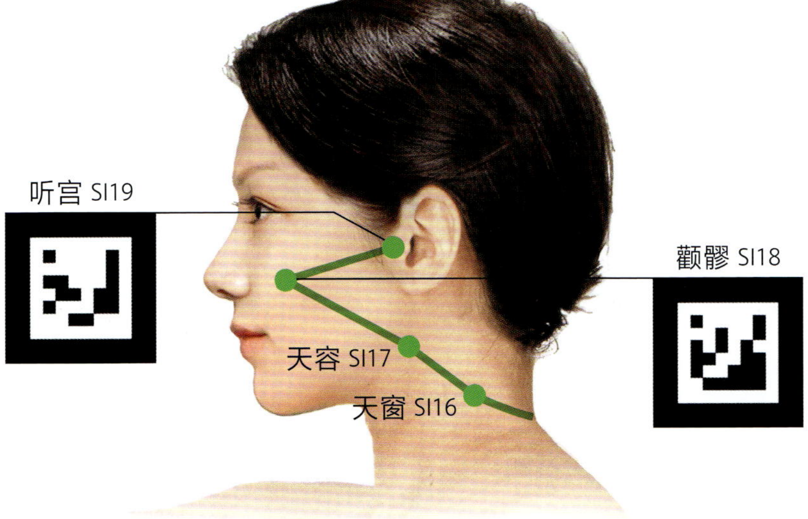

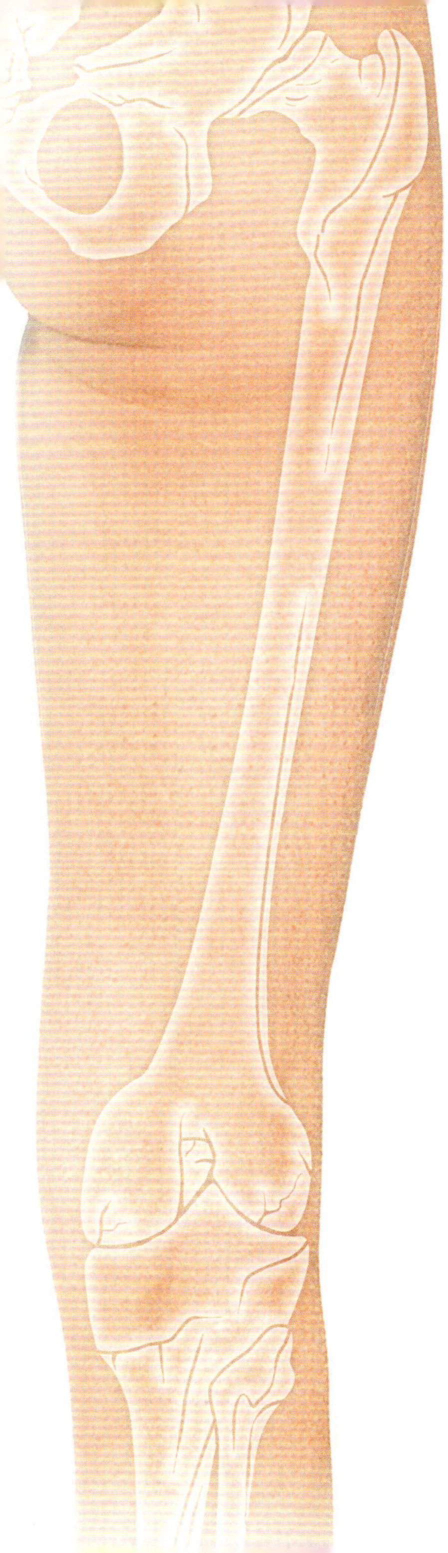

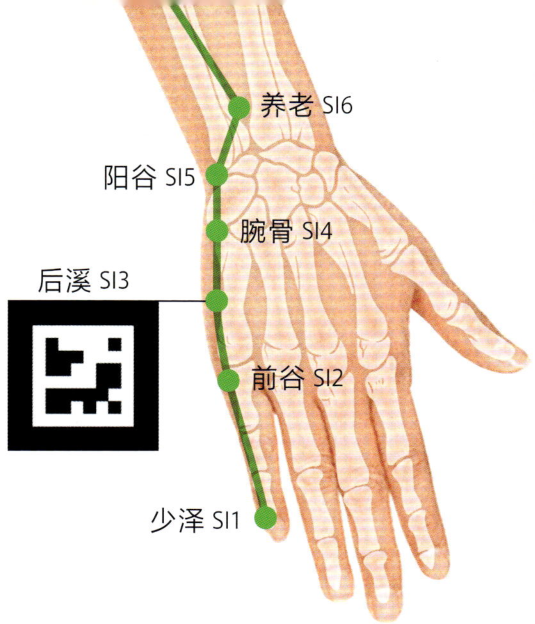

Small Intestine Meridian of Hand-Taiyang, SI.

Small Intestine Meridian of Hand-Taiyang emerges from Shaoze (SI1) in the little finger, runs along the lateral side of arm to the neck and terminates at Tinggong (SI19) in the ear.

Small Intestine Meridian mainly treats the ear diseases including deafness, tinnitus and otitis media; diseases of parts of running courses of meridian including cerebrovascular accident sequelae, facial pain, facial paralysis, stiff neck, cervical spondylopathy, shoulder periarthritis, back pain and lower back pain.

SI	Acupoints	Indications
1	Shàozé	Swelling and pain of breast; lack of breast milk; coma; febrile diseases; headache; cataract; swelling and pain in throat
2	Qiángǔ	Febrile diseases; swelling and pain of breast; lack of breast milk; headache; eyes pain; tinnitus; swelling and pain in throat
★ 3	Hòuxī	Stiffness and pain of head and neck; lumbago and back pain; spasm and pain of finger; spasm and pain of elbow and arm; deafness and red eyes; manic and depressive psychosis; chill and fever
4	Wàngǔ	Spasm of finger and wrist pain; stiffness and pain of head and neck; cataract; jaundice; febrile diseases; chill and fever
5	Yánggǔ	Swelling of neck and jaw; pain in lateral side of arm; wrist pain; headache; dizziness; tinnitus; deafness; febrile diseases; manic and depressive psychosis
6	Yǎnglǎo	Blurry vision; soreness in shoulder, back, elbow and arm

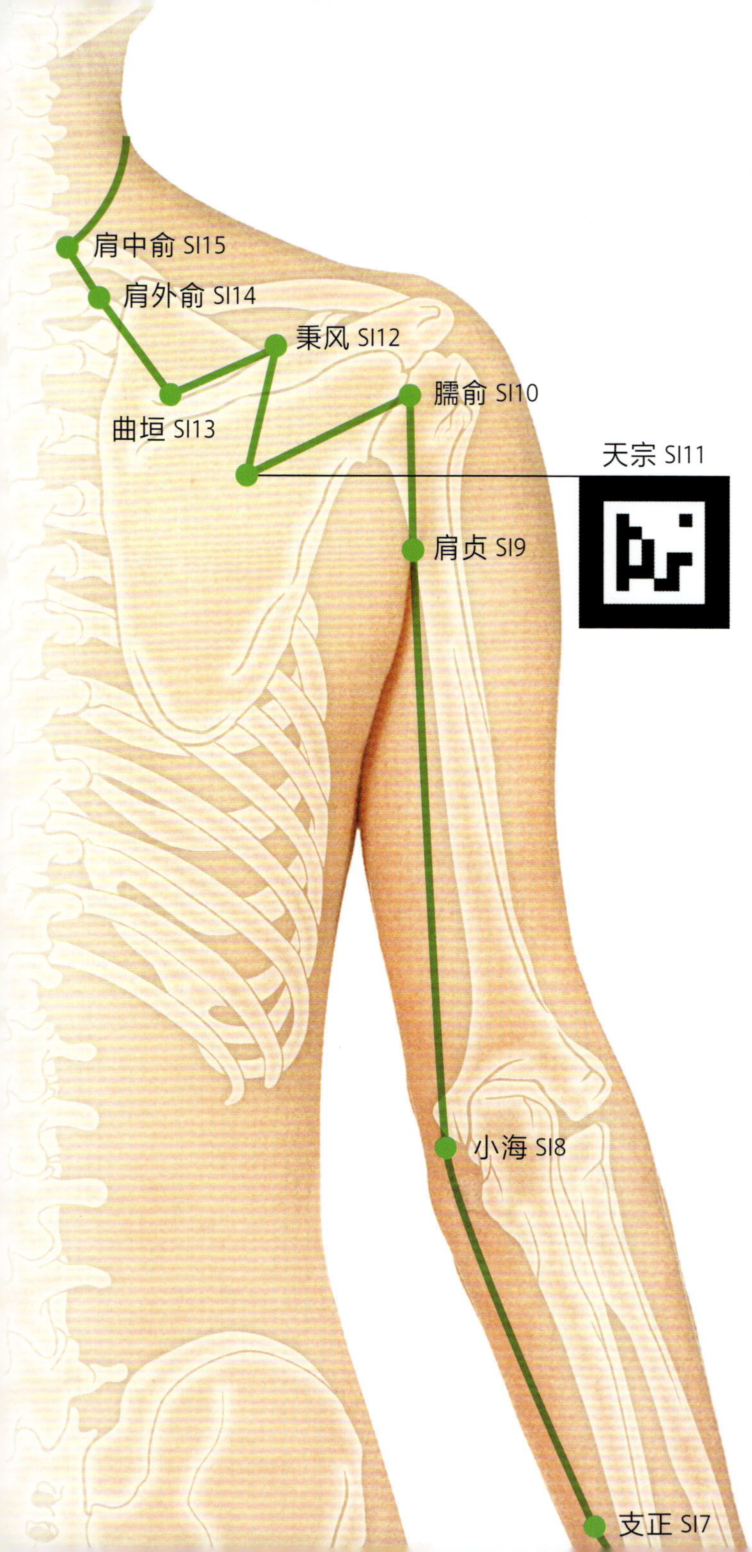

续表

SI	穴 名	主 治
7	支正	头痛、项强、肘臂酸痛、热病、癫狂、疣
8	小海	肘臂疼痛、麻木、癫痫
9	肩贞	肩周炎、上肢不遂、颈淋巴结结核
10	臑俞	肩周炎、颈淋巴结结核
★ 11	天宗	肩胛疼痛、肩背部损伤、气喘
12	秉风	肩胛疼痛、上肢酸麻
13	曲垣	肩胛疼痛
14	肩外俞	肩背疼痛、颈项强急
15	肩中俞	咳嗽、气喘、肩背疼痛
16	天窗	耳鸣、耳聋、咽喉肿痛、急性咽喉炎、颈项强痛
17	天容	耳鸣、耳聋、咽喉肿痛、头痛、颈项强痛
★ 18	颧髎	口眼歪斜、眼睑瞤动、齿痛、三叉神经痛
★ 19	听宫	耳鸣、耳聋、齿痛

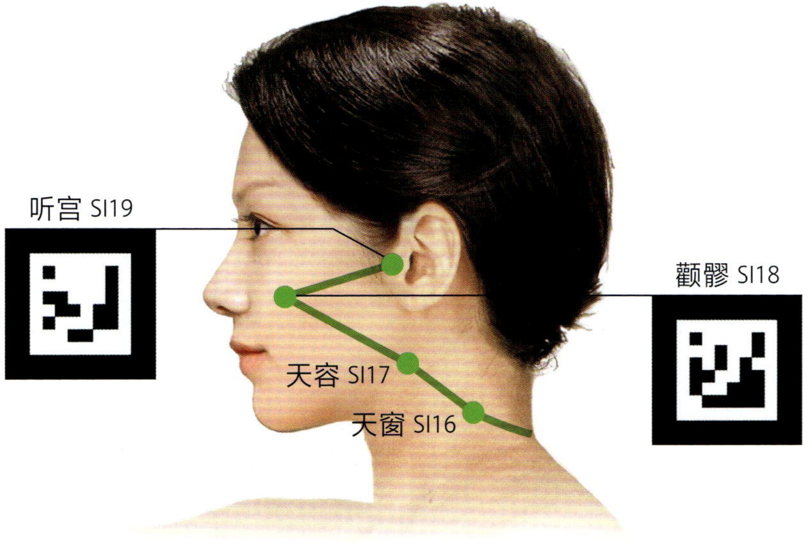

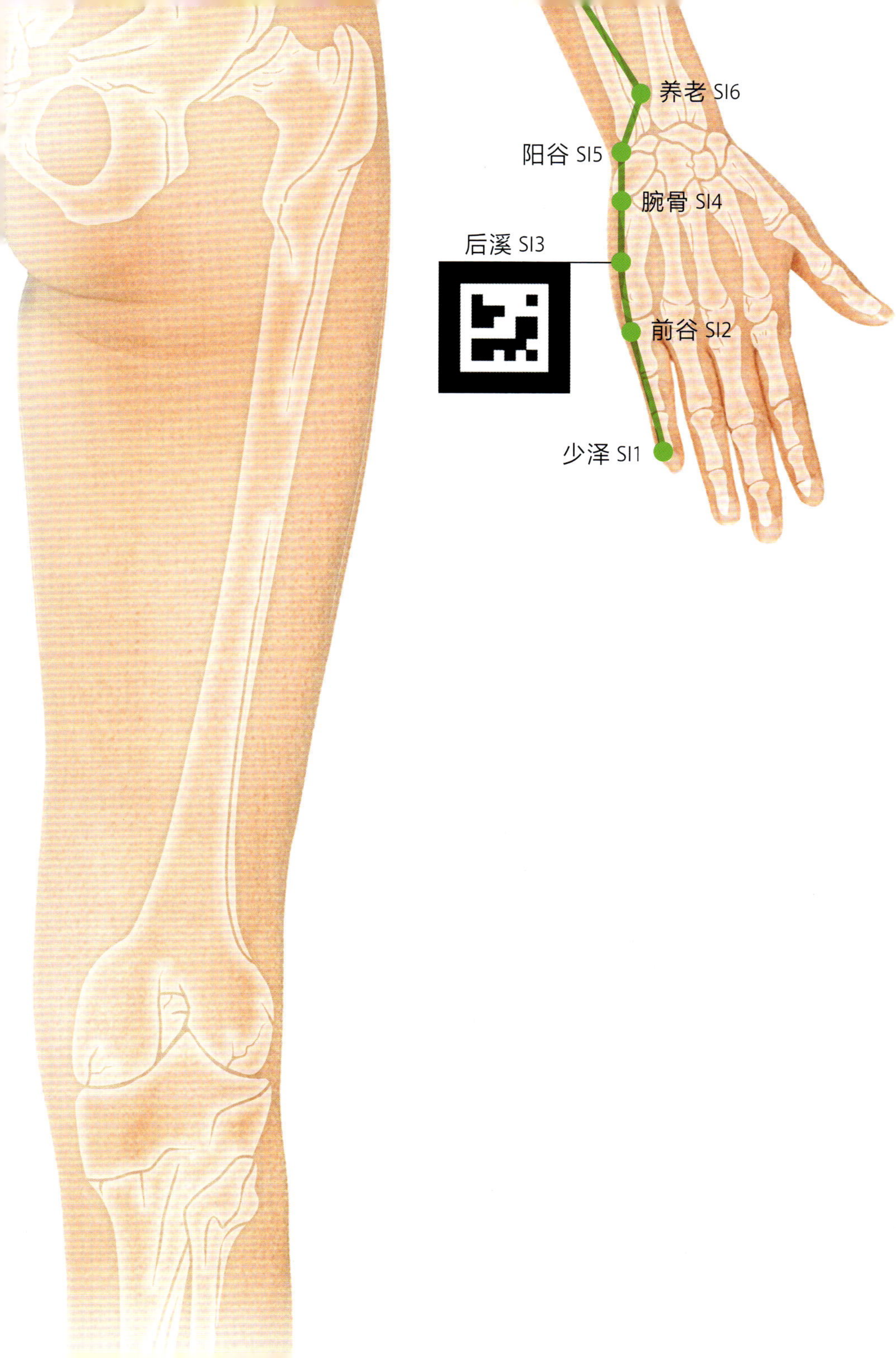

Continued

SI	Acupoints	Indications
7	Zhīzhèng	Headache; stiff neck; soreness of elbow and arm; febrile diseases; manic and depressive psychosis; wart
8	Xiǎohǎi	Elbow and arm pain; numbness of elbow and arm; manic and depressive psychosis
9	Jiānzhēn	Shoulder periarthritis; motor impairment of upper limbs; cervical lymph node tuberculosis
10	Nàoshū	Shoulder periarthritis; cervical lymph node tuberculosis
★ 11	Tiānzōng	Scapular pain; shoulder and back injury; asthma
12	Bǐngfēng	Shoulder periarthritis; soreness and numbness of upper limbs
13	Qūyuán	Scapular pain
14	Jiānwàishū	Shoulder and back pain; neck stiffness
15	Jiānzhōngshū	Cough; asthma; shoulder and back pain
16	Tiānchuāng	Tinnitus; deafness; swelling and pain in throat; acute sphagitis; neck stiffness and pain
17	Tiānróng	Tinnitus; deafness; swelling and pain in throat; headache; neck stiffness and pain
★ 18	Quánliáo	Deviation of mouth and eye; eyelid twitching; toothache; prosopalgia
★ 19	Tīnggōng	Tinnitus; deafness; toothache

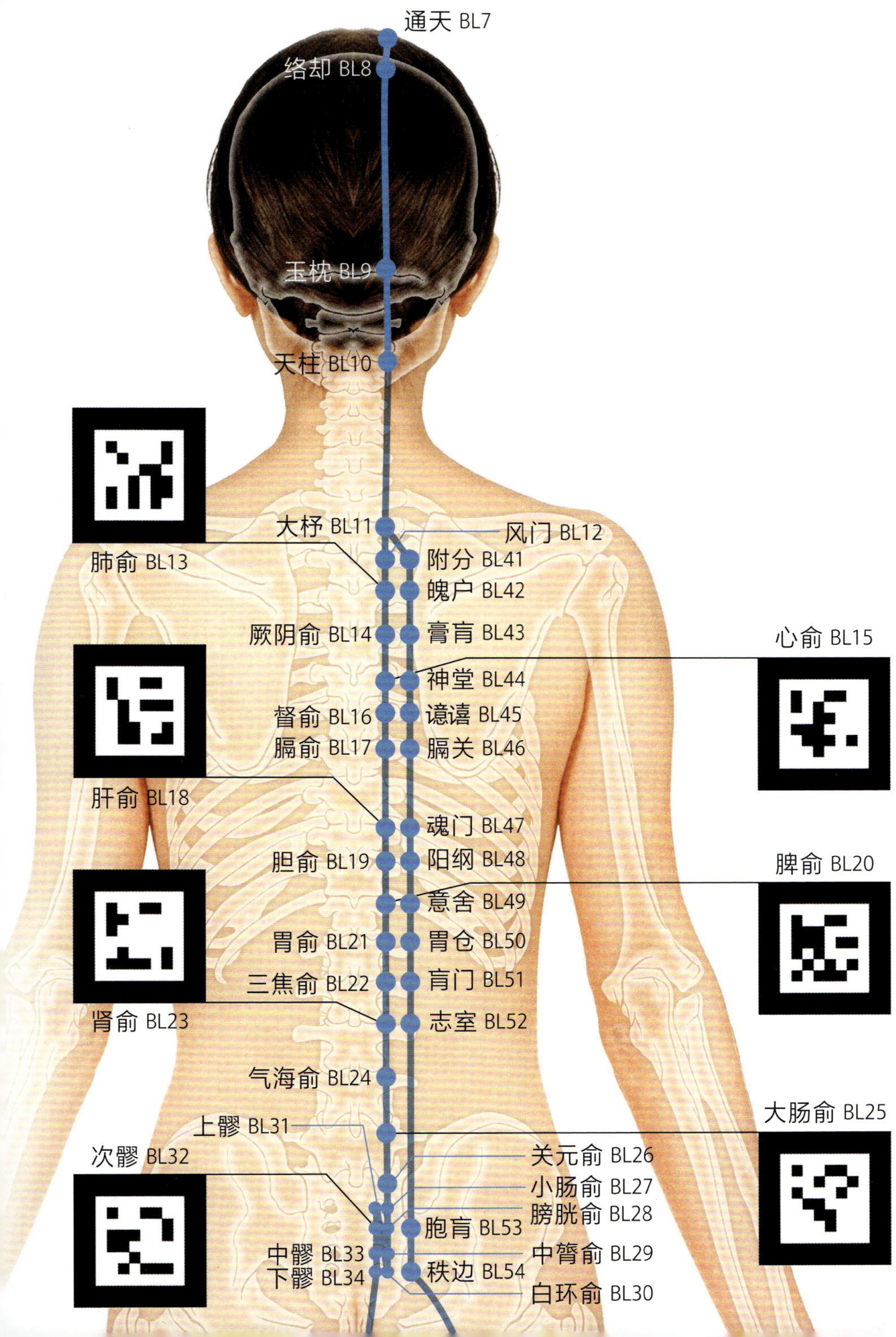

足太阳膀胱经

足太阳膀胱经起于眼睛内侧的睛明，经头顶、颈椎至足小趾外侧的至阴。

膀胱经主治病症：感冒、上呼吸道感染等呼吸系统疾患；失眠、癫狂等神经精神疾患；迎风流泪、头痛、颈椎病、腰背痛、膝关节炎、痔疮、脱肛等经脉循行部位的疾患。

BL	穴 名	主 治
★ 1	睛明	目赤肿痛、流泪、视物不明、目眩、近视、夜盲、色盲、急性腰扭伤、坐骨神经痛、心动过速
2	攒竹	头痛、眉棱骨痛、眼睑瞤动、眼睑下垂、口眼歪斜、目视不明、流泪、目赤肿痛、呃逆
3	眉冲	头痛、目眩、鼻塞、鼻出血
4	曲差	头痛、目眩、鼻塞、鼻出血

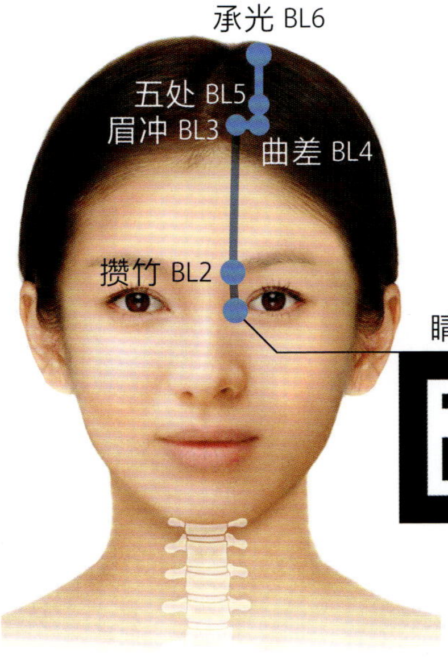

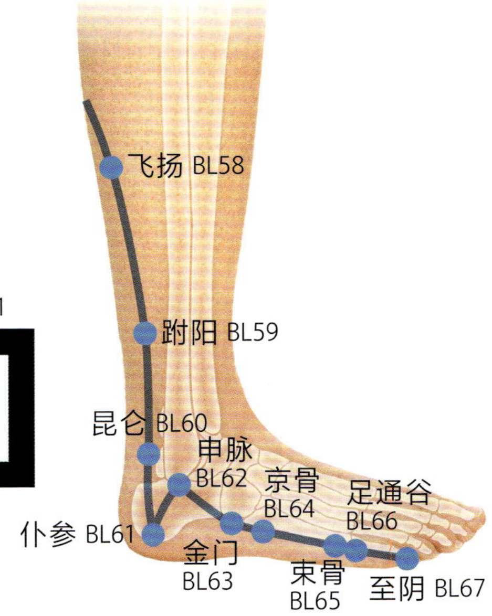

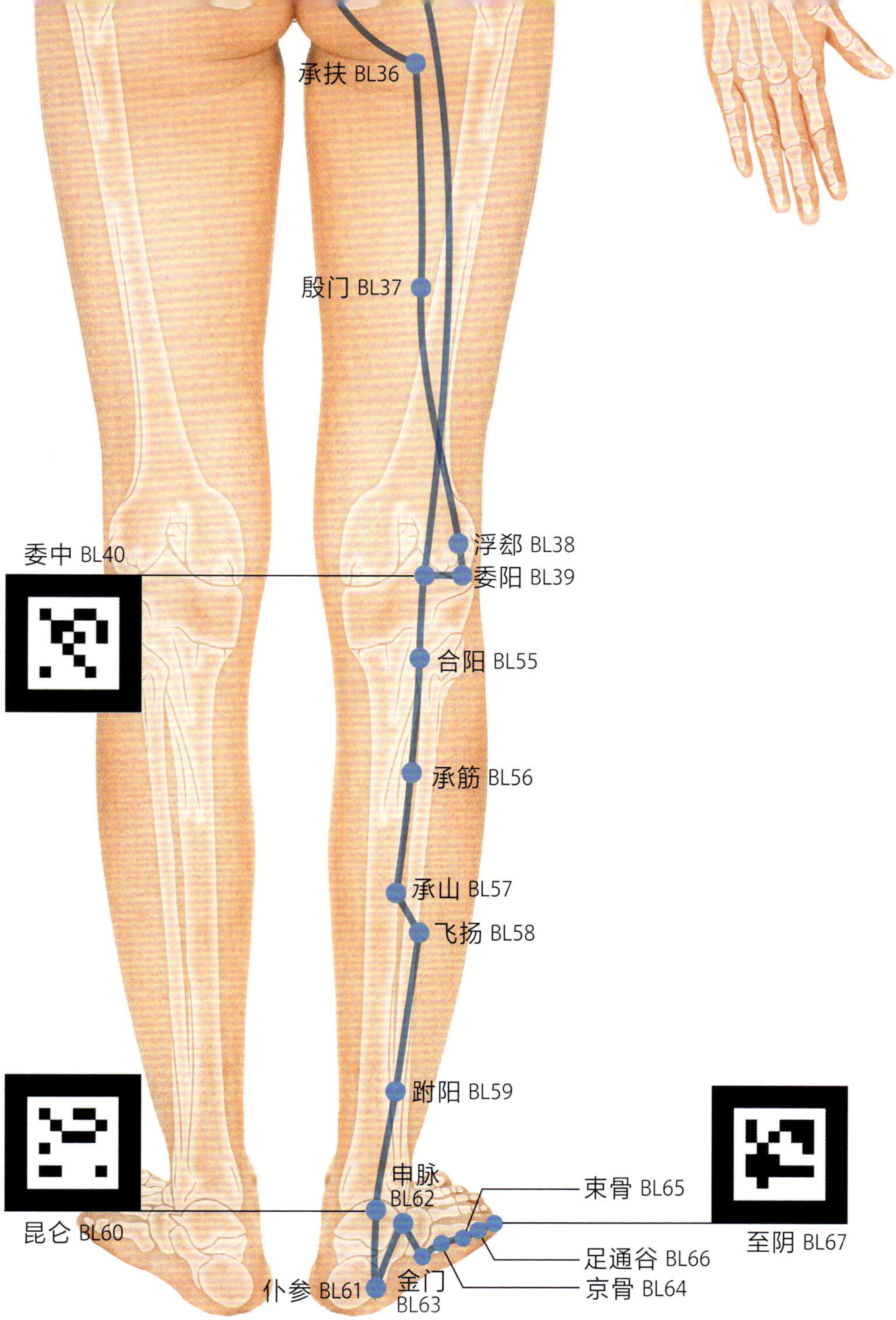

Bladder Meridian of Foot-Taiyang, BL.

Bladder Meridian of Foot-Taiyang emerges from Jingming (BL1) in medial side of eyes, runs through the top of the head and terminates at Zhiyin (BL67) in lateral side of the little toe of the foot.

Bladder Meridian mainly treats diseases of respiratory system including cold and infection of upper respiratory; diseases of nervous system including insomnia and manic and depressive psychosis; diseases of running courses of meridian including tearing induced by the wind, headache, cervical spondylopathy, lumbago and back pain, knee arthritis, hemorrhoids and prolapse of the rectum.

BL	Acupoints	Indications
★ 1	Jīngmíng	Redness, swelling and pain of eye; tearing; blurry vision; dizziness; myopia; nyctalopia; color blindness; acute sprain of lower back ; sciatica; tachycardia
2	Cuánzhú	Headache; supraorbital bone pain; eyelid twitching; blepharoptosis; deviation of mouth and eye; blurry vision; tearing; redness, swelling and pain of eye; hiccup
3	Méichōng	Headache; dizziness; nasal obstruction; nose bleeding
4	Qūchā	Headache; dizziness; nasal obstruction; nose bleeding

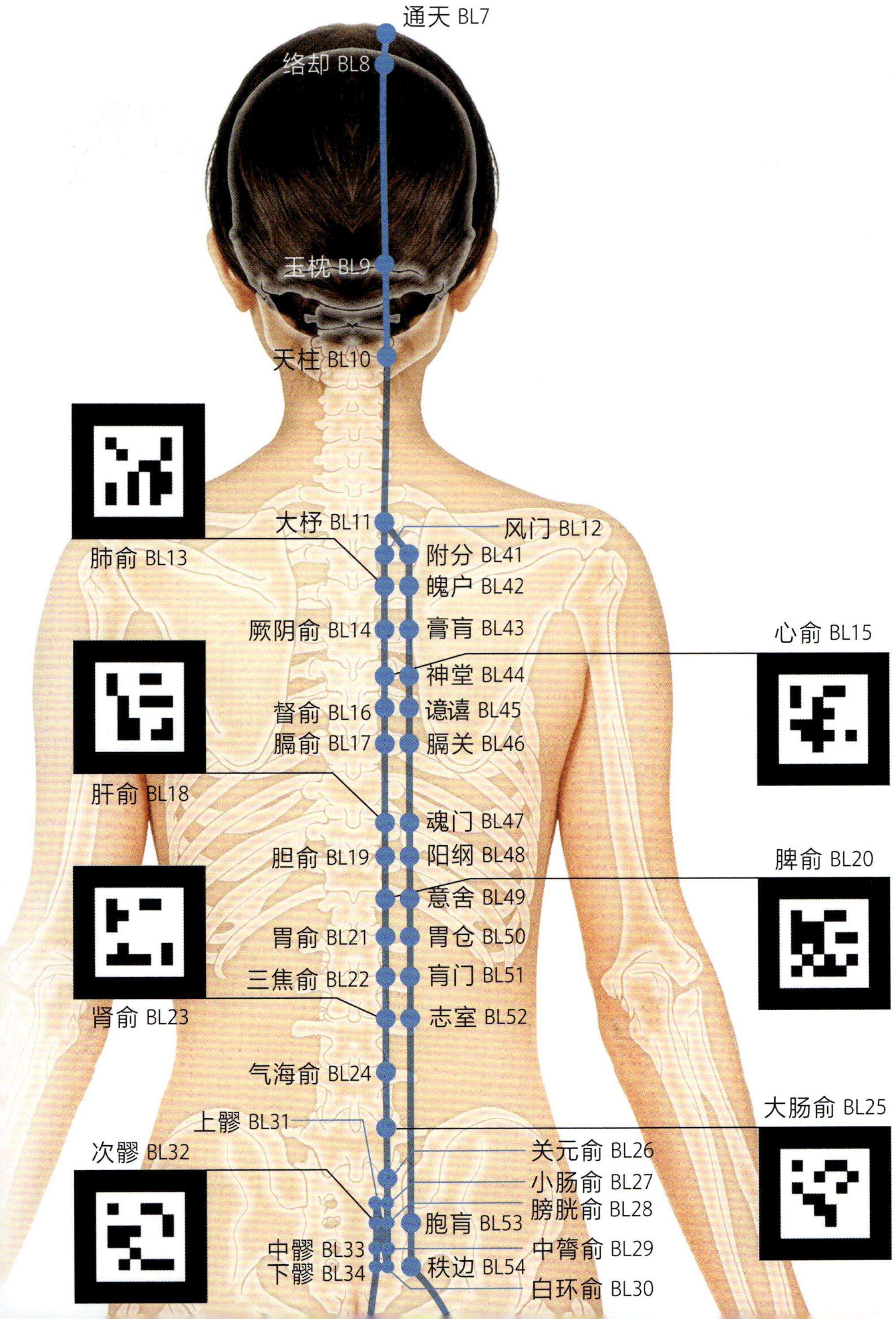

续表

BL	穴名	主治
5	五处	头痛、目眩、癫痫
6	承光	头痛、目眩、鼻塞、热病
7	通天	头痛、眩晕、鼻塞、鼻出血、鼻窦炎
8	络却	头晕、目视不明、耳鸣
9	玉枕	头项痛、目痛、鼻塞
10	天柱	后头痛、项强、肩背腰痛、鼻塞、癫狂、热病
11	大杼	咳嗽、发热、头痛、肩背痛、颈项拘急
12	风门	感冒、咳嗽、发热、头痛、项强、胸背痛
★ 13	肺俞	咳嗽、气喘、咯血、骨蒸潮热、盗汗
14	厥阴俞	心痛、心悸、咳嗽、胸闷、呕吐
★ 15	心俞	心痛、惊悸、失眠、健忘、癫狂、咳嗽、吐血、盗汗、遗精

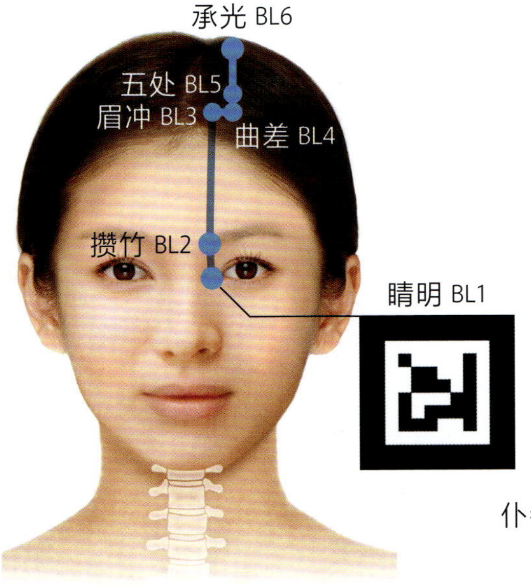

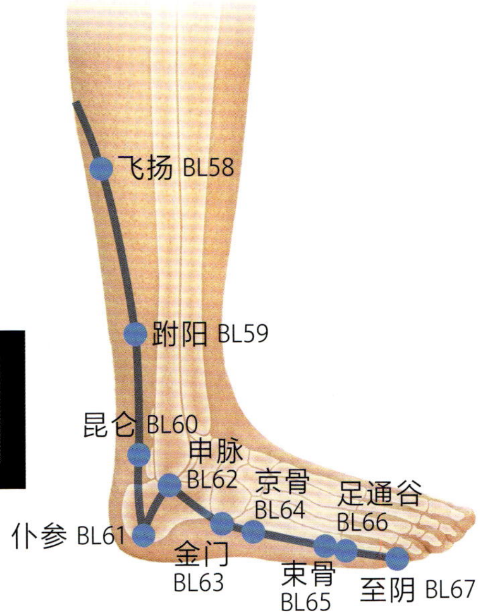

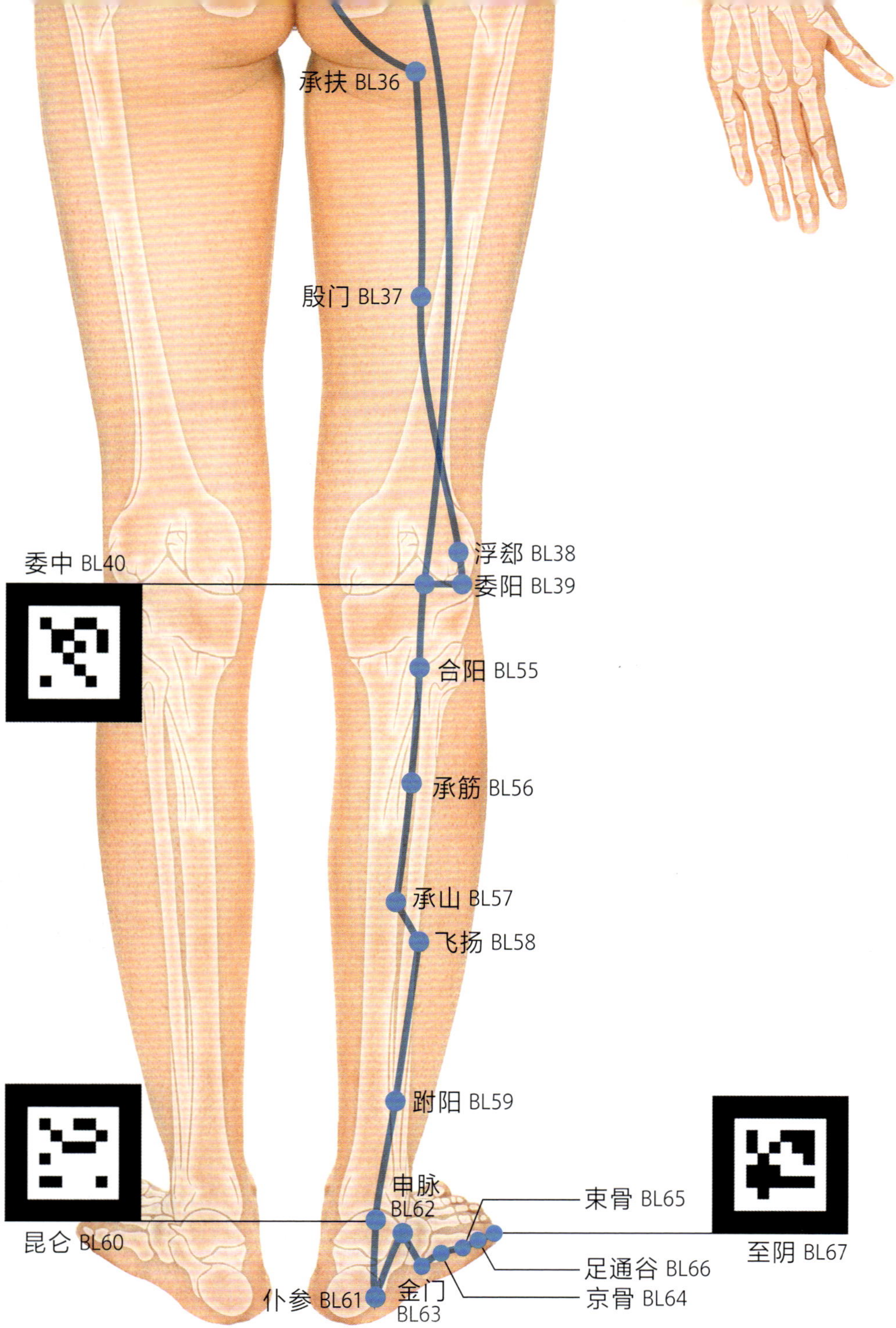

Continued

BL	Acupoints	Indications
5	Wǔchù	Headache; dizziness; epilepsy
6	Chéngguāng	Headache; dizziness; nasal obstruction; febrile diseases
7	Tōngtiān	Headache; dizziness; nasal obstruction; nose bleeding; sinusitis
8	Luòquè	Dizziness; blurry vision; tinnitus
9	Yùzhěn	Head and neck pain; eyes pain; nasal obstruction
10	Tiānzhù	Occipital headache; neck stiffness; shoulder, back and lower back pain; nasal obstruction; manic and depressive psychosis; febrile diseases
11	Dàzhù	Cough; fever; headache; shoulder and back pain; spastic neck
12	Fēngmén	Cold; cough; fever; headache; neck stiffness; chest and back pain
★ 13	Fèishū	Cough; asthma; hematemesis; tidal fever and steaming bone ; night sweat
14	Juéyīnshū	Cardiac pain; palpitation; cough; chest congestion; vomiting
★ 15	Xīnshū	Cardiac pain; palpitation due to fright; insomnia; amnesia; manic and depressive psychosis; cough; night sweat; seminal emission

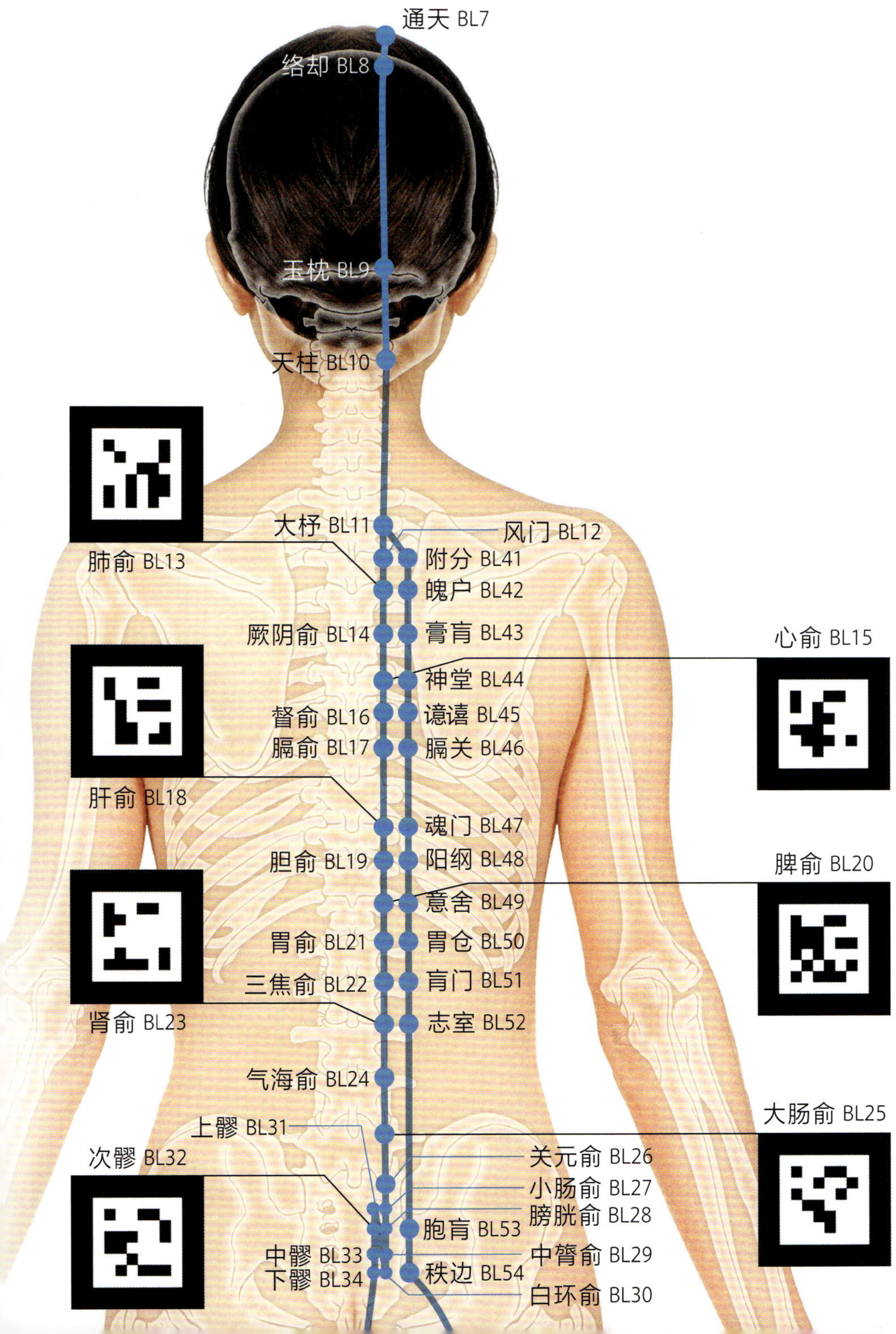

续表

BL	穴名	主治
16	督俞	心痛、胸闷、气喘、腹胀、腹痛、肠鸣、呃逆
17	膈俞	呕吐、呃逆、气喘、吐血、贫血、荨麻疹、皮肤瘙痒、潮热、盗汗
★ 18	肝俞	胁痛、黄疸、目赤、目视不明、夜盲、迎风流泪、癫狂、脊背痛
19	胆俞	黄疸、口苦、胁痛、肺结核、潮热
★ 20	脾俞	腹胀、纳呆、呕吐、腹泻、痢疾、便血、水肿、背痛
21	胃俞	胃脘痛、呕吐、腹胀、肠鸣
22	三焦俞	肠鸣、腹胀、呕吐、腹泻、痢疾、小便不利、水肿、腰背强痛
★ 23	肾俞	头晕、耳鸣、耳聋、腰酸痛、遗尿、遗精、阳痿、早泄、不育、月经不调、带下

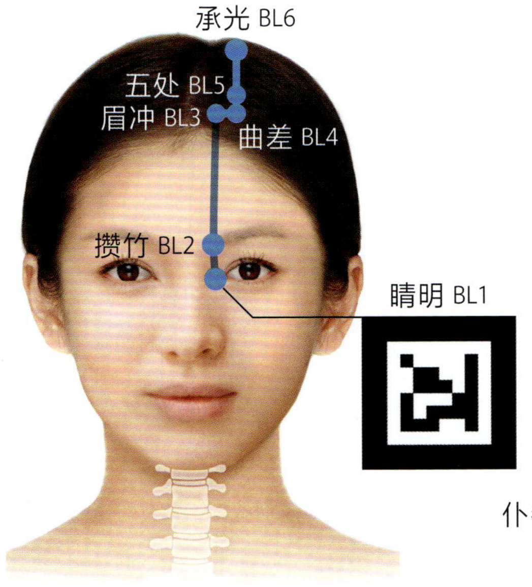

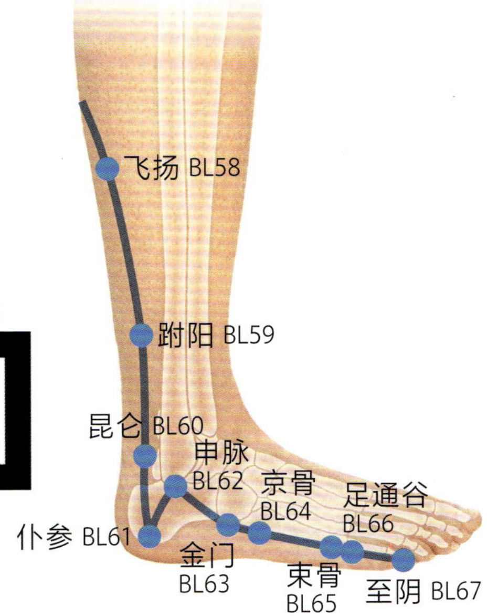

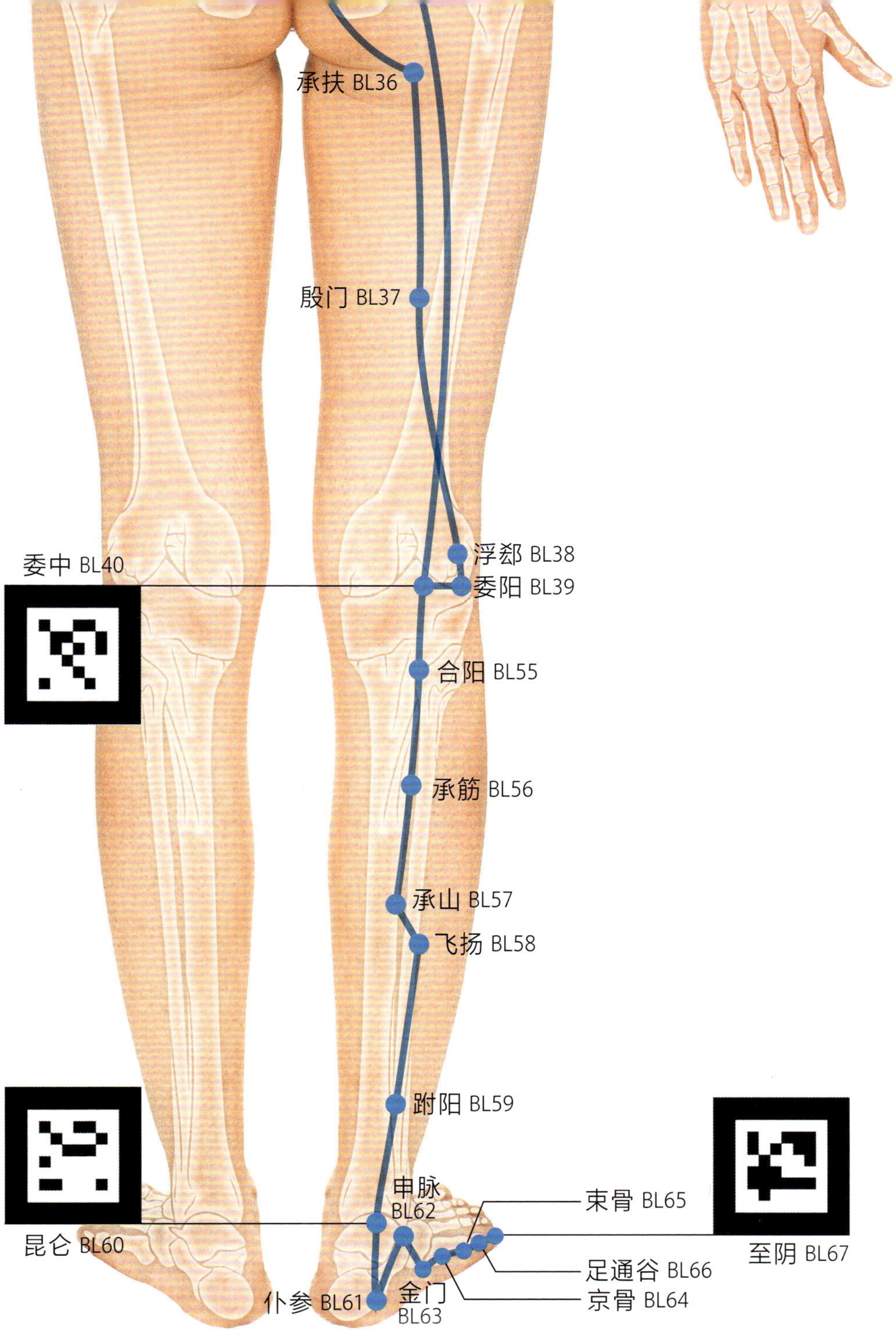

Continued

BL	Acupoints	Indications
16	Dūshū	Cardiac pain; chest congestion; asthma; distention of abdomen; abdominal pain; borborygmus; hiccup
17	Géshū	Vomiting; hiccup; asthma; hematemesis; anemia; measles; itchy skin; tidal fever; night sweat
★ 18	Gānshū	Hypochondrium pain; jaundice; red eyes; blurry vision; nyctalopia; tearing induced by the wind; manic and depressive psychosis; spine and back pain
19	Dǎnshū	Jaundice; bitter taste in mouth; hypochondrium pain; pulmonary tuberculosis; tidal fever
★ 20	Píshū	Distention of abdomen; loss of appetite; vomiting; diarrhea; dysentery; bloody stool; edema; back pain
21	Wèishū	Epigastric pain; vomiting; distention of abdomen; borborygmus
22	Sānjiāoshū	Borborygmus; distention of abdomen; vomiting; diarrhea; dysentery; dysuria; edema; stiffness and pain of lower back and back
★ 23	Shènshū	Dizziness; tinnitus; deafness; lower back soreness; enuresis; seminal emission; impotence; premature ejaculation; infertility; irregular menstruation; leukorrheal diseases

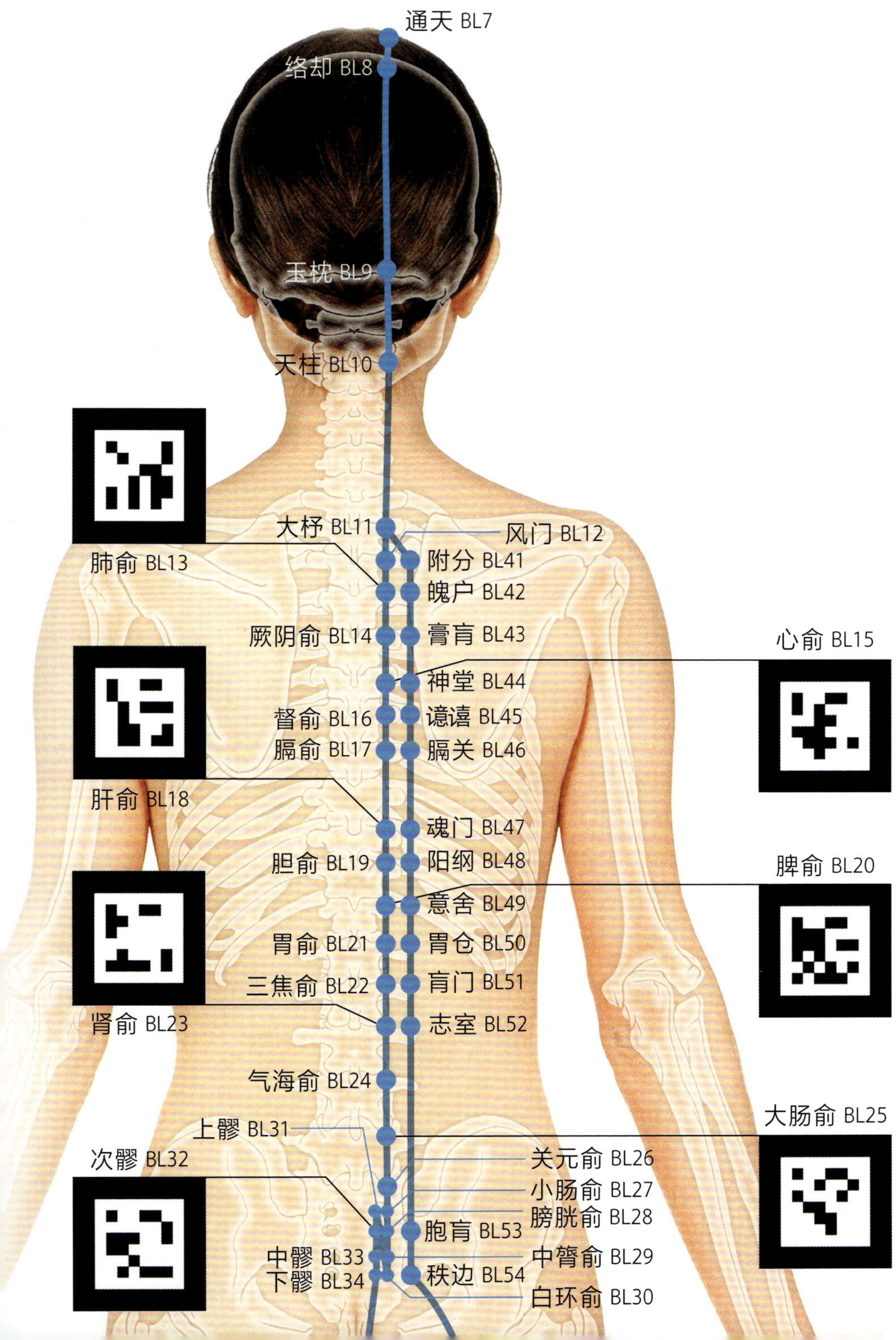

续表

BL	穴名	主治
24	气海俞	肠鸣腹胀、痛经、腰痛
★ 25	大肠俞	腰腿痛、腹胀、腹泻、便秘
26	关元俞	腹胀、腹泻、腰骶痛、小便频数、小便不利、遗尿
27	小肠俞	遗精、遗尿、尿血、尿痛、带下、腹泻、痢疾、疝气、腰骶痛
28	膀胱俞	小便不利、遗尿、腰骶痛、腹泻、便秘
29	中膂俞	腹泻、疝气、腰骶痛
30	白环俞	遗尿、遗精、月经不调、带下、疝气、腰骶痛
31	上髎	大小便不利、月经不调、带下、子宫或阴道脱垂、遗精、阳痿、腰骶痛
★ 32	次髎	月经不调、痛经、带下、小便不利、遗精、疝气、腰骶痛、下肢痿痹

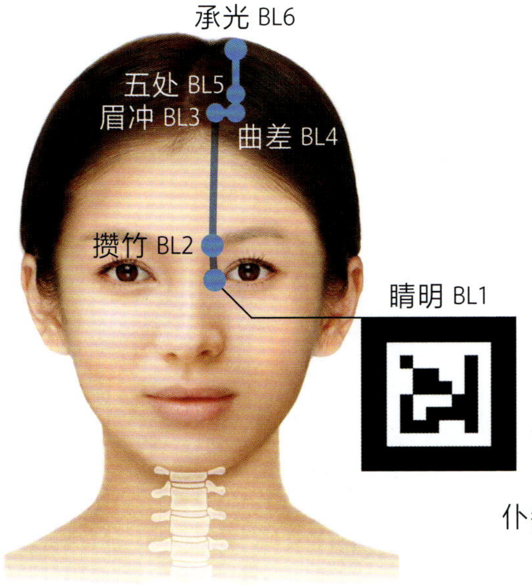

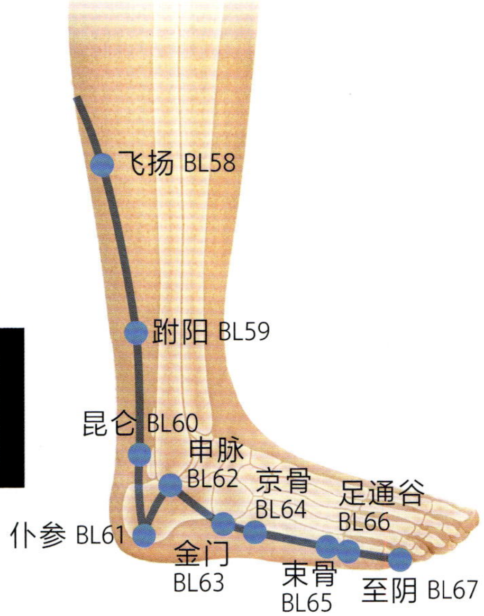

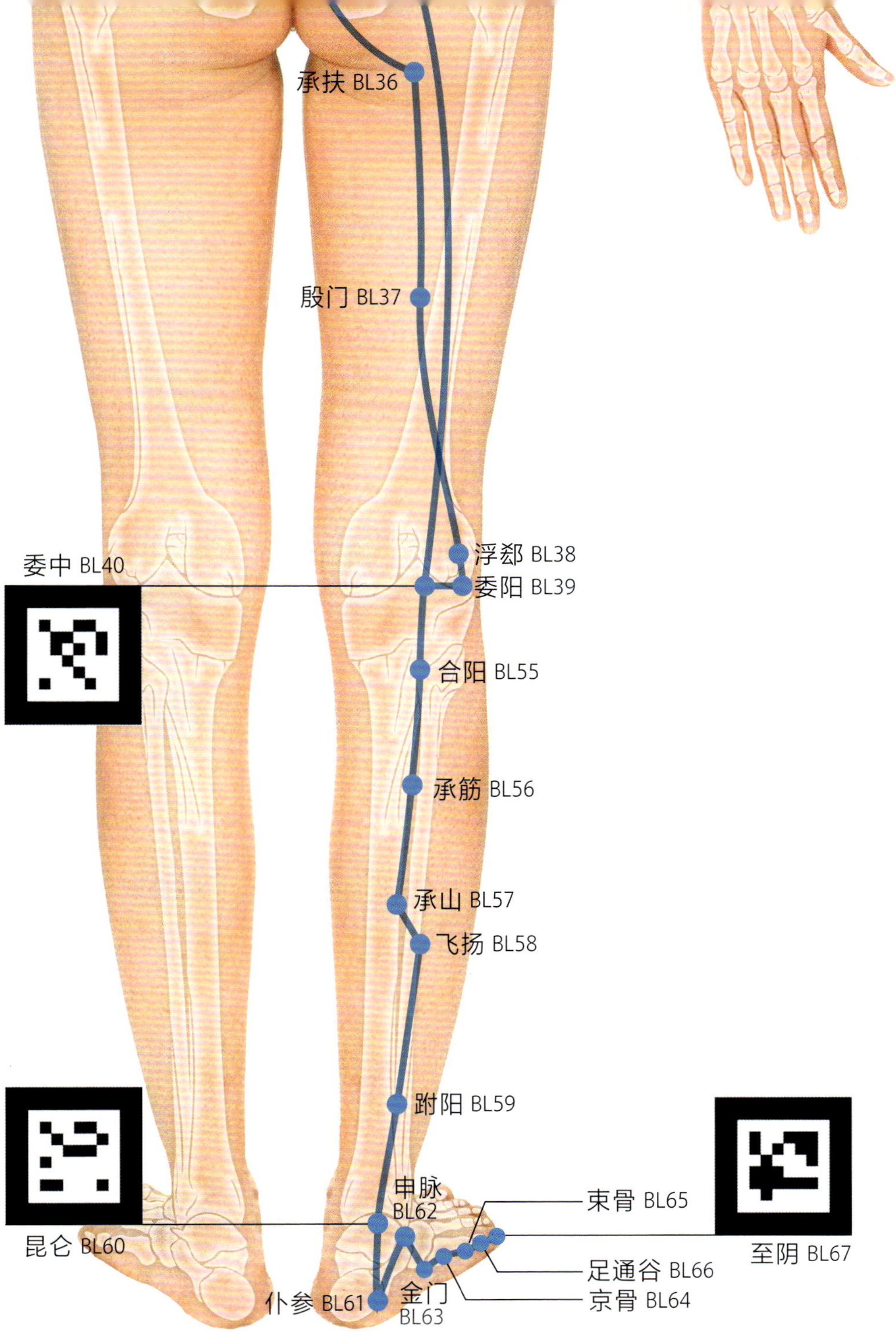

Continued

BL	Acupoints	Indications
24	Qìhǎishū	Borborygmus and distention of abdomen; dysmenorrhea; lower back pain
★ 25	Dàchángshū	Lower back and leg pain; distention of abdomen; diarrhea; constipation
26	Guānyuánshū	Distention of abdomen; diarrhea; lumbosacral pain; frequent and urgent urination; dysuria; enuresis
27	Xiǎochángshū	Seminal emission; enuresis; hematuria; pain during urination; leukorrheal diseases; diarrhea; dysentery; hernia; lumbosacral pain
28	Pángguāngshū	Dysuria; enuresis; lumbosacral pain; diarrhea; constipation
29	Zhōnglǚshū	Diarrhea; hernia; lumbosacral pain
30	Báihuánshū	Enuresis; seminal emission; irregular menstruation; leukorrheal diseases; hernia; lumbosacral pain
31	Shàngliáo	Difficulty in urination and stool; irregular menstruation; leukorrheal diseases; uterus prolapse and vagina prolapse; seminal emission; impotence; lumbosacral pain
★ 32	Cìliáo	Irregular menstruation; dysmenorrhea; leukorrheal diseases; dysuria; seminal emission; hernia; lumbosacral pain; flaccidity and motor impairment of lower limbs

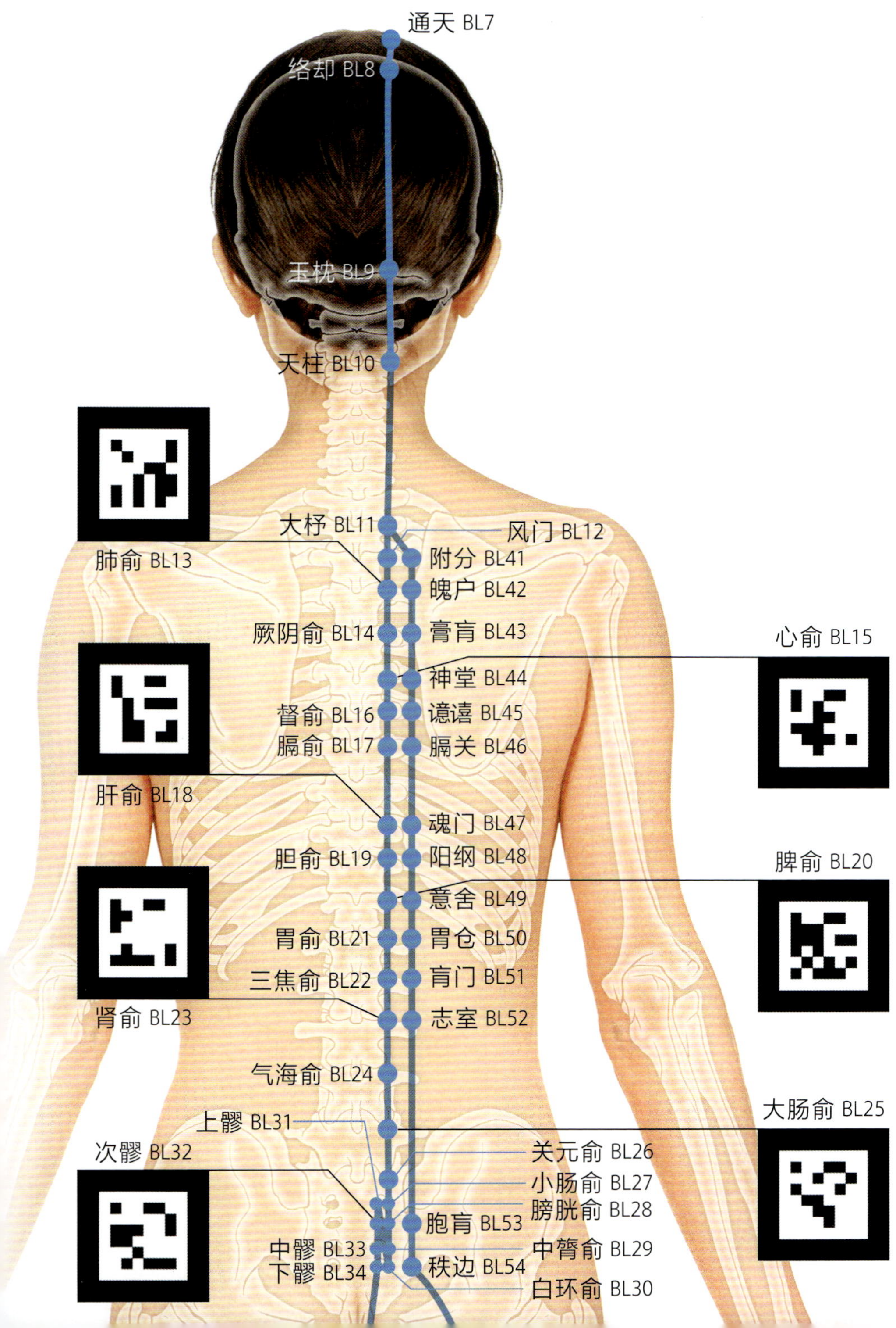

续表

BL	穴 名	主 治
33	中髎	便秘、腹泻、小便不利、月经不调、带下、腰骶痛
34	下髎	腹痛、便秘、小便不利、带下、腰骶痛
35	会阳	痔疮、腹泻、阳痿、带下
36	承扶	腰或骶疼痛、臀或大腿部疼痛、痔疮
37	殷门	腰痛、下肢痿痹
38	浮郄	膝部疼痛或麻木、便秘
39	委阳	腹满、小便不利、腰强痛、腿足挛痛
★ 40	委中	腰背痛、下肢痿痹、腹痛、急性吐泻、小便不利、遗尿、丹毒
41	附分	颈项强痛、肩周炎、背拘急、肘臂麻木
42	魄户	咳嗽、气喘、肺结核、项强、肩周炎、背痛

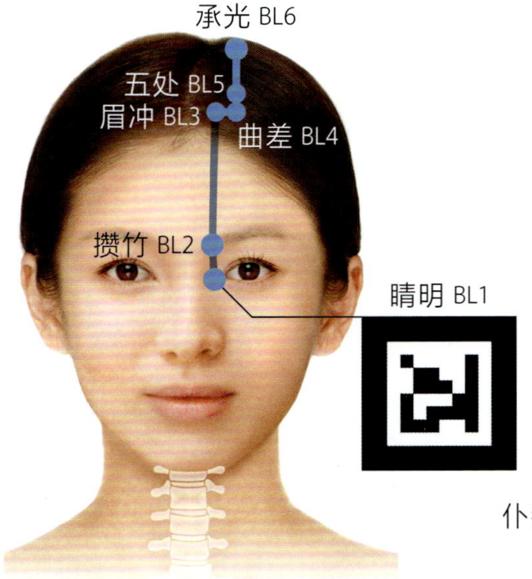

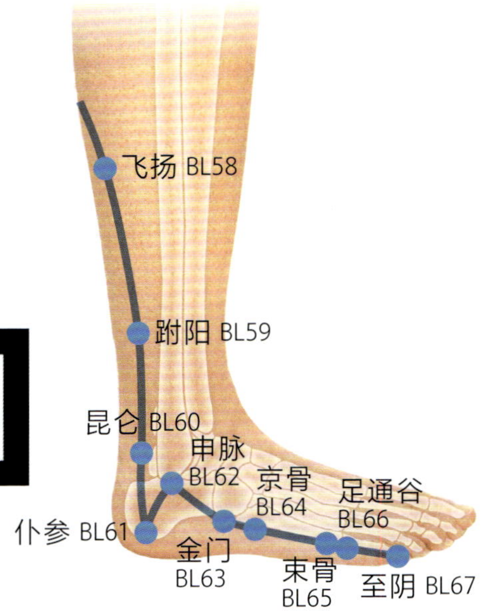

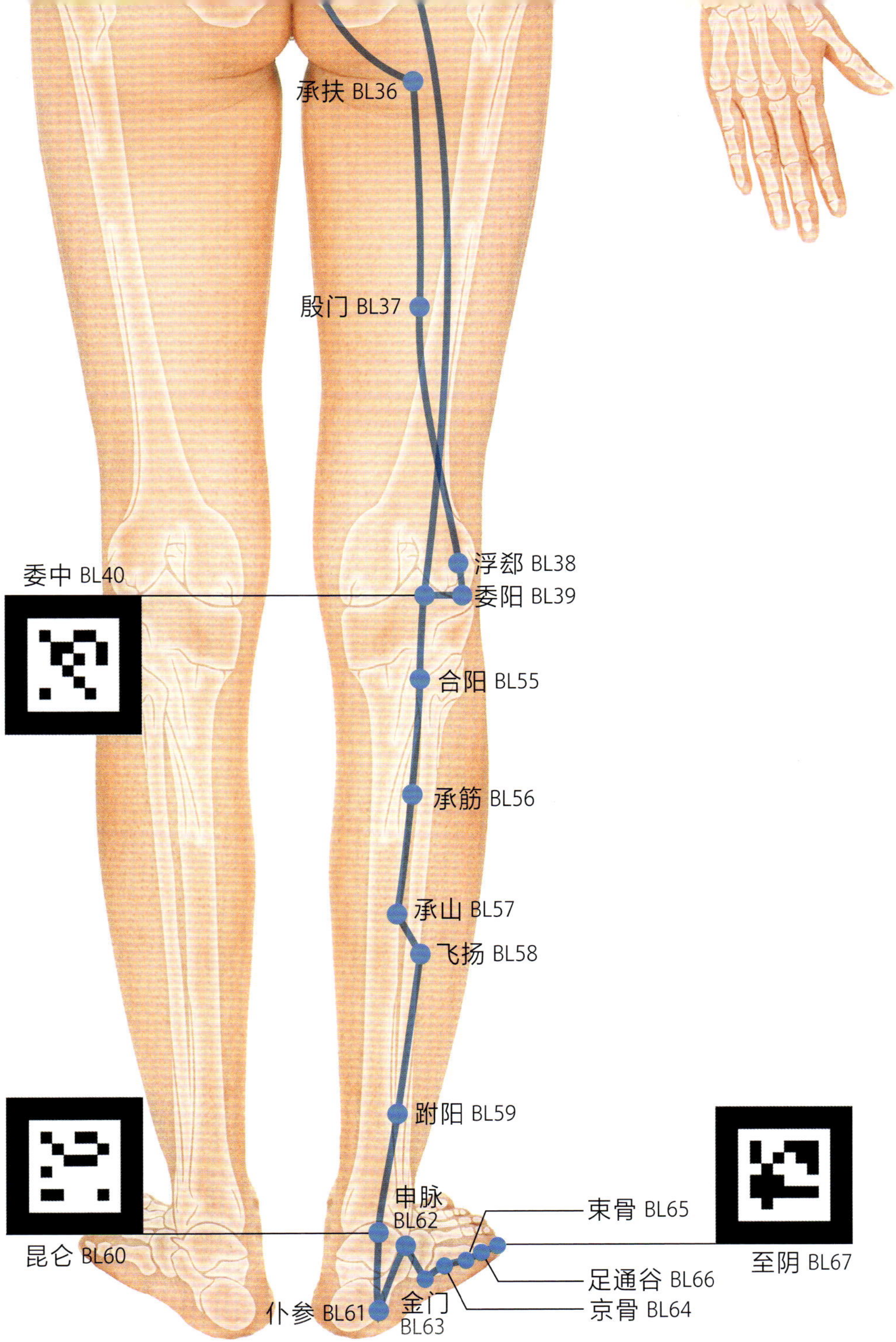

Continued

BL	Acupoints	Indications
33	Zhōngliáo	Constipation; diarrhea; dysuria; irregular menstruation; leukorrheal diseases; lumbosacral pain
34	Xiàliáo	Abdominal pain; constipation; dysuria; leukorrheal diseases; lumbosacral pain
35	Huìyáng	Hemorrhoids; diarrhea; impotence; leukorrheal diseases
36	Chéngfú	Pain in lower back, sacrum, buttocks and thigh; hemorrhoids
37	Yīnmén	Lower back pain; flaccidity and motor impairment of lower limbs
38	Fúxì	Knees pain; numb knees; constipation
39	Wěiyáng	Fullness in abdomen; dysuria; lower back stiffness and pain; spasm and pain of legs and foot
★ 40	Wěizhōng	Lumbago and back pain; flaccidity and motor impairment of lower limbs; abdominal pain; acute vomiting and diarrhea; dysuria; enuresis; erysipelas
41	Fùfēn	Neck stiffness and pain; shoulder periarthritis; spastic back; numb elbow and arm
42	Pòhù	Cough; asthma; pulmonary tuberculosis; neck stiffness; shoulder periarthritis; back pain

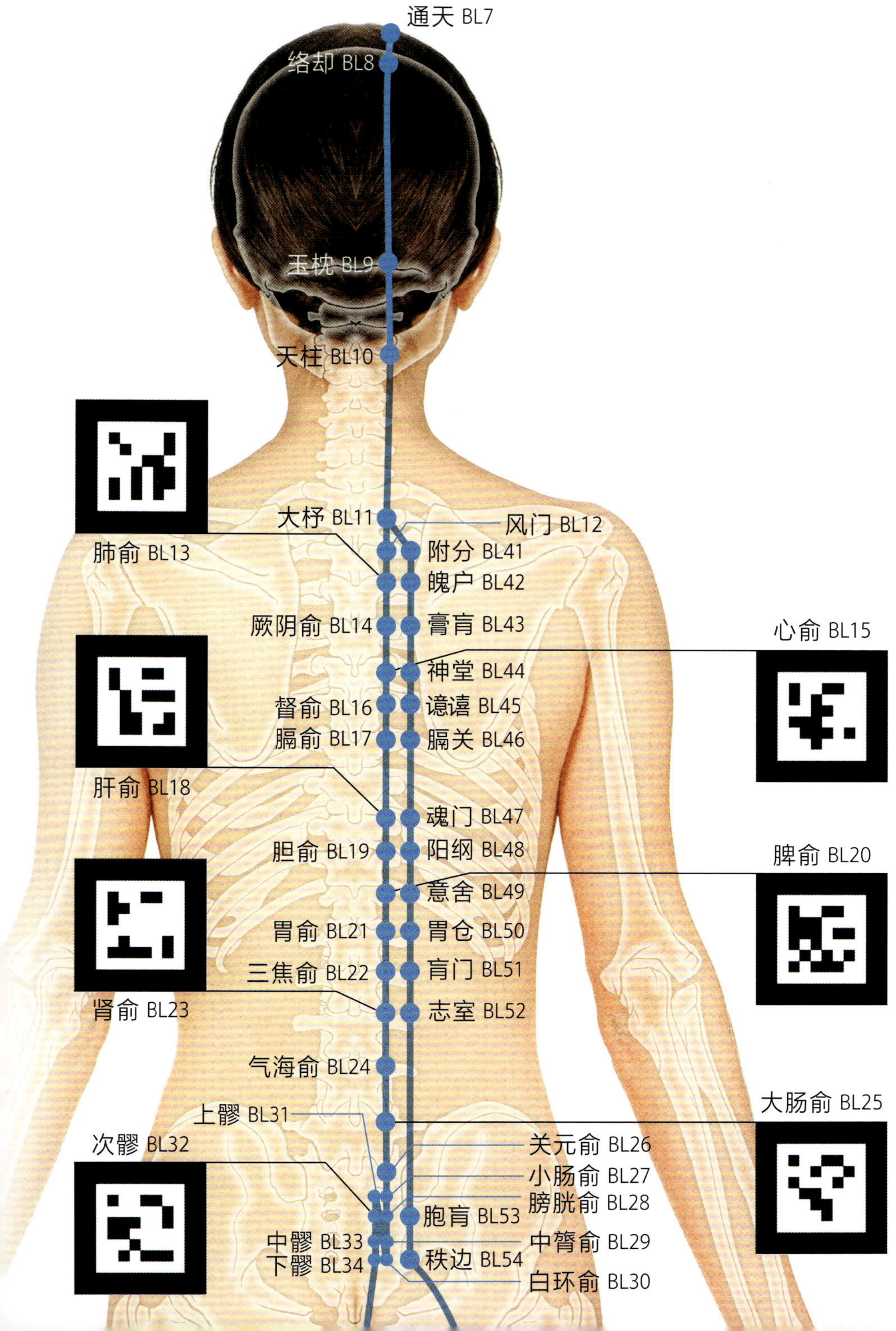

续表

BL	穴名	主治
43	膏肓	咳嗽、气喘、肺结核、肩胛痛、健忘、遗精、盗汗
44	神堂	咳嗽、气喘、胸闷、脊背强痛
45	譩譆	咳嗽、气喘、肩周炎、背痛、疟疾、热病
46	膈关	胸闷、嗳气、呕吐、脊背强痛
47	魂门	胸胁痛、背痛、呕吐、腹泻
48	阳纲	肠鸣、腹痛、腹泻、黄疸、1 型糖尿病
49	意舍	腹胀、肠鸣、呕吐、腹泻
50	胃仓	胃脘痛、腹胀、小儿食积、水肿、背脊痛
51	肓门	腹痛、痞块、便秘、乳房肿痛、乳腺疾病
52	志室	遗精、阳痿、小便不利、水肿、腰背强痛

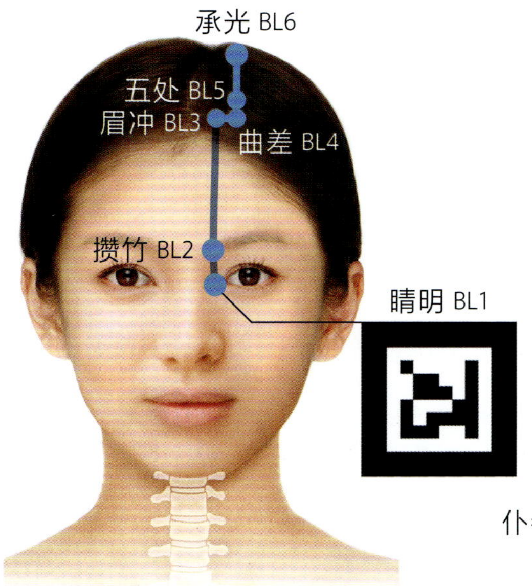

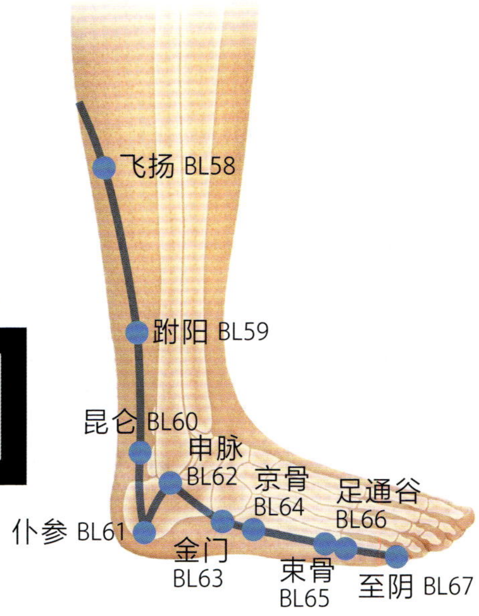

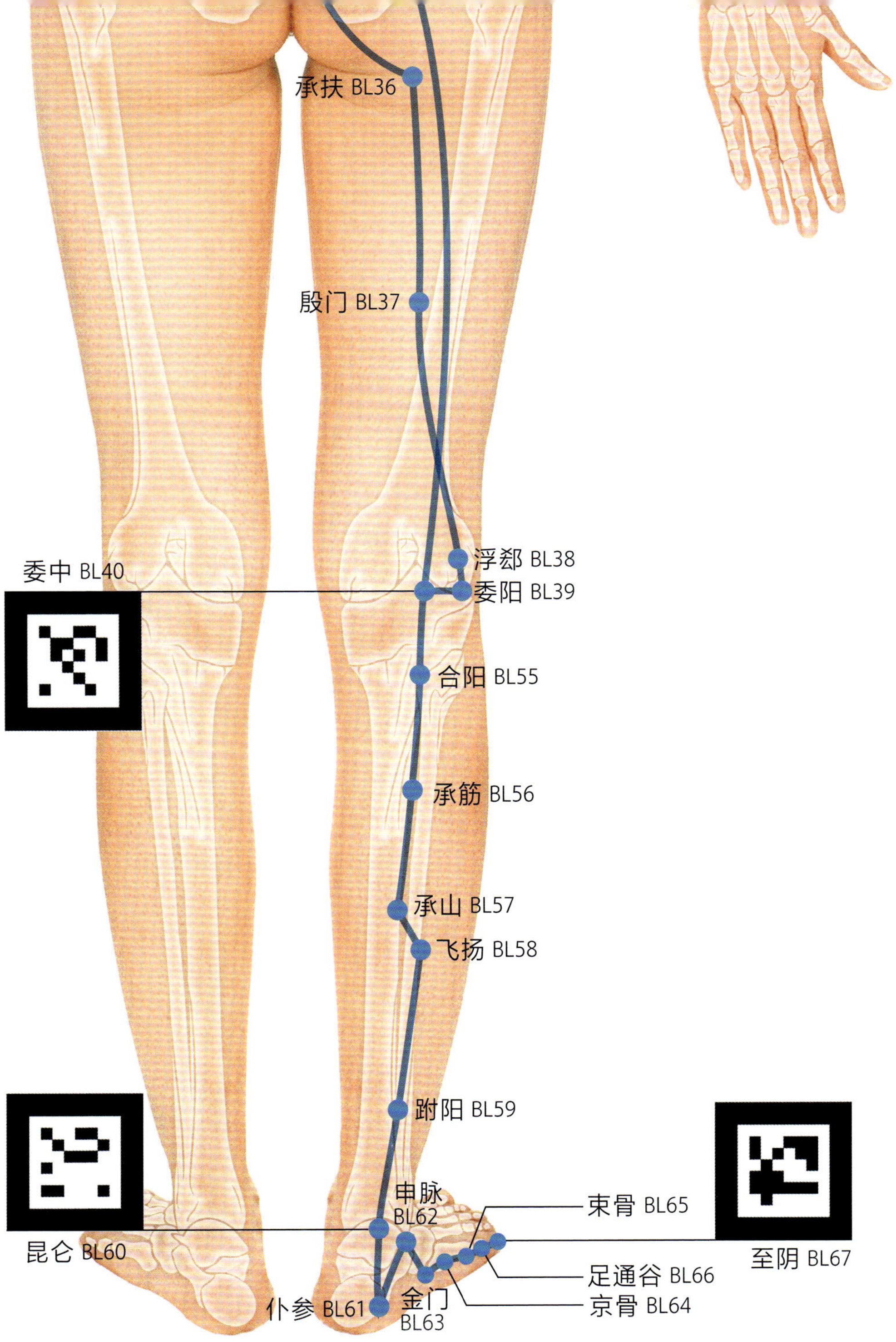

Continued

BL	Acupoints	Indications
43	Gāohuāng	Cough; asthma; pulmonary tuberculosis; scapular pain; amnesia; seminal emission; night sweat
44	Shéntáng	Cough; asthma; chest congestion; spine and back stiffness and pain
45	Yìxǐ	Cough; asthma; shoulder periarthritis; back pain; malaria; febrile diseases
46	Géguān	Chest congestion; belching; vomiting; spine and back stiffness and pain
47	Húnmén	Chest and hypochondrium pain; back pain; vomiting; diarrhea
48	Yánggāng	Borborygmus; abdominal pain; diarrhea; jaundice; diabetes mellitus type 1
49	Yìshè	Distention of abdomen; borborygmus; vomiting; diarrhea
50	Wèicāng	Epigastric pain; distention of abdomen; infantile indigestion with food retention; edema; back and spine pain
51	Huāngmén	Abdominal pain; abdominal mass; constipation; swelling and pain of breast; breast diseases
52	Zhìshì	Seminal emission; impotence; dysuria; edema; stiffness and pain of lower back and back

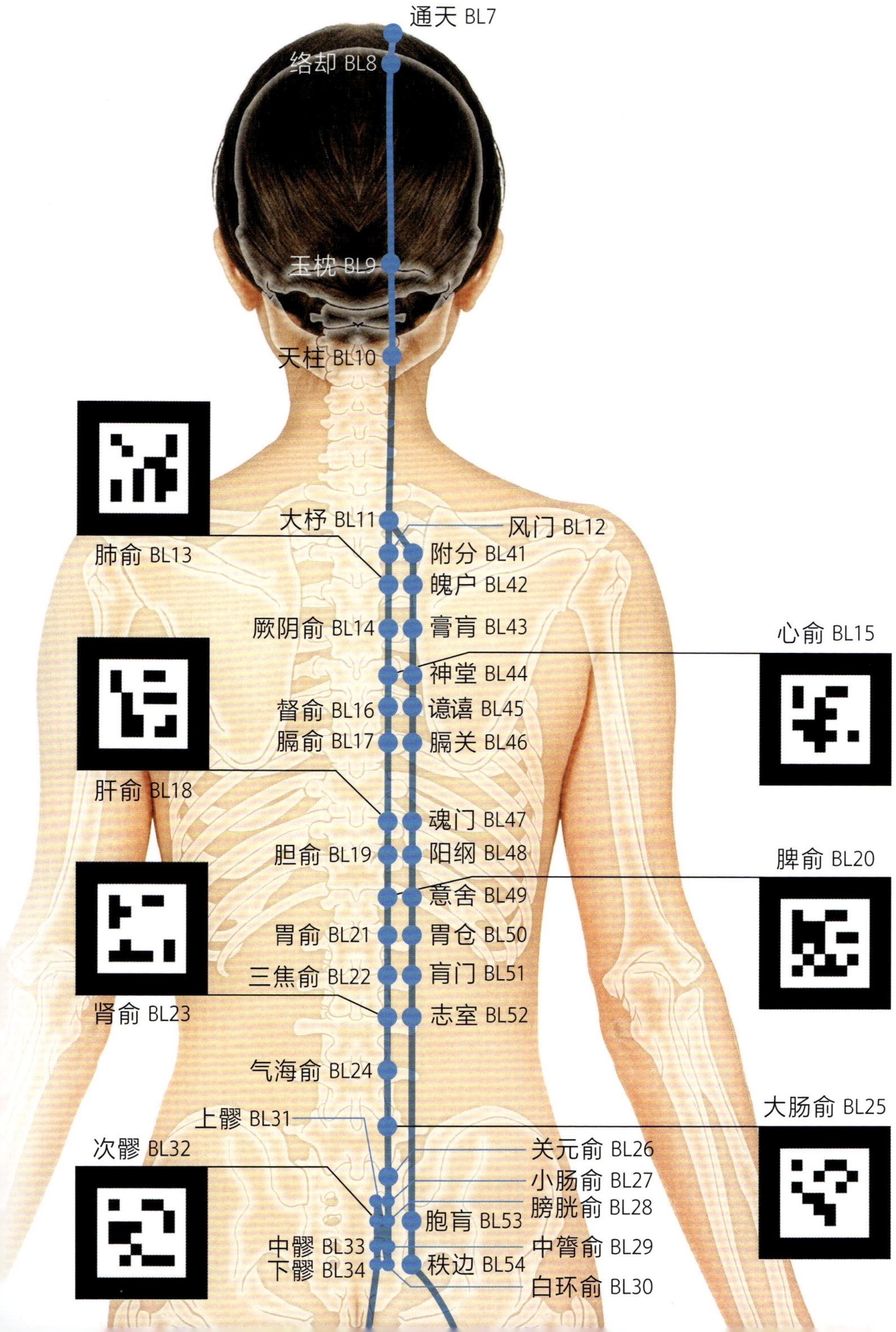

续表

BL	穴名	主治
53	胞肓	肠鸣、腹胀、便秘、癃闭、腰背强痛
54	秩边	腰骶痛、下肢痿痹、小便不利、便秘、痔疮、阴痛
55	合阳	腰背强痛、下肢痿痹、疝气、崩漏
56	承筋	小腿痛、肌肉痉挛、腰背拘急、痔疮
57	承山	腰背痛、小腿肌肉痉挛、痔疮、便秘
58	飞扬	头痛、目眩、鼻塞、鼻出血、腰背痛、腿软无力、痔疮
59	跗阳	腰骶痛、外踝肿痛、头痛
★ 60	昆仑	后头痛、项强、腰骶疼痛、足踝肿痛、癫狂、滞产

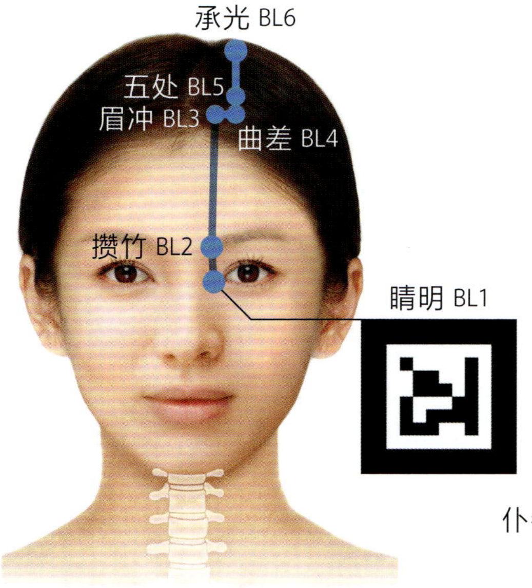

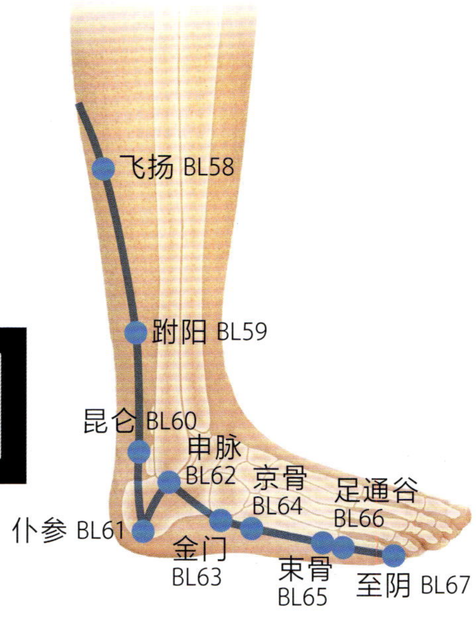

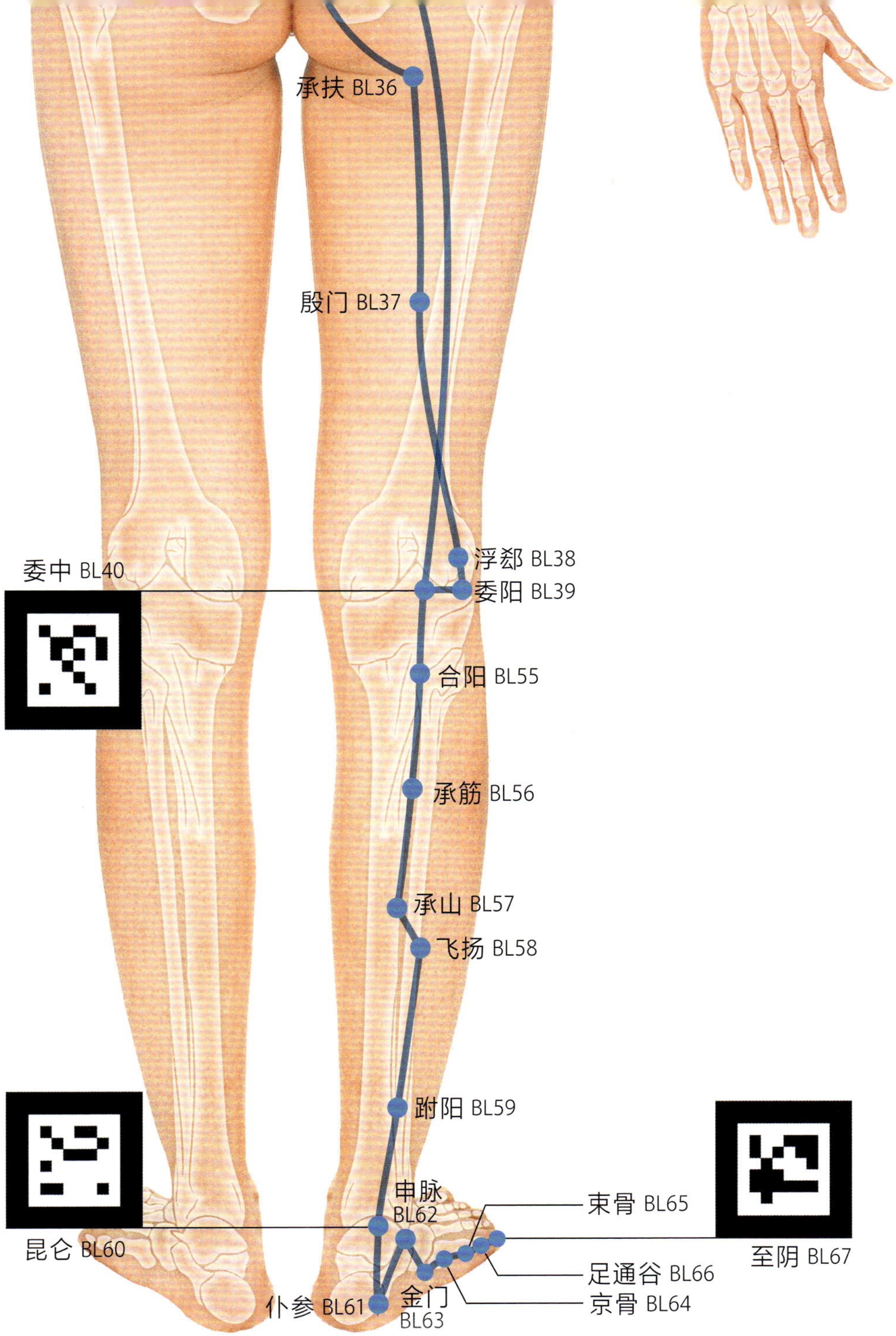

Continued

BL	Acupoints	Indications
53	Bāohuāng	Borborygmus; distention of abdomen; constipation; retention of urine; stiffness and pain of lower back and back
54	Zhìbiān	lumbosacral pain; flaccidity and motor impairment of lower limbs; dysuria; constipation; hemorrhoids; genitalia pain
55	Héyáng	Stiffness and pain in lower back and back; flaccidity and motor impairment of lower limbs; hernia; metrorrhagia and metrostaxis
56	Chéngjīn	Lower leg pain; spasm of muscles; spasm of lower back and back; hemorrhoids
57	Chéngshān	Lumbago and back pain; spasm of muscles in lower leg; hemorrhoids; constipation
58	Fēiyáng	Headache; dizziness; nasal obstruction; nose bleeding; lumbago and back pain; softness and flaccidity of legs; hemorrhoids
59	Fūyáng	lumbosacral pain; swelling and pain in lateral malleolus; headache
★ 60	Kūnlún	Occipital headache; neck stiffness; lumbosacral pain; swelling and pain in malleolus; manic and depressive psychosis; prolonged delivery

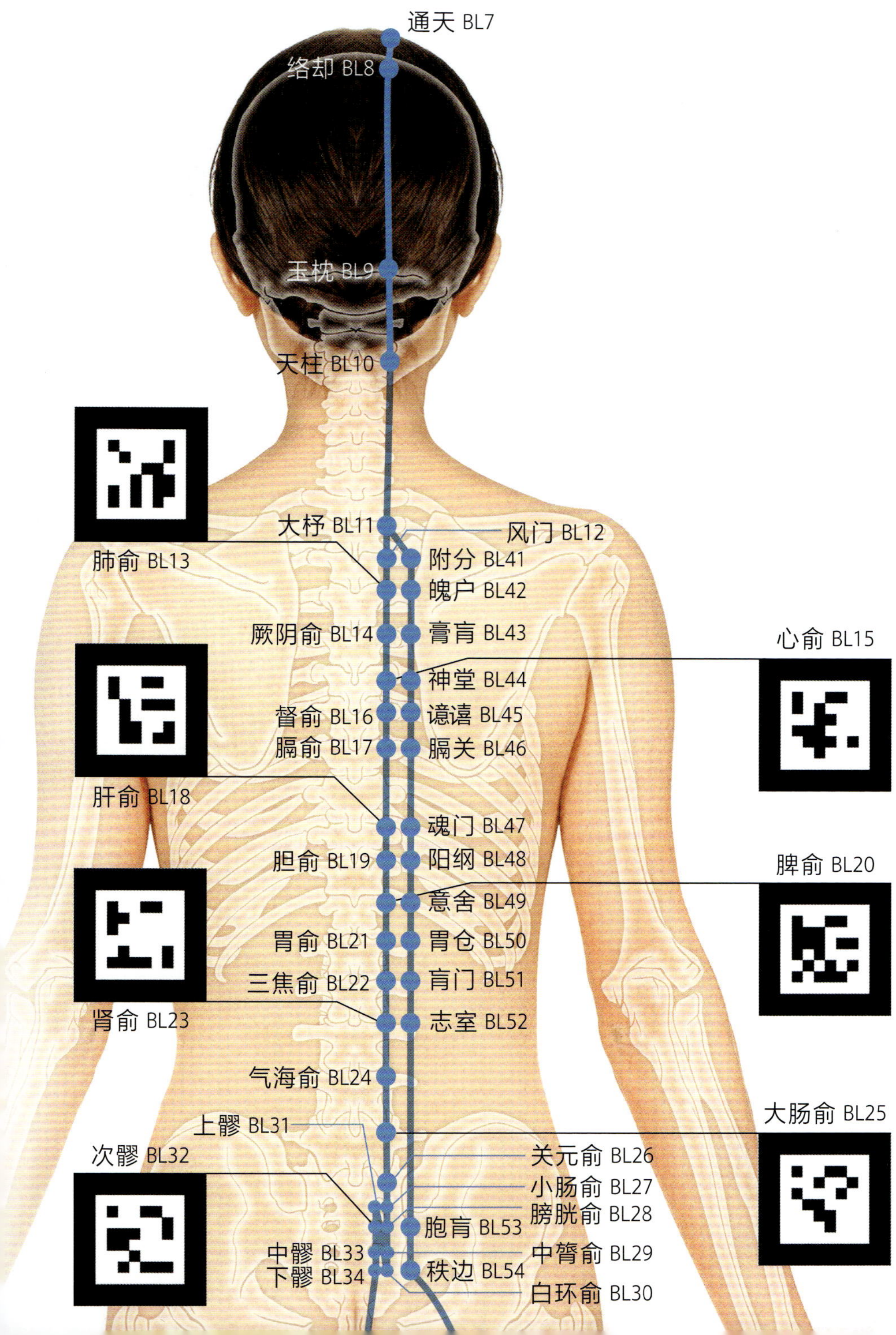

续表

BL	穴名	主治
61	仆参	下肢痿痹、足跟痛、癫狂
62	申脉	头痛、眩晕、癫狂、失眠、腰腿酸痛
63	金门	头痛、腰痛、下肢痿痹、外踝痛、痹证、癫狂、小儿惊风
64	京骨	头痛、项强、腰腿痛、癫狂
65	束骨	头痛、项强、目眩、腰腿痛、癫狂
66	足通谷	头痛、项强、鼻出血、癫狂
★ 67	至阴	胎位不正、滞产、头痛、目痛、鼻塞、鼻出血

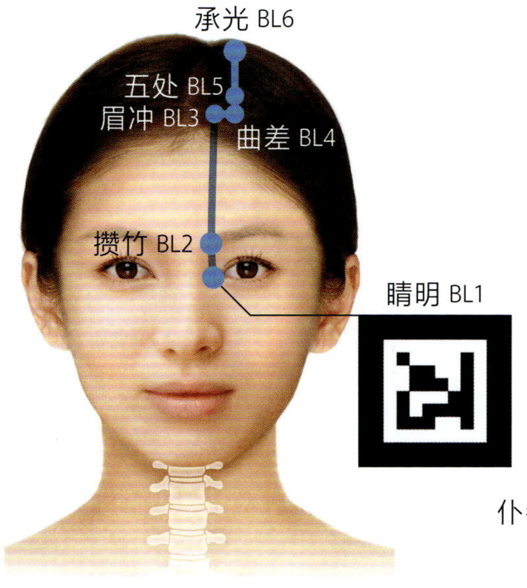

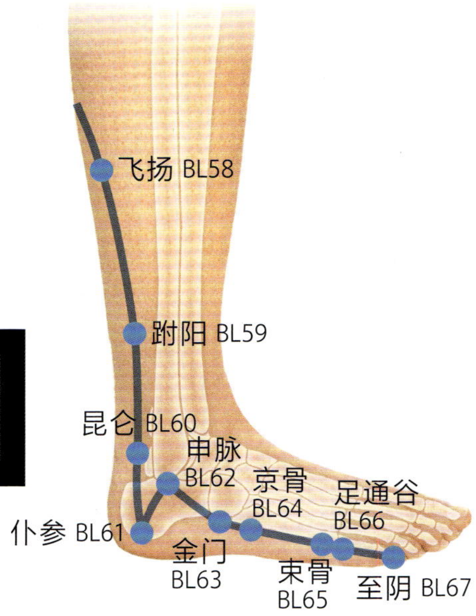

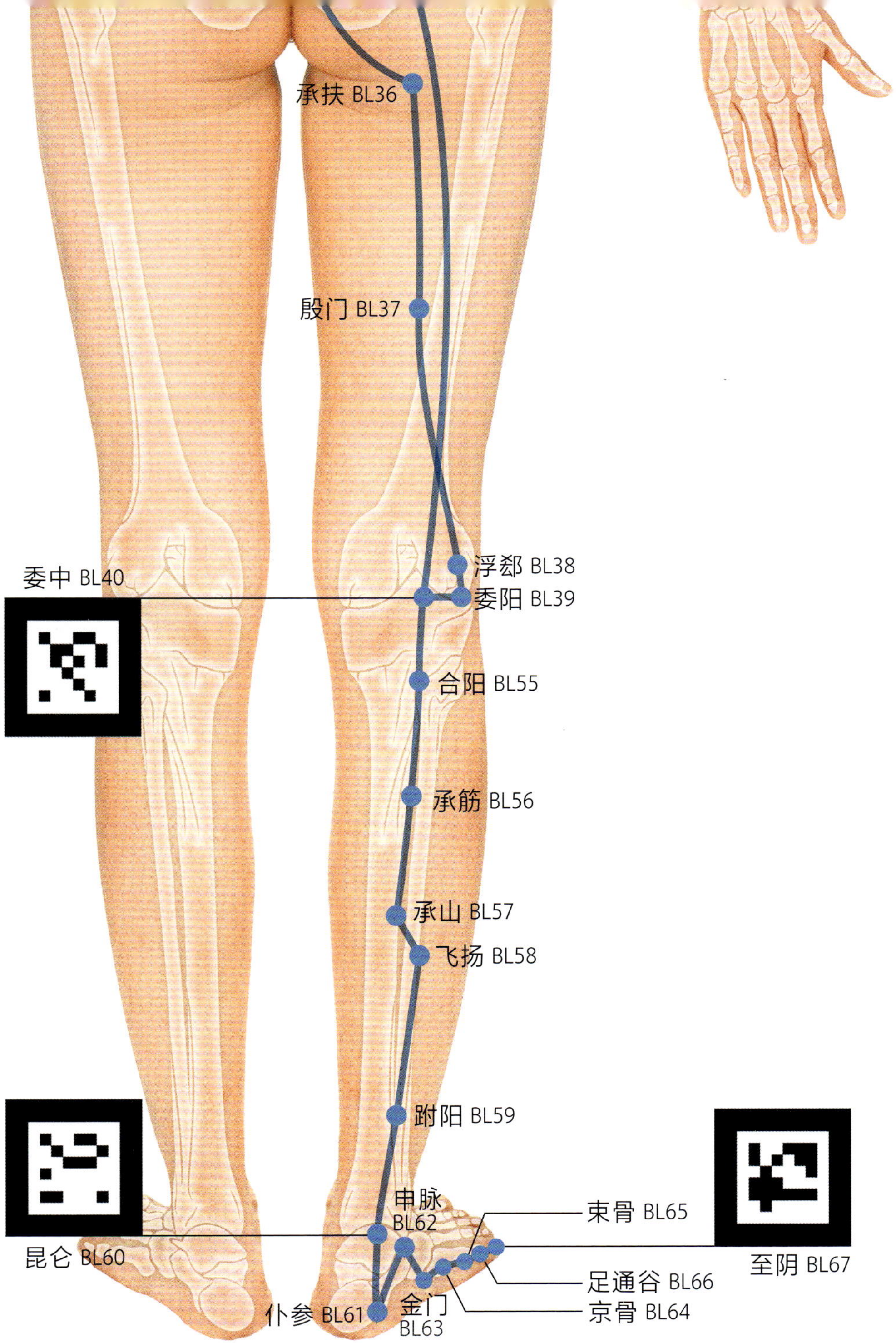

Continued

BL	Acupoints	Indications
61	Púcān	Flaccidity and motor impairment of lower limbs; heel pain; manic and depressive psychosis
62	Shēnmài	Headache; dizziness; manic and depressive psychosis; insomnia; soreness in lower back and leg
63	Jīnmén	Headache; lower back pain; flaccidity and motor impairment of lower limbs; lateral malleolus pain; Bi syndrome (sourness, pain and spasm of knees or muscles); manic and depressive psychosis; infantile convulsion
64	Jīnggǔ	Headache; neck stiffness; lower back and leg pain; manic and depressive psychosis
65	Shùgǔ	Headache; neck stiffness; dizziness; lower back and leg pain; manic and depressive psychosis
66	Zútōnggǔ	Headache; neck stiffness; nose bleeding; manic and depressive psychosis
★ 67	Zhìyīn	Malposition of fetus; prolonged delivery; headache; eyes pain; nasal obstruction; nose bleeding

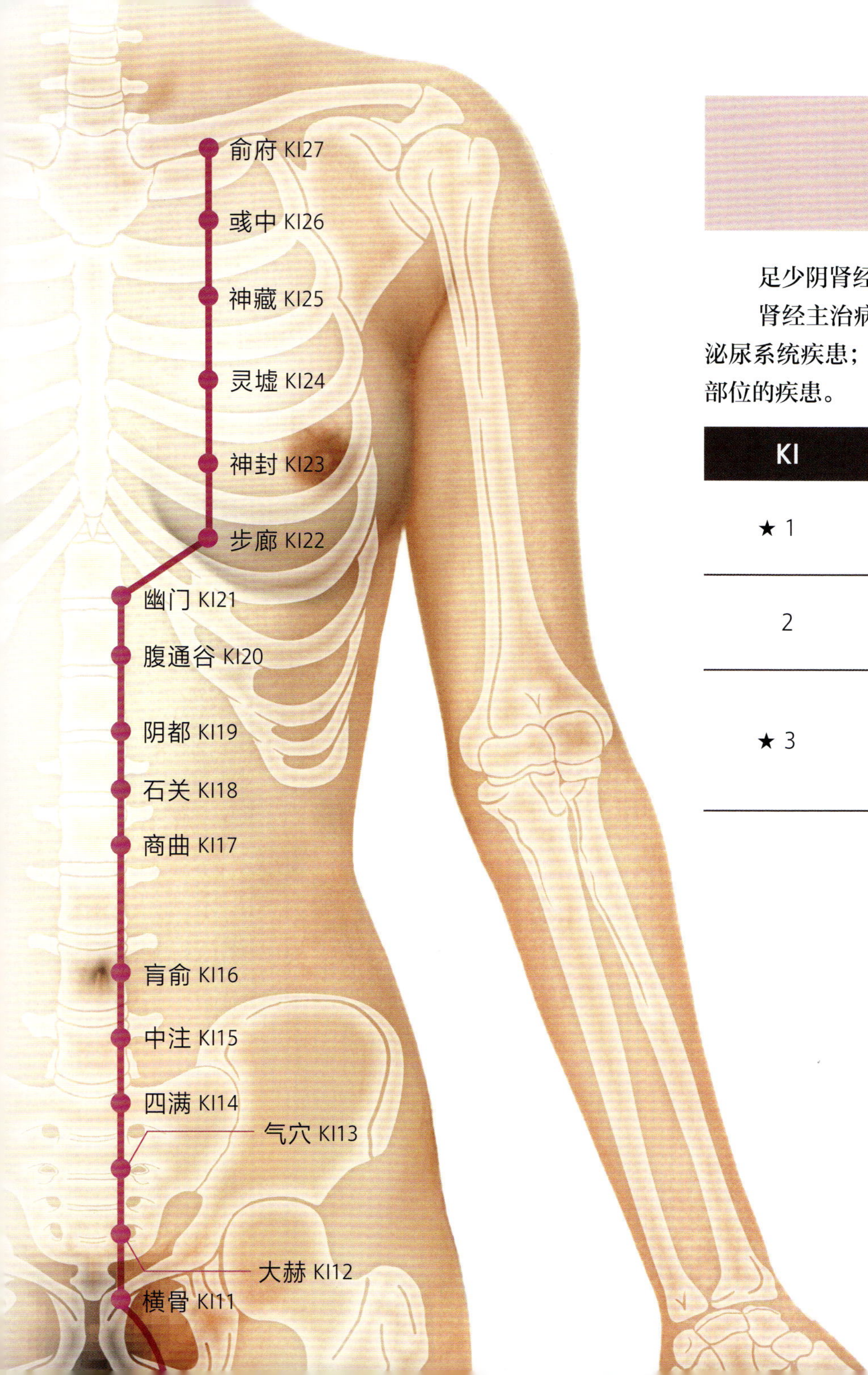

足少阴肾经

足少阴肾经起于足掌心的涌泉，经腿部内侧上达胸前的俞府。

肾经主治病症：月经不调、带下病、遗精、阳痿、早泄等生殖系统疾患；尿潴留、小儿遗尿等泌尿系统疾患；头晕、腰膝酸软、耳聋耳鸣等与肾相关疾患；下肢内侧后缘疼痛、腰痛等经脉循行部位的疾患。

KI	穴名	主治
★ 1	涌泉	昏厥、中暑、小儿惊风、癫狂、头痛、头晕、目眩、失眠、咯血、咽喉肿痛、大便难、小便不利
2	然谷	月经不调、子宫或阴道脱垂、外阴瘙痒、白浊、遗精、阳痿、小便不利、咯血、咽喉肿痛、1 型糖尿病、腹泻
★ 3	太溪	头痛、目眩、失眠、健忘、遗精、咽喉肿痛、齿痛、耳鸣、耳聋、咳嗽、气喘、咯血、胸痛、1 型糖尿病、小便频数、便秘、月经不调、腰脊痛、下肢厥冷

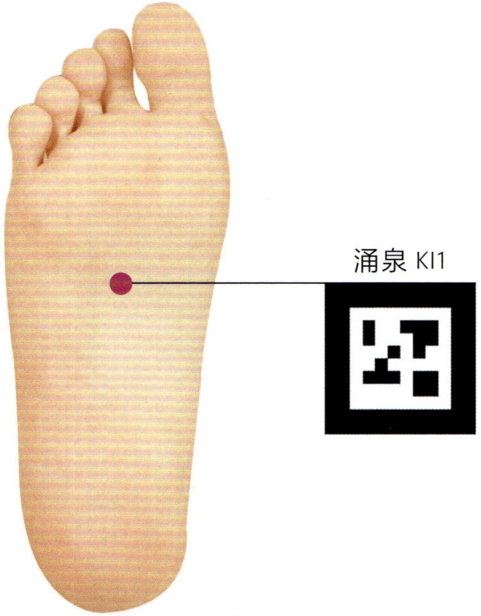

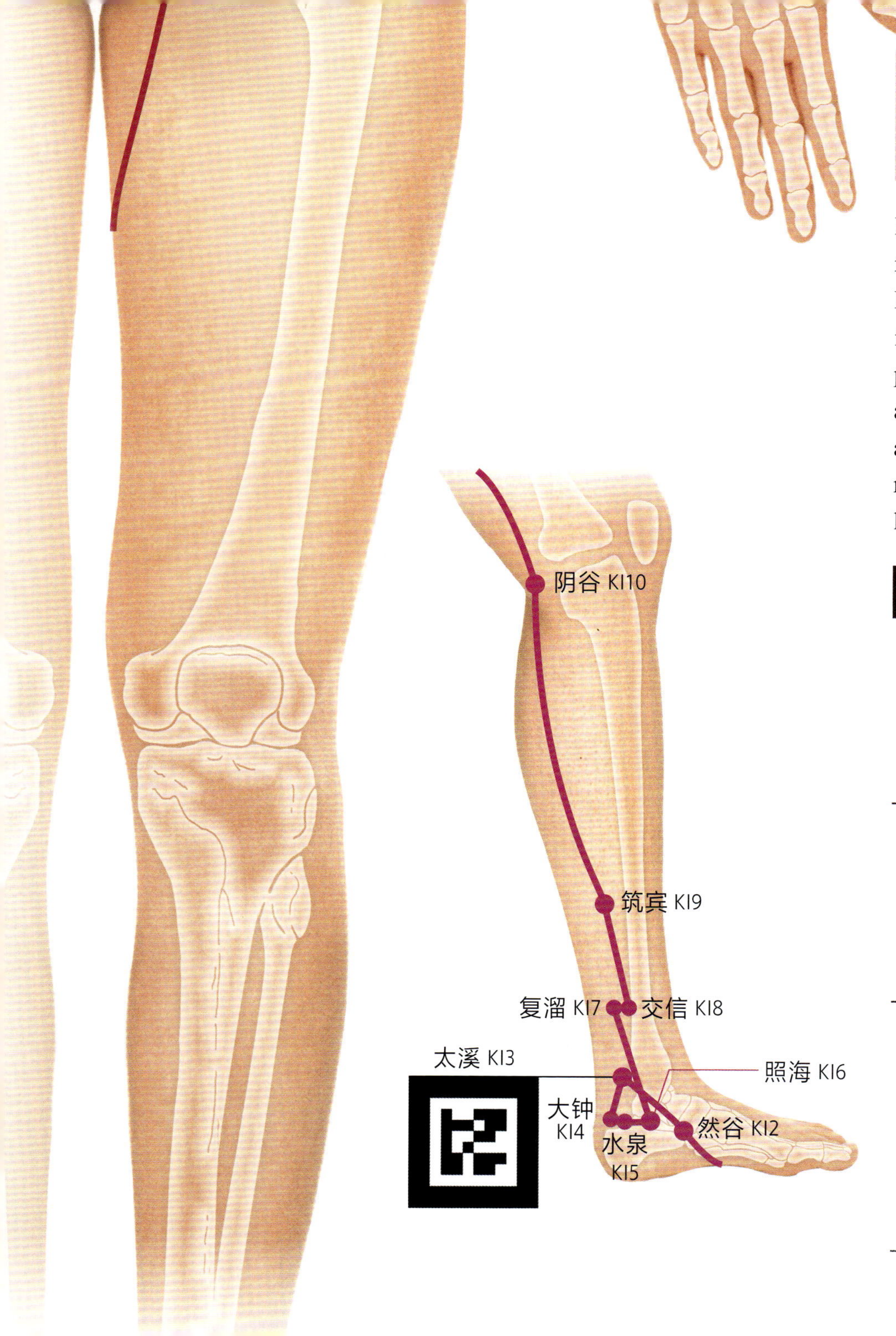

Kidney Meridian of Foot-Shaoyin, KI.

Kidney Meridian of Foot-Shaoyin emerges from Yongquan (KI1) in soles and runs along medial side of legs upwardly to Yufu (KI27) in the chest.

Kidney meridian mainly treats diseases of reproductive system including irregular menstruation,leukorrheal diseases, seminal emission, impotence and premature ejaculation; diseases of urinary system including retention of urine and infantile enuresis; diseases related to kidney including dizziness, soreness and weakness of lower back and knee, deafness and tinnitus; diseases of running courses of meridian including pain in medial posterior side of lower limbs and lower back pain.

KI	Acupoints	Indications
★ 1	Yǒngquán	Syncope; heat stroke; infantile convulsion; manic and depressive psychosis; headache; dizziness; vertigo; insomnia; hemoptysis; swelling and pain in throat; constipation;dysuria
2	Rángǔ	Irregular menstruation; uterus prolapse and vagina prolapse; external genitalia itch; turbid leukorrhea; seminal emission; impotence; dysuria; hemoptysis; swelling and pain in throat; diabetes mellitus type 1; diarrhea
★ 3	Tàixī	Headache; dizziness; insomnia; amnesia; seminal emission; swelling and pain in throat; toothache; tinnitus; deafness; cough; asthma; hemoptysis; chest pain; diabetes mellitus type 1; frequent and urgent urine; constipation; irregular menstruation; lower back and spine pain; stiffness and coldness of lower limbs

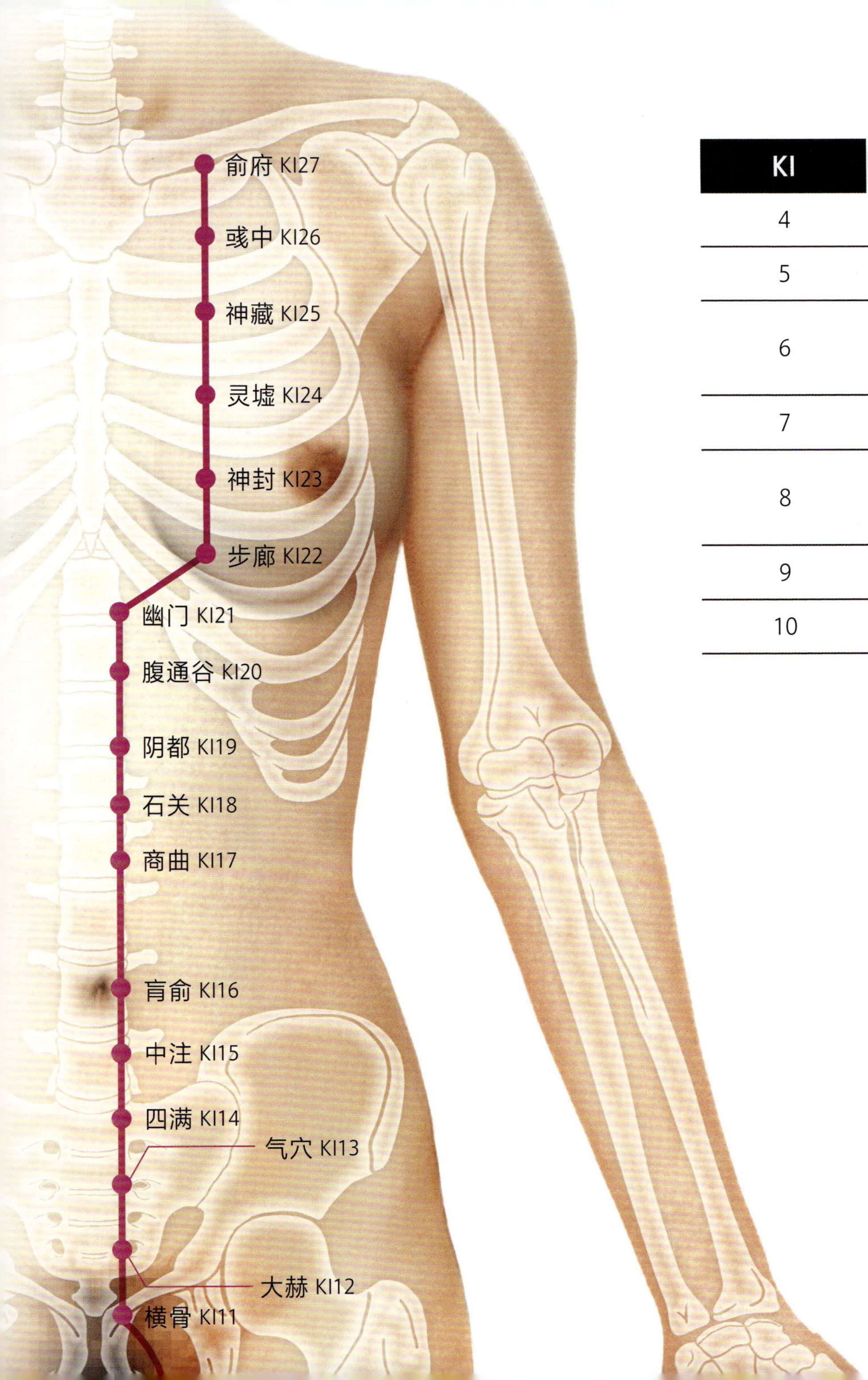

续表

KI	穴名	主治
4	大钟	癃闭、遗尿、便秘、月经不调、气喘、腰脊强痛、足跟痛
5	水泉	月经不调、痛经、经闭、子宫或阴道脱垂、小便不利
6	照海	失眠、癫痫、咽喉干痛、目赤肿痛、月经不调、带下、子宫或阴道脱垂、小便频数、癃闭
7	复溜	水肿、汗证、腹胀、腹泻、腰背强痛、下肢痿痹
8	交信	月经不调、崩漏、子宫或阴道脱垂、外阴瘙痒、疝气、淋证、腹泻、便秘、痢疾
9	筑宾	癫狂、疝气、呕吐涎沫、吐舌、小腿内侧痛
10	阴谷	癫狂、阳痿、小便不利、月经不调、崩漏、膝及大腿内侧痛

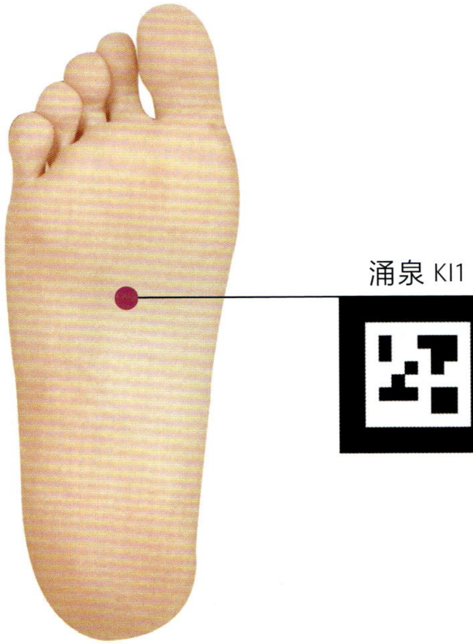

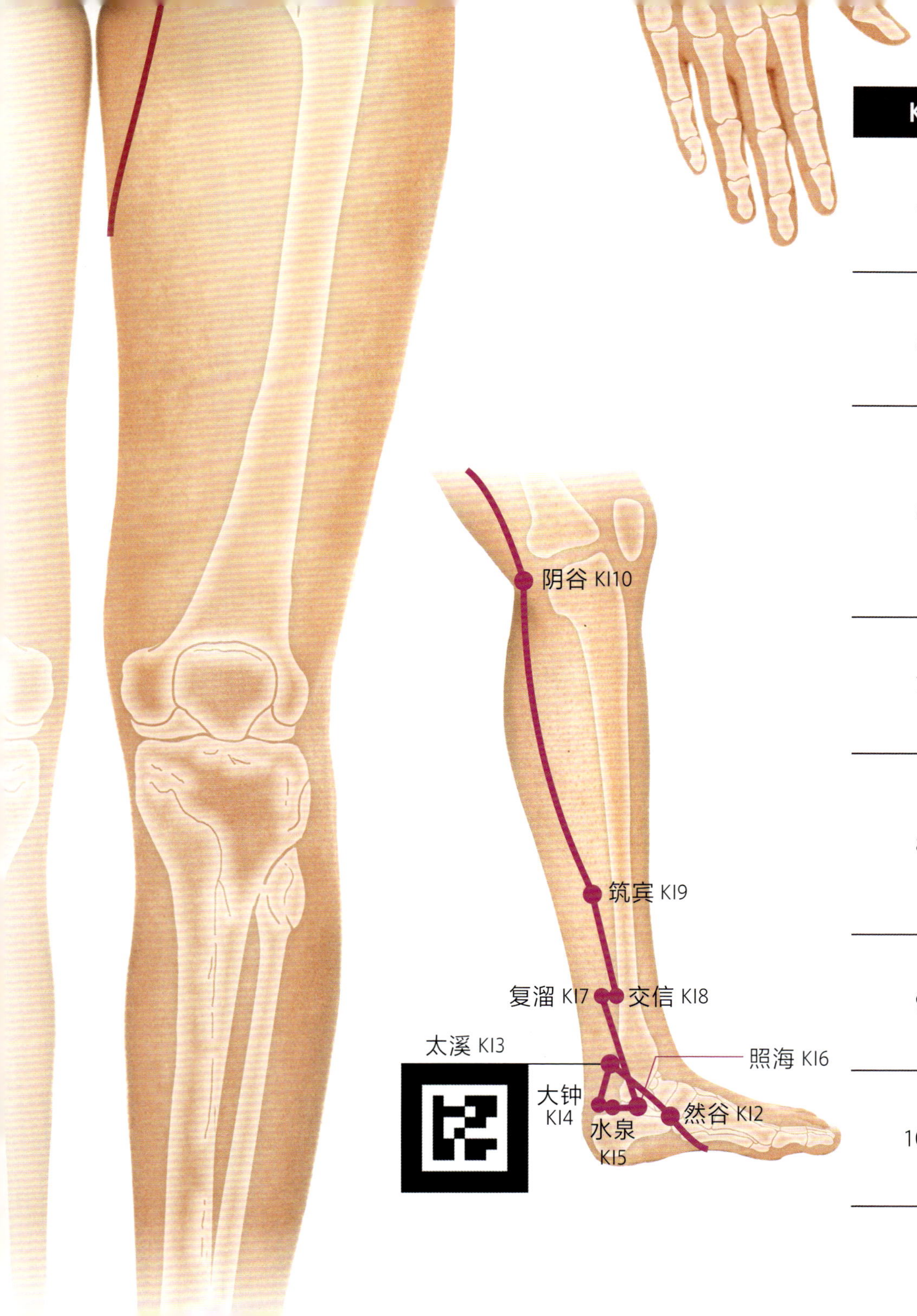

Continued

KI	Acupoints	Indications
4	Dàzhōng	Retention of urine; enuresis; constipation; irregular menstruation; asthma; stiffness and pain of lower back and spine; heel pain
5	Shuǐquán	Irregular menstruation; dysmenorrhea; amenorrhea; uterus prolapse and vagina prolapse; dysuria
6	Zhàohǎi	Insomnia; manic and depressive psychosis; dry and pain throat; redness, swelling and pain of eyes; irregular menstruation; leukorrheal diseases; uterus prolapse and vagina prolapse; frequent and urgent urine; retention of urine
7	Fùliū	Edema; sweat syndrome; distention of abdomen; diarrhea; stiffness and pain of lower back and back; flaccidity and motor impairment of lower limbs
8	Jiāoxìn	Irregular menstruation; metrorrhagia and metrostaxis; uterus prolapse and vagina prolapse; external genitalia itch; hernia; stranguria syndrome; diarrhea; constipation; dysentery
9	Zhùbīn	Manic and depressive psychosis; hernia; vomiting saliva; tongue protrusion; pain in medial side of lower legs
10	Yīngǔ	Manic and depressive psychosis; impotence; dysuria; irregular menstruation; metrorrhagia and metrostaxis; pain in medial side of knee and thigh

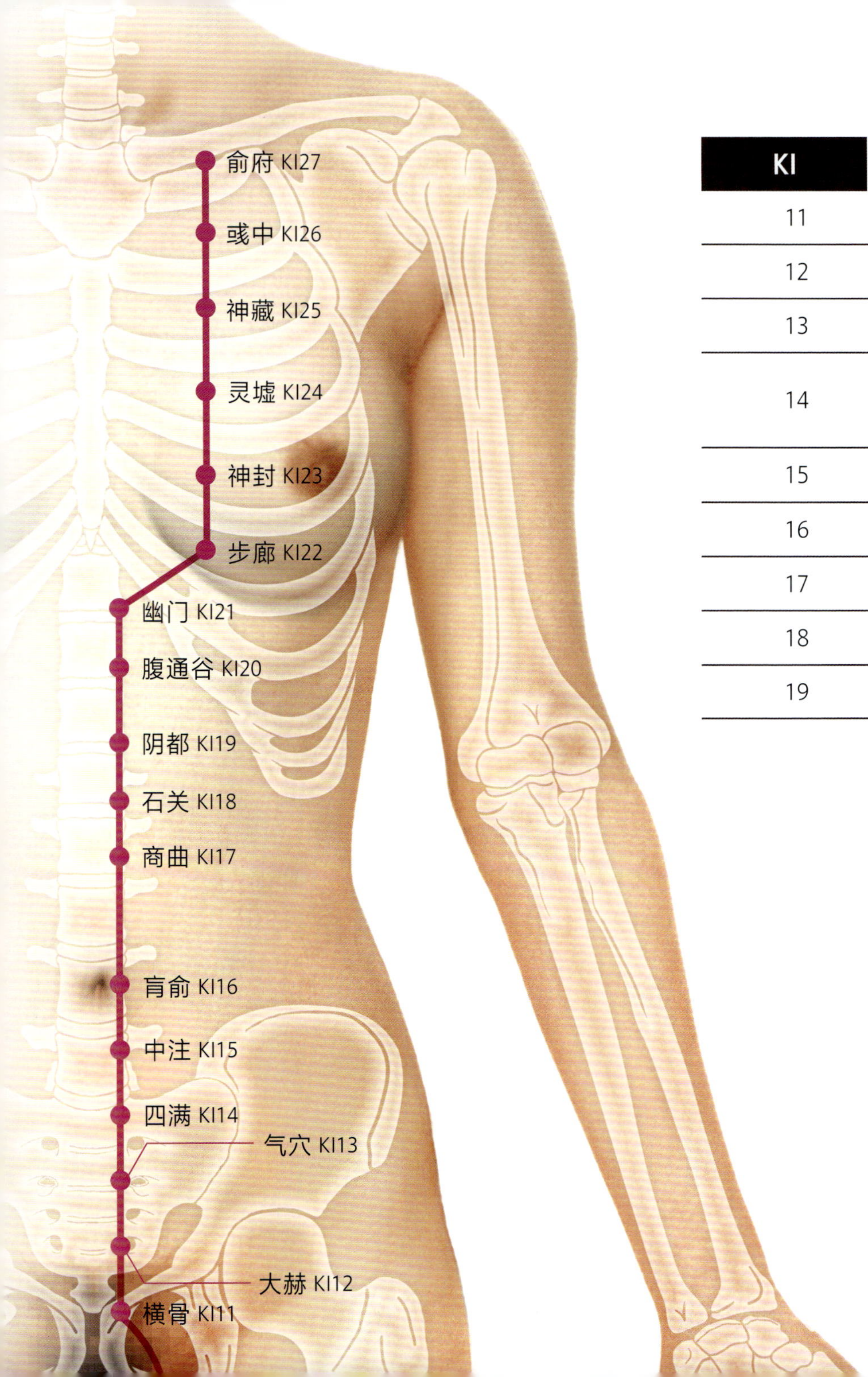

续表

KI	穴名	主治
11	横骨	下腹胀痛、小便不利、遗尿、遗精、阳痿、疝气
12	大赫	遗精、阳痿、子宫或阴道脱垂、带下
13	气穴	奔豚气、月经不调、带下、小便不利、腹泻
14	四满	月经不调、崩漏、带下、产后恶露不净、遗精、遗尿、小腹痛、便秘、水肿
15	中注	月经不调、腹痛、便秘、腹泻
16	肓俞	腹痛、腹胀、腹泻、便秘、月经不调、疝气
17	商曲	胃痛、腹痛、腹胀、腹泻、便秘、腹中积聚
18	石关	胃痛、呕吐、腹痛、腹胀、便秘、不孕
19	阴都	胃痛、腹胀、便秘

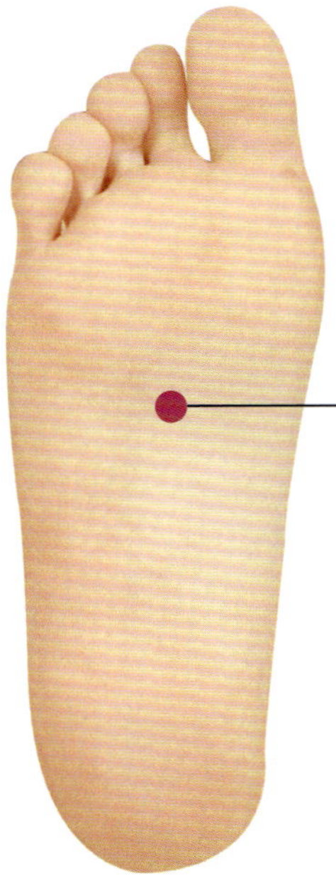

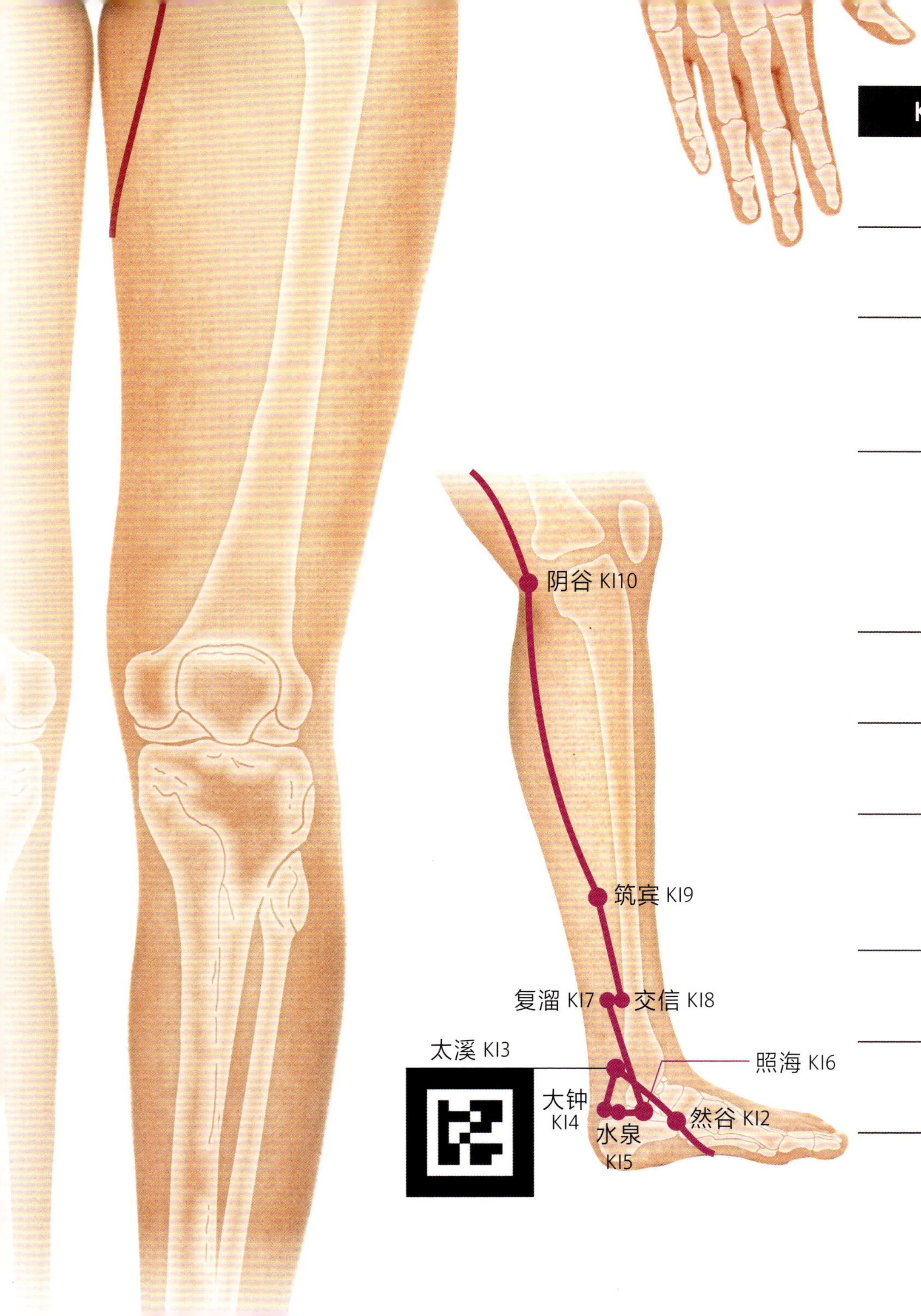

Continued

KI	Acupoints	Indications
11	Hénggǔ	Distending pain of lower abdomen; dysuria; enuresis; seminal emission; impotence; hernia
12	Dàhè	Seminal emission; impotence; uterus prolapse and vagina prolapse; leukorrheal diseases
13	Qìxué	Sensation of gas rushing like a running pig; irregular menstruation; leukorrheal diseases; dysuria; diarrhea
14	Sìmǎn	Irregular menstruation; metrorrhagia and metrostaxis; leukorrheal diseases; lochiorrhagia after delivery; seminal emission; enuresis; lower abdominal pain; constipation; edema
15	Zhōngzhù	Irregular menstruation; abdominal pain; constipation; diarrhea
16	Huāngshū	Abdominal pain; distention of abdomen; diarrhea; constipation; irregular menstruation; hernia
17	Shāngqū	Stomachache; abdominal pain; distention of abdomen; diarrhea; constipation; abdominal mass
18	Shíguān	Stomachache; vomiting; abdominal pain; distention of abdomen; constipation; sterility
19	Yīndū	Stomachache; distention of abdomen; constipation

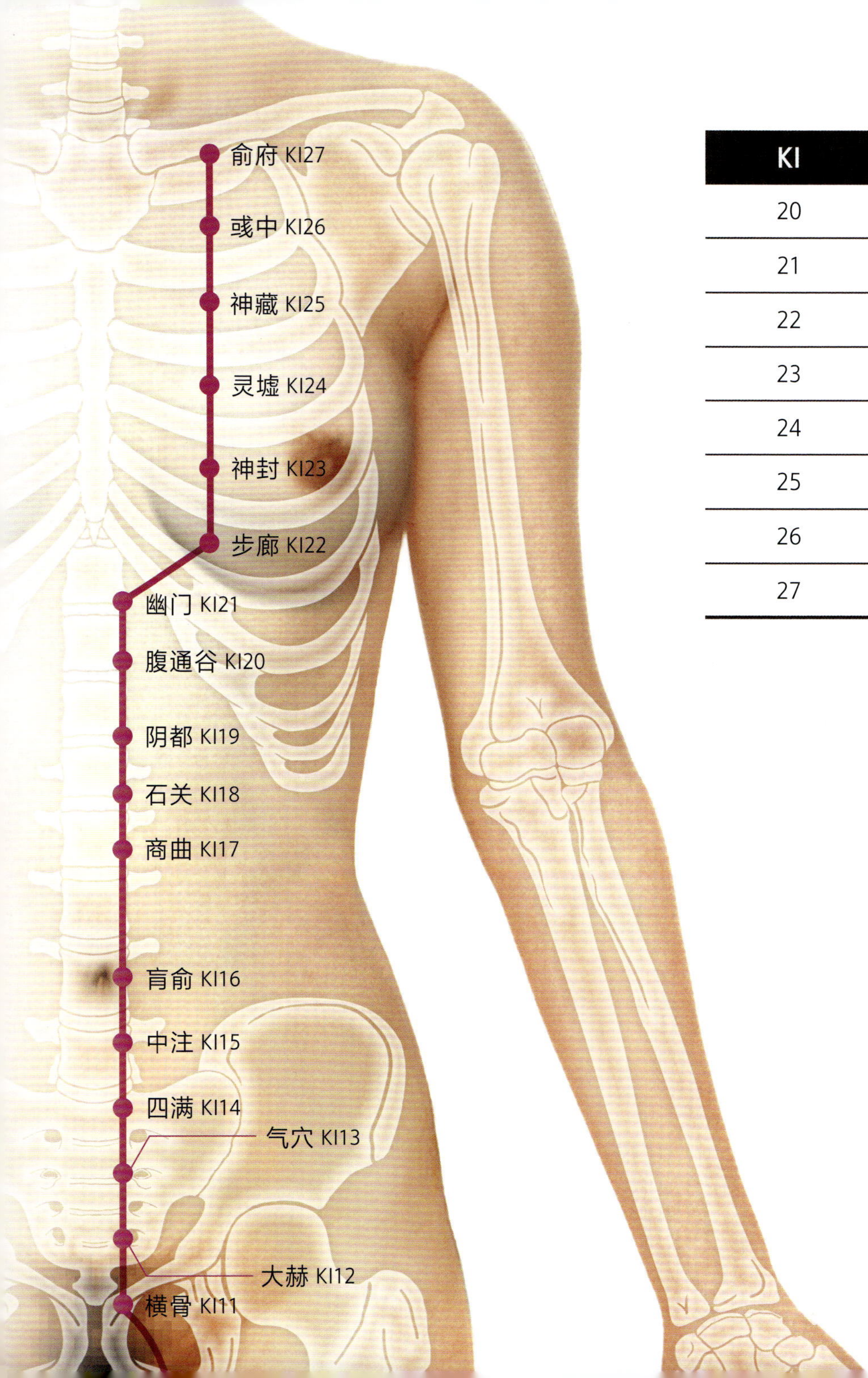

续表

KI	穴 名	主 治
20	腹通谷	腹痛、腹胀、胃痛、呕吐、心悸、胸痛
21	幽门	呕吐、腹痛、腹胀、腹泻
22	步廊	胸痛、咳嗽、气喘、乳房肿痛
23	神封	胸胁支满、咳嗽、气喘、乳房肿痛、呕吐、不嗜食
24	灵墟	胸胁支满、咳嗽、气喘、乳房肿痛、呕吐
25	神藏	胸胁支满、咳嗽、气喘、呕吐、不嗜食
26	彧中	胸胁支满、咳嗽、气喘
27	俞府	咳嗽、气喘、胸痛

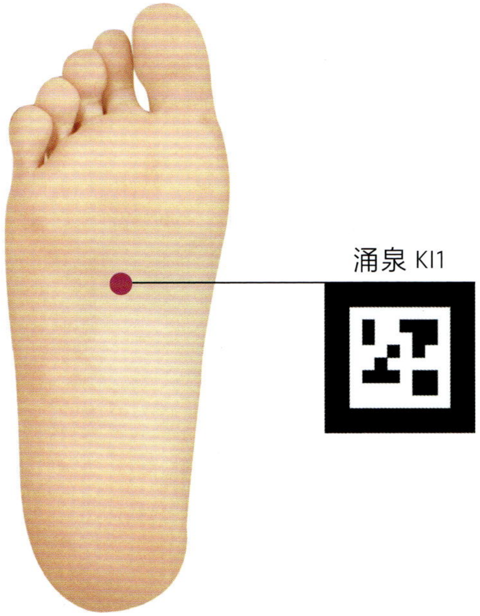

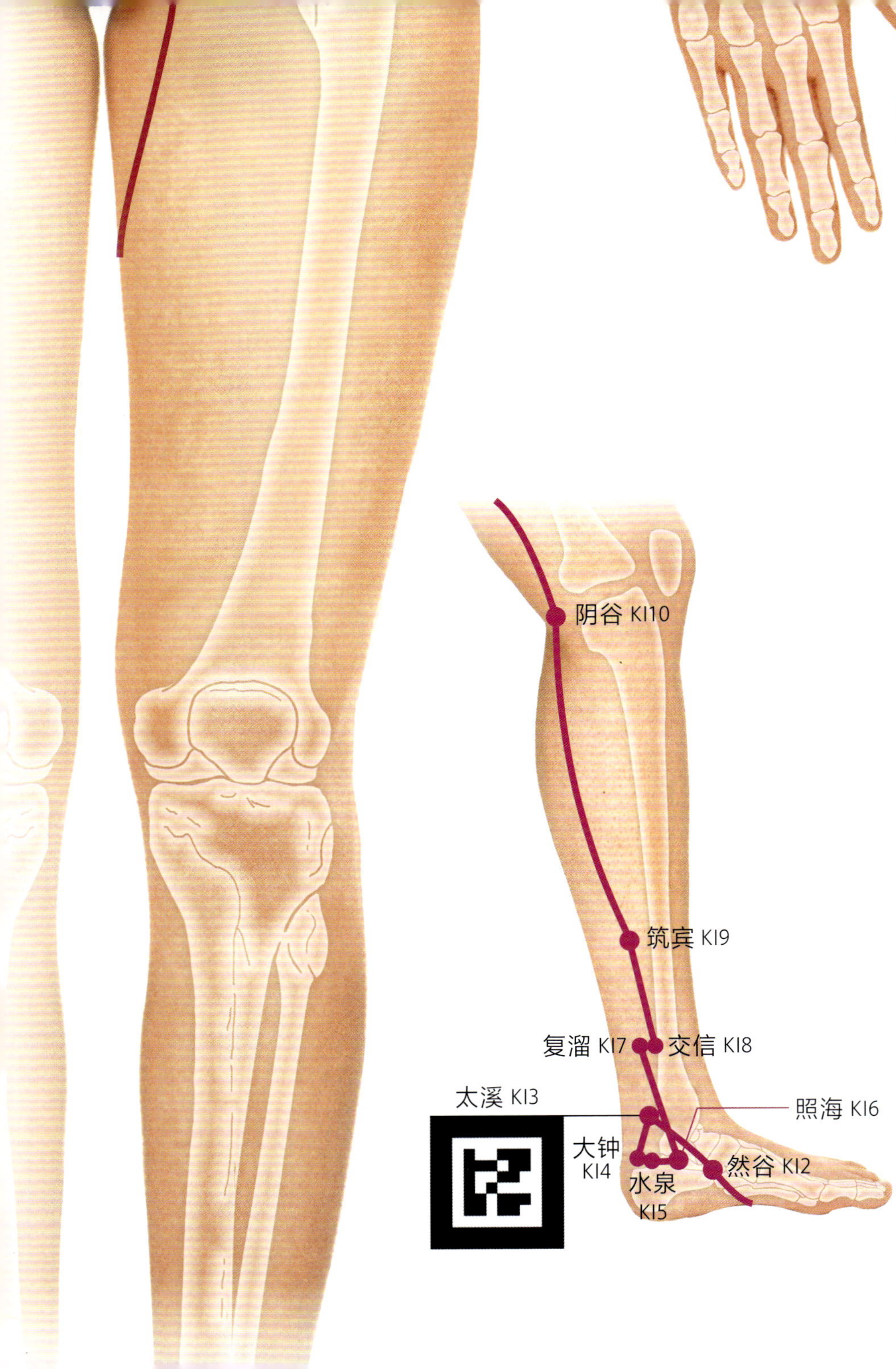

Continued

KI	Acupoints	Indications
20	Fùtōnggǔ	Abdominal pain; distention of abdomen; stomachache; vomiting; palpitation; chest pain
21	Yōumén	Vomiting; abdominal pain; distention of abdomen; diarrhea
22	Bùláng	Chest pain; cough; asthma; swelling and pain of breast
23	Shénfēng	Fullness of chest and hypochondrium; cough; asthma; swelling and pain of breast; vomiting; anorexia
24	Língxū	Fullness of chest and hypochondrium; cough; asthma; swelling and pain of breast; vomiting
25	Shéncáng	Fullness of chest and hypochondrium; cough; asthma; vomiting; anorexia
26	Yùzhōng	Fullness of chest and hypochondrium; cough; asthma
27	Shūfǔ	Cough; asthma; chest pain

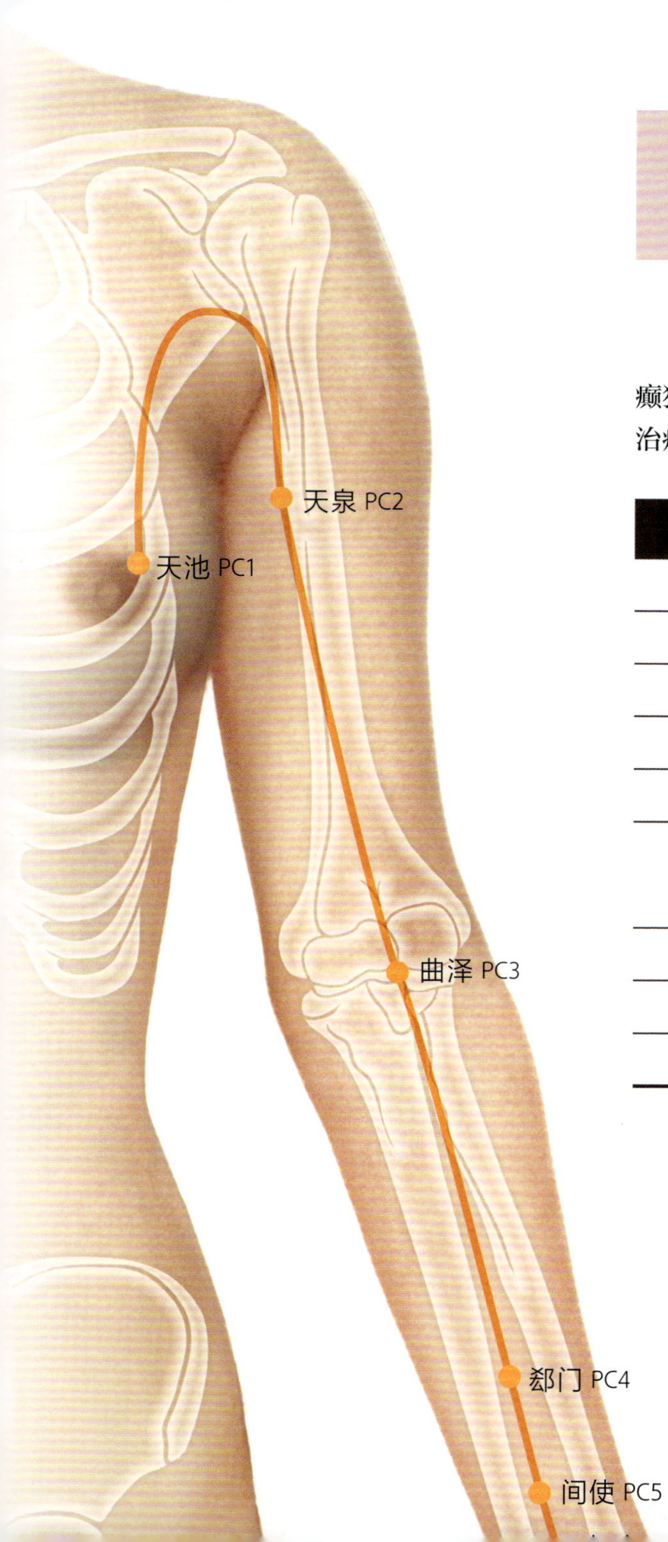

手厥阴心包经

手厥阴心包经起于乳房外侧的天池，经手臂内侧，止于手中指的中冲。

心包经主治病症：胸痛咳喘、乳房胀痛、心慌心烦、呃逆呕吐、胃脘胀痛、腹痛、腹泻等胸腹部疾患；心中恐惧、癫狂、小儿夜啼等神经精神疾患；手臂、肘关节疼痛不适，腋下肿痛，胸胁疼痛等经脉循行部位的疾患。本经还可治疗小儿夜啼等儿童疾患。

PC	穴名	主治
1	天池	咳嗽、痰多、胸闷、气喘、胸痛、乳房肿痛
2	天泉	心痛、咳嗽、胸胁胀满、胸背及上臂内侧痛
3	曲泽	心痛、心悸、胃痛、呕血、呕吐、热病、肘臂挛痛
4	郄门	急性心痛、心悸、心烦、胸痛、咯血、呕血、黏膜出血、疔疮、癫痫
5	间使	心痛、心悸、胃痛、呕吐、热病、寒战发热、癫狂
6	内关	心痛、胸闷、心动过速或过缓、胃痛、呕吐、呃逆、中风、失眠、郁证、癫狂、晕车、晕船、耳源性眩晕、肘臂挛痛
7	大陵	心痛、心悸、胸胁满痛、胃痛、呕吐、口臭、失眠、癫狂、手臂挛痛
★ 8	劳宫	中风昏迷、中暑、心痛、烦闷、癫狂、口疮、口臭、鹅掌风
9	中冲	中风昏迷、舌强不语、中暑、昏厥、小儿惊风

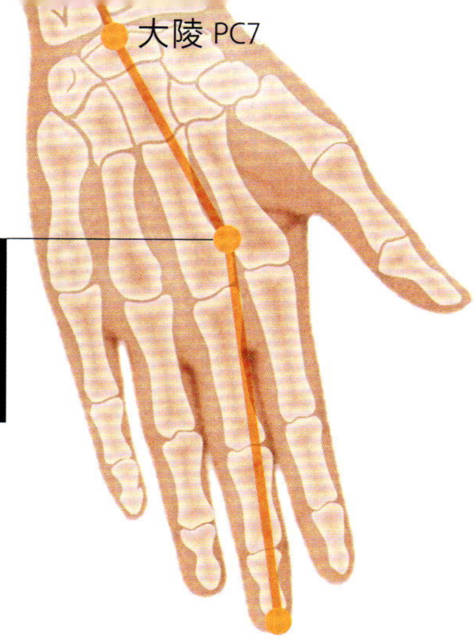

Pericardium Meridian of Hand-Jueyin, PC.

Pericardium Meridian of Hand-Jueyin emerges from Tianchi (PC1) in the lateral side of breast, runs along the medial side of arm and terminates at Zhongchong (PC9) in the middle finger. Pericardium Meridian mainly treats diseases of chest and abdomen including chest pain with cough and asthma, distending pain of breast, flusteredness and upset, hiccup and vomiting, distending pain of epigastrium, abdominal pain and diarrhea; diseases of nervous system including fear, manic and depressive psychosis and morbid night crying of children; diseases of running courses of meridian including pain and discomfort of arm and elbow joint, swelling and pain of armpit and pain of chest and hypochondrium. Pericardium Meridian can also cure children diseases including morbid night crying.

PC	Acupoints	Indications
1	Tiānchí	Cough; profuse phlegm; chest congestion; asthma; chest pain; swelling and pain of breast
2	Tiānquán	Cardiac pain; cough; distention and fullness of chest and hypochondrium; pain in chest, back and medial side of upper arm
3	Qūzé	Cardiac pain; palpitation; stomachache; hematemesis; vomiting; febrile diseases; spasm and pain of elbow and arm
4	Xìmén	Acute cardiac pain; palpitation; upset; chest pain; hemoptysis; hematemesis; mucosa bleeding; furuncle; manic and depressive psychosis
5	Jiānshǐ	Cardiac pain; palpitation; stomachache; vomiting; febrile diseases; chill and fever; manic and depressive psychosis
6	Nèiguān	Cardiac pain; chest congestion; tachycardia or bradycardia; stomachache; vomiting; hiccup; wind stroke; insomnia; depression syndrome; manic and depressive psychosis; car sickness; boat sickness; aural dizziness; spasm and pain of elbow and arm
7	Dàlíng	Cardiac pain; palpitation; fullness and pain of chest and hypochondrium; stomachache; vomiting; halitosis; insomnia; manic and depressive psychosis; spasm and pain of hand and arm
★ 8	Láogōng	Apoplectic coma; heat stroke; cardiac pain; upset; manic and depressive psychosis; mouth sores; halitosis; tinea unguium
9	Zhōngchōng	Apoplectic coma; aphasia due to tongue stiffness; heat stroke; syncope; infantile convulsion

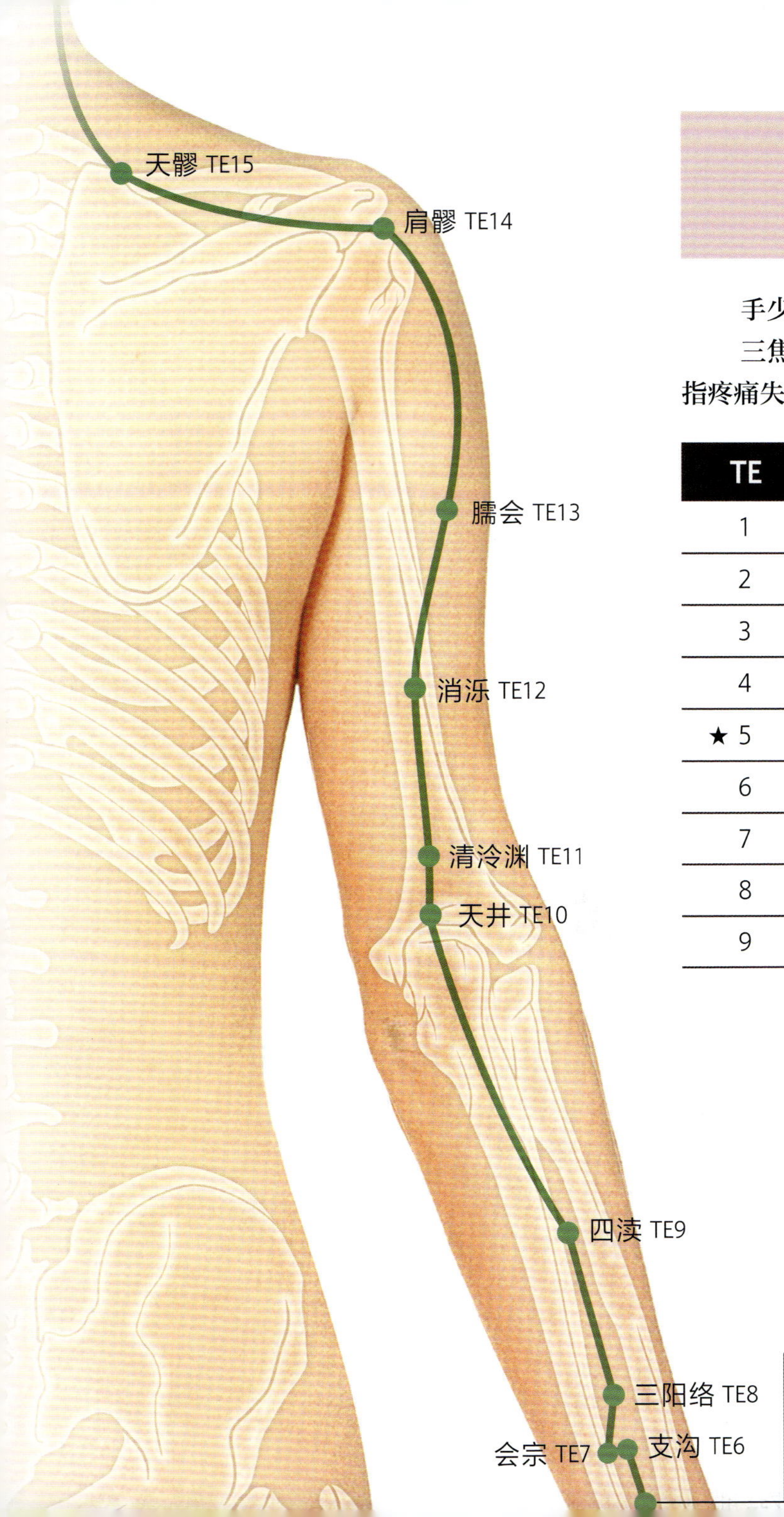

手少阳三焦经

手少阳三焦经从无名指关冲，经手臂外侧、耳后，止于眉梢的丝竹空。

三焦经主治病症：耳聋、耳鸣、耳痛、耳痒、耳流脓等耳部疾患；肩部、臂部、肘部疼痛，手小指、次指疼痛失用等经脉循行部位的疾患。

TE	穴 名	主 治
1	关冲	头痛、目赤、耳鸣、耳聋、扁桃体炎、舌强、热病、中暑
2	液门	头痛、目赤、耳鸣、耳聋、扁桃体炎、寒战发热、手臂痛
3	中渚	头痛、目赤、耳鸣、耳聋、扁桃体炎、热病、肘臂酸痛、手指屈伸不利
4	阳池	目赤肿痛、耳聋、扁桃体炎、1 型糖尿病、口干、腕痛、肩周炎、臂痛
★ 5	外关	热病、头痛、目赤肿痛、耳鸣、耳聋、颈淋巴结结核、胁肋痛、上肢痿痹不遂
6	支沟	便秘、耳鸣、耳聋、急性咽喉炎、颈淋巴结结核、胁肋痛、热病
7	会宗	耳聋、痫证、上肢痹痛
8	三阳络	耳聋、急性咽喉炎、齿痛、手臂痛
9	四渎	耳聋、急性咽喉炎、齿痛、咽喉肿痛、手臂痛

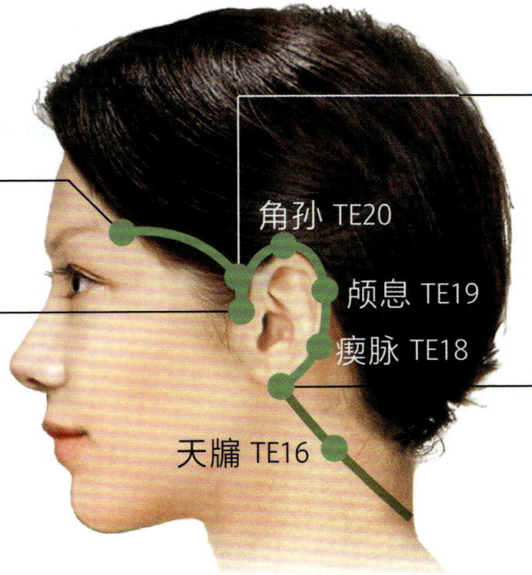

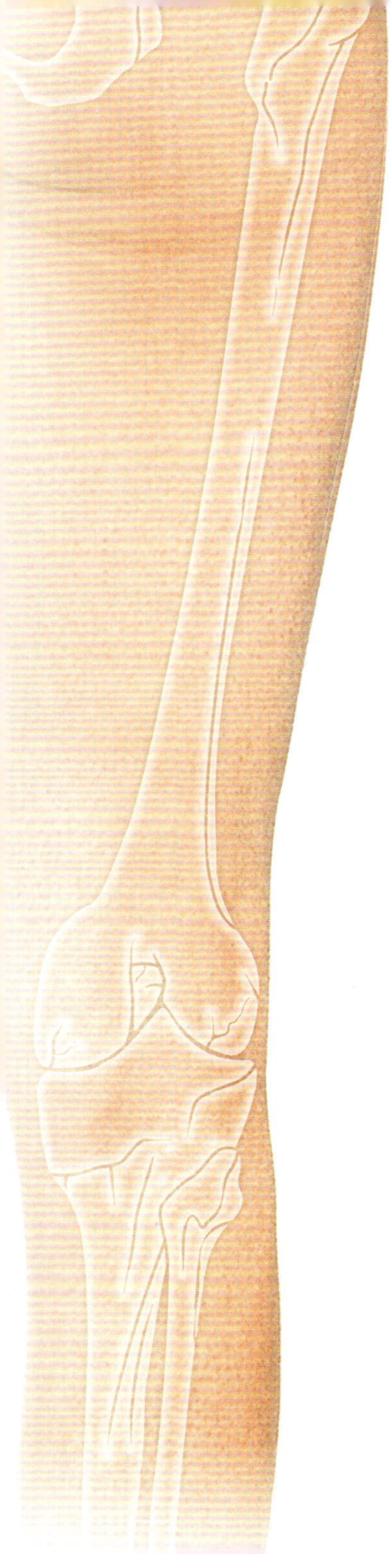

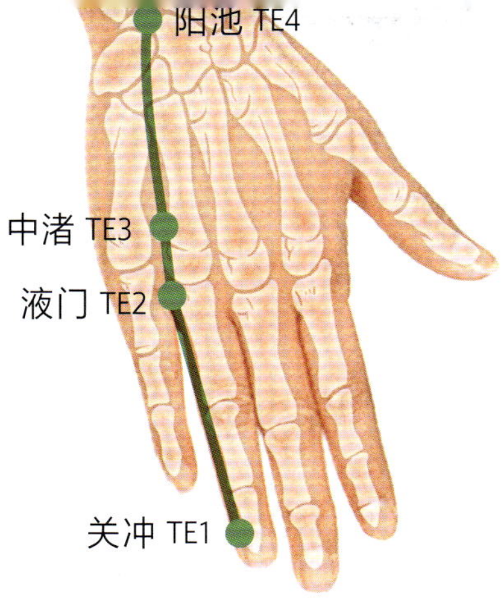

Triple Energizer Meridian of Hand-Shaoyang, TE.

Triple Energizer Meridian of Hand-Shaoyang emerges from Guanchong (TE1) at the ring finger, runs along lateral side of arm and under the ear, then it terminates at Sizhukong (TE23) at the tip of the brow.

Triple Energizer Meridian mainly treats ear diseases including deafness, tinnitus, earache, itching in ear and otorrhea; diseases of running courses of meridian including pain in shoulder, arm and elbow as well as pain and apraxia of the little finger and ring finger.

TE	Acupoints	Indications
1	Guānchōng	Headache; red eyes; tinnitus; deafness; tonsillitis; tongue stiffness; febrile diseases; heat stroke
2	Yèmén	Headache; red eyes; tinnitus; deafness; tonsillitis; chill and fever; hand and arm pain
3	Zhōngzhǔ	Headache; red eyes; tinnitus; deafness; tonsillitis; febrile diseases;soreness in elbow and arm; difficulty in finger bending and stretching
4	Yángchí	Redness, swelling and pain of eyes; deafness; tonsillitis; diabetes mellitus type 1; dry mouth; wrist pain; shoulder periarthritis; arm pain
★ 5	Wàiguān	Febrile diseases; headache; redness, swelling and pain of eyes; tinnitus; deafness; cervical lymph node tuberculosis; hypochondriun and rib pain; flaccidity and motor impairment of upper limbs
6	ZhīGōu	Constipation; tinnitus; deafness; acute sphagitis; cervical lymph node tuberculosis; hypochondriun and rib pain; febrile diseases
7	Huìzōng	Deafness; epilepsy; arthralgia of upper limbs
8	Sānyángluò	Deafness; acute sphagitis; toothache; hand and arm pain
9	Sìdú	Deafness; acute sphagitis; toothache; swelling and pain in throat; hand and arm pain

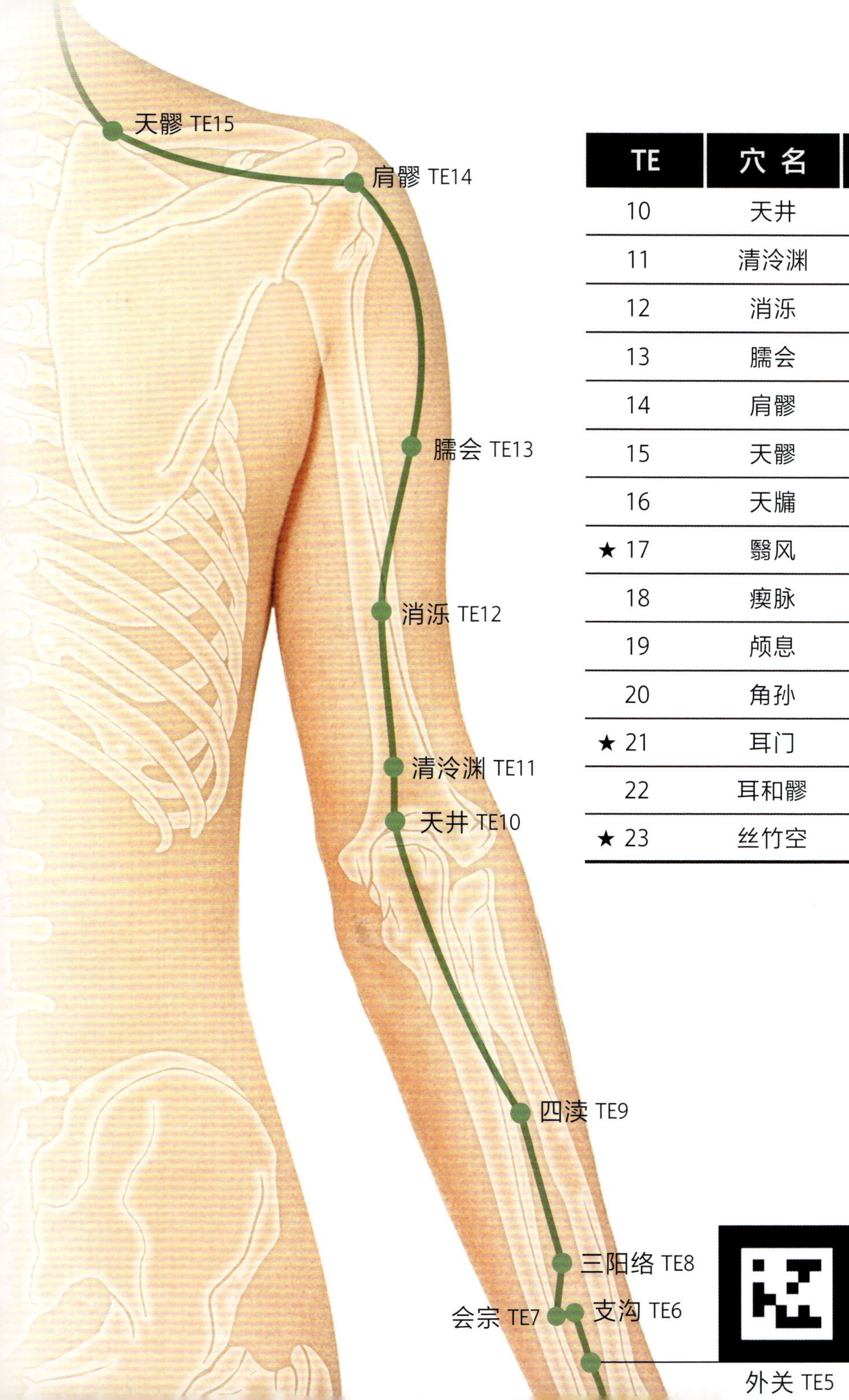

续表

TE	穴 名	主 治
10	天井	耳聋、癫狂、颈淋巴结结核、甲状腺肿大、偏头痛、胁肋痛、肩周炎、臂痛、颈项痛
11	清泠渊	头痛、目痛、胁痛、肩周炎、臂痛
12	消泺	头痛、齿痛、项背痛
13	臑会	颈淋巴结结核、甲状腺肿大、上肢痹痛
14	肩髎	肩臂挛痛
15	天髎	肩周炎、臂痛、颈项强急
16	天牖	头痛、头眩、项强、目不明、暴聋、鼻出血、扁桃体炎、颈淋巴结结核、肩周炎、背痛
★ 17	翳风	耳鸣、耳聋、口眼歪斜、面风、牙关紧闭、颊肿、颈淋巴结结核
18	瘈脉	头痛、耳鸣、耳聋、小儿惊风
19	颅息	头痛、耳鸣、耳聋、小儿惊风
20	角孙	头痛、项强、目赤肿痛、白内障、齿痛、颊肿
★ 21	耳门	耳鸣、耳聋、中耳炎、齿痛、颈颔痛
22	耳和髎	头痛、耳鸣、牙关紧闭、口歪
★ 23	丝竹空	癫狂、头痛、目眩、目赤肿痛、眼睑瞤动、齿痛

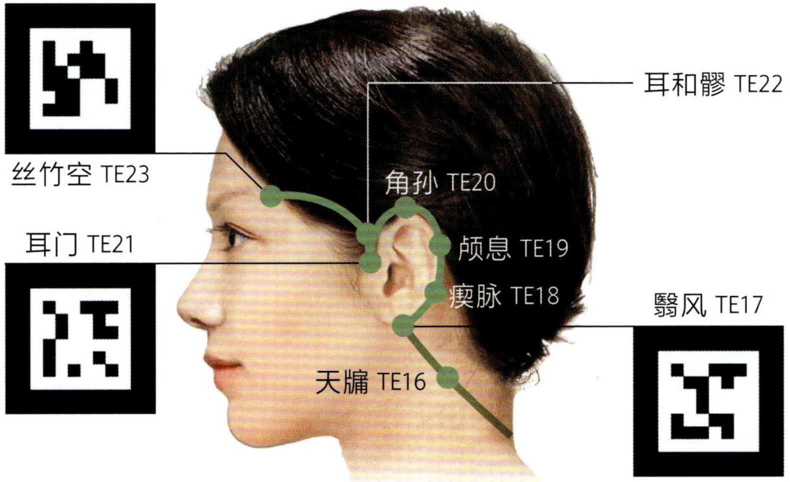

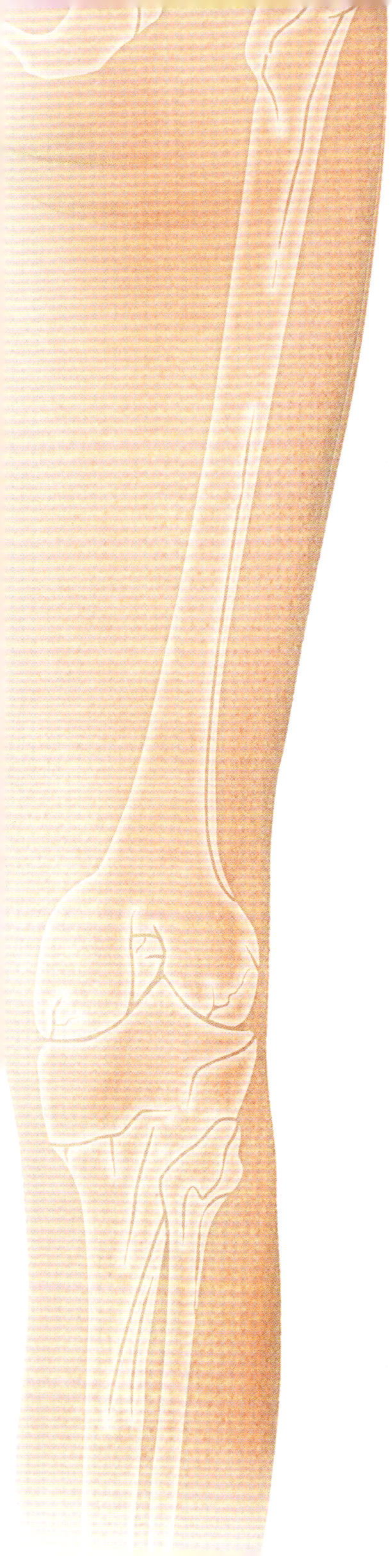

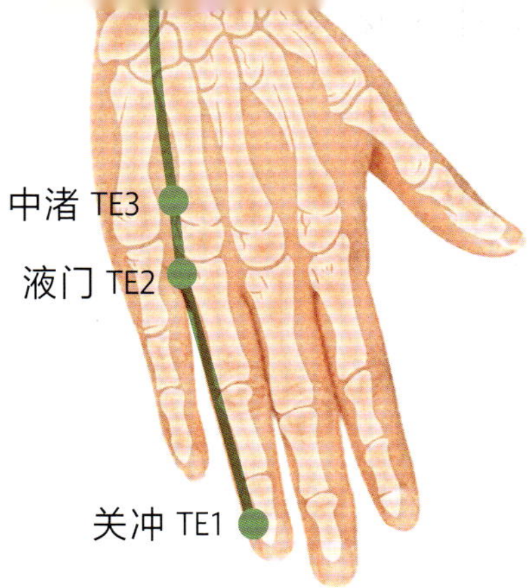

Continued

TE	Acupoints	Indications
10	Tiānjǐng	Deafness; manic and depressive psychosis; cervical lymph node tuberculosis; goiter; migraine; hypochondriun and rib pain; shoulder periarthritis; arm pain; neck pain
11	Qīnglíngyuān	Headache; eyes pain; hypochondrium pain; shoulder periarthritis; arm pain
12	Xiāoluò	Headache; toothache; neck and back pain
13	Nàohuì	Cervical lymph node tuberculosis; goiter; arthralgia of upper limbs
14	Jiānliáo	Spasm and pain of shoulder and arm
15	Tiānliáo	Shoulder periarthritis; arm pain; neck stiffness
16	Tiānyǒu	Headache; dizziness; neck stiffness; blurry vision; sudden deafness; nose bleeding; tonsillitis; cervical lymph node tuberculosis; shoulder periarthritis; back pain
★ 17	Yìfēng	Tinnitus; deafness; deviation of mouth and eye; facial muscle twitching; lockjaw; swollen cheek; cervical lymph node tuberculosis
18	Chìmài	Headache; tinnitus; deafness; infantile convulsion
19	Lúxī	Headache; tinnitus; deafness; infantile convulsion
20	Jiǎosūn	Headache; neck stiffness; redness, swelling and pain of eyes; cataract; toothache; swollen cheek
★ 21	Ěrmén	Tinnitus; deafness; otitis media; toothache; neck and jaw pain
22	Ěrhéliáo	Headache; tinnitus; lockjaw; deviation of the mouth
★ 23	Sīzhúkōng	Manic and depressive psychosis; headache; dizziness; redness, swelling and pain of eyes; eyelid twitching; toothache

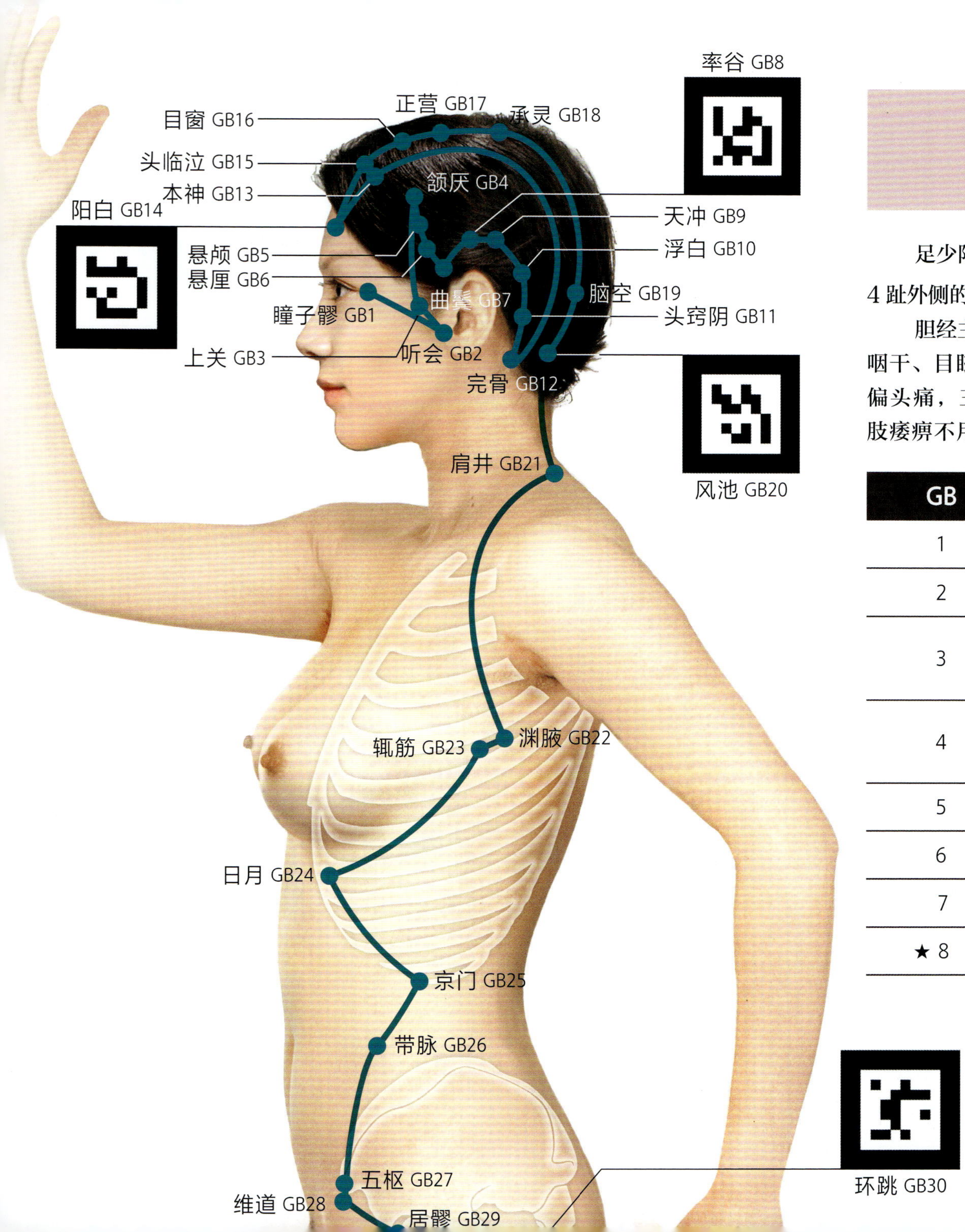

足少阳胆经

足少阳胆经起于眼睛外侧的瞳子髎，经耳后、颈、腿部外侧，止于第4趾外侧的足窍阴。

胆经主治病症：胆囊炎、胆结石、胆道蛔虫症等胆腑病症；口苦、咽干、目眩、往来寒热、胸胁苦满、心烦、食欲不振、呕吐等少阳证；偏头痛，三叉神经痛，耳聋、耳鸣，目疾，落枕，胸胁痛，膝痛，下肢痿痹不用等经脉循行部位的病症。

GB	穴名	主治
1	瞳子髎	头痛、目赤肿痛、羞明流泪、白内障
2	听会	耳鸣、耳聋、中耳炎、齿痛、口眼歪斜
3	上关	耳鸣、耳聋、中耳炎、齿痛、面痛、口眼歪斜、口噤
4	颔厌	偏头痛、眩晕、惊痫、耳鸣、目外眦痛、齿痛
5	悬颅	偏头痛、目赤肿痛、齿痛
6	悬厘	偏头痛、目赤肿痛、耳鸣
7	曲鬓	头痛连齿、颊颔肿、口噤
★ 8	率谷	头痛、眩晕、小儿惊风

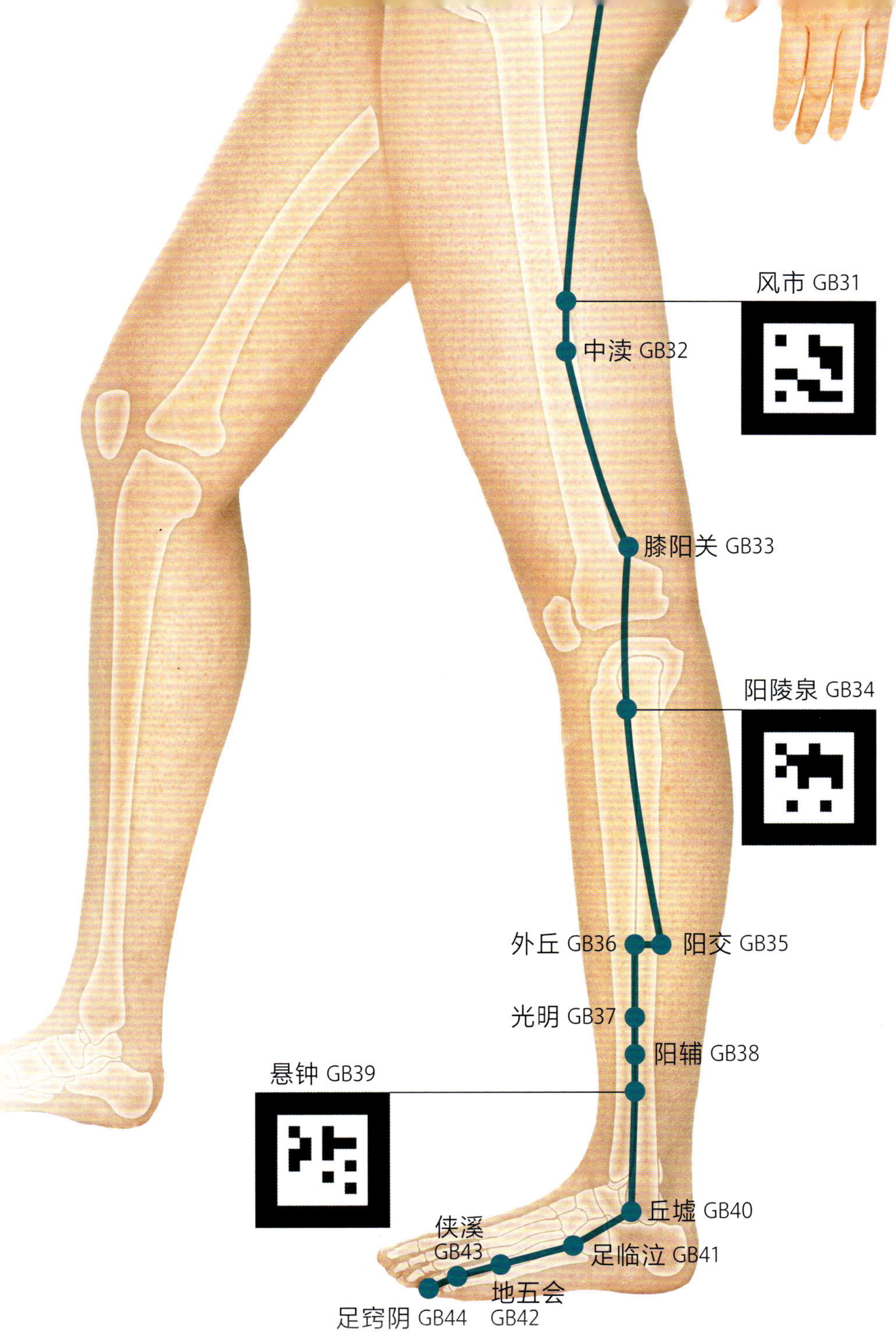

Gallbladder Meridian of Foot-Shaoyang, GB.

Gallbladder Meridian of Foot-Shaoyang emerges from Tongziliao (GB1) in the lateral side of eyes, runs behind the ears and along the neck and the lateral side of legs, it terminates at Zuqiaoyin (GB44) in the lateral side of the 4th toe.

Gallbladder Meridian mainly treats gallbladder diseases including cholecystitis, gallstones and biliary ascariasis; Shaoyang syndromes including bitter taste in mouth, dry throat, dizziness, alternate attacks of chill and fever; fullness and discomfort in chest and hypochondrium, upset, poor appetite and vomiting; diseases of running courses of meridian including migraine, prosopalgia, deafness, tinnitus, eye diseases, stiff neck, chest and hypochondrium pain, knee pain and flaccidity and motor impairment of lower limbs.

GB	Acupoints	Indications
1	Tóngzǐliáo	Headache; redness, swelling and pain of eyes; photophobia and tearing; cataract
2	Tīnghuì	Tinnitus; deafness; otitis media; toothache; deviation of mouth and eye
3	Shàngguān	Tinnitus; deafness; otitis media; toothache; face pain; deviation of mouth and eye; lockjaw
4	Hànyàn	Migraine; dizziness; fright epilepsy; tinnitus; outer canthus pain; toothache
5	Xuánlú	Migraine; redness, swelling and pain of eyes; toothache
6	Xuánlí	Migraine; redness, swelling and pain of eyes; tinnitus
7	Qūbìn	Headache radiating to tooth; swollen cheek and jaw; lockjaw
★ 8	Shuàigǔ	Headache; dizziness; infantile convulsion

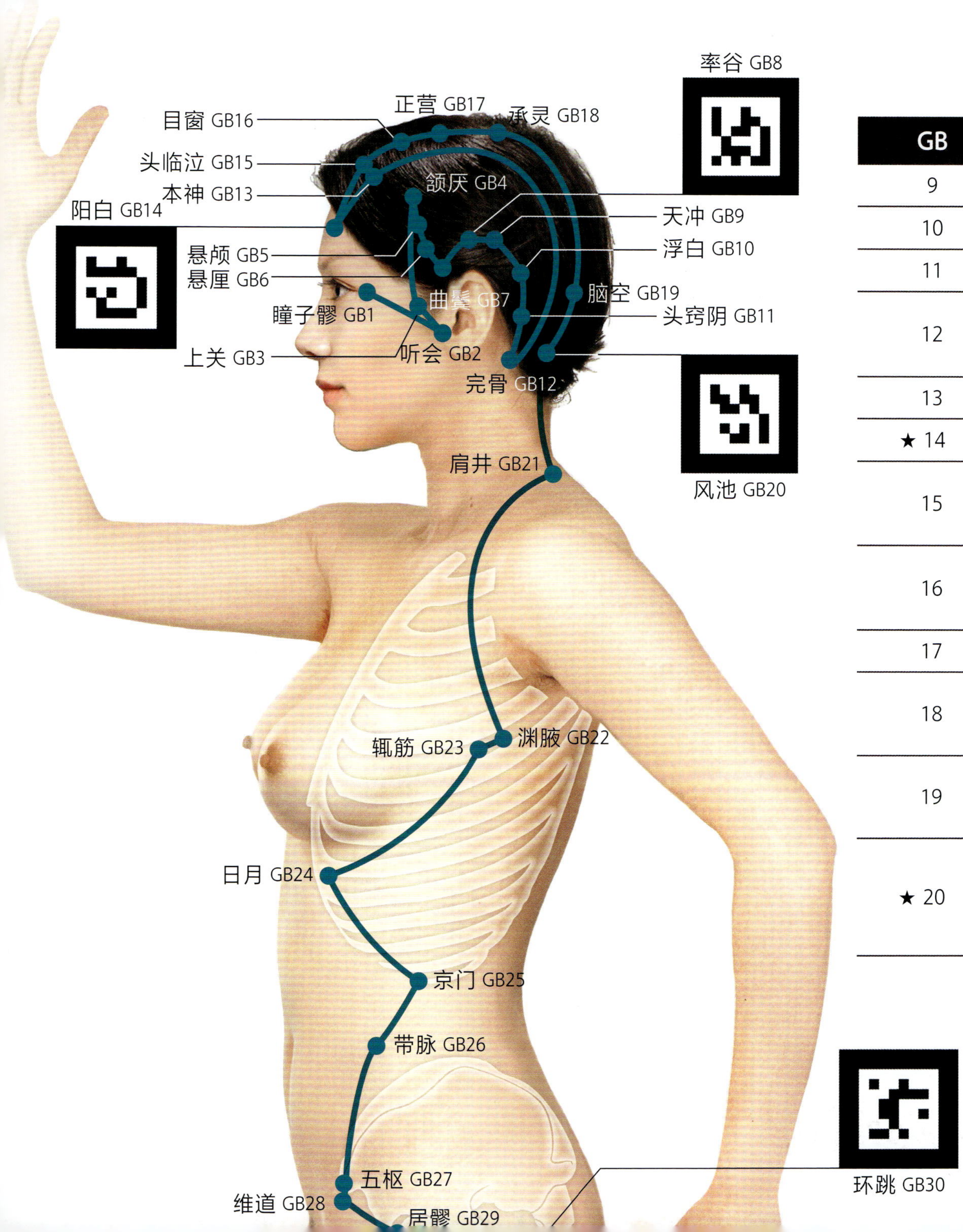

续表

GB	穴 名	主 治
9	天冲	头痛、癫痫、牙龈肿痛
10	浮白	头痛、耳鸣、耳聋、齿痛、甲状腺肿大
11	头窍阴	头痛、眩晕、颈项强痛、耳鸣、耳聋
12	完骨	癫痫、头痛、颈项强痛、扁桃体炎、颊肿、齿痛、口歪
13	本神	癫痫、小儿惊风、中风、头痛、目眩
★ 14	阳白	前头痛、目痛、视物模糊、眼睑瞤动
15	头临泣	头痛、目痛、目眩、流泪、目翳、鼻塞、鼻窦炎、小儿惊风
16	目窗	头痛、目痛、目眩、远视、近视、小儿惊风
17	正营	头痛、头晕、目眩
18	承灵	头痛、眩晕、目痛、鼻窦炎、鼻出血、多涕
19	脑空	热病、头痛、颈项强痛、目眩、目赤肿痛、鼻痛、耳聋、惊悸、癫狂
★ 20	风池	中风、癫狂、头痛、眩晕、耳鸣、耳聋、感冒、鼻塞、鼻出血、目赤肿痛、口眼歪斜、颈项强痛

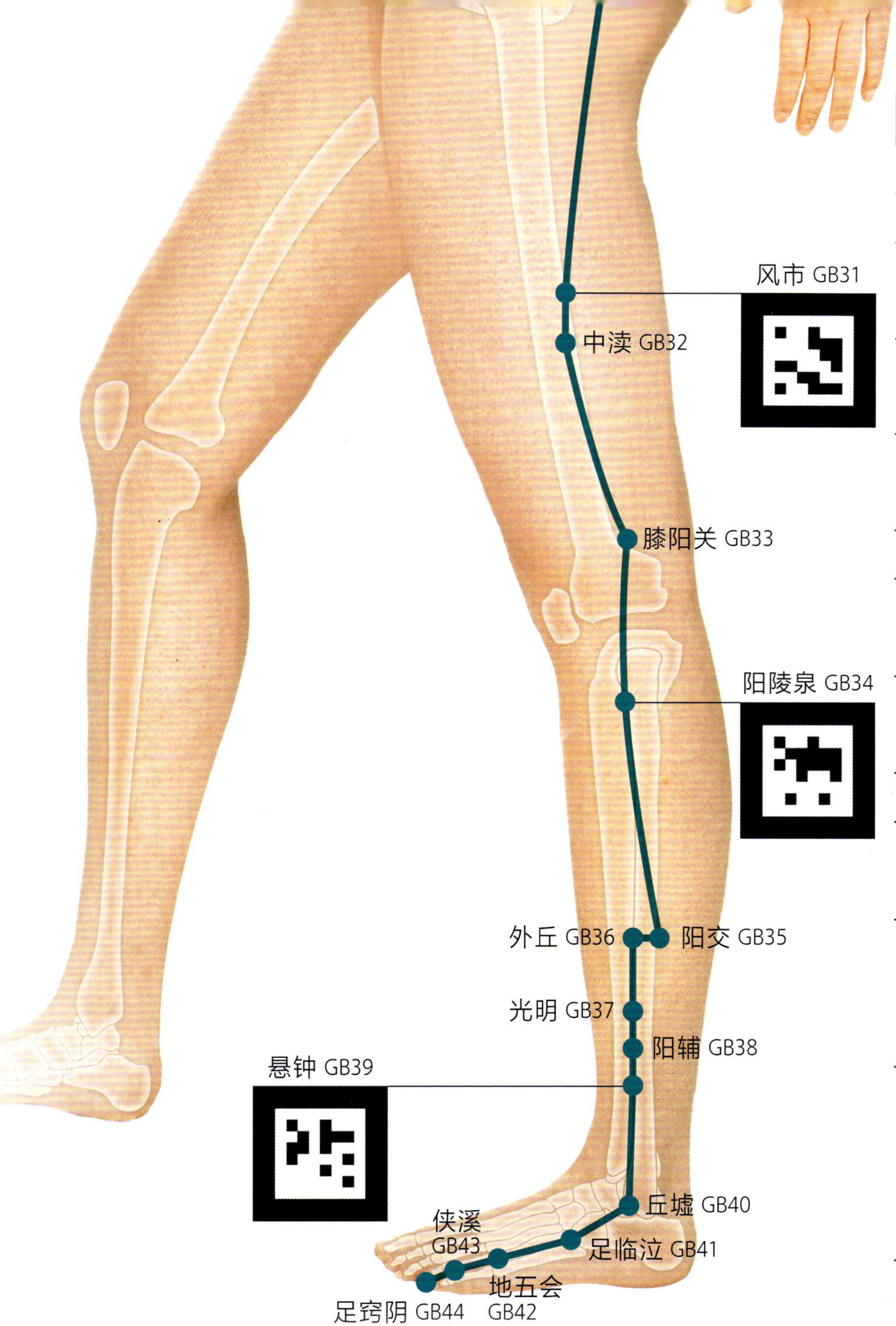

Continued

GB	Acupoints	Indications
9	Tiānchōng	Headache; epilepsy; swelling and pain of gums
10	Fúbái	Headache; tinnitus; deafness; toothache; goiter
11	Tóuqiàoyīn	Headache; dizziness; neck stiffness and pain; tinnitus; deafness
12	Wángǔ	Epilepsy; headache; neck stiffness and pain; tonsillitis; swollen cheek; toothache; mouth deviation
13	Běnshén	Epilepsy; infantile convulsion; wind stroke; headache; dizziness
★ 14	Yángbái	Forehead pain; eyes pain; blurry vision; eyelid twitching
15	Tóulínqì	Headache; eyes pain; dizziness; tearing; nephelium; nasal obstruction; sinusitis; infantile convulsion
16	Mùchuāng	Headache; eyes pain; dizziness; hyperopia; myopia; infantile convulsion
17	Zhèngyíng	Headache; dizziness; vertigo
18	Chénglíng	Headache; dizziness; eyes pain; sinusitis; nose bleeding; profuse running nose
19	Nǎokōng	Febrile diseases; headache; neck stiffness and pain; dizziness; redness, swelling and pain of eyes; nose pain; deafness; palpitation; manic and depressive psychosis
★ 20	Fēngchí	Wind stroke; manic and depressive psychosis; headache; dizziness; tinnitus; deafness; cold; nasal obstruction; nose bleeding; redness, swelling and pain of eyes; deviation of mouth and eye; neck stiffness and pain

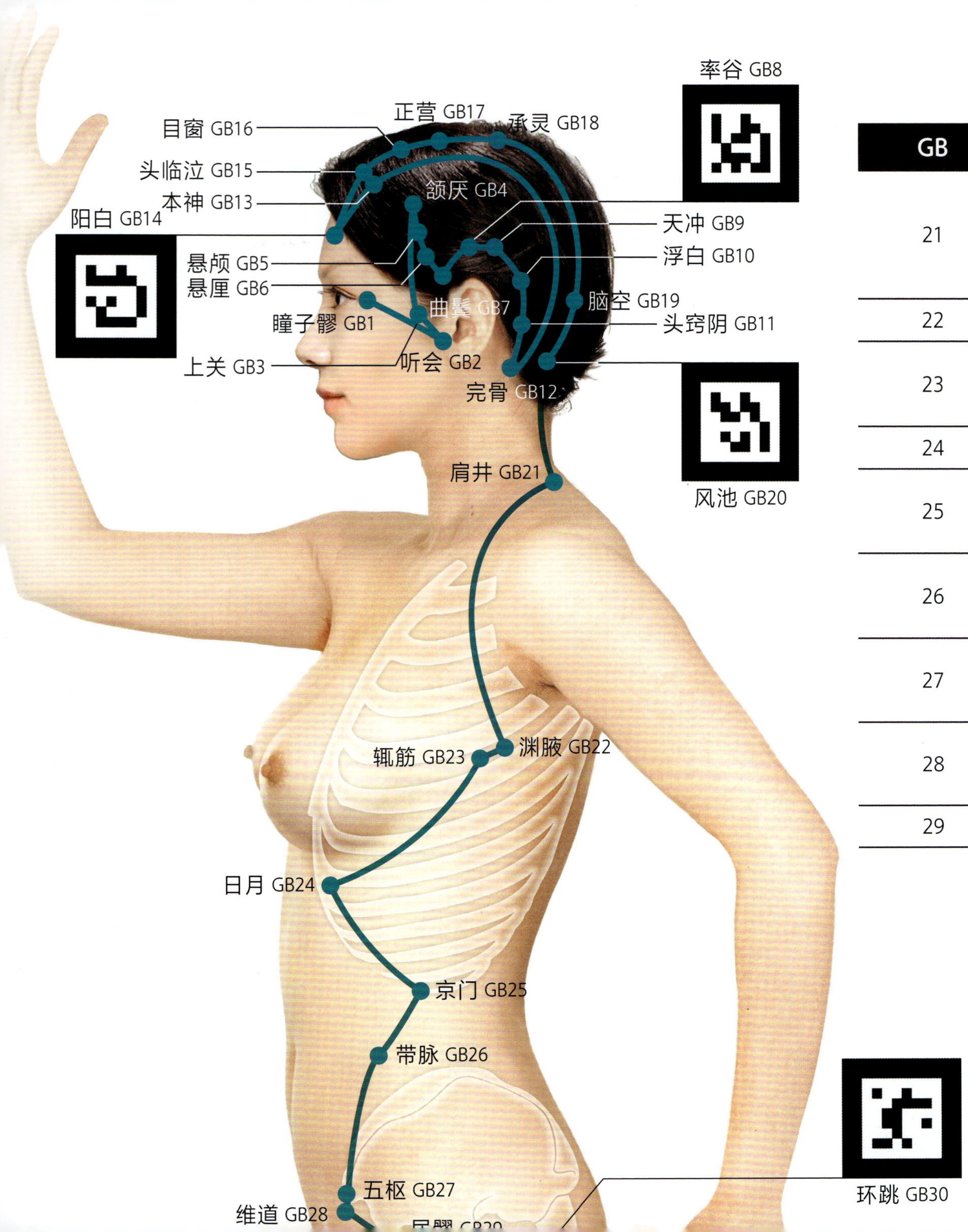

续表

GB	穴 名	主 治
21	肩井	颈项强痛、肩周炎、背疼痛、上肢不遂、难产、乳房肿痛、乳汁不下、乳房肿块、颈淋巴结结核（炎）
22	渊腋	胸满、胁痛、上肢痹痛、腋下肿痛
23	辄筋	胸满、气喘、呕吐、吞酸、胁痛、腋下肿、肩周炎、背痛
24	日月	黄疸、胁肋疼痛、呕吐、吞酸、呃逆
25	京门	小便不利、水肿、腹胀、肠鸣、腹泻、腰痛、胁痛
26	带脉	月经不调、闭经、赤白带下、疝气、腰痛、胁痛
27	五枢	子宫或阴道脱垂、赤白带下、月经不调、少腹痛、腰胯痛
28	维道	子宫或阴道脱垂、赤白带下、月经不调、少腹痛、腰胯痛
29	居髎	腰腿痹痛、瘫痪、疝气、少腹痛

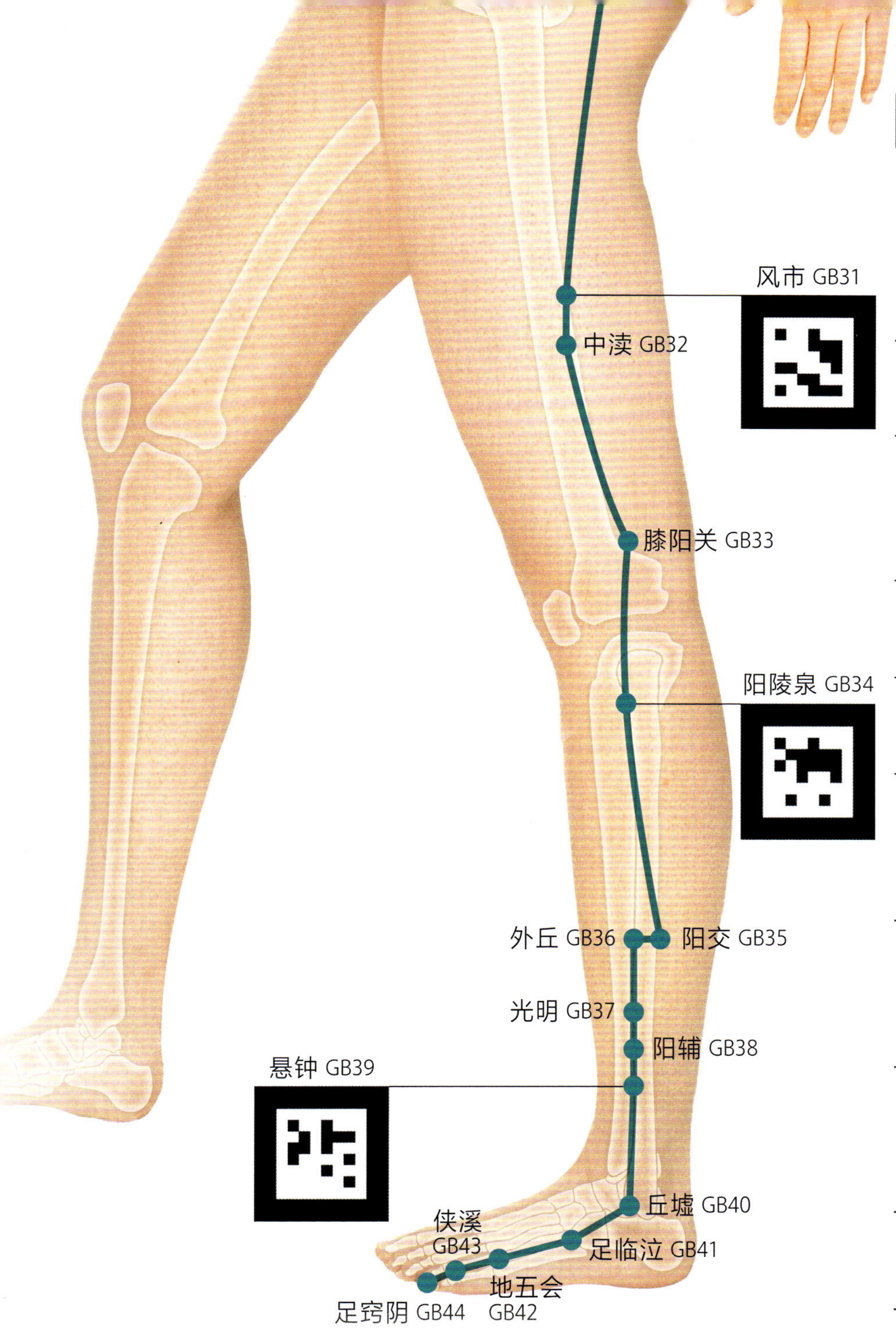

Continued

GB	Acupoints	Indications
21	Jiānjǐng	Neck stiffness and pain; shoulder periarthritis; back pain; motor impairment of upper limbs; difficult delivery; breast swelling and pain; agalactia; breast mass; cervical lymph node tuberculosis
22	Yuānyè	Chest fullness; hypochondrium pain; arthralgia of upper limbs; armpit swelling and pain
23	Zhéjīn	Chest fullness; asthma; vomiting; acid swallow; hypochondrium pain; armpit swelling; shoulder periarthritis; back pain
24	Rìyuè	Jaundice; chest and hypochondrium pain; vomiting; acid swallow; hiccup
25	Jīngmén	Dysuria; edema; abdominal distention; borborygmus; diarrhea; lower back pain; hypochondrium pain
26	Dàimài	Irregular menstruation; amenorrhea; leukorrhea with reddish discharge; hernia; lower back pain; hypochondrium pain
27	Wǔshū	Uterus prolapse and vagina prolapse; leukorrhea with reddish discharge; irregular menstruation; lower abdominal pain; lower back and hip pain
28	Wéidào	Uterus prolapse and vagina prolapse; leukorrhea with reddish discharge; irregular menstruation; lower abdominal pain; lower back and hip pain
29	Jūliáo	Arthralgia of lower back and legs; paralysis; hernia; lower abdominal pain

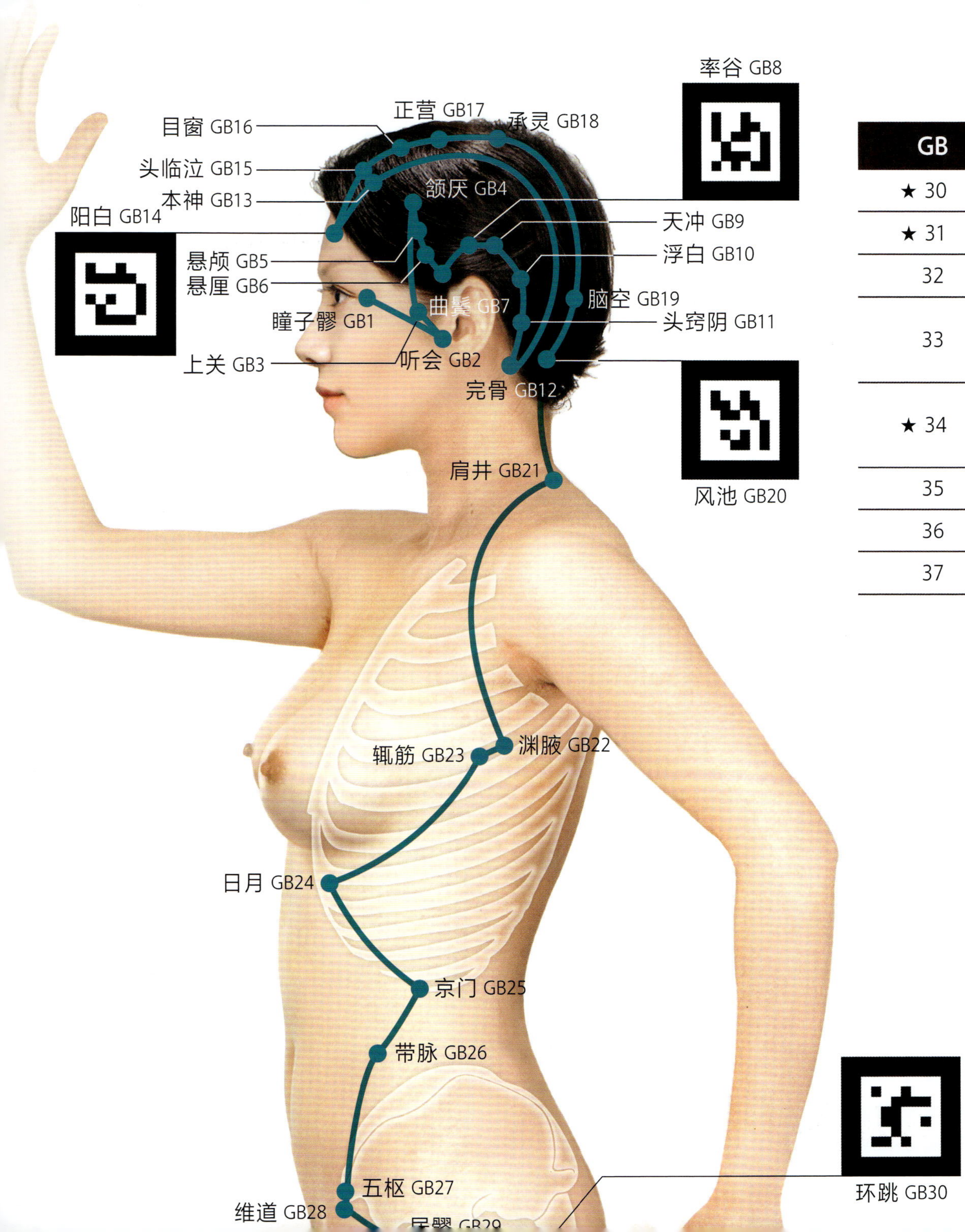

续表

GB	穴名	主治
★ 30	环跳	腰胯疼痛、下肢痿痹、半身不遂、风疹
★ 31	风市	下肢痿痹、麻木、半身不遂、遍身瘙痒
32	中渎	下肢痿痹、麻木、半身不遂
33	膝阳关	膝腘肿痛、挛急、小腿麻木、膝关节疾患
★ 34	阳陵泉	黄疸、胁痛、口苦、呕吐、吞酸、膝肿痛、下肢痿痹、膝关节疾患、小儿惊风
35	阳交	惊狂、癫痫、胸胁满痛、下肢痿痹
36	外丘	癫狂、胸胁胀满、下肢痿痹
37	光明	目痛、夜盲、乳房胀痛、下肢痿痹

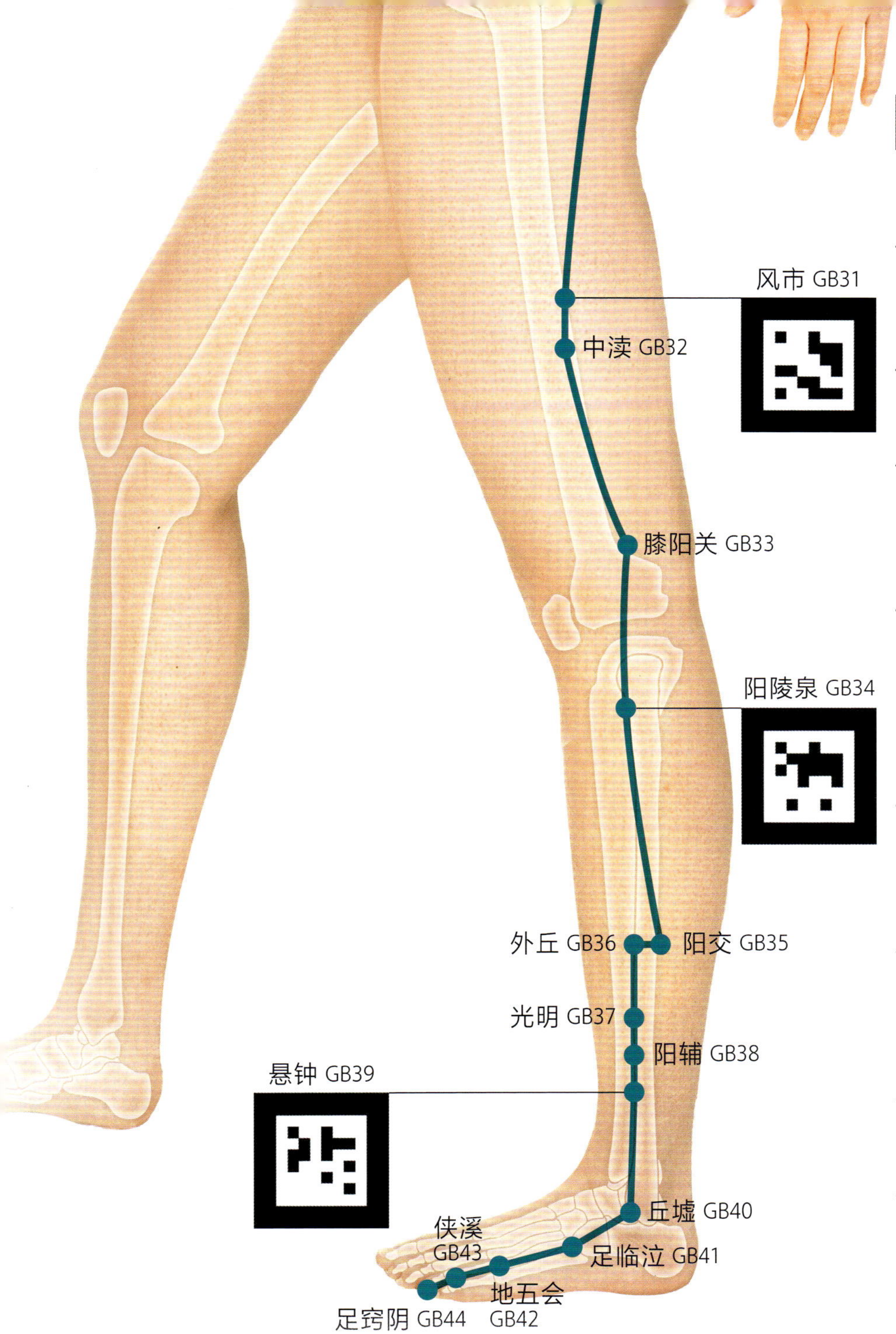

Continued

GB	Acupoints	Indications
★ 30	Huántiào	Lower back and hip pain; flaccidity and motor impairment of lower limbs; hemiplegia; rubella
★ 31	Fēngshì	Flaccidity and motor impairment of lower limbs; numb lower limbs; hemiplegia; itching all over the body
32	Zhōngdú	Flaccidity and pain of lower limbs; numb lower limbs; hemiplegia
33	Xīyángguāng	Swelling and pain of knee and popliteal fossa; spasm of knee and popliteal fossa; numbness of lower legs; knee joint diseases
★ 34	Yánglíngquán	Jaundice; hypochondrium pain; bitter taste in the mouth; vomiting; acid swallow; knee swelling and pain; flaccidity and motor impairment of lower limbs; knee joint diseases; infantile convulsion
35	Yángjiāo	Mania due to fright; epilepsy; fullness and pain of chest and hypochondrium; flaccidity and motor impairment of lower limbs
36	Wàiqiū	Manic and depressive psychosis; fullness and pain of chest and hypochondrium; flaccidity and motor impairment of lower limbs
37	Guāngmíng	Eyes pain; nyctalopia; distending pain of breast; flaccidity and motor impairment of lower limbs

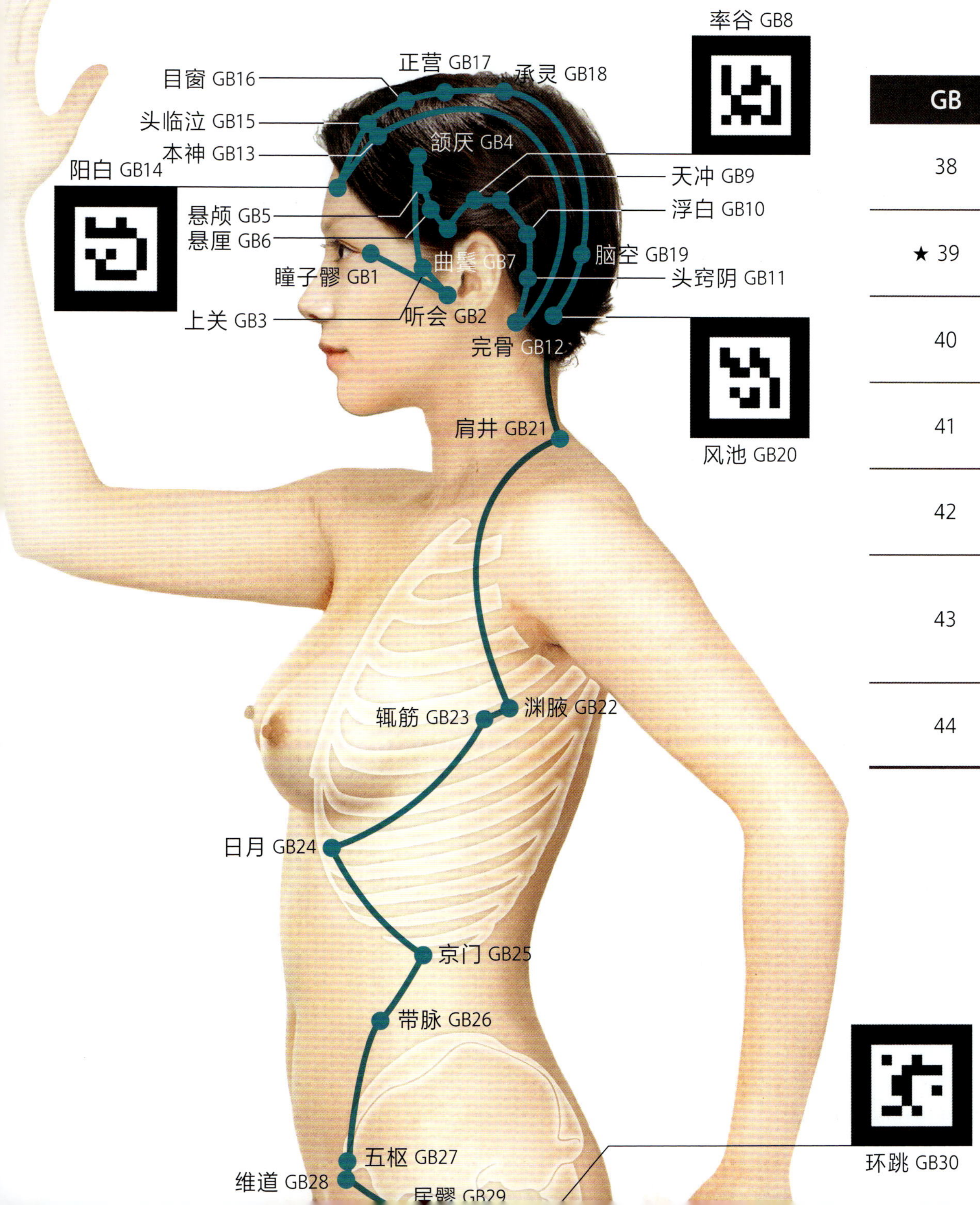

续表

GB	穴 名	主 治
38	阳辅	偏头痛、目外眦痛、咽喉肿痛、腋下肿痛、胸胁满痛、下肢痿痹
★ 39	悬钟	痴呆、中风、颈项强痛、胸胁满痛、下肢痿痹
40	丘墟	目赤肿痛、白内障、颈项痛、腋下肿痛、胸胁痛、外踝肿痛、足内翻、足下垂
41	足临泣	偏头痛、目赤肿痛、胁肋疼痛、足跟疼痛、月经不调、乳房肿痛
42	地五会	头痛、目赤肿痛、胁痛、足跟肿痛、耳鸣、耳聋、乳房肿痛
43	侠溪	惊悸、头痛、眩晕、颊肿、耳鸣、耳聋、目赤肿痛、胁肋疼痛、膝股痛、足跟肿痛、乳房肿痛、热病
44	足窍阴	头痛、目赤肿痛、耳鸣、耳聋、咽喉肿痛、胸胁痛、足跟肿痛

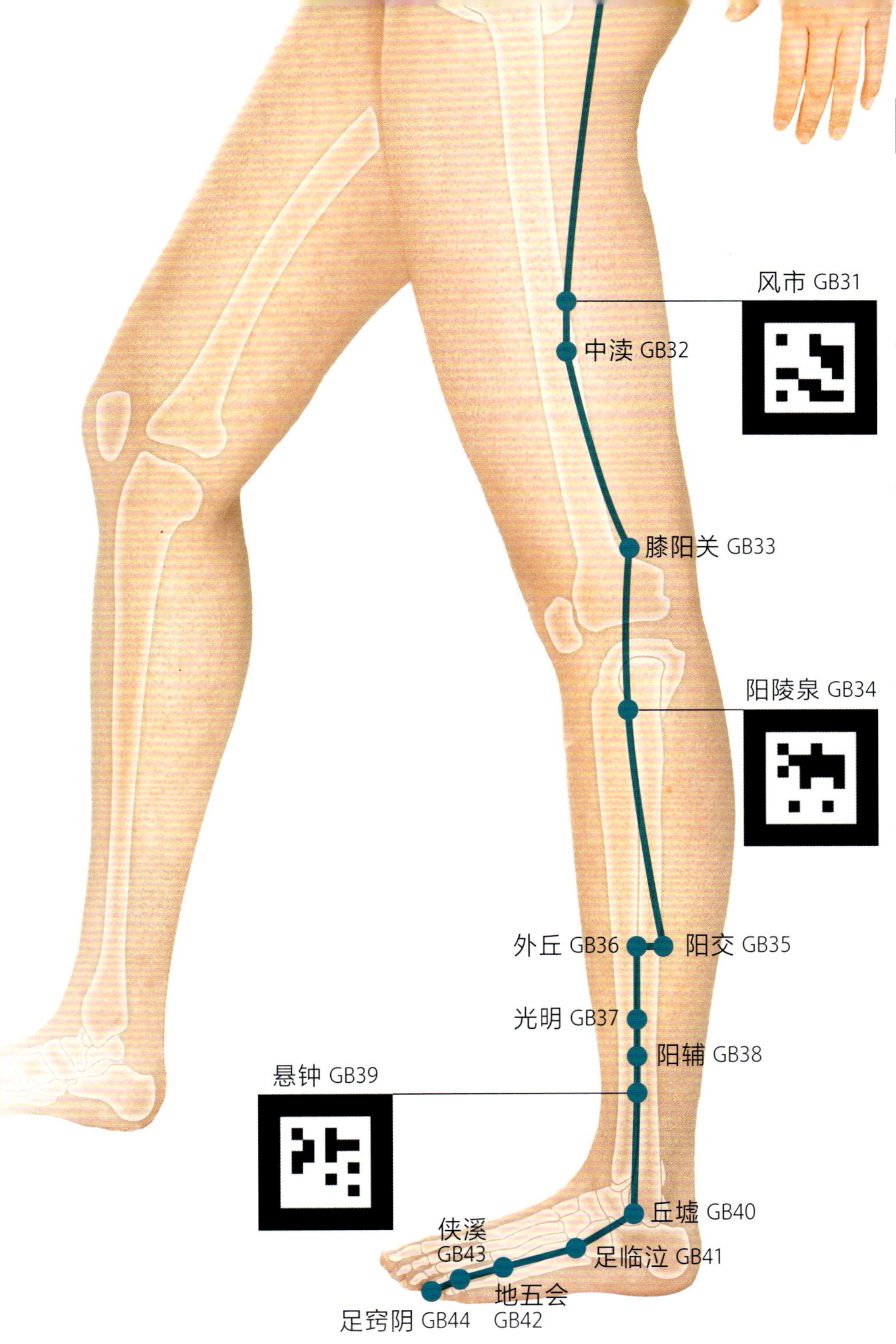

Continued

GB	Acupoints	Indications
38	Yángfǔ	Migraine; outer canthus pain; swelling and pain in throat; armpit swelling and pain; fullness and pain of chest and hypochondrium; flaccidity and motor impairment of lower limbs
★ 39	Xuánzhōng	Dementia; wind stroke; neck stiffness and pain; fullness and pain of chest and hypochondrium; flaccidity and motor impairment of lower limbs
40	Qiūxū	Redness, swelling and pain of eyes; cataract; neck pain; armpit swelling and pain; chest and hypochondrium pain; lateral malleolus swelling and pain; strephenopodia; drooping foot
41	Zúlínqì	Migraine; redness, swelling and pain of eyes; pain in hypochondrium and rib; heel pain; irregular menstruation; breast swelling and pain
42	Dìwǔhuì	Headache; redness, swelling and pain of eyes; hypochondrium pain; heel swelling and pain; tinnitus; deafness; breast swelling and pain
43	Xiáxī	Palpitation due to fright; headache; dizziness; swollen cheek; tinnitus; deafness; redness, swelling and pain of eyes; pain in hypochondrium and rib; knee and thigh pain; heel swelling and pain; breast swelling and pain; febrile diseases
44	Zúqiàoyīn	Headache; redness, swelling and pain of eyes; tinnitus; deafness; swelling and pain in throat; chest and hypochondrium pain; heel swelling and pain

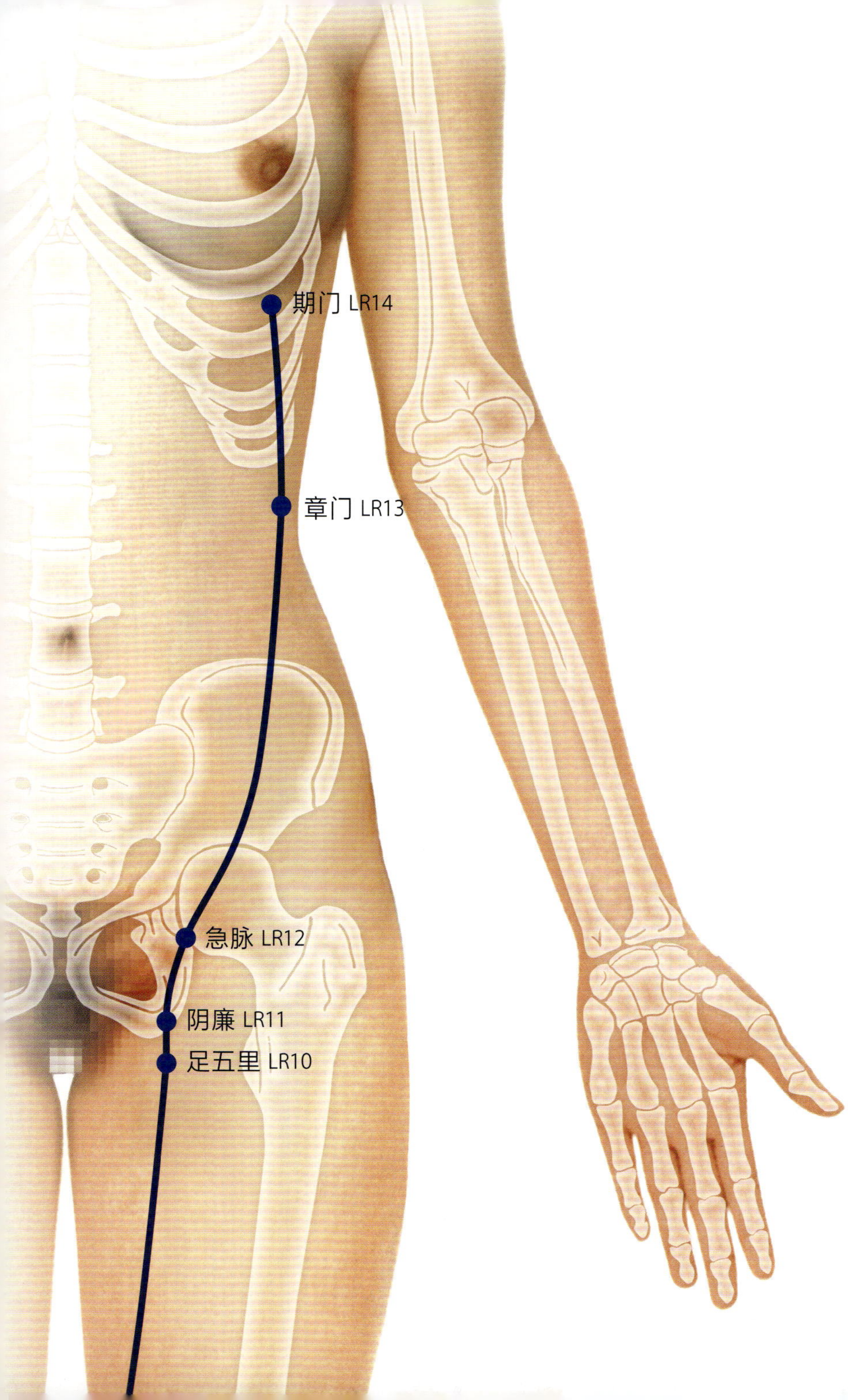

足厥阴肝经

足厥阴肝经起于足跗趾外侧的大敦，沿腿部内侧往上，经腹部，止于乳房下方的期门。

肝经所治病症：肝炎、胆囊炎、胃痛等肝胆脾胃疾患；女性阴道脱垂、阴部瘙痒或湿疹、排尿困难、遗尿等前阴病；咽干、咽痛、咽中异物感、青光眼、近视、视网膜病变，面瘫、三叉神经痛、面肌痉挛，头顶胀痛等头面五官疾患；下肢内侧麻木、痿痹等经脉循行部位的疾患。

LR	穴 名	主 治
1	大敦	疝气、遗尿、癃闭、五淋、尿血、月经不调、崩漏、子宫或阴道脱垂、癫痫、善寐
2	行间	中风、癫狂、头痛、目眩、目赤肿痛、口歪、月经不调、痛经、闭经、崩漏、带下、疝气、遗尿、癃闭、五淋、胸胁满痛
★ 3	太冲	中风、癫狂、小儿惊风、头痛、眩晕、耳鸣、目赤肿痛、口歪、咽痛、月经不调、痛经、经闭、崩漏、带下、黄疸、胁痛、腹胀、呕逆、癃闭、遗尿、下肢痿痹、足跟肿痛

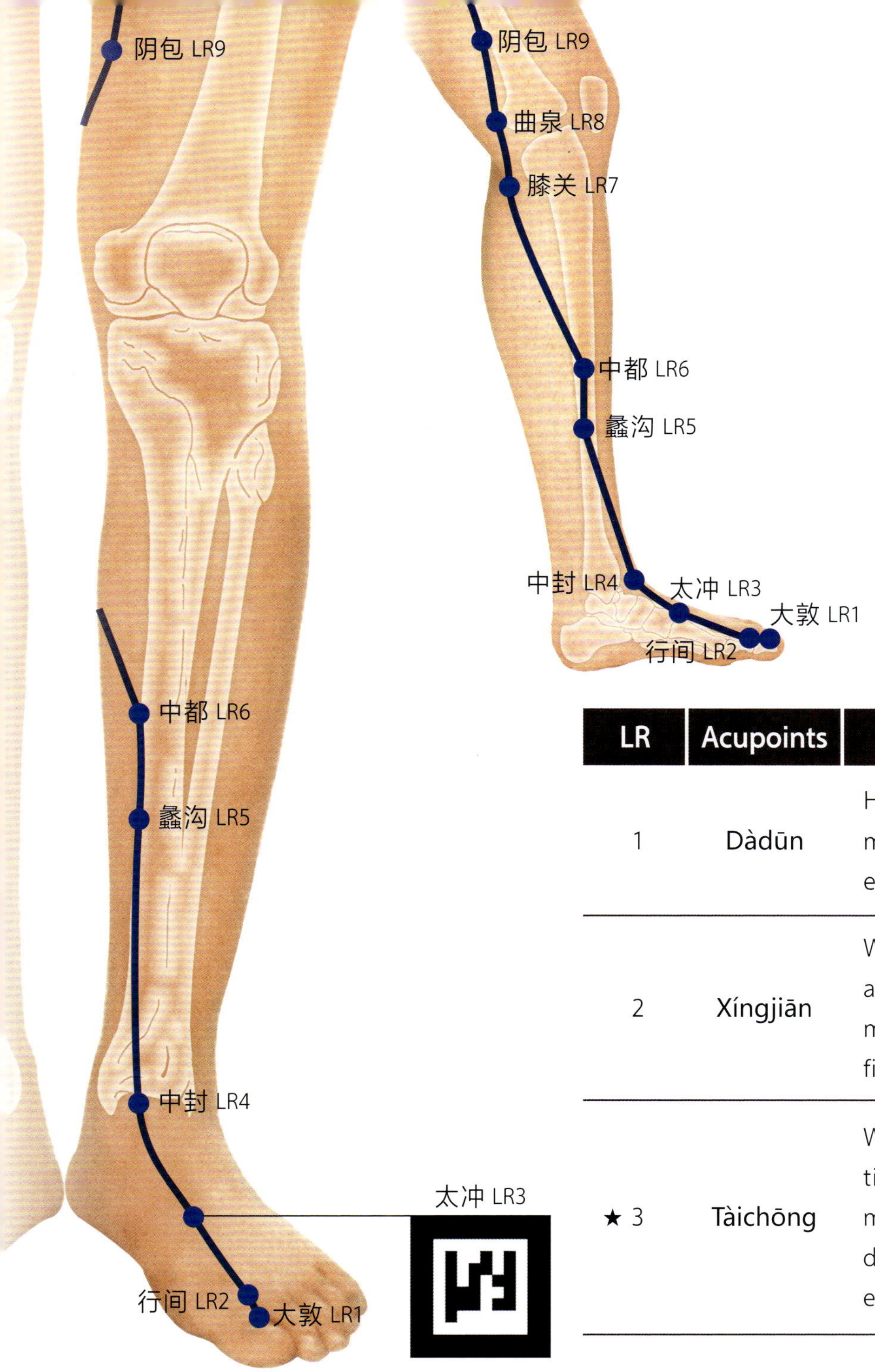

Liver Meridian of Foot-Jueyin, LR.

Liver Meridian of Foot-Jueyin emerges from Dadun (LR1) in lateral side of the foot great toe, runs upwardly along medial side of the legs and through abdomen, then it terminates at Qimen (LR14) under the breast.

Liver Meridian treats diseases of liver, gallbladder, spleen and stomach including hepatitis, cholecystitis and stomachache; external genitalia diseases including prolapsed vagina, itching vagina, eczema, difficult urination and enuresis; diseases of head, face and five sensory organs including dry throat, throat pain, foreign body sensation in throat, glaucoma, myopia, retinopathy, facial paralysis, prosopalgia, spasm of facial muscles and distending pain in the top of head; diseases of parts that meridian is running along including numbness, flaccidity and motor impairment in medial side of lower limbs.

LR	Acupoints	Indications
1	Dàdūn	Hernia; enuresis; retention of urine; five stranguries diseases; bloody urine; irregular menstruation; metrorrhagia and metrostaxis; uterus prolapse and vagina prolapse; epilepsy; lethargy
2	Xíngjiān	Wind stroke; manic and depressive psychosis; headache; dizziness; redness, swelling and pain of eyes; mouth deviation; irregular menstruation; dysmenorrhea; amenorrhea; metrorrhagia and metrostaxis; leukorrheal diseases; hernia; enuresis; retention of urine; five stranguries diseases; fullness and pain of chest and hypochondrium
★ 3	Tàichōng	Wind stroke; manic and depressive psychosis; infantile convulsion; headache; dizziness; tinnitus; redness, swelling and pain of eyes; mouth deviation; throat pain; irregular menstruation; dysmenorrhea; amenorrhea; metrorrhagia and metrostaxis; leukorrheal diseases; jaundice; hypochondrium pain; abdominal distention; hiccup; retention of urine; enuresis; flaccidity and motor impairment of lower limbs; heel swelling and pain

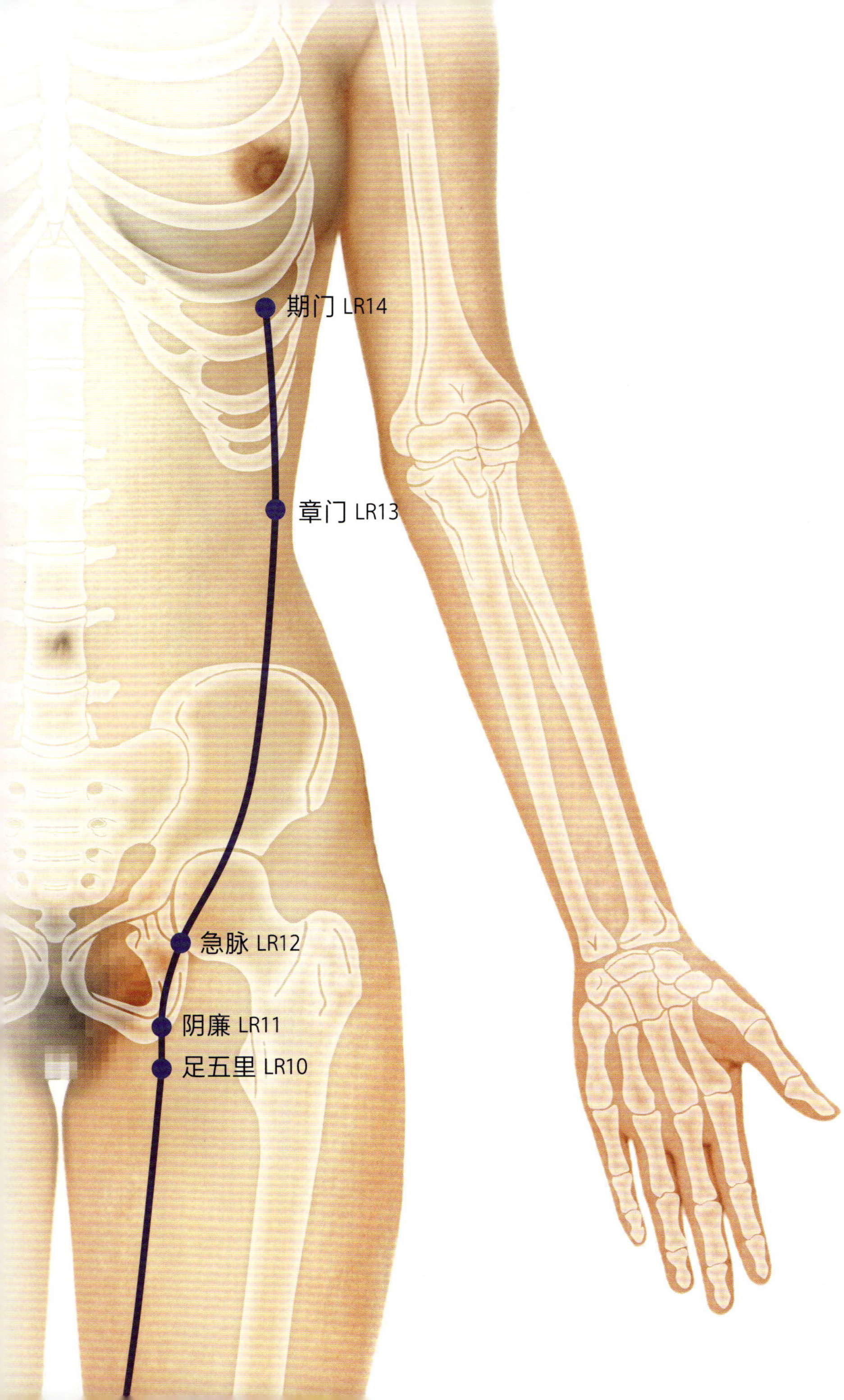

续表

LR	穴名	主治
4	中封	疝气、遗精、小便不利、腰痛、少腹痛、内踝肿痛
5	蠡沟	月经不调、赤白带下、子宫或阴道脱垂、外阴瘙痒、小便不利、疝气、睾丸肿痛
6	中都	疝气、小腹痛、崩漏、恶露不尽、泄泻
7	膝关	膝部肿痛、下肢痿痹
8	曲泉	月经不调、痛经、带下、子宫或阴道脱垂、外阴瘙痒、产后腹痛、遗精、阳痿、疝气、小便不利、膝部肿痛、下肢痿痹
9	阴包	月经不调、小便不利、遗尿、腰骶痛引少腹
10	足五里	少腹痛、小便不通、子宫或阴道脱垂、睾丸肿痛、颈淋巴结结核
11	阴廉	月经不调、带下、少腹痛
12	急脉	少腹痛、疝气、子宫或阴道脱垂
13	章门	腹痛、腹胀、肠鸣、腹泻、呕吐、胁痛、黄疸、肝脾肿大
14	期门	胸胁胀痛、呕吐、吞酸、腹胀、腹泻、气上冲心、乳房肿痛

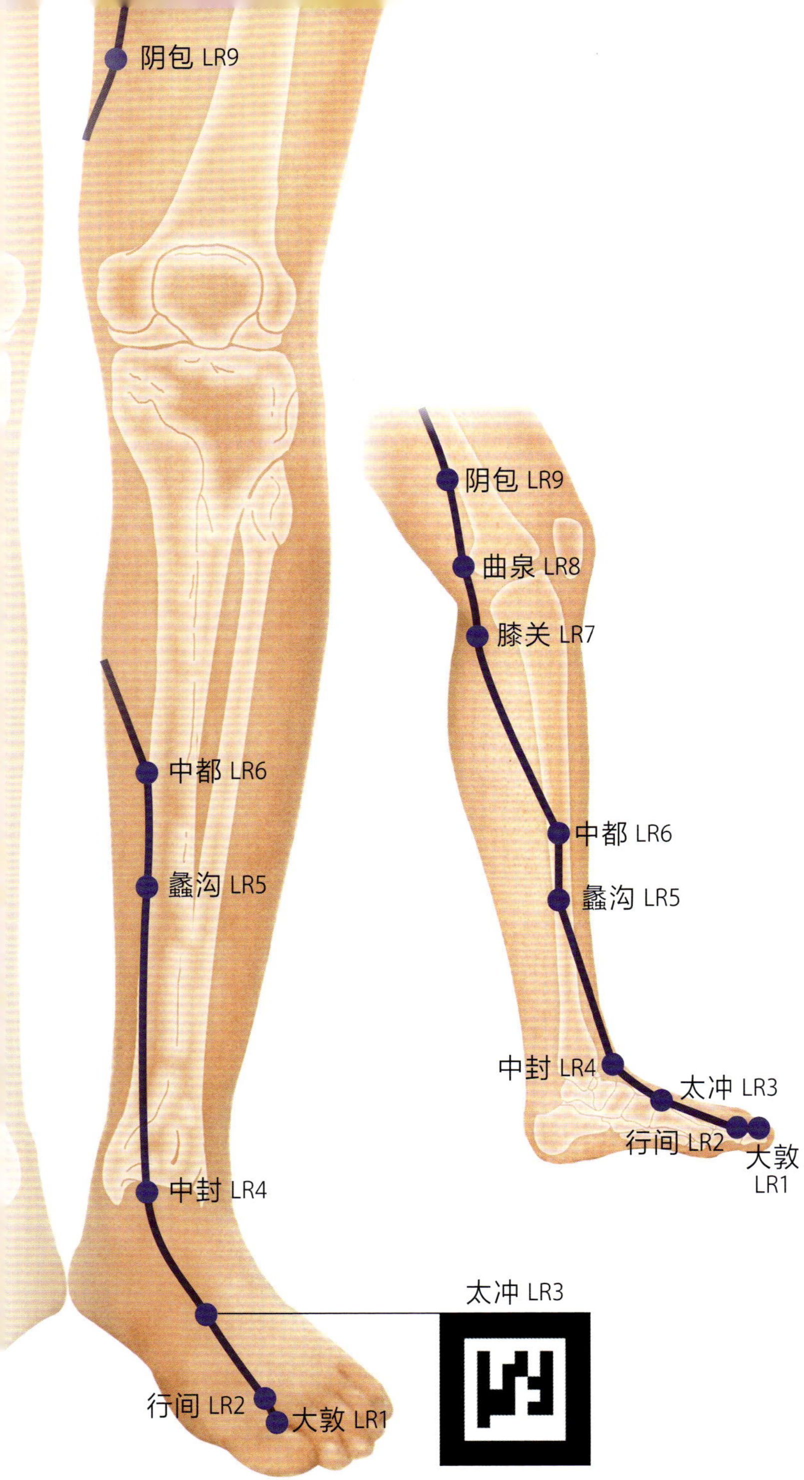

Continued

LR	Acupoints	Indications
4	Zhōngfēng	Hernia; seminal emission; dysuria; lower back pain; lower abdominal pain; interior malleolus swelling and pain
5	Lígōu	Irregular menstruation; leukorrhea with reddish discharge; uterus prolapse and vagina prolapse; outer genitalia itching; dysuria; hernia; swelling and pain of testicle
6	Zhōngdū	Hernia; little abdominal pain; metrorrhagia and metrostaxis; lochiorrhea; diarrhea
7	Xīguān	Swelling and pain of knees; flaccidity and motor impairment of lower limbs
8	Qūquán	Irregular menstruation; dysmenorrhea; leukorrheal diseases; uterus prolapse and vagina prolapse; outer genitalia itching; abdominal pain after delivery; seminal emission; impotence; hernia; dysuria; swelling and pain of knee; flaccidity and motor impairment of lower limbs
9	Yīnbāo	Irregular menstruation; dysuria; enuresis; lumbosacral pain radiating to lower abdomen
10	Zúwǔlǐ	Lower abdominal pain; retention of urine; uterus prolapse and vagina prolapse; swelling and pain of testicle; cervical lymph node tuberculosis
11	Yīnlián	Irregular menstruation; leukorrheal diseases; lower abdominal pain
12	Jímài	Lower abdominal pain; hernia; uterus prolapse and vagina prolapse
13	Zhāngmén	Abdominal pain; abdominal distention; borborygmus; diarrhea; vomiting; hypochondrium pain; jaundice; hepatosplenomegaly
14	Qīmén	Distending pain of chest and hypochondrium; vomiting; acid swallow; abdominal distention; diarrhea; reflux of Qi to the heart; swelling and pain of breast

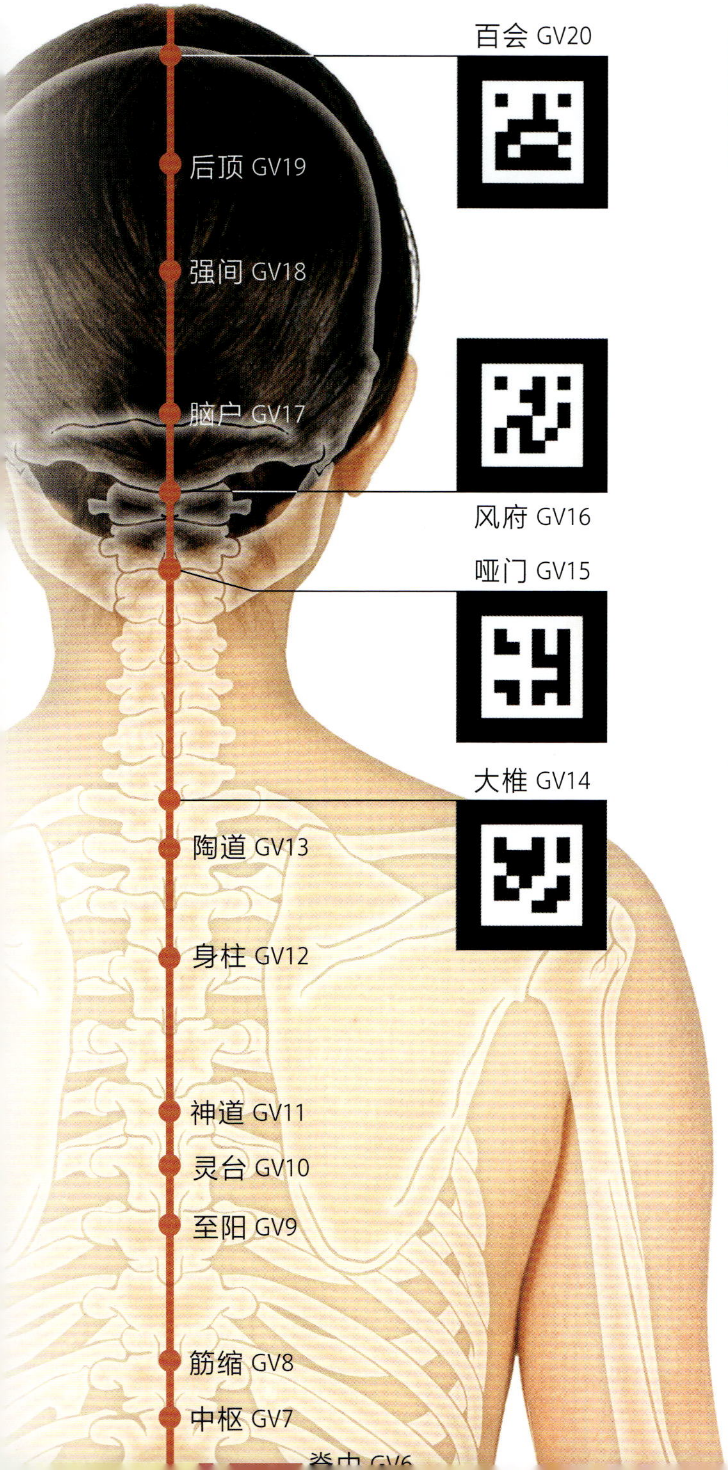

督脉

督脉起于腹部，下出于会阴部，向后行于脊柱，上至头顶，沿前额下行鼻柱。

督脉主治病症：头痛、头晕、健忘、耳鸣、目眩、失眠、颈部强直疼痛等头面五官疾患；颈椎病、急性腰扭伤、强直性脊柱炎等脊柱病变；癫、狂、痫等神志疾患。

GV	穴 名	主 治
1	长强	腹泻、痢疾、便血、便秘、痔疮、脱肛、癫狂、腰脊和尾骶部疼痛
2	腰俞	腹泻、痢疾、便血、便秘、痔疮、脱肛、月经不调、经闭、腰脊强痛、下肢痿痹、痫证
3	腰阳关	腰骶疼痛、下肢痿痹、月经不调、赤白带下、遗精、阳痿
★ 4	命门	腰脊强痛、下肢痿痹、月经不调、赤白带下、痛经、经闭、不孕、遗精、阳痿、精冷不育、小便频数、小腹冷痛、腹泻

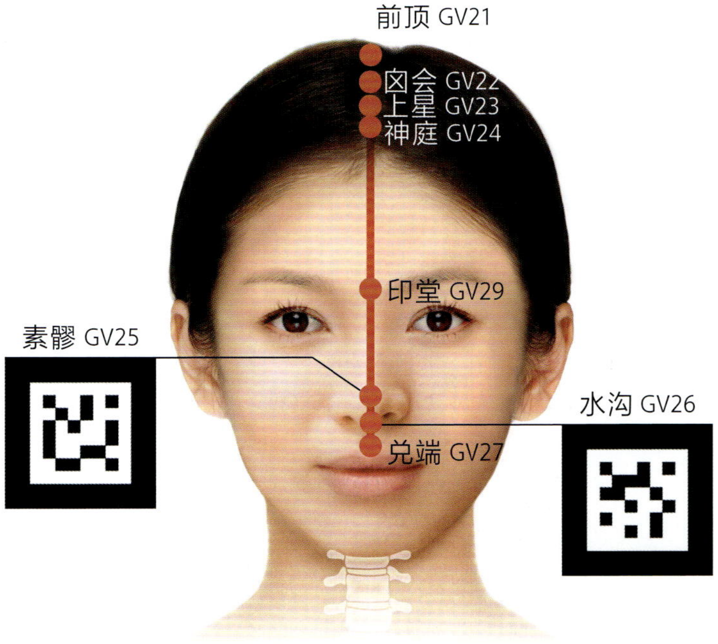

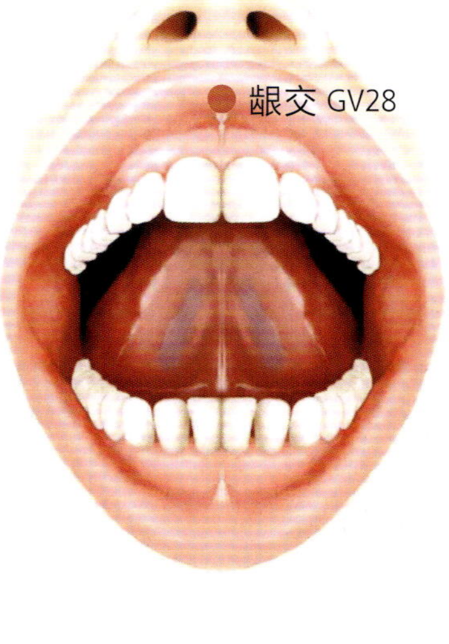

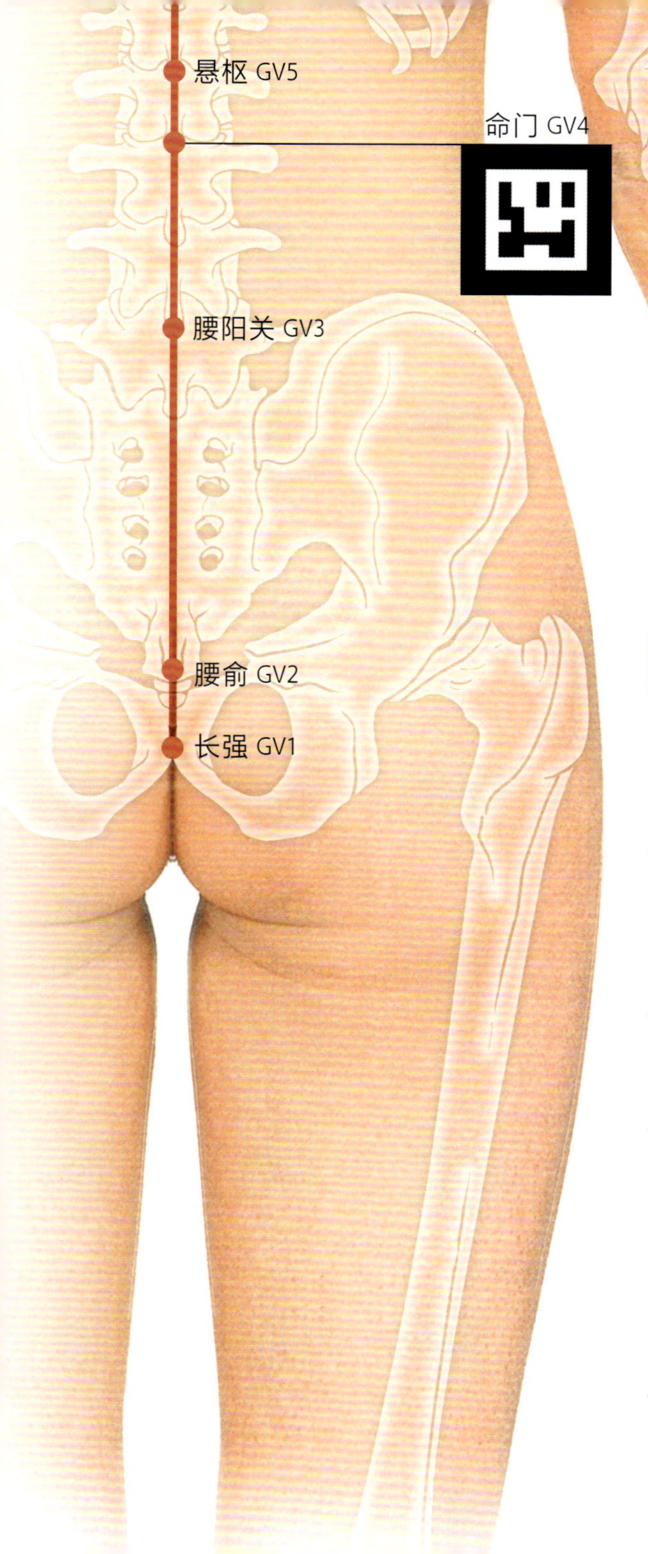

Governor Vessel Meridian, GV.

Governor Vessel Meridian emerges from the abdomen, upwardly comes out of perineum, backwardly runs along the spine upward to the top of head and downward to nasal septum along the forehead.

Governor Vessel Meridian mainly treats diseases of head, face and five sensory organs including headache, dizziness, amnesia, tinnitus, vertigo, insomnia and stiffness and pain of neck; spine diseases including cervical spondylopathy, acute sprain of lower back and ankylosing spondylitis; mental diseases including depressive psychosis, mania and epilepsy.

GV	Acupoints	Indications
1	Chángqiáng	Diarrhea; dysentery; bloody stool; constipation; hemorrhoids; prolapse of rectum; manic and depressive psychosis; pain in lower back, spine, coccygis and sacrum
2	Yāoshū	Diarrhea; dysentery; bloody stool; constipation; hemorrhoids; prolapse of rectum; irregular menstruation; amenorrhea; stiffness and pain of lower back and spine; flaccidity and motor impairment of lower limbs; epilepsy
3	Yāoyángguān	Lumbosacral pain; flaccidity and motor impairment of lower limbs; irregular menstruation; leukorrhea with reddish discharge; seminal emission; impotence
★ 4	Mìngmén	Stiffness and pain of lower back and spine; flaccidity and motor impairment of lower limbs; irregular menstruation; leukorrhea with reddish discharge; dysmenorrhea; amenorrhea; sterility; seminal emission; impotence; infertility due to cold sperm; frequent urination; lower abdominal coldness and pain; diarrhea

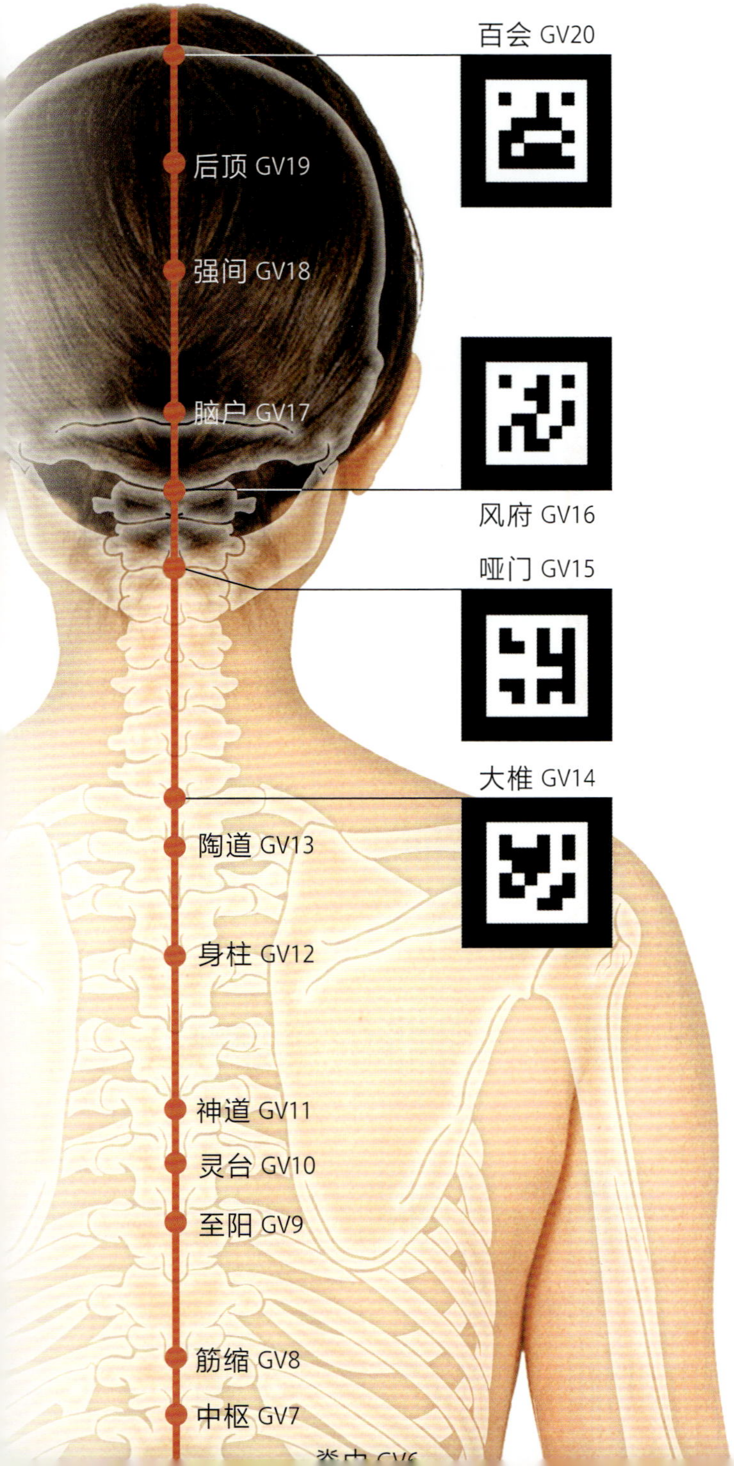

续表

GV	穴名	主治
5	悬枢	腰脊强痛、腹胀、腹痛、完谷不化、腹泻、痢疾
6	脊中	癫狂、黄疸、腹泻、痢疾、痔疮、脱肛、便血、腰脊强痛、小儿疳积
7	中枢	黄疸、呕吐、腹满、胃痛、食欲不振、腰背疼痛
8	筋缩	癫狂、抽搐、脊强、四肢不收、筋挛拘急、胃痛、黄疸
9	至阳	黄疸、胸胁胀满、咳嗽、气喘、腰背疼痛、脊强
10	灵台	咳嗽、气喘、脊痛、项强、疔疮
11	神道	心痛、心悸、怔忡、失眠、健忘、中风不语、痫证、神志病、咳嗽、气喘、腰脊强、肩周炎、背痛
12	身柱	身热、头痛、咳嗽、气喘、惊厥、癫狂、腰脊强痛、疔疮发背
13	陶道	热病、寒战发热、恶寒发热、咳嗽、气喘、骨蒸潮热、癫狂、脊强

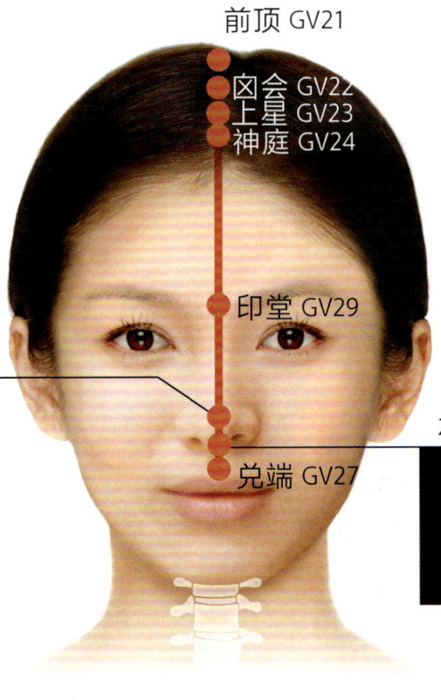

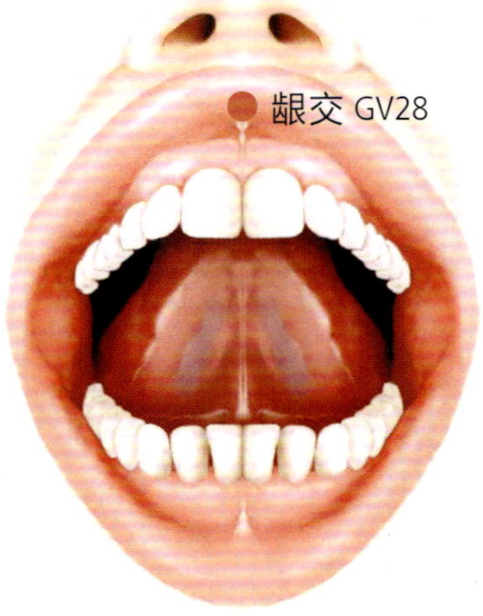

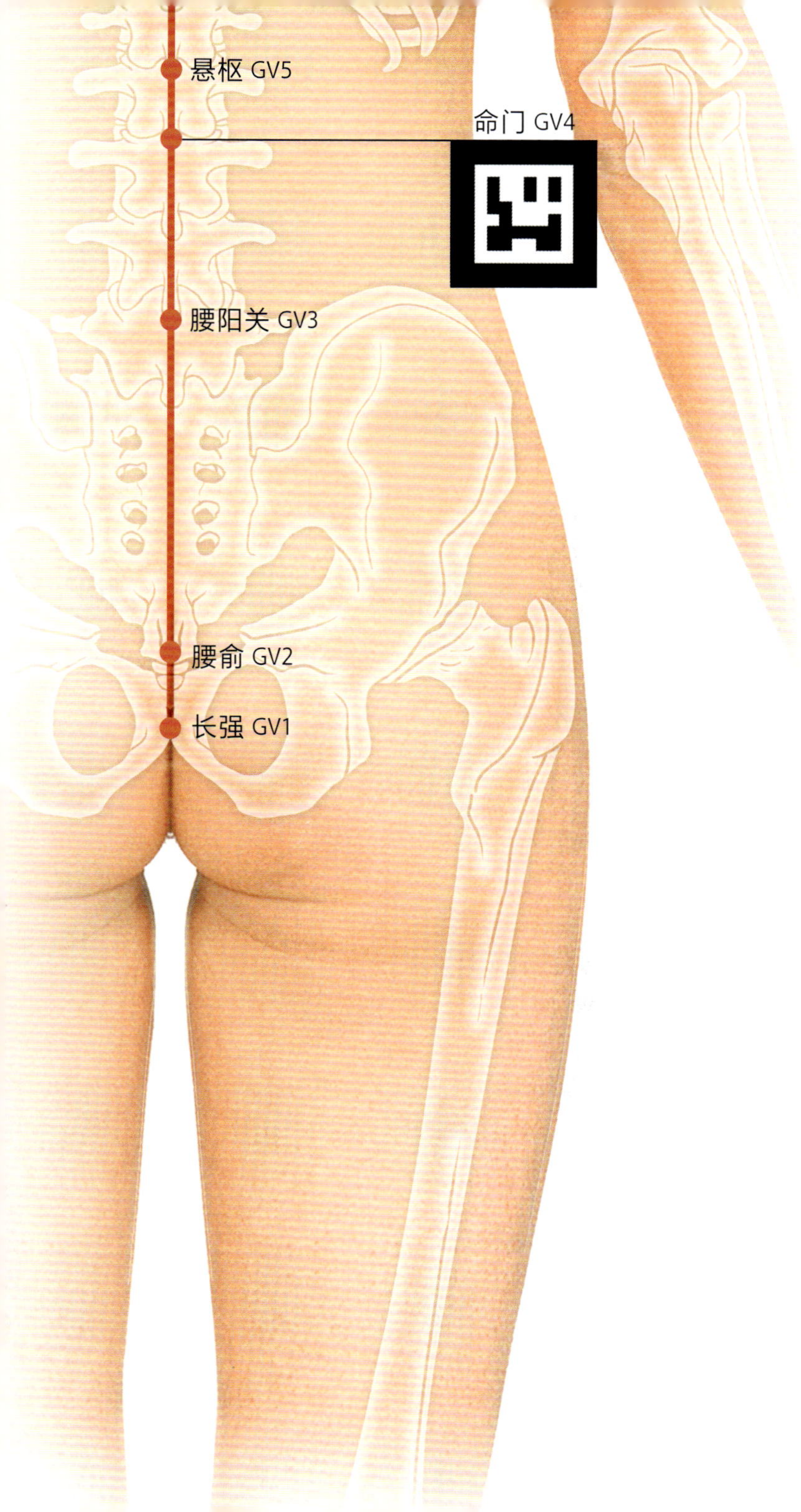

Continued

GV	Acupoints	Indications
5	Xuánshū	Stiffness and pain of lower back and spine; abdominal distention; abdominal pain; indigestion; diarrhea; dysentery
6	Jǐzhōng	Manic and depressive psychosis; jaundice; diarrhea; dysentery; hemorrhoids; prolapse of rectum; bloody stool; stiffness and pain of lower back and spine; infantile malnutrition
7	Zhōngshū	Jaundice; vomiting; abdominal fullness; stomachache; poor appetite; lumbago and back pain
8	Jīnsuō	Manic and depressive psychosis; convulsion; spine stiffness; flaccidity of four extremities; spasm of sinew; stomachache; jaundice
9	Zhìyáng	Jaundice; distention and fullness of chest and hypochondrium; cough; asthma; lumbago and back pain; spine stiffness
10	Língtái	Cough; asthma; spine pain; neck stiffness; deep-rooted boil
11	Shéndào	Cardiac pain; palpitation; severe palpitation; insomnia; amnesia; aphasia from wind stroke; manic and depressive psychosis; mental disorder; cough; asthma; lower back and spine pain; shoulder periarthritis; back pain
12	Shēnzhù	Fever; headache; cough; asthma; syncope due to fright; manic and depressive psychosis; stiffness and pain of lower back and spine; deep-rooted boil in the back
13	Táodào	Febrile diseases; chill and fever; cough; asthma; tidal fever and steaming bone; manic and depressive psychosis; spine stiffness

续表

GV	穴 名	主 治
★ 14	大椎	热病、寒战发热、恶寒发热、咳嗽、气喘、骨蒸潮热、癫狂、小儿惊风、项强、脊痛、风疹、痤疮
★ 15	哑门	急性咽喉炎、舌缓不语、癫狂、癫痫、癔症、头痛、颈项强痛
★ 16	风府	中风、癫狂、癫痫、癔症、头痛、眩晕、颈项强痛、咽喉肿痛、失音、目痛、鼻出血
17	脑户	头晕、项强、失音、癫狂
18	强间	头痛、目眩、项强、癫狂
19	后顶	头痛、眩晕、癫狂
★ 20	百会	痴呆、中风、失语、失眠、健忘、癫狂、癔症、头风、头痛、眩晕、耳鸣、脱肛、子宫或阴道脱垂、胃下垂
21	前顶	头痛、眩晕、鼻窦炎、癫狂
22	囟会	头痛、眩晕、鼻窦炎、癫狂

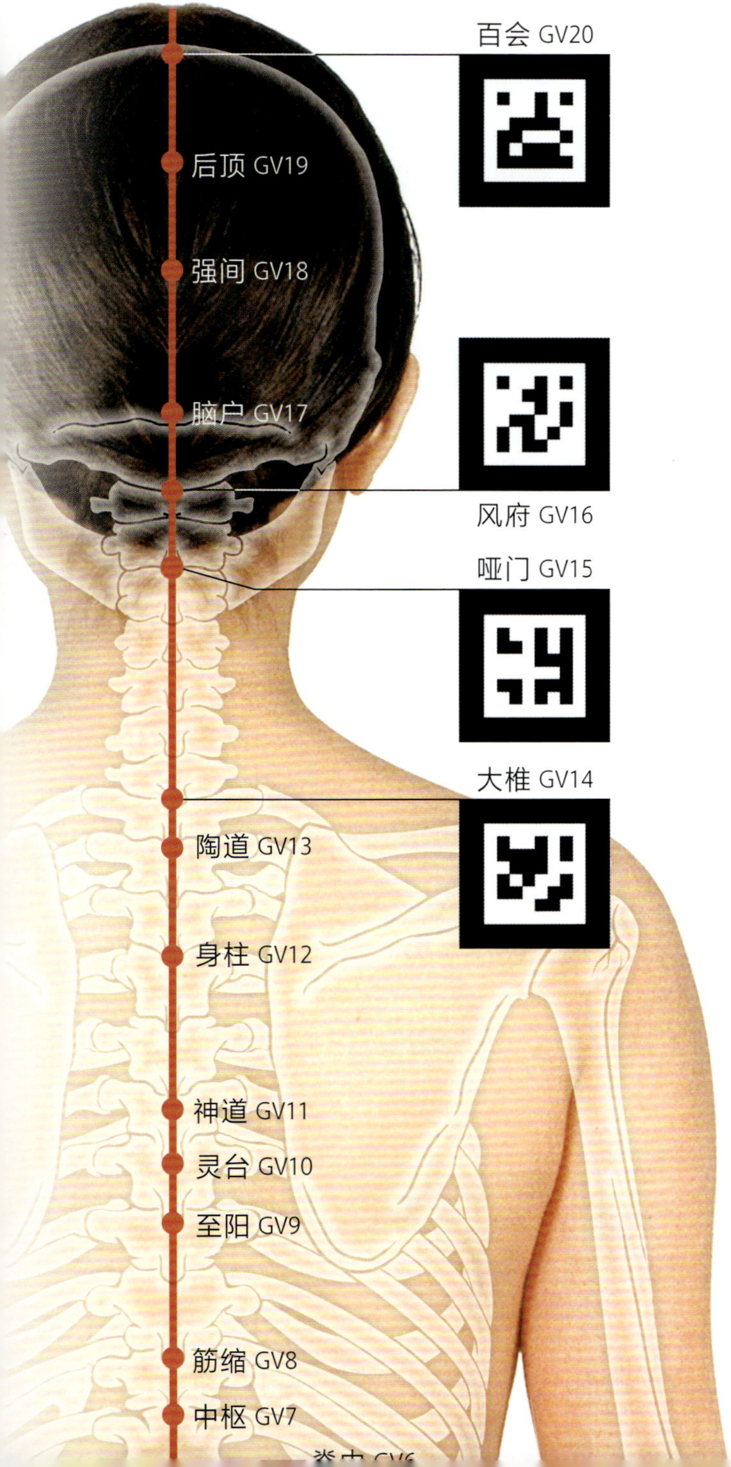

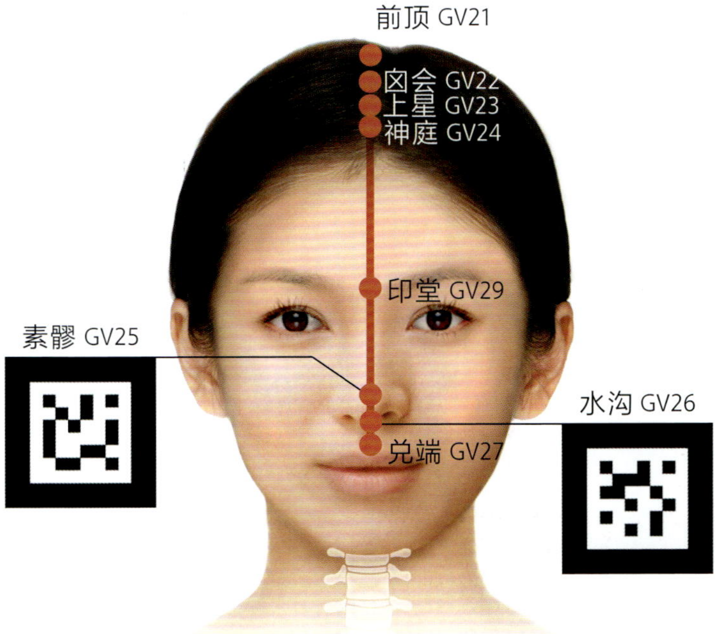

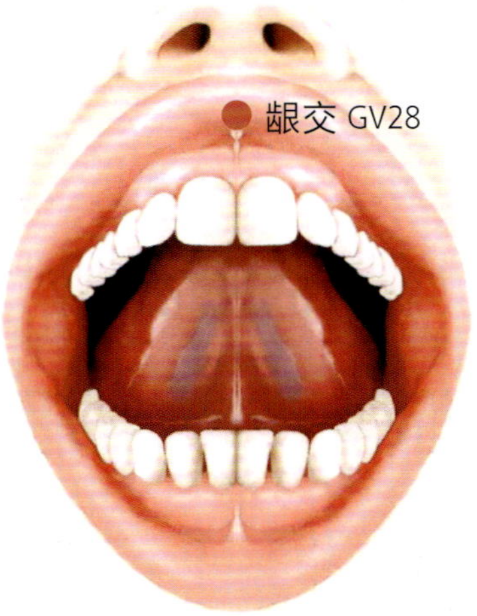

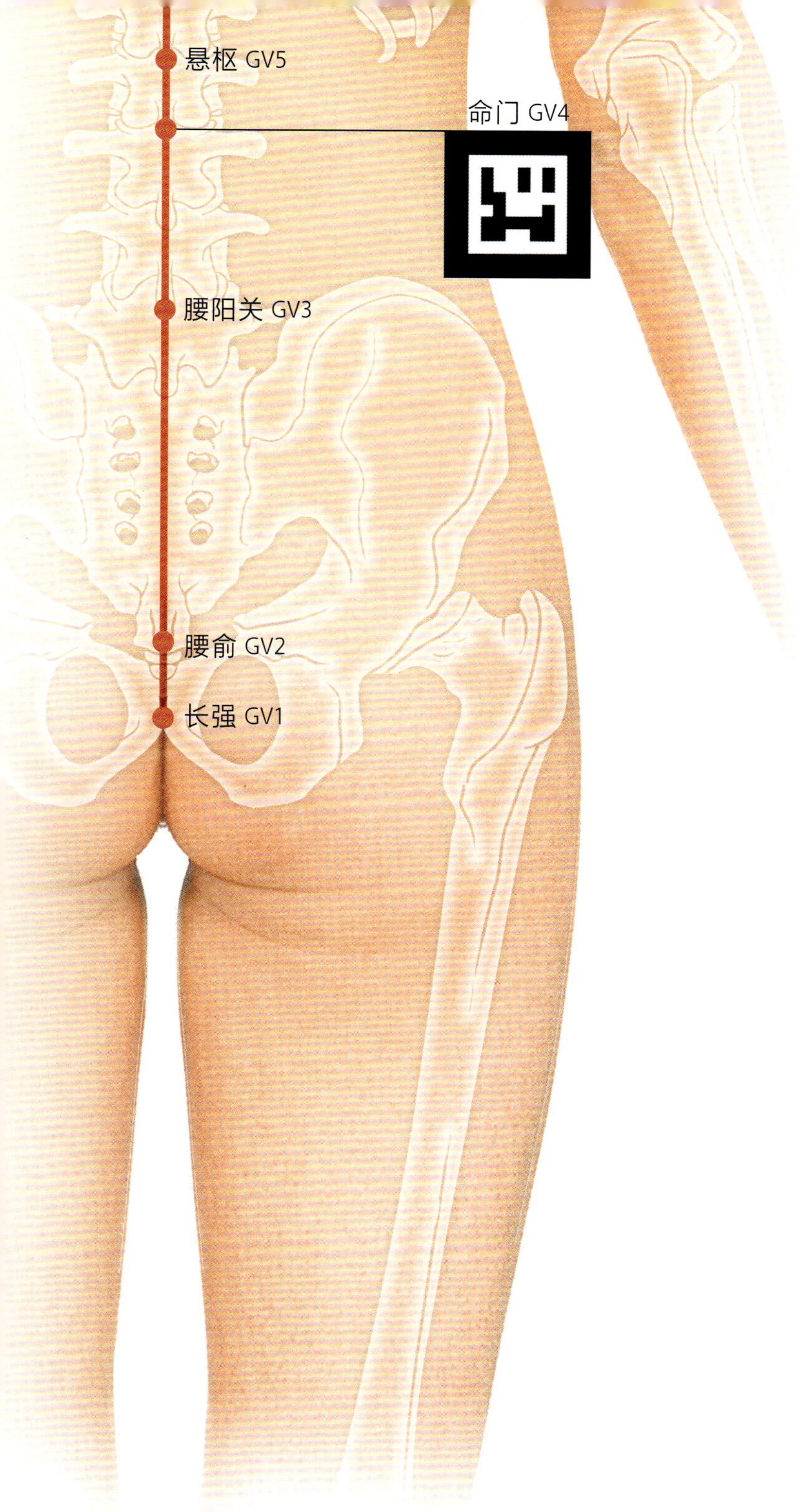

Continued

GV	Acupoints	Indications
★ 14	Dàzhuī	Febrile diseases; chill and fever; aversion to cold with fever; cough; asthma; tidal fever and steaming bone; manic and depressive psychosis; infantile convulsion; neck stiffness; spine pain; rubella; hemorrhoids
★ 15	Yǎmén	Acute sphagitis; aphasia due to flaccid tongue; manic and depressive psychosis; epilepsy; hysteria; headache; neck stiffness and pain
★ 16	Fēngfǔ	Wind stroke; manic and depressive psychosis; epilepsy; hysteria; headache; dizziness; neck stiffness and pain;swelling and pain in throat; loss of voice; eyes pain; nose bleeding
17	Nǎohù	Dizziness; neck stiffness; loss of voice; manic and depressive psychosis
18	Qiángjiān	Headache; dizziness; neck stiffness; manic and depressive psychosis
19	Hòudǐng	Headache; dizziness; manic and depressive psychosis
★ 20	Bǎihuì	Dementia; wind stroke; aphasia; insomnia; amnesia; manic and depressive psychosis; hysteria; recurrent headache; headache; dizziness; tinnitus; prolapse of rectum; uterus prolapse and vagina prolapse; drooping stomach
21	Qiándǐng	Headache; dizziness; sinusitis; manic and depressive psychosis
22	Xìnhuì	Headache; dizziness; sinusitis; manic and depressive psychosis

续表

GV	穴 名	主 治
23	上星	头痛、目痛、鼻窦炎、鼻出血、热病、寒战发热、癫狂
24	神庭	癫狂、失眠、惊悸、头痛、目眩、目赤、白内障、鼻窦炎、鼻出血
★ 25	素髎	昏迷、惊厥、新生儿窒息、休克、呼吸衰竭、鼻窦炎、鼻出血
★ 26	水沟	昏迷、晕厥、中风、中暑、休克、呼吸衰竭、癔症、癫狂、急慢惊风、鼻塞、鼻出血、面肿、口歪、齿痛、牙关紧闭、闪挫腰痛，是急救要穴之一
27	兑端	昏迷、晕厥、癫狂、癔症、口歪、口噤、口臭、齿痛
28	龈交	口歪、口噤、口臭、齿衄、齿痛、鼻出血、面赤颊肿、癫狂
29	印堂	头痛、眩晕、失眠、小儿惊风、鼻塞、鼻渊、眉棱骨痛、目痛

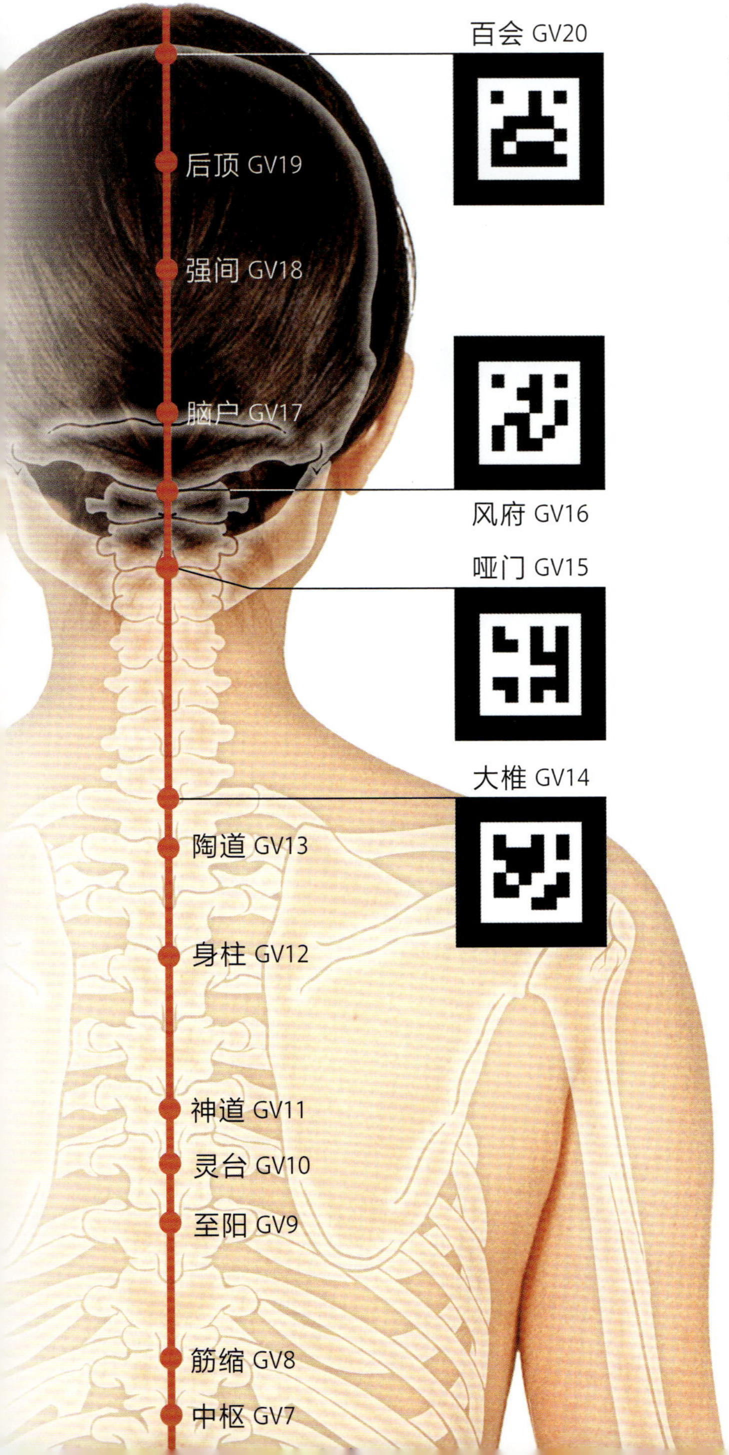

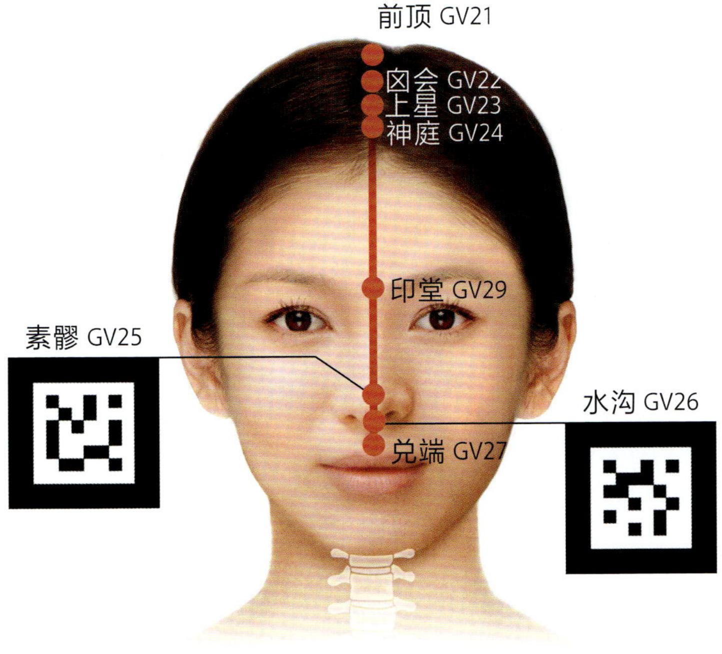

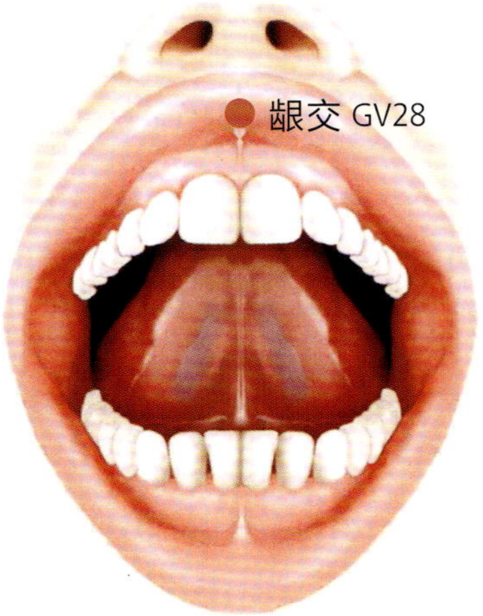

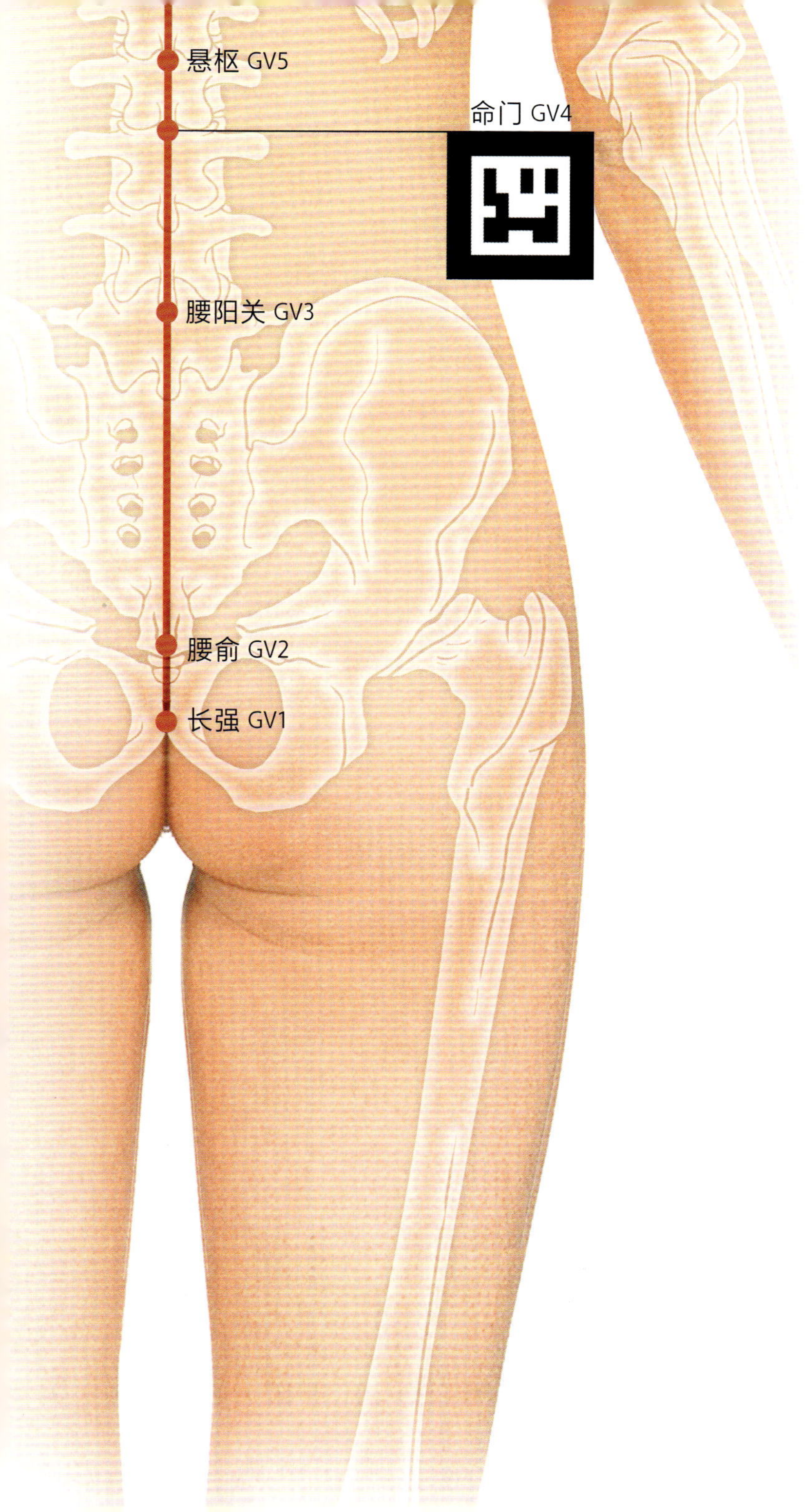

Continued

GV	Acupoints	Indications
23	Shàngxīng	Headache; eyes pain; sinusitis; nose bleeding; febrile diseases; chill and fever; manic and depressive psychosis
24	Shéntíng	Manic and depressive psychosis;insomnia; palpitation due to fright; headache; dizziness; red eyes; cataract; sinusitis; nose bleeding
★ 25	Sùliáo	Coma; syncope due to fright; asphyxia neonatorum; shock; respiratory failure; sinusitis; nose bleeding
★ 26	Shuǐgōu	Coma; syncope; wind stroke; heat stroke; shock; respiratory failure; hysteria; manic and depressive psychosis; acute and chronic convulsion; hysteria; nasal obstruction; nose bleeding; swollen face; mouth deviation; toothache; lockjaw; lower back pain due to sudden sprain or contusion; used for emergency treatment
27	Duìduān	Coma; syncope; manic and depressive psychosis; hysteria; mouth deviation; lockjaw; halitosis; toothache
28	Yínjiāo	Mouth deviation; lockjaw; halitosis; gum bleeding; toothache; nose bleeding; red face and swollen cheek; manic and depressive psychosis
29	Yìntáng	Headache; dizziness; insomnia; infantile convulsion; nasal obstruction; sinusitis; supraorbital ridge pain; eyes pain

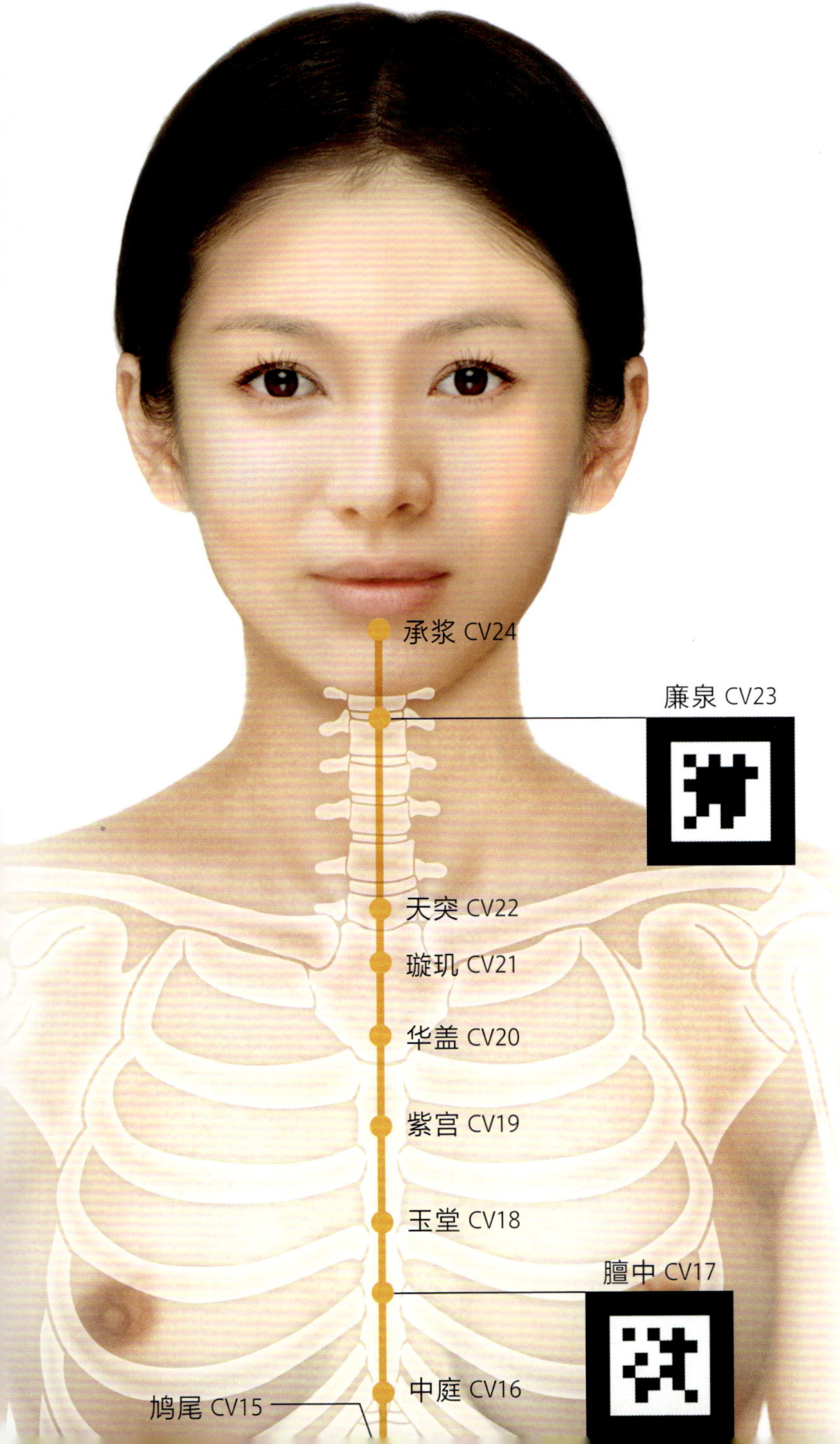

任脉

任脉起于小腹内，下出会阴，沿着腹部正中线到达咽喉部，再上行环绕口唇，经过面部，进入眼眶下。

任脉主治病症：尿道阻塞、遗尿、疝气、月经不调、痛经、白带异常、不孕、子宫肌瘤、卵巢囊肿等泌尿生殖系统疾患；胃脘痛、呕吐、打嗝、腹胀、厌食、反酸等脾胃疾患；胸痛、咳嗽、哮喘、心慌、气短等心肺疾患；癫、狂、痫等神志疾患。本经还可治疗前列腺增生、阳痿、遗精、不育等男性疾患。

CV	穴名	主治
1	会阴	溺水窒息、昏迷、小便不利、遗尿、阴痛、外阴瘙痒、脱肛、子宫或阴道脱垂、痔疮、遗精、月经不调
2	曲骨	小便不利、遗尿、遗精、阳痿、阴囊湿痒、月经不调、痛经、赤白带下
★ 3	中极	遗尿、癃闭、遗精、阳痿、不育、月经不调、阴道脱垂、不孕、产后恶露不尽
★ 4	关元	虚劳冷惫、羸瘦无力、少腹疼痛、疝气、腹泻、脱肛、尿血、尿闭、尿频、遗精、阳痿、早泄、月经不调、子宫或阴道脱垂、恶露不尽、胞衣不下

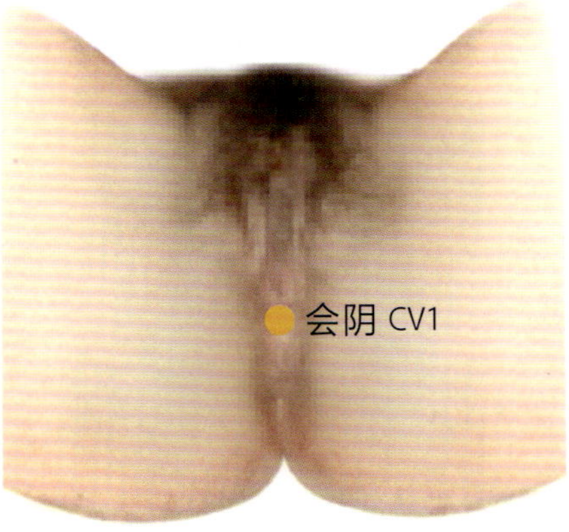

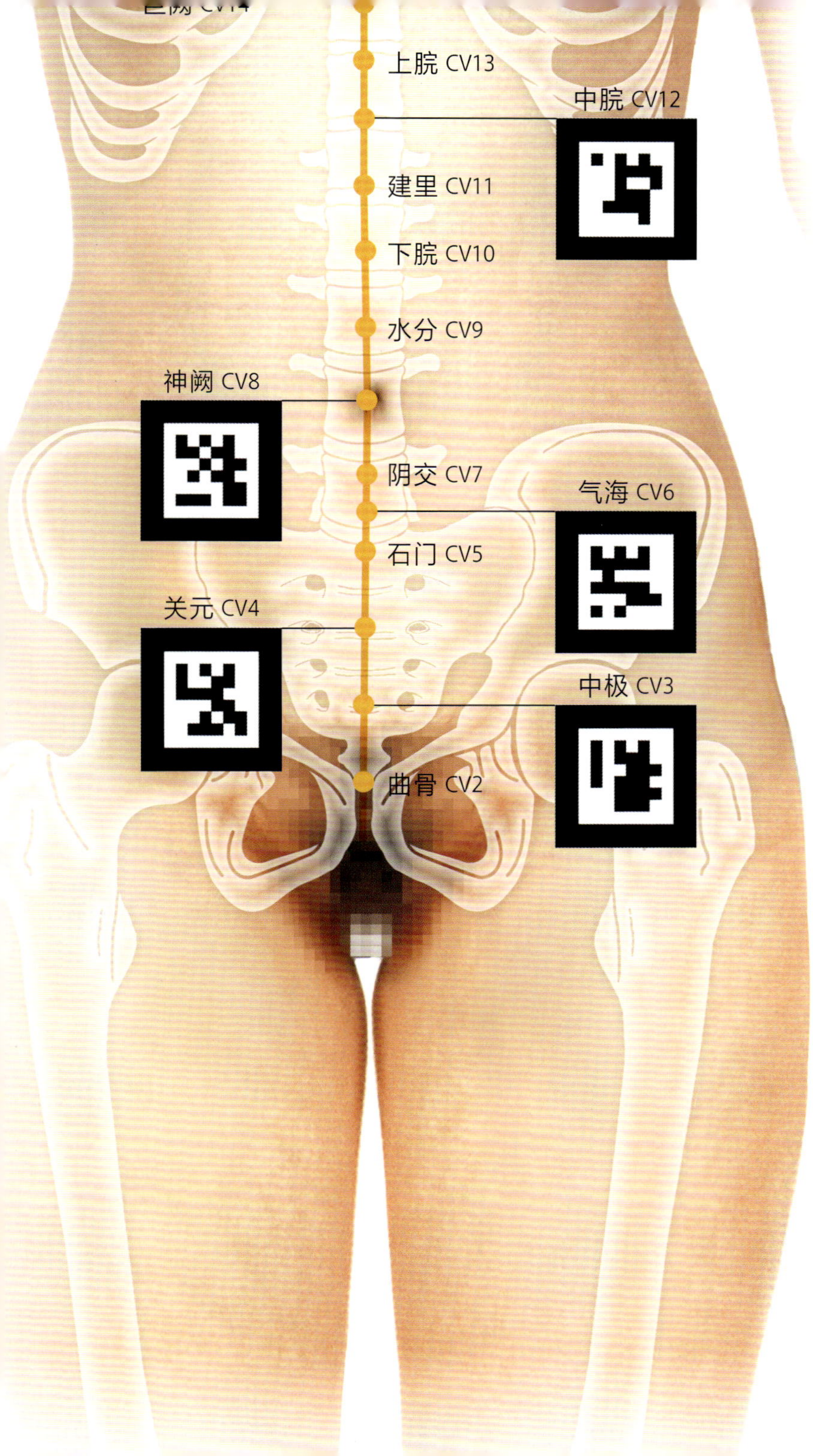

Conception Vessel Meridian, CV.

Conception Vessel Meridian emerges within the lower abdomen, comes out from the perineum below, runs along the middle line of abdomen to the throat and upward around the mouth and lips, then it enters the region under orbit.

Conception Vessel Meridian mainly treats diseases of urogenital system including obstruction of urethra, enuresis, hernia, irregular menstruation, dysmenorrhea, abnormal vaginal discharge, sterility, uterine fibroids and ovarian cysts; diseases of intestine and stomach including epigastric pain, vomiting, belching, distention of abdomen, anorexia and acid regurgitation; diseases of heart and lung including chest pain, cough, asthma, flusteredness and short of breath; mental diseases including depressive psychosis, mania and epilepsy. It can also treats diseases of andrology including benign prostatic hyperplasia, impotence, seminal emission and inferlity.

CV	Acupoints	Indications
1	Huìyīn	Suffocation due to drowning; coma; dysuria; genitalia pain; external genitalia itching; prolapse of rectum; uterus prolapse and vagina prolapse; hemorrhoids; seminal emission; irregular menstruation
2	Qūgǔ	Dysuria; enuresis; seminal emission; impotence; scrotum dampness and itching; irregular menstruation; dysmenorrhea; leukorrhea with reddish discharge
★ 3	Zhōngjí	Enuresis; retention of urine; seminal emission; impotence; infertility; irregular menstruation; uterus prolapse and vagina prolapse; sterility; lochiorrhea after delivery
★ 4	Guānyuán	Consumptive disease and fatigue of cold type; emaciation and weakness; lower abdomen pain; hernia; diarrhea; prolapse of rectum; hematuria; anuresis; frequent urine; seminal emission; impotence; premature ejaculation; irregular menstruation; uterus prolapse and vagina prolapse; lochiorrhea; retention of placenta

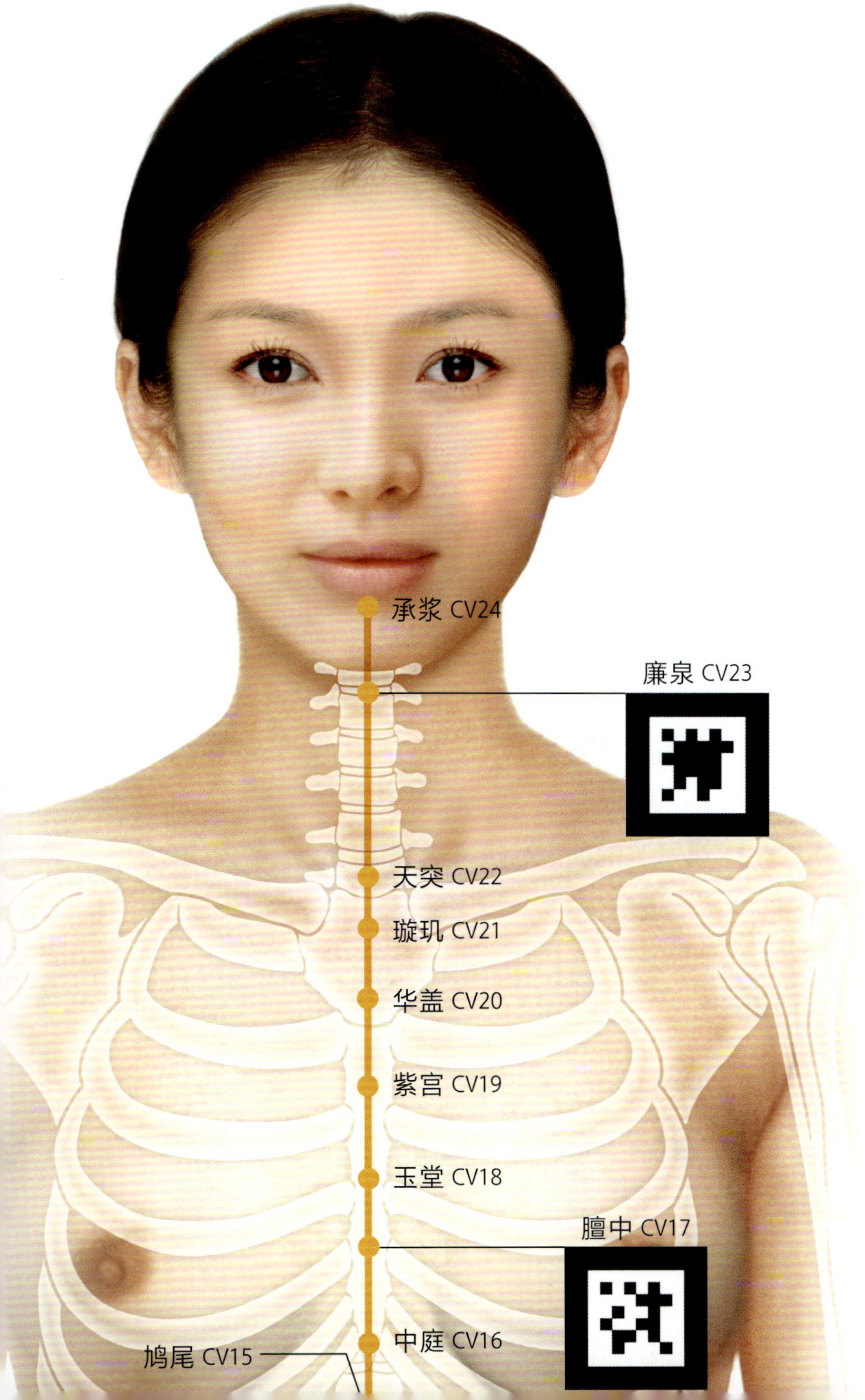

续表

CV	穴 名	主 治
5	石门	腹胀、腹泻、痢疾、绕脐疼痛、疝气、水肿、小便不利、遗精、阳痿、经闭、带下、崩漏、产后恶露不尽
★ 6	气海	虚脱、形体羸瘦、乏力、水谷不化、绕脐疼痛、腹泻、便秘、小便不利、遗尿、遗精、阳痿、疝气、月经不调、带下、子宫或阴道脱垂、产后恶露不止、胞衣不下
7	阴交	疝气、水肿、小便不利、月经不调、带下
★ 8	神阙	虚脱、中风脱证、腹痛、腹胀、腹泻、痢疾、便秘、脱肛、水肿、小便不利
9	水分	水肿、小便不利、腹痛、腹泻、反胃吐食
10	下脘	腹痛、腹胀、腹泻、呕吐、食谷不化、小儿疳积、痞块
11	建里	胃痛、呕吐、食欲不振、腹胀、腹痛、水肿
★ 12	中脘	胃痛、腹胀、纳呆、呕吐、吞酸、呃逆、小儿疳积、黄疸、脏躁
13	上脘	胃痛、呕吐、呃逆、腹胀、癫狂

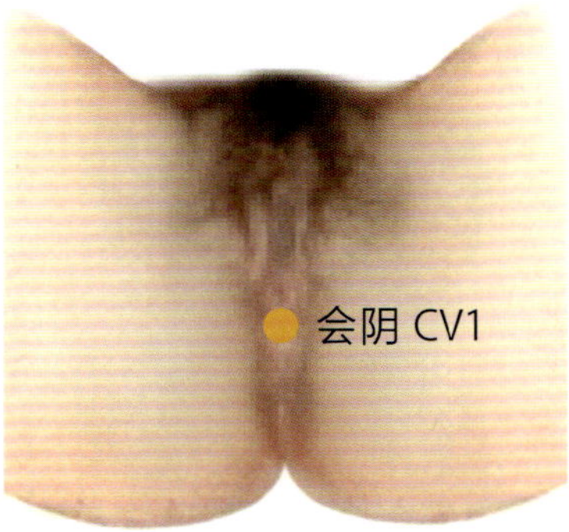

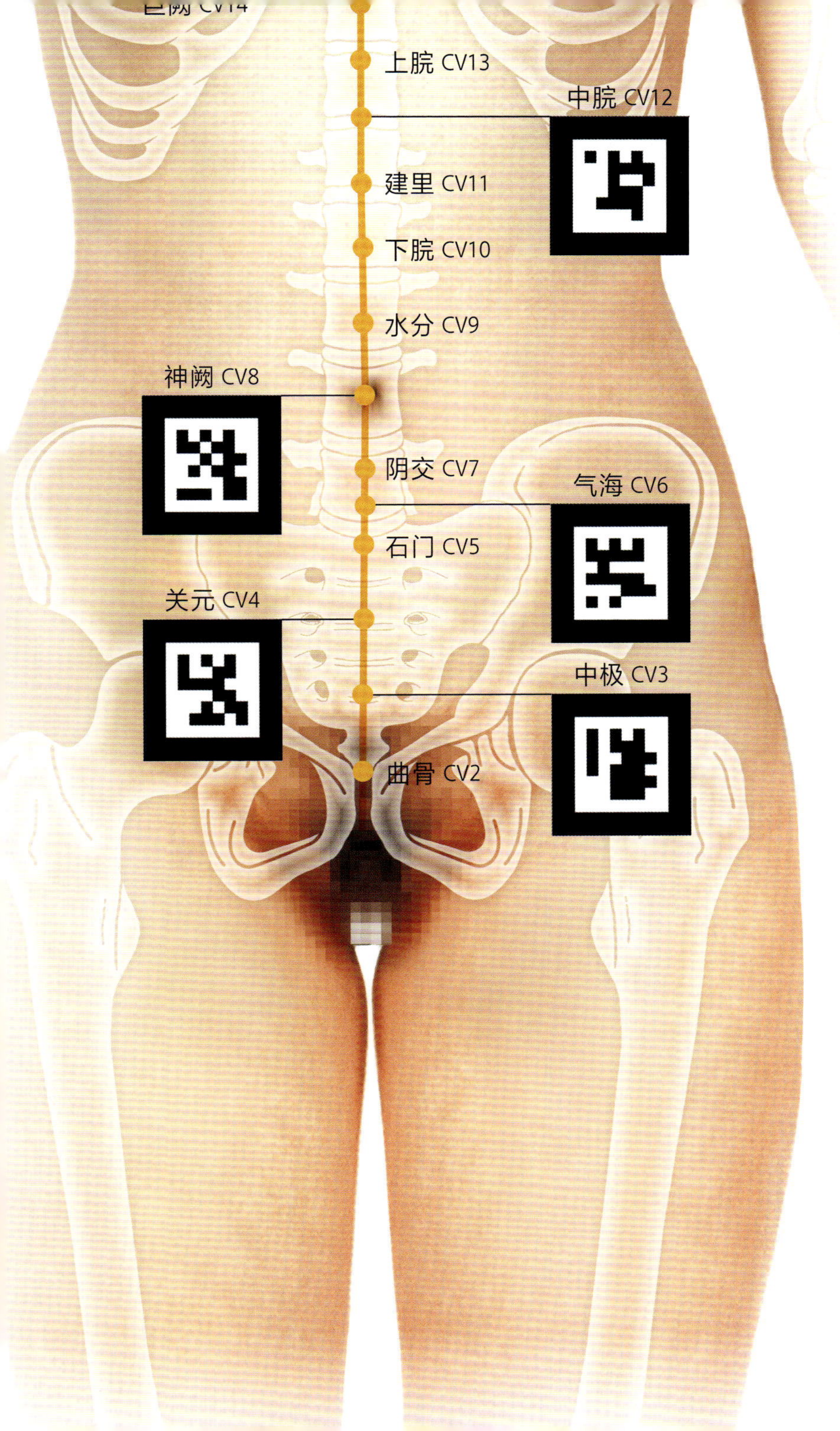

Continued

CV	Acupoints	Indications
5	Shímén	Abdominal distention; diarrhea; dysentery; pain around navel; hernia; edema; dysuria; seminal emission; impotence; amenorrhea; leukorrheal diseases; metrorrhagia and metrostaxis; lochiorrhea after delivery
★ 6	Qìhǎi	Collapse; emaciation; fatigue; indigestion; pain around navel; diarrhea; constipation; dysuria; enuresis; seminal emission; impotence; hernia; irregular menstruation; leukorrheal diseases; uterus prolapse and vagina prolapse; lochiorrhea after delivery; retention of placenta
7	Yīnjiāo	Hernia; edema; dysuria; irregular menstruation; leukorrheal diseases
★ 8	Shénquè	Collapse; collapse syndrome due to wind stroke; abdominal pain; abdominal distention; diarrhea; dysentery; constipation; prolapse of rectum; edema; dysuria
9	Shuǐfēn	Edema; dysuria; abdominal pain; diarrhea; nausea and vomiting
10	Xiàwǎn	Abdominal pain; abdominal distention; diarrhea; vomiting; indigestion; infantile malnutrition; mass
11	Jiànlǐ	Stomachache; vomiting; poor appetite; distention of abdomen; abdominal pain; edema
★ 12	Zhōngwǎn	Stomachache; abdominal distention; poor appetite; vomiting; acid swallow; hiccup; infantile malnutrition; jaundice; hysteria
13	Shàngwǎn	Stomachache; vomiting; hiccup; abdominal distention; manic and depressive psychosis

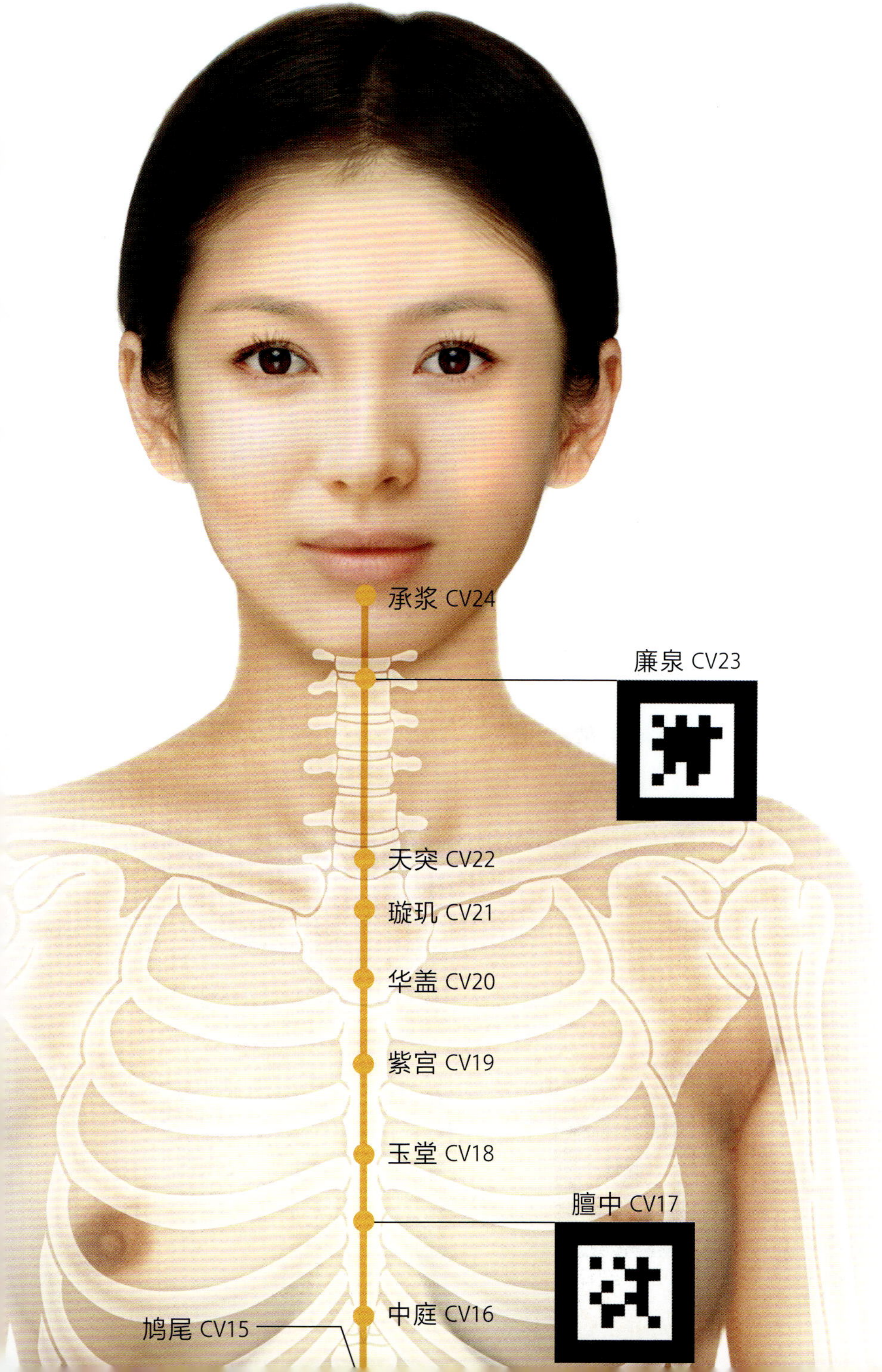

续表

CV	穴名	主治
14	巨阙	癫狂、胸痛、心悸、呕吐、吞酸
15	鸠尾	癫狂、胸痛、腹胀、呃逆
16	中庭	胸胁胀痛、心痛、呕吐、小儿吐乳
★ 17	膻中	咳嗽、气喘、胸闷、心痛、呃逆、产后乳少、乳房肿痛、乳房肿块
18	玉堂	咳嗽、气喘、胸闷、胸痛、乳房胀痛、呕吐
19	紫宫	咳嗽、气喘、胸痛
20	华盖	咳嗽、气喘、胸痛
21	璇玑	咳嗽、气喘、胸痛、咽喉肿痛、积食
22	天突	咳嗽、哮喘、胸痛、咽喉肿痛、急性咽喉炎、甲状腺肿大、梅核气、呃逆
★ 23	廉泉	中风失语、急性咽喉炎、吞咽困难、舌缓流涎、舌下肿痛、口舌生疮、扁桃体炎
24	承浆	口歪、齿龈肿痛、流涎、急性咽喉炎、癫狂

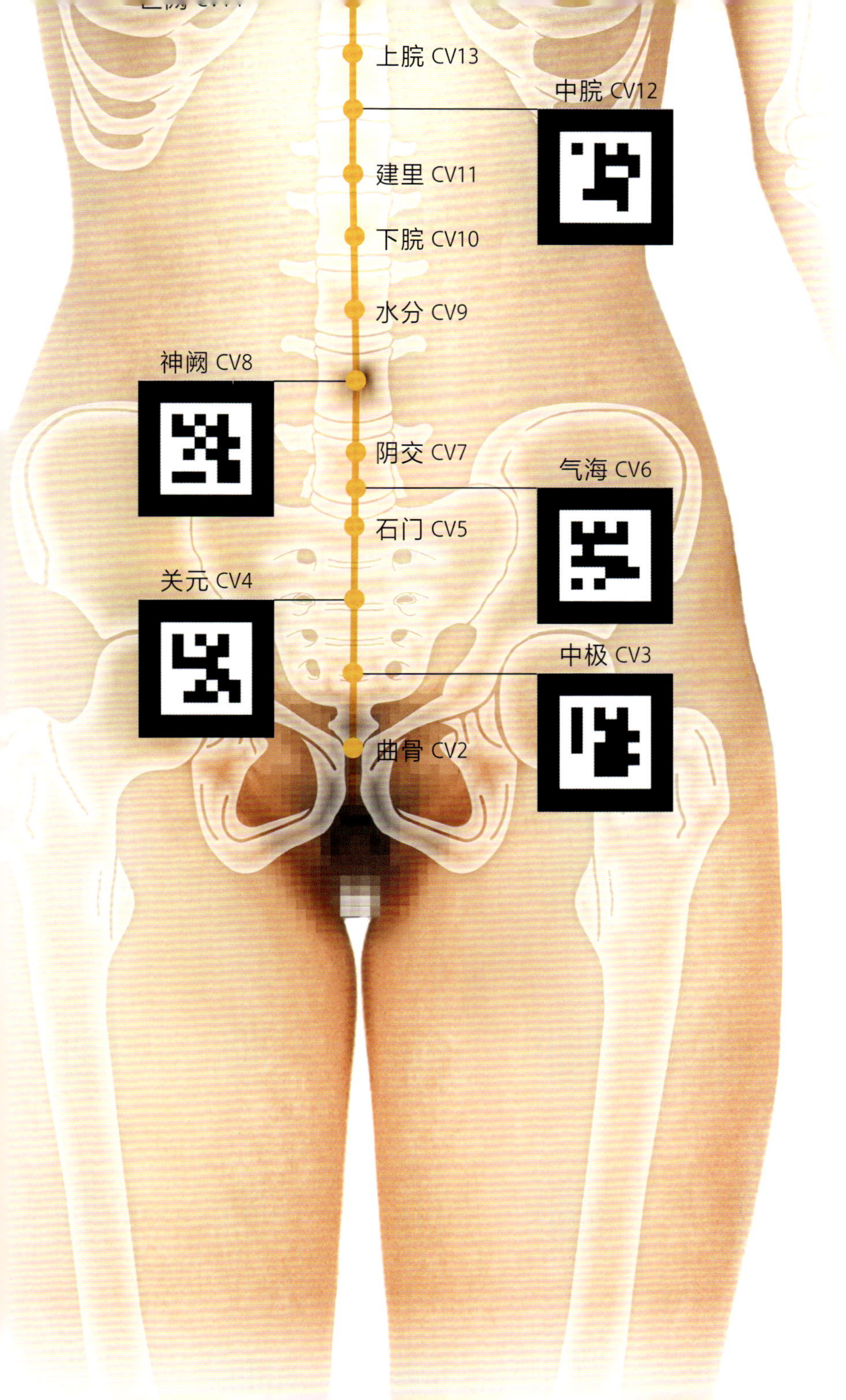

Continued

CV	Acupoints	Indications
14	Jùquè	Manic and depressive psychosis; chest pain; palpitation; vomiting; acid swallow
15	jiūwěi	Manic and depressive psychosis; chest pain; abdominal distention; hiccup
16	Zhōngtíng	Distending pain of chest and hypochondrium; cardiac pain; vomiting; vomiting of milk in children
★ 17	Dànzhōng	Cough; asthma; chest congestion; cardiac pain; hiccup; lack of milk after delivery; swelling and pain of breast; breast mass
18	Yùtáng	Cough; asthma; chest congestion; chest pain; distending pain of breast; vomiting
19	Zǐgōng	Cough; asthma; chest pain
20	Huágài	Cough; asthma; chest pain
21	Xuánjī	Cough; asthma; chest pain; swelling and pain in throat; food retention
22	Tiāntū	Cough; asthma; chest pain; swelling and pain in throat; acute sphagitis; goiter; plum-stone Qi (globus hystericus); hiccup
★ 23	Liánquán	Aphasia due to wind stroke; acute sphagitis; dysphagia; tongue flaccidity and salivation; swelling and pain under the tongue; sores in mouth and tongue; tonsillitis
24	Chéngjiāng	Mouth deviation; swelling and pain of teeth and gum; sallivation; acute sphagitis; manic and depressive psychosis

第二章 穴位分部图解

Chapter 2: Diagrams of Acupoints in Different Divisions

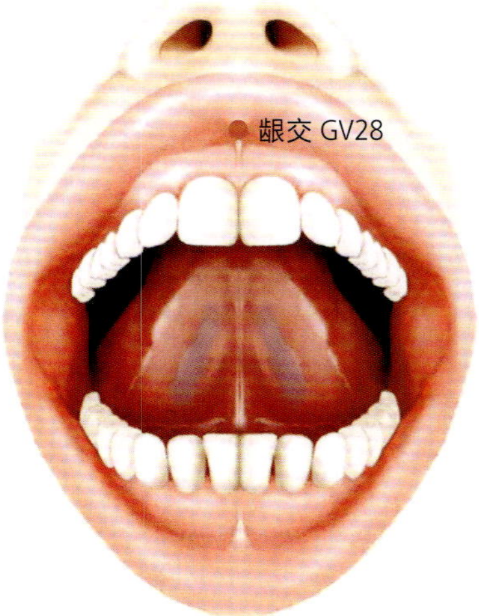

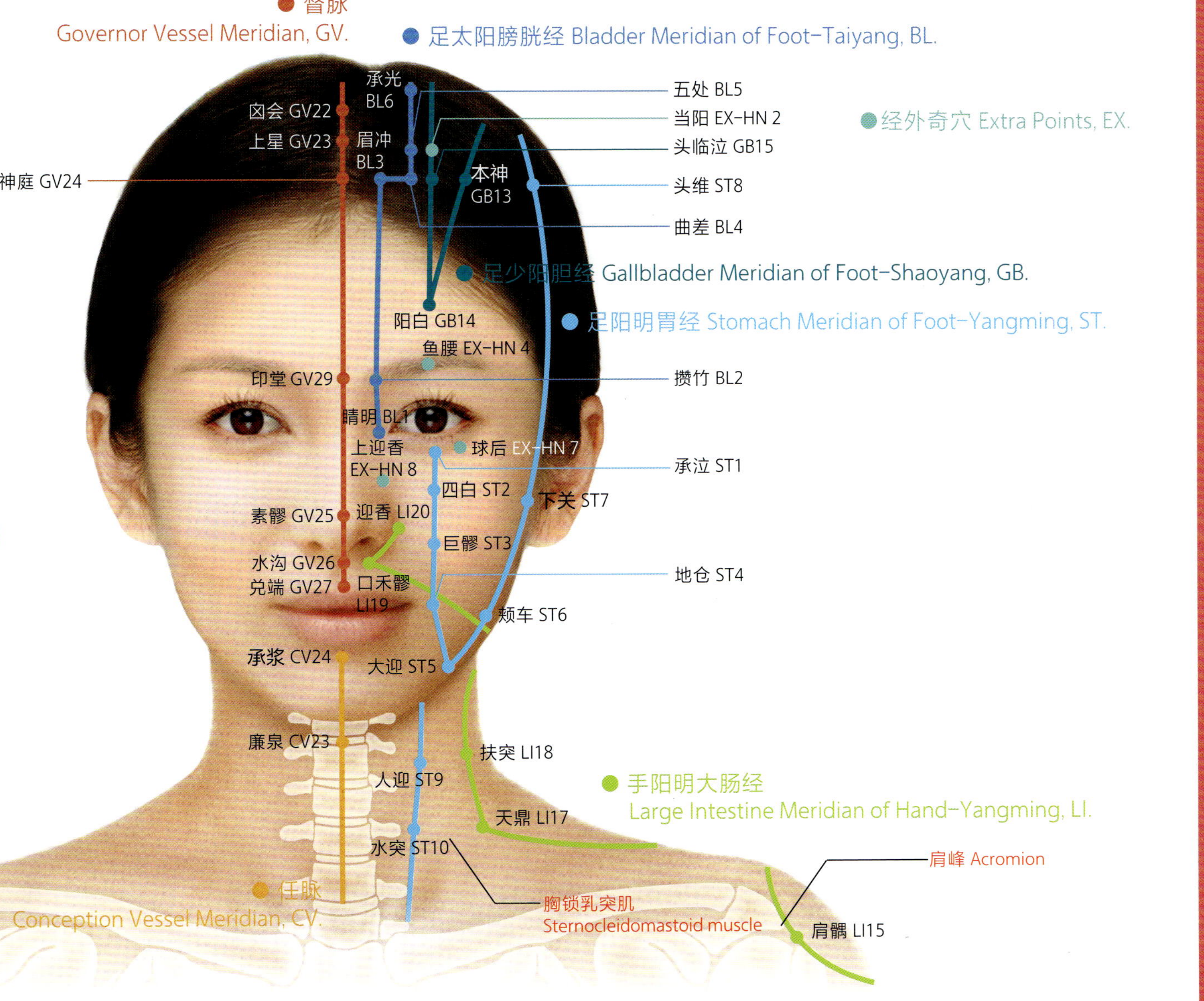

续表

穴位	定位	穴位	定位
肩髃	在三角肌区，肩峰外侧缘前端与肱骨大结节两骨间凹陷中	巨髎	在面部，横平鼻翼下缘，瞳孔直下
天鼎	在颈部，横平环状软骨，胸锁乳突肌后缘	地仓	在面部，口角旁开 0.4 寸
扶突	在胸锁乳突肌区，横平喉结，胸锁乳突肌前、后缘中间	大迎	在面部，下颌角前方，咬肌附着部的前缘凹陷中，面动脉搏动处
口禾髎	在面部，横平人中沟上 1/3 与下 2/3 交点，鼻孔外缘直下	颊车	在面部，下颌角前上方一横指（中指）
迎香	在面部，鼻翼外缘中点旁，鼻唇沟中	下关	在面部，颧弓下缘中央与下颌切迹之间凹陷中
承泣	在面部，眼球与眶下缘之间，瞳孔直下	头维	在头部，额角发际直上 0.5 寸，头正中线旁开 4.5 寸
四白	在面部，眶下孔处		

Acupoints	Location
Jiānyú(LI15)	In deltoid muscle area, in the depression of anterior lateral margin of acromion and humerus greater tuberosity
Tiāndǐng(LI17)	On the neck, horizontal to cricoid cartilage, in the posterior border of the sternocleidomastoid muscle
Fútū(LI18)	In the area of sternocleidomastoid muscle, horizontal to the tip of the Adam's apple, at the midpoint between anterior and posterior border of sternocleidomastoid muscle
Kǒuhéliáo(LI19)	On the face, horizontal to the junction of upper 1/3 and lower 2/3 of the philtrum, directly below the lateral margin of the nostril
Yíngxiān(LI20)	On the face, beside the midpoint of the lateral side of the ala nasi, in the nasolabial groove
Chéngqì(ST1)	On the face, between the eyeball and the infraorbital ridge, directly below the pupil
Sìbái(ST2)	On the face, at the infraorbital foramen
Jùliáo(ST3)	On the face, at the level of the lower border of the ala nasi, directly below the pupil
Dìcāng(ST4)	On the face, 0.4 cun lateral to the corner of the mouth
Dàyíng(ST5)	On the face, anterior to the angle of the mandible, in the depression of the anterior border of the attached portion of the masseter muscle, on the pulsation place of facial artery
Jiáchē(ST6)	On the face, one finger breadth(middle finger) anterior and superior to the lower angle of the mandible
Xiàguān(ST7)	On the face, in the depression of midpoint of lower border of the zygomatic arch and mandibular notch
Tóuwéi(ST8)	On the head, 0.5 cun within the anterior hairline at the corner of the forehead, 4.5 cun lateral to middle line of the head

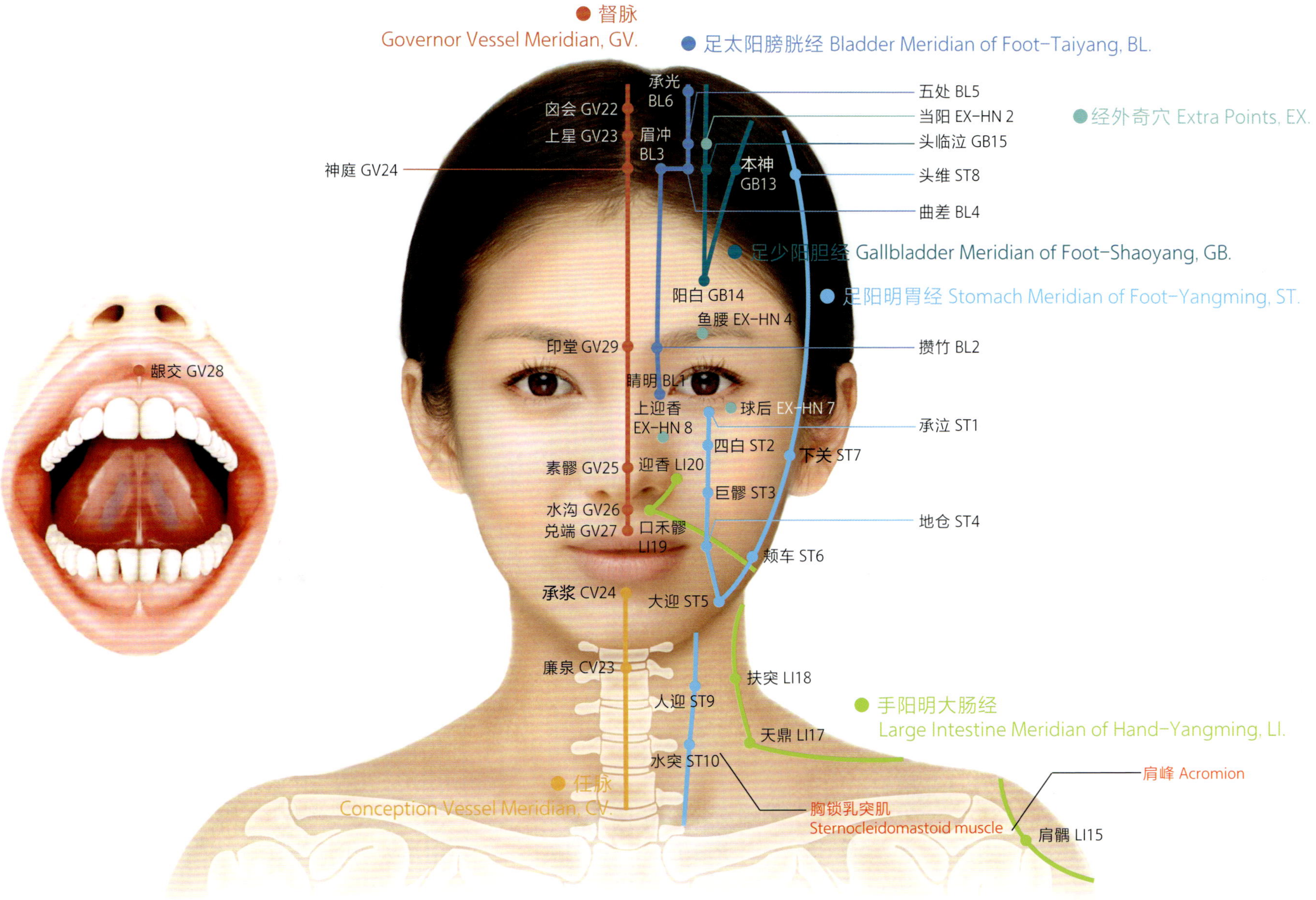
督脉
Governor Vessel Meridian, GV.
足太阳膀胱经 Bladder Meridian of Foot-Taiyang, BL.
经外奇穴 Extra Points, EX.
足少阳胆经 Gallbladder Meridian of Foot-Shaoyang, GB.
足阳明胃经 Stomach Meridian of Foot-Yangming, ST.
手阳明大肠经
Large Intestine Meridian of Hand-Yangming, LI.
任脉
Conception Vessel Meridian, CV.
承光 BL6
囟会 GV22
上星 GV23
眉冲 BL3
神庭 GV24
本神 GB13
五处 BL5
当阳 EX-HN 2
头临泣 GB15
头维 ST8
曲差 BL4
阳白 GB14
鱼腰 EX-HN 4
印堂 GV29
攒竹 BL2
龈交 GV28
睛明 BL1
上迎香 EX-HN 8
球后 EX-HN 7
承泣 ST1
四白 ST2
下关 ST7
素髎 GV25
迎香 LI20
巨髎 ST3
水沟 GV26
地仓 ST4
兑端 GV27
口禾髎 LI19
颊车 ST6
承浆 CV24
大迎 ST5
廉泉 CV23
扶突 LI18
人迎 ST9
天鼎 LI17
水突 ST10
肩峰 Acromion
胸锁乳突肌
Sternocleidomastoid muscle
肩髃 LI15

续表

穴 位	定 位	穴 位	定 位
人迎	在颈部，横平喉结，胸锁乳突肌前缘，颈总动脉搏动处	承光	在头部，前发际正中直上 2.5 寸，旁开 1.5 寸
水突	在颈部，横平环状软骨，胸锁乳突肌前缘	本神	在头部，前发际上 0.5 寸，头正中线旁开 3 寸
睛明	在面部，目内眦内上方眶内侧壁凹陷中	阳白	在头部，眉上 1 寸，瞳孔直上
攒竹	在面部，眉头凹陷中，额切迹处	头临泣	在头部，前发际上 0.5 寸，瞳孔直上
眉冲	在头部，额切际直上入发际 0.5 寸	囟会	在头部，前发际正中直上 2 寸
曲差	在头部，前发际正中直上 0.5 寸，旁开 1.5 寸	上星	在头部，前发际正中直上 1 寸
五处	在头部，前发际正中直上 1 寸，旁开 1.5 寸	神庭	在头部，前发际正中直上 0.5 寸

Continued

Acupoints	Location
Rényíng(ST9)	On the neck, horizontal to the tip of the Adam's apple, in the anterior border of sternocleidomastoid muscle, on the pulsation place of arteria carotis communis
Shuǐtū(ST10)	On the neck, horizontal to cricoid cartilage, in the anterior border of the sternocleidomastoid muscle
Jīngmíng(BL1)	On the face, in the depression of medial orbital wall in the medial and superior border of inner canthus
Cuánzhú(BL2)	On the face, in the depression of medial extermity of the eyebrow, on the supraorbital notch
Méichōng(BL3)	On the head, 0.5 cun within the hairline that is directly above supraorbital notch
Qūchā(BL4)	On the head, 0.5 cun directly within the midpoint of anterior hairline, 1.5 cun lateral to the middle line of head
Wǔchù(BL5)	On the head, 1 cun directly within the midpoint of anterior hairline , 1.5 cun lateral to the middle line of head
Chéngguāng(BL6)	On the head, 2.5 cun directly within the midpoint of anterior hairline, 1.5 cun lateral to the middle line of head
Běnshén(GB13)	On the head, 0.5 cun above the anterior hairline, 3 cun lateral to middle line of head
Yángbái(GB14)	On the head, 1 cun above the eyebrow, directly above the pupil
Tóulínqì(GB15)	On the head, 0.5 cun above the anterior hairline, directly above the pupil
Xìnhuì(GV22)	On the head, 2 cun directly above the midpoint of the anterior hairline
Shàngxīng(GV23)	On the head, 1 cun directly above the midpoint of the anterior hairline
Shéntíng(GV24)	On the head, 0.5 cun directly above the midpoint of the anterior hairline

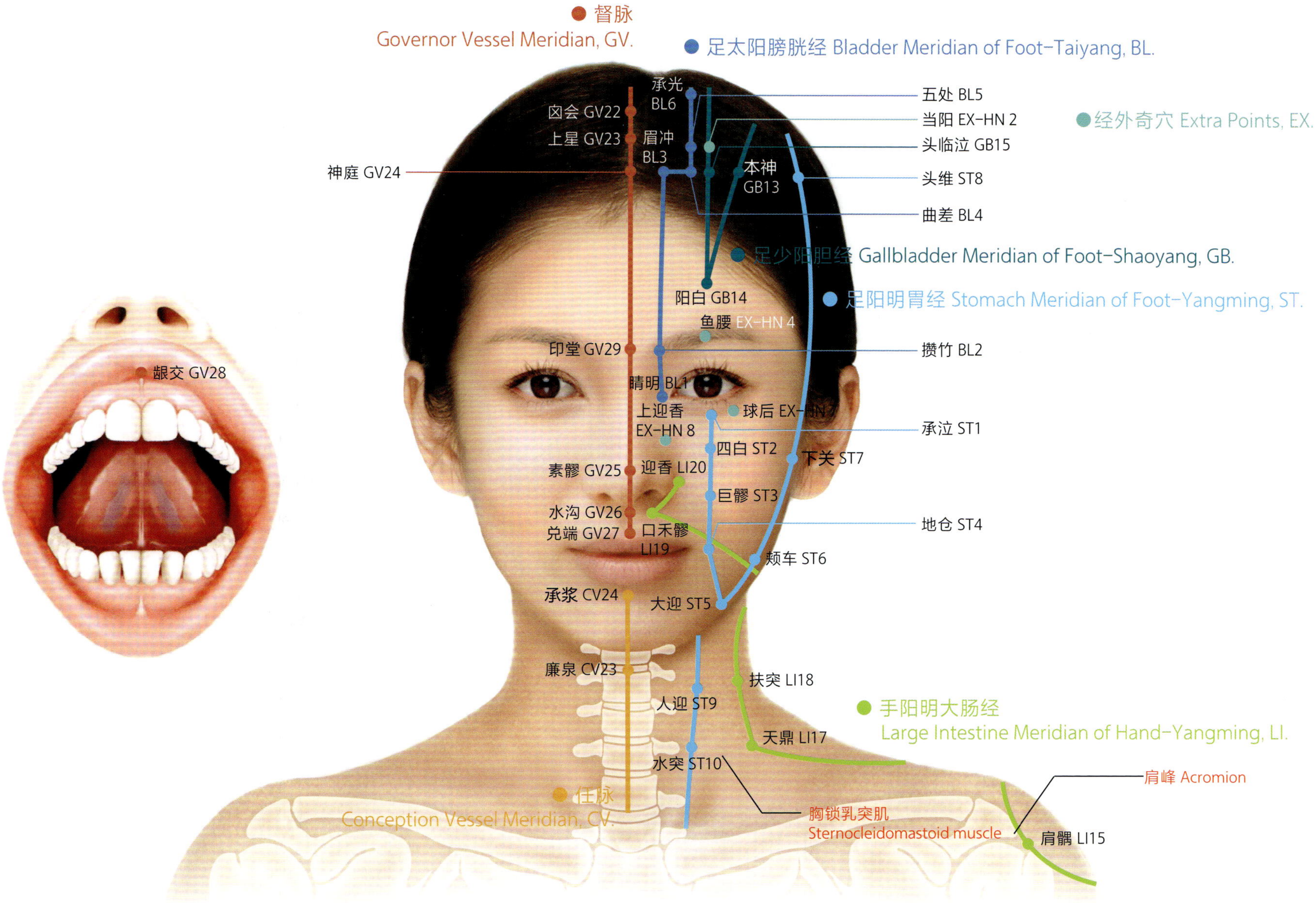

督脉
Governor Vessel Meridian, GV.
足太阳膀胱经 Bladder Meridian of Foot-Taiyang, BL.
承光 BL6
囟会 GV22
上星 GV23
眉冲 BL3
神庭 GV24
本神 GB13
五处 BL5
当阳 EX-HN 2
经外奇穴 Extra Points, EX.
头临泣 GB15
头维 ST8
曲差 BL4
足少阳胆经 Gallbladder Meridian of Foot-Shaoyang, GB.
阳白 GB14
足阳明胃经 Stomach Meridian of Foot-Yangming, ST.
鱼腰 EX-HN 4
印堂 GV29
攒竹 BL2
龈交 GV28
睛明 BL1
上迎香 EX-HN 8
球后 EX-HN 7
承泣 ST1
四白 ST2
下关 ST7
素髎 GV25
迎香 LI20
巨髎 ST3
水沟 GV26
兑端 GV27
口禾髎 LI19
地仓 ST4
颊车 ST6
承浆 CV24
大迎 ST5
廉泉 CV23
扶突 LI18
人迎 ST9
手阳明大肠经
Large Intestine Meridian of Hand-Yangming, LI.
天鼎 LI17
水突 ST10
肩峰 Acromion
任脉
Conception Vessel Meridian, CV.
胸锁乳突肌
Sternocleidomastoid muscle
肩髃 LI15

续表

穴位	定位
素髎	在面部，鼻尖的正中央
水沟	在面部，人中沟的上 1/3 与中 1/3 交点处
兑端	在面部，上唇结节的中点
龈交	在上唇内，上唇系带与上齿龈的交点
印堂	在头部，两眉毛内侧端中间的凹陷中
廉泉	在颈前区，喉结上方，舌骨上缘凹陷中，前正中线上

穴位	定位
承浆	在面部，颏唇沟的正中凹陷处
当阳	在头前部，当瞳孔直上，前发际上 1 寸。
鱼腰	在额部，瞳孔直上，眉毛中。
球后	球后在面部，当眶下缘外 1/4 与内 3/4 交界处。
上迎香	在面部，当鼻翼软骨与鼻甲的交界处，近鼻唇沟上端处。

Continued

Acupoints	Location
Sùliáo(GV25)	On the face, on the tip of the nose
Shuǐgōu(GV26)	On the face, at the junction of upper 1/3 and lower 1/3 of the philtrum
Duìduān(GV27)	On the face, on the median tubercle of the upper lip
Yínjiāo(GV28)	Within the upper lip, at the junction of frenulum of the upper lip and the upper gum
Yìntáng(GV29)	On the head, in the depression of midpoint of medial margin of two eyebrows
Liánquán(CV23)	In the anterior neck region, above the Adam' s apple, in the depression of the superior border of the hyoid bone, on the anterior middle line of the body
Chéngjiāng(CV24)	On the face, in the depression of the midpoint of the mentolabial groove
Dāngyáng(EX-HN2)	On the lateral head, directly above the pupil, 1 cun within the anterior hairline
Yúyāo(EX-HN4)	On the forehead, directly above the pupil, inside the eyebrow
Qiúhòu(EX-HN7)	On the face, on the junction of outer 1/4 and inner 3/4 of the infraorbital margin
Shàngyíngxiāng(EX-HN8)	On the face, at the junction of cartilage of ala nasi and turbinate, near the superior border of nasolabial groove

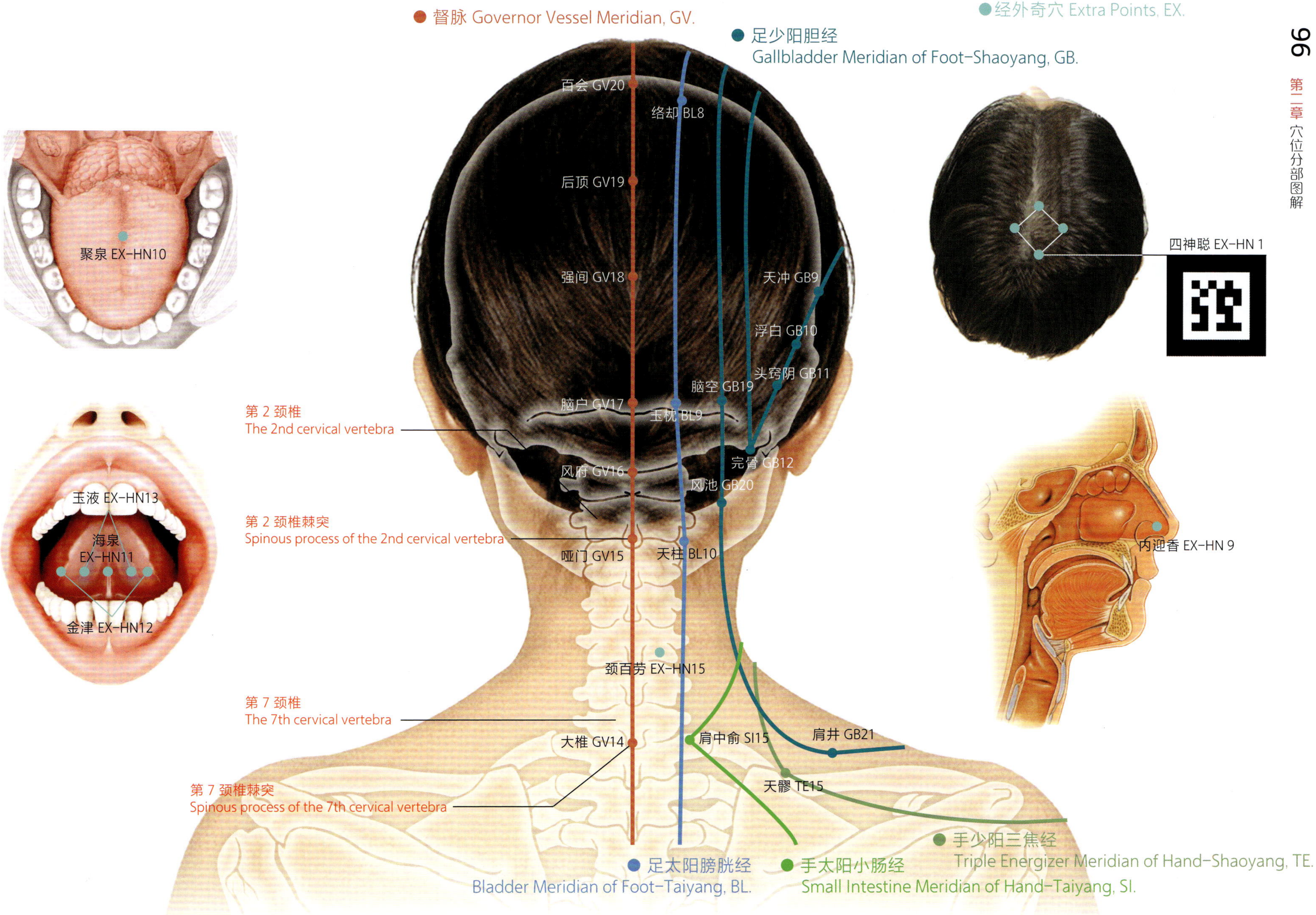
督脉 Governor Vessel Meridian, GV.
足少阳胆经
Gallbladder Meridian of Foot-Shaoyang, GB.
经外奇穴 Extra Points, EX.
百会 GV20
络却 BL8
后顶 GV19
强间 GV18
天冲 GB9
浮白 GB10
头窍阴 GB11
脑空 GB19
脑户 GV17
玉枕 BL9
完骨 GB12
风府 GV16
风池 GB20
哑门 GV15
天柱 BL10
颈百劳 EX-HN15
大椎 GV14
肩中俞 SI15
肩井 GB21
天髎 TE15
第 2 颈椎
The 2nd cervical vertebra
第 2 颈椎棘突
Spinous process of the 2nd cervical vertebra
第 7 颈椎
The 7th cervical vertebra
第 7 颈椎棘突
Spinous process of the 7th cervical vertebra
聚泉 EX-HN10
玉液 EX-HN13
海泉
EX-HN11
金津 EX-HN12
四神聪 EX-HN 1
内迎香 EX-HN 9
足太阳膀胱经
Bladder Meridian of Foot-Taiyang, BL.
手太阳小肠经
Small Intestine Meridian of Hand-Taiyang, SI.
手少阳三焦经
Triple Energizer Meridian of Hand-Shaoyang, TE.

续表

穴位	定位
肩中俞	在脊柱区，第 7 颈椎棘突下，后正中线旁开 2 寸
络却	在头部，前发际正中直上 5.5 寸，旁开 1.5 寸
玉枕	在头部，横平枕外隆凸上缘，后发际正中线旁开 1.3 寸
天柱	在颈后区，横平第 2 颈椎棘突上际，斜方肌外缘凹陷中
天髎	在肩胛区，肩胛骨上角骨际凹陷中
天冲	在头部，耳根后缘直上，入发际 2 寸

穴位	定位
浮白	在头部，耳后乳突的后上方，从天冲至完骨的弧形连线（其弧度与耳廓弧度相应）的上 1/3 与下 2/3 交点处
头窍阴	在头部，耳后乳突的后下方，从天冲至完骨的弧形连线（其弧度与耳廓弧度相应）的上 2/3 与下 1/3 交点处
完骨	在头部，耳后乳突的后下方凹陷中
脑空	在头部，横平枕外隆凸的上缘，风池直上
风池	在颈后区，枕骨之下，胸锁乳突肌上端与斜方肌上端之间的凹陷中

Acupoints	Location
Jiānzhōngshū(SI15)	In the spinal region, below spinous process of the 7th cervical vertebra, 2 cun lateral to posterior midline of head
Luòquè(BL8)	On the head, 5.5 cun directly above the midpoint of the anterior hairline, 1.5 cun lateral to midline of head
Yùzhěn(BL9)	On the head, horizontal to the superior border of external occipital protuberance, 1.3 cun lateral to midline of head
Tiānzhù(BL10)	In the posterior neck region, horizontal to superior border of spinous process of the 2nd cervical vertebra, in the depression of the lateral border of the muscle trapezius
Tiānliáo(TE15)	In the scapular region, in the depression of the superior angle of scapula
Tiānchōng(GB9)	On the head, directly above the posterior border of the root of auricle, 2 cun within the hairline
Fúbái(GB10)	On the head, posterior and superior to the mastoid process, at the junction of upper 1/3 and lower 2/3 on the curved line (the curved line corresponding to that of auricle) drawn from Tianchong (GB9) to Wangu (GB12)
Tóuqiàoyīn(GB11)	On the head, posterior and superior to the mastoid process, at the junction of upper 2/3 and lower 1/3 on the curved line (the curved line corresponding to that of auricle) drawn from Tianchong (GB9) to Wangu (GB12)
Wángǔ(GB12)	On the head, in the depression posterior and inferior to the mastoid process
Nǎokōng(GB19)	On the head, horizontal to the superior border of external occipital protuberance, directly above Fengchi (GB20)
Fēngchí(GB20)	In the posterior neck region, below the occipital, in the depression between the upper portion of sternocleidomastoid muscle and the muscle trapezius

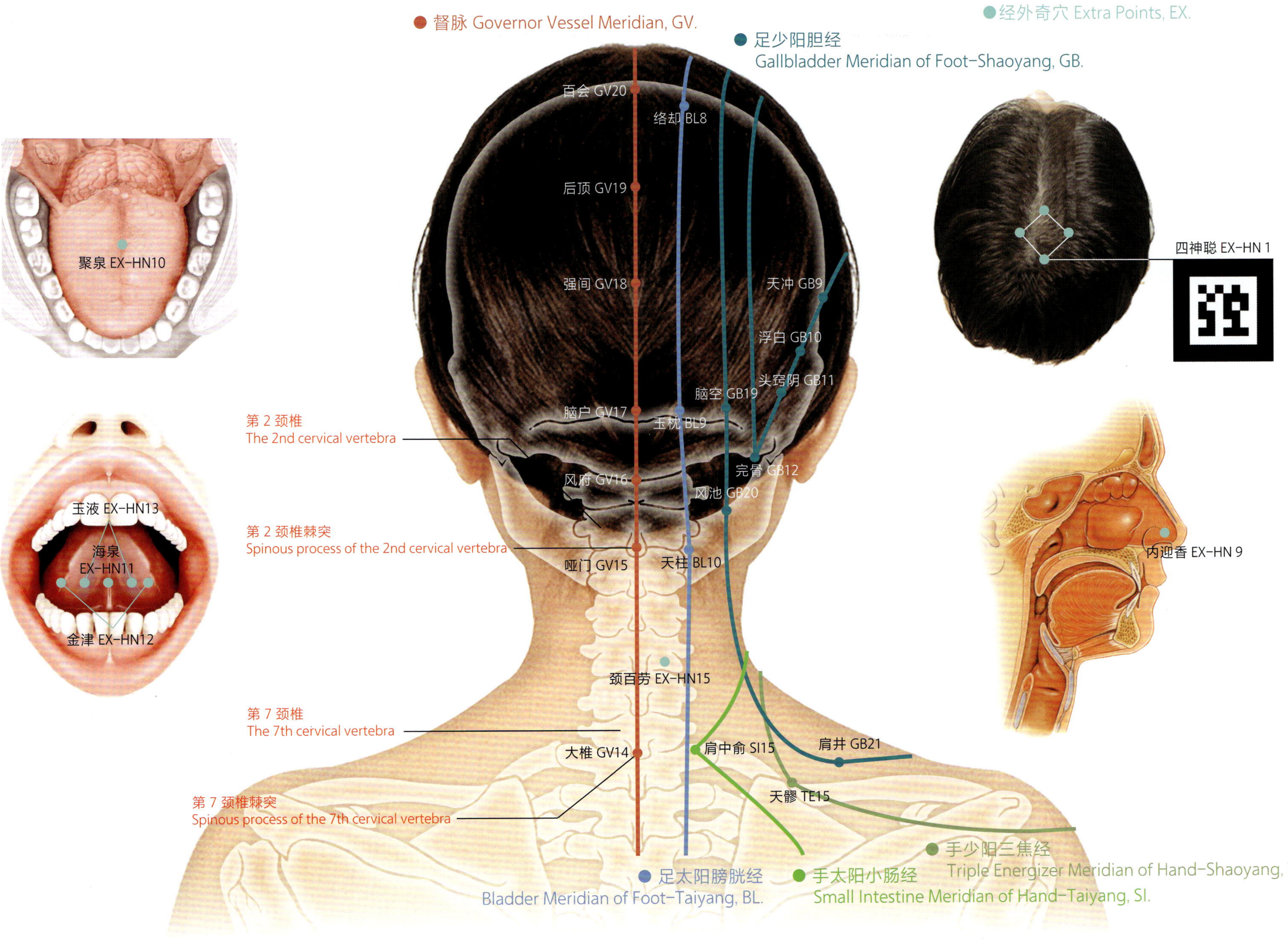
督脉 Governor Vessel Meridian, GV.
足少阳胆经
Gallbladder Meridian of Foot-Shaoyang, GB.
经外奇穴 Extra Points, EX.
百会 GV20
络却 BL8
后顶 GV19
强间 GV18
天冲 GB9
浮白 GB10
头窍阴 GB11
脑空 GB19
脑户 GV17
玉枕 BL9
完骨 GB12
风府 GV16
风池 GB20
哑门 GV15
天柱 BL10
颈百劳 EX-HN15
大椎 GV14
肩中俞 SI15
肩井 GB21
天髎 TE15
第 2 颈椎
The 2nd cervical vertebra
第 2 颈椎棘突
Spinous process of the 2nd cervical vertebra
第 7 颈椎
The 7th cervical vertebra
第 7 颈椎棘突
Spinous process of the 7th cervical vertebra
聚泉 EX-HN10
玉液 EX-HN13
海泉
EX-HN11
金津 EX-HN12
四神聪 EX-HN 1
内迎香 EX-HN 9
手少阳三焦经
Triple Energizer Meridian of Hand-Shaoyang, TE.
足太阳膀胱经
Bladder Meridian of Foot-Taiyang, BL.
手太阳小肠经
Small Intestine Meridian of Hand-Taiyang, SI.

续表

穴位	定位
肩井	在肩胛区，第 7 颈椎棘突与肩峰最外侧点连线的中点
大椎	在脊柱区，第 7 颈椎棘突下凹陷中，后正中线上
哑门	在项后区，第 2 颈椎棘突上际凹陷中，后正中线上
风府	在项后区，枕外隆凸直下，两侧斜方肌之间凹陷中
脑户	在头部，枕外隆凸的上缘凹陷中
强间	在头部，后发际正中直上 4 寸
后顶	在头部，后发际正中直上 5.5 寸
百会	在头部，前发际正中直上 5 寸
四神聪	在头顶部，当百会前后左右各 1 寸，共 4 穴
内迎香	在鼻孔内，当鼻翼软骨与鼻甲交界的黏膜处
聚泉	口腔内，当舌背正中缝的中点处
海泉	位于口腔内，当舌下系带中点处
金津、玉液	在口腔内，当舌下系带左右两侧的静脉上
颈百劳	在项部，当大椎直上 2 寸，后正中线旁开 1 寸

Continued

Acupoints	Location
Jiānjǐng(GB21)	In the scapular region, at the midpoint of spinous process of the 7th cervical vertebra and the outer point of the acromion
Dàzhuī(GV14)	In the scapular region, in the depression of spinous process of the 7th cervical vertebra, on the posterior middle line
Yǎmén(GV15)	In the posterior neck region, in the depression of superior border of spinous process of the 2nd cervical vertebra, on the posterior middle line
Fēngfǔ(GV16)	In the posterior neck region, directly below the external occipital protuberance, in the depression between muscle trapezius
Nǎohù(GV17)	On the head, in the depression of the superior border of external occipital protuberance
Qiángjiān(GV18)	On the head, 4 cun directly above the midpoint of the posterior hairline
Hòudǐng(GV19)	On the head, 5.5 cun directly above the midpoint of the posterior hairline
Bǎihuì(GV20)	On the head, 5 cun directly above the midpoint of the posterior hairline
Sìshéncōng(EX-HN1)	On the head, 1 cun respectively posterior, anterior and lateral to Baihui (GV20), altogether 4 points
Nèiyíngxiāng(EX-HN9)	Inside nostril, at the conjunctive mucosa of cartilage of ala nasi and turbinate
Jùquán(EX-HN10)	In the mouth, at the midpoint of median raphe of back of the tongue
Hǎiquán(EX-HN11)	In the mouth, at the midpoint of the frenulum of the tongue
Jīnjīn(EX-HN12) Yùyè(EX-HN13)	In the mouth, on the veins on left and right sides of the frenulum of the tongue
Jìngbǎiláo(EX-HN15)	On the neck, 2 cun directly above Dazhui (GV14), 1 cun lateral to posterior median line

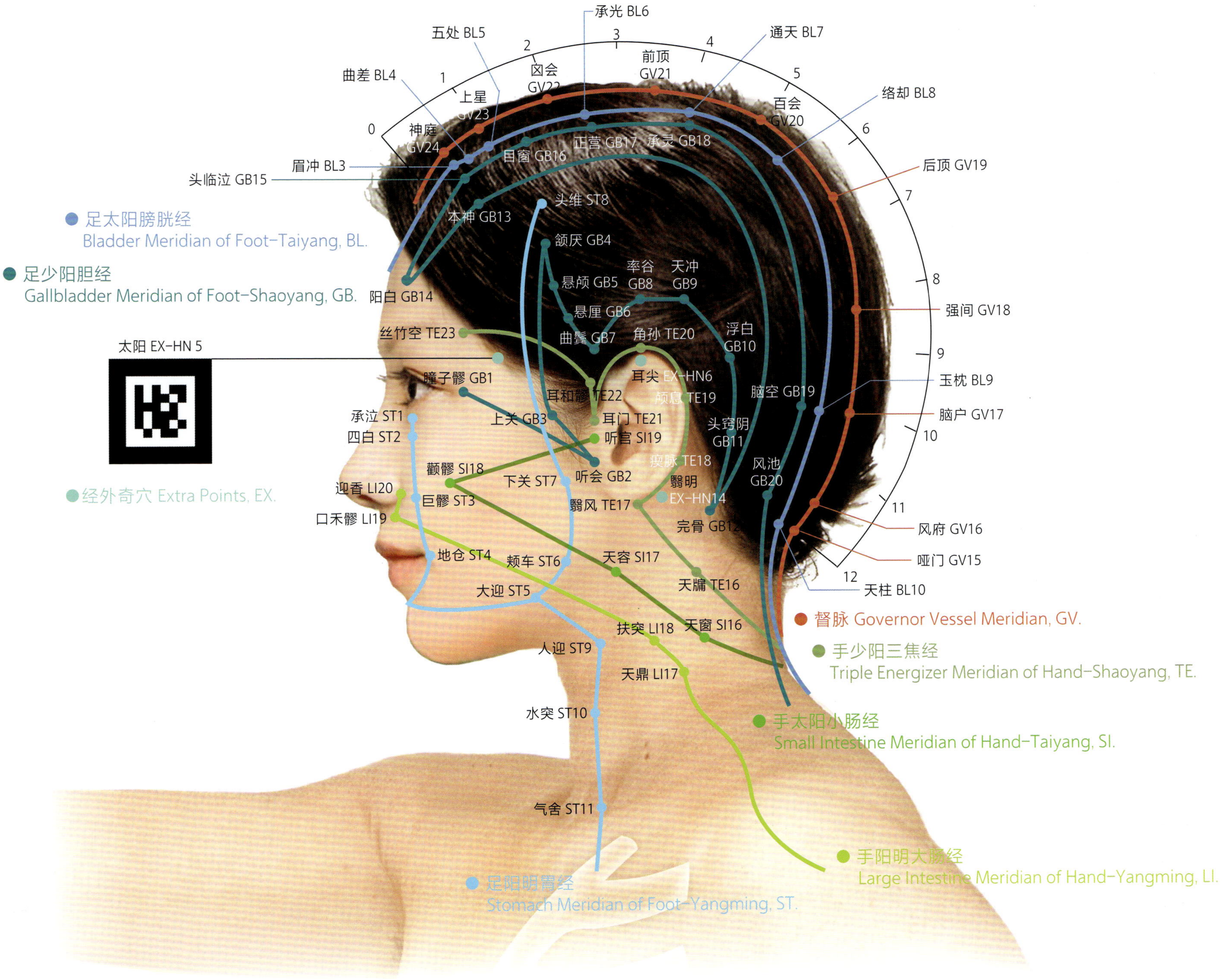
承光 BL6
五处 BL5
通天 BL7
曲差 BL4
前顶
GV21
囟会
GV22
上星
GV23
百会
GV20
络却 BL8
神庭
GV24
正营 GB17
承灵 GB18
目窗 GB16
眉冲 BL3
头临泣 GB15
后顶 GV19
足太阳膀胱经
Bladder Meridian of Foot-Taiyang, BL.
头维 ST8
本神 GB13
颔厌 GB4
足少阳胆经
Gallbladder Meridian of Foot-Shaoyang, GB.
悬颅 GB5
率谷
GB8
天冲
GB9
阳白 GB14
强间 GV18
悬厘 GB6
丝竹空 TE23
曲鬓 GB7
角孙 TE20
浮白
GB10
太阳 EX-HN 5
耳尖 EX-HN6
玉枕 BL9
瞳子髎 GB1
耳和髎 TE22
颅息 TE19
脑空 GB19
脑户 GV17
承泣 ST1
上关 GB3
耳门 TE21
头窍阴
GB11
四白 ST2
听宫 SI19
颧髎 SI18
瘈脉 TE18
风池
GB20
下关 ST7
听会 GB2
翳明
迎香 LI20
经外奇穴 Extra Points, EX.
EX-HN14
巨髎 ST3
翳风 TE17
口禾髎 LI19
完骨 GB12
风府 GV16
地仓 ST4
颊车 ST6
天容 SI17
哑门 GV15
天牖 TE16
大迎 ST5
天柱 BL10
督脉 Governor Vessel Meridian, GV.
扶突 LI18
天窗 SI16
人迎 ST9
手少阳三焦经
Triple Energizer Meridian of Hand-Shaoyang, TE.
天鼎 LI17
水突 ST10
手太阳小肠经
Small Intestine Meridian of Hand-Taiyang, SI.
气舍 ST11
手阳明大肠经
Large Intestine Meridian of Hand-Yangming, LI.
足阳明胃经
Stomach Meridian of Foot-Yangming, ST.

续表

穴位	定位	穴位	定位
天鼎	在颈部，横平环状软骨，胸锁乳突肌后缘	地仓	在面部，口角旁开 0.4 寸（指寸）
扶突	在胸锁乳突肌区，横平喉结，胸锁乳突肌前、后缘中间	大迎	在面部，下颌角前方，咬肌附着部的前缘凹陷中，面动脉搏动处
口禾髎	在面部，横平人中沟上 1/3 与下 2/3 交点，鼻孔外缘直下		
迎香	在面部，鼻翼外缘中点旁，鼻唇沟中	颊车	在面部，下颌角前上方一横指（中指）
承泣	在面部，眼球与眶下缘之间，瞳孔直下	下关	在面部，颧弓下缘中央与下颌切迹之间凹陷中
四白	在面部，眶下孔处	头维	在头部，额角发际直上 0.5 寸，正中线旁开 4.5 寸
巨髎	在面部，横平鼻翼下缘，瞳孔直下	人迎	在颈部，横平喉结，胸锁乳突肌前缘，颈总动脉搏动处

Acupoints	Location
Tiāndǐng(LI17)	On the neck, horizontal to cricoid cartilage, in the posterior border of the sternocleidomastoid muscle
Fútū(LI18)	In the area of sternocleidomastoid muscle, horizontal to the tip of the Adam's apple, at the midpoint between anterior and posterior of sternocleidomastoid muscle
Kǒuhéliáo(LI19)	On the face, horizontal to the junction of upper 1/3 and lower 2/3 of the philtrum, just below the lateral margin of the nostril
Yíngxiāng(LI20)	On the face, beside the midpoint of the lateral side of the ala nasi, in the nasolabial groove
Chéngqì(ST1)	On the face, between the eyeball and the infraorbital ridge, directly below the pupil
Sìbái(ST2)	On the face, at the infraorbital foramen
Jùliáo(ST3)	On the face, horizontal to the lower border of the ala nasi, directly below the pupil
Dìcāng(ST4)	On the face, 0.4 cun lateral to the corner of the mouth
Dàyíng(ST5)	On the face, anterior to the angle of the mandible, in the depression of the anterior border of the attached portion of the masseter muscle, on the pulsation place of facial artery
Jiáchē(ST6)	On the face, one finger breadth(middle finger) anterior and superior to the lower angle of the mandible
Xiàguān(ST7)	On the face, in the depression of mandibular notch and midpoint of lower border of the zygomatic arch
Tóuwéi(ST8)	On the head, 0.5 cun within the anterior hairline at the corner of the forehead, 4.5 cun lateral to middle line of the head
Rényíng(ST9)	On the neck, horizontal to the tip of the Adam's apple, in the anterior border of sternocleidomastoid muscle, on the pulsation place of arteria carotis communis

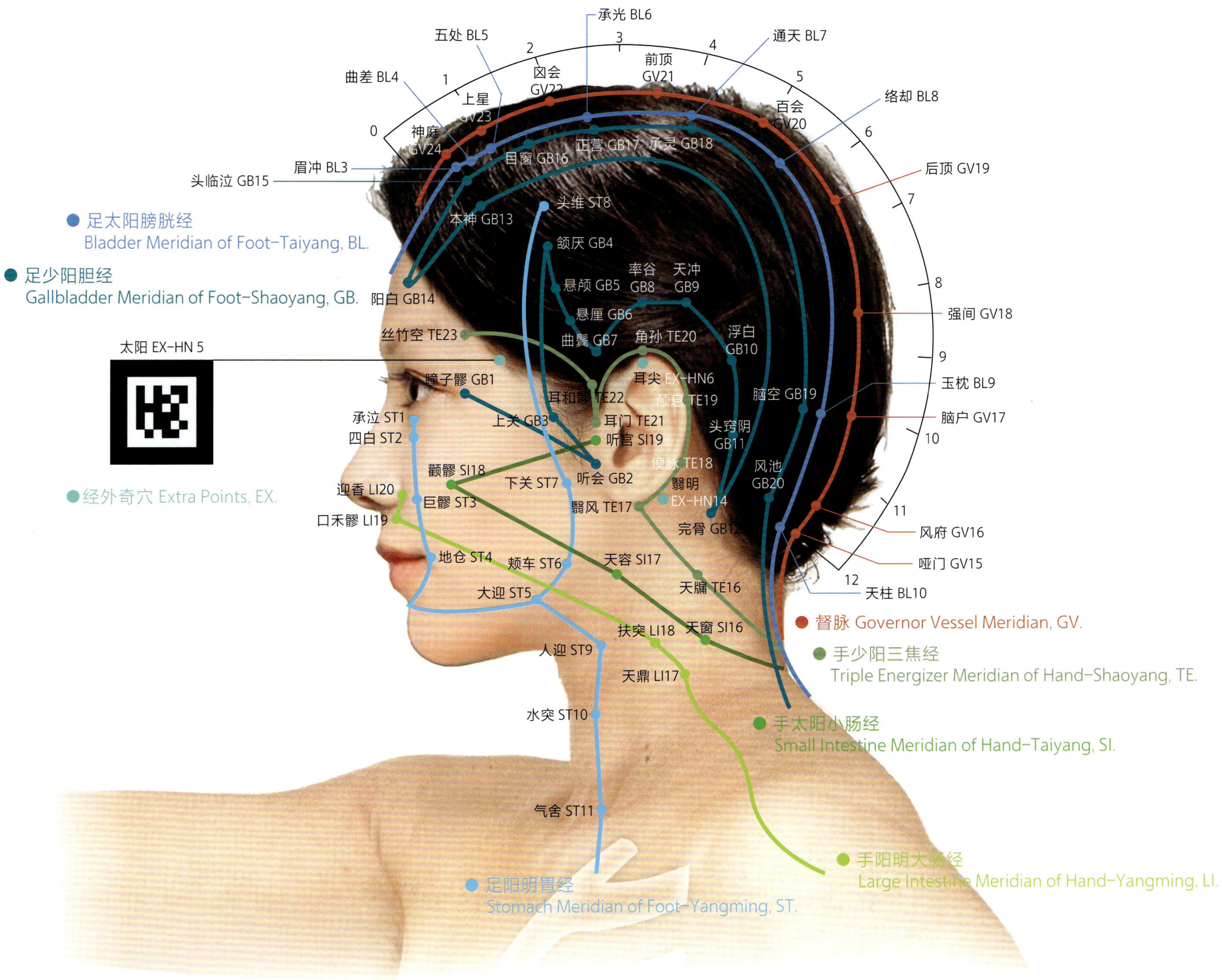
承光 BL6
五处 BL5
通天 BL7
曲差 BL4
囟会
GV22
前顶
GV21
络却 BL8
上星
GV23
百会
GV20
神庭
GV24
正营 GB17
承灵 GB18
目窗 GB16
眉冲 BL3
头临泣 GB15
后顶 GV19
头维 ST8
本神 GB13
足太阳膀胱经
Bladder Meridian of Foot-Taiyang, BL.
颔厌 GB4
率谷
GB8
天冲
GB9
足少阳胆经
Gallbladder Meridian of Foot-Shaoyang, GB.
悬颅 GB5
阳白 GB14
悬厘 GB6
强间 GV18
丝竹空 TE23
曲鬓 GB7
角孙 TE20
浮白
GB10
太阳 EX-HN 5
瞳子髎 GB1
耳尖 EX-HN6
玉枕 BL9
耳和髎 TE22
颅息 TE19
脑空 GB19
脑户 GV17
承泣 ST1
上关 GB3
耳门 TE21
头窍阴
GB11
四白 ST2
听宫 SI19
颧髎 SI18
瘈脉 TE18
风池
GB20
下关 ST7
听会 GB2
翳明
EX-HN14
迎香 LI20
巨髎 ST3
翳风 TE17
经外奇穴 Extra Points, EX.
口禾髎 LI19
完骨 GB12
风府 GV16
地仓 ST4
颊车 ST6
天容 SI17
哑门 GV15
天牖 TE16
天柱 BL10
大迎 ST5
督脉 Governor Vessel Meridian, GV.
扶突 LI18
天窗 SI16
手少阳三焦经
Triple Energizer Meridian of Hand-Shaoyang, TE.
人迎 ST9
天鼎 LI17
水突 ST10
手太阳小肠经
Small Intestine Meridian of Hand-Taiyang, SI.
气舍 ST11
手阳明大肠经
Large Intestine Meridian of Hand-Yangming, LI.
足阳明胃经
Stomach Meridian of Foot-Yangming, ST.
0
1
2
3
4
5
6
7
8
9
10
11
12

续表

穴位	定位
水突	在颈部，横平环状软骨，胸锁乳突肌前缘
气舍	在胸锁乳突肌区，锁骨上小窝，锁骨胸骨端上缘，胸锁乳突肌胸骨头与锁骨头中间的凹陷中
天窗	在颈部，横平喉结，胸锁乳突肌的后缘
天容	在颈部，下颌角后方，胸锁乳突肌的前缘凹陷中
颧髎	在面部，颧骨下缘，目外眦直下凹陷中
听宫	在面部，耳屏正中与下颌骨髁突之间的凹陷中

穴位	定位
眉冲	在头部，额切迹直上入发际 0.5 寸
曲差	在头部，前发际正中直上 0.5 寸，旁开 1.5 寸
五处	在头部，前发际正中直上 1 寸，旁开 1.5 寸
承光	在头部，前发际正中直上 2.5 寸，旁开 1.5 寸
通天	在头部，前发际正中直上 4 寸，旁开 1.5 寸
络却	在头部，前发际正中直上 5.5 寸，旁开 1.5 寸
玉枕	在头部，横平枕外隆凸上缘，后发际正中线旁开 1.3 寸

Continued

Acupoints	Location
Shuǐtū(ST10)	On the neck, horizontal to cricoid cartilage, in the anterior border of the sternocleidomastoid muscle
Qìshè(ST11)	In the region of sternocleidomastoid muscle, at the clavicular fossa, in the superior border of the sternal extremity, in the depression of the sternal head and the clavicular head of the sternocleidomastoid muscle
Tiānchuāng(SI16)	On the neck, horizontal to the tip of the Adam' s apple, in the posterior border of sternocleidomastoid muscle
Tiānróng(SI17)	On the neck, posterior to lower angle of the mandible, in the depression of anterior border of sternocleidomastoid muscle
Quánliáo(SI18)	On the face, in the lower border of zygoma, in the depression directly below the outer canthus
Tīnggōng(SI19)	On the face, in the depression between the midpoint of the tragus and the condyloid process of the mandible
Méichōng(BL3)	On the head, 0.5 cun within the hairline, directly above supraorbital notch
Qūchā(BL4)	On the head, 0.5 cun directly within the midpoint of anterior hairline, 1.5 cun lateral to the midpoint of anterior hairline
Wǔchù(BL5)	On the head, 1 cun directly within the midpoint of anterior hairline, 1.5 cun lateral to the midpoint of anterior hairline
Chéngguāng(BL6)	On the head, 2.5 cun directly within the midpoint of anterior hairline, 1.5 cun lateral to the midpoint of anterior hairline
Tōngtiān(BL7)	On the head, 4 cun directly within the midpoint of anterior hairline, 1.5 cun lateral to the midpoint of anterior hairline
Luòquè(BL8)	On the head, 5.5 cun within the midpoint of the anterior hairline, 1.5 cun lateral to midpoint of anterior hairline
Yùzhěn(BL9)	On the head, horizontal to the lateral border of external occipital protuberance, 1.3 cun lateral to posterior hairline

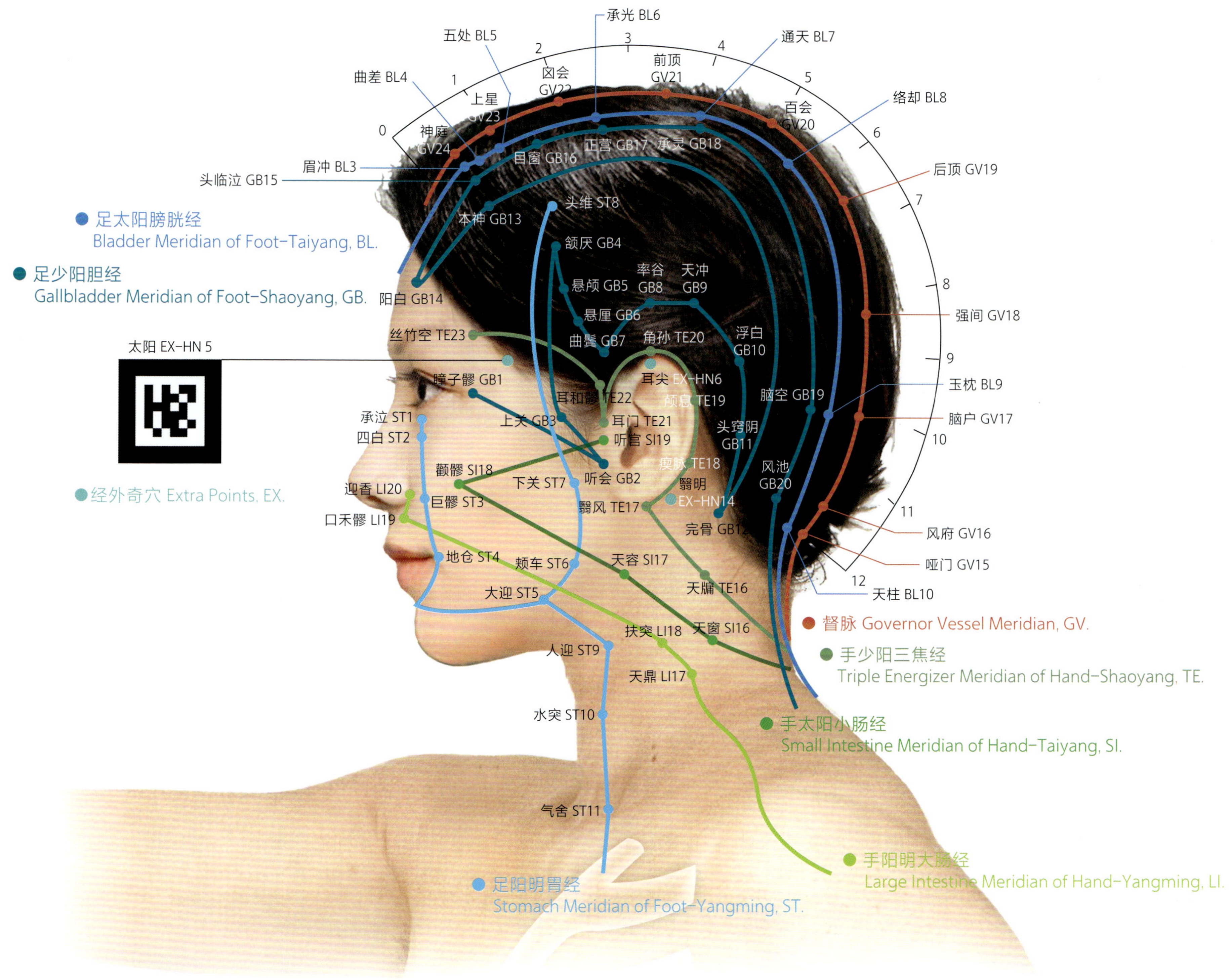
承光 BL6
五处 BL5
通天 BL7
曲差 BL4
前顶 GV21
囟会 GV22
上星 GV23
百会 GV20
络却 BL8
神庭 GV24
正营 GB17
承灵 GB18
目窗 GB16
后顶 GV19
眉冲 BL3
头临泣 GB15
头维 ST8
本神 GB13
足太阳膀胱经
Bladder Meridian of Foot-Taiyang, BL.
颔厌 GB4
足少阳胆经
Gallbladder Meridian of Foot-Shaoyang, GB.
悬颅 GB5
率谷 GB8
天冲 GB9
阳白 GB14
悬厘 GB6
强间 GV18
丝竹空 TE23
曲鬓 GB7
角孙 TE20
浮白 GB10
太阳 EX-HN 5
瞳子髎 GB1
耳尖 EX-HN6
玉枕 BL9
耳和髎 TE22
颅息 TE19
脑空 GB19
脑户 GV17
承泣 ST1
上关 GB3
耳门 TE21
头窍阴 GB11
四白 ST2
听宫 SI19
瘈脉 TE18
颧髎 SI18
下关 ST7
听会 GB2
翳明 EX-HN14
风池 GB20
迎香 LI20
经外奇穴 Extra Points, EX.
巨髎 ST3
翳风 TE17
口禾髎 LI19
完骨 GB12
风府 GV16
地仓 ST4
颊车 ST6
天容 SI17
哑门 GV15
大迎 ST5
天牖 TE16
天柱 BL10
督脉 Governor Vessel Meridian, GV.
扶突 LI18
天窗 SI16
人迎 ST9
手少阳三焦经
Triple Energizer Meridian of Hand-Shaoyang, TE.
天鼎 LI17
水突 ST10
手太阳小肠经
Small Intestine Meridian of Hand-Taiyang, SI.
气舍 ST11
手阳明大肠经
Large Intestine Meridian of Hand-Yangming, LI.
足阳明胃经
Stomach Meridian of Foot-Yangming, ST.

续表

穴 位	定 位
天柱	在颈后区，横平第 2 颈椎棘突上际，斜方肌外缘凹陷中
天牖	在颈部，横平下颌角，胸锁乳突肌的后缘凹陷中
翳风	在颈部，耳垂后方，乳突下端前方凹陷中
瘈脉	在头部，乳突中央，角孙与翳风沿耳轮弧形连线的上 2/3 与下 1/3 的交点处
颅息	在头部，角孙与翳风沿耳轮弧形连线的上 1/3 与下 2/3 的交点处
角孙	在头部，耳尖正对发际处
耳门	在耳区，耳屏上切迹的与下颌骨髁突之间的凹陷中
耳和髎	在头部，鬓发后缘，耳廓根的前方，颞浅动脉的后缘
丝竹空	在面部，眉梢凹陷中
瞳子髎	在面部，目外眦外侧 0.5 寸凹陷中
听会	在面部，耳屏间切迹与下颌骨髁突之间的凹陷中
上关	在面部，颧弓上缘中央凹陷中

Continued

Acupoints	Location
Tiānzhù(BL10)	In the posterior neck region, horizontal to superior border of spinous process of the 2nd cervical vertebra, in the depression of the lateral border of the muscle trapezius
Tiānyǒu(TE16)	On the neck, horizontal to lower angle of the mandible, in the depression of the posterior border of the sternocleidomastoid muscle
Yìfēng(TE17)	On the neck, posterior to the lobule of the ear, in the anterior depression of the lower portion of the mastoid process
Chìmài(TE18)	On the head, at the midpoint of the mastoid process, at the junction of upper 2/3 and lower 1/3 on the curved line along the helix drawn from Jiaosun (TE20) to Yifeng (TE17)
Lúxī(TE19)	On the head, at the junction of upper 1/3 and lower 2/3 on the curved line along the helix drawn from Jiaosun (TE20) to Yifeng (TE17)
Jiǎosūn(TE20)	On the head, within the hairline, horizontal to the ear apex
Ěrmén(TE21)	In the ear region, in the depression between supratragic notch of the tragus and the condyloid process of the mandible
Ěrhéliáo(TE22)	On the head, in the posterior border of the hairline of the temple, anterior to the root of the auricle, in the posterior border of superficial temporal artery
Sīzhúkōng(TE23)	On the face, in the depression at the lateral end of the eyebrow
Tóngzǐliáo(GB1)	On the face, in the depression 0.5 cun lateral to the outer canthus
Tīnghuì(GB2)	On the face, in the depression between intertragic notch and condyloid process of mandible
Shàngguān(GB3)	On the face, in the middle depression superior to the upper margin of the zygomatic arch

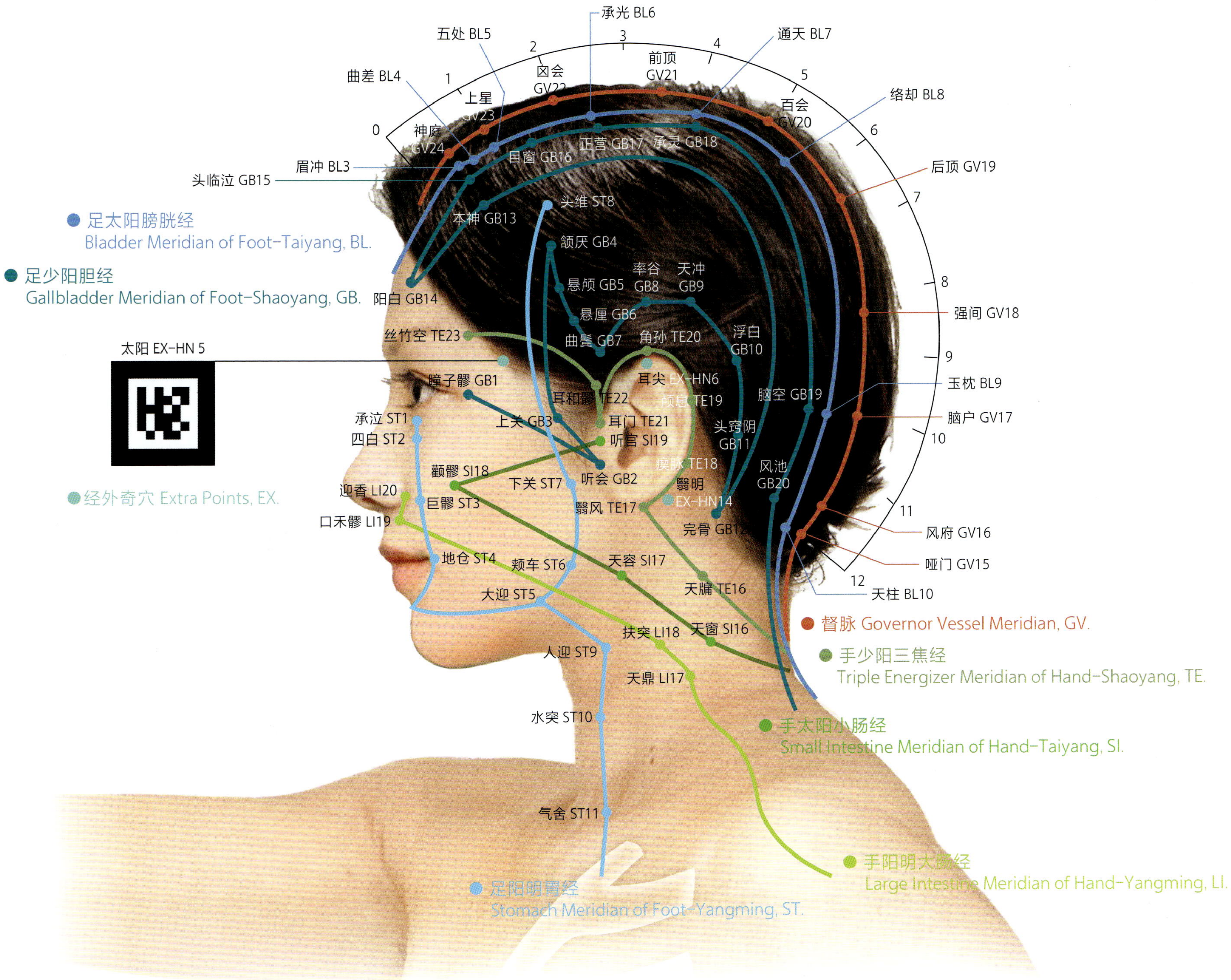
承光 BL6
五处 BL5
通天 BL7
曲差 BL4
前顶 GV21
囟会 GV22
上星 GV23
百会 GV20
络却 BL8
神庭 GV24
0
1
2
3
4
5
6
7
8
9
10
11
12
正营 GB17
承灵 GB18
目窗 GB16
眉冲 BL3
头临泣 GB15
后顶 GV19
本神 GB13
头维 ST8
足太阳膀胱经
Bladder Meridian of Foot-Taiyang, BL.
颔厌 GB4
足少阳胆经
Gallbladder Meridian of Foot-Shaoyang, GB.
阳白 GB14
悬颅 GB5
率谷 GB8
天冲 GB9
悬厘 GB6
强间 GV18
丝竹空 TE23
曲鬓 GB7
角孙 TE20
浮白 GB10
太阳 EX-HN 5
耳尖 EX-HN6
瞳子髎 GB1
耳和髎 TE22
颅息 TE19
脑空 GB19
玉枕 BL9
承泣 ST1
上关 GB3
耳门 TE21
头窍阴 GB11
脑户 GV17
四白 ST2
听宫 SI19
颧髎 SI18
瘈脉 TE18
风池 GB20
迎香 LI20
下关 ST7
听会 GB2
翳明 EX-HN14
经外奇穴 Extra Points, EX.
巨髎 ST3
翳风 TE17
口禾髎 LI19
完骨 GB12
风府 GV16
地仓 ST4
颊车 ST6
天容 SI17
哑门 GV15
天牖 TE16
大迎 ST5
天柱 BL10
督脉 Governor Vessel Meridian, GV.
扶突 LI18
天窗 SI16
手少阳三焦经
Triple Energizer Meridian of Hand-Shaoyang, TE.
人迎 ST9
天鼎 LI17
水突 ST10
手太阳小肠经
Small Intestine Meridian of Hand-Taiyang, SI.
气舍 ST11
手阳明大肠经
Large Intestine Meridian of Hand-Yangming, LI.
足阳明胃经
Stomach Meridian of Foot-Yangming, ST.

续表

穴 位	定 位
颔厌	在头部，从头维至曲鬓的弧形连线（其弧度与鬓发弧度相应）的上 1/4 与下 3/4 交点处
悬颅	在头部，从头维至曲鬓的弧形连线（其弧度与鬓发弧度相应）的中点处
悬厘	在头部，从头维至曲鬓的弧形连线（其弧度与鬓发弧度相应）的上 3/4 与下 1/4 交点处
曲鬓	在头部，耳前鬓角发际后缘与耳尖水平线的交点处
率谷	在头部，耳尖直上入发际 1.5 寸
天冲	在头部，耳根后缘直上，入发际 2 寸
浮白	在头部，耳后乳突的后上方，从天冲至完骨的弧形连线（其弧度与耳郭弧度相应）的上 1/3 与下 2/3 交点处
头窍阴	在头部，耳后乳突的后上方，从天冲至完骨的弧形连线（其弧度与耳郭弧度相应）的上 2/3 与下 1/3 交点处
完骨	在头部，耳后乳突的后下方凹陷中
本神	在头部，前发际上 0.5 寸，头正中线旁开 3 寸
阳白	在头部，眉上 1 寸，瞳孔直上

Continued

Acupoints	Location
Hànyàn(GB4)	On the head, at the junction of upper 1/4 and lower 3/4 of the curved line joining Touwei(ST8) and Qubin(GB7)
Xuánlú(GB5)	On the head, at the midpoint of the curved line joining Touwei(ST8) and Qubin(GB7)
Xuánlí(GB6)	On the head, at the junction of upper 3/4 and lower 1/4 of the curved line joining Touwei(ST8) and Qubin(GB7)
Qūbìn(GB7)	On the head, at the junction of posterior margin of the temple and horizontal line of ear apex
Shuàigǔ(GB8)	On the head, directly above the apex of the ear and 1.5 cun within the hairline
Tiānchōng(GB9)	On the head, directly above the posterior border of the ear and 2 cun within the hairline
Fúbái(GB10)	On the head, posterior and superior to the mastoid process, at the junction of upper 1/3 and lower 2/3 of the curved line joining Tianchong(GB9) and Wangu(GB12)
Tóuqiàoyīn(GB11)	On the head, posterior and superior to the mastoid process, at the junction of upper 2/3 and lower 1/3 of the curved line joining Tianchong(GB9) and Wangu(GB12)
Wángǔ(GB12)	On the head, in the depression posterior and inferior to the mastoid process
Běnshén(GB13)	On the head, 0.5 cun above the anterior hairline, 3 cun lateral to the midline of the head
Yángbái(GB14)	On the head, 1 cun superior to the eyebrow, directly above the pupil

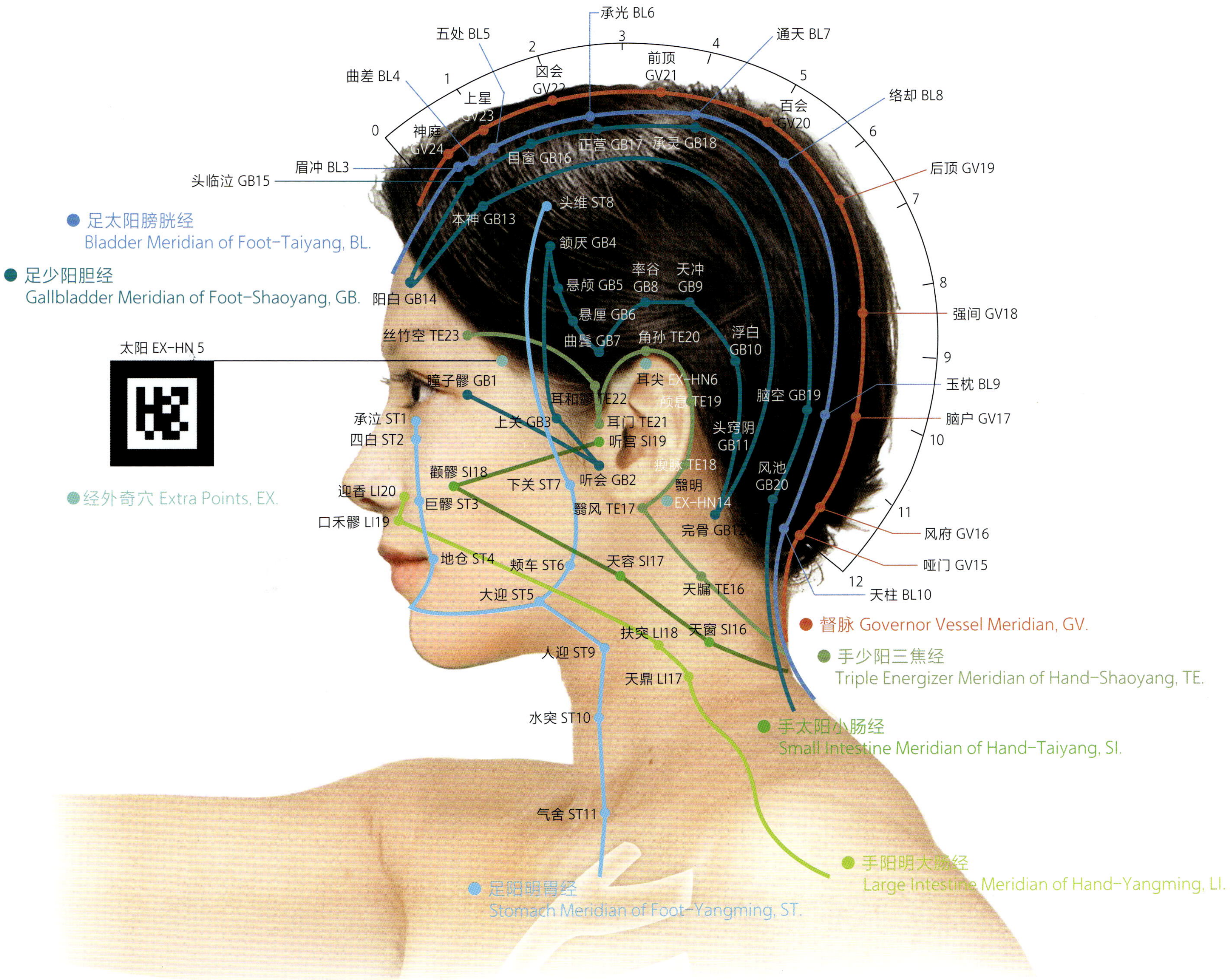
承光 BL6
五处 BL5
通天 BL7
曲差 BL4
前顶 GV21
囟会 GV22
络却 BL8
上星 GV23
百会 GV20
神庭 GV24
正营 GB17
承灵 GB18
目窗 GB16
眉冲 BL3
头临泣 GB15
后顶 GV19
头维 ST8
本神 GB13
足太阳膀胱经
Bladder Meridian of Foot-Taiyang, BL.
颔厌 GB4
足少阳胆经
Gallbladder Meridian of Foot-Shaoyang, GB.
率谷 GB8
天冲 GB9
悬颅 GB5
阳白 GB14
悬厘 GB6
强间 GV18
丝竹空 TE23
曲鬓 GB7
角孙 TE20
浮白 GB10
太阳 EX-HN 5
瞳子髎 GB1
耳尖 EX-HN6
耳和髎 TE22
颅息 TE19
脑空 GB19
玉枕 BL9
承泣 ST1
上关 GB3
耳门 TE21
头窍阴 GB11
脑户 GV17
四白 ST2
听宫 SI19
颧髎 SI18
瘈脉 TE18
风池 GB20
下关 ST7
听会 GB2
瘛明
EX-HN14
迎香 LI20
经外奇穴 Extra Points, EX.
巨髎 ST3
翳风 TE17
口禾髎 LI19
完骨 GB12
风府 GV16
地仓 ST4
颊车 ST6
天容 SI17
哑门 GV15
天牖 TE16
天柱 BL10
大迎 ST5
督脉 Governor Vessel Meridian, GV.
扶突 LI18
天窗 SI16
手少阳三焦经
Triple Energizer Meridian of Hand-Shaoyang, TE.
人迎 ST9
天鼎 LI17
水突 ST10
手太阳小肠经
Small Intestine Meridian of Hand-Taiyang, SI.
气舍 ST11
手阳明大肠经
Large Intestine Meridian of Hand-Yangming, LI.
足阳明胃经
Stomach Meridian of Foot-Yangming, ST.
0
1
2
3
4
5
6
7
8
9
10
11
12

续表

穴位	定位
头临泣	在头部，前发际上 0.5 寸，瞳孔直上
目窗	在头部，前发际上 1.5 寸，瞳孔直上
正营	在头部，前发际上 2.5 寸，瞳孔直上
承灵	在头部，前发际上 4 寸，瞳孔直上
脑空	在头部，横平枕外隆凸的上缘，风池直上
风池	在颈后区，枕骨之下，胸锁乳突肌上端与斜方肌上端之间的凹陷中

穴位	定位
哑门	在项后区，第 2 颈椎棘突上际凹陷中，后正中线上
风府	在项后区，枕外隆凸直下，两侧斜方肌之间凹陷中
脑户	在头部，枕外隆凸的上缘凹陷中
强间	在头部，后发际正中直上 4 寸
后顶	在头部，后发际正中直上 5.5 寸
百会	在头部，前发际正中直上 5 寸

Continued

Acupoints	Location
Tóulínqì(GB15)	On the head, 0.5 cun superior to the anterior hairline, directly above the pupil
Mùchuāng(GB16)	On the head, 1.5 cun superior to the anterior hairline, directly above the pupil
Zhèngyíng(GB17)	On the head, 2.5 cun superior to the anterior hairline, directly above the pupil
Chénglíng(GB18)	On the head, 4 cun superior to the anterior hairline, directly above the pupil
Nǎokōng(GB19)	On the head, horizontal to superior border of external occipital protuberance, directly above Fengchi(GB20)
Fēngchí(GB20)	In the posterior region of neck, inferior to the occipital bone, in the depression between superior margin of sternocleidomastoid muscle and superior margin of trapezius
Yǎmén(GV15)	In the posterior region of neck, in the depression of superior border of the 2nd cervical vertebra, on the posterior midline
Fēngfǔ(GV16)	In the posterior region of neck, directly below external occipital protuberance, in the depression between bilateral trapezius
Nǎohù(GV17)	On the head, in the depression of the superior border of external occipital protuberance
Qiángjiān(GV18)	On the head, 4 cun directly above the midpoint of posterior hairline
Hòudǐng(GV19)	On the head, 5.5 cun directly above the midpoint of posterior hairline
Bǎihuì(GV20)	On the head, 5 cun directly above the midpoint of anterior hairline

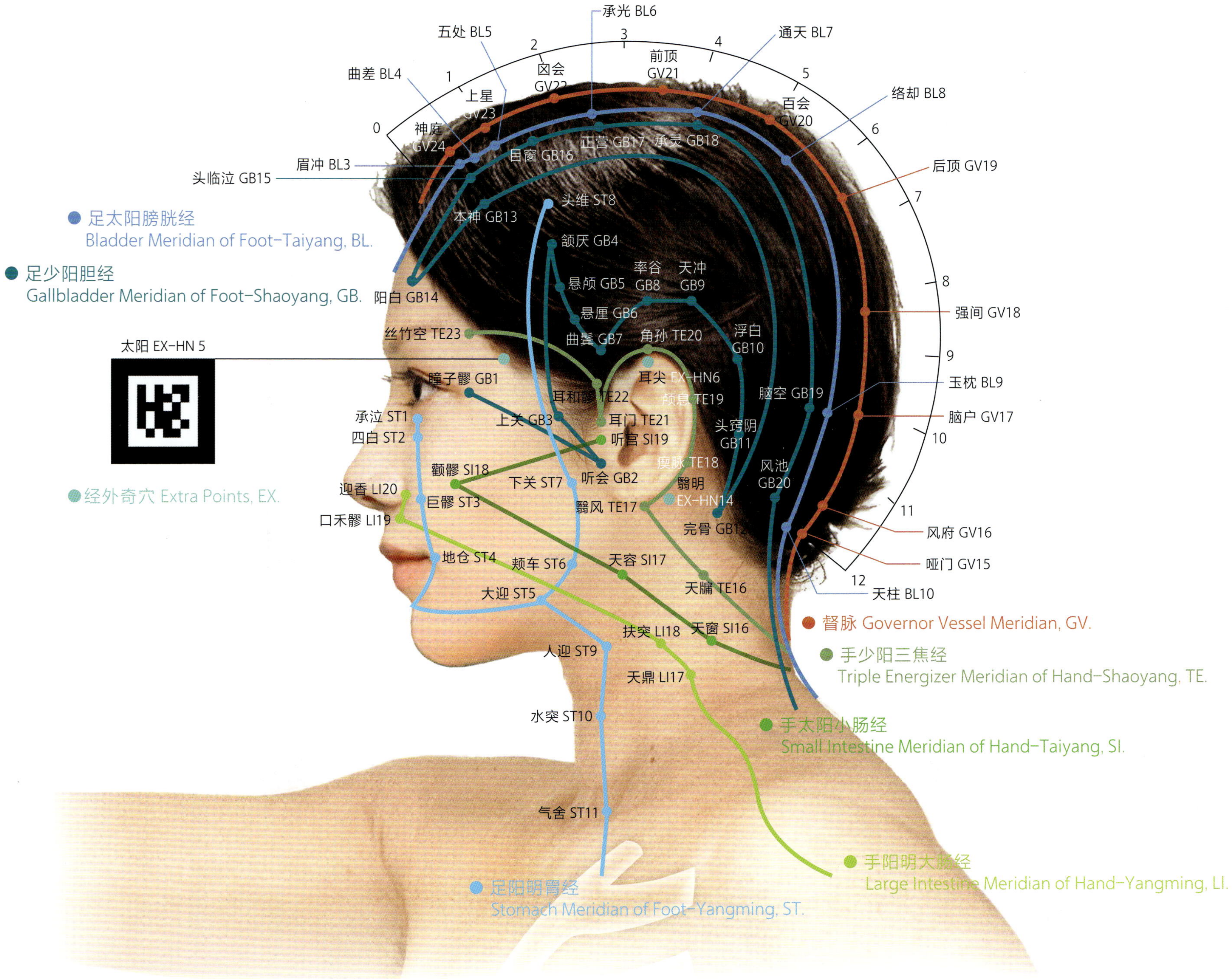

承光 BL6
五处 BL5
通天 BL7
曲差 BL4
囟会 GV22
前顶 GV21
络却 BL8
上星 GV23
百会 GV20
神庭 GV24
正营 GB17
承灵 GB18
目窗 GB16
眉冲 BL3
后顶 GV19
头临泣 GB15
本神 GB13
头维 ST8
足太阳膀胱经
Bladder Meridian of Foot-Taiyang, BL.
颔厌 GB4
足少阳胆经
Gallbladder Meridian of Foot-Shaoyang, GB.
阳白 GB14
悬颅 GB5
率谷 GB8
天冲 GB9
悬厘 GB6
强间 GV18
丝竹空 TE23
曲鬓 GB7
角孙 TE20
浮白 GB10
太阳 EX-HN 5
瞳子髎 GB1
耳尖 EX-HN6
耳和髎 TE22
颅息 TE19
脑空 GB19
玉枕 BL9
承泣 ST1
上关 GB3
耳门 TE21
头窍阴 GB11
脑户 GV17
四白 ST2
听宫 SI19
颧髎 SI18
瘈脉 TE18
风池 GB20
下关 ST7
听会 GB2
翳明 EX-HN14
迎香 LI20
经外奇穴 Extra Points, EX.
巨髎 ST3
翳风 TE17
口禾髎 LI19
完骨 GB12
风府 GV16
地仓 ST4
颊车 ST6
天容 SI17
哑门 GV15
天牖 TE16
天柱 BL10
大迎 ST5
督脉 Governor Vessel Meridian, GV.
扶突 LI18
天窗 SI16
人迎 ST9
手少阳三焦经
Triple Energizer Meridian of Hand-Shaoyang, TE.
天鼎 LI17
手太阳小肠经
Small Intestine Meridian of Hand-Taiyang, SI.
水突 ST10
气舍 ST11
手阳明大肠经
Large Intestine Meridian of Hand-Yangming, LI.
足阳明胃经
Stomach Meridian of Foot-Yangming, ST.

续表

穴位	定位
前顶	在头部，前发际正中直上 3.5 寸
囟会	在头部，前发际正中直上 2 寸
上星	在头部，前发际正中直上 1 寸
神庭	在头部，前发际正中直上 0.5 寸
太阳	在颞部，当眉梢与目外眦之间，向后约 1 横指的凹陷处
耳尖	在耳郭的上方，当折耳向前，耳郭上方的尖端处
翳明	在项部，当翳风后 1 寸

Continued

Acupoints	Location
Qiándǐng(GV21)	On the head, 3.5 cun directly above the midpoint of anterior hairline
Xìnhuì(GV22)	On the head, 2 cun directly above the midpoint of anterior hairline
Shàngxīng(GV23)	On the head, 1 cun directly above the midpoint of anterior hairline
Shénting(GV24)	On the head, 0.5 cun directly above the midpoint of anterior hairline
Tàiyáng(EX-HN5)	In the temporal region, between the eyebrow and outer canthus, in the depression around one finger breadth backward
Ěrjiān(EX-HN6)	Superior to the auricle, when you are folding the auricle forward, this point lies at the apex of the ear
Yìmíng(EX-HN14)	On the neck, 1 cun posterior to Yifeng (TE17)

胸腹部穴位
Acupoints of Chest and Abdomen

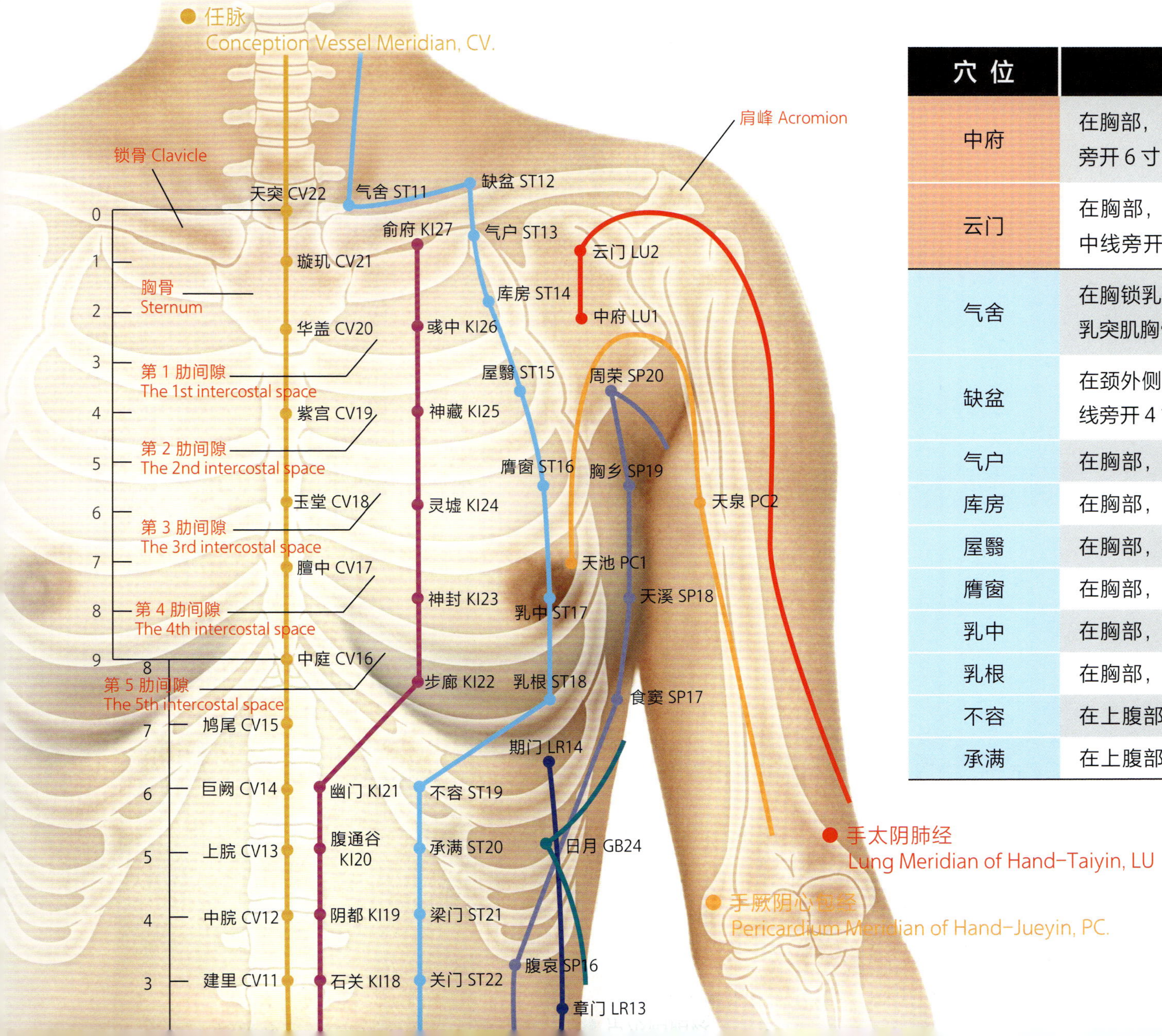

穴 位	定 位
中府	在胸部，横平第 1 肋间隙，锁骨下窝外侧，前正中线旁开 6 寸
云门	在胸部，锁骨下窝凹陷中，肩胛骨喙突内缘，前正中线旁开 6 寸
气舍	在胸锁乳突区，锁骨上小窝，锁骨胸骨端上缘，胸锁乳突肌胸骨头与锁骨头中间的凹陷中
缺盆	在颈外侧区，锁骨上大窝，锁骨上缘凹陷中，前正中线旁开 4 寸
气户	在胸部，锁骨下缘，前正中线旁开 4 寸
库房	在胸部，第 1 肋间隙，前正中线旁开 4 寸
屋翳	在胸部，第 2 肋间隙，前正中线旁开 4 寸
膺窗	在胸部，第 3 肋间隙，前正中线旁开 4 寸
乳中	在胸部，乳头中央
乳根	在胸部，第 5 肋间隙，前正中线旁开 4 寸
不容	在上腹部，脐中上 6 寸，前正中线旁开 2 寸
承满	在上腹部，脐中上 5 寸，前正中线旁开 2 寸

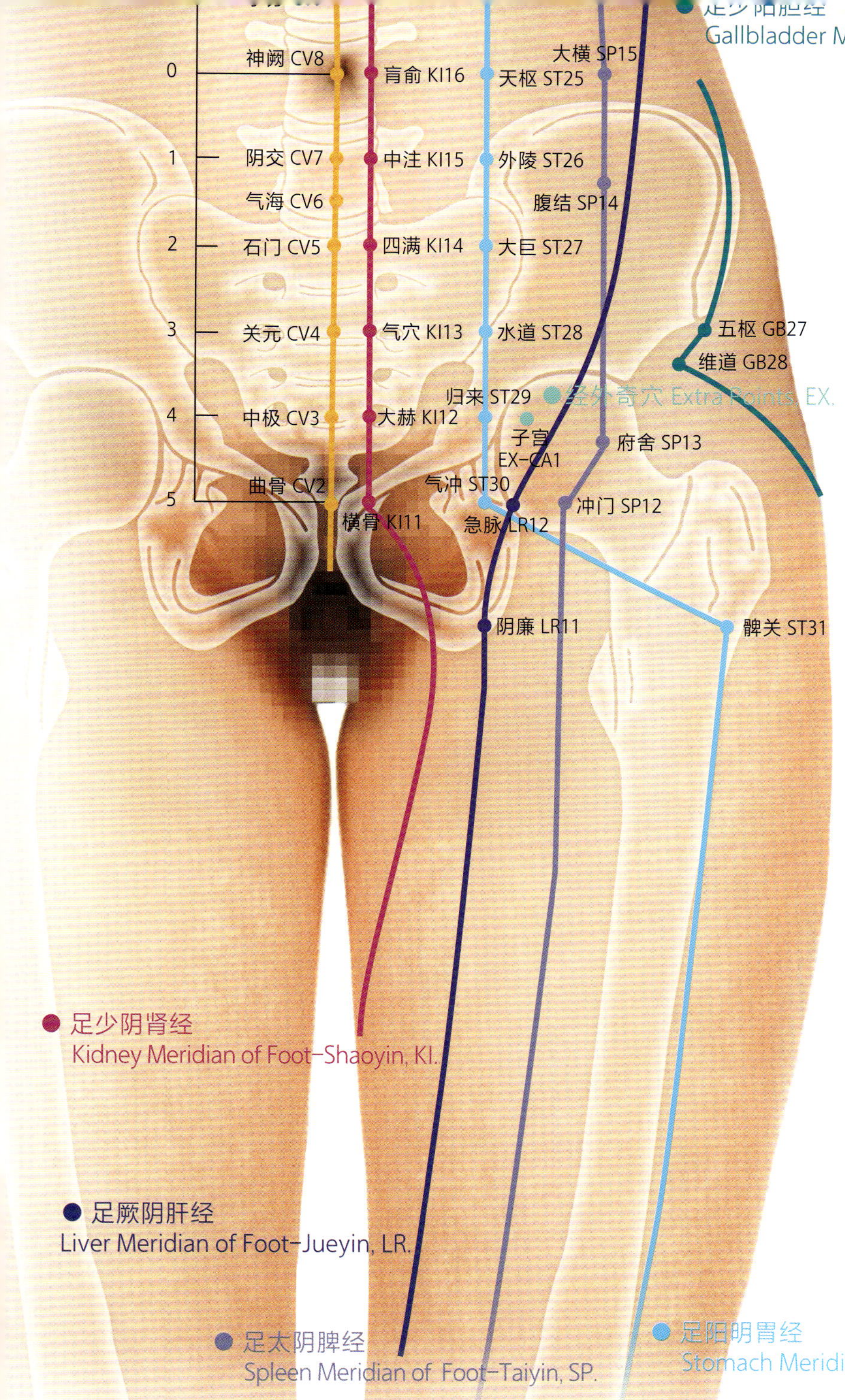

Acupoints	Location
Zhōngfǔ(LU1)	On the chest, horizontal to the 1st intercostal space, in the lateral side of the infraclavicular fossa, 6 cun lateral to the anterior midline
Yúnmén(LU2)	On the chest, in the depression of infraclavicular fossa, in the interior margin of scapular coracoid process, 6 cun lateral to the anterior midline
Qìshè(ST11)	In the sternoclavicular mastoid region, in the lesser supraclavicular fossa, in the superior border of sternal end of clavicle, in depression between the sternal head and clavicular head of sternocleidomastoid muscle
Quēpén(ST12)	In the lateral region of neck, in the greater supraclavicular fossa, in the depression of the upper border of clavicle, 4 cun lateral to the anterior midline
Qìhù(ST13)	On the chest, in the inferior border of clavicle, 4 cun lateral to the anterior midline
Kùfáng(ST14)	On the chest, in the 1st intercostal space,4 cun lateral to the anterior midline
Wūyì(ST15)	On the chest, in the 2nd intercostal space, 4 cun lateral to the anterior midline
Yīngchuāng(ST16)	On the chest, in the 3rd intercostal space, 4 cun lateral to the anterior midline
Rǔzhōng(ST17)	On the chest, in center of nipple
Rǔgēn(ST18)	On the chest, in the 5th intercostal space, 4 cun lateral to the anterior midline
Bùróng(ST19)	On the upper abdomen, 6 cun superior to the navel, 2 cun lateral to the anterior midline
Chéngmǎn(ST20)	On the upper abdomen, 5 cun superior to the navel, 2 cun lateral to the anterior midline

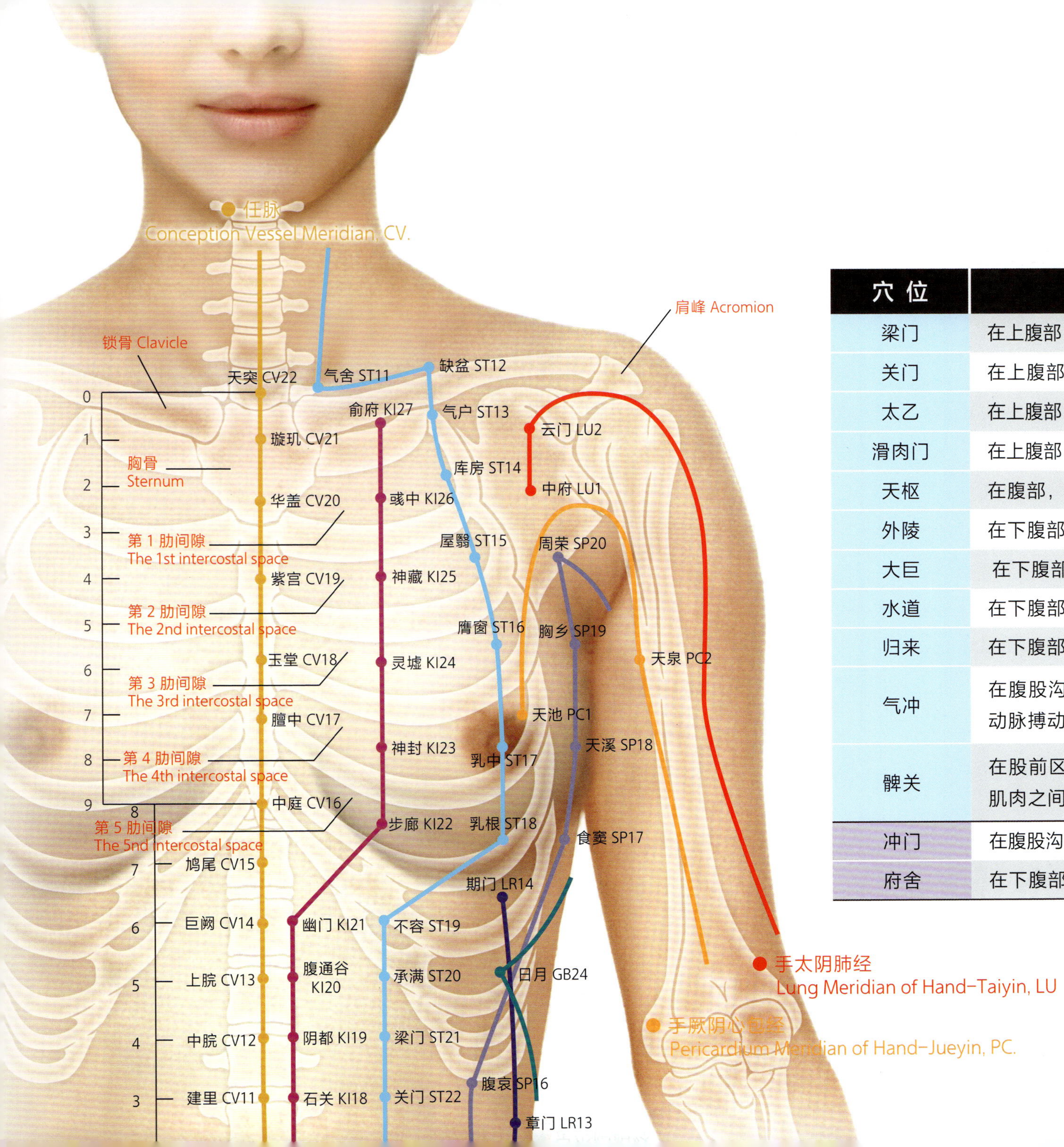

续表

穴 位	定 位
梁门	在上腹部，脐中上 4 寸，前正中线旁开 2 寸
关门	在上腹部，脐中上 3 寸，前正中线旁开 2 寸
太乙	在上腹部，脐中上 2 寸，前正中线旁开 2 寸
滑肉门	在上腹部，脐中上 1 寸，前正中线旁开 2 寸
天枢	在腹部，横平脐中，前正中线旁开 2 寸
外陵	在下腹部，脐中下 1 寸，前正中线旁开 2 寸
大巨	在下腹部，脐中下 2 寸，前正中线旁开 2 寸
水道	在下腹部，脐中下 3 寸，前正中线旁开 2 寸
归来	在下腹部，脐中下 4 寸，前正中线旁开 2 寸
气冲	在腹股沟区，耻骨联合上缘，前正中线旁开 2 寸，动脉搏动处
髀关	在股前区，股直肌近端，缝匠肌与阔筋膜张肌 3 条肌肉之间凹陷中
冲门	在腹股沟区，腹股沟斜纹中，髂外动脉搏动处的外侧
府舍	在下腹部，脐中下 4.3 寸，前正中线旁开 4 寸

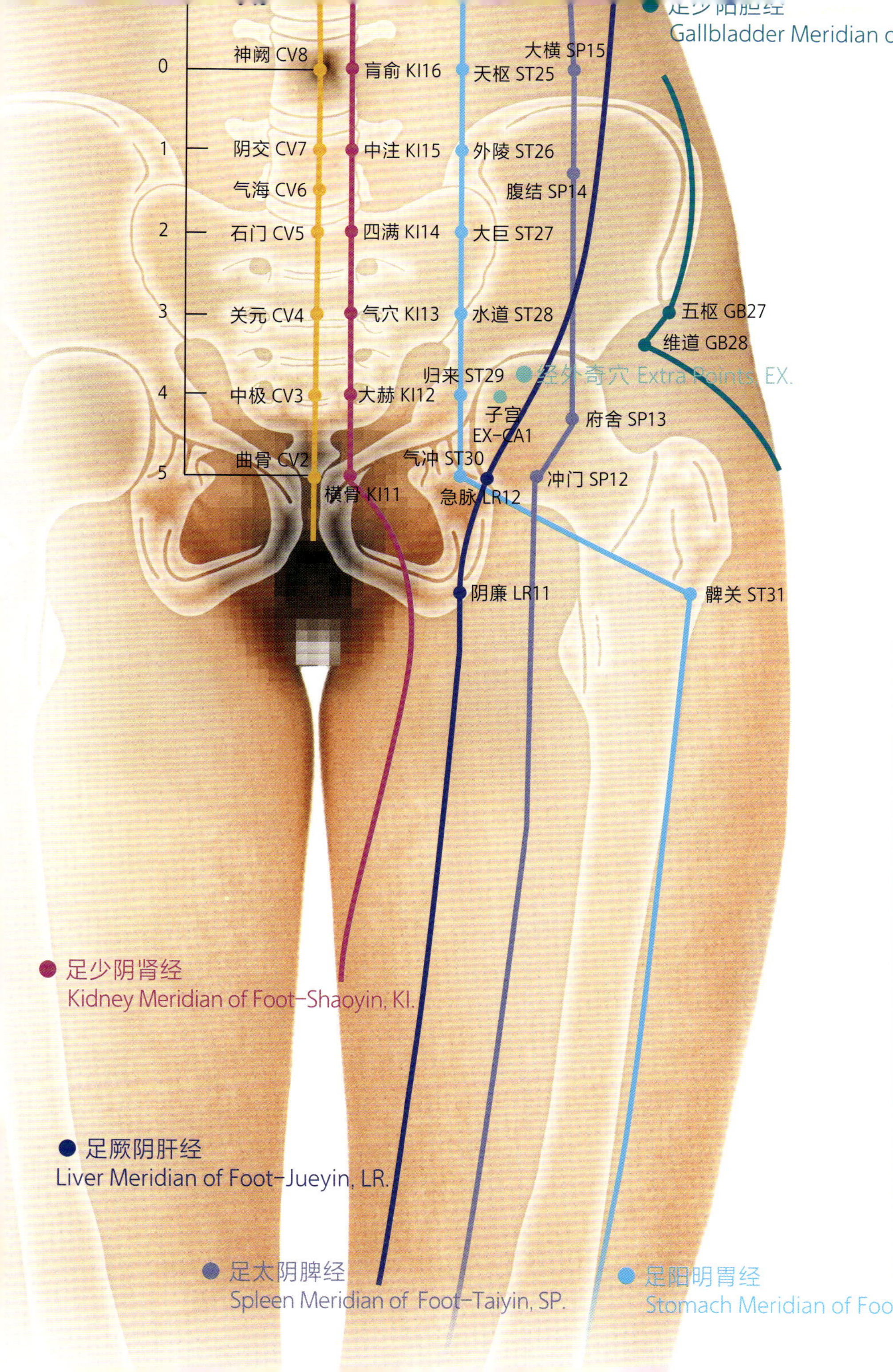

Continued

Acupoints	Location
Liángmén(ST21)	On the upper abdomen, 4 cun superior to the navel, 2 cun lateral to the anterior midline
Guānmén(ST22)	On the upper abdomen, 3 cun superior to the navel, 2 cun lateral to the anterior midline
Tàiyǐ(ST23)	On the upper abdomen, 2 cun superior to the navel, 2 cun lateral to the anterior midline
Huáròumén(ST24)	On the upper abdomen, 1 cun superior to the navel, 2 cun lateral to the anterior midline
Tiānshū(ST25)	On the abdomen, horizontal to navel, 2 cun lateral to the anterior midline
Wàilíng(ST26)	On the lower abdomen, 1 cun inferior to the navel, 2 cun lateral to the anterior midline
Dàjù(ST27)	On the lower abdomen, 2 cun inferior to the navel, 2 cun lateral to the anterior midline
Shuǐdào(ST28)	On the lower abdomen, 3 cun inferior to the navel, 2 cun lateral to the anterior midline
Guīlái(ST29)	On the lower abdomen, 4 cun inferior to the navel, 2 cun lateral to the anterior midline
Qìchōng(ST30)	In the inguinal region, in the superior margin of symphysis pubis, 2 cun lateral to the anterior midline, in the arterial pulse palpated
Bìguān(ST31)	In the anterior region of thigh, proximal to rectus femoris, In the depression between sartorius and three muscles of tensor fasciae latae
Chōngmén(SP12)	In the inguinal region, in the inguinal twill, in the exterior side of the external iliac artery pulse
Fǔshè(SP13)	On the lower abdomen, 4.3 cun inferior to the navel, 4 cun lateral to the anterior midline

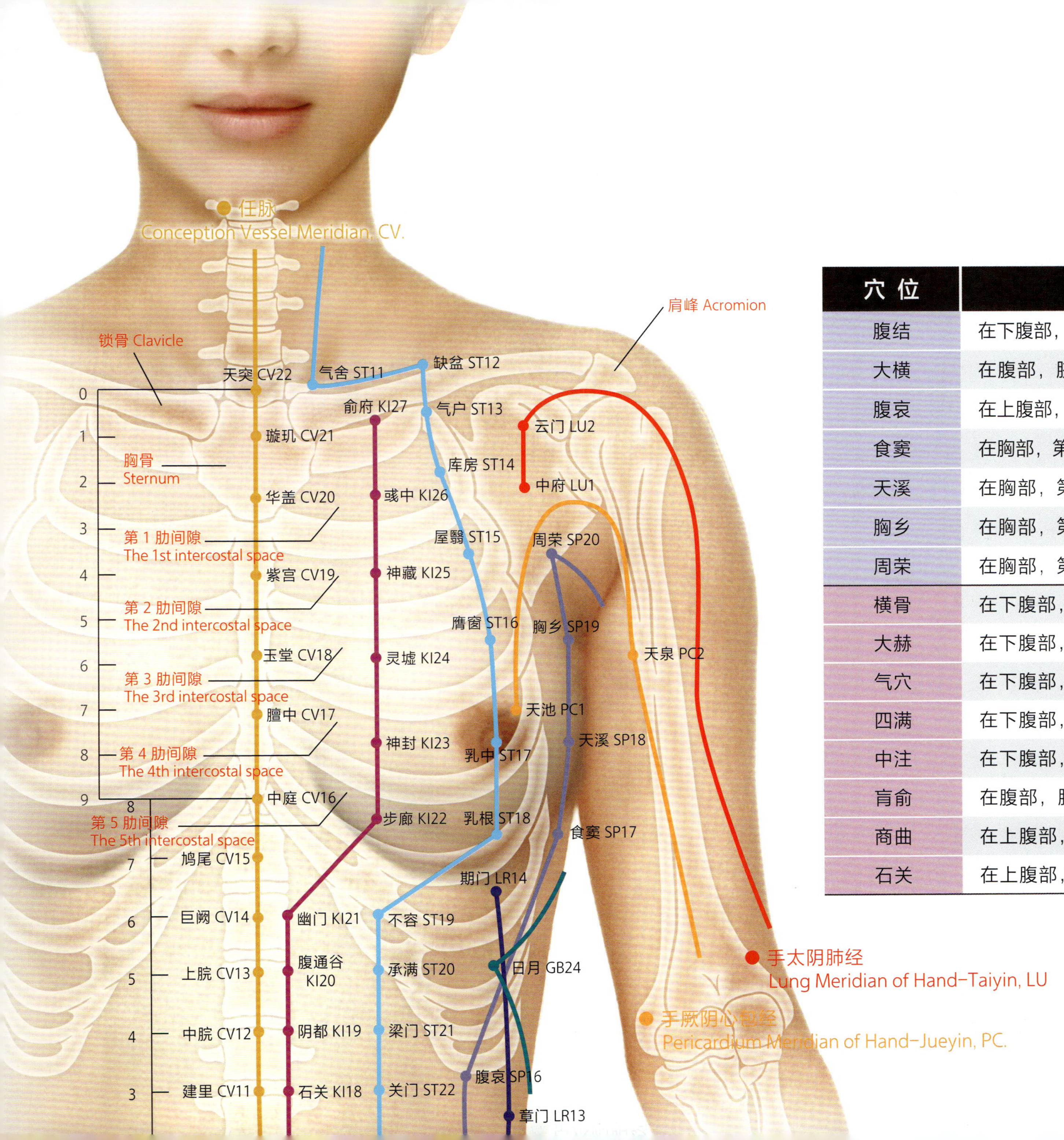

续表

穴 位	定 位
腹结	在下腹部，脐中下 1.3 寸，前正中线旁开 4 寸
大横	在腹部，脐中旁开 4 寸
腹哀	在上腹部，脐中上 3 寸，前正中线旁开 4 寸
食窦	在胸部，第 5 肋间隙，前正中线旁开 6 寸
天溪	在胸部，第 4 肋间隙，前正中线旁开 6 寸
胸乡	在胸部，第 3 肋间隙，前正中线旁开 6 寸
周荣	在胸部，第 2 肋间隙，前正中线旁开 6 寸
横骨	在下腹部，脐中下 5 寸，前正中线旁开 0.5 寸
大赫	在下腹部，脐中下 4 寸，前正中线旁开 0.5 寸
气穴	在下腹部，脐中下 3 寸，前正中线旁开 0.5 寸
四满	在下腹部，脐中下 2 寸，前正中线旁开 0.5 寸
中注	在下腹部，脐中下 1 寸，前正中线旁开 0.5 寸
肓俞	在腹部，脐中旁开 0.5 寸
商曲	在上腹部，脐中上 2 寸，前正中线旁开 0.5 寸
石关	在上腹部，脐中上 3 寸，前正中线旁开 0.5 寸

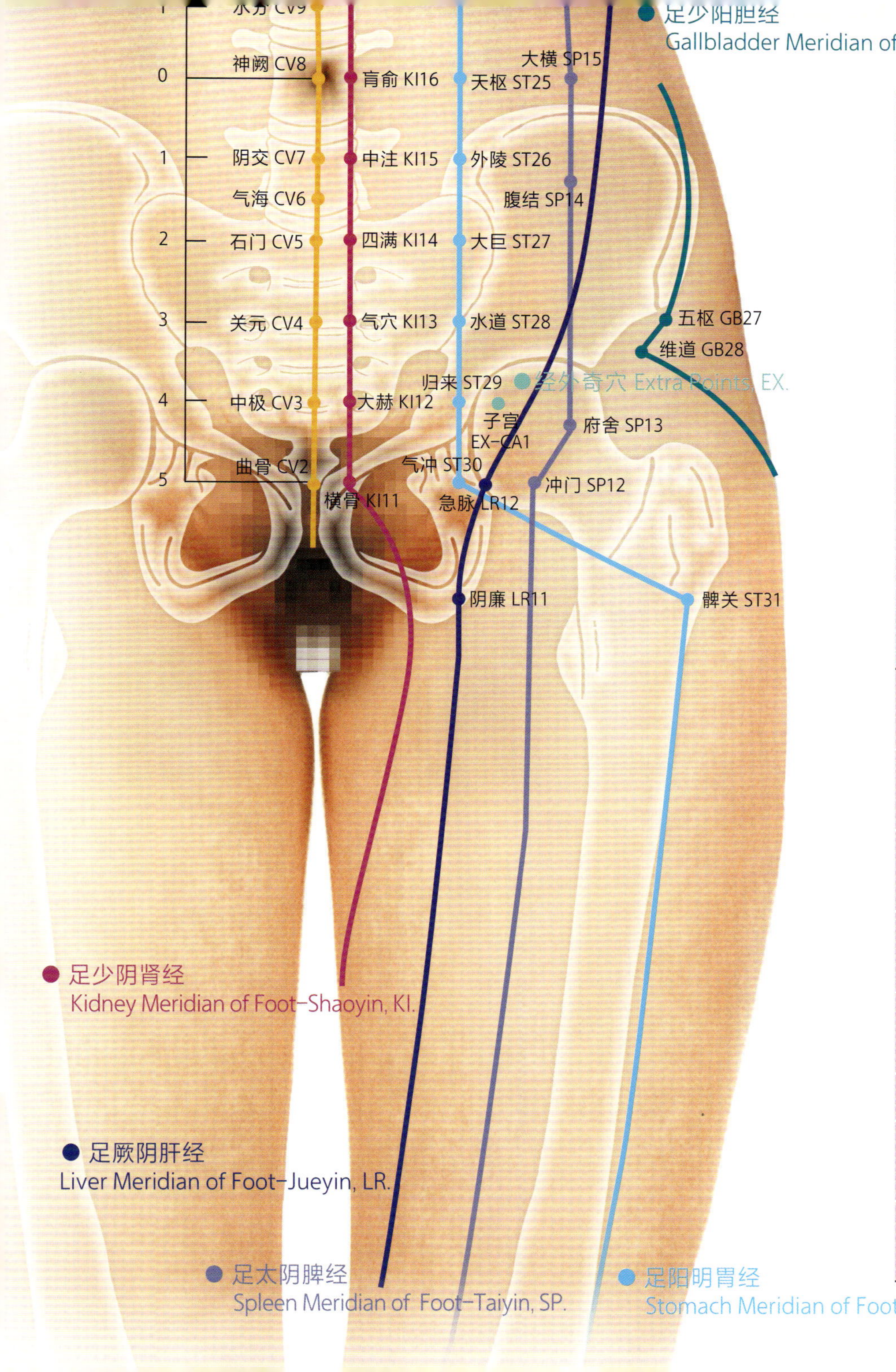

Continued

Acupoints	Location
Fùjié(SP14)	On the lower abdomen, 1.3 cun inferior to the navel, 4 cun lateral to the anterior midline
Dàhéng(SP15)	On the abdomen, 4 cun lateral to the navel
Fù'āi(SP16)	On the upper abdomen, 3 cun superior to the navel, 4 cun lateral to the anterior midline
Shídòu(SP17)	On the chest, in the 5th intercostal space, 6 cun lateral to the anterior midline
Tiānxī(SP18)	On the chest, in the 4th intercostal space, 6 cun lateral to the anterior midline
Xiōngxiāng(SP19)	On the chest, in the 3rd intercostal space, 6 cun lateral to the anterior midline
Zhōuróng(SP20)	On the chest, in the 2nd intercostal space, 6 cun lateral to the anterior midline
Hénggǔ(KI11)	On the lower abdomen, 5 cun inferior to the navel, 0.5 cun lateral to the anterior midline
Dàhè(KI12)	On the lower abdomen, 4 cun inferior to the navel, 0.5 cun lateral to the anterior midline
Qìxué(KI13)	On the lower abdomen, 3 cun inferior to the navel, 0.5 cun lateral to the anterior midline
Sìmǎn(KI14)	On the lower abdomen, 2 cun inferior to the navel, 0.5 cun lateral to the anterior midline
Zhōngzhù(KI15)	On the lower abdomen, 1 cun inferior to the navel, 0.5 cun lateral to the anterior midline
Huāngshū(KI16)	On the abdomen, 0.5 cun lateral to the navel
Shāngqū(KI17)	On the upper abdomen, 2 cun superior to the navel, 0.5 cun lateral to the anterior midline
Shíguān(KI18)	On the upper abdomen, 3 cun superior to the navel, 0.5 cun lateral to the anterior midline

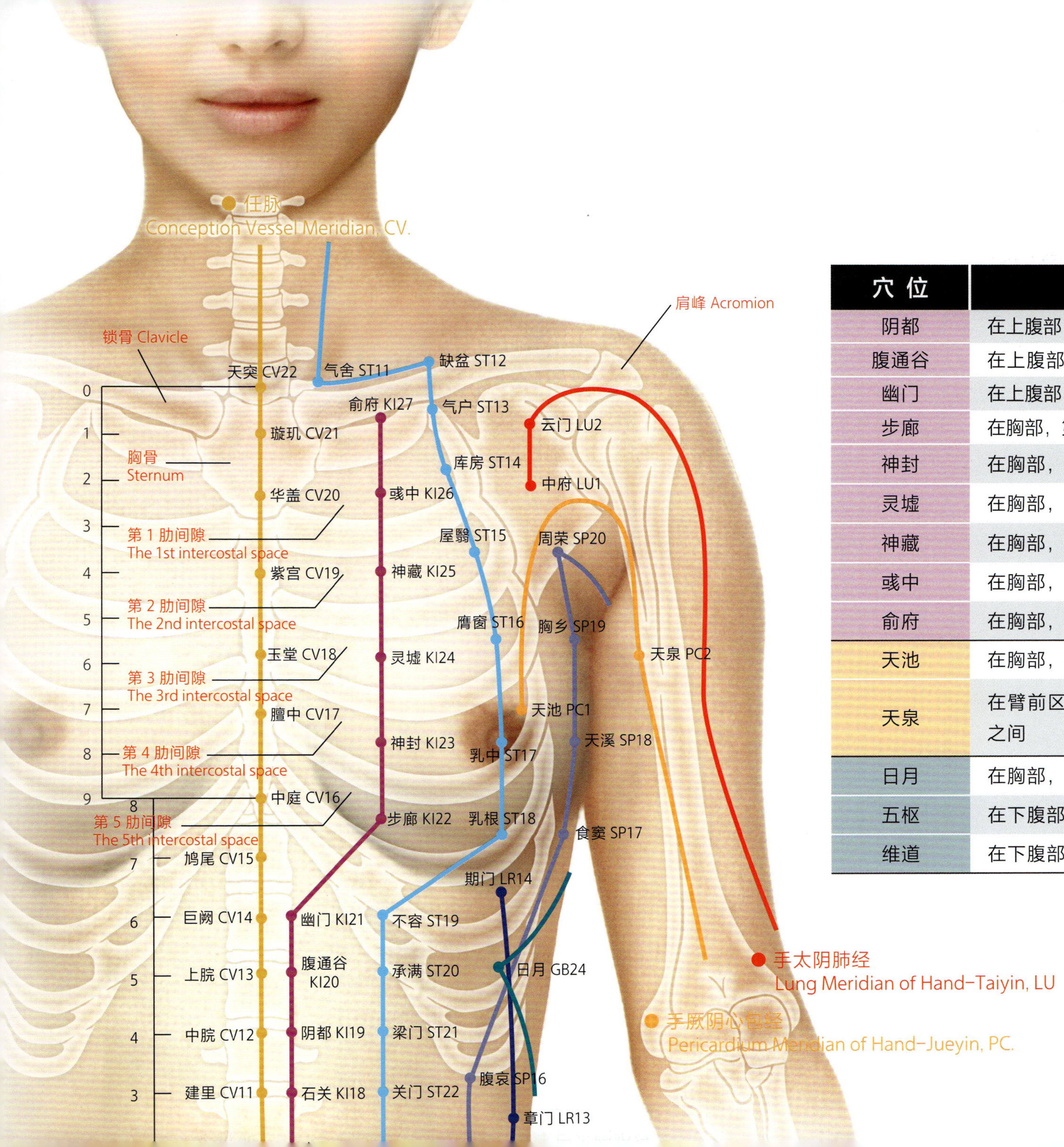

续表

穴 位	定 位
阴都	在上腹部，脐中上 4 寸，前正中线旁开 0.5 寸
腹通谷	在上腹部，脐中上 5 寸，前正中线旁开 0.5 寸
幽门	在上腹部，脐中上 6 寸，前正中线旁开 0.5 寸
步廊	在胸部，第 5 肋间隙，前正中线旁开 2 寸
神封	在胸部，第 4 肋间隙，前正中线旁开 2 寸
灵墟	在胸部，第 3 肋间隙，前正中线旁开 2 寸
神藏	在胸部，第 2 肋间隙，前正中线旁开 2 寸
彧中	在胸部，第 1 肋间隙，前正中线旁开 2 寸
俞府	在胸部，锁骨下缘，前正中线旁开 2 寸
天池	在胸部，第 4 肋间隙，前正中线旁开 5 寸
天泉	在臂前区，腋前纹头下 2 寸，肱二头肌的长、短头之间
日月	在胸部，第 7 肋间隙中，前正中线旁开 4 寸
五枢	在下腹部，横平脐下 3 寸，髂前上棘内侧
维道	在下腹部，髂前上棘内下 0.5 寸

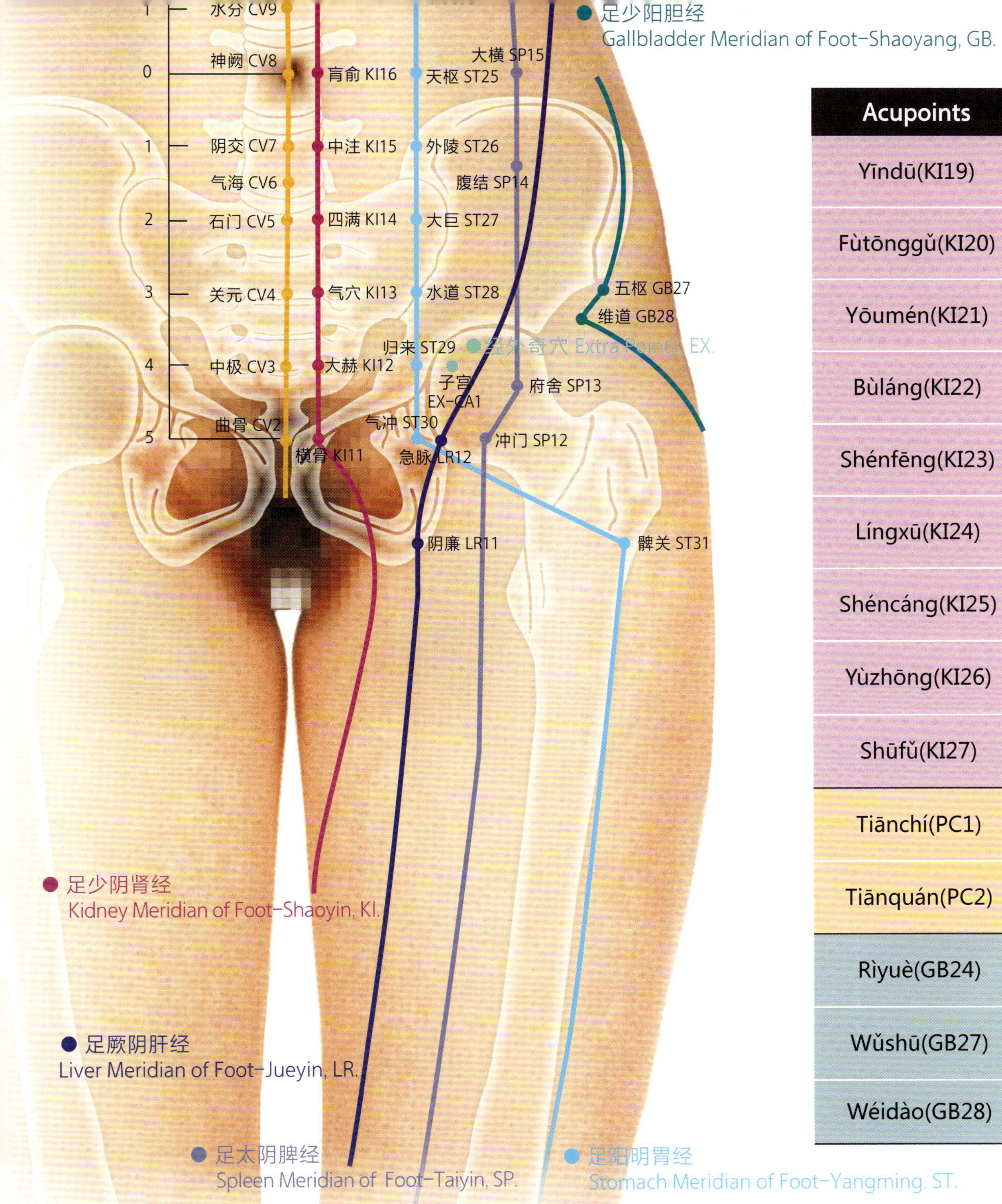

Continued

Acupoints	Location
Yīndū(KI19)	On the upper abdomen, 4 cun superior to the navel, 0.5 cun lateral to the anterior midline
Fùtōnggǔ(KI20)	On the upper abdomen, 5 cun superior to the navel, 0.5 cun lateral to the anterior midline
Yōumén(KI21)	On the upper abdomen, 6 cun superior to the navel, 0.5 cun lateral to the anterior midline
Bùláng(KI22)	On the chest, in the 5th intercostal space, 2 cun lateral to the anterior midline
Shénfēng(KI23)	On the chest, in the 4th intercostal space, 2 cun lateral to the anterior midline
Língxū(KI24)	On the chest, in the 3rd intercostal space, 2 cun lateral to the anterior midline
Shéncáng(KI25)	On the chest, in the 2nd intercostal space, 2 cun lateral to the anterior midline
Yùzhōng(KI26)	On the chest, in the 1st intercostal space, 2 cun lateral to the anterior midline
Shūfǔ(KI27)	On the chest, in the inferior margin of the clavicle, 2 cun lateral to the anterior midline
Tiānchí(PC1)	On the chest, in the 4th intercostal space, 5 cun lateral to the anterior midline
Tiānquán(PC2)	In the anterior region of arm, 2 cun below the anterior axillary fold, between the two heads of the biceps brachii muscle
Rìyuè(GB24)	On the chest, in the 7th intercostal space, 4 cun lateral to the anterior midline
Wǔshū(GB27)	On the lower abdomen, 3 cun below the navel, in the interior side of the anterior superior iliac spine
Wéidào(GB28)	On the lower abdomen, 0.5 cun interior and inferior to the anterior superior iliac spine

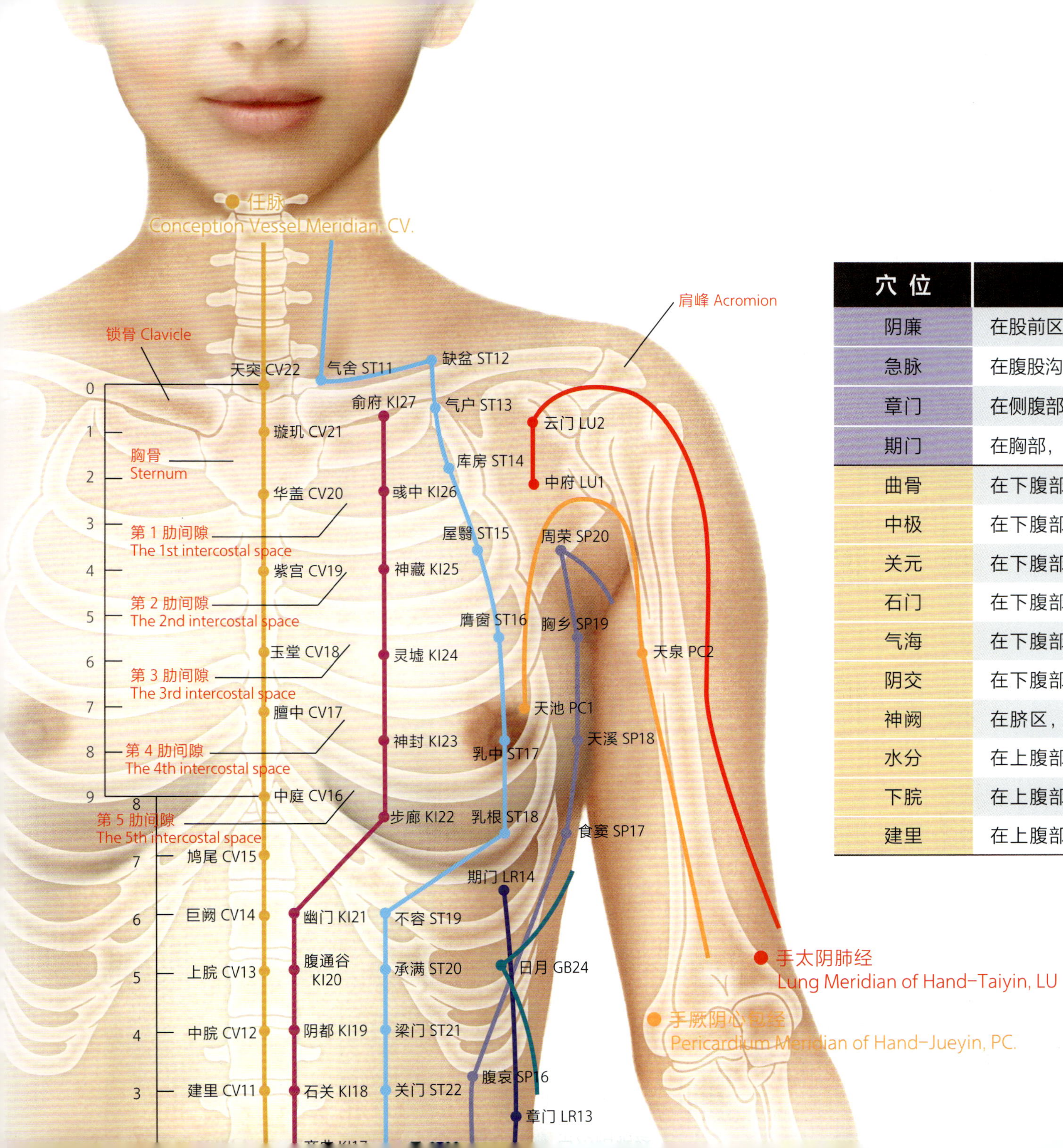

续表

穴 位	定 位
阴廉	在股前区，气冲直下 2 寸
急脉	在腹股沟区，横平耻骨联合上缘，前正中线旁开 2.5 寸
章门	在侧腹部，在第 11 肋游离端的下际
期门	在胸部，第 6 肋间隙，前正中线旁开 4 寸
曲骨	在下腹部，耻骨联合上缘，前正中线上
中极	在下腹部，脐中下 4 寸，前正中线上
关元	在下腹部，脐中下 3 寸，前正中线上
石门	在下腹部，脐中下 2 寸，前正中线上
气海	在下腹部，脐中下 1.5 寸，前正中线上
阴交	在下腹部，脐中下 1 寸，前正中线上
神阙	在脐区，脐中央
水分	在上腹部，脐中上 1 寸，前正中线上
下脘	在上腹部，脐中上 2 寸，前正中线上
建里	在上腹部，脐中上 3 寸，前正中线上

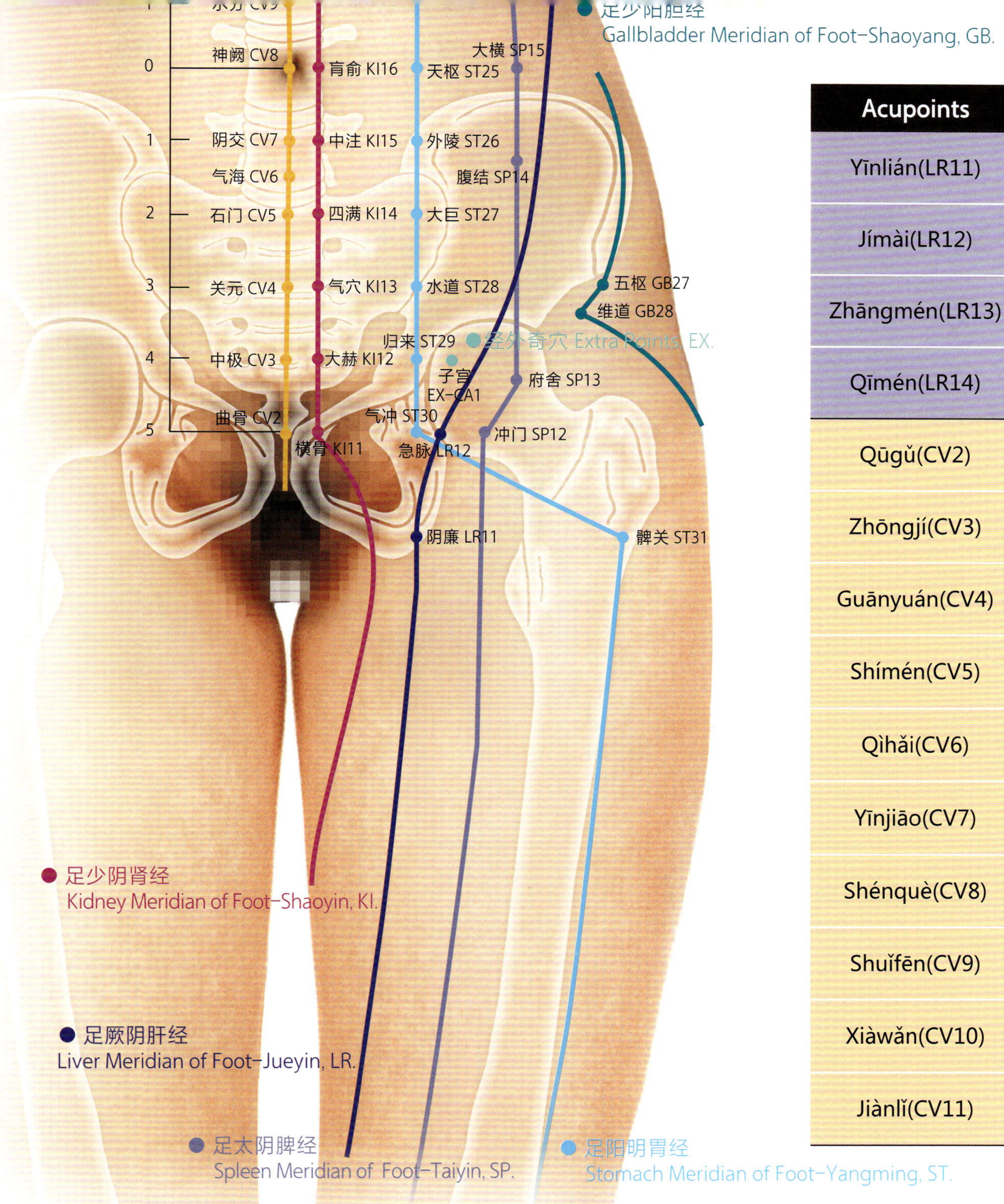

Continued

Acupoints	Location
Yīnlián(LR11)	In the anterior region of thigh, 2 cun directly below the Qichong (ST30)
Jímài(LR12)	In the region of groin, horizontal to the superior margin of the symphysis pubis, 2.5 cun lateral to the anterior midline
Zhāngmén(LR13)	On the lateral abdomen, in the inferior border of the free end of thd 11th rib
Qīmén(LR14)	On the chest, in the 6th intercostal space, 4 cun lateral to the anterior midline
Qūgǔ(CV2)	On the lower abdomen, superior to pubic symphysis, on the anterior midline
Zhōngjí(CV3)	On the lower abdomen, 4 cun inferior to the navel, on the anterior midline
Guānyuán(CV4)	On the lower abdomen, 3 cun inferior to the navel, on the anterior midline
Shímén(CV5)	On the lower abdomen, 2 cun inferior to the navel, on the anterior midline
Qìhǎi(CV6)	On the lower abdomen, 1.5 cun inferior to the navel, on the anterior midline
Yīnjiāo(CV7)	On the lower abdomen, 1 cun inferior to the navel, on the anterior midline
Shénquè(CV8)	In the umbilical region, in the center of navel
Shuǐfēn(CV9)	On the upper abdomen, 1 cun superior to the navel, on the anterior midline
Xiàwǎn(CV10)	On the upper abdomen, 2 cun superior to the navel, on the anterior midline
Jiànlǐ(CV11)	On the upper abdomen, 3 cun superior to the navel, on the anterior midline

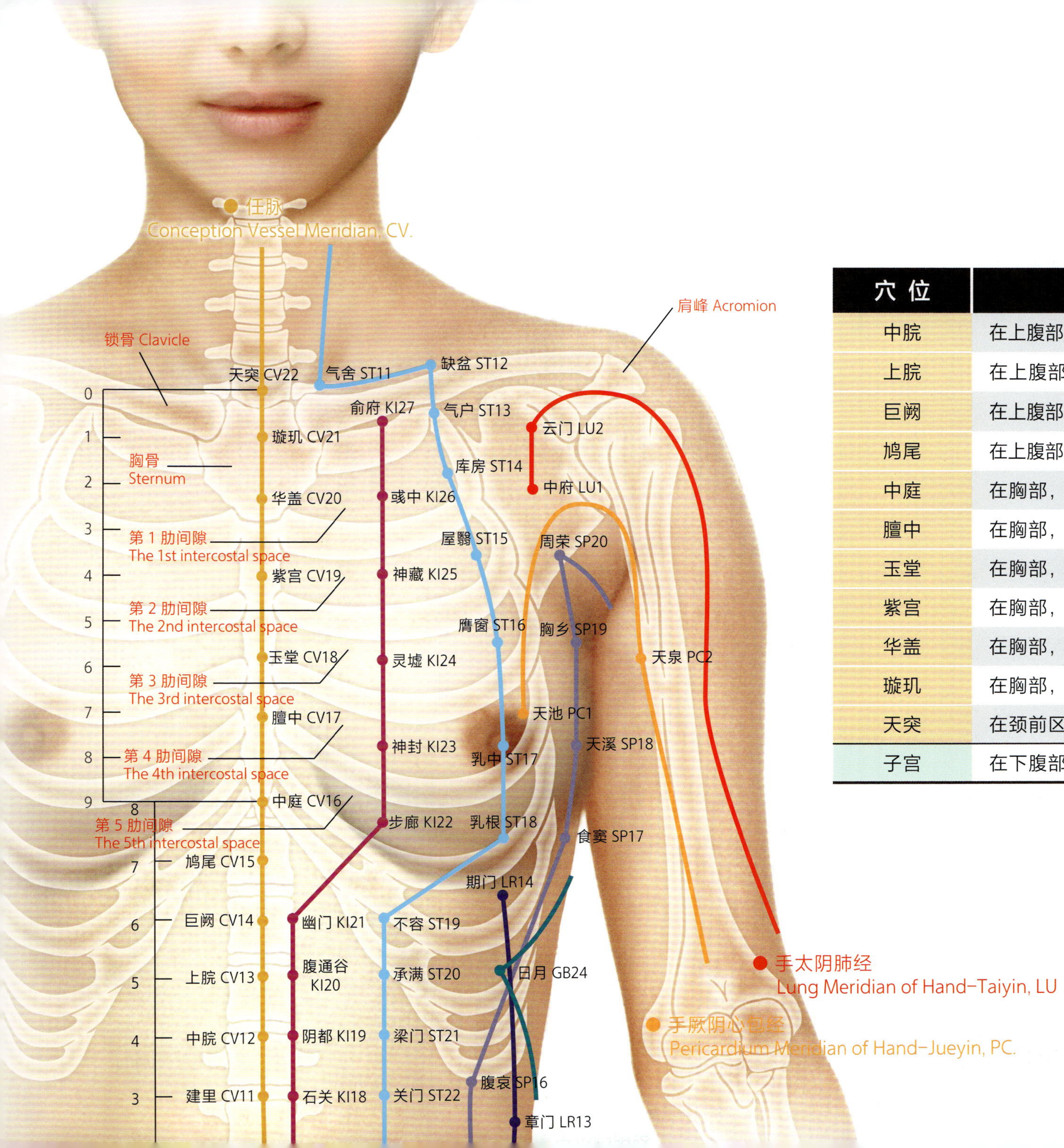

续表

穴 位	定 位
中脘	在上腹部，脐中上 4 寸，前正中线上
上脘	在上腹部，脐中上 5 寸，前正中线上
巨阙	在上腹部，脐中上 6 寸，前正中线上
鸠尾	在上腹部，剑胸结合部下 1 寸，前正中线上
中庭	在胸部，胸剑结合中点处，前正中线上
膻中	在胸部，横平第 4 肋间隙，前正中线上
玉堂	在胸部，横平第 3 肋间隙，前正中线上
紫宫	在胸部，横平第 2 肋间隙，前正中线上
华盖	在胸部，横平第 1 肋间隙，前正中线上
璇玑	在胸部，胸骨上窝下 1 寸，前正中线上
天突	在颈前区，胸骨上窝中央，前正中线上
子宫	在下腹部，当脐中下 4 寸，前正中线旁开 3 寸

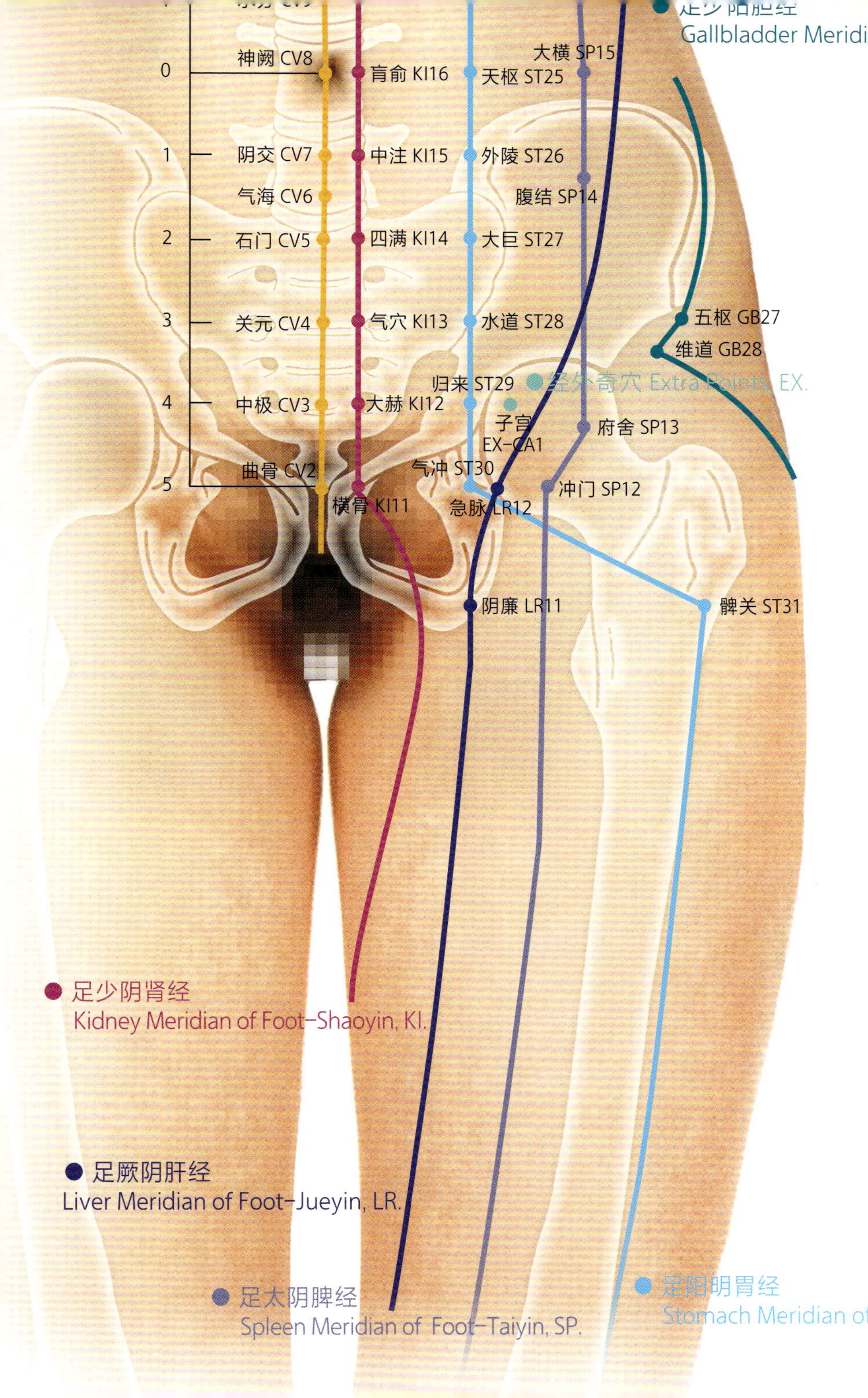

Continued

Acupoints	Location
Zhōngwǎn(CV12)	On the upper abdomen, 4 cun superior to the navel, on the anterior midline
Shàngwǎn(CV13)	On the upper abdomen, 5 cun superior to the navel, on the anterior midline
Jùquè(CV14)	On the upper abdomen, 6 cun superior to the navel, on the anterior midline
Jiūwěi(CV15)	On the upper abdomen, 1 cun inferior to xiphosternal synchondrosis, on the anterior midline
Zhōngtíng(CV16)	On the chest, at the midpoint of xiphosternal synchondrosis, on the anterior midline
Dànzhōng(CV17)	On the chest, horizontal to the 4th intercostal space, on the anterior midline
Yùtáng(CV18)	On the chest, horizontal to the 3rd intercostal space, on the anterior midline
Zǐgōng(CV19)	On the chest, horizontal to the 2nd intercostal space, on the anterior midline
Huágài(CV20)	On the chest, horizontal to the 1st intercostal space, on the anterior midline
Xuánjī(CV21)	On the chest, 1 cun inferior to the suprasternal fossa, on the anterior midline
Tiāntū(CV22)	In the anterior region of neck, in the center of sterna fossa, on the anterior midline
Zǐgōng(EX-CA1)	On the lower abdomen, 4 cun inferior to the navel, 3 cun lateral to the anterior midline

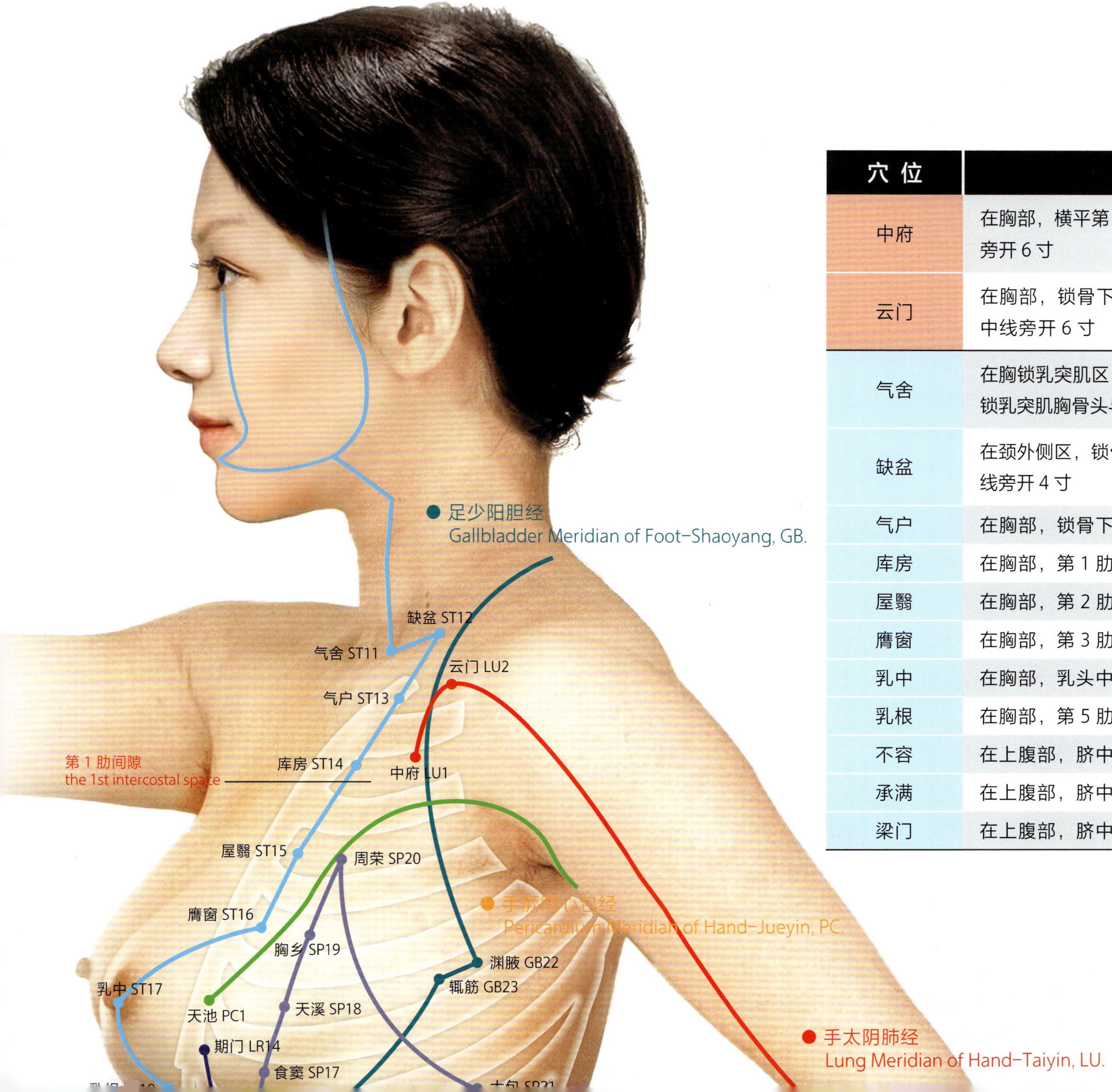

穴 位	定 位
中府	在胸部，横平第 1 肋间隙，锁骨下窝外侧，前正中线旁开 6 寸
云门	在胸部，锁骨下窝凹陷中，肩胛骨喙突内缘，前正中线旁开 6 寸
气舍	在胸锁乳突肌区，锁骨上小窝，锁骨胸骨端上缘，胸锁乳突肌胸骨头与锁骨头中间的凹陷中
缺盆	在颈外侧区，锁骨上大窝，锁骨上缘凹陷中，前正中线旁开 4 寸
气户	在胸部，锁骨下缘，前正中线旁开 4 寸
库房	在胸部，第 1 肋间隙，前正中线旁开 4 寸
屋翳	在胸部，第 2 肋间隙，前正中线旁开 4 寸
膺窗	在胸部，第 3 肋间隙，前正中线旁开 4 寸
乳中	在胸部，乳头中央
乳根	在胸部，第 5 肋间隙，前正中线旁开 4 寸
不容	在上腹部，脐中上 6 寸，前正中线旁开 2 寸
承满	在上腹部，脐中上 5 寸，前正中线旁开 2 寸
梁门	在上腹部，脐中上 4 寸，前正中线旁开 2 寸

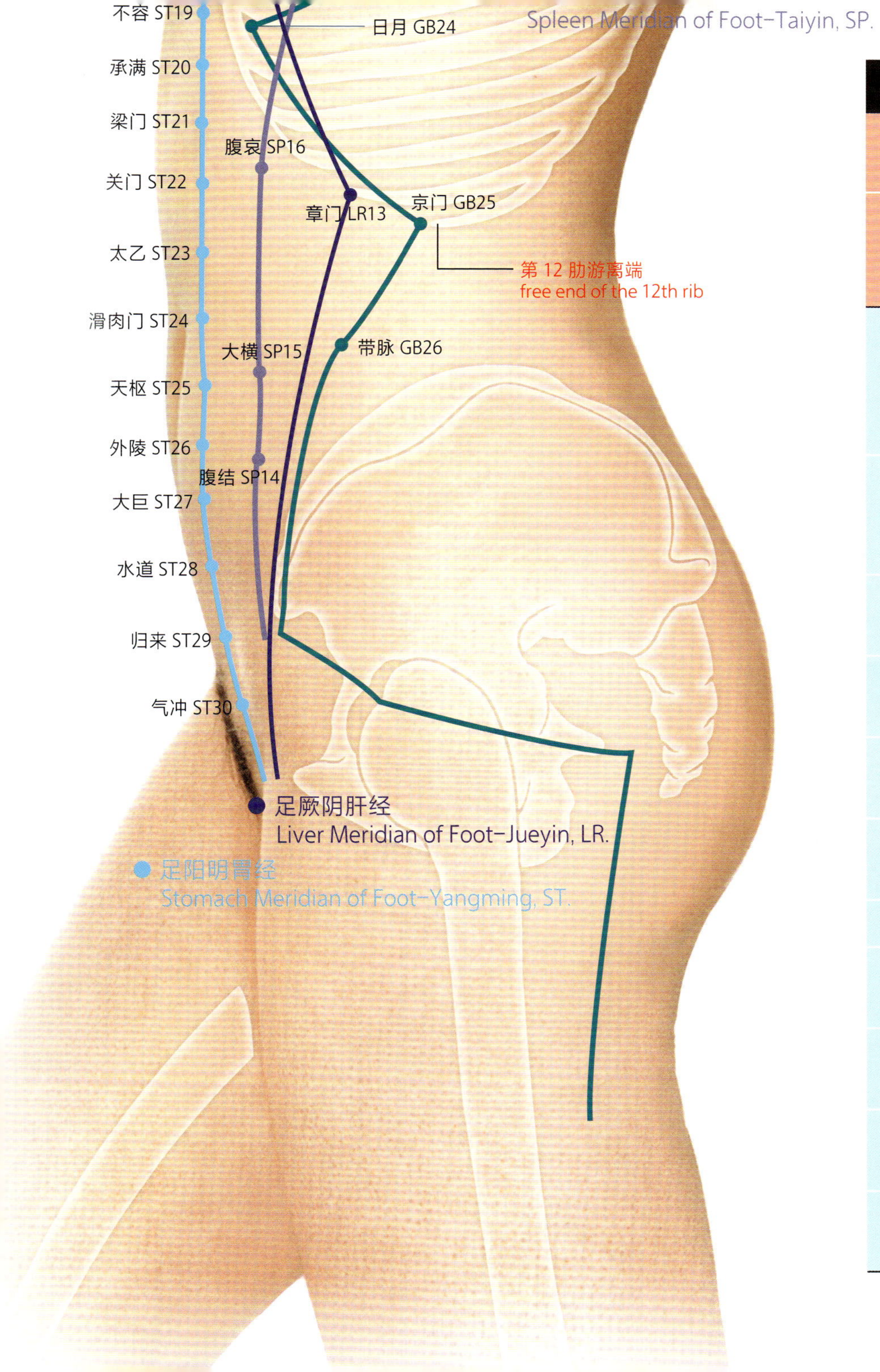

Acupoints	Location
Zhōngfǔ(LU1)	On the chest, horizontal to the 1st intercostal space, 6 cun lateral to the anterior midline
Yúnmén(LU2)	On the chest, in the depression of infraclavicular fossa, in the interior margin of coracoid process, 6 cun lateral to the anterior midline
Qìshè(ST11)	In the sternoclavicular mastoid region, in the lesser supraclavicular fossa, in the superior border of sternal end of clavicle, in the depression between the sterna head and clavicular head of sternocleidomastoid
Quēpén(ST12)	In lateral region of neck, in the greater supraclavicular fossa and the depression of the superior border of clavicle, 4 cun lateral to the anterior midline
Qìhù(ST13)	On the chest, in the inferior border of clavicle, 4 cun lateral to the anterior midline
Kùfáng(ST14)	On the chest, in the 1st intercostal space,4 cun lateral to the anterior midline
Wūyì(ST15)	On the chest, in the 2nd intercostal space, 4 cun lateral to the anterior midline
Yīngchuāng(ST16)	On the chest, in the 3rd intercostal space, 4 cun lateral to the anterior midline
Rǔzhōng(ST17)	On the chest, in the center of nipple
Rǔgēn(ST18)	On the chest, in the 5th intercostal space, 4 cun lateral to the anterior midline
Bùróng(ST19)	On the upper abdomen, 6 cun superior to the navel, 2 cun lateral to the anterior midline
Chéngmǎn(ST20)	On the upper abdomen, 5 cun superior to the navel, 2 cun lateral to the anterior midline
Liángmén(ST21)	On the upper abdomen, 4 cun superior to the navel, 2 cun lateral to the anterior midline

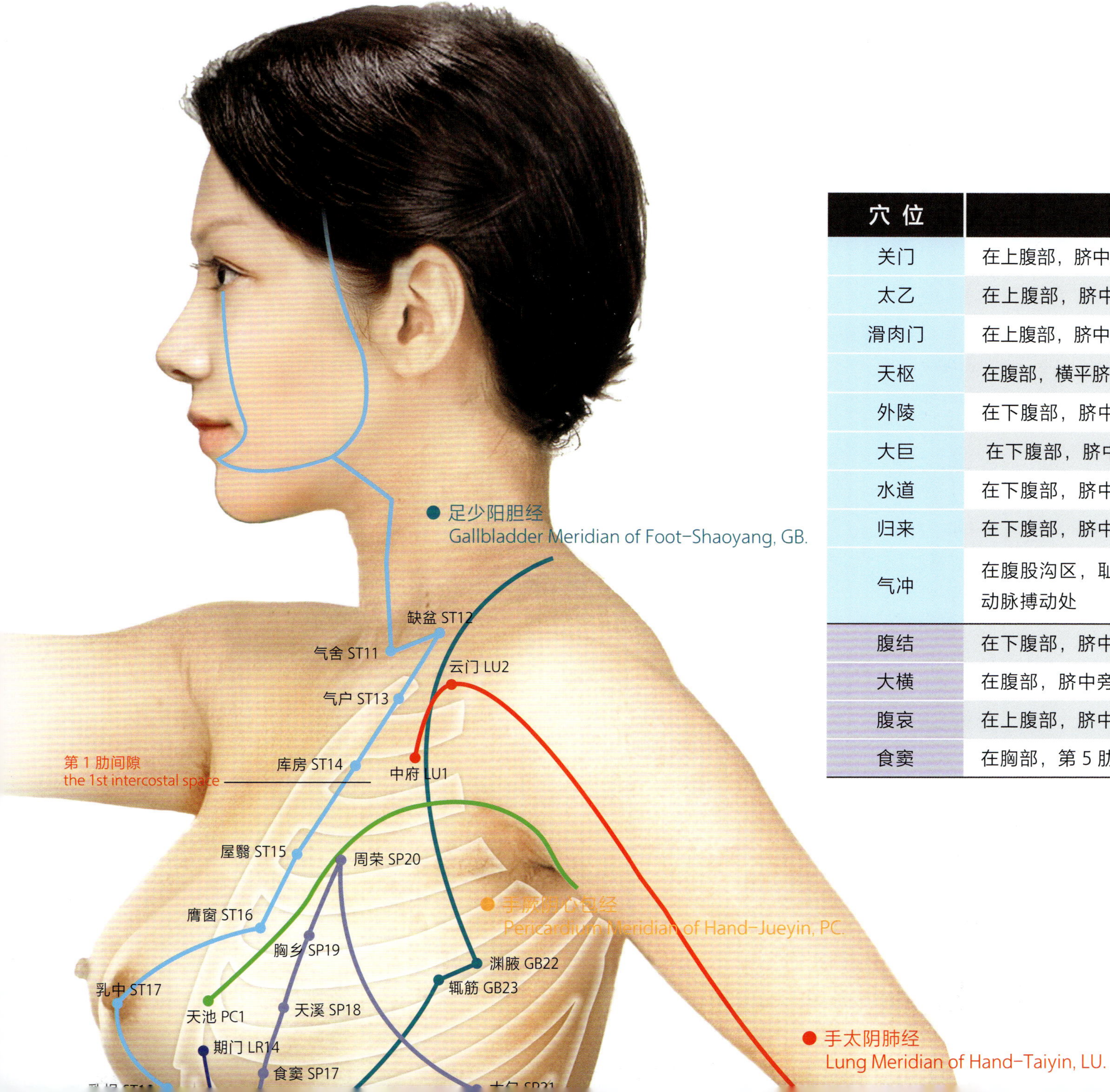

续表

穴位	定位
关门	在上腹部，脐中上 3 寸，前正中线旁开 2 寸
太乙	在上腹部，脐中上 2 寸，前正中线旁开 2 寸
滑肉门	在上腹部，脐中上 1 寸，前正中线旁开 2 寸
天枢	在腹部，横平脐中，前正中线旁开 2 寸
外陵	在下腹部，脐中下 1 寸，前正中线旁开 2 寸
大巨	在下腹部，脐中下 2 寸，前正中线旁开 2 寸
水道	在下腹部，脐中下 3 寸，前正中线旁开 2 寸
归来	在下腹部，脐中下 4 寸，前正中线旁开 2 寸
气冲	在腹股沟区，耻骨联合上缘，前正中线旁开 2 寸，动脉搏动处
腹结	在下腹部，脐中下 1.3 寸，前正中线旁开 4 寸
大横	在腹部，脐中旁开 4 寸
腹哀	在上腹部，脐中上 3 寸，前正中线旁开 4 寸
食窦	在胸部，第 5 肋间隙，前正中线旁开 6 寸

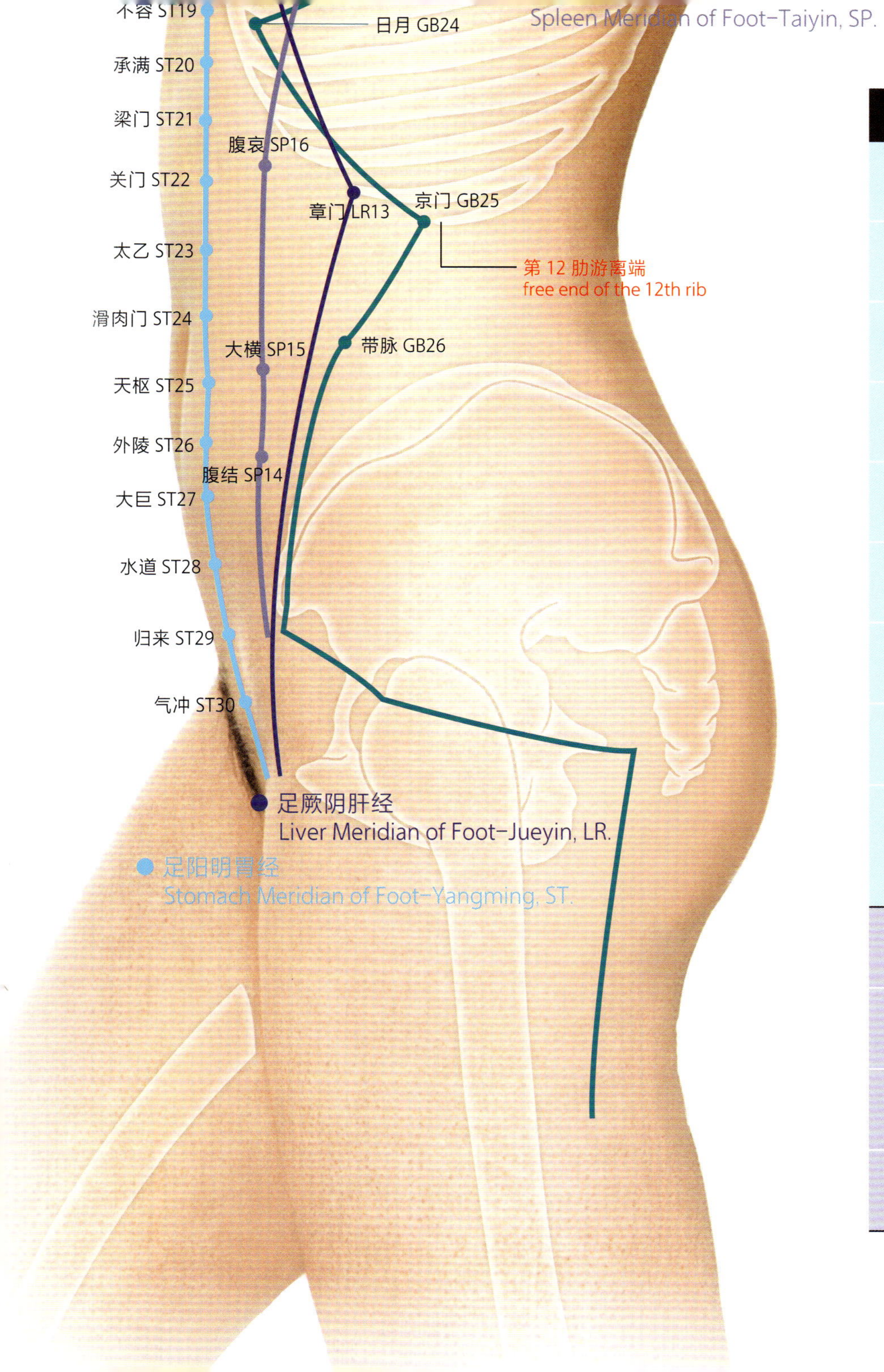

Continued

Acupoints	Location
Guānmén(ST22)	On the upper abdomen, 3 cun superior to the navel, 2 cun lateral to the anterior midline
Tàiyǐ(ST23)	On the upper abdomen, 2 cun superior to the navel, 2 cun lateral to the anterior midline
Huáròumén(ST24)	On the upper abdomen, 1 cun superior to the navel, 2 cun lateral to the anterior midline
Tiānshū(ST25)	On the abdomen, horizontal to navel, 2 cun lateral to the anterior midline
Wàilíng(ST26)	On the lower abdomen, 1 cun inferior to the navel, 2 cun lateral to the anterior midline
Dàjù(ST27)	On the lower abdomen, 2 cun inferior to the navel, 2 cun lateral to the anterior midline
Shuǐdào(ST28)	On the lower abdomen, 3 cun inferior to the navel, 2 cun lateral to the anterior midline
Guīlái(ST29)	On the lower abdomen, 4 cun inferior to the navel, 2 cun lateral to the anterior midline
Qìchōng(ST30)	In the inguinal region, in the superior margin of symphysis pubis, 2 cun lateral to the anterior midline, on the position of arterial pulsation
Fùjié(SP14)	On the lower abdomen, 1.3 cun inferior to the navel, 4 cun lateral to the anterior midline
Dàhéng(SP15)	On the abdomen, 4 cun lateral to the navel
Fù' āi(SP16)	On the upper abdomen, 3 cun superior to the navel, 4 cun lateral to the anterior midline
Shídòu(SP17)	On the chest, in the 5th intercostal space, 6 cun lateral to the anterior midline

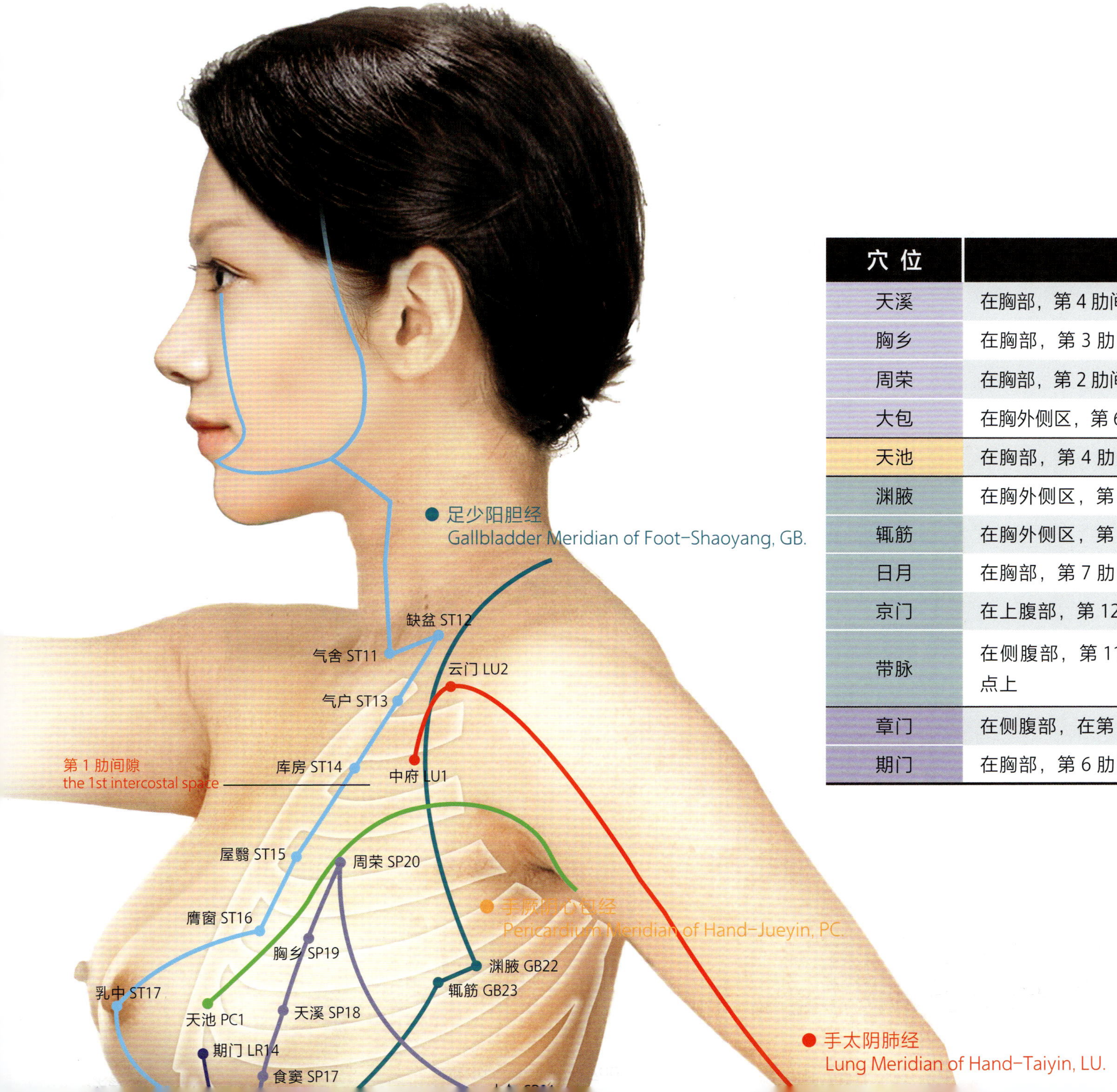

续表

穴 位	定 位
天溪	在胸部，第 4 肋间隙，前正中线旁开 6 寸
胸乡	在胸部，第 3 肋间隙，前正中线旁开 6 寸
周荣	在胸部，第 2 肋间隙，前正中线旁开 6 寸
大包	在胸外侧区，第 6 肋间隙，在腋中线上
天池	在胸部，第 4 肋间隙，前正中线旁开 5 寸
渊腋	在胸外侧区，第 4 肋间隙中，在腋中线上
辄筋	在胸外侧区，第 4 肋间隙中，腋中线前 1 寸
日月	在胸部，第 7 肋间隙中，前正中线旁开 4 寸
京门	在上腹部，第 12 肋骨游离端的下际
带脉	在侧腹部，第 11 肋骨游离端垂线与脐水平线的交点上
章门	在侧腹部，在第 11 肋游离端的下际
期门	在胸部，第 6 肋间隙，前正中线旁开 4 寸

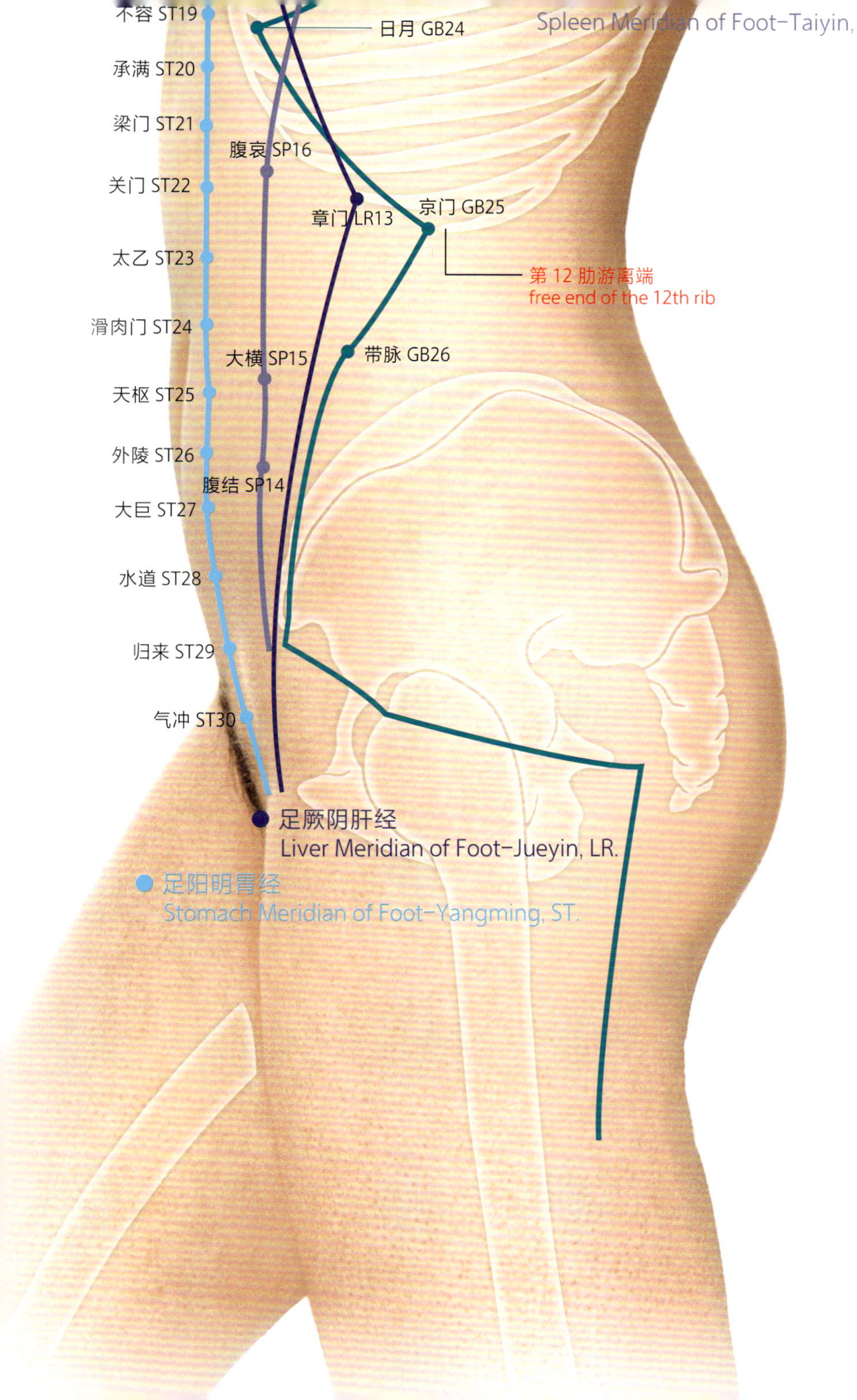

Continued

Acupoints	Location
Tiānxī(SP18)	On the chest, in the 4th intercostal space, 6 cun lateral to the anterior midline
Xiōngxiāng(SP19)	On the chest, in the 3rd intercostal space, 6 cun lateral to the anterior midline
Zhōuróng(SP20)	On the chest, in the 2nd intercostal space, 6 cun lateral to the anterior midline
Dàbāo(SP21)	In the exterior region of the chest, in the 6th intercostal space, on the midaxillary line
Tiānchí(PC1)	On the chest, in the 4th intercostal space, 5 cun lateral to the anterior midline
Yuānyè(GB22)	In the exterior region of the chest, in the 4th intercostal space, on the midaxillary line
Zhéjīn(GB23)	In the exterior region of the chest, in the 4th intercostal space, 1 cun anterior to the midaxillary line
Rìyuè(GB24)	On the chest, in the 7th intercostal space, 4 cun lateral to the anterior midline
Jīngmén(GB25)	On the upper abdomen, in the inferior border of free end of the 12th rib
Dàimài(GB26)	On the lateral abdomen, at the junction of the vertical line of free end of the 11th rib and horizontal line of the navel
Zhāngmén(LR13)	On the lateral abdomen, in the inferior border of free end of the 11th rib
Qīmén(LR14)	On the chest, in the 6th intercostal space, 4 cun lateral to the anterior midline

腰背臀部穴位

Acupoints of Waist, Back and Buttock

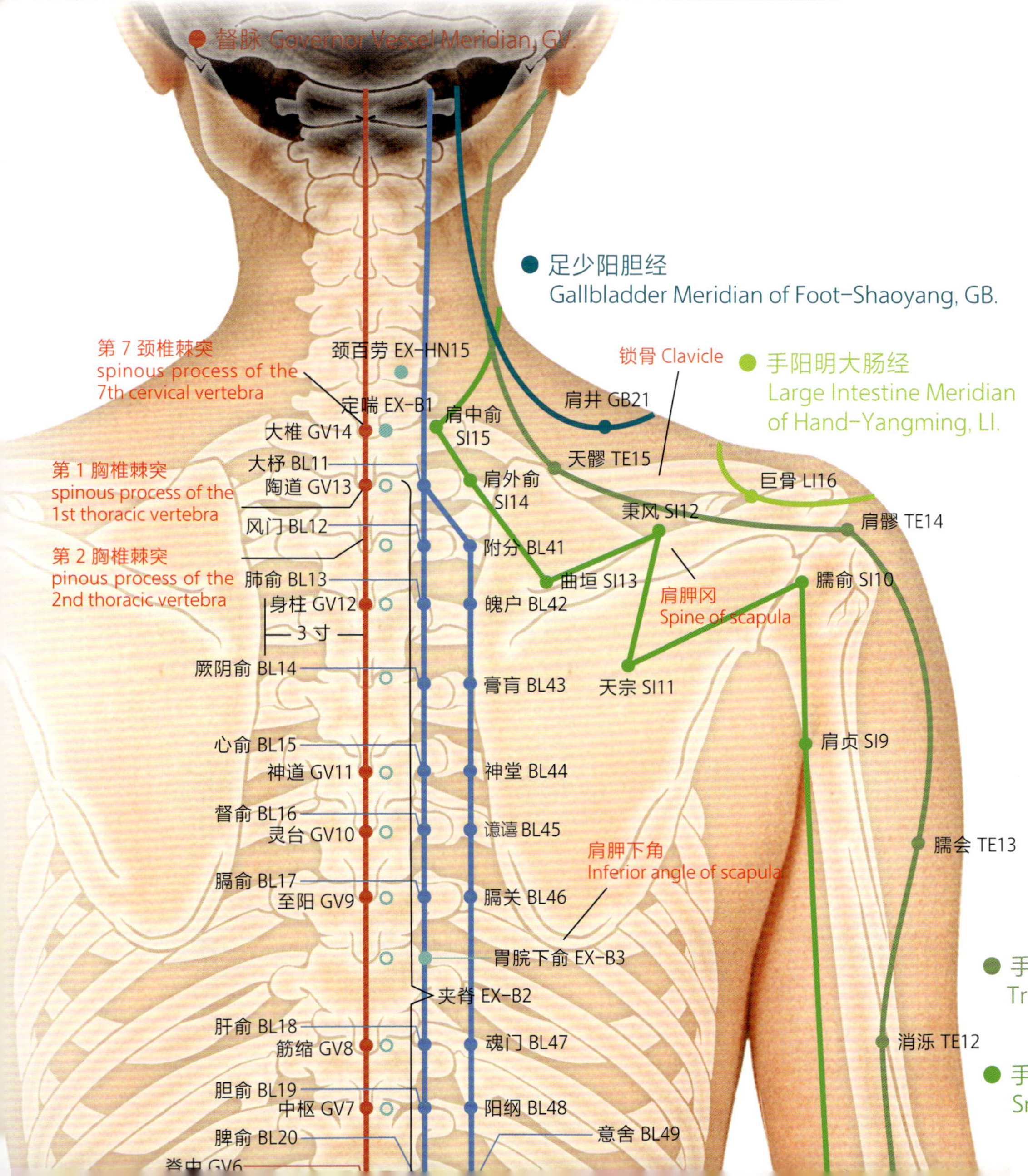

穴位	定位
巨骨	在肩胛区，锁骨肩峰端与肩胛冈之间凹陷中
肩贞	在肩胛区，肩关节后下方，腋后纹头直上 1 寸
臑俞	在肩胛区，腋后纹头直上，肩胛冈下缘凹陷中
天宗	在肩胛区，肩胛冈中点与肩胛下角连线上 1/3 与下 2/3 交点凹陷中
秉风	在肩胛区，肩胛冈中点上方冈上窝中
曲垣	在肩胛区，肩胛冈内侧端上缘凹陷中
肩外俞	在脊柱区，第 1 胸椎棘突下，后正中线旁开 3 寸
肩中俞	在脊柱区，第 7 颈椎棘突下，后正中线旁开 2 寸
大杼	在脊柱区，第 1 胸椎棘突下，后正中线旁开 1.5 寸
风门	在脊柱区，第 2 胸椎棘突下，后正中线旁开 1.5 寸
肺俞	在脊柱区，第 3 胸椎棘突下，后正中线旁开 1.5 寸
厥阴俞	在脊柱区，第 4 胸椎棘突下，后正中线旁开 1.5 寸
心俞	在脊柱区，第 5 胸椎棘突下，后正中线旁开 1.5 寸

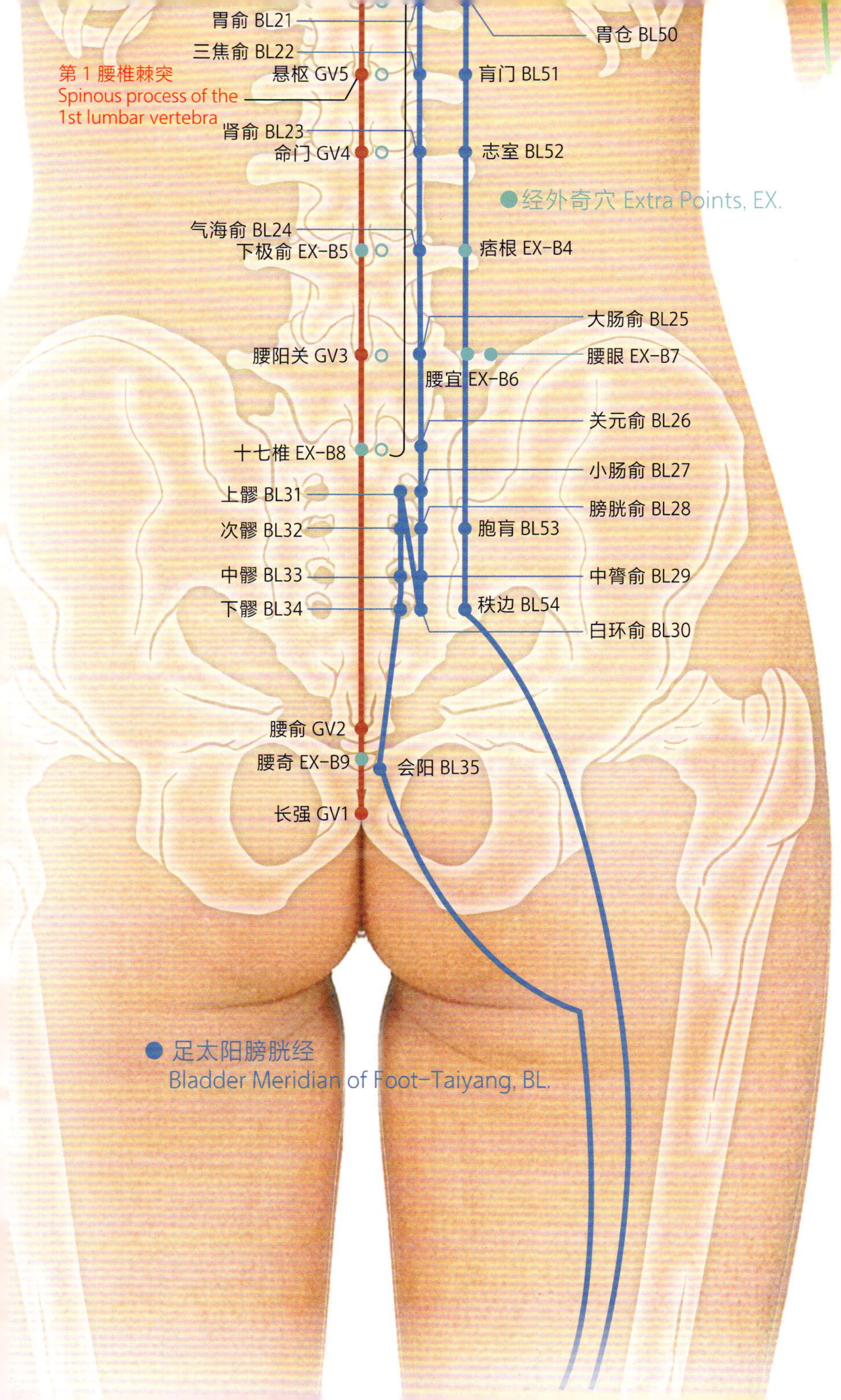

Acupoints	Location
Jùgǔ(LI16)	In the scapular region, in the depression between acromion end of clavicle and spine of scapula
Jiānzhēn(SI9)	In the scapular region, posterior and inferior to shoulder joint, 1 cun directly above the posterior axillary fold
Nàoshū(SI10)	In the scapular region, directly above the posterior axillary fold, in the depression of inferior border of scapular spine
Tiānzōng(SI11)	In the scapular region, at the junction of upper 1/3 and lower 2/3 of joining line between midpoint of scapular spine and inferior angle of scapula
Bǐngfēng(SI12)	In the scapular region, in the supraspinous fossa above the midpoint of scapular spine
Qūyuán(SI13)	In the scapular region, in the depression of superior border of interior end of scapular spine
Jiānwàishū(SI14)	In the spinal region, inferior to the 1st spinous process of thoracic vertebra, 3 cun lateral to the posterior midline
Jiānzhōngshū(SI15)	In the spinal region, inferior to the 1st spinous process of cervical vertebra, 2 cun lateral to the posterior midline
Dàzhù(BL11)	In the spinal region, inferior to the 1st spinous process of thoracic vertebra, 1.5 cun lateral to the posterior midline
Fēngmén(BL12)	In the spinal region, inferior to the 2nd spinous process of thoracic vertebra, 1.5 cun lateral to the posterior midline
Fèishū(BL13)	In the spinal region, inferior to the 3rd spinous process of thoracic vertebra, 1.5 cun lateral to the posterior midline
Juéyīngshū(BL14)	In the spinal region, inferior to the 4th spinous process of thoracic vertebra, 1.5 cun lateral to the posterior midline
Xīnshū(BL15)	In the spinal region, inferior to the 5th spinous process of thoracic vertebra, 1.5 cun lateral to the posterior midline

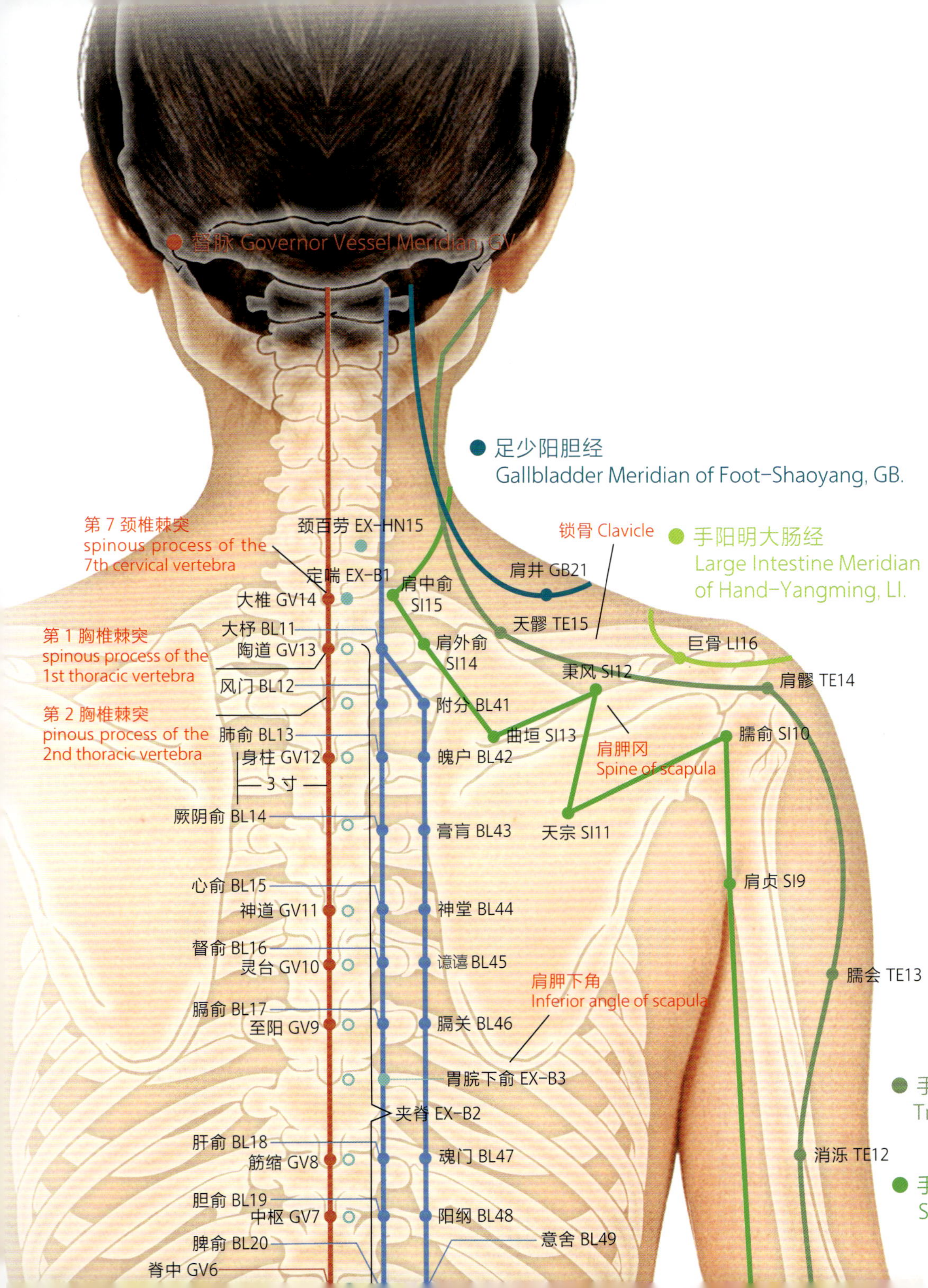

续表

穴 位	定 位
督俞	在脊柱区，第 6 胸椎棘突下，后正中线旁开 1.5 寸
膈俞	在脊柱区，第 7 胸椎棘突下，后正中线旁开 1.5 寸
肝俞	在脊柱区，第 9 胸椎棘突下，后正中线旁开 1.5 寸
胆俞	在脊柱区，第 10 胸椎棘突下，后正中线旁开 1.5 寸
脾俞	在脊柱区，第 11 胸椎棘突下，后正中线旁开 1.5 寸
胃俞	在脊柱区，第 12 胸椎棘突下，后正中线旁开 1.5 寸
三焦俞	在脊柱区，第 1 腰椎棘突下，后正中线旁开 1.5 寸
肾俞	在脊柱区，第 2 腰椎棘突下，后正中线旁开 1.5 寸
气海俞	在脊柱区，第 3 腰椎棘突下，后正中线旁开 1.5 寸
大肠俞	在脊柱区，第 4 腰椎棘突下，后正中线旁开 1.5 寸
关元俞	在脊柱区，第 5 腰椎棘突下，后正中线旁开 1.5 寸
小肠俞	在骶区，横平第 1 骶后孔，骶正中嵴旁开 1.5 寸
膀胱俞	在骶区，横平第 2 骶后孔，骶正中嵴旁开 1.5 寸

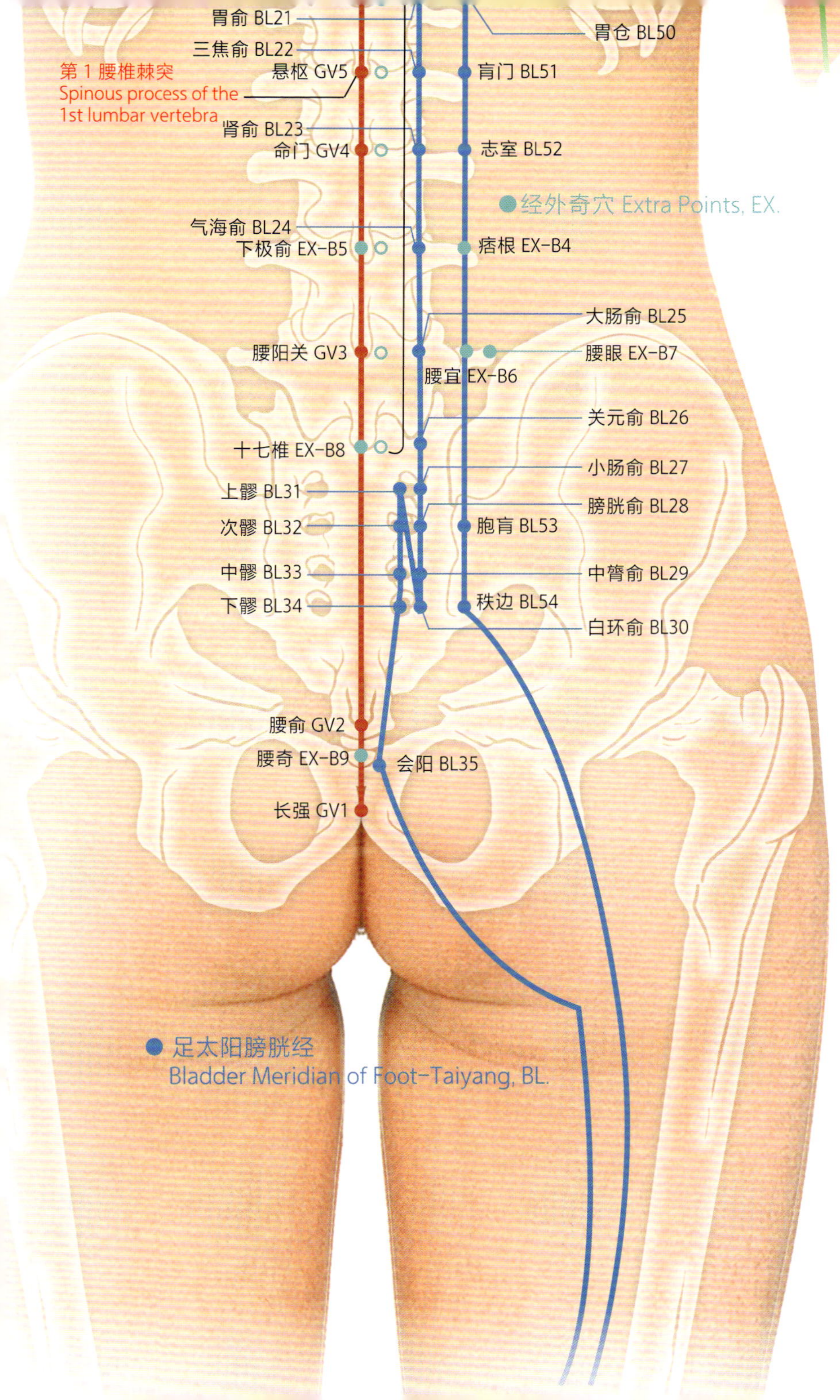

Continued

Acupoints	Location
Dūshū(BL16)	In the spinal region, inferior to the 6th spinous process of thoracic vertebra, 1.5 cun lateral to the posterior midline
Géshū(BL17)	In the spinal region, inferior to the 7th spinous process of thoracic vertebra, 1.5 cun lateral to the posterior midline
Gānshū(BL18)	In the spinal region, inferior to the 9th spinous process of thoracic vertebra, 1.5 cun lateral to the posterior midline
Dǎnshū(BL19)	In the spinal region, inferior to the 10th spinous process of thoracic vertebra, 1.5 cun lateral to the posterior midline
Píshū(BL20)	In the spinal region, inferior to the 11th spinous process of thoracic vertebra, 1.5 cun lateral to the posterior midline
Wèishū(BL21)	In the spinal region, inferior to the 12th spinous process of thoracic vertebra, 1.5 cun lateral to the posterior midline
Sānjiāoshū(BL22)	In the spinal region, inferior to the 1st spinous process of lumbar vertebra, 1.5 cun lateral to the posterior midline
Shènshū(BL23)	In the spinal region, inferior to the 2nd spinous process of lumbar vertebra, 1.5 cun lateral to the posterior midline
Qìhǎishū(BL24)	In the spinal region, inferior to the 3rd spinous process of lumbar vertebra, 1.5 cun lateral to the posterior midline
Dàchángshū(BL25)	In the spinal region, inferior to the 4th spinous process of lumbar vertebra, 1.5 cun lateral to the posterior midline
Guānyuánshū(BL26)	In the spinal region, inferior to the 5th spinous process of lumbar vertebra, 1.5 cun lateral to the posterior midline
Xiǎochángshū(BL27)	In the sacral region, horizontal to the 1st posterior sacral foramina, 1.5 cun lateral to median sacral crest
Pángguāngshū(BL28)	In the sacral region, horizontal to the 2nd posterior sacral foramina, 1.5 cun lateral to median sacral crest

续表

穴 位	定 位
中膂俞	在骶区，横平第 3 骶后孔，骶正中嵴旁开 1.5 寸
白环俞	在骶区，横平第 4 骶后孔，骶正中嵴旁开 1.5 寸
上髎	在骶区，正对第 1 骶后孔中
次髎	在骶区，正对第 2 骶后孔中
中髎	在骶区，正对第 3 骶后孔中
下髎	在骶区，正对第 4 骶后孔中
会阳	在骶区，尾骨端旁开 0.5 寸
附分	在脊柱区，第 2 胸椎棘突下，后正中线旁开 3 寸
魄户	在脊柱区，第 3 胸椎棘突下，后正中线旁开 3 寸
膏肓	在脊柱区，第 4 胸椎棘突下，后正中线旁开 3 寸
神堂	在脊柱区，第 5 胸椎棘突下，后正中线旁开 3 寸
譩譆	在脊柱区，第 6 胸椎棘突下，后正中线旁开 3 寸
膈关	在脊柱区，第 7 胸椎棘突下，后正中线旁开 3 寸

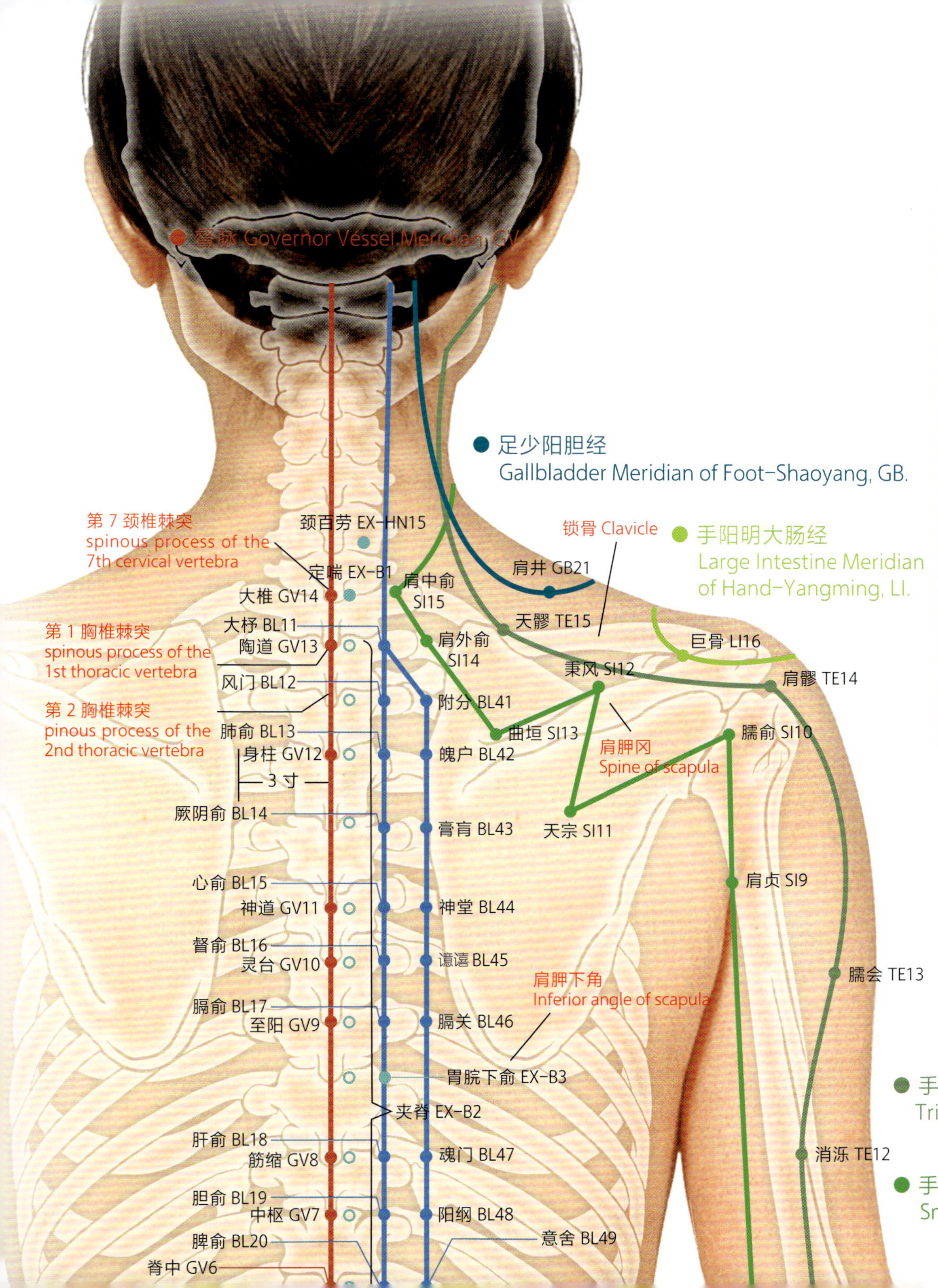

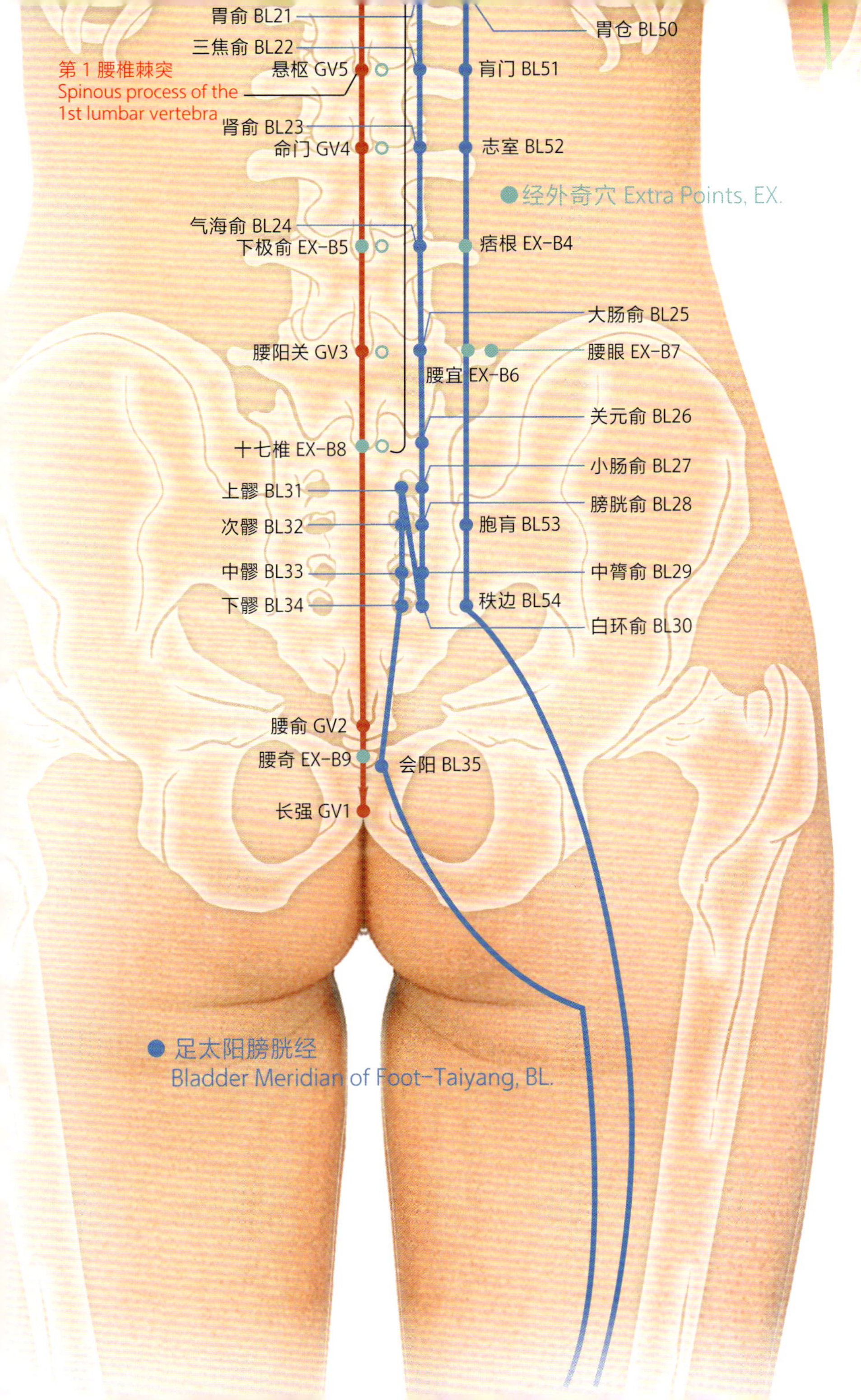

Continued

Acupoints	Location
Zhōnglǚshū(BL29)	In the sacral region, horizontal to the 3rd posterior sacral foramina, 1.5 cun lateral to median sacral crest
Báihuánshū(BL30)	In the sacral region, horizontal to the 4th posterior sacral foramina, 1.5 cun lateral to median sacral crest
Shàngliáo(BL31)	In the sacral region, directly faced with the 1st posterior sacral foramina
Cìliáo(BL32)	In the sacral region, directly faced with the 2nd posterior sacral foramina
Zhōngliáo(BL33)	In the sacral region, directly faced with the 3rd posterior sacral foramina
Xiàliáo(BL34)	In the sacral region, directly faced with the 4th posterior sacral foramina
Huìyáng(BL35)	In the sacral region, 0.5 cun lateral to coccyx end
Fùfēn(BL41)	In the spinal region, inferior to the process of the 2nd thoracic spine, 3 cun lateral to the posterior midline
Pòhù(BL42)	In the spinal region, inferior to the process of the 3rd thoracic spine, 3 cun lateral to the posterior midline
Gāohuāng(BL43)	In the spinal region, inferior to the process of the 4th thoracic spine, 3 cun lateral to the posterior midline
Shéntáng(BL44)	In the spinal region, inferior to the process of the 5th thoracic spine, 3 cun lateral to the posterior midline
Yìxǐ(BL45)	In the spinal region, inferior to the process of the 6th thoracic spine, 3 cun lateral to the posterior midline
Géguān(BL46)	In the spinal region, inferior to spinous process of the 7th thoracic vertebra, 3 cun lateral to the posterior midline

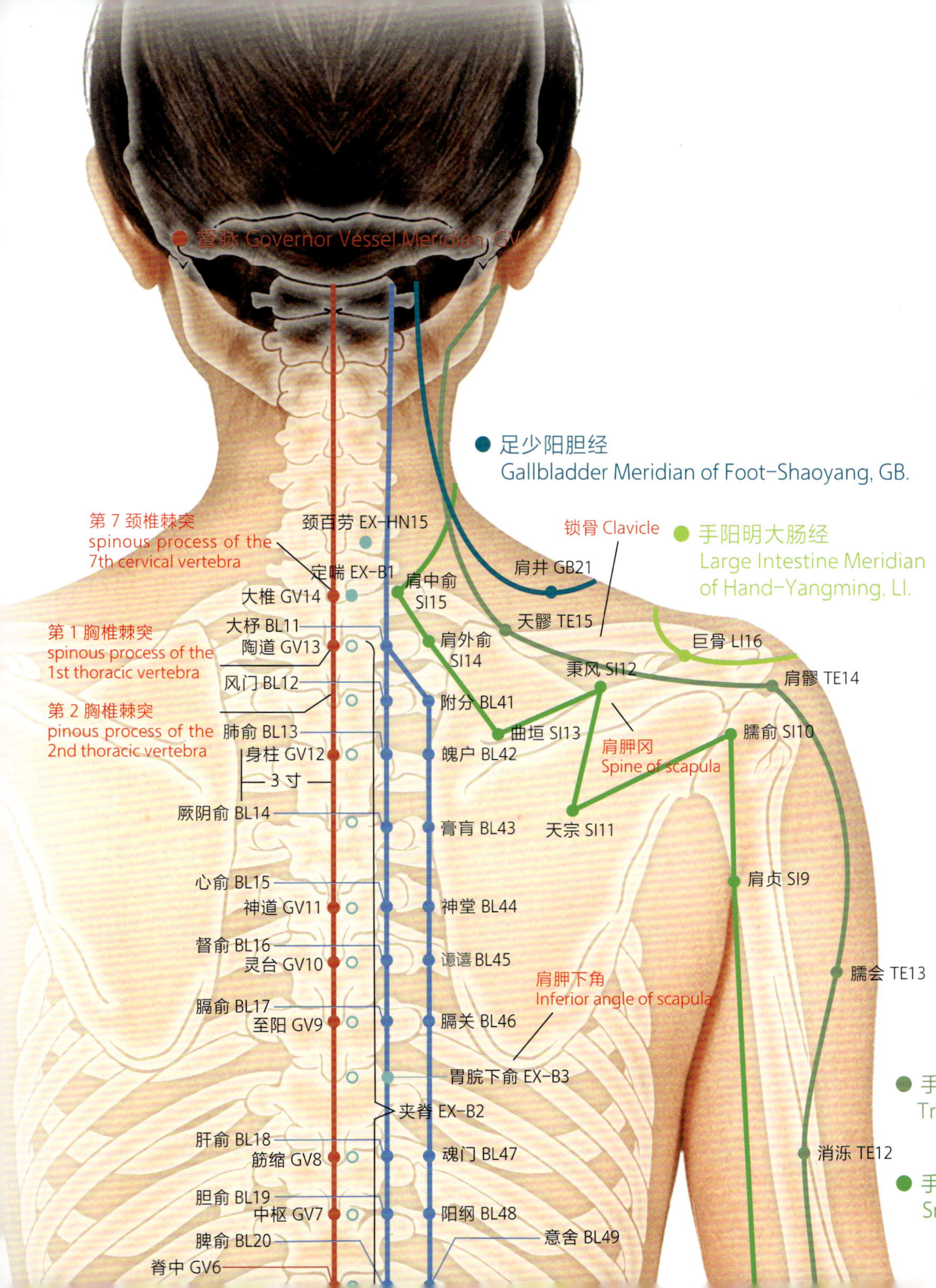

续表

穴位	定位
魂门	在脊柱区，第 9 胸椎棘突下，后正中线旁开 3 寸
阳纲	在脊柱区，第 10 胸椎棘突下，后正中线旁开 3 寸
意舍	在脊柱区，第 11 胸椎棘突下，后正中线旁开 3 寸
胃仓	在脊柱区，第 12 胸椎棘突下，后正中线旁开 3 寸
肓门	在腰区，第 1 腰椎棘突下，后正中线旁开 3 寸
志室	在腰区，第 2 腰椎棘突下，后正中线旁开 3 寸
胞肓	在骶区，横平第 2 骶后孔，骶正中嵴旁开 3 寸
秩边	在骶区，横平第 4 骶后孔，骶正中嵴旁开 3 寸
消泺	在臂后区，肘尖与肩峰角连线上，肘尖上 5 寸
臑会	在臂后区，肩峰角下 3 寸，三角肌的后下缘
肩髎	在三角肌区，肩峰角与肱骨大结节两骨间凹陷中
天髎	在肩胛区，肩胛骨上角骨际凹陷中
肩井	在肩胛区，第 7 颈椎棘突与肩峰最外侧点连线的中点

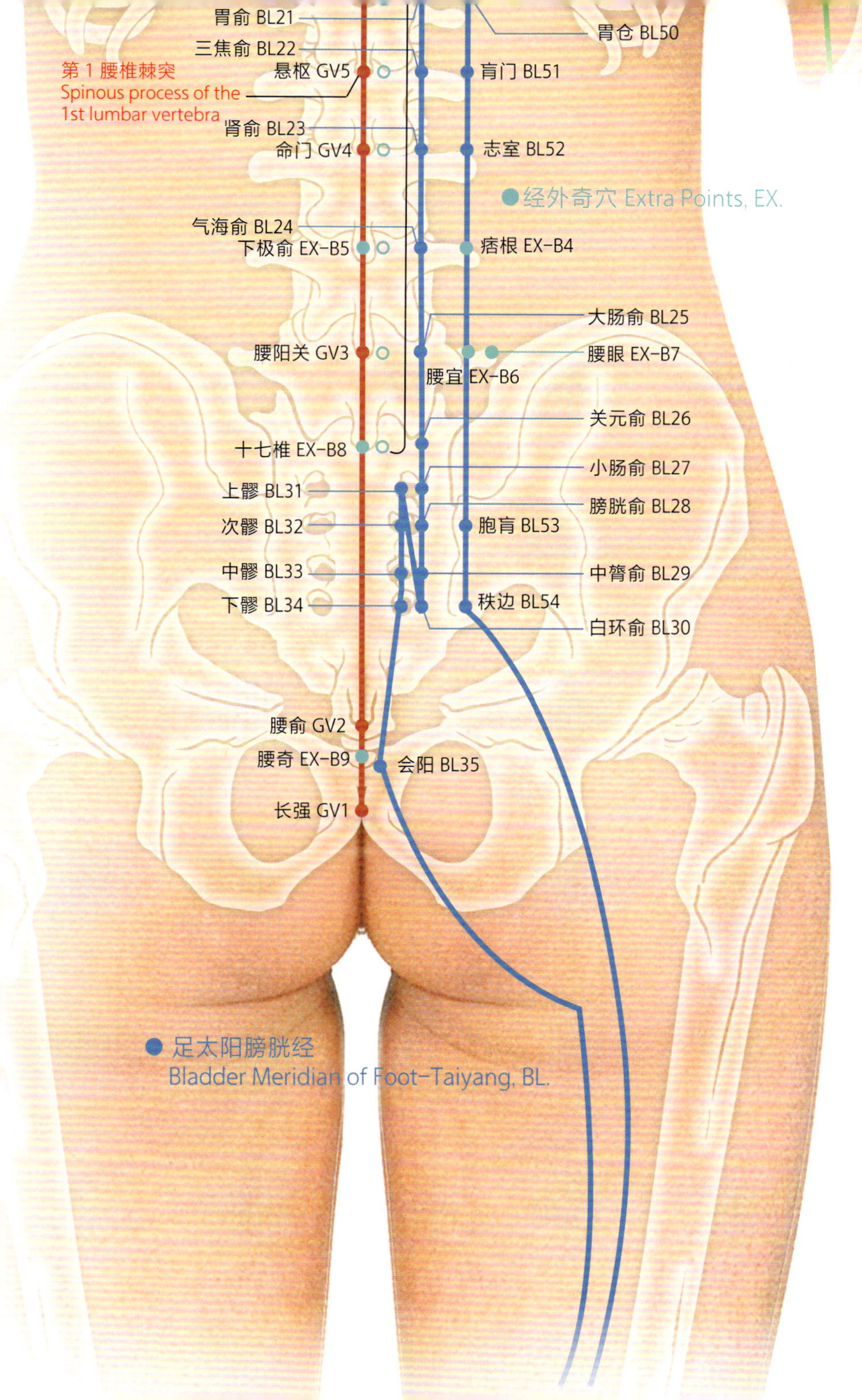

Continued

Acupoints	Location
Húnmén(BL47)	In the spinal region, inferior to spinous process of the 9th thoracic vertebra, 3 cun lateral to the posterior midline
Yánggāng(BL48)	In the spinal region, inferior to spinous process of the 10th thoracic vertebra, 3 cun lateral to the posterior midline
Yìshè(BL49)	In the spinal region, inferior to spinous process of the 11th thoracic vertebra, 3 cun lateral to the posterior midline
Wèicāng(BL50)	In the spinal region, inferior to spinous process of the 12th thoracic vertebra, 3 cun lateral to the posterior midline
Huāngmén(BL51)	In the lumbar region, inferior to spinous process of the 1st lumbar vertebra, 3 cun lateral to the posterior midline
Zhìshǐ(BL52)	In the lumbar region, inferior to spinous process of the 2nd lumbar vertebra, 3 cun lateral to the posterior midline
Bāohuāng(BL53)	In the sacral region, horizontal to the 2nd posterior sacral foramina, 3 cun lateral to the median sacral crest
Zhìbiān(BL54)	In the sacral region, horizontal to the 4th posterior sacral foramina, 3 cun lateral to the median sacral crest
Xiāoluò(TE12)	In the posterior brachial region, on the joining line of the tip of the elbow and acromial angle, 5 cun superior to the tip of the elbow
Nàohuì(TE13)	In the posterior brachial region, 3 cun inferior to the acromial angle, posterior and inferior to the deltoid
Jiānliáo(TE14)	In the deltoid region, in the depression between acromial angle and greater tuberosity of humerus
Tiānliáo(TE15)	In the scapular region, in the skeletal depression of superior angle of scapula
Jiānjǐng(GB21)	In the scapular region, at the midpoint of the joining line of the spinous process of the 7th cervical vertebra and the outmost point of acromion

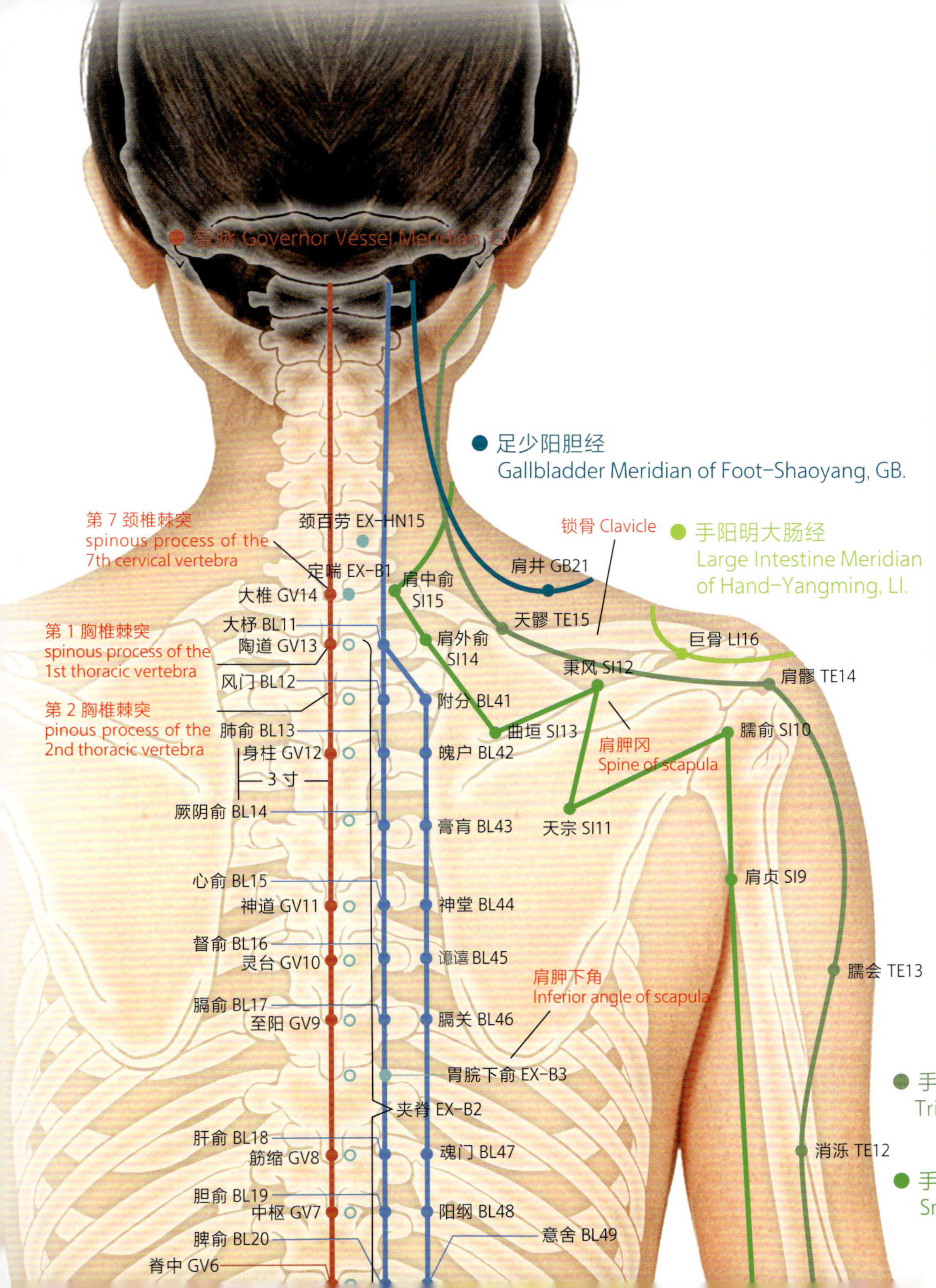

续表

穴 位	定 位
长强	在会阴部，尾骨下方，尾骨端与肛门连线的中点处
腰俞	在骶区，正对骶管裂孔，后正中线上
腰阳关	在脊柱区，第 4 腰椎棘突下凹陷中，后正中线上
命门	在脊柱区，第 2 腰椎棘突下凹陷中，后正中线上
悬枢	在脊柱区，第 1 腰椎棘突下凹陷中，后正中线上
脊中	在脊柱区，第 11 胸椎棘突下凹陷中，后正中线上
中枢	在脊柱区，第 10 胸椎棘突下凹陷中，后正中线上
筋缩	在脊柱区，第 9 胸椎棘突下凹陷中，后正中线上
至阳	在脊柱区，第 7 胸椎棘突下凹陷中，后正中线上
灵台	在脊柱区，第 6 胸椎棘突下凹陷中，后正中线上
神道	在脊柱区，第 5 胸椎棘突下凹陷中，后正中线上

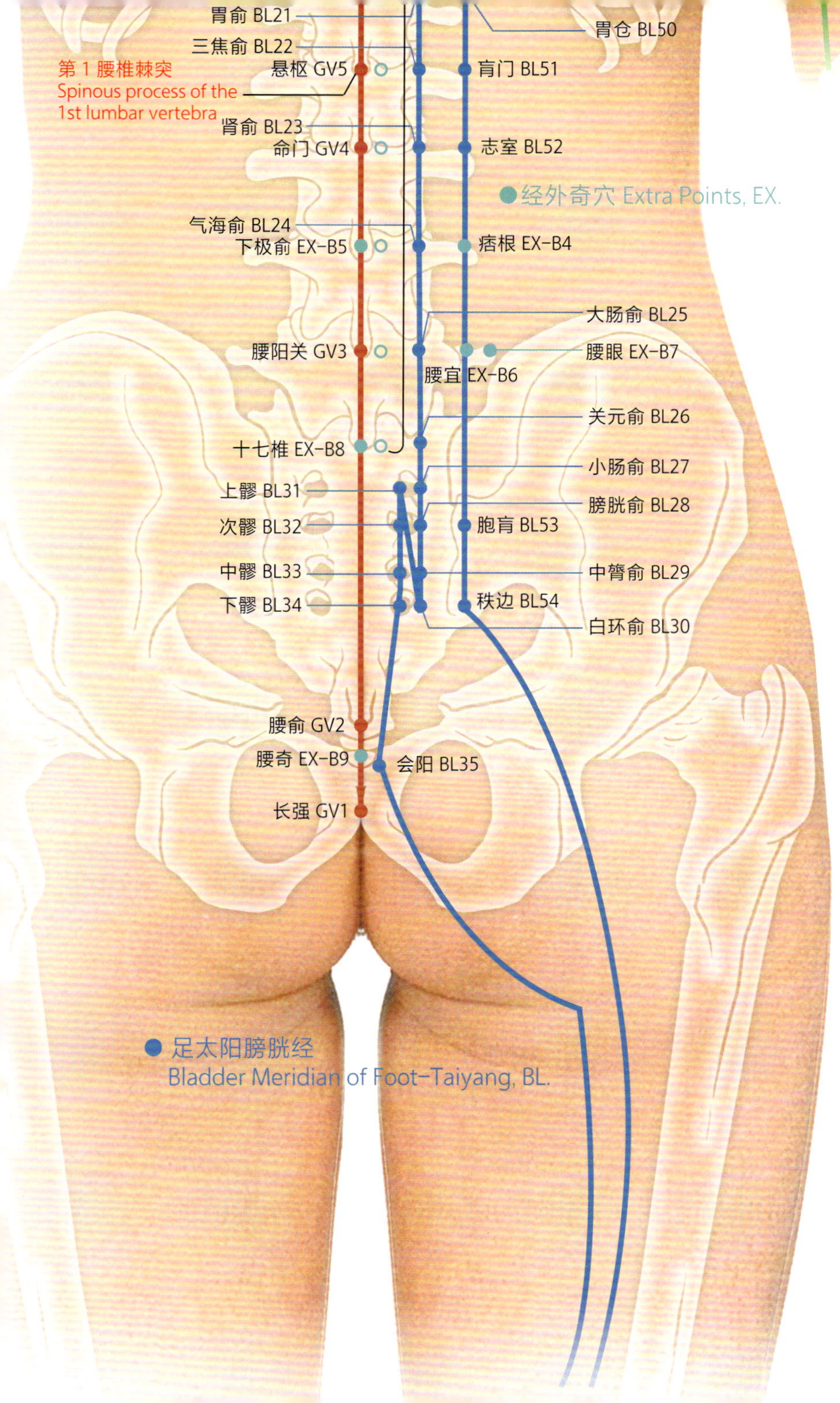

Continued

Acupoints	Location
Chángqiáng(GV1)	In the perineum region, inferior to coccyx, at the midpoint of coccyx end and anus
Yāoshū(GV2)	In the sacral region, directly faced with sacral hiatus, on the posterior midline
Yāoyángguān(GV3)	On the spinal region, in the depression inferior to spinous process of the 4th lumbar vertebra, on the posterior midline
Mìngmén(GV4)	On the spinal region, in the depression inferior to spinous process of the 2nd lumbar vertebra, on the posterior midline
Xuánshū(GV5)	On the spinal region, in the depression inferior to spinous process of the 1st lumbar vertebra, on the posterior midline
Jǐzhōng(GV6)	On the spinal region, in the depression inferior to spinous process of the 11th thoracic vertebra, on the posterior midline
Zhōngshū(GV7)	On the spinal region, in the depression inferior to spinous process of the 10th thoracic vertebra, on the posterior midline
Jīnsuō(GV8)	On the spinal region, in the depression inferior to spinous process of the 9th thoracic vertebra, on the posterior midline
Zhìyáng(GV9)	On the spinal region, in the depression inferior to spinous process of the 7th thoracic vertebra, on the posterior midline
Língtái(GV10)	On the spinal region, in the depression inferior to spinous process of the 6th thoracic vertebra, on the posterior midline
Shéndào(GV11)	On the spinal region, in the depression inferior to spinous process of the 5th thoracic vertebra, on the posterior midline

续表

穴 位	定 位
身柱	在脊柱区，第 3 胸椎棘突下凹陷中，后正中线上
陶道	在脊柱区，第 1 胸椎棘突下凹陷中，后正中线上
大椎	在脊柱区，第 7 颈椎棘突下凹陷中，后正中线上
颈百劳	在项部，第 7 颈椎棘突直上 2 寸，后正中线旁开 1 寸
定喘	在脊柱区，横平第 7 颈椎棘突下，后正中线旁开 0.5 寸
夹脊	在脊柱区，第 1 胸椎至第 5 腰椎棘突下两侧，后正中线旁开 0.5 寸，一侧 17 穴
胃脘下俞	在脊柱区，横平第 8 胸椎棘突下，后正中线旁开 1.5 寸
痞根	在腰区，横平第 1 腰椎棘突下，后正中线旁开 3.5 寸
下极俞	在腰区，第 3 腰椎棘突下
腰宜	在腰区，横平第 4 腰椎棘突下，后正中线旁开 3 寸
腰眼	在腰区，横平第 4 腰椎棘突下，后正中线旁开约 3.5 寸凹陷中
十七椎	在腰区，第 5 腰椎棘突下凹陷中
腰奇	在骶区，尾骨端直上 2 寸，骶角之间凹陷中

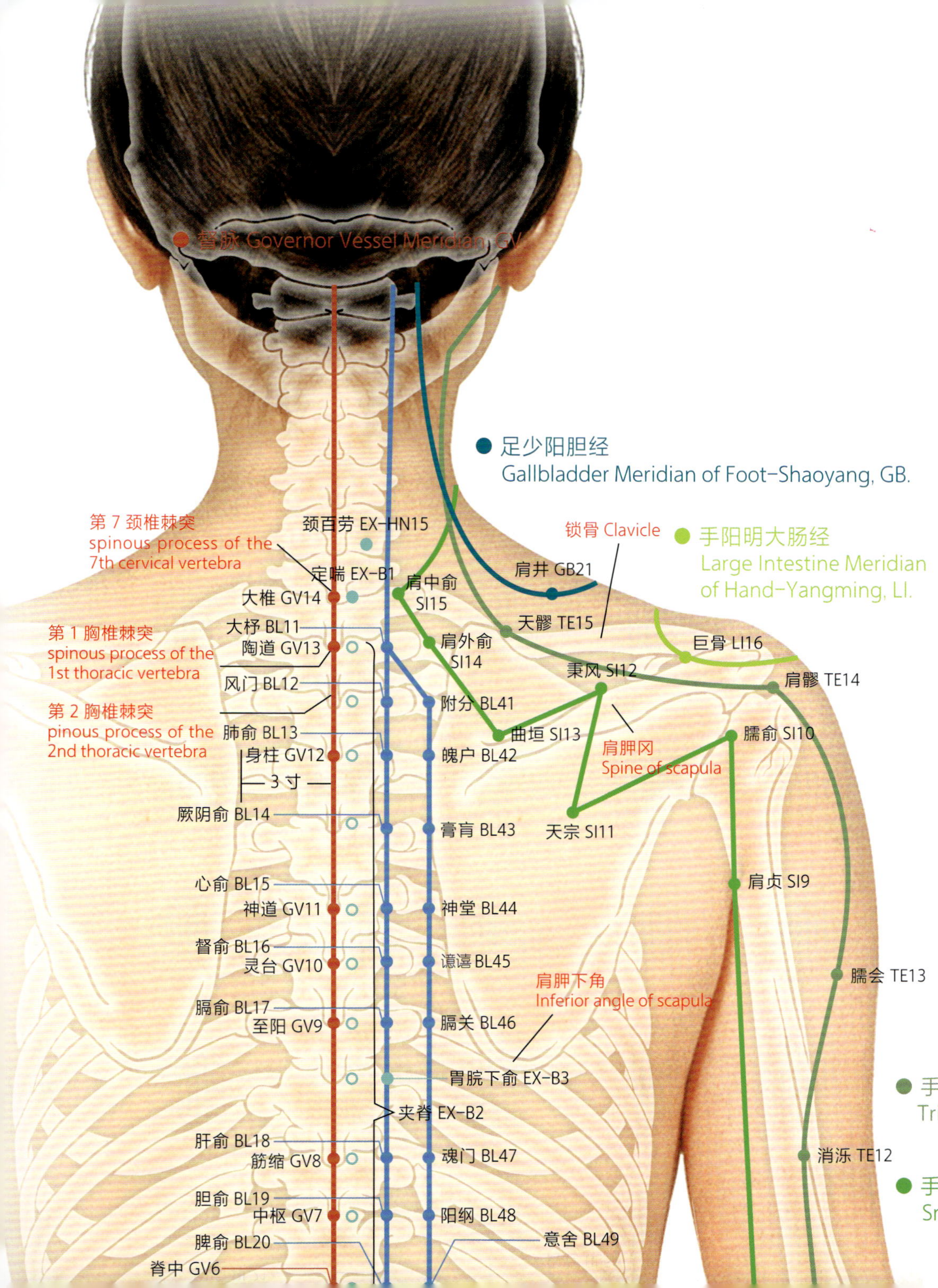

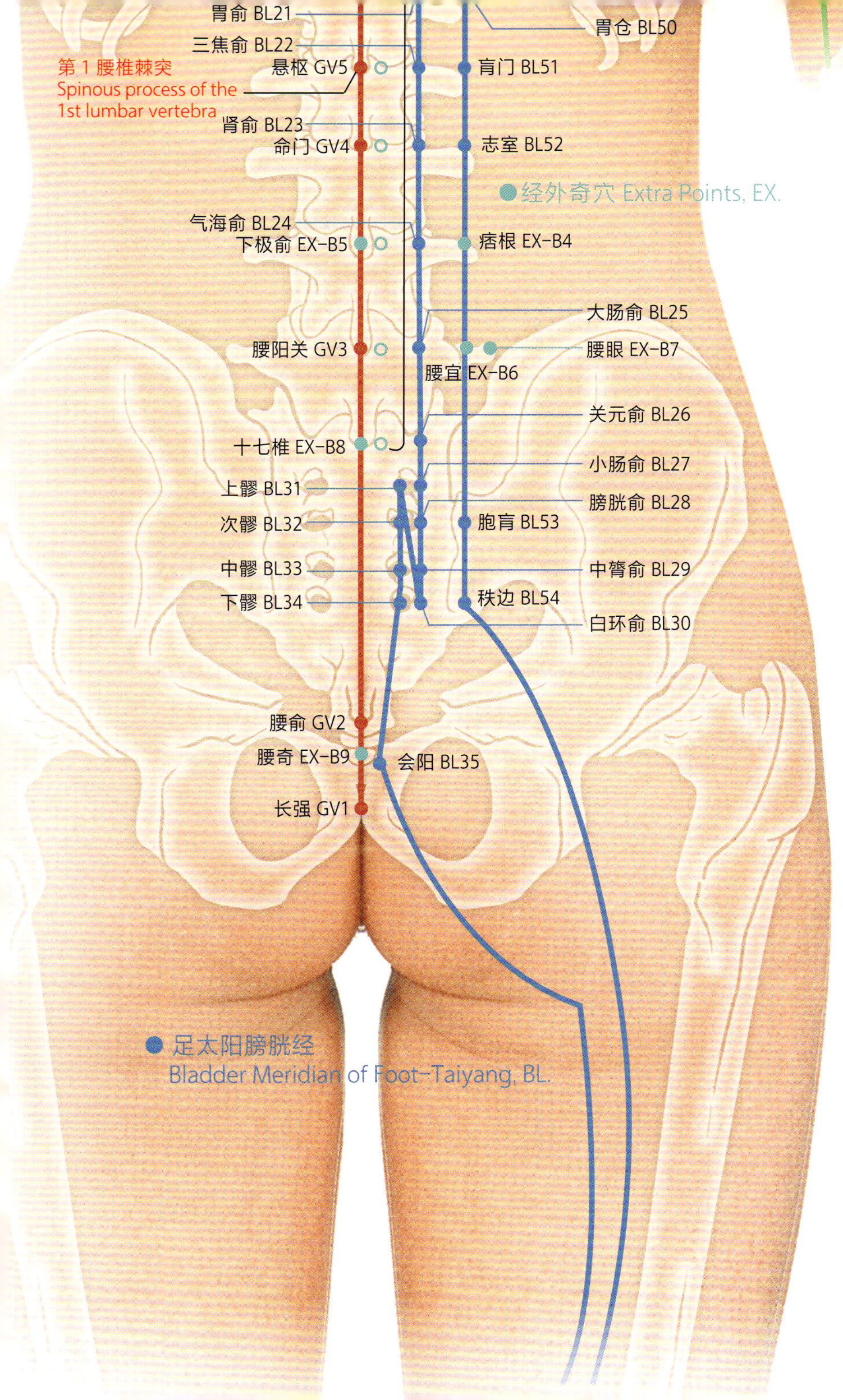

Continued

Acupoints	Location
Shēnzhù(GV12)	On the spinal region, in the depression inferior to spinous process of the 3th thoracic vertebra, on the posterior midline
Táodào(GV13)	On the spinal region, in the depression inferior to spinous process of the 1st thoracic vertebra, on the posterior midline
Dàzhuī(GV14)	On the spinal region, in the depression inferior to spinous process of the 7th cervical vertebra, on the posterior midline
Jìngbǎiláo(EX-HN15)	On the nape, 2 cun above the spinous process of the 7th cervical vertebra, 1 cun lateral to the posterior midline
Dìngchuǎn(EX-B1)	In the spinal region, horizontal to the spinous process of the 7th cervical vertebra, 0.5 cun lateral to the posterior midline
Jiájǐ(EX-B2)	In the spinal region, in two sides of spinous process of the 1st thoracic vertebra to the 5th lumbar vertebra, 0.5 cun lateral to the posterior midline, with 17 acupoints in each side
Wèiwǎnxiàshū(EX-B3)	In the spinal region, horizontal to the spinous process of the 8th thoracic vertebra, 1.5 cun lateral to the posterior midline
Pǐgēn(EX-B4)	In the lumbar region, horizontal to the spinous process of the 1st lumbar vertebra, 3.5 cun lateral to the posterior midline
Xiàjíshū(EX-B5)	In the lumbar region, inferior to spinous process of the 3rd lumbar vertebra
Yāoyí(EX-B6)	In the lumbar region, horizontal to the spinous process of the 4th lumbar vertebra, 3 cun lateral to the posterior midline
Yāoyǎn(EX-B7)	In the lumbar region, horizontal to the spinous process of the 4th lumbar vertebra, in the depression about 3.5 cun lateral to the posterior midline
Shíqīzhuī(EX-B8)	In the lumbar region, in the depression inferior to the spinous process of the 5th lumbar vertebra
Yāoqí(EX-B9)	In the sacral region, 2 cun above the coccyx end, in the depression between the sacral angle

上肢部穴位

Acupoints of Upper Limbs

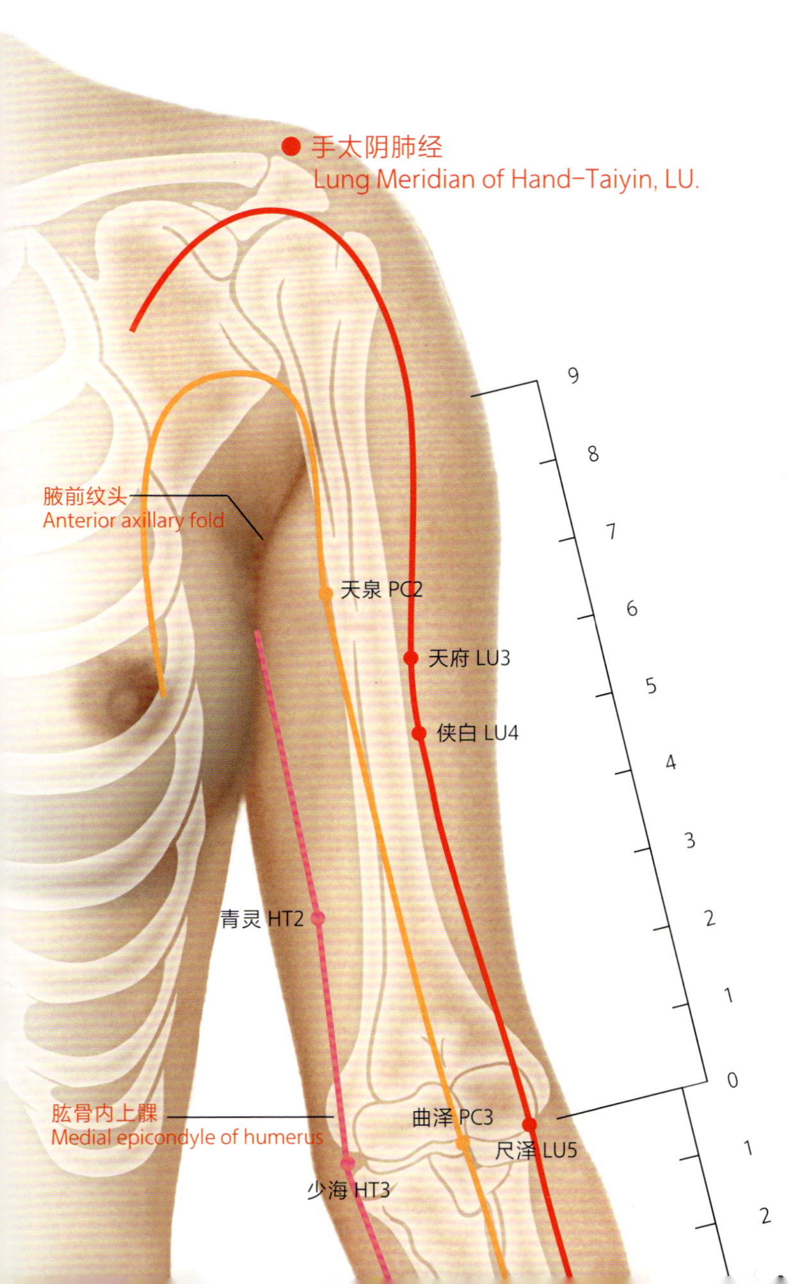

穴 位	定 位
天府	在臂前区，腋前纹头下 3 寸，肱二头肌桡侧缘处
侠白	在臂前区，腋前纹头下 4 寸，肱二头肌桡侧缘处
尺泽	在肘区，肘横纹上，肱二头肌腱桡侧缘凹陷中
孔最	在前臂前区，腕掌侧远端横纹上 7 寸，尺泽与太渊连线上
列缺	在前臂，腕掌侧远端横纹上 1.5 寸，拇短伸肌腱与拇长展肌腱之间，拇长展肌腱沟的凹陷中
经渠	在前臂前区，腕掌侧远端横纹上 1 寸，桡骨茎突与桡动脉之间
太渊	在腕前区，桡骨茎突与舟状骨之间，拇长展肌腱尺侧凹陷中
鱼际	在手外侧，第 1 掌骨桡侧中点赤白肉际处
少商	在手指，拇指末节桡侧，指甲根角侧上方 0.1 寸

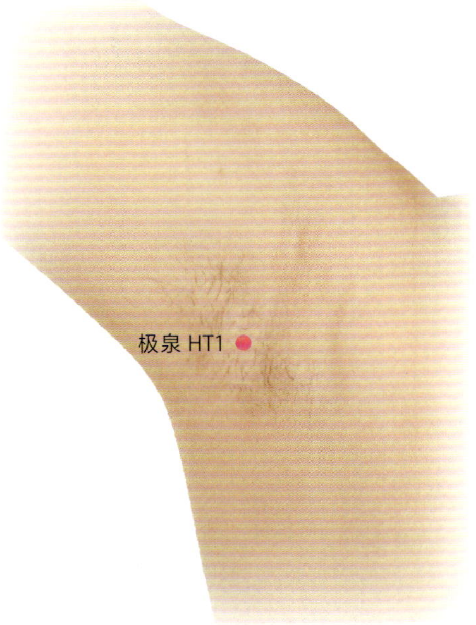

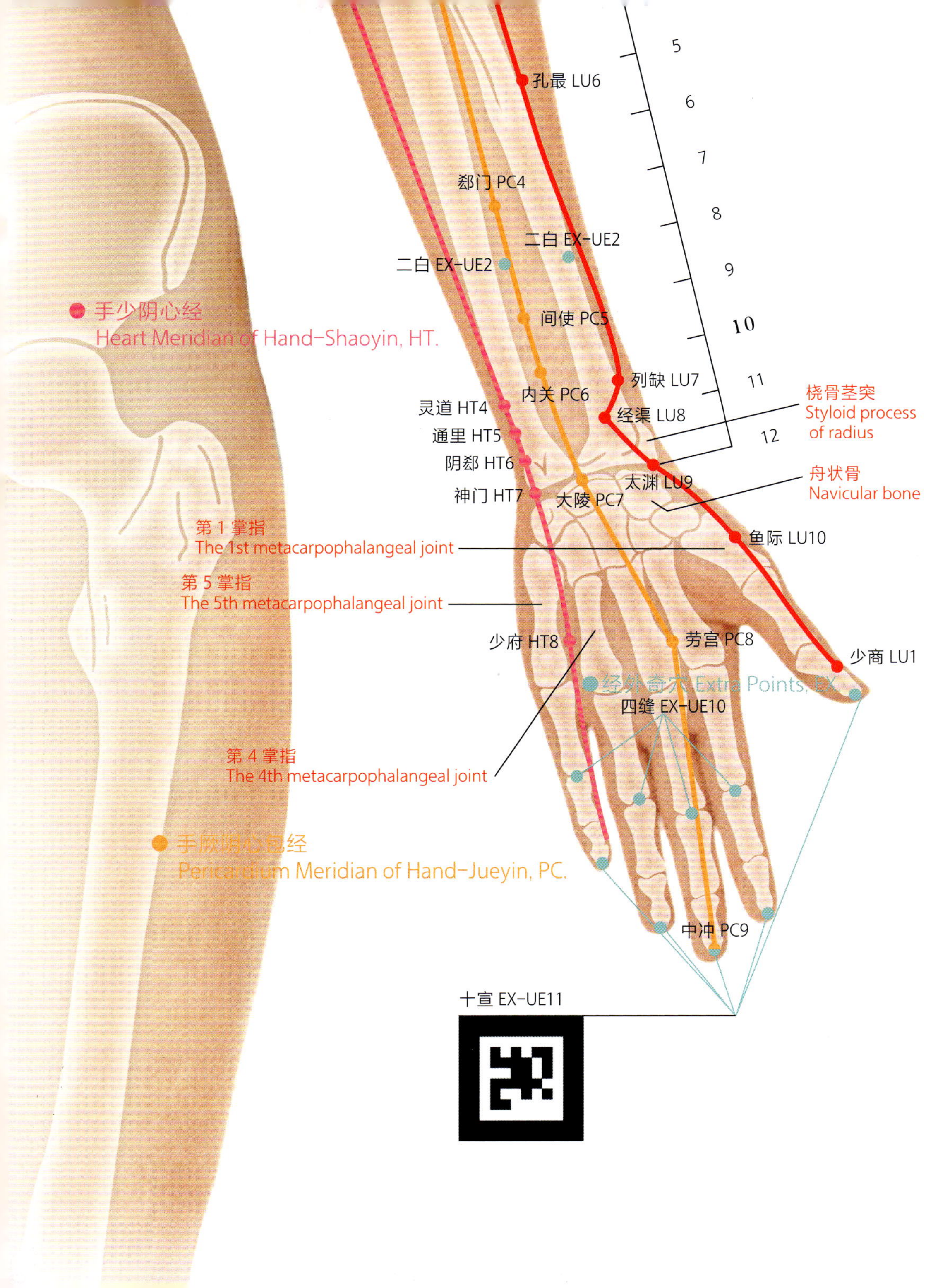

Acupoints	Location
Tiānfǔ(LU3)	In the anterior region of the arm, 3 cun inferior to anterior axillary fold, in the radial margin of biceps brachii
Xiábái(LU4)	In the anterior region of the arm, 4 cun inferior to anterior axillary fold, in the radial margin of biceps brachii
Chǐzé(LU5)	In the elbow region, on the cubital crease, in the depression of the radial border of biceps brachii tendon
Kǒngzuì(LU6)	In the anterior region of forearm, 7 cun superior to the distal transverse crease of the palmar wrist, on the line of Chize(LU5) and Taiyuan(LU9)
Lièquē(LU7)	On the forearm, 1.5 cun superior to the distal transverse crease of the palmar wrist, between tendon of extensor pollicis brevis and tendon of abductor pollicis longus, in the depression of tendon groove of abductor pollicis longus
Jīngqú(LU8)	In the anterior region of forearm, 1 cun superior to the distal transverse crease of the palmar wrist, between styloid process of radius and radial artery
Tàiyuān(LU9)	In the anterior region of the wrist, between styloid process of radius and navicular bone, in the ulnar depression of tendon of abductor pollicis longus
Yújì(LU10)	In the exterior region of the hand, at the midpoint of the first metacarpal bone, at the junction of the red and white skin of the hand
Shàoshāng(LU11)	On the finger, in radial end of the thumb, 0.1 cun from the corner of the nail

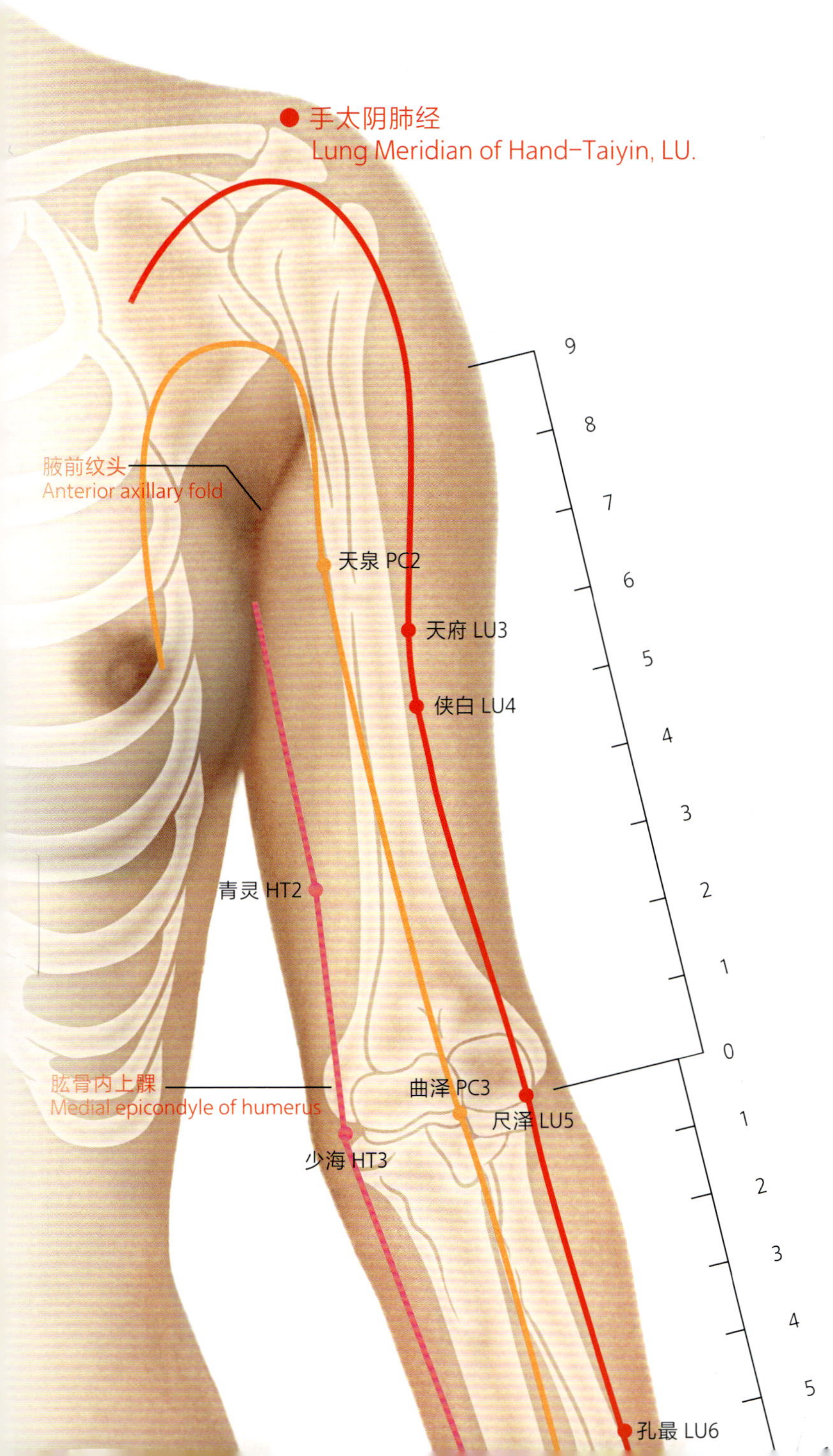

续表

穴 位	定 位
极泉	在腋区，腋窝中央，腋动脉搏动处
青灵	在臂前区，肘横纹上 3 寸，肱二头肌的内侧沟中
少海	在肘前区，横平肘横纹，肱骨内上髁前缘
灵道	在前臂前区，腕掌侧远端横纹上 1.5 寸，尺侧腕屈肌腱的桡侧缘
通里	在前臂前区，腕掌侧远端横纹上 1 寸，尺侧腕屈肌腱的桡侧缘
阴郄	在前臂前区，腕掌侧远端横纹上 0.5 寸，尺侧腕屈肌腱的桡侧缘
神门	在腕前区，腕掌侧远端横纹尺侧端，尺侧腕屈肌腱的桡侧缘
少府	在手掌，横平第 5 掌指关节近端，第 4，5 掌骨之间
天泉	在臂前区，腋前纹头下 2 寸，肱二头肌的长、短头之间
曲泽	在肘前区，肘横纹上，肱二头肌腱的尺侧缘凹陷中

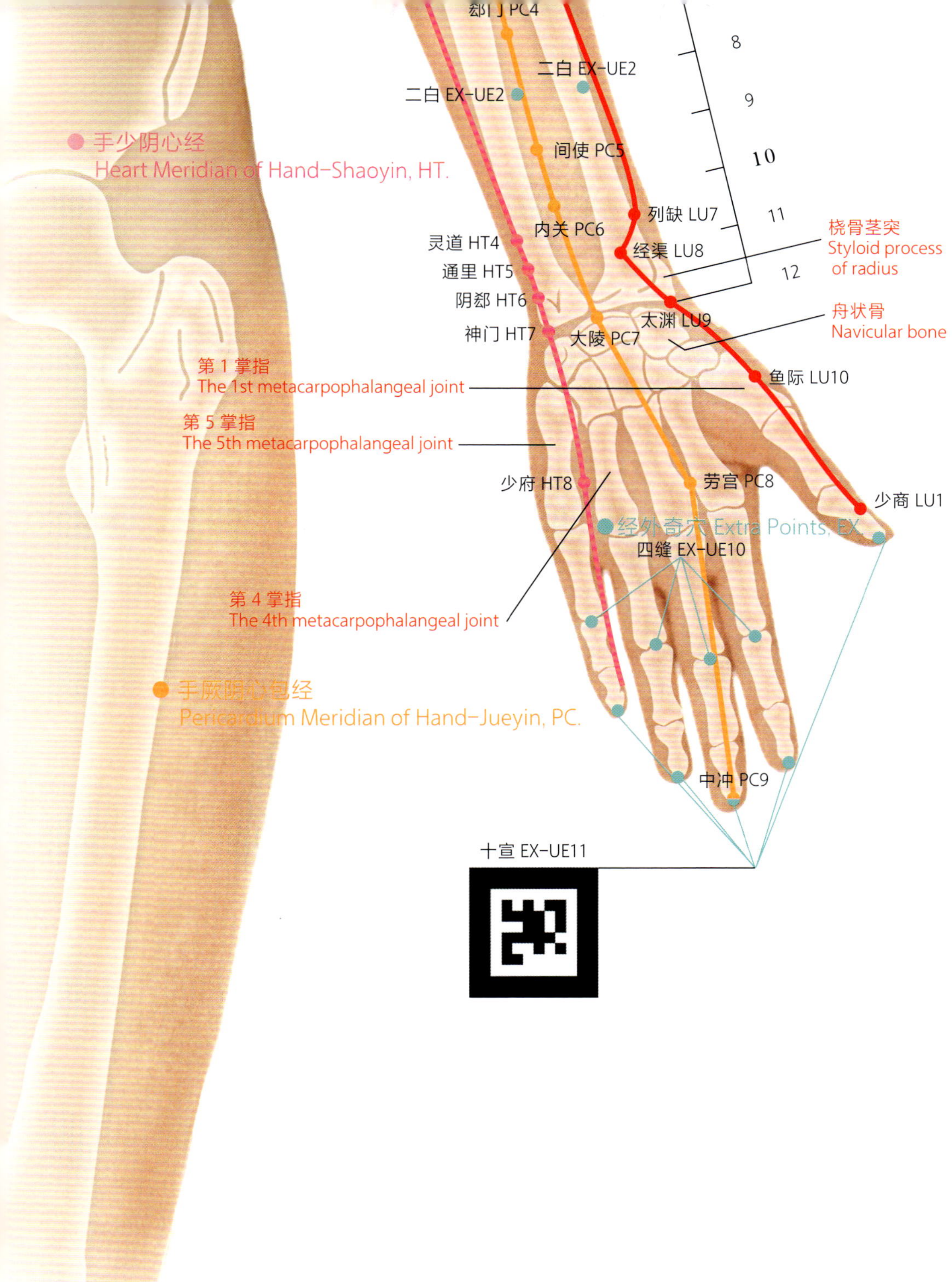

Continued

Acupoints	Location
Jíquán(HT1)	In the axillary region, in the center of the armpit where axillary artery pulses
Qīnglíng(HT2)	In the anterior region of arm, 3 cun superior to the transverse crease of the elbow, in medial groove of biceps
Shàohǎi(HT3)	In the anterior region of the elbow, horizontal to transverse crease of the elbow, in the anterior border of medial epicondyle of humerus
Língdào(HT4)	In the anterior region of the forearm, 1.5 cun superior to distal transverse crease of the palmar wrist, in the radial border of tendon of flexor carpi ulnaris
Tōnglǐ(HT5)	In the anterior region of the forearm, 1 cun superior to distal transverse crease of the palmar wrist, in the radial border of tendon of flexor carpi ulnaris
Yīnxì(HT6)	In the anterior region of the forearm, 0.5 cun superior to distal transverse crease of the palmar wrist, in the radial border of tendon of flexor carpi ulnaris
Shénmén(HT7)	In the anterior region of the wrist, in the ulnar border of distal transverse crease of palmar wrist, in the radial border of tendon of flexor carpi ulnaris
Shàofǔ(HT8)	On the palm, level with proximal end of the 5th metacarpophalangeal joint, between the 4th and the 5th metacarpal bone
Tiānquán(PC2)	In the anterior region of arm, 2 cun inferior to anterior axillary fold, between longus and brevis of biceps
Qūzé(PC3)	In the anterior region of the elbow, on the transverse crease of the elbow, in the depression of ulnar border of biceps tendon

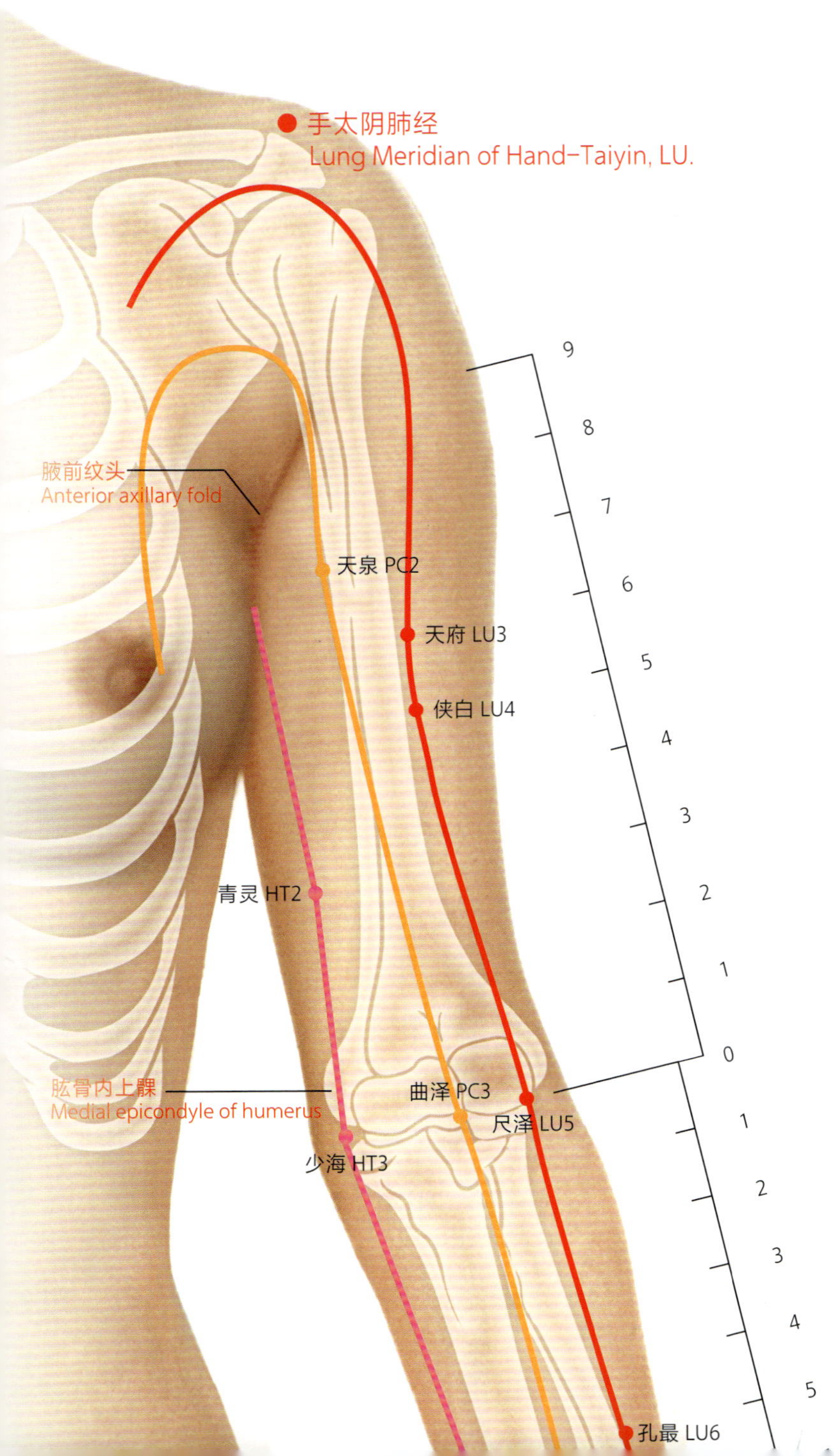

续表

穴 位	定 位
郄门	在前臂前区，腕掌侧远端横纹上 5 寸，掌长肌腱与桡侧腕屈肌腱之间
间使	在前臂前区，腕掌侧远端横纹上 3 寸，掌长肌腱与桡侧腕屈肌腱之间
内关	在前臂前区，腕掌侧远端横纹上 2 寸，掌长肌腱与桡侧腕屈肌腱之间
大陵	在腕前区，腕掌侧远端横纹中，掌长肌腱与桡侧腕屈肌腱之间
劳宫	在掌区，横平第 3 掌指关节近端，第 2、3 掌骨之间偏于第 3 掌骨
中冲	在手指，中指末端最高点
二白	在前臂前区，腕掌侧远端横纹上 4 寸，桡侧腕屈肌腱的两侧，一肢 2 穴
四缝	在手指，第 2~5 指掌面的近侧指间关节横纹的中央，一手 4 穴
十宣	在手指，十指尖端，距指甲游离缘 0.1 寸，左右共 10 穴

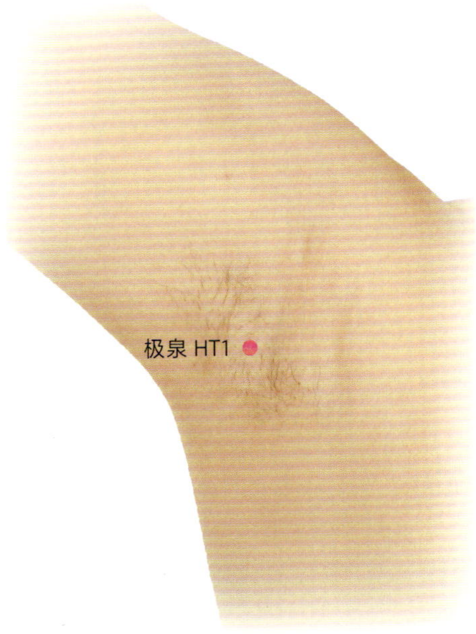

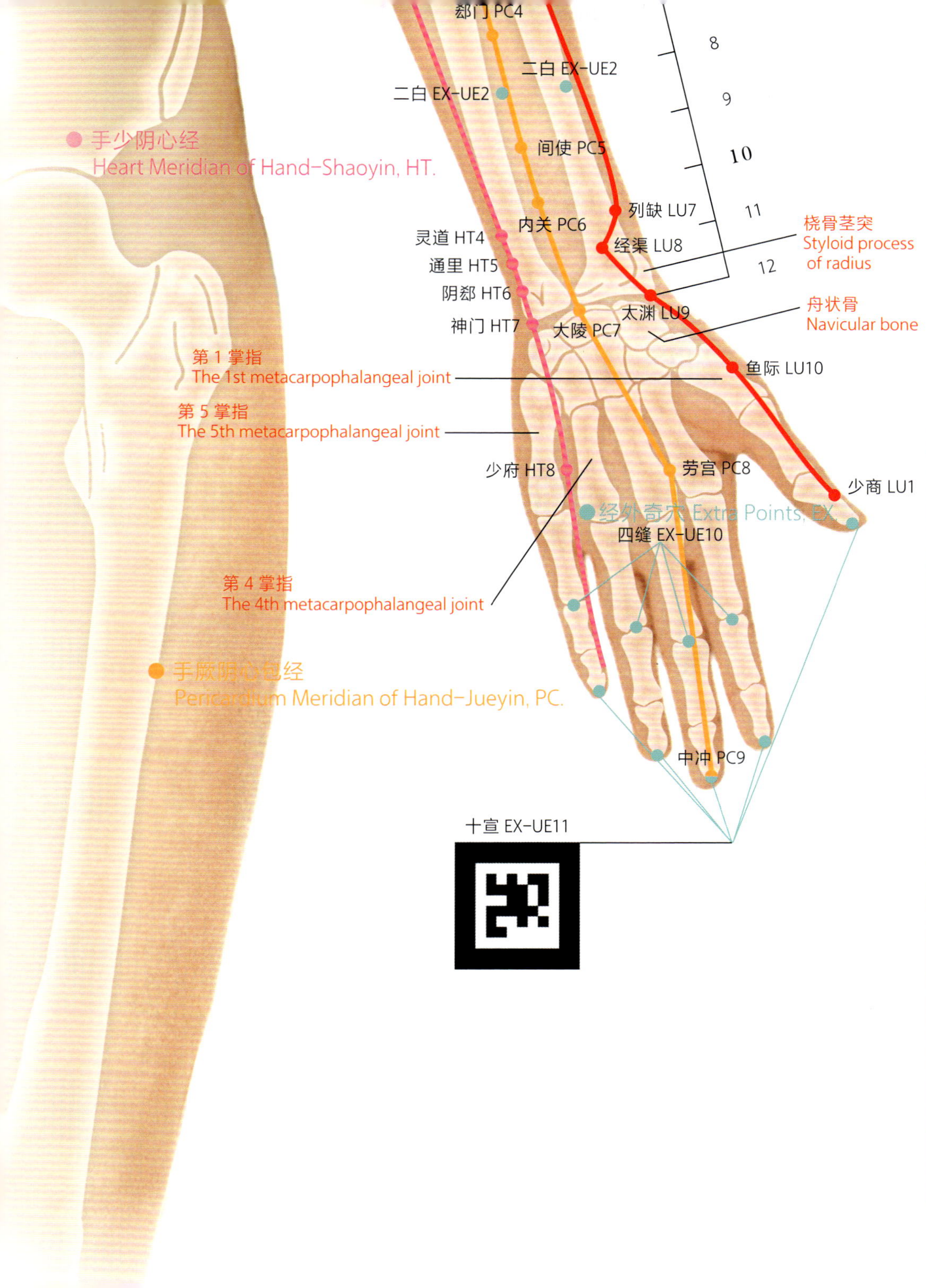

Continued

Acupoints	Location
Xìmén(PC4)	In the anterior region of the forearm, 5 cun superior to distal transverse crease of palmar wrist, in the depression between tendon palmaris longus and radial flexor tendon of wrist
Jiānshǐ(PC5)	In the anterior region of the forearm, 3 cun superior to distal transverse crease of palmar wrist, in the depression between tendon palmaris longus and radial flexor tendon of wrist
Nèiguān(PC6)	In the anterior region of the forearm, 2 cun superior to distal transverse crease of palmar wrist, in the depression between tendon palmaris longus and radial flexor tendon of wrist
Dàlíng(PC7)	In the anterior region of the wrist, on the distal transverse crease of palmar wrist, between tendon palmaris longus and radial flexor tendon of wrist
Láogōng(PC8)	In the region of palm, horizontal to distal end of the 3rd metacarpophalangeal joint, between the 2nd and the 3rd metacarpal bone, near the 3rd metacarpal bone
Zhōngchōng(PC9)	On the finger, at the apex of the middle finger
Èrbái(EX-UE2)	In the anterior region of the forearm, 4 cun superior to the distal transverse crease of the palmar wrist, lateral to radial flexor tendon of the wrist
Sìfèng(EX-UE10)	On the finger, in the middle of the transverse crease of interphalangeal joint proximal to the 2nd to the 5th finger on the palmar side, with 4 points of each hand
Shíxuān(EX-UE11)	On the finger, at the tip of ten fingers, 0.1 cun from the free edge of the nails, with 10 points in total

穴 位	定 位
商阳	在手指，食指末节桡侧，指甲根角侧上方 0.1 寸
二间	在手指，第 2 掌指关节桡侧远端赤白肉际处
三间	在手背，第 2 掌指关节桡侧近端凹陷处
合谷	在手背，第 2 掌骨桡侧的中点处
阳溪	在腕区，腕背侧远端横纹桡侧，桡骨茎突远端，解剖学“鼻烟窝”凹陷中
偏历	在前臂，腕背侧远端横纹上 3 寸，阳溪与曲池连线上
温溜	在前臂，腕背侧远端横纹上 5 寸，阳溪与曲池连线上
下廉	在前臂，肘横纹下 4 寸，阳溪与曲池连线上
上廉	在前臂，肘横纹下 3 寸，阳溪与曲池连线上
手三里	在前臂，肘横纹下 2 寸，阳溪与曲池连线上

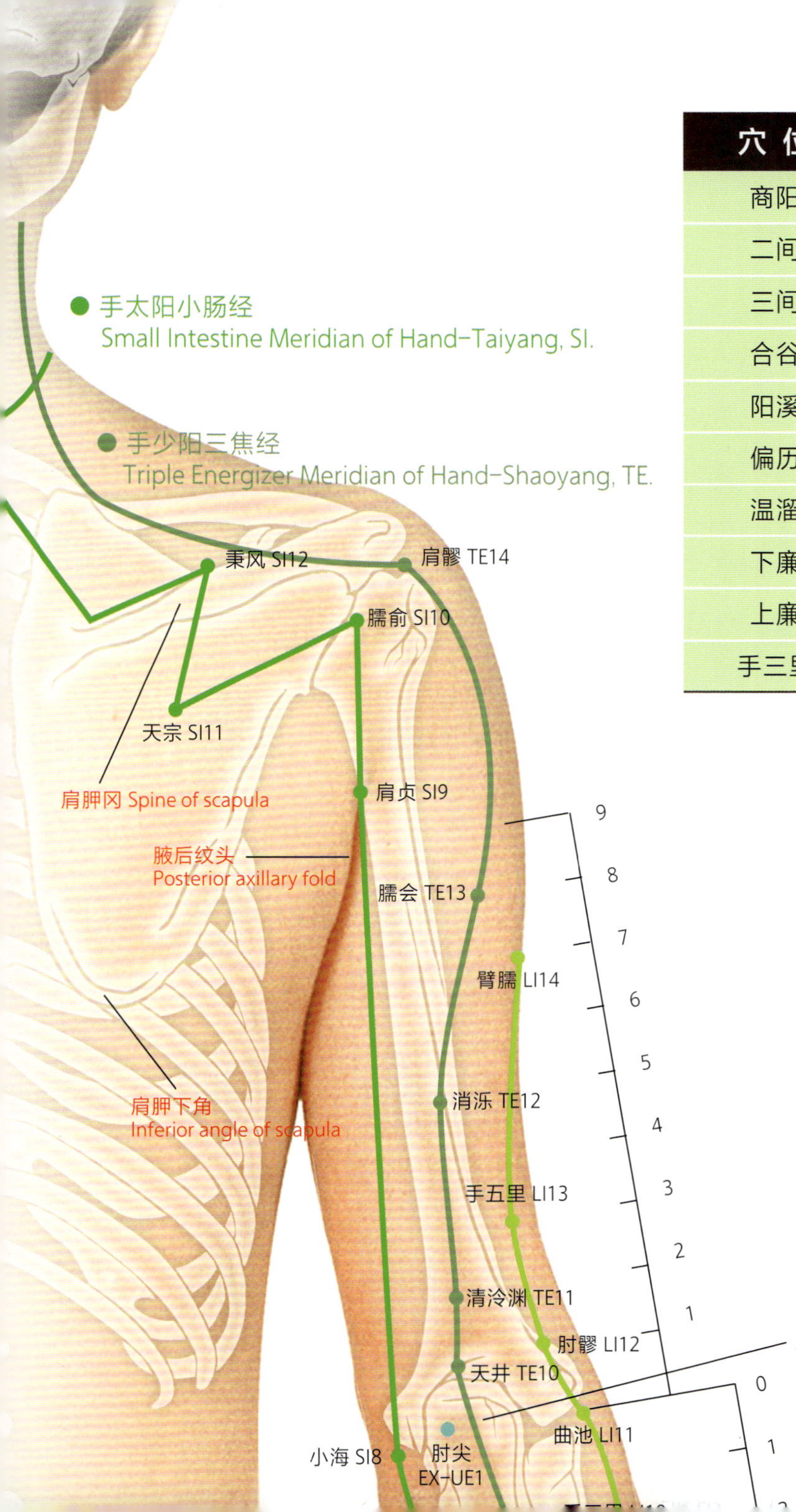

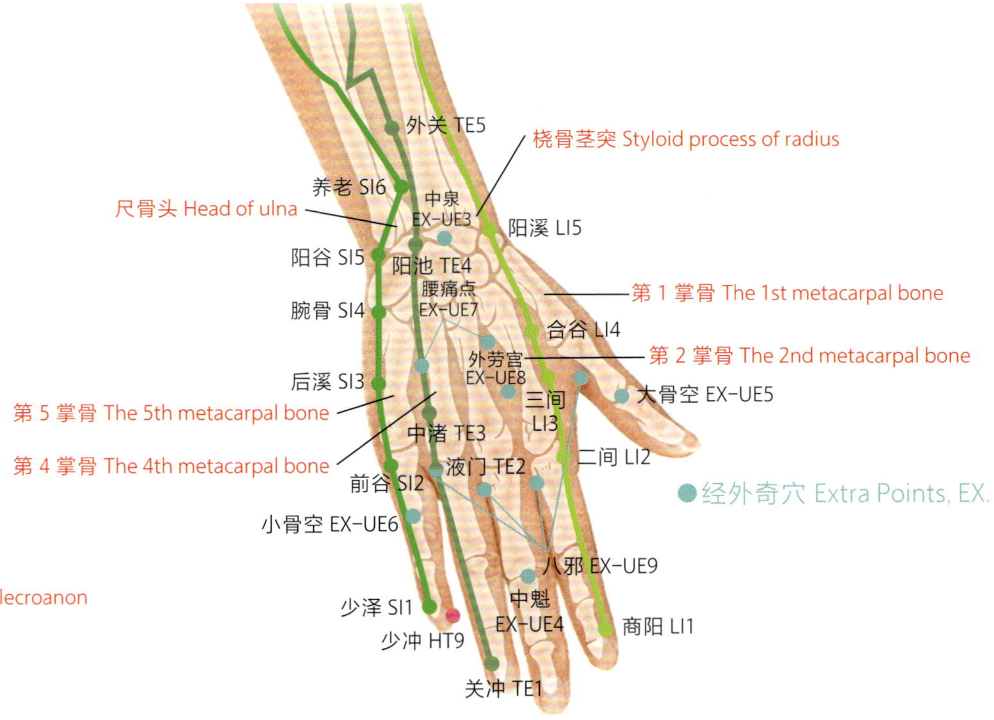

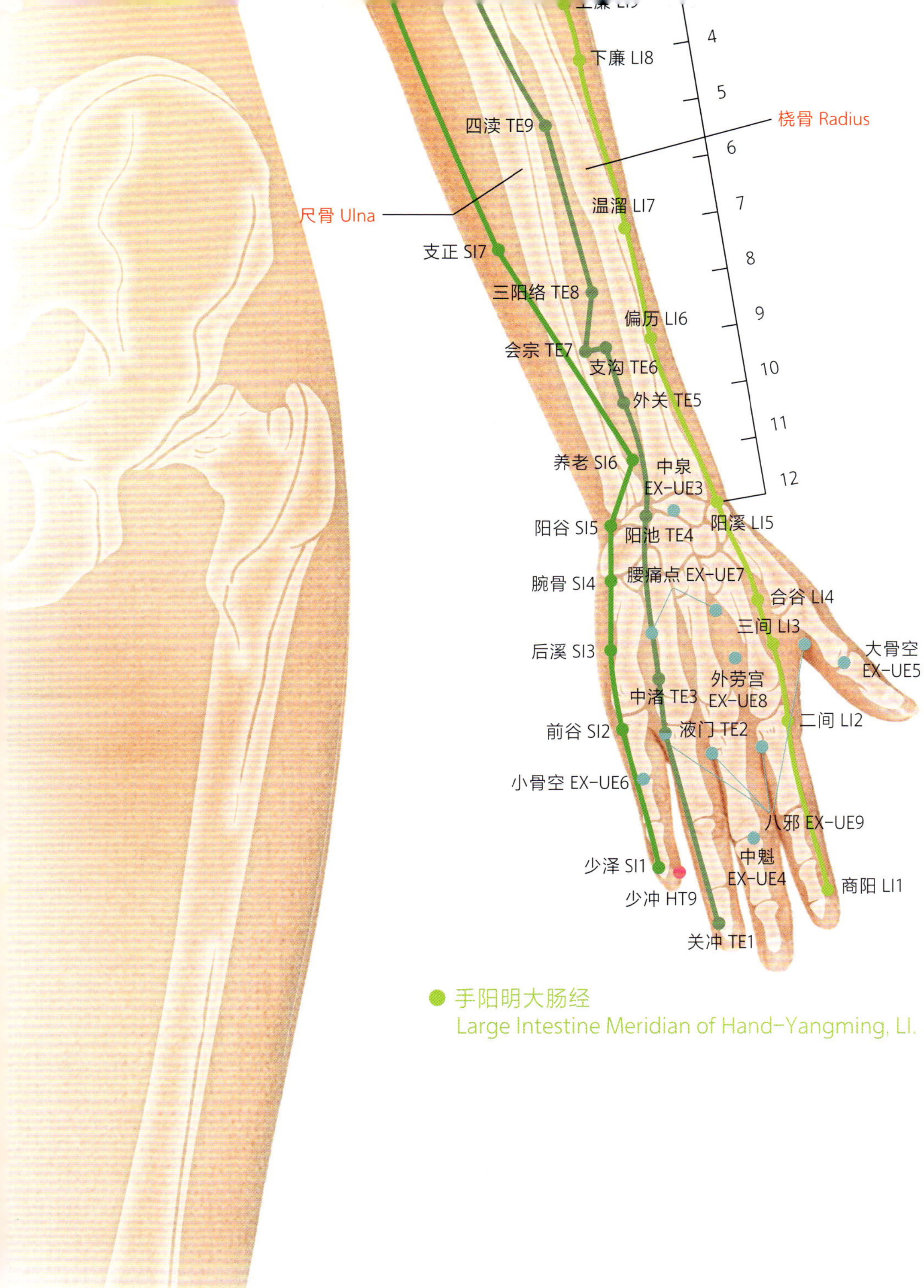

● 手阳明大肠经
Large Intestine Meridian of Hand-Yangming, LI.

Acupoints	Location
Shāngyáng(LI1)	On the finger, in the radial border of the index finger, 0.1 cun from the corner of the nail
Èrjiān (LI2)	On the finger, in the distal radial side of the 2nd metacarpophalangeal joint, at the junction of the red and white skin of the hand
Sānjiān(LI3)	On the dorsum of the hand, in the depression of proximal radial side of the 2nd metacarpophalangeal joint
Hégǔ(LI4)	On the dorsum of the hand, at the midpoint of the 2nd metacarpal bone on the radial side
Yángxī(LI5)	On the wrist, in the radial side of the distal end of transverse crease on the dorsal wrist, in the distal end of styloid process of radius, in the depression of anatomical snuffbox
Piānlì(LI6)	On the forearm, 3 cun superior to the the distal end of transverse crease on dorsal wrist, along the line of Yangxi(LI5) and Quchi(LI11)
Wēnliū(LI7)	On the forearm, 5 cun superior to the the distal end of transverse crease on the dorsal wrist, along the line connecting Yangxi(LI5) and Quchi(LI11)
Xiàlián(LI8)	On the forearm, 4 cun inferior to the transverse crease of the elbow, along the line conneting Yangxi(LI5) and Quchi(LI11)
Shànglián(LI9)	On the forearm, 3 cun inferior to the transverse crease of the elbow, along the line conneting Yangxi(LI5) and Quchi(LI11)
Shǒusānlǐ(LI10)	On the forearm, 2 cun inferior to the transverse crease of the elbow, along the line conneting Yangxi(LI5) and Quchi(LI11)

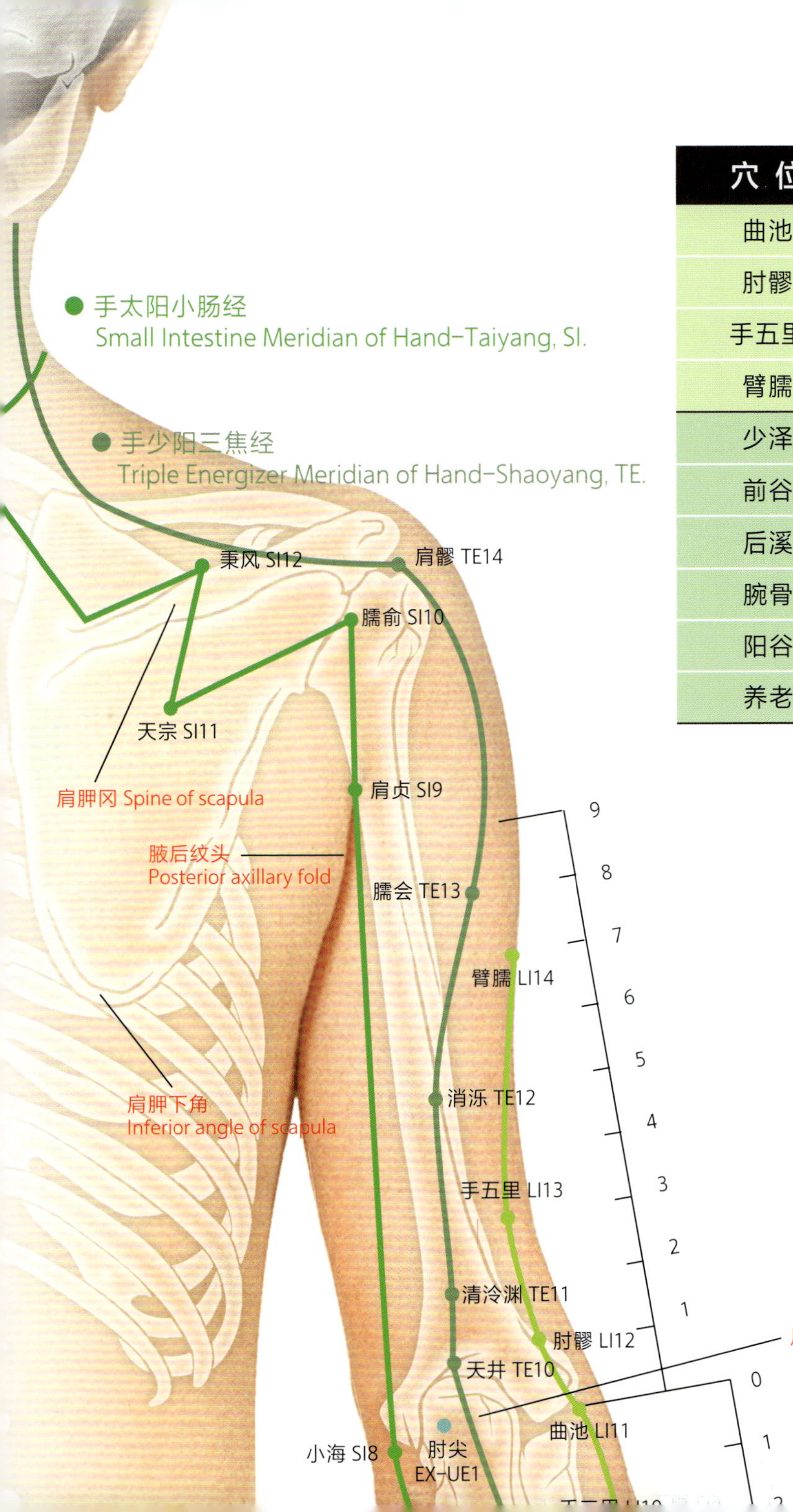

续表

穴位	定位
曲池	在肘区，尺泽与肱骨外上髁连线的中点处
肘髎	在肘区，肱骨外上髁上缘，髁上嵴的前缘
手五里	在臂部，肘横纹上 3 寸处，曲池与肩髃连线上
臂臑	在臂部，曲池上 7 寸，三角肌前缘处
少泽	在手指，小指末节尺侧，指甲根角侧上方 0.1 寸
前谷	在手指，第 5 掌指关节尺侧远端赤白肉际凹陷中
后溪	在手内侧，第 5 掌指关节尺侧近端赤白肉际凹陷中
腕骨	在腕区，第 5 掌骨底与三角骨之间的赤白肉际凹陷中
阳谷	在腕后区，尺骨茎突与三角骨之间的凹陷中
养老	在前臂后区，腕背横纹上 1 寸，尺骨头桡侧凹陷中

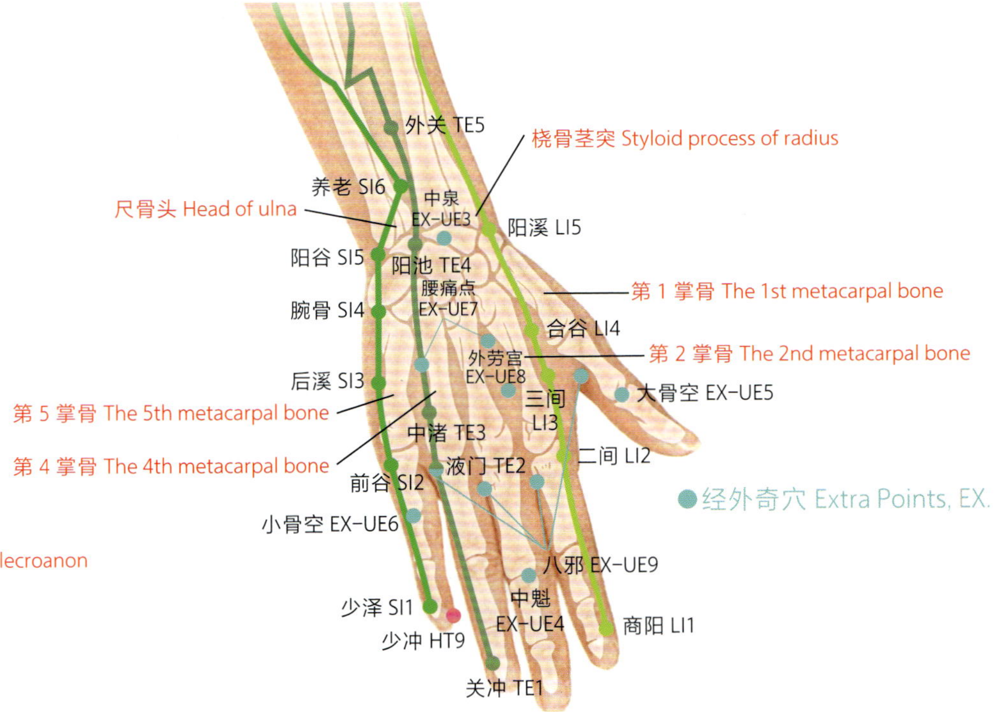

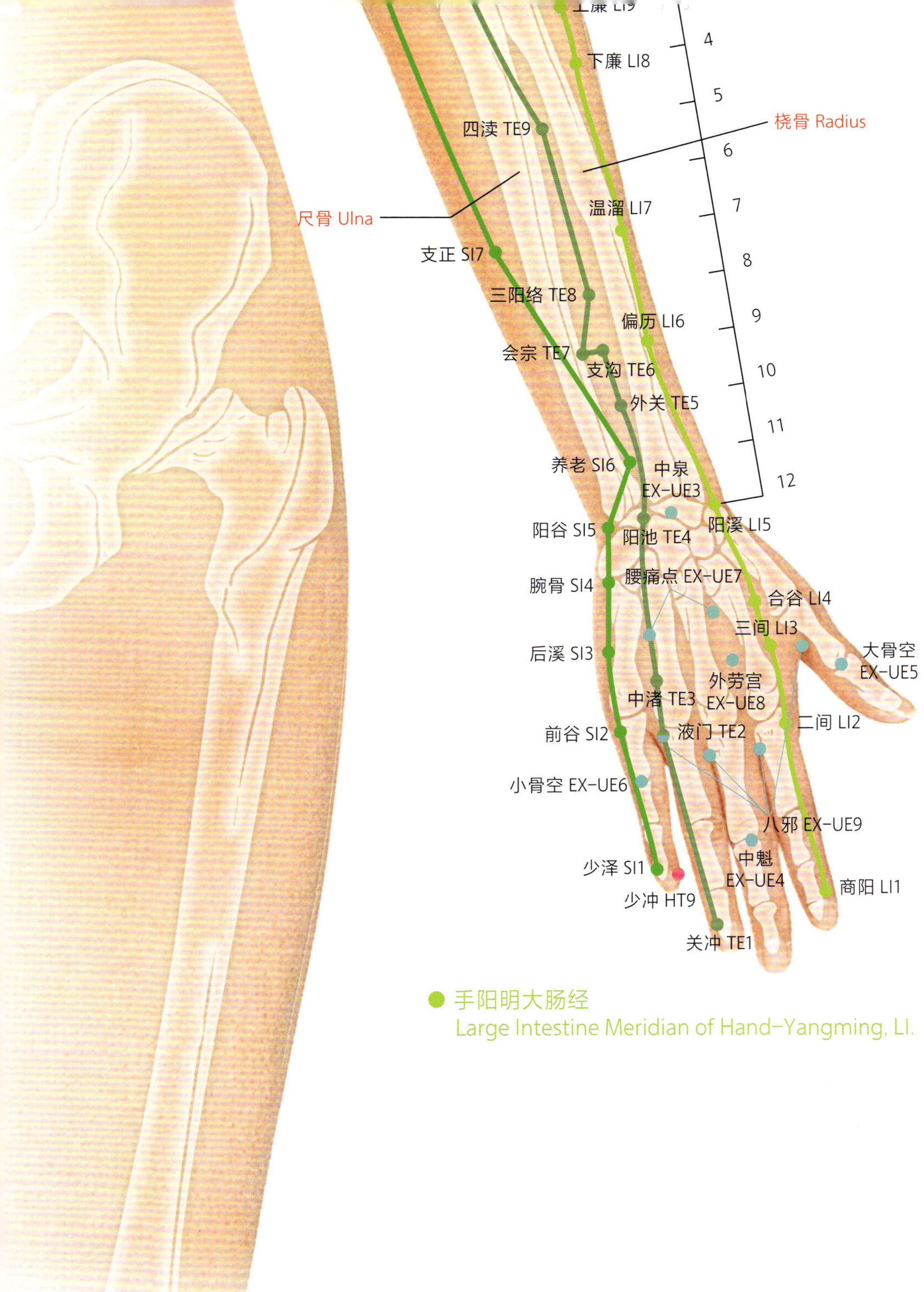

● 手阳明大肠经
Large Intestine Meridian of Hand-Yangming, LI.

Continued

Acupoints	Location
Qūchí(LI11)	In the elbow region, at the midpoint of the line joining Chize(LU5) and external epicondyle of humerus
Zhǒuliáo(LI12)	In the elbow region, in the superior border of external epicondyle of humerus, in the anterior border of supracondylar ridge
Shǒuwǔiǐ(LI13)	On the arm, 3 cun superior to the transverse crease of the elbow, along the line connecting Quchi(LI11) and Jianyu(LI15)
Bìnào(LI14)	On the arm, 7 cun superior to Quchi(LI11), in the anterior border of the deltoid
Shàozé(SI1)	On the finger, in the ulnar end of the little finger, 0.1 cun from the corner of the nail
Qiángǔ(SI2)	On the finger, in depression of the junction of the red and white skin at ulnar distal end of the 5th metacarpophalangeal joint
Hòuxī(SI3)	In the interior region of the hand, in the depression of the junction of the red and white skin at ulnar proximal end of the 5th metacarpophalangeal joint
Wàngǔ(SI4)	On the wrist, in the depression of the junction of the red and white skin of the hand between the basis of the 5th metacarpal bone and triangular bone
Yánggǔ(SI5)	In the posterior region of the wrist, in the depression between the styloid process of ulna and triangular bone
Yǎnglǎo(SI6)	In the posterior region of the forearm, 1 cun superior to the transverse crease of dorsal wrist, in the radial depression of the ulna head

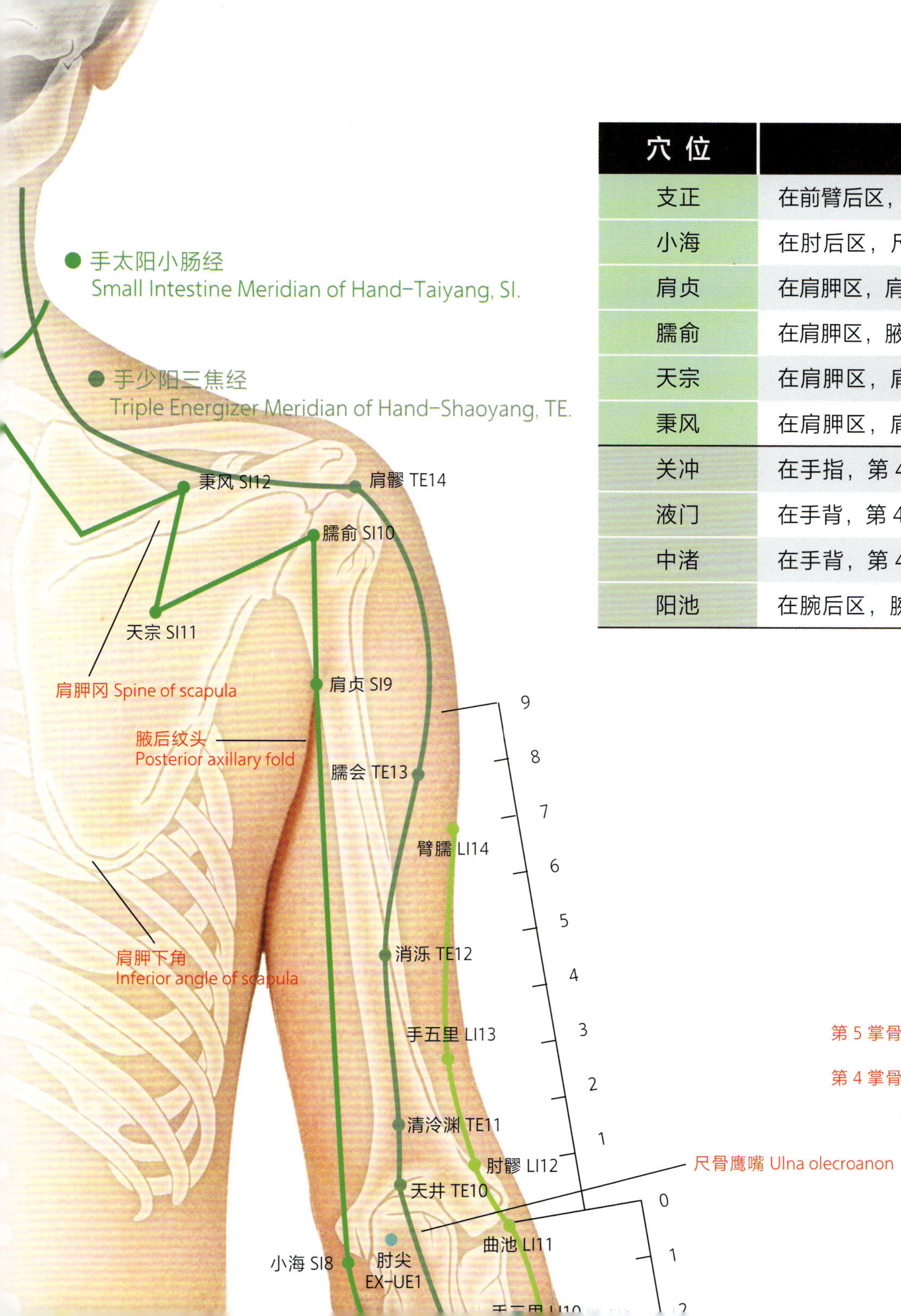

续表

穴位	定位
支正	在前臂后区，腕背侧远端横纹上 5 寸，尺骨尺侧与尺侧腕屈肌之间
小海	在肘后区，尺骨鹰嘴与肱骨内上髁之间凹陷中
肩贞	在肩胛区，肩关节后下方，腋后纹头直上 1 寸
臑俞	在肩胛区，腋后纹头直上，肩胛冈下缘凹陷中
天宗	在肩胛区，肩胛冈中点与肩胛下角连线上 1/3 与下 2/3 交点凹陷中
秉风	在肩胛区，肩胛冈中点上方冈上窝中
关冲	在手指，第 4 指末节尺侧，指甲根角侧上方 0.1 寸
液门	在手背，第 4、5 指间，指蹼缘上方赤白肉际凹陷中
中渚	在手背，第 4、5 掌骨间，第 4 掌指关节近端凹陷中
阳池	在腕后区，腕背侧远端横纹上，指伸肌腱的尺侧缘凹陷中

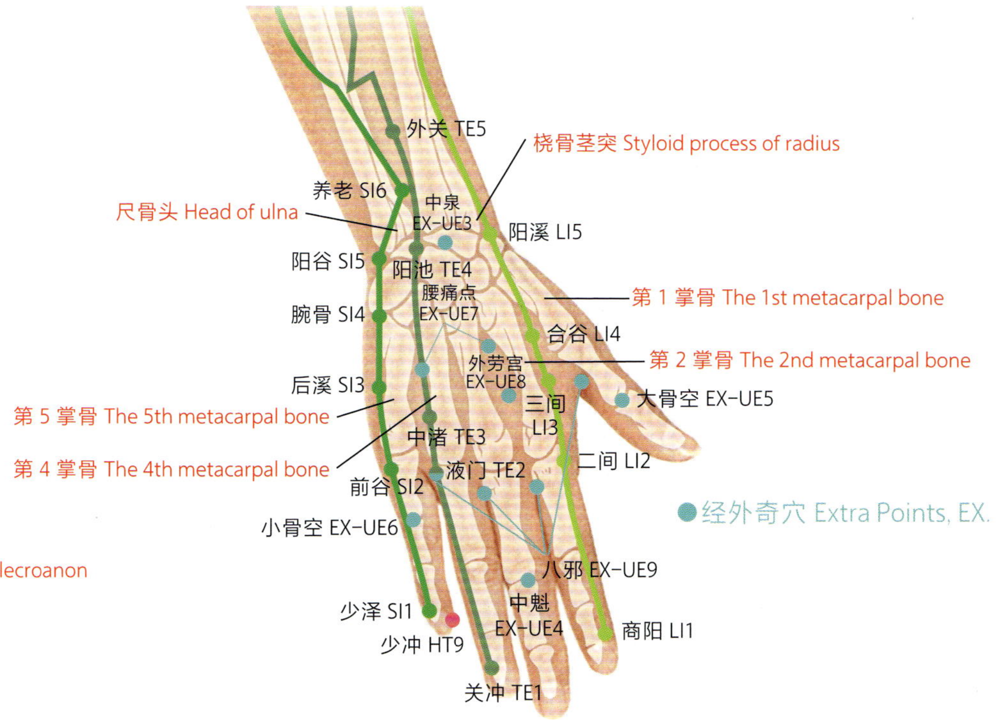

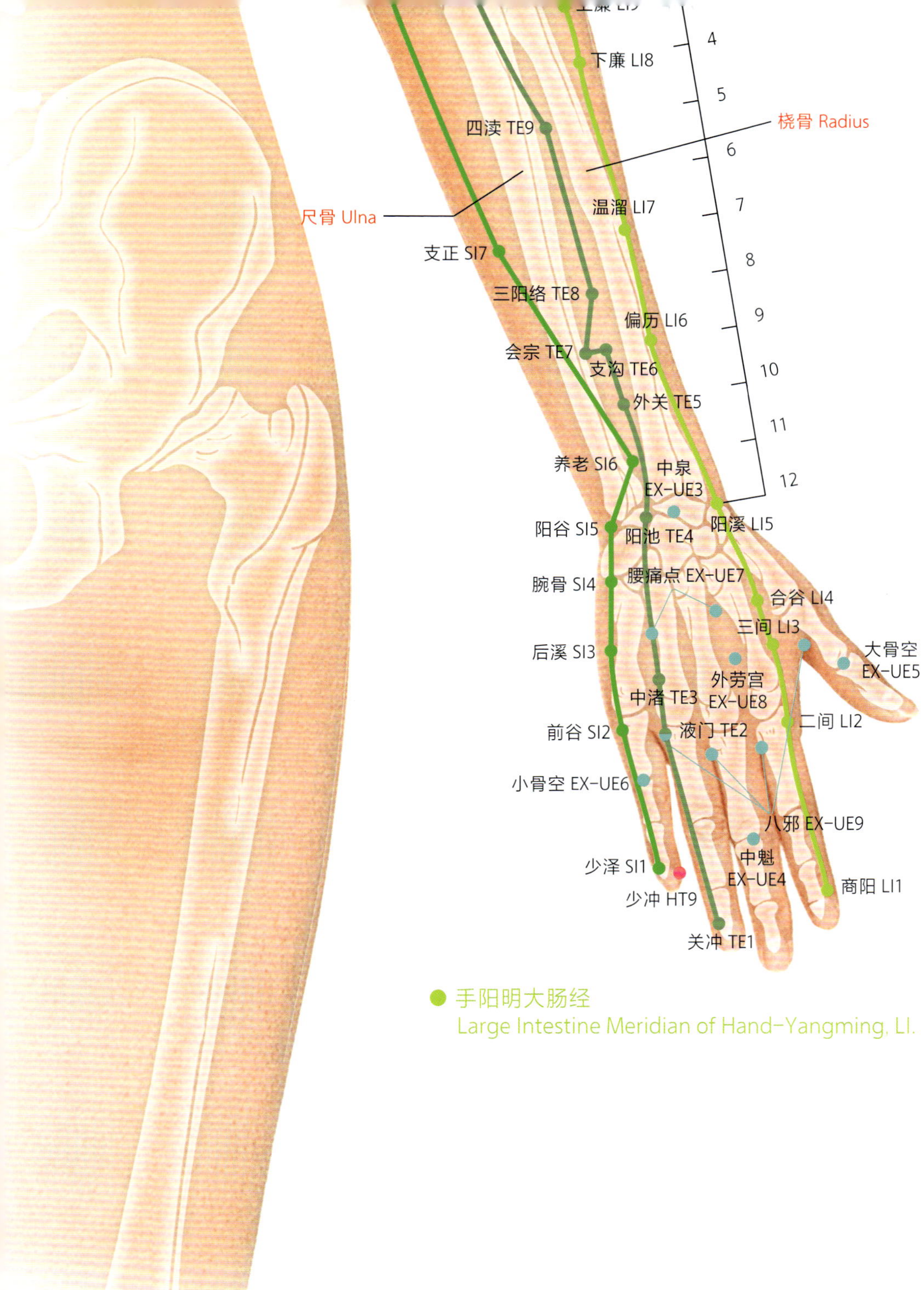

● 手阳明大肠经
Large Intestine Meridian of Hand-Yangming, LI.

Continued

Acupoints	Location
Zhīzhèng(SI7)	In the posterior region of the forearm, 5 cun superior to distal transverse crease of dorsal wrist, between ulnar side of the ulna and ulnar flexor of wrist
Xiǎohǎi(SI8)	In the posterior region of the elbow, in the depression between ulna olecroanon and medial epicondyle of humerus
Jiānzhēn(SI9)	In the scapular region, posterior and inferior to shoulder joint, 1 cun directly above the posterior axillary fold
Nàoshū(SI10)	In the scapular region, directly above the posterior axillary fold, in the depression of inferior border of scapular spine
Tiānzōng(SI11)	In the scapular region, in the depression of the junction of upper 1/3 and lower 2/3 of the line joining the midpoint of scapular spine and inferior angle of scapula
Bǐngfēng(SI12)	In the scapular region, in the supraspinous fossa above the midpoint of scapular spine
Guānchōng(TE1)	On the finger, in the ulnar end of the ring finger, 0.1 cun from the corner of the nail
Yèmén(TE2)	On the dorsum of the hand, between the ring finger and little finger, above the web border, in the depression at the junction of the red and white skin
Zhōngzhǔ(TE3)	On the dorsum of the hand, between the the 4th and the 5th metacarpal bone, in proximal depression of the 4th metacarpophalangeal joint
Yángchí(TE4)	In the posterior region of wrist, on distal transverse crease of the dorsal wrist, in the ulnar depression of the tendon of extensor digitorum

续表

穴 位	定 位
外关	在前臂后区，腕背侧远端横纹上 2 寸，尺骨与桡骨间隙中点
支沟	在前臂后区，腕背侧远端横纹上 3 寸，尺骨与桡骨间隙中点
会宗	在前臂后区，腕背侧远端横纹上 3 寸，尺骨的桡侧缘
三阳络	在前臂后区，腕背侧远端横纹上 4 寸，尺骨与桡骨间隙中点
四渎	在前臂后区，肘尖下 5 寸，尺骨与桡骨间隙中点
天井	在肘后区，肘尖上 1 寸凹陷中
清泠渊	在臂后区，肘尖与肩峰角连线上，肘尖上 2 寸
消泺	在臂后区，肘尖与肩峰角连线上，肘尖上 5 寸
臑会	在臂后区，肩峰角下 3 寸，三角肌的后下缘

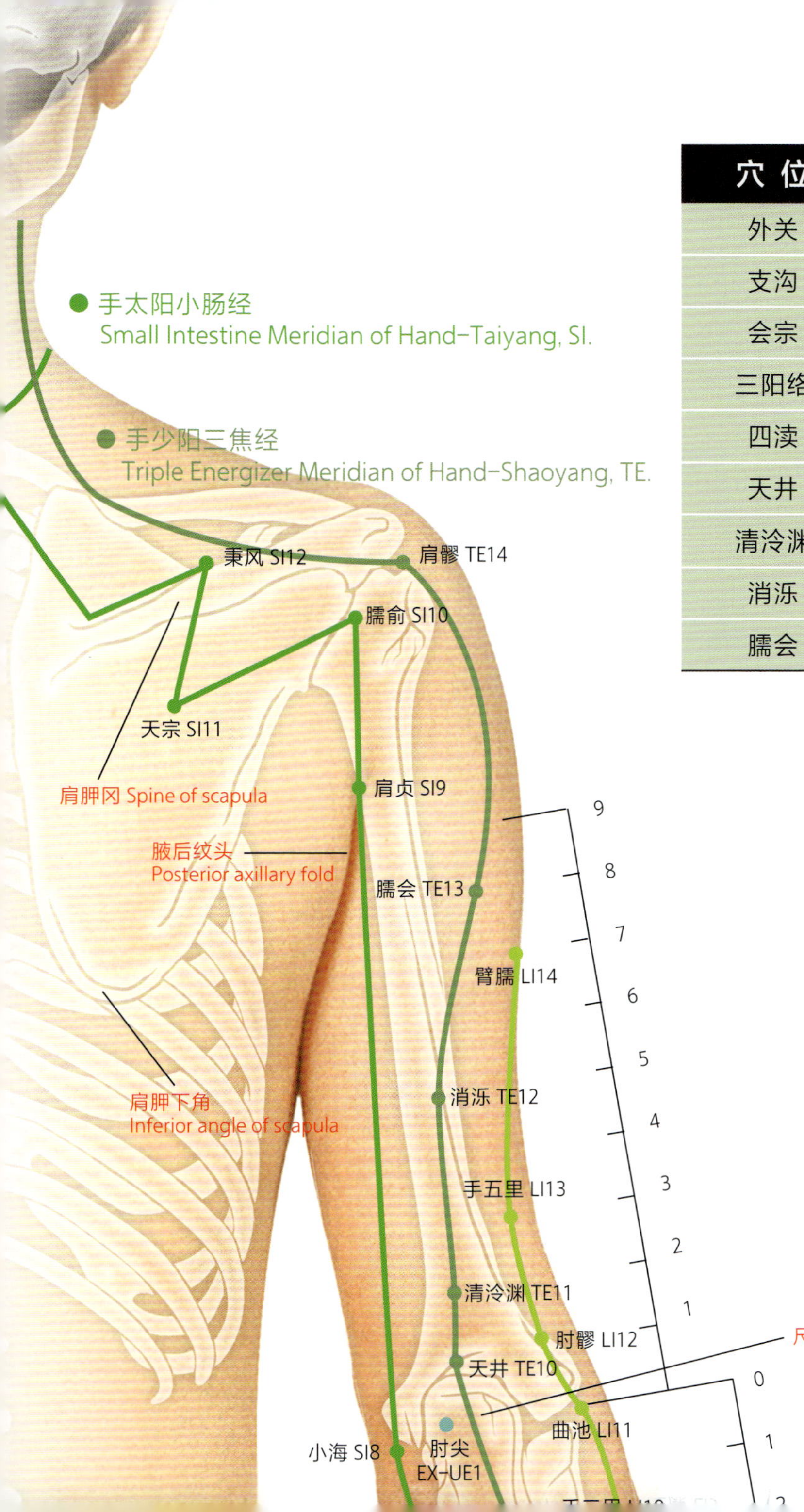

尺骨鹰嘴 Ulna olecroanon

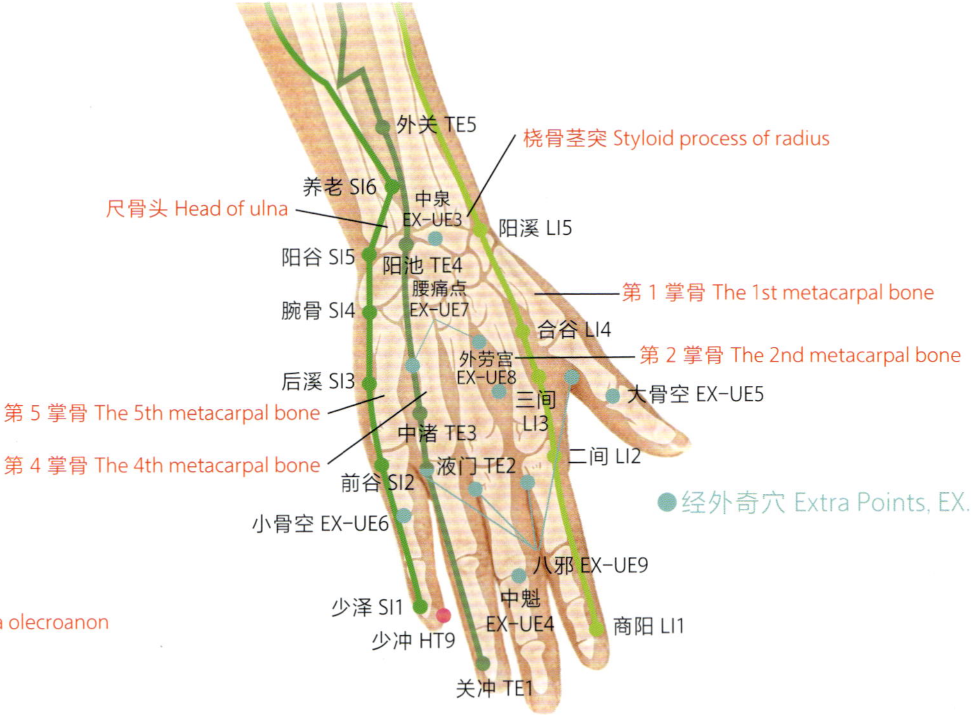

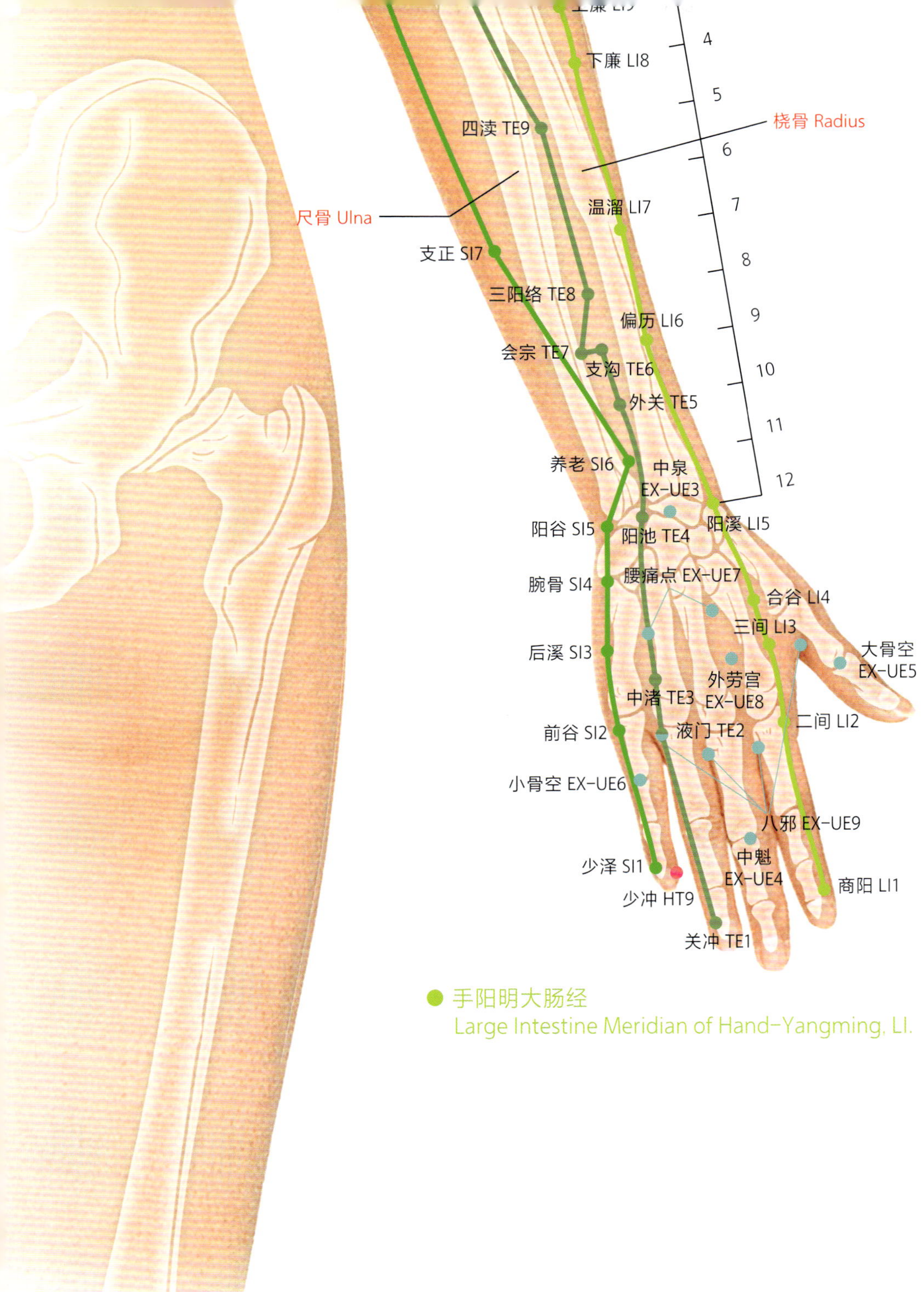

● 手阳明大肠经
Large Intestine Meridian of Hand-Yangming, LI.

Continued

Acupoints	Location
Wàiguān(TE5)	In the posterior region of the forearm, 2 cun superior to the distal transverse crease of dorsal wrist, at the midpoint of the depression between ulna and radius
Zhīgōu(TE6)	In the posterior region of the forearm, 3 cun superior to the distal transverse crease of dorsal wrist, at the midpoint of the depression between ulna and radius
Huìzōng(TE7)	In the posterior region of the forearm, 3 cun superior to the distal transverse crease of dorsal wrist, in the radial border of the ulna
Sānyángluò(TE8)	In the posterior region of the forearm, 4 cun superior to the distal transverse crease of dorsal wrist, at the midpoint of the depression between ulna and radius
Sìdú(TE9)	In the posterior region of the forearm, 5 cun below the tip of the elbow, between the ulna and radius
Tiānjǐng(TE10)	On the dorsum of the elbow, in the depression 1 cun above the tip of the elbow
Qīnglíngyuān(TE11)	In posterior region of the arm, along the line joining the tip of the elbow and acromial angle, 2 cun above the tip of the elbow
Xiāoluò(TE12)	In posterior region of the arm, along the line joining the tip of the elbow and acromial angle, 5 cun above the tip of the elbow
Nàohuì(TE13)	In posterior region of the arm, 3 cun below the acromial angle, in the posterior and inferior border of the deltoid

续表

穴 位	定 位
肩髎	在三角肌区，肩峰角与肱骨大结节两骨间凹陷中
少冲	在手指，小指末节桡侧，指甲根角侧上方 0.1 寸（指寸）
肘尖	在肘后区，尺骨鹰嘴的尖端
中泉	在前臂后区，腕背侧远端横纹上，指总伸肌腱桡侧的凹陷中
中魁	在手指，中指背面，近侧指间关节的中点处
大骨空	在手指，拇指背面，指间关节的中点处
小骨空	在手指，小指背面，近侧指间关节的中点处
腰痛点	在手背，第 2、3 掌骨间及第 4、5 掌骨间，腕背侧远端横纹与掌指关节的中点处，一手 2 穴
外劳宫	在手背，第 2、3 掌骨间，掌指关节后 0.5 寸（指寸）凹陷中
八邪	在手背，第 1~5 指间，指蹼缘后方赤白肉际处，左右共 8 穴

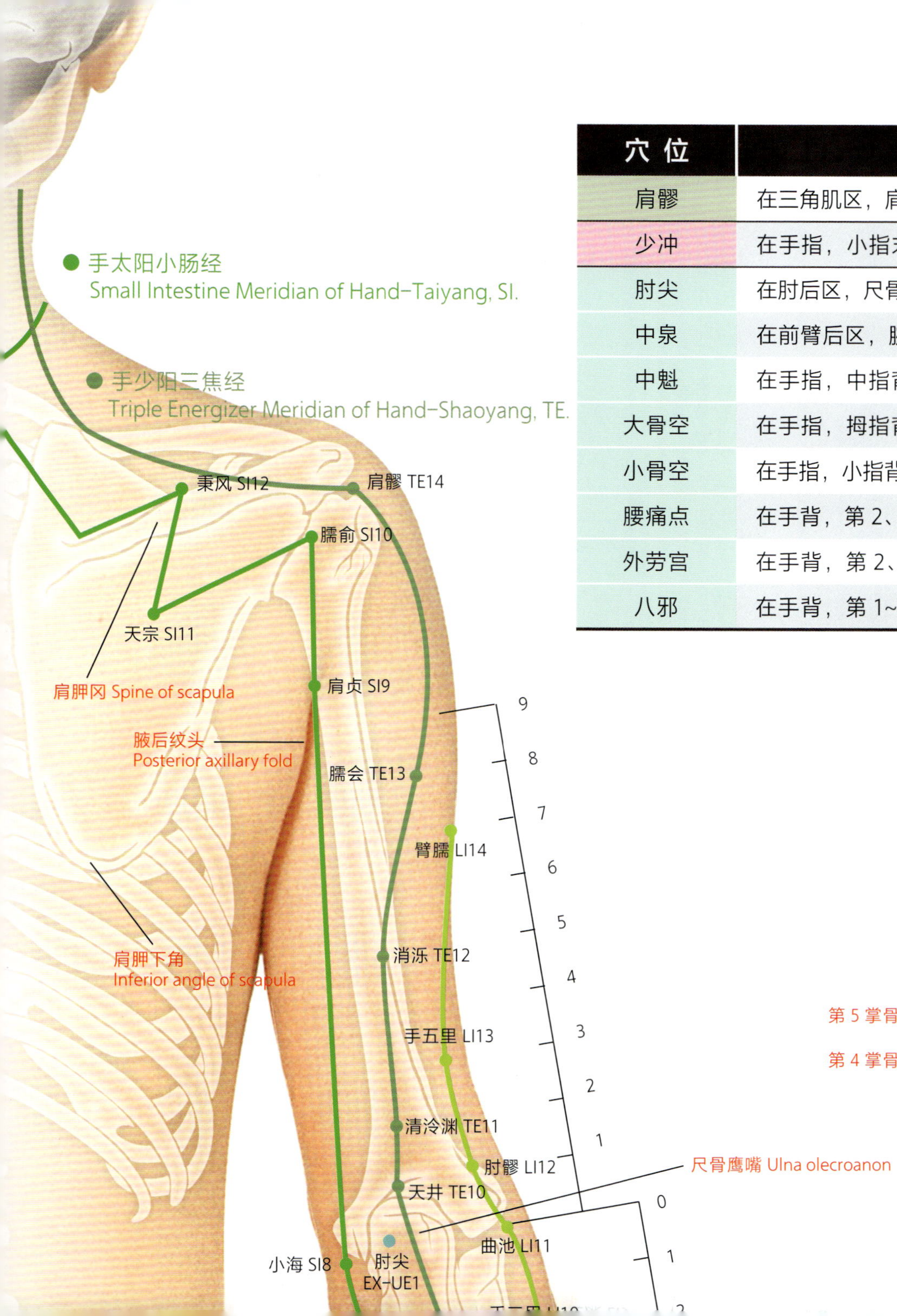

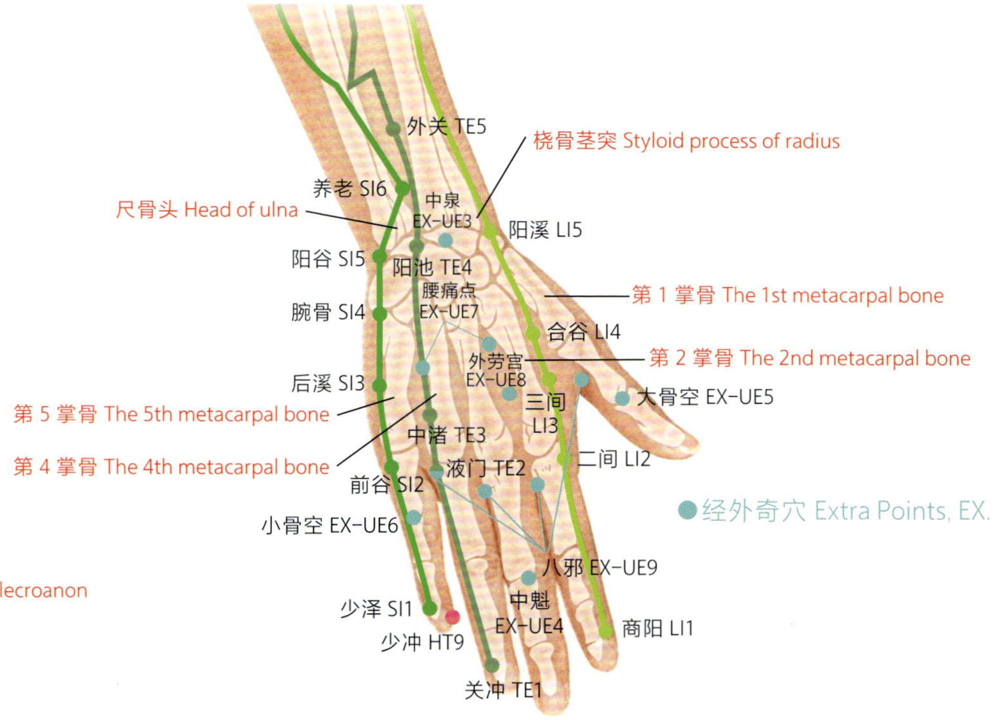

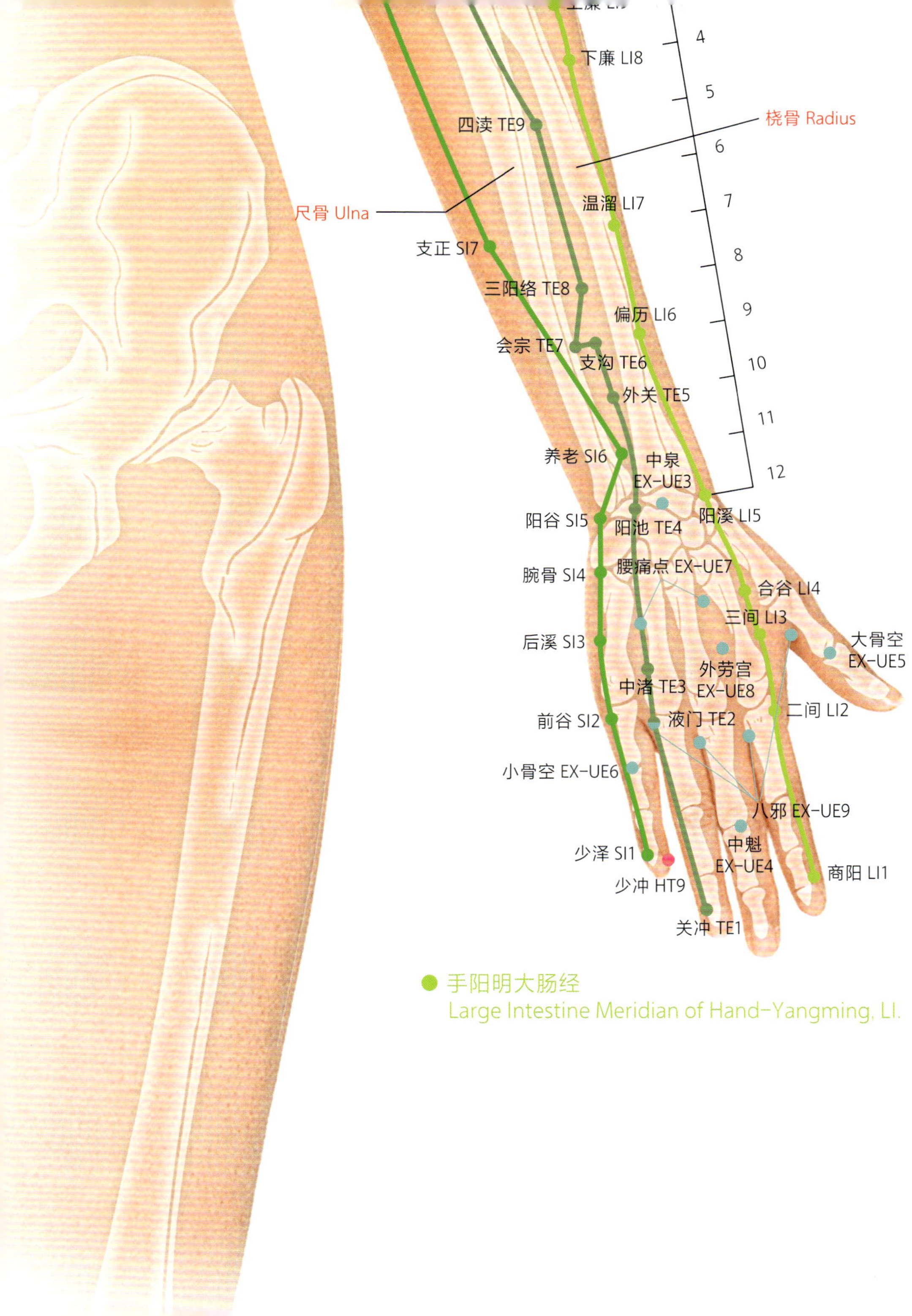

Continued

Acupoints	Location
Jiānliáo(TE14)	In the deltoid region, In depression between acromial angle and greater tuberosity of humerus
Shàochōng(HT9)	On the finger, In radial end of little finger, 0.1 cun from the corner of the nail
Zhǒujiān(EX-UE1)	On the posterior region of the elbow, at the tip of ulna olecroanon
Zhōngquán(EX-UE3)	In the posterior region of the forearm, on distal transverse crease of the dorsal wrist, in the depression of radial tendon of extensor digitorum communis
Zhōngkuí(EX-UE4)	On the finger, on dorsum of middle finger, at the midpoint of proximal interphalangeal joint
Dàgǔkōng(EX-UE5)	On the finger, on dorsum of thumb, at the midpoint of interphalangeal joint
Xiǎogǔkōng(EX-UE6)	On the finger, on the dorsum of little finger, at the midpoint of proximal interphalangeal joint
Yāotòngdiǎn(EX-UE7)	On the dorsum of the hand, between the 2nd and the 3rd metacarpal bone as well as the 4th and the 5th metacarpal bone, at the midpoint of distal transverse crease of dorsal wrist and metacarpophalangeal joint, with 2 points on each hand
Wàiláogōng(EX-UE8)	On the dorsum of the hand, between the 2nd and the 3rd metacarpal bone, in the depression 0.5 cun posterior to metacarpophalangeal joint
Bāxié(EX-UE9)	On the dorsum of the hand, between the fingers, at the junction of the red and white skin posterior to the web, with 8 points on two hands in total

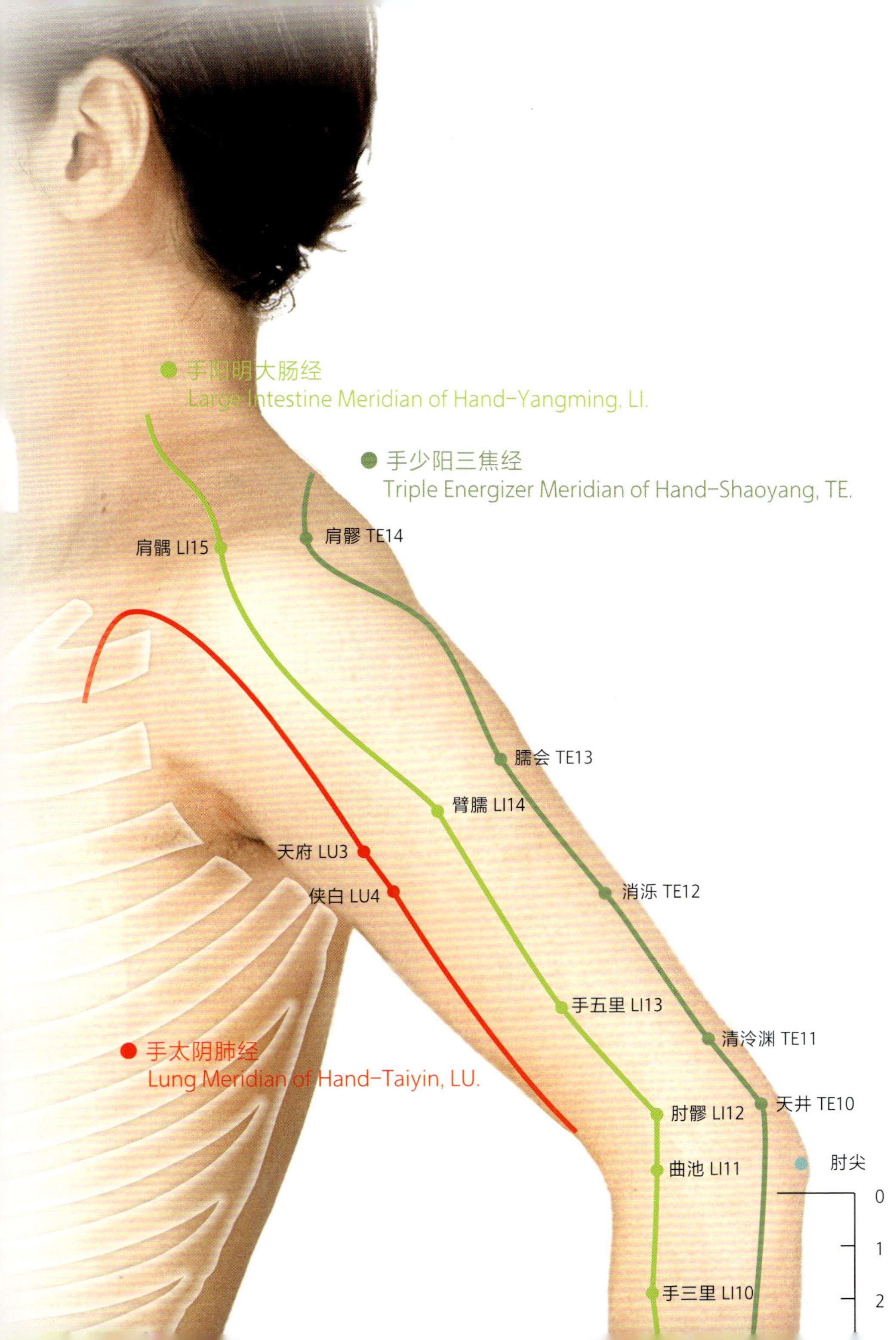

穴 位	定 位
天府	在臂前区，腋前纹头下 3 寸，肱二头肌桡侧缘处
侠白	在臂前区，腋前纹头下 4 寸，肱二头肌桡侧缘处
商阳	在手指，食指末节桡侧，指甲根角侧上方 0.1 寸
二间	在手指，第 2 掌指关节桡侧远端赤白肉际处
三间	在手背，第 2 掌指关节桡侧近端凹陷处
合谷	在手背，第 2 掌骨桡侧的中点处
阳溪	在腕区，腕背侧远端横纹桡侧，桡骨茎突远端，解剖学“鼻烟窝”凹陷中
偏历	在前臂，腕背侧远端横纹上 3 寸，阳溪与曲池连线上
温溜	在前臂，腕背侧远端横纹上 5 寸，阳溪与曲池连线上
下廉	在前臂，肘横纹下 4 寸，阳溪与曲池连线上
上廉	在前臂，肘横纹下 3 寸，阳溪与曲池连线上

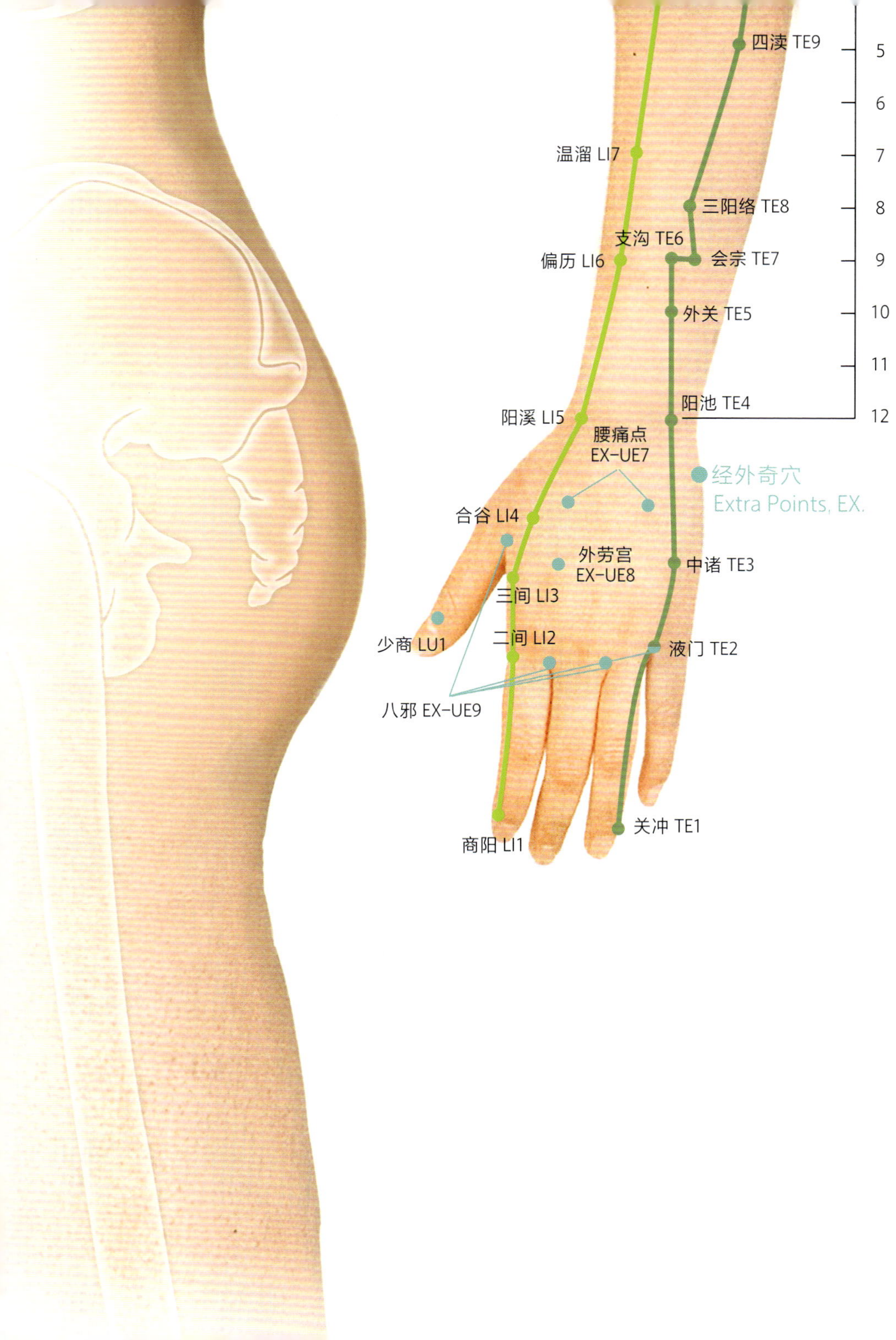

Acupoints	Location
Tiānfǔ(LU3)	In the anterior region of the arm, 3 cun inferior to anterior axillary fold, in the radial border of biceps
Xiábái(LU4)	In the anterior region of the arm, 4 cun inferior to anterior axillary fold, in the radial border of biceps
Shāngyáng(LI1)	On the finger, in the radial side of the index finger, 0.1 cun lateral and superior to the nail
Èrjiān(LI2)	On the finger, in the distal radial side of the 2nd metacarpophalangeal joint, at the junction of the red and white skin of the hand
Sānjiān(LI3)	On the dorsum of the hand, in the depression of proximal radial side of the 2nd metacarpophalangeal joint
Hégǔ(LI4)	On the dorsum of the hand, at the midpoint of the 2nd metacarpal bone on the radial side
Yángxī(LI5)	On the wrist, in the radial side of the distal end of transverse crease on the dorsal wrist, in the distal end of styloid process of radius, in the depression of anatomical snuffbox
Piānlì(LI6)	On the forearm, 3 cun superior to the the distal end of transverse crease on dorsal wrist, along the line of Yangxi(LI5) and Quchi(LI11)
Wēnliū(LI7)	On the forearm, 5 cun superior to the the distal end of transverse crease on the dorsal wrist, along the line connecting Yangxi(LI5) and Quchi(LI11)
Xiàlián(LI8)	On the forearm, 4 cun inferior to the transverse crease of the elbow, along the line conneting Yangxi(LI5) and Quchi(LI11)
Shànglián(LI9)	On the forearm, 3 cun inferior to the transverse crease of the elbow, along the line conneting Yangxi(LI5) and Quchi(LI11)

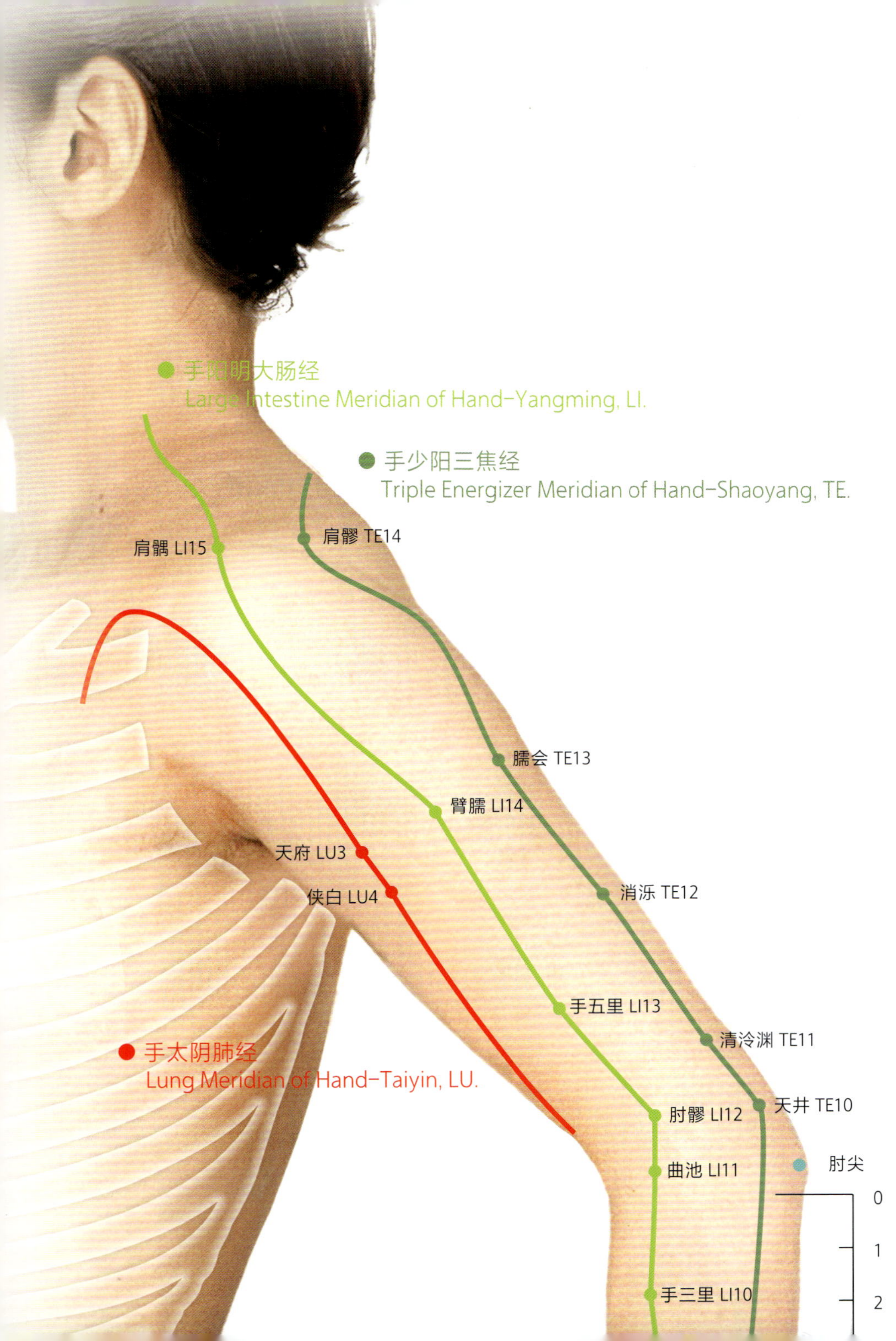

续表

穴 位	定 位
手三里	在前臂，肘横纹下 2 寸，阳溪与曲池连线上
曲池	在肘区，尺泽与肱骨外上髁连线的中点处
肘髎	在肘区，肱骨外上髁上缘，髁上嵴的前缘
手五里	在臂部，肘横纹上 3 寸处，曲池与肩髃连线上。
臂臑	在臂部，曲池上 7 寸，三角肌前缘处
肩髃	在三角肌区，肩峰外侧缘前端与肱骨大结节两骨间凹陷中
关冲	在手指，第 4 指末节尺侧，指甲根角侧上方 0.1 寸
液门	在手背，第 4、5 指间，指蹼缘上方赤白肉际凹陷中
中渚	在手背，第 4、5 掌骨间，第 4 掌指关节近端凹陷中
阳池	在腕后区，腕背侧远端横纹上，指伸肌腱的尺侧缘凹陷中
外关	在前臂后区，腕背侧远端横纹上 2 寸，尺骨与桡骨间隙中点

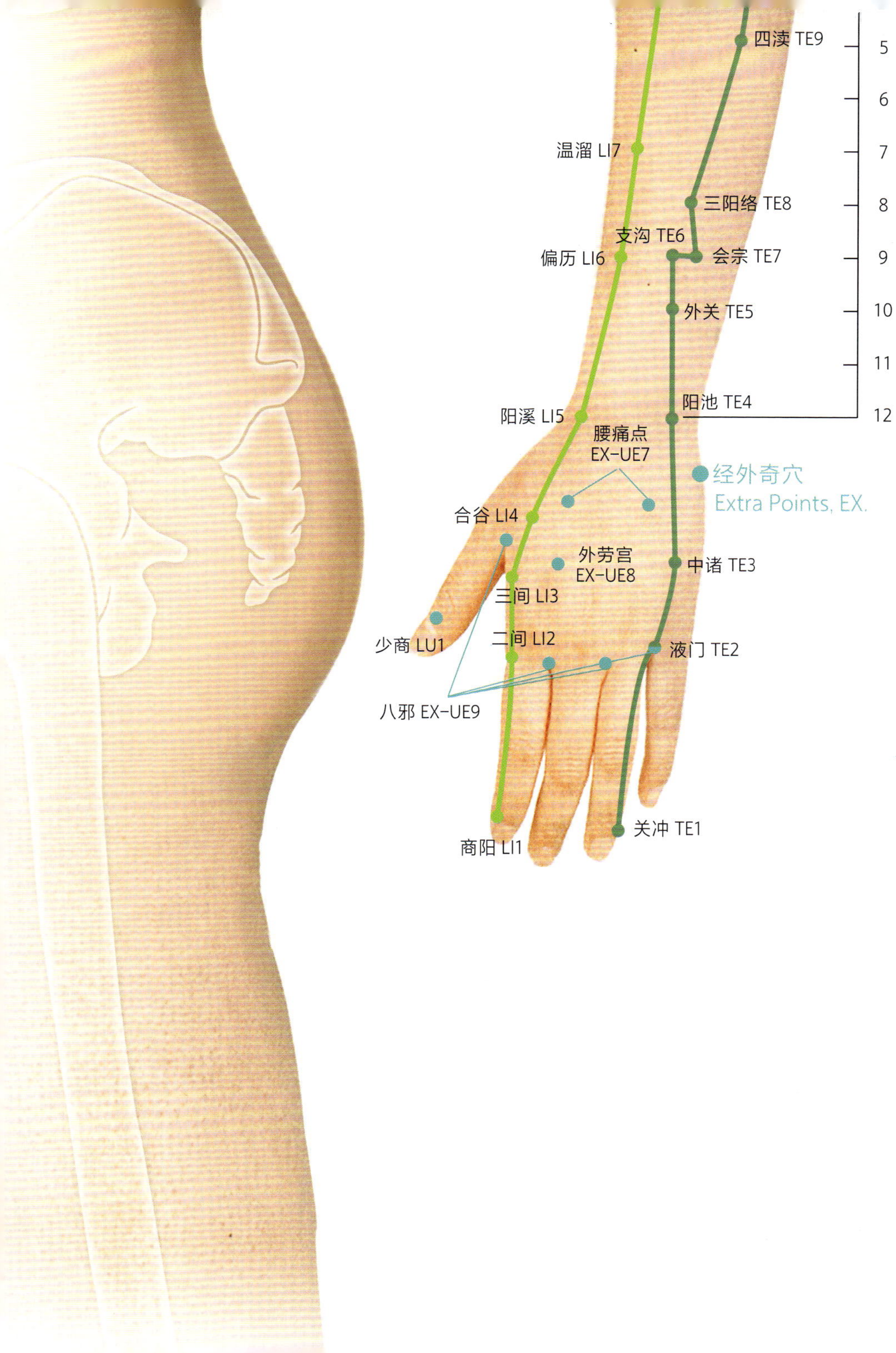

Continued

Acupoints	Location
Shǒusānlǐ(LI10)	On the forearm, 2 cun inferior to the transverse crease of the elbow, along the line connecting Yangxi(LI5) and Quchi(LI11)
Qūchí(LI11)	In the elbow region, at the midpoint of the line joining Chize(LU5) and external epicondyle of humerus
Zhǒuliáo(LI12)	In the elbow region, in the superior border of external epicondyle of humerus and the anterior border of supracondylar ridge
Shǒuwǔlǐ(LI13)	On the arm, 3 cun superior to the transverse crease of the elbow, along the line connecting Quchi(LI11) and Jianyu(LI15)
Bìnào(LI14)	On the arm, 7 cun above Quchi(LI11), in the anterior border of deltoid
Jiānyú(LI15)	In the deltoid region, in the depression between anterior end of lateral border of acromion and greater tuberosity of humerus
Guānchōng(TE1)	On the finger, in the ulnar end of the ring finger, 0.1 cun from the corner of the base of the nail
Yèmén(TE2)	On the back of the hand, between the ring finger and little finger, above the fingerweb border, at the junction of the red and white skin
Zhōngzhǔ(TE3)	On the back of the hand, between the the 4th and the 5th metacarpal bone, in the proximal depression of the 4th metacarpophalangeal joint
Yángchí(TE4)	In the posterior region of wrist, on the distal transverse crease of the dorsal wrist, in the ulnar depression of the tendon of extensor digitorum
Wàiguān(TE5)	In the posterior region of the forearm, 2 cun superior to the distal transverse crease of dorsal wrist, at the midpoint of the depression between ulna and radius

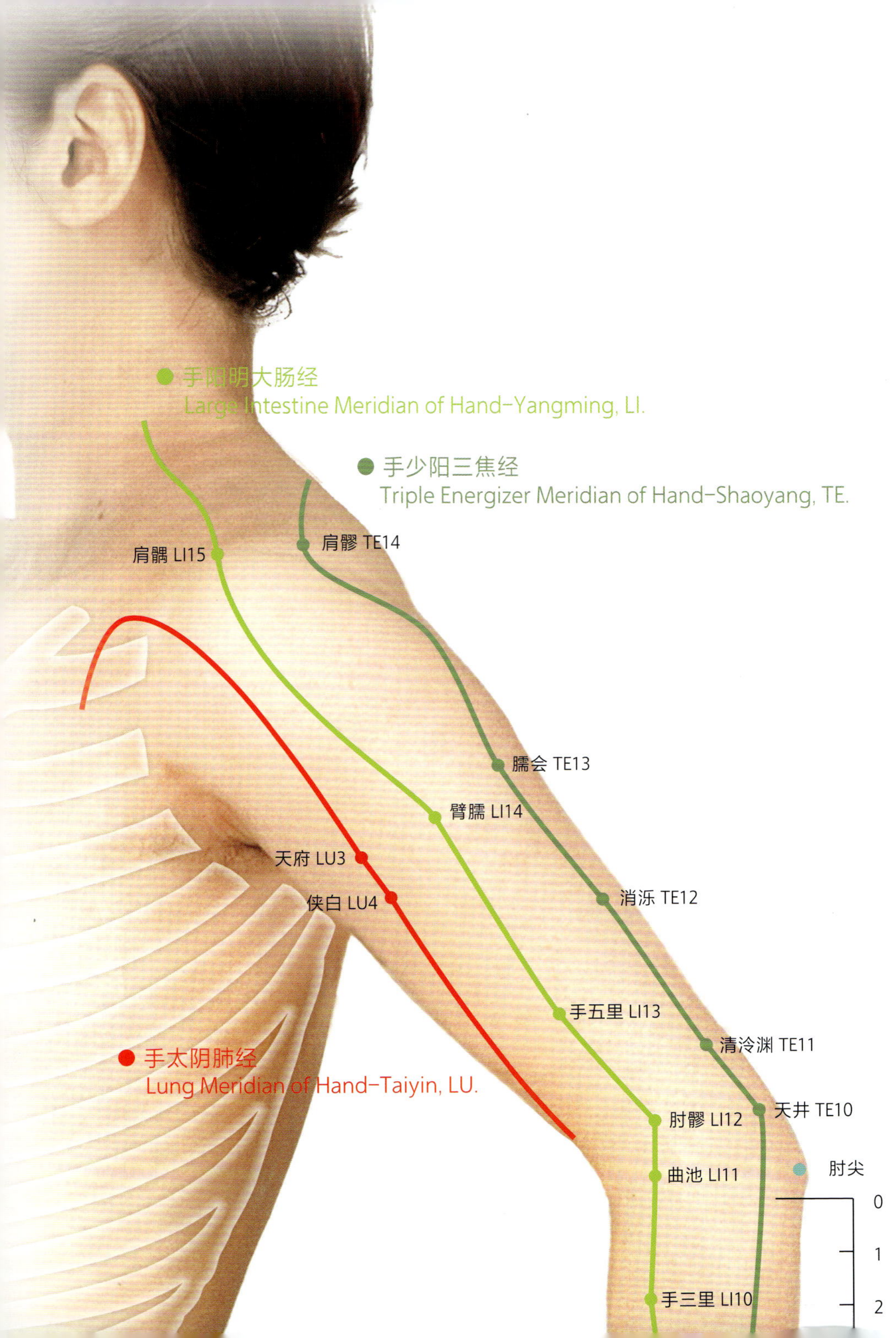

续表

穴 位	定 位
支沟	在前臂后区，腕背侧远端横纹上 3 寸，尺骨与桡骨间隙中点
会宗	在前臂后区，腕背侧远端横纹上 3 寸，尺骨的桡侧缘
三阳络	在前臂后区，腕背侧远端横纹上 4 寸，尺骨与桡骨间隙中点
四渎	在前臂后区，肘尖下 5 寸，尺骨与桡骨间隙中点
天井	在肘后区，肘尖上 1 寸凹陷中
清泠渊	在臂后区，肘尖与肩峰角连线上，肘尖上 2 寸
消泺	在臂后区，肘尖与肩峰角连线上，肘尖上 5 寸
臑会	在臂后区，肩峰角下 3 寸，三角肌的后下缘
肩髎	在三角肌区，肩峰角与肱骨大结节两骨间凹陷中
腰痛点	在手背，第 2、3 掌骨间及第 4、5 掌骨间，腕背侧远端横纹与掌指关节的中点处，一手 2 穴
外劳宫	在手背，第 2、3 掌骨间，掌指关节后 0.5 寸（指寸）凹陷中
八邪	在手背，第 1~5 指间，指蹼缘后方赤白肉际处，左右共 8 穴

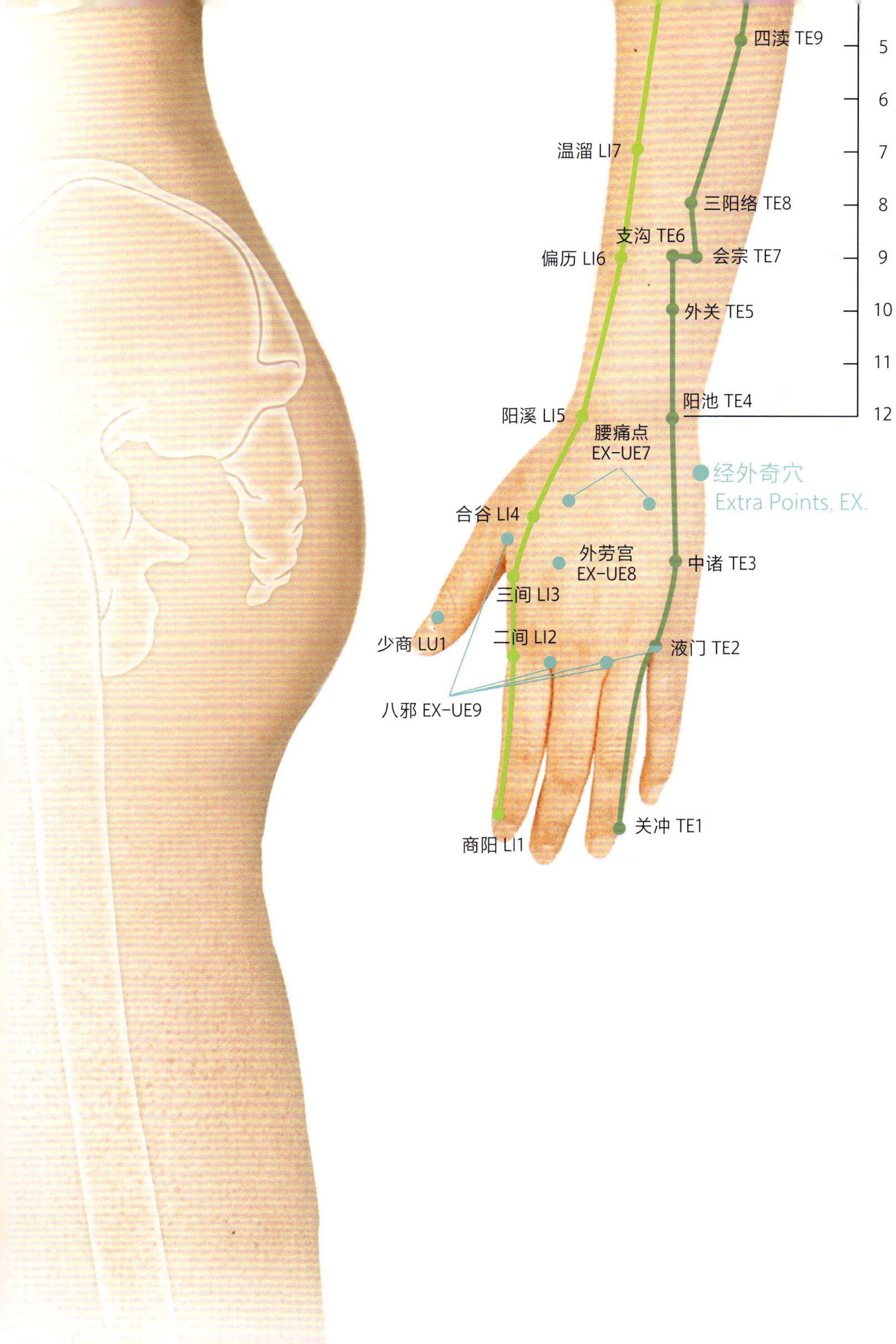

Continued

Acupoints	Location
Zhīgōu(TE6)	In the posterior region of the forearm, 3 cun superior to the distal transverse crease of dorsal wrist, at the midpoint of the depression between ulna and radius
Huìzōng(TE7)	In the posterior region of the forearm, 3 cun superior to the distal transverse crease of dorsal wrist, in the radial border of the ulna
Sānyángluò(TE8)	In the posterior region of the forearm, 4 cun superior to the distal transverse crease of dorsal wrist, at the midpoint of the depression between ulna and radius
Sìdú(TE9)	In the posterior region of the forearm, 5 cun below the tip of the elbow, between the ulna and radius
Tiānjǐng(TE10)	On the dorsum of the elbow, in the depression 1 cun above the tip of the elbow
Qīnglíngyuān (TE11)	In posterior region of the arm, along the line joining the tip of the elbow and acromial angle, 2 cun above the tip of the elbow
Xiāoluò(TE12)	In posterior region of the arm, along the line joining the tip of the elbow and acromial angle, 5 cun above the tip of the elbow
Nàohuì(TE13)	In posterior region of the arm, 3 cun below the acromial angle, in the posterior and inferior border of the deltoid
Jiānliáo(TE14)	On the deltoid region, in the depression between acromial angle and greater tuberosity of humerus
Yāotòngdiǎn (EX-UE7)	On the dorsum of the hand, between the 2nd and the 3rd metacarpal bone as well as the 4th and the 5th metacarpal bone, at the midpoint of distal transverse crease of dorsal wrist and metacarpophalangeal joint, with 2 points on each hand
Wàiláogōng (EX-UE8)	On the dorsum of the hand, between the 2nd and the 3rd metacarpal bone, in the depression 0.5 cun posterior to metacarpophalangeal joint
Bāxié(EX-UE9)	On the dorsum of the hand, between the fingers, at the junction of the red and white skin posterior to the web, with 8 points on two hands in total

下肢部穴位

Acupoints of Lower Limbs

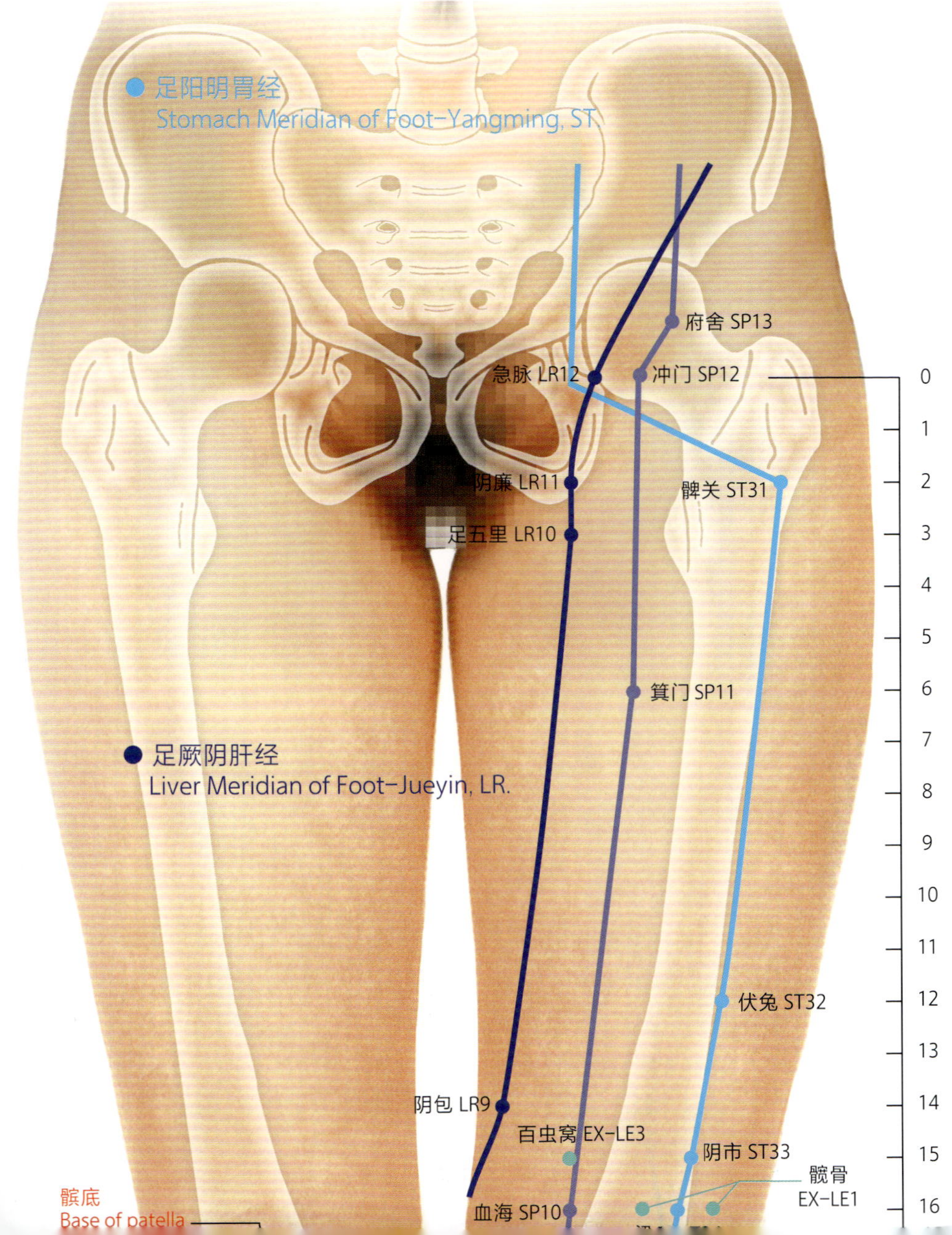

穴 位	定 位
髀关	在股前区，股直肌近端，缝匠肌与阔筋膜张肌 3 条肌肉之间凹陷中
伏兔	在股前区，髌底上 6 寸，髂前上棘与髌底外侧端的连线上
阴市	在股前区，髌底上 3 寸，股直肌肌腱外侧缘
梁丘	在股前区，髌底上 2 寸，股外侧肌与股直肌肌腱之间
犊鼻	在膝前区，髌韧带外侧凹陷中
足三里	在小腿前外侧，犊鼻下 3 寸，犊鼻与解溪连线上
上巨虚	在小腿外侧，犊鼻下 6 寸，犊鼻与解溪连线上
条口	在小腿外侧，犊鼻下 8 寸，犊鼻与解溪连线上
下巨虚	在小腿外侧，犊鼻下 9 寸，犊鼻与解溪连线上
丰隆	在小腿外侧，外踝尖上 8 寸，胫骨前肌的外侧
解溪	在踝部，踝关节前面中央凹陷中，当拇长伸肌腱与趾长伸肌腱之间
冲阳	在足背，第 2 跖骨基底部与中间楔状骨关节处，可触及足背动脉

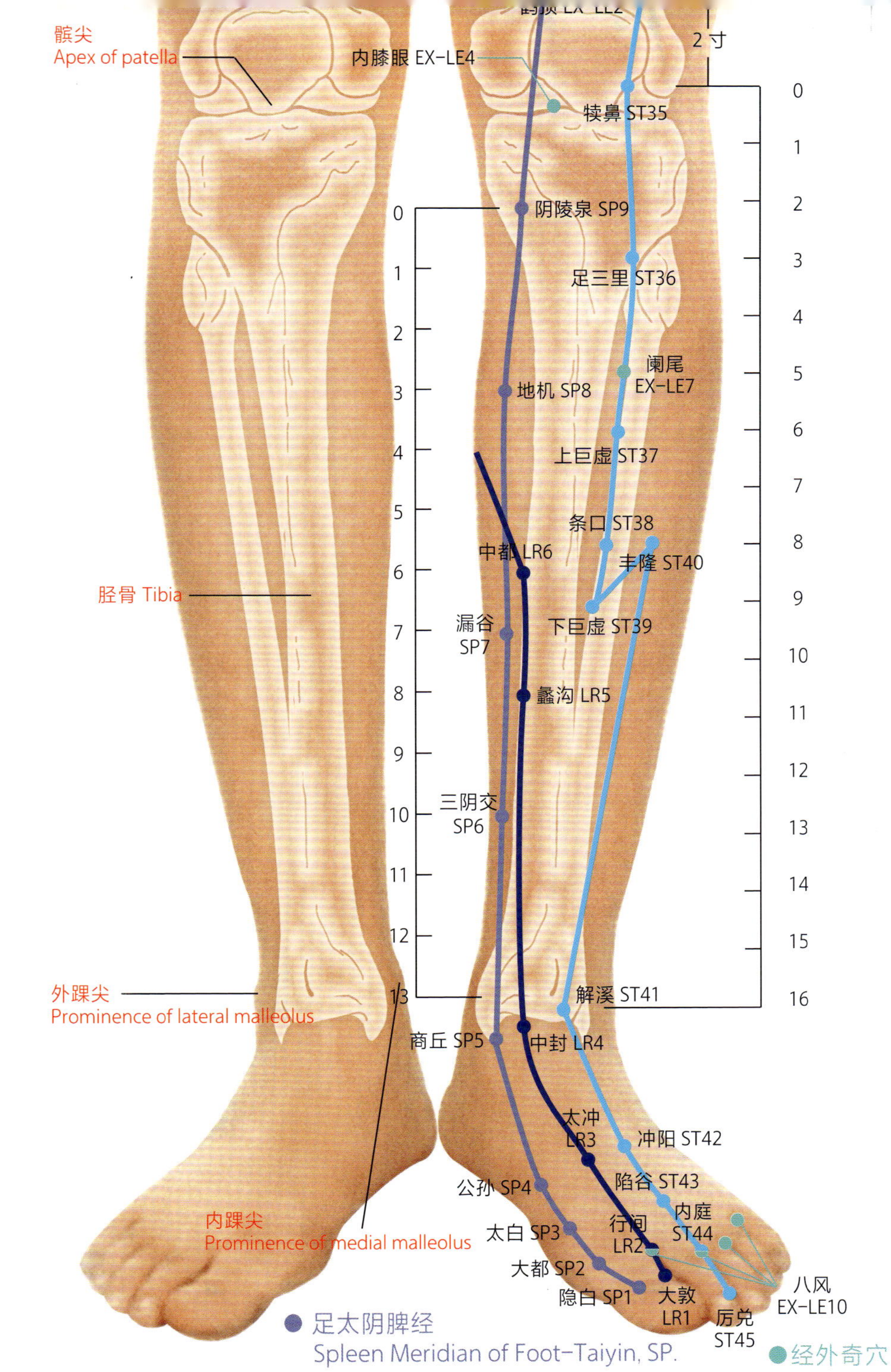

经外奇穴 Extra Points, EX.

Acupoints	Location
Bìguān(ST31)	In the anterior region of thigh, in the proximal end of rectus femoris, in the depression between sartorius and three muscles of tensor fasciae latae
Fútù(ST32)	In the anterior region of thigh, 6 cun superior to the base of patella, along the line joining anterior superior iliac spine and lateral end of the base of patella
Yīnshì(ST33)	In the anterior region of thigh, 3 cun superior to the base of patella, in the lateral border of tendon of rectus femoris
Liángqiū(ST34)	In the anterior region of thigh, 2 cun superior to the base of patella, between vastus lateralis and tendon of rectus femoris
Dúbí(ST35)	In the anterior region of knee, in the lateral depression of patellar tendon
Zúsānlǐ(ST36)	Anterior and lateral to the crus, 3 cun below Dubi (ST35), on the line connecting Dubi (ST35) and Jiexi (ST41)
Shàngjùxū(ST37)	Lateral to the crus, 6 cun below Dubi (ST35), on the line connecting Dubi (ST35) and Jiexi (ST41)
Tiáokǒu(ST38)	Lateral to the crus, 8 cun below Dubi (ST35), on the line connecting Dubi (ST35) and Jiexi (ST41)
Xiàjùxū(ST39)	Lateral to the crus, 9 cun below Dubi (ST35), on the line connecting Dubi (ST35) and Jiexi (ST41)
Fēnglóng(ST40)	Lateral to the crus, 8 cun above the prominence of the lateral malleolus, lateral to the anterior tibial muscle
Jiěxī(ST41)	On the ankle, in the middle depression of anterior ankle joint, between the tendon of extensor pollicis longus and the tendon of extensor digitorum longus
Chōngyáng(ST42)	On the dorsum of foot, between the base of the 2nd metatarsal bone and the joint of middle cuneiform bone, in the place where dorsal artery of foot can be palpated

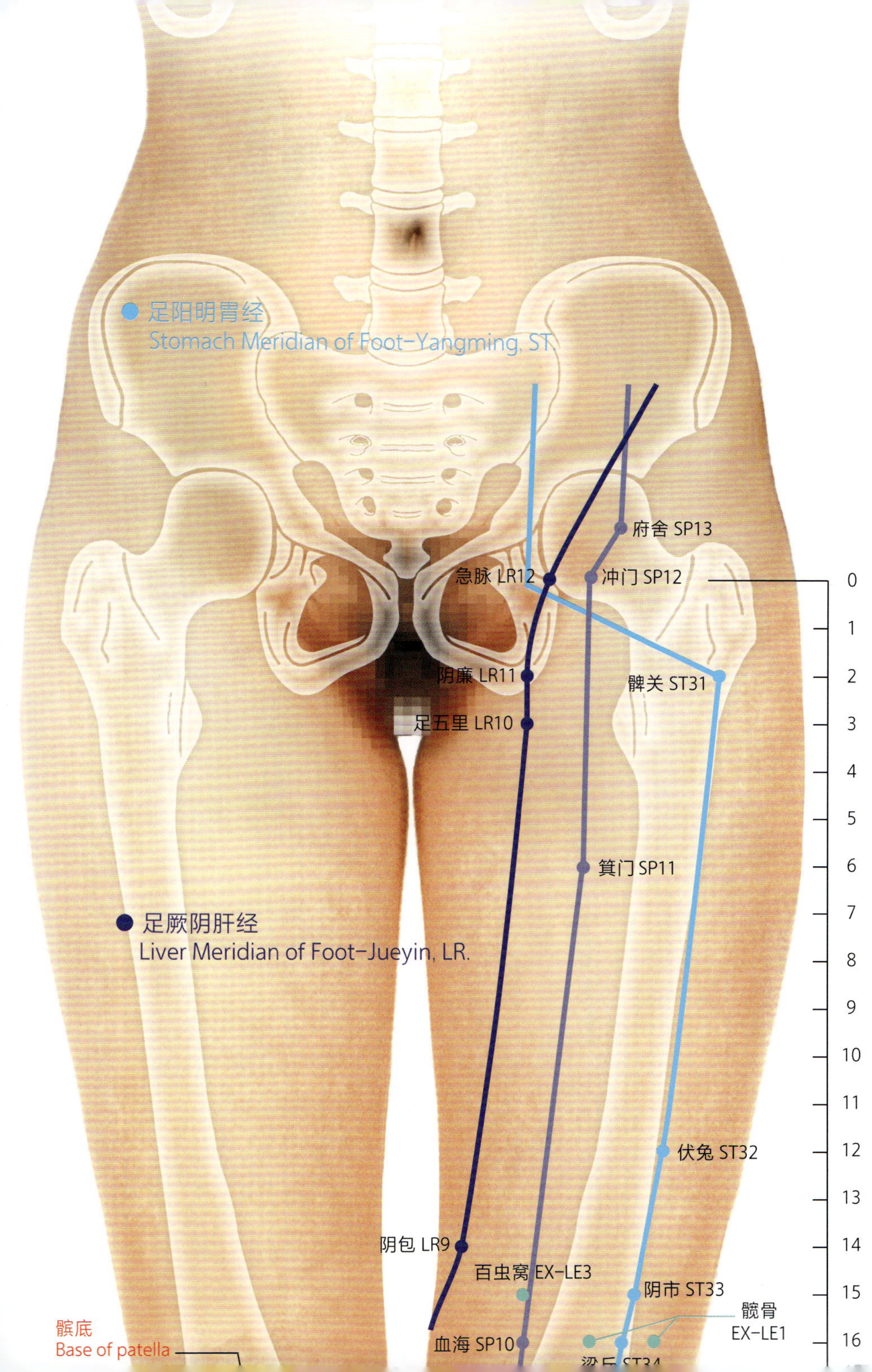

续表

穴位	定位
陷谷	在足背，当第 2、3 跖骨间，第 2 跖趾关节近端凹陷中
内庭	在足背，第 2、3 趾间，趾蹼缘后方赤白肉际处
厉兑	在足趾，第 2 趾末节外侧，趾甲根角侧后方 0.1 寸
隐白	在足趾，大趾末节内侧，趾甲根角侧后方 0.1 寸
大都	在足趾，第 1 跖趾关节远端赤白肉际凹陷中
太白	在跖区，第 1 跖趾关节近端赤白肉际凹陷中
公孙	在跖区，第 1 跖骨底的前下缘赤白肉际处
商丘	在踝区，内踝前下方，舟骨粗隆与内踝尖连线中点凹陷中
三阴交	在小腿内侧，内踝尖上 3 寸，胫骨内侧缘后际
漏谷	在小腿内侧，内踝尖上 6 寸，胫骨内侧缘后际
地机	在小腿内侧，阴陵泉下 3 寸，胫骨内侧缘后际
阴陵泉	在小腿内侧，胫骨内侧髁下缘与胫骨内侧缘之间的凹陷中

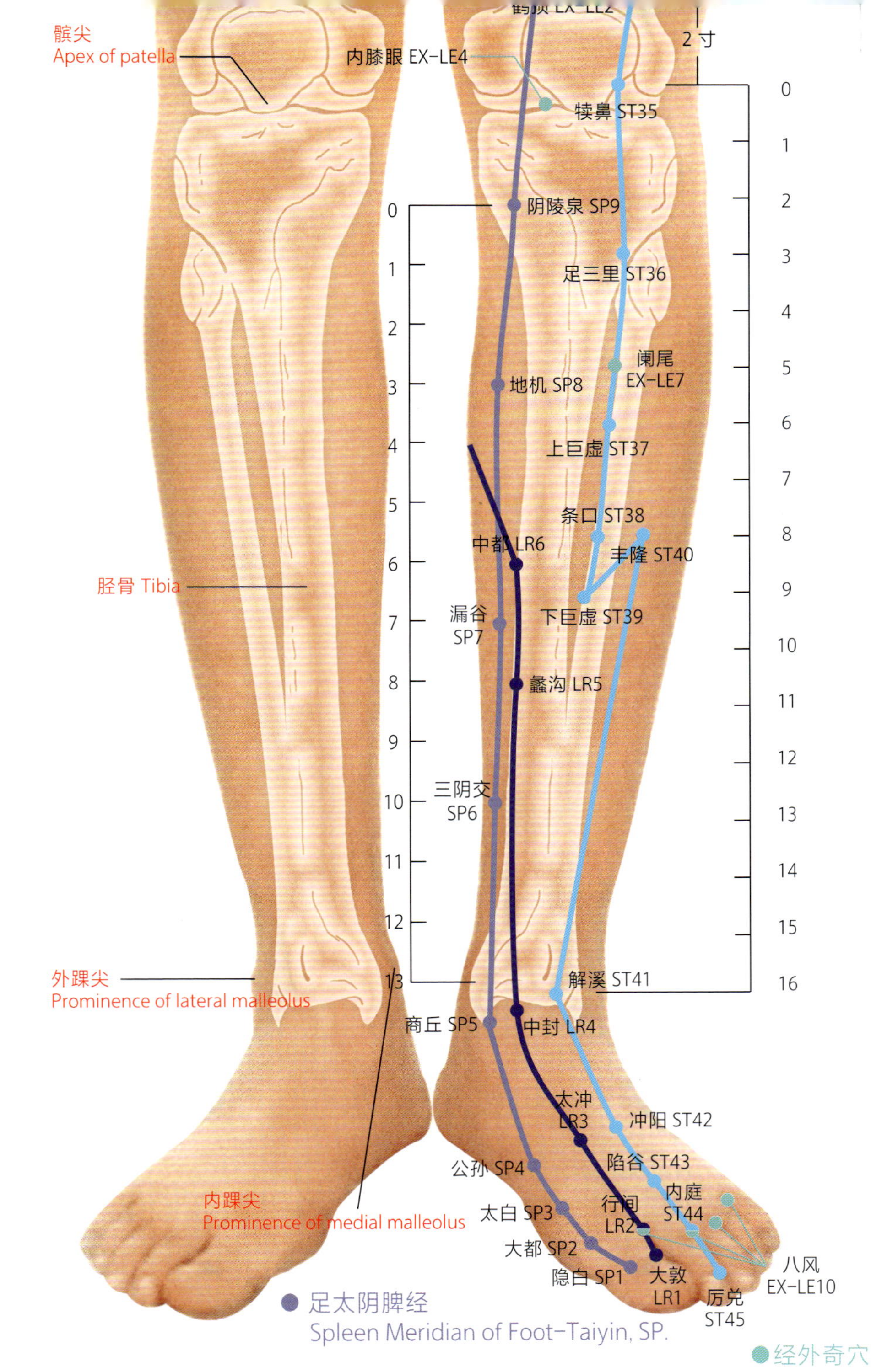

Continued

Acupoints	Location
Xiàngǔ(ST43)	On the dorsum of foot, between the 2nd and the 3rd metatarsal bone, in the proximal depression of the 2nd metatarsophalangeal joint
Nèitíng(ST44)	On the dorsum of foot, between the 2nd and the 3rd toe, at the junction of the red and white skin posterior to the border of web
Lìduì(ST45)	On the toe, lateral to the end of the 2nd toe, 0.1 cun lateral and posterior to the corner of the nail
Yǐnbái(SP1)	On the toe, in the medial side of the end of the 1st toe, 0.1 cun lateral and posterior to the corner of the nail
Dàdū(SP2)	On the toe, in the depression at the junction of the red and white skin of the distal end of the 1st metatarsophalangeal joint
Tàibái(SP3)	On the sole of the foot, in the depression at the junction of the red and white skin of the proximal end of the 1st metatarsophalangeal joint
Gōngsūn(SP4)	On the sole of the foot, at the junction of the red and white skin anterior and inferior to the base of the 1st metatarsal bone
Shāngqiū(SP5)	In the ankle region, anterior and inferior to medial malleolus, In depression at the midpoint of the line joining tuberosity of navicular bone and the prominence of medial malleolus
Sānyīnjiāo(SP6)	On the medial crus, 3 cun above the prominence of medial malleolus, posterior to medial margin of tibia
Lòugǔ(SP7)	On the medial crus, 6 cun above the prominence of medial malleolus, posterior to medial margin of tibia
Dìjī(SP8)	On the medial crus, 3 cun below Yinlingquan (SP9), posterior to medial margin of tibia
Yīnlíngquán(SP9)	On the medial crus, in the depression between inferior border of medial tibial condyle and medial border of tibia

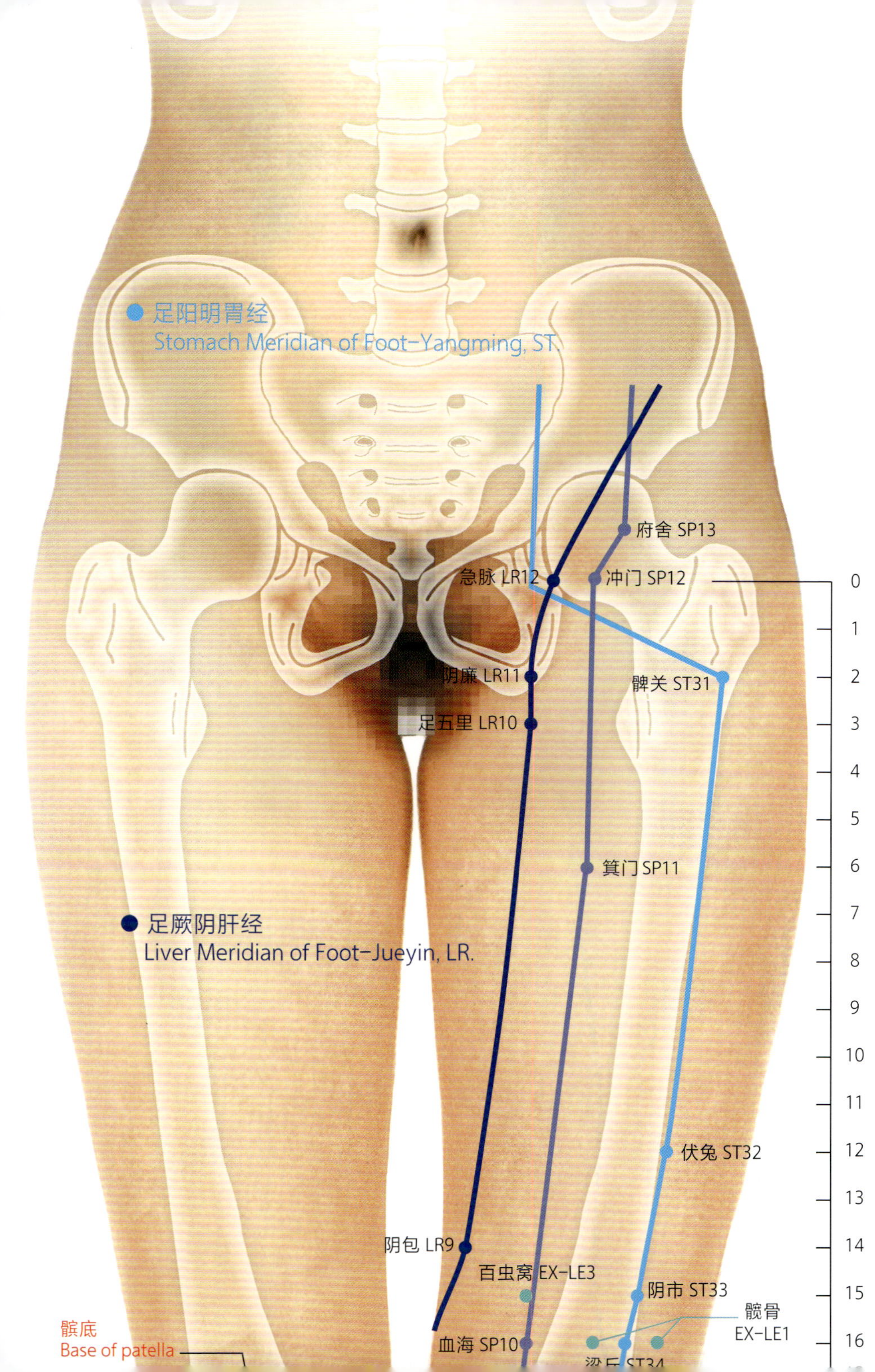

续表

穴 位	定 位
血海	在股前区，髌底内侧端上 2 寸，股内侧肌隆起处
箕门	在股前区，髌底内侧端与冲门的连线上 1/3 与下 2/3 交点，长收肌和缝匠肌交角的动脉搏动处
冲门	在腹股沟区，腹股沟斜纹中，髂外动脉搏动处的外侧
府舍	在下腹部，脐中下 4.3 寸，前正中线旁开 4 寸
大敦	在足趾，大趾末节外侧，趾甲根角侧后方 0.1 寸
行间	在足背，第 1、2 趾间，趾蹼缘后方赤白肉际处
太冲	在足背，第 1、2 跖骨间，跖骨底结合部前方凹陷中，或触及动脉搏动
中封	在踝区，内踝前，胫骨前肌肌腱的内侧缘凹陷中
蠡沟	在小腿内侧，内踝尖上 5 寸，胫骨内侧面的中央
中都	在小腿内侧，内踝尖上 7 寸，胫骨内侧面的中央
阴包	在股前区，髌底上 4 寸，股薄肌与缝匠肌之间
足五里	在股前区，气冲直下 3 寸，动脉搏动处

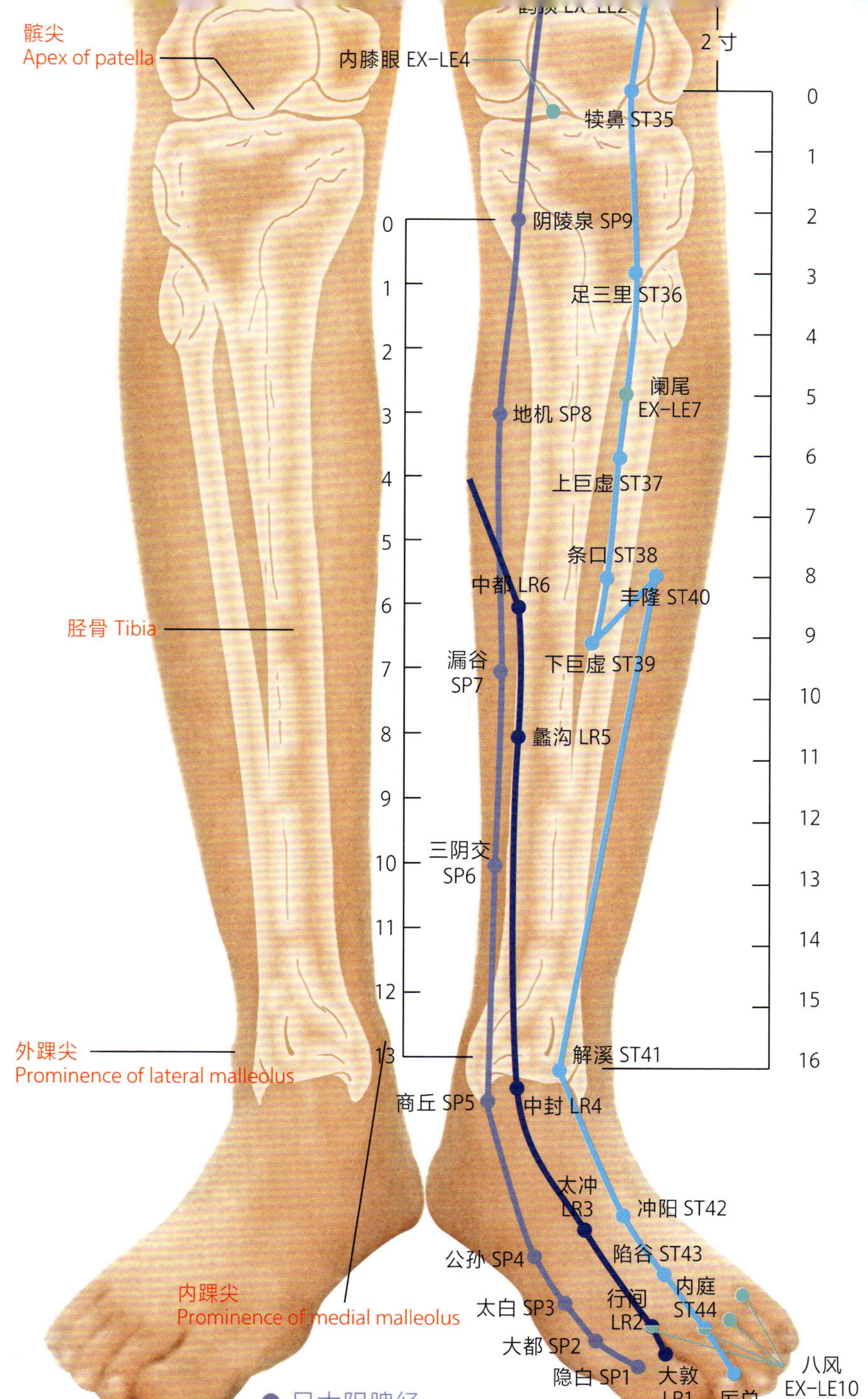

● 足太阴脾经
Spleen Meridian of Foot-Taiyin, SP.

● 经外奇穴 Extra Points, EX.

Continued

Acupoints	Location
Xuèhǎi(SP10)	In the anterior region of thigh, 2 cun superior to medial end of the base of patella, in the bump of medial vastus muscle
Jīmén(SP11)	In the anterior region of thigh, at the junction of upper 1/3 and lower 2/3 of the line joining medial base of patella and Chongmen(SP12), on the angle of intersection of adductor longus and sartorius where the arterial pulse can be palpated
Chōngmén(SP12)	In the inguinal region, on the inguinal twill, lateral to the pulse of external illiac artery
Fǔshè(SP13)	On the lower abdomen, 4.3 cun below the lavel, 4 cun lateral to the anterior midline
Dàdūn(LR1)	On the toe, in the lateral side of the end of the toe, 0.1 cun lateral and posterior to the corner of the base of the nail
Xíngjiān(LR2)	On the dorsum of the foot, between the 1st and the 2nd toe, at the junction of the red and white skin posterior to the web
Tàichōng(LR3)	On the dorsum of the foot, between the 1st and the 2nd metatarsal bone, in the depression anterior to the junction of the base of metatarsal bone where the arterial pulse can be palpated
Zhōngfēng(LR4)	In the ankle region, anterior to the medial malleolus, in the depression of medial border of tendon of anterior tibial muscle
Lígōu(LR5)	On the medial crus, 5 cun above the prominence of medial malleolus, in the center of medial surface of tibia
Zhōngdū(LR6)	On the medial crus, 7 cun above the prominence of medial malleolus, in the center of medial surface of tibia
Yīnbāo(LR9)	In the anterior region of thigh, 4 cun superior to the patellar base, between gracilis and sartorius
Zúwǔlǐ(LR10)	In the anterior region of thigh, 3 cun directly below Qichong(ST 30) where arterial pulse can be palpated

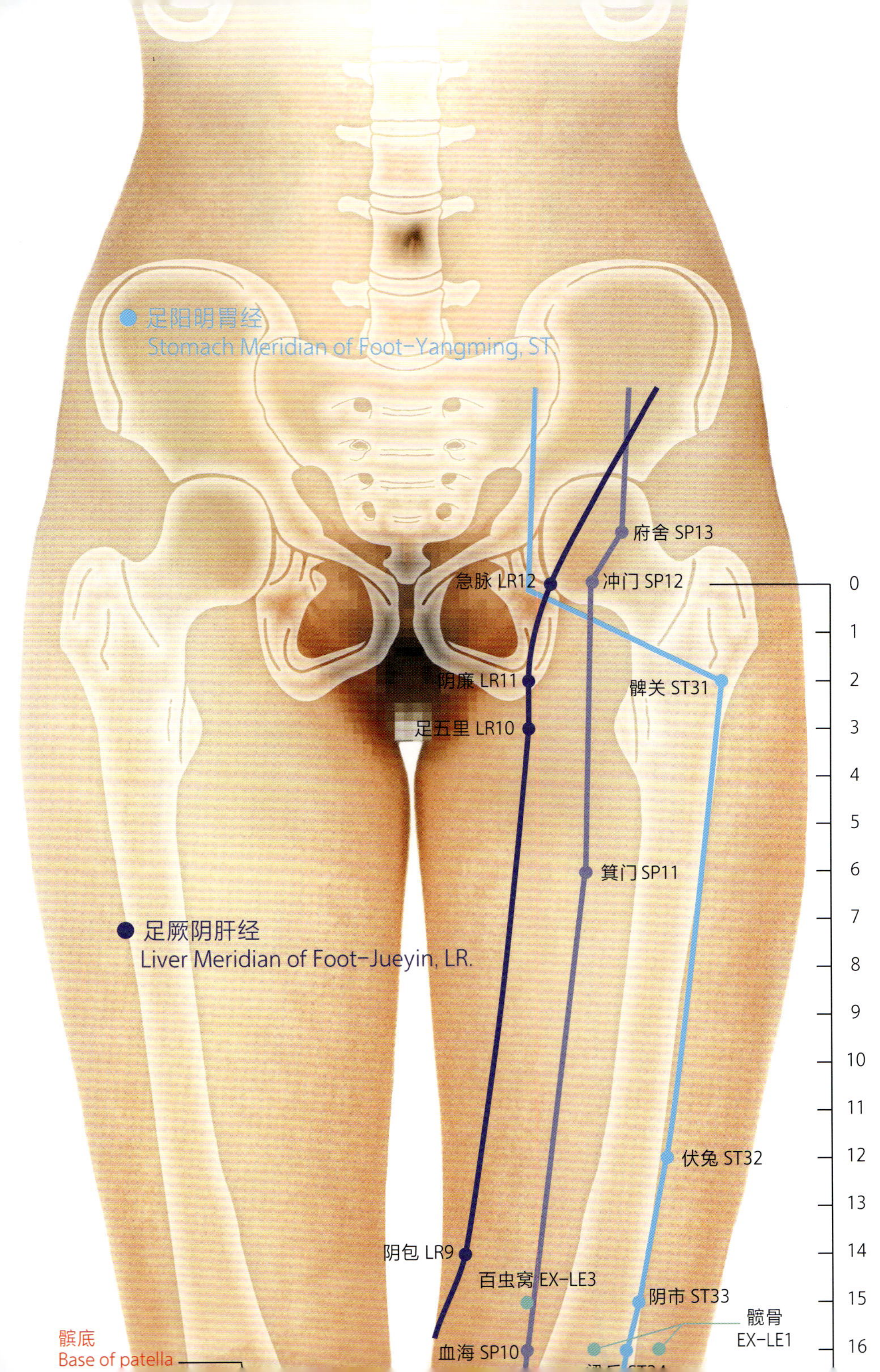

续表

穴位	定位
阴廉	在股前区，气冲直下 2 寸
急脉	在腹股沟区，横平耻骨联合上缘，前正中线旁开 2.5 寸
会阴	在会阴区，在大阴唇后联合与肛门连线的中点
髋骨	在股前区，梁丘两旁各 1.5 寸，一肢 2 穴
鹤顶	在膝前区，髌底中点的上方凹陷中
百虫窝	在股前区，髌底内侧端上 3 寸
内膝眼	在膝部，髌韧带内侧凹陷处的中央
阑尾	在小腿外侧，髌韧带外侧凹陷下 5 寸，胫骨前嵴外一横指（中指）
八风	在足背，第 1~5 趾间，趾蹼缘后方赤白肉际处，左右共 8 穴

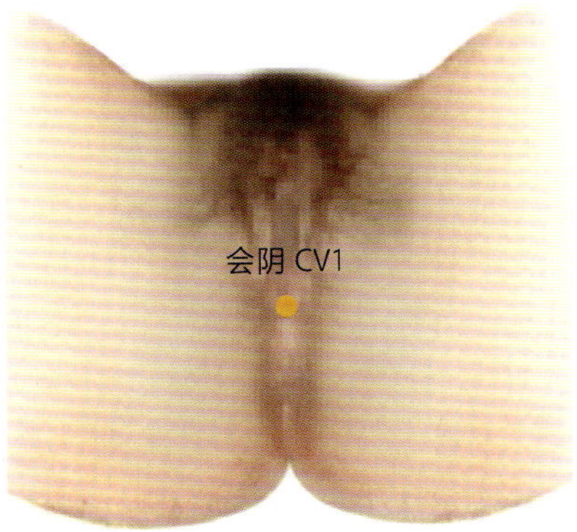

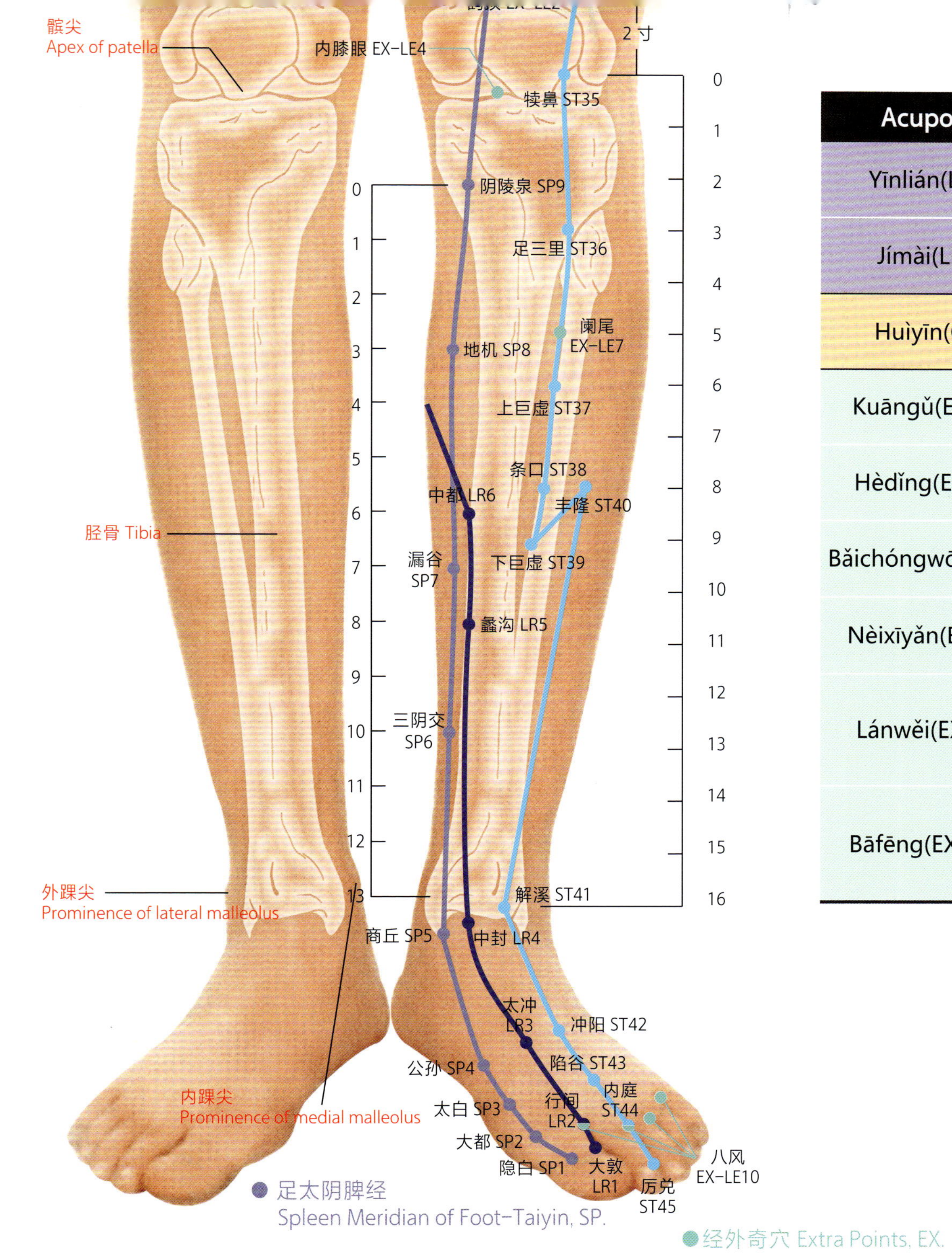

Continued

Acupoints	Location
Yīnlián(LR11)	In the anterior region of thigh, 2 cun directly below Qichong(ST30)
Jímài(LR12)	In the inguinal region, horizontal to superior border of pubic symphysis, 2.5 cun lateral to the anterior midline
Huìyīn(CV1)	In the perineum region, at the midpoint of the line joining posterior commissure of labia majora and anus
Kuāngǔ(EX-LE1)	In the anterior region of thigh, respectively 1.5 cun beside Liangqiu(ST34), with 2 points on each limb
Hèdǐng(EX-LE2)	In the anterior region of knee, in the depression superior to the midpoint of petallar base
Bǎichóngwō(EX-LE3)	In the anterior region of thigh, 3 cun superior to medial base of patella
Nèixīyǎn(EX-LE4)	On the knee, in the middle of the medial depression of patellar ligament
Lánwěi(EX-LE7)	Lateral to crus, 5 cun below the lateral depression of patellar ligament, one finger breadth(middle finger) exterior to tibial eminence
Bāfēng(EX-LE10)	On the dorsum of the foot, between the 1st to the 5th toe, at the junction of the red and white skin posterior to the web, with 8 points in total

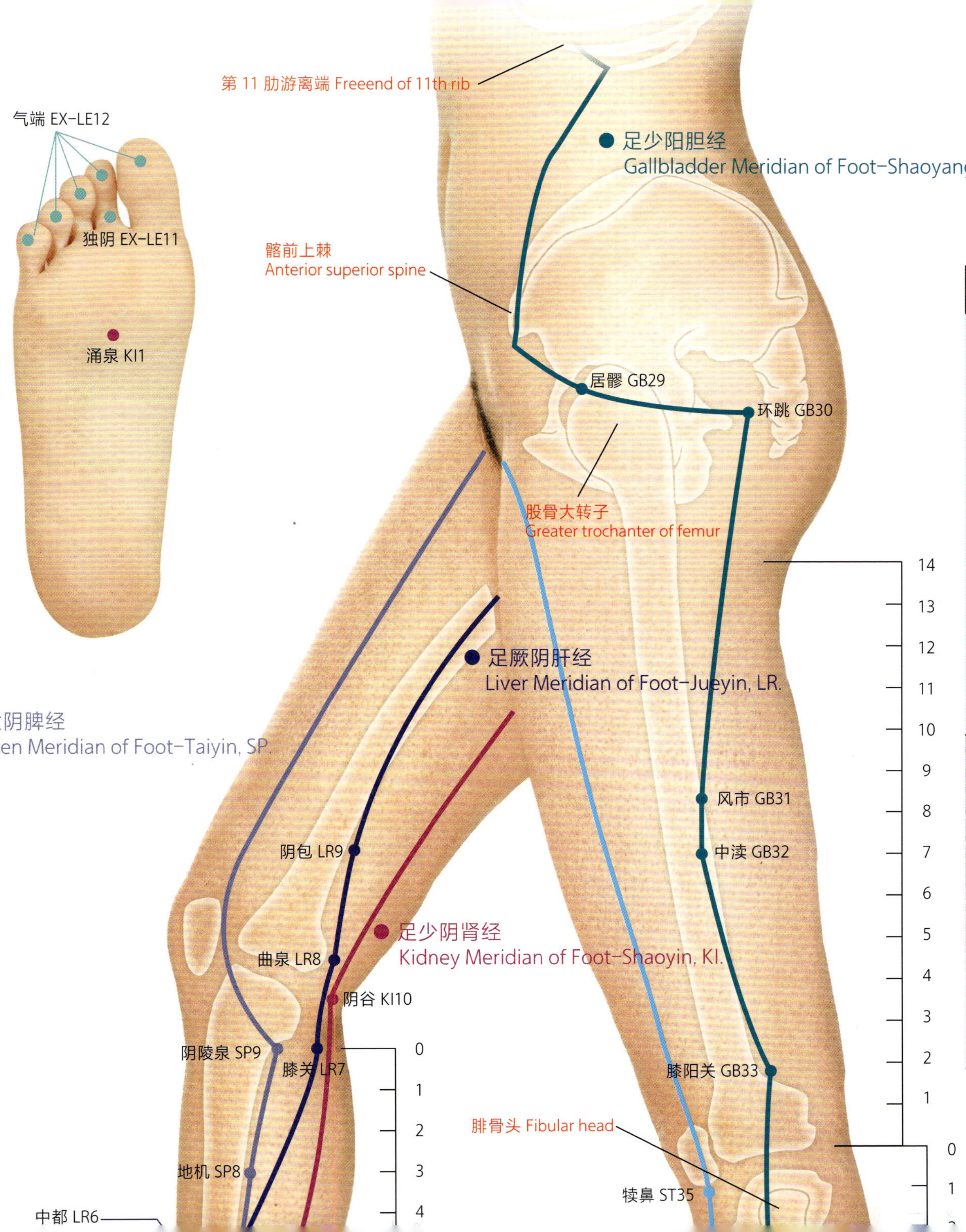

穴 位	定 位
犊鼻	在膝前区，髌韧带外侧凹陷中
丰隆	在小腿外侧，外踝尖上 8 寸，胫骨前肌的外侧
陷谷	在足背，当第 2、3 跖骨间，第 2 跖趾关节近端凹陷中
内庭	在足背，第 2、3 趾间，趾蹼缘后方赤白肉际处
厉兑	在足趾，第 2 趾末节外侧，趾甲根角侧后方 0.1 寸
隐白	在足趾，大趾末节内侧，趾甲根角侧后方 0.1 寸
大都	在足趾，第 1 跖趾关节远端赤白肉际凹陷中
太白	在跖区，第 1 跖趾关节近端赤白肉际凹陷中
公孙	在跖区，第 1 跖骨底的前下缘赤白肉际处

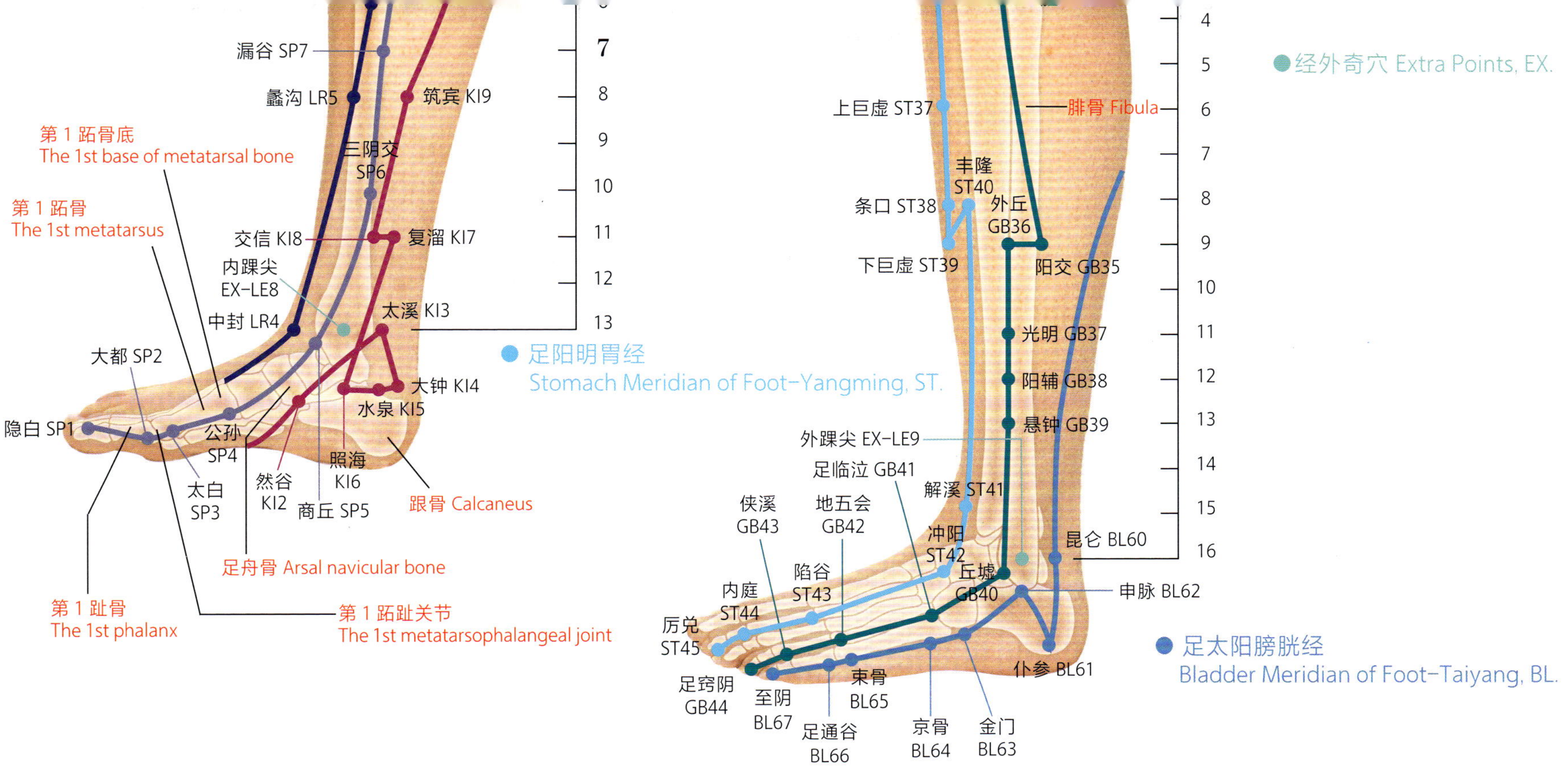

Acupoints	Location
Dúbí(ST35)	In the anterior region of the knee, in the lateral depression of the ligamentum patellae
Fēnglóng(ST40)	In the ectocnemial, 8 cun above the Waihuaijian (EX-LE9), lateral to the tibialis anterior muscle
Xiàngǔ(ST43)	On the dorsum of foot, between the 2nd and 3rd metatarsus, in the proximal depression of the 2nd metatarsophalangeal joint
Nèitíng(ST44)	On the dorsum of foot, between the 2nd and 3rd toes, at the junction of the red and white skin posterior to the edge of toe-web
Lìduì(ST45)	On the toe, lateral to the tip of the 2nd toe, 0.1 cun posterior and lateral to the corner of the toenail
Yǐnbái(SP1)	On the toe, interior to the tip of the big toe, 0.1 cun lateral and posterior to the corner of toenail
Dàdū(SP2)	On the toe, in the depression of the junction of the red and white skin of the distal end of 1st metatarsophalangeal joint
Tàibái(SP3)	In the metatarsal region, in the depression of the junction of the red and white skin of the proximal end of first metatarsophalangeal joint
Gōngsūn(SP4)	In the metatarsal region, at the junction of red and white skin anterior and inferior to the base of the 1st metatarsal bone

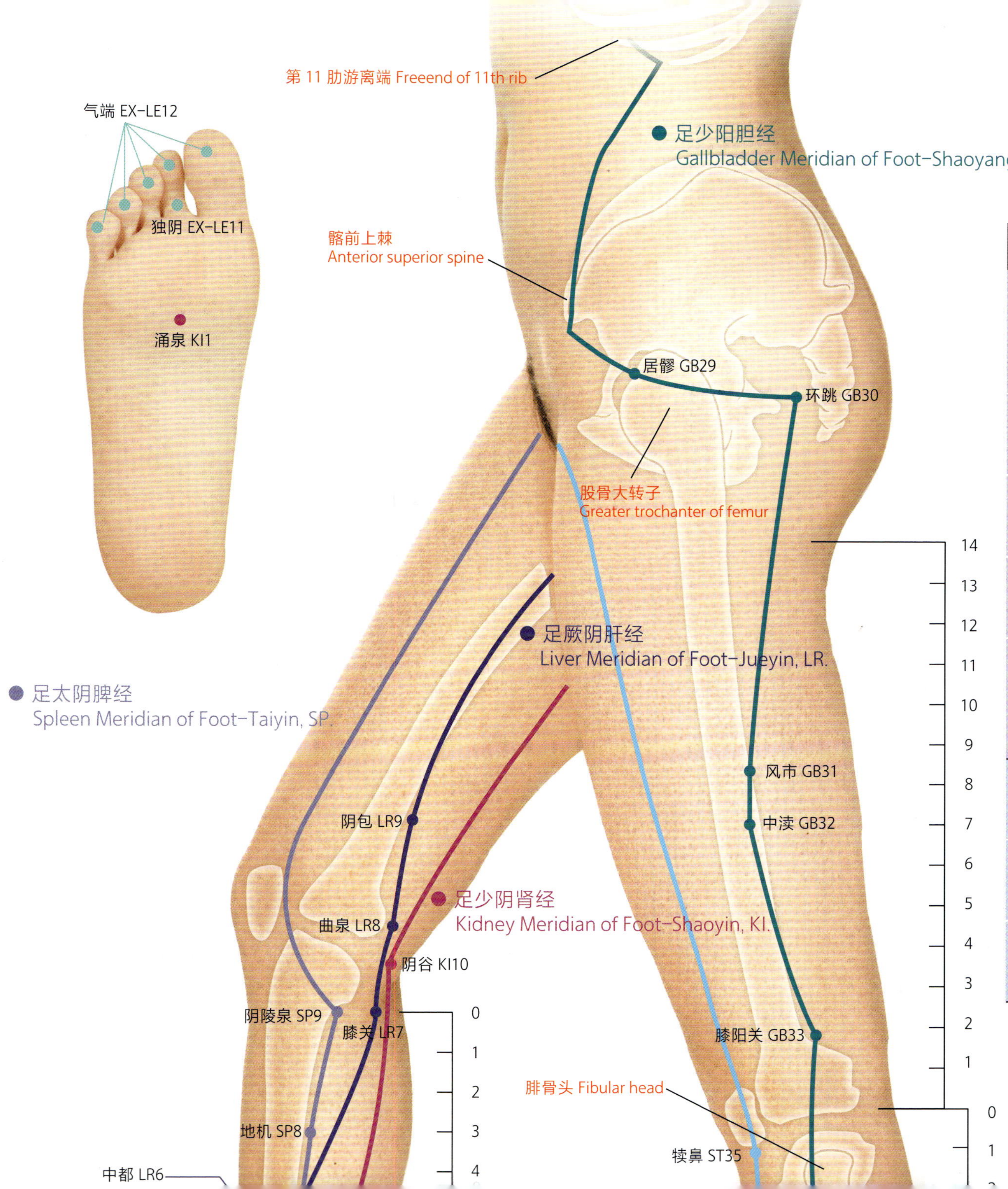

续表

穴 位	定 位
商丘	在踝区，内踝前下方，舟骨粗隆与内踝尖连线中点凹陷中
三阴交	在小腿内侧，内踝尖上 3 寸，胫骨内侧缘后际
漏谷	在小腿内侧，内踝尖上 6 寸，胫骨内侧缘后际
地机	在小腿内侧，阴陵泉下 3 寸，胫骨内侧缘后际
阴陵泉	在小腿内侧，胫骨内侧髁下缘与胫骨内侧缘之间的凹陷中
昆仑	在踝区，外踝尖与跟腱之间的凹陷中
仆参	在跟区，昆仑直下，跟骨外侧，赤白肉际处
申脉	在踝区，外踝尖直下，外踝下缘与跟骨之间凹陷中

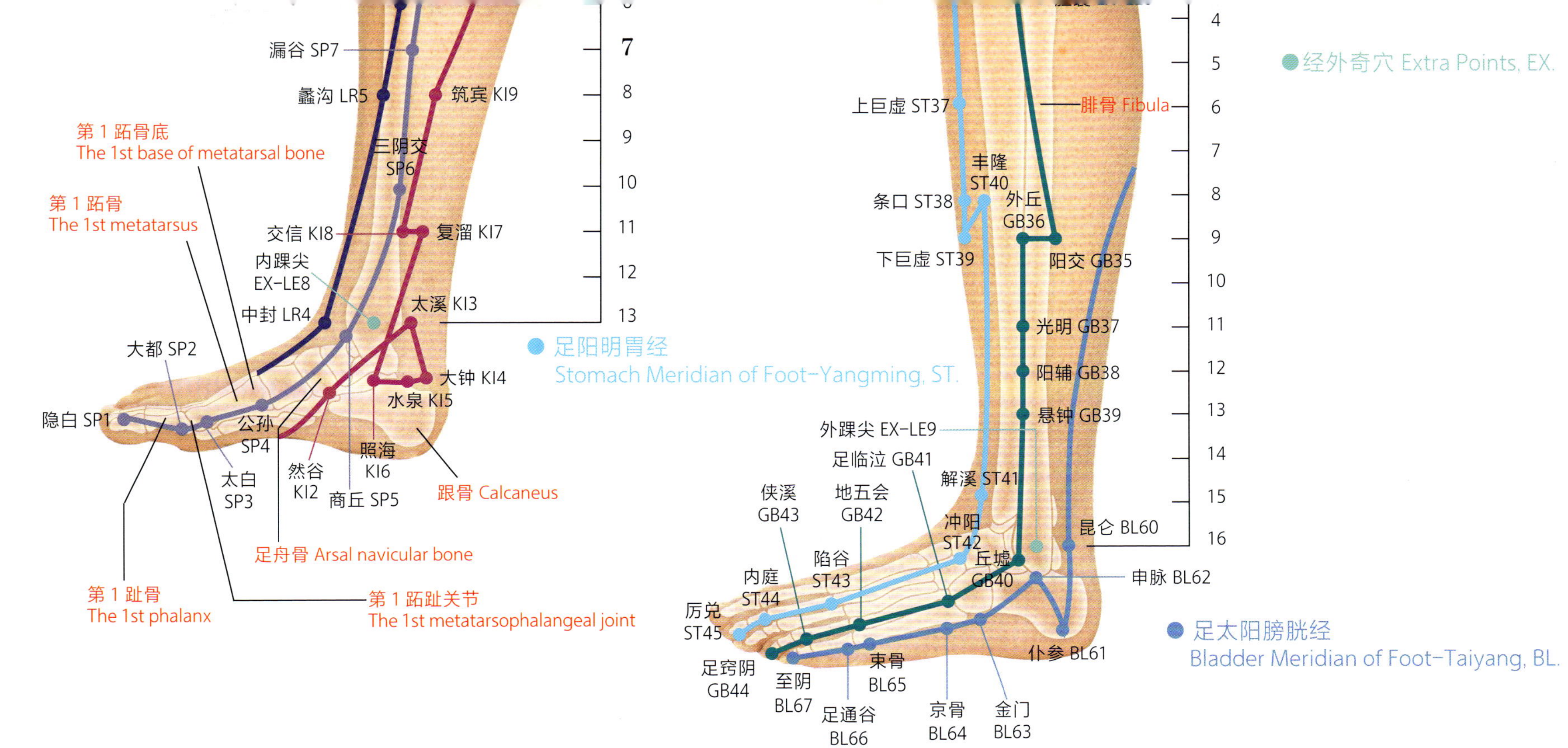

Continued

Acupoints	Location
Shāngqiū(SP5)	In the ankle region, anterior inferior to the medial malleolus, in the depression of the midpoint of the line joining tuberosity of navicular bone and prominence of the medial malleolus
Sānyīnjiāo(SP6)	Interior to the crus, 3 cun above the Neihuaijian (EX-LE8), in the posterior side of the medial tibia
Lòugǔ(SP7)	Interior to the crus, 6 cun above the Neihuaijian (EX-LE8), in the posterior side of the medial tibia
Dìjī(SP8)	Interior to the crus, 3 cun below Yinlingquan (SP9), in the posterior side of the medial tibia
Yīnlíngquán(SP9)	Interior to the crus, in the depression between the inferior margin of the medial tibia and the interior side of the medical tibia
Kūnlún(BL60)	In the ankle region, in the depression between Waihuaijian (EX-LE9) and achilles tendon
Púcān(BL61)	In the calcaneal region, right under Kunlun (BL60), lateral to the calcaneus, at the junction of red and white skin
Shēnmài(BL62)	In the ankle region, right under the Waihuaijian (EX-LE9), in the depression between the inferior margin of the lateral malleolus and the calcaneus

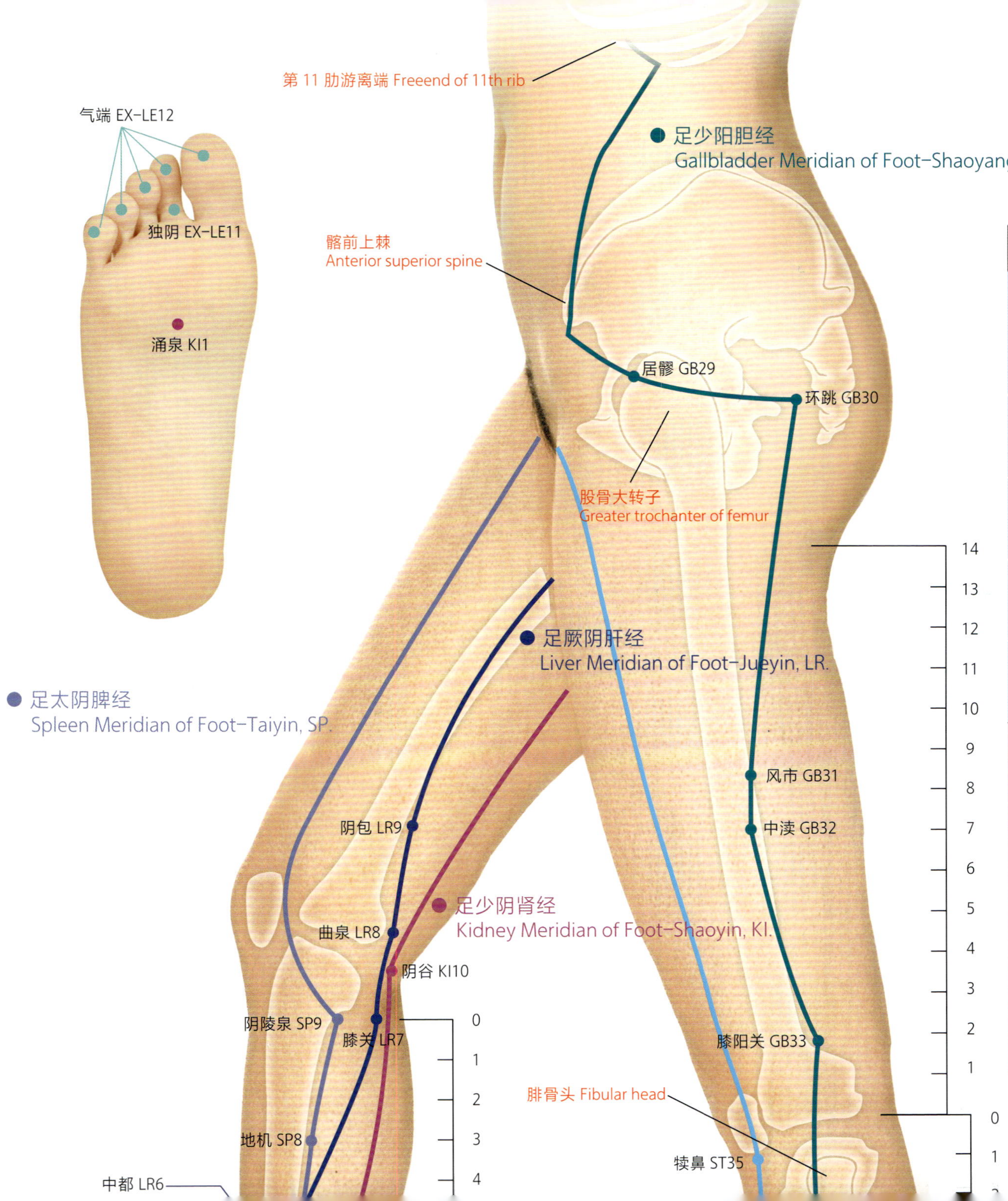

续表

穴 位	定 位
金门	在足背，外踝前缘直下。第 5 跖骨粗隆后方，骰骨下缘凹陷中
京骨	在跖区，第 5 跖骨粗隆前下方，赤白肉际处
束骨	在跖区，第 5 跖趾关节的近端，赤白肉际处
足通谷	在足趾，第 5 跖趾关节的远端，赤白肉际处
至阴	在足趾，小趾末节外侧，趾甲根角侧后方 0.1 寸
涌泉	在足底，屈足卷趾时足心最凹陷中
然谷	在足内侧，足舟骨粗隆下方，赤白肉际处
太溪	在踝区，内踝尖与跟腱之间的凹陷中
大钟	在跟区，内踝后下方，跟骨上缘，跟腱附着部前缘凹陷中

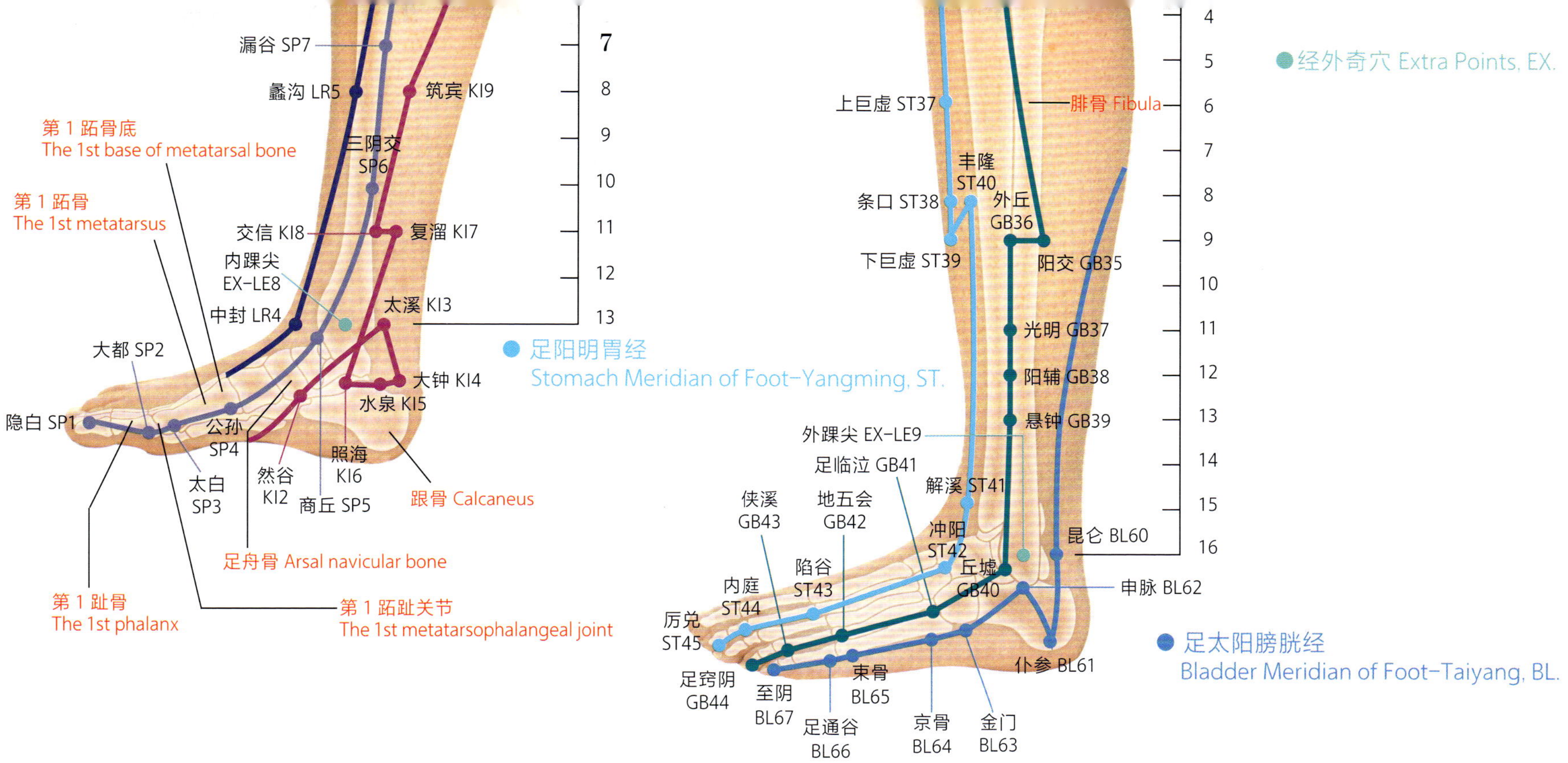

Continued

Acupoints	Location
Jīnmén(BL63)	On the dorsum of foot, right below the anterior side of the lateral malleolus, posterior to the tuberosity of the 5th metatarsal bone, in the depression in the inferior margin of cuboid bone
Jīnggǔ(BL64)	In the metatarsal region, anterior inferior to the tuberosity of the 5th metatarsal bone, at the junction of red and white skin
Shùgǔ (BL65)	In the metatarsal region, in the proximal side of the 5th metatarsophalangeal joint, at the junction of the red and white skin
Zútōnggǔ(BL66)	On the toe, in the distal side of the 5th metatarsophalangeal joint, at the junction of the red and white skin
Zhìyīn(BL67)	On the toe, lateral to the tip of the little toe, 0.1 cun lateral and posterior to the corner of the toenail
Yǒngquán(KI1)	On the sole, right in the depression appearing when you bend the leg and toes
Rángǔ(KI2)	In medial region of the foot, under the tuberosity of navicular bone, at the junction of the red and white skin
Tàixī(KI3)	In the ankle region, in the depression between Neihuaijian (EX-LE8) and achilles tendon
Dàzhōng(KI4)	In the calcaneal region, inferior and posterior to the interior malleolus, in the upper margin of the calcaneus, in the depression of the anterior margin of the adhesion of achilles tendon

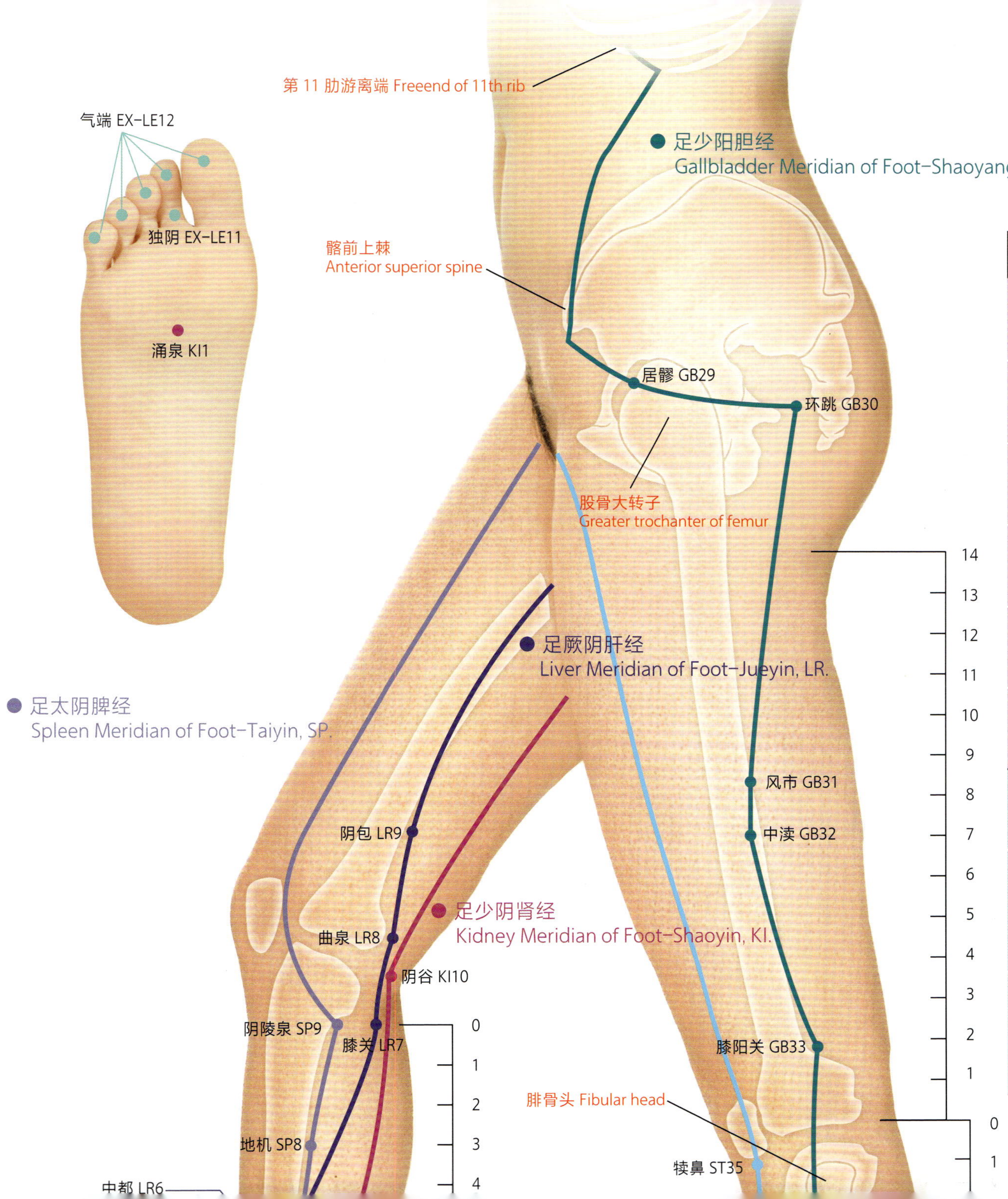

续表

穴 位	定 位
水泉	在跟区，太溪直下 1 寸，跟骨结节内侧凹陷中
照海	在踝区，内踝尖下 1 寸，内踝下缘边际凹陷中
复溜	在小腿内侧，内踝尖直上 2 寸，跟腱的前缘
交信	在小腿内侧，内踝尖上 2 寸，胫骨内侧缘后际凹陷中
筑宾	在小腿内侧，太溪直上 5 寸，比目鱼肌与跟腱之间
阴谷	在膝后区，腘横纹上，半腱肌肌腱外侧缘
居髎	在臀区，髂前上棘与股骨大转子最凸点连线的中点处
环跳	在臀区，股骨大转子最凸点与骶管裂孔连线的外 1/3 与内 2/3 交点处
风市	在股部，直立垂手，掌心贴于大腿时，中指尖所指凹陷中，髂胫束后缘

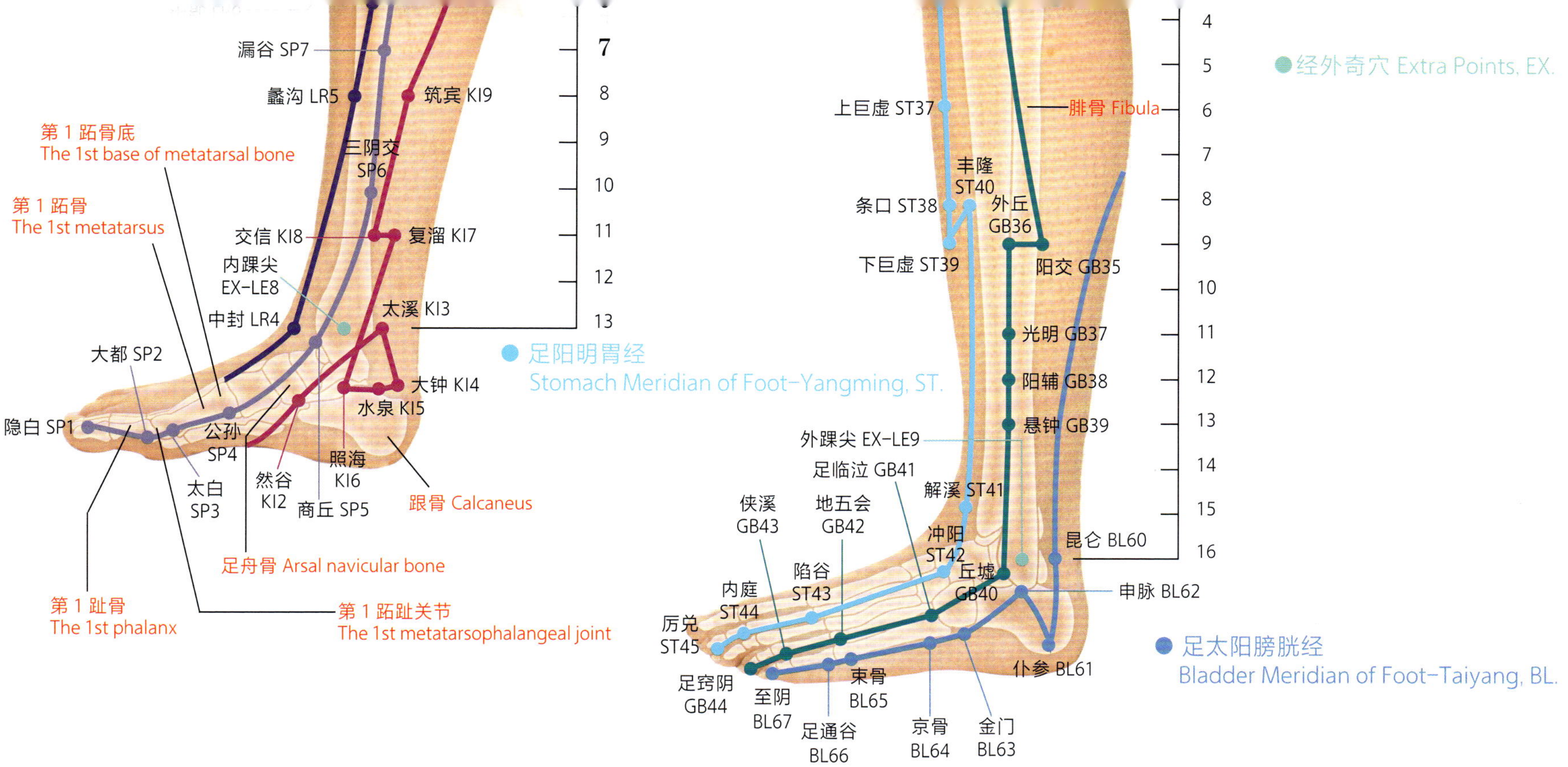

Continued

Acupoints	Location
Shuǐquán(KI5)	In the calcaneal region, 1 cun below Taixi (KI3), in the depression of the interior tuber calcanei
Zhàohǎi(KI6)	In the ankle region, 1 cun below Neihuaijian (EX-LE8), in the depression of the inferior margin of medial malleolus
Fùliū(KI7)	Interior to the crus, 2 cun above Neihuaijian (EX-LE8), in the lateral margin of the achilles tendon
Jiāoxìn(KI8)	Interior to the crus, 2 cun above Neihuaijian (EX-LE8), in the depression posterior to the medial margin of tibia
Zhùbīn(KI9)	Interior to the crus, 5 cun above Taixi (KI3), between soleus and achilles tendon
Yīngǔ(KI10)	In the posterior region of knee, on popliteal crease, in lateral border of semitendinosus tendon
Jūliáo(GB29)	In the gluteal region, at the middle point of the line joining the prominence of the greater trochanter of femur and anterior superior illiac spine
Huántiào(GB30)	In the gluteal region, at the junction of the middle 2/3 and lateral 1/3 of the line joining the prominence of the greater trochanter of femur and the sacral hiatus
Fēngshì(GB31)	In the femoral region, stand with hands down, palm affixed to the thigh, in the depression pointed by the middle finger, in the posterior margin of iliotibial tract

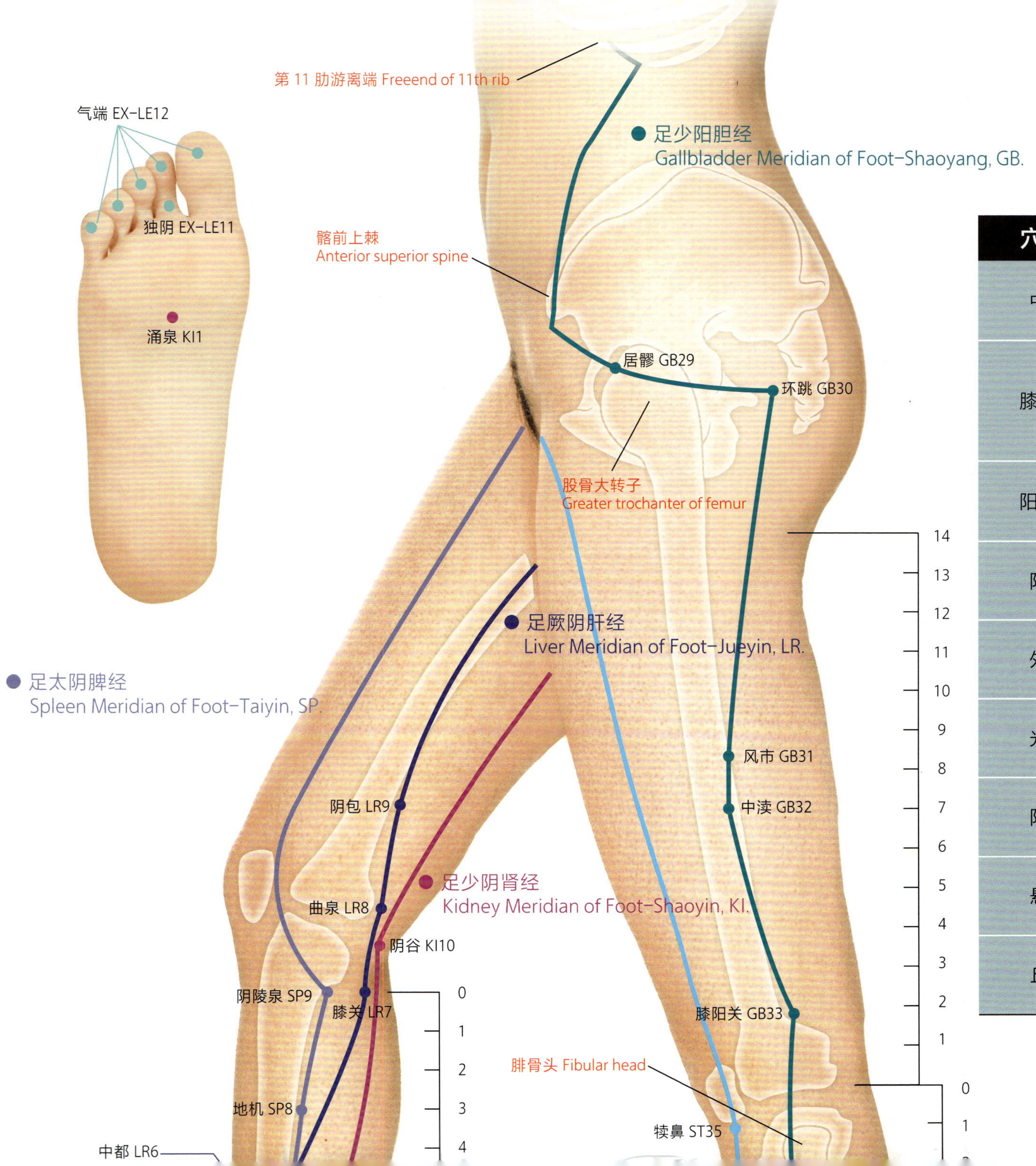

续表

穴 位	定 位
中渎	在股部，腘横纹上 7 寸，髂胫束后缘
膝阳关	在膝部，股骨外上髁后上缘，股二头肌腱与髂胫束之间的凹陷中
阳陵泉	在小腿外侧，腓骨头前下方凹陷中
阳交	在小腿外侧，外踝尖上 7 寸，腓骨后缘
外丘	在小腿外侧，外踝尖上 7 寸，腓骨前缘
光明	在小腿外侧，外踝尖上 5 寸，腓骨前缘
阳辅	在小腿外侧，外踝尖上 4 寸，腓骨前缘
悬钟	在小腿外侧，外踝尖上 3 寸，腓骨前缘
丘墟	在踝区，外踝的前下方，趾长伸肌腱的外侧凹陷中

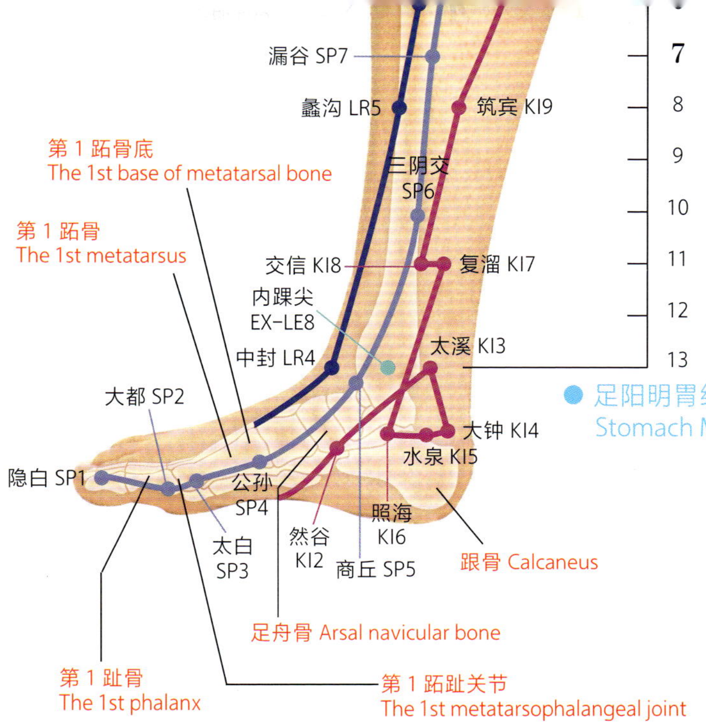

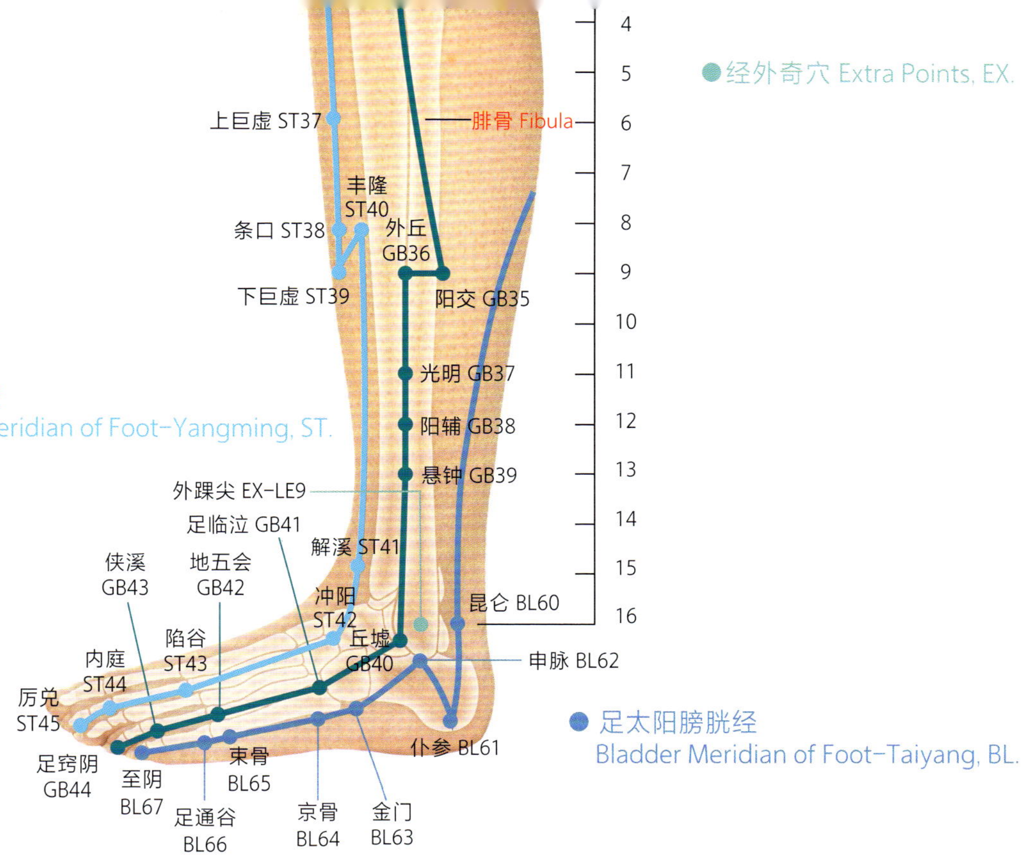

Continued

Acupoints	Location
Zhōngdú(GB32)	In the femoral region, 7 cun above popliteal crease, in the posterior side of iliotibial tract
Xīyángguān(GB33)	In the knee, in the superior and posterior margin of lateral femoral epicondyle, in the depression between biceps femoris tendon and iliotibial tract
Yánglíngquán(GB34)	In the lateral side of crus, in the anterior inferior depression of fibula head
Yángjiāo(GB35)	In the lateral side of crus, 7 cun above the Waihuaijian (EX–LE9), in the posterior margin of the fibula
Wàiqiū(GB36)	In the lateral side of crus, 7 cun above the Waihuaijian (EX–LE9), in the anterior margin of the fibula
Guāngmíng (GB37)	In the lateral side of crus, 5 cun above the Waihuaijian (EX–LE9), in the anterior margin of the fibula
Yángfǔ(GB38)	In the lateral side of crus, 4 cun above the Waihuaijian (EX–LE9), in the anterior margin of the fibula
Xuánzhōng(GB39)	In the lateral side of crus, 3 cun above the Waihuaijian (EX–LE9), in the anterior margin of the fibula
Qiūxū(GB40)	In the ankle region, anterior and inferior to the lateral malleolus, in the depression lateral to the toe's extensor hallucis longus tendon

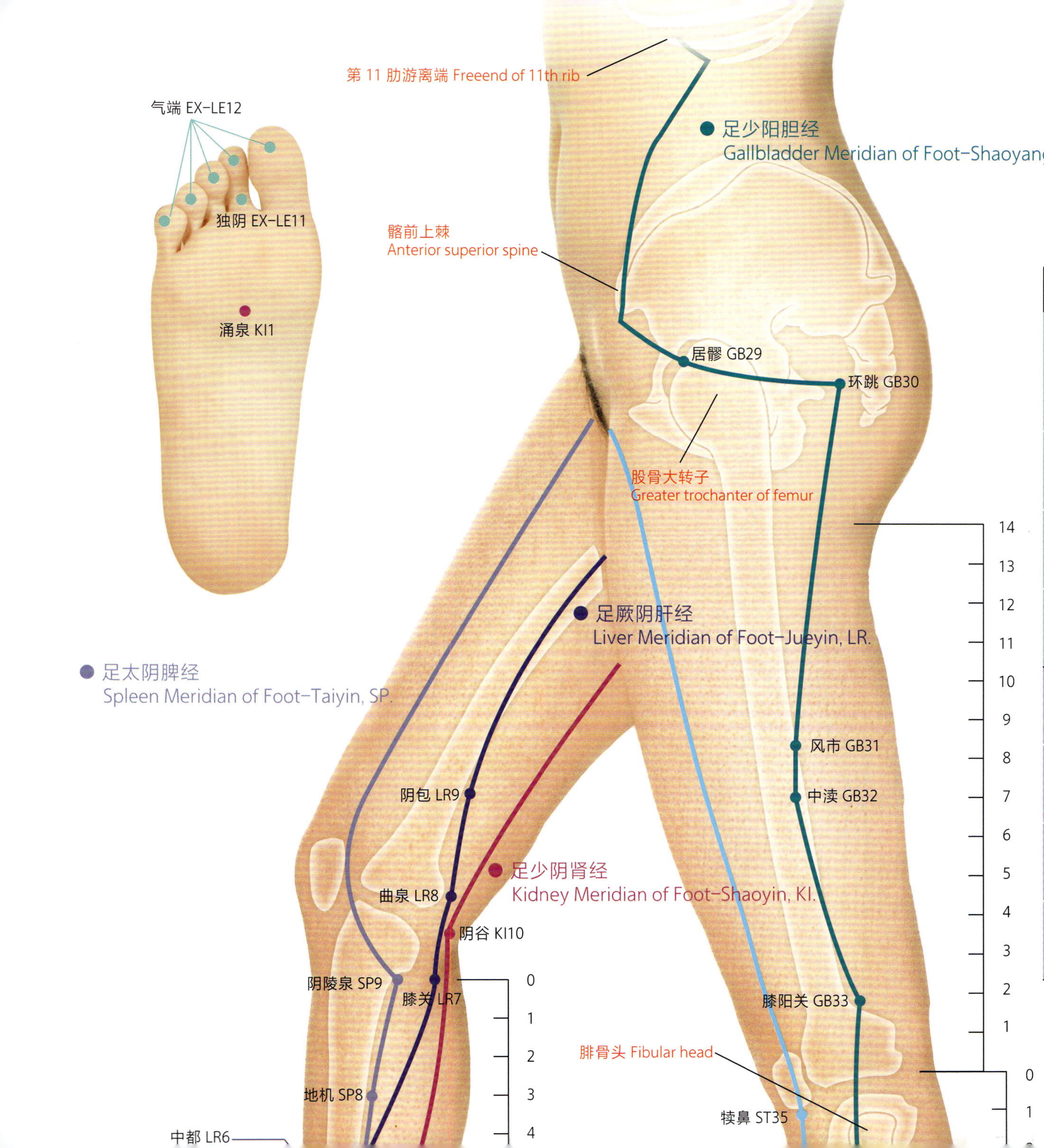

续表

穴 位	定 位
足临泣	在足背，第 4、5 跖骨底结合部的前方，第 5 趾长伸肌腱外侧凹陷中
地五会	在足背，第 4、5 跖骨间，第 4 跖趾关节近端凹陷中
侠溪	在足背，第 4、5 趾间，趾蹼缘后方赤白肉际处
足窍阴	在足趾，第 4 趾末节外侧，趾甲根角侧后方 0.1 寸
中封	在踝区，内踝前，胫骨前肌肌腱的内侧缘凹陷中
蠡沟	在小腿内侧，内踝尖上 5 寸，胫骨内侧面的中央
中都	在小腿内侧，内踝尖上 7 寸，胫骨内侧面的中央
膝关	在膝部，胫骨内侧髁的下方，阴陵泉后 1 寸

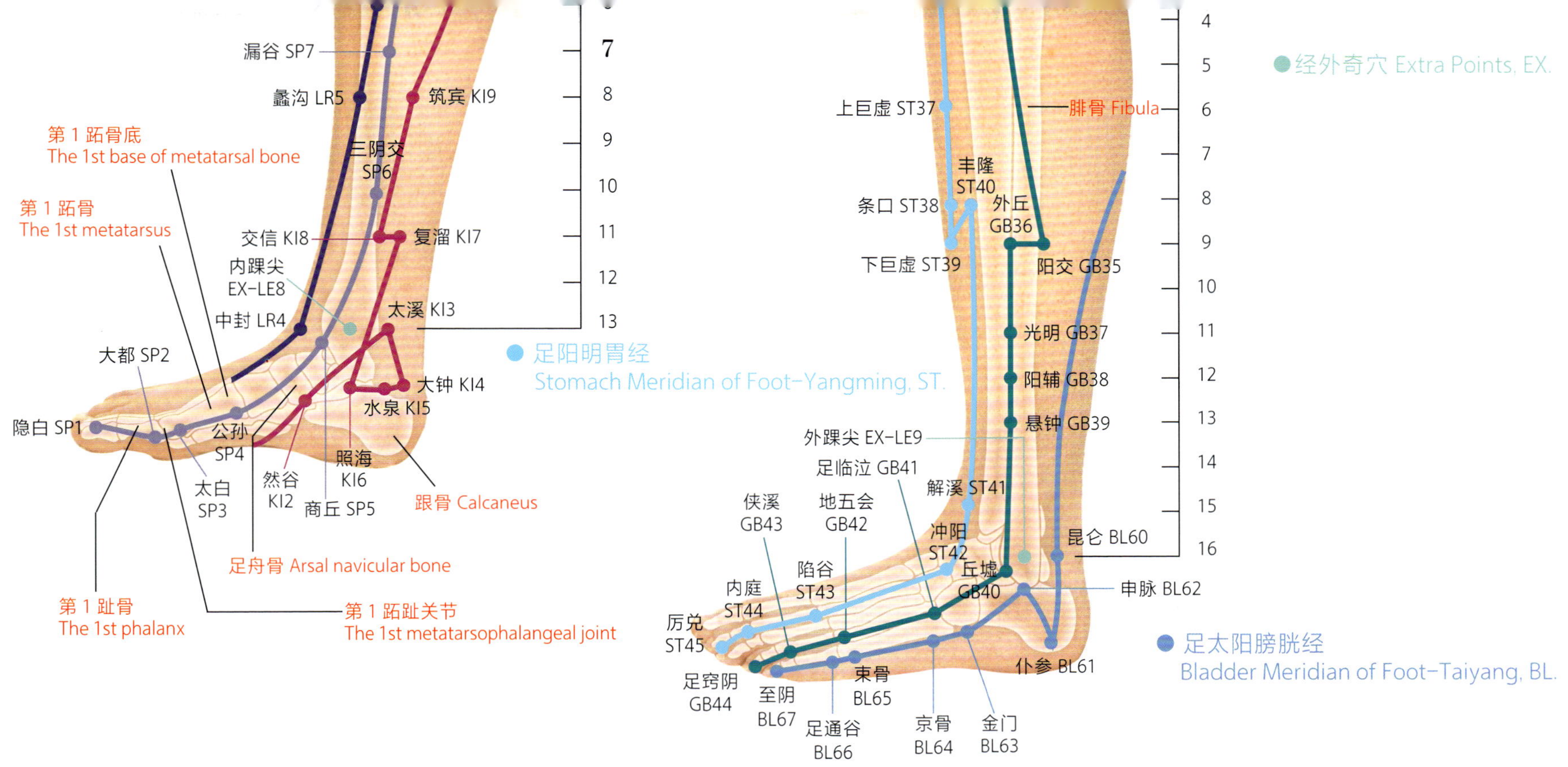

Continued

Acupoints	Location
Zúlínqì(GB41)	On the dorsum of foot, anterior to the junction of the 4th and 5th base of metatarsal bone , in the depression lateral to the 5th toe's extensor hallucis longus tendon
Dìwǔhuì(GB42)	On the dorsum of foot, between the 4th and the 5th metatarsal bone, right in the depression of the proximal end of the 4th metatarsophalangeal joint
Xiáxī(GB43)	On the dorsum of foot, between the 4th and 5th toe, right in the junction of red and white skin posterior to toe-web
Zúqiàoyīn(GB44)	On the toe, lateral to the tip of the 4th toe, 0.1 cun posterior and lateral to the corner of the toenail
Zhōngfēng(LR4)	In the ankle region, before medial malleolus, in the interior depression of tendon of anterior tibialis
Lígōu(LR5)	Interior to the crus, 5 cun above Neihuaijian (EX-LE8), in the center of facies medialis tibiae
Zhōngdū (LR6)	Inside of the crus, 7 cun above Neihuaijian (EX-LE8), in the center of facies medialis tibiae
Xīguān(LR7)	In the knee, down the tibial medial condyle and 1 cun posterior to Yinlingquan (SP9)

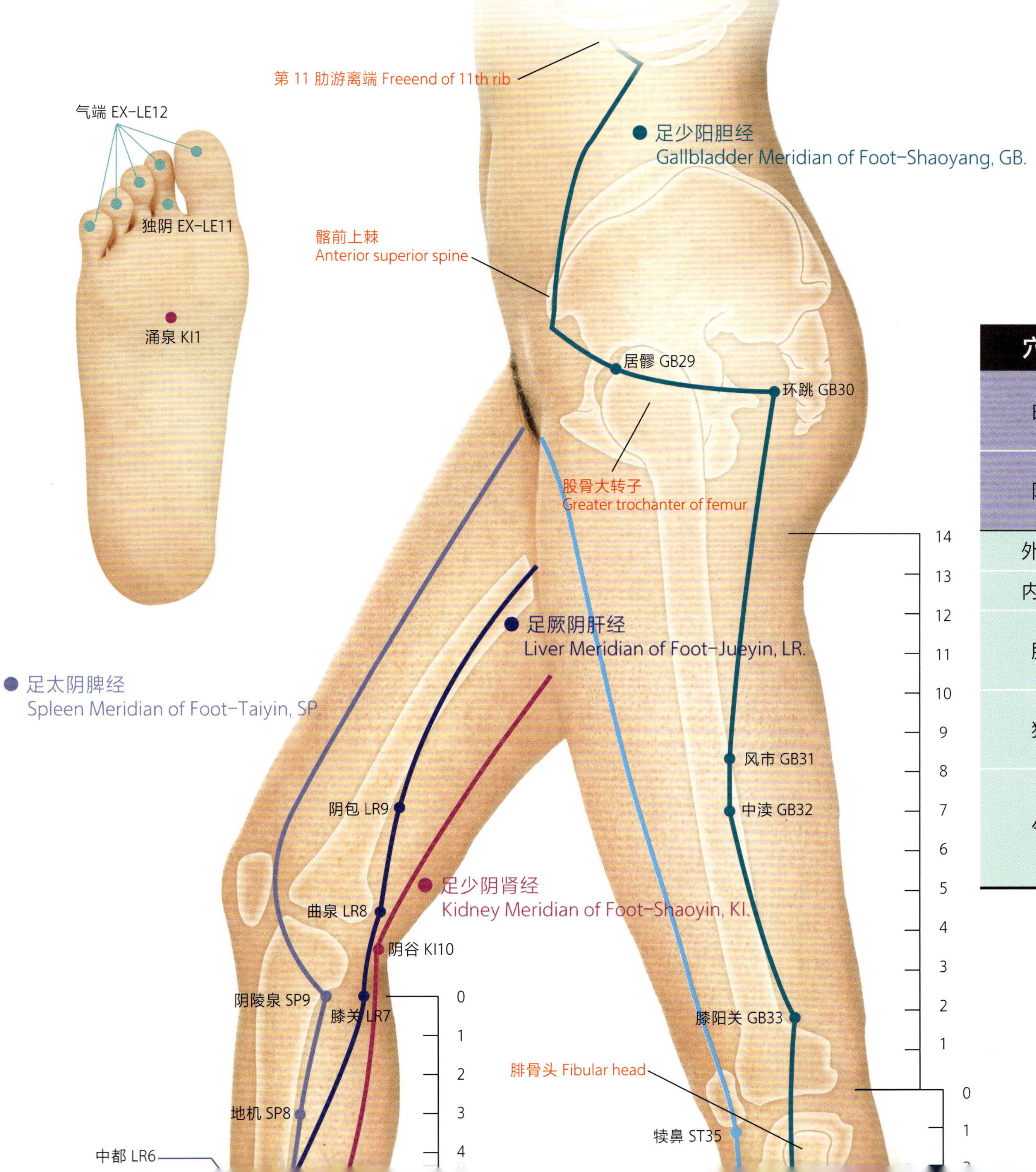

续表

穴 位	定 位
曲泉	在膝部，腘横纹内侧端，半腱肌肌腱内缘凹陷中
阴包	在股前区，髌底上 4 寸，股薄肌与缝匠肌之间
外踝尖	在踝区，外踝的最凸起处
内踝尖	在踝区，内踝的最凸起处
胆囊	在小腿外侧，腓骨小头直下 2 寸
独阴	在足底，第 2 趾的跖侧远端趾间关节
气端	在足趾，十趾端的中央，距趾甲游离缘 0.1 寸，左右共 10 穴

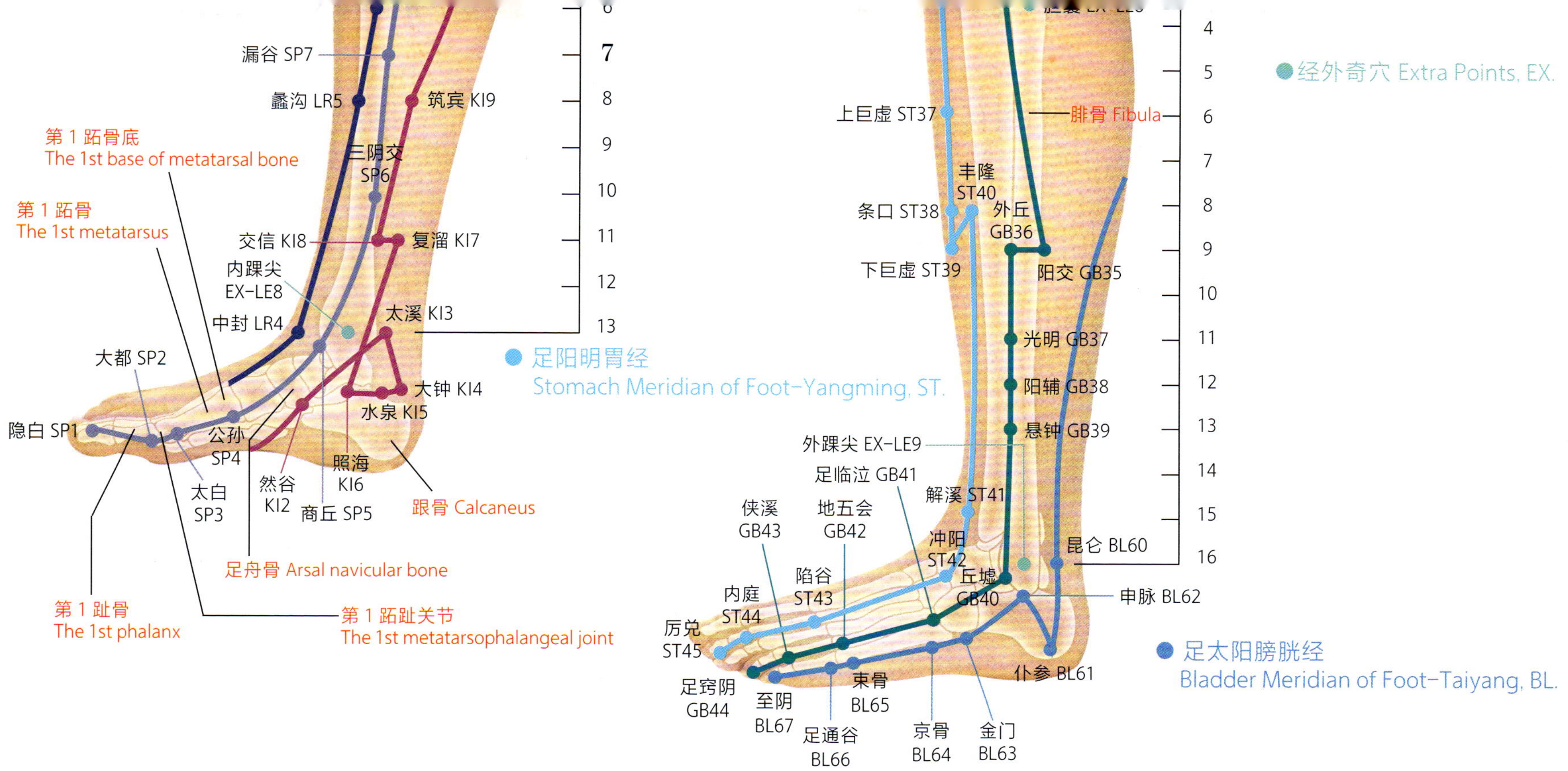

Continued

Acupoints	Location
Qūquán(LR8)	In the knee, in popliteal stripes medial side, in the depression of the interior edge of semitendinosus tendon
Yīnbāo(LR9)	In anterior region of thigh, 4 cun above base of patella, between gracilis and sartorius
Wàihuáijiān(EX-LE9)	In the ankle region, in the most obvious embossment of lateral malleolus
Nèihuáijiān(EX-LE8)	In the ankle region, in the most obvious embossment of medial malleolus
Dǎnnáng(EX-LE6)	Lateral to the crus, 2 cun directly below fibular head
Dúyīn(EX-LE11)	On the sole of the foot, in the interphalangeal joint on the distal end of metatarsal side of the 2nd toe
Qìduān(EX-LE12)	On the toe, in the center of ten toes tip, 0.1 cun away from the free edge of the toenails, with 10 acupoints in both sides

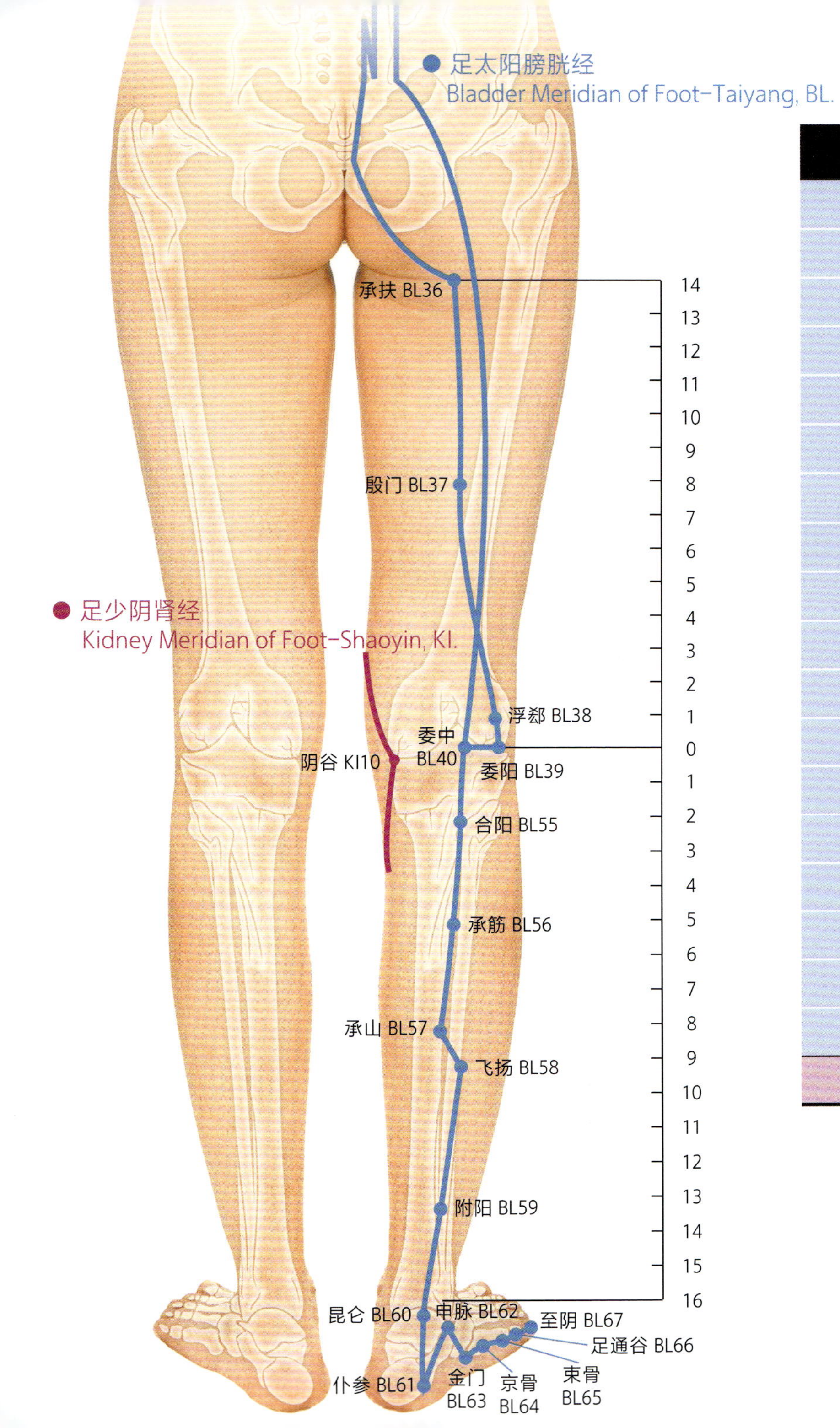

穴 位	定 位
承扶	在股后区，臀沟的中点
殷门	在股后区，臀沟下 6 寸，股二头肌与半腱肌之间
浮郄	在膝后区，腘横纹上 1 寸，股二头肌腱的内侧缘
委阳	在膝部，腘横纹上，股二头肌腱的内侧缘
委中	在膝后区，腘横纹中点
合阳	在小腿后区，腘横纹下 2 寸，腓肠肌内、外侧头之间
承筋	在小腿后区，腘横纹下 5 寸，腓肠肌两肌腹之间
承山	在小腿后区，腓肠肌两肌腹与肌腱交角处
飞扬	在小腿后区，昆仑直上 7 寸，腓肠肌外下缘与跟腱移行处
跗阳	在小腿后区，昆仑直上 3 寸，腓骨与跟腱之间
昆仑	在踝区，外踝尖与跟腱之间的凹陷中
仆参	在跟区，昆仑直下，跟骨外侧，赤白肉际处
申脉	在踝区，外踝尖直下，外踝下缘与跟骨之间凹陷中
金门	在足背，外踝前缘直下，第 5 跖骨粗隆后方，骰骨下缘凹陷中
京骨	在跖区，第 5 跖骨粗隆前下方，赤白肉际处
束骨	在跖区，第 5 跖趾关节的近端，赤白肉际处
足通谷	在足趾，第 5 跖趾关节的远端，赤白肉际处
至阴	在足趾，小趾末节外侧，趾甲根角侧后方 0.1 寸
阴谷	在膝后区，腘横纹上，半腱肌肌腱外侧缘

Acupoints	Location
Chéngfú(BL36)	In posterior region of thigh, at the midpoint of the gluteal fold
Yīnmén(BL37)	In posterior region of thigh, 6 cun below the gluteal fold, between biceps femoris muscle and semitendinosus
Fúxì(BL38)	In the posterior region of knee, 1 cun above popliteal crease, in medial margin of biceps femoris tendon
Wěiyáng(BL39)	In the knee, above popliteal crease, in medial margin of biceps femoris tendon
Wěizhōng(BL40)	In the posterior region of knee, at the midpoint of popliteal crease
Héyáng(BL55)	In the posterior crural region, 2 cun below popliteal crease, between lateral head and medial head of musculus gastrocnemius
Chéngjīn(BL56)	In the posterior crural region,5 cun below popliteal crease, between the two muscle bellys of musculus gastrocnemius
Chéngshān(BL57)	In the posterior crural region, in the corner between the two muscle bellys of musculus gastrocnemius and tendon
Fēiyáng(BL58)	In the posterior crural region, 7 cun above Kunlun (BL60), right in the junction between lateral and inferior margin of musculus gastrocnemius and tendon
Fūyáng(BL59)	In the posterior crural region, 7 cun above Kunlun (BL60), between fibula and tendon
Kūnlún(BL60)	In the ankle region, in the depression between Waihuaijian (EX–LE9) and tendon
Púcān(BL61)	In the calcaneal region, right below Kunlun (BL60), lateral to the calcaneus, at the junction of red and white skin
Shēnmài(BL62)	In the ankle region, right below Waihuaijian (EX–LE9), in the depression of inferior border of lateral malleolus and calcaneus
Jīnmén(BL63)	On the dorsum of foot, right below the anterior margin of the lateral malleolus, posterior to tuberosity of the 5th metatarsal bones, in the depression of the edge of cuboid
Jīnggǔ(BL64)	In the metatarsal region, anterior and inferior to the tuberosity of the 5th metatarsal bones, at the junction of red and white skin
Shùgǔ(BL65)	In the metatarsal region, in the proximal end of the 5th metatarsophalangeal joint, at the junction of red and white skin
Zútōnggǔ(BL66)	In the toe, in the distal end of the 5th metatarsophalangeal joint, at the junction of red and white skin
Zhìyīn(BL67)	In the toe, in the lateral side of the tip of the little toe, 0.1 cun lateral and posterior to the corner of the toenail
Yīngǔ(KI10)	In the posterior region of knee, on popliteal crease, in lateral border of semitendinosus tendon

第三章　超速效三步对症按摩法

1 黑眼圈

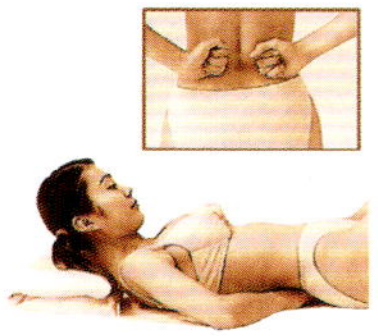

肾俞 仰卧、握拳，用拳头上突出的关节顶住穴位，利用体重按压穴位。

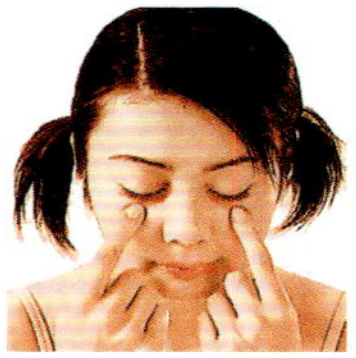

四白 双手食指同时按压同侧穴位。

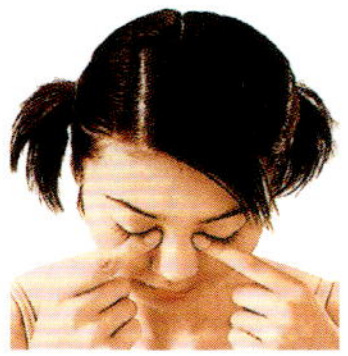

睛明 双手食指同时按压同侧穴位。

2 去皱防皱

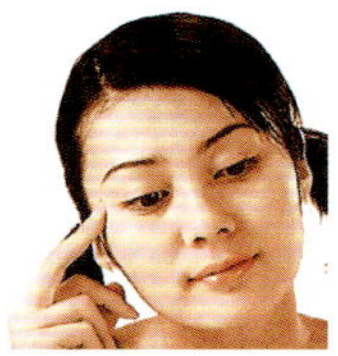

瞳子髎 用中指按压穴位。

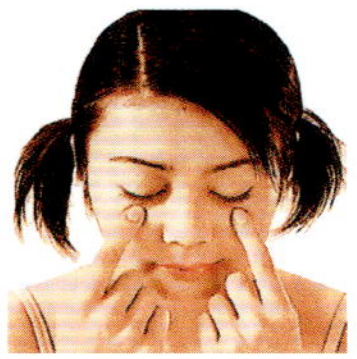

四白 两手食指放到同侧穴位上，闭上眼睛，头部前倾按压穴位。

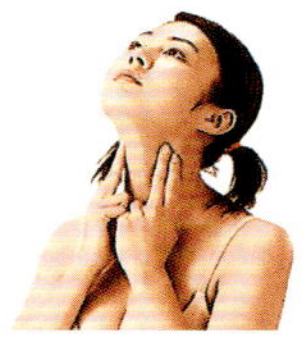

人迎 中指和食指并拢按同侧穴位，以穴位为中心用指腹平推。

3 美白祛斑

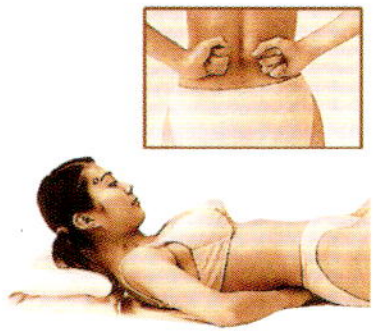

肾俞 仰卧，双手握拳，用拳头突出的关节顶住穴位，利用体重按压穴位。

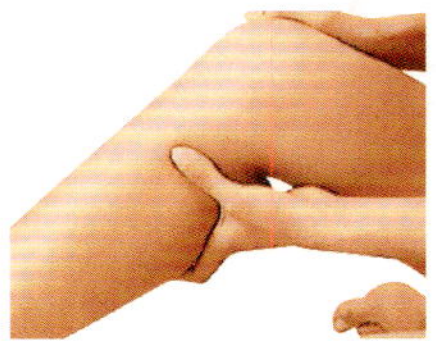

阴陵泉 一手固定膝盖，另一只手拇指垂直按压穴位。

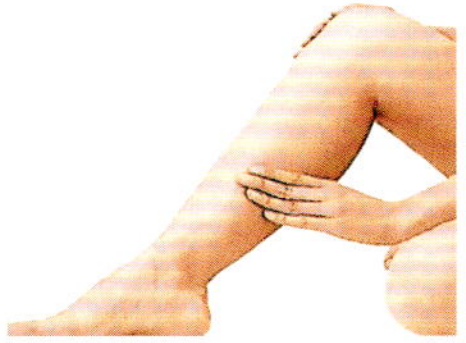

三阴交 用除拇指外的四指，以穴位为中心，从下向上平推。

4 乌发美发

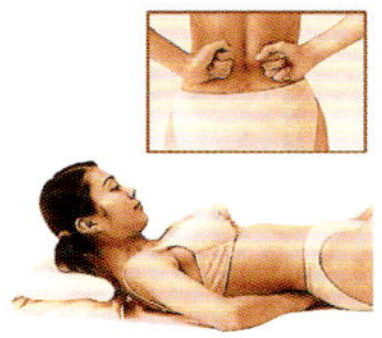

肾俞 仰卧，双手握拳，用拳头突出的关节顶住穴位，利用体重按压穴位。

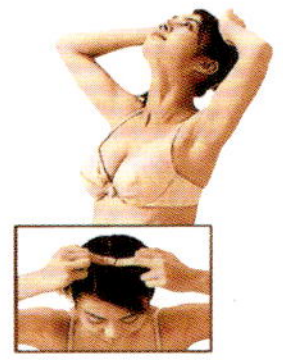

百会 双手中指叠放在穴位上按压。

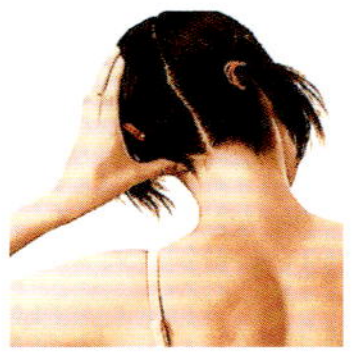

风池 用拇指按压同侧穴位。

5 减肥减脂

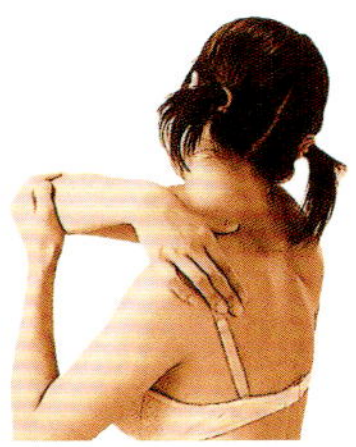

肩井 拇指按对侧穴位。

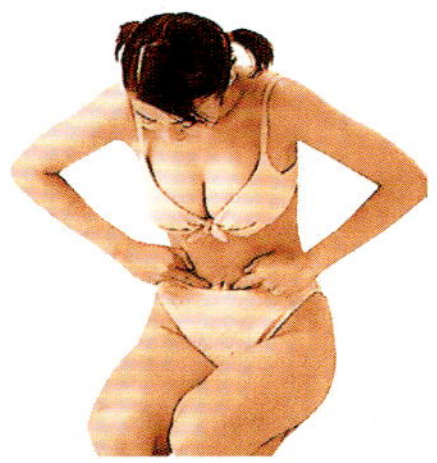

天枢 双手中指同时按压同侧穴位。

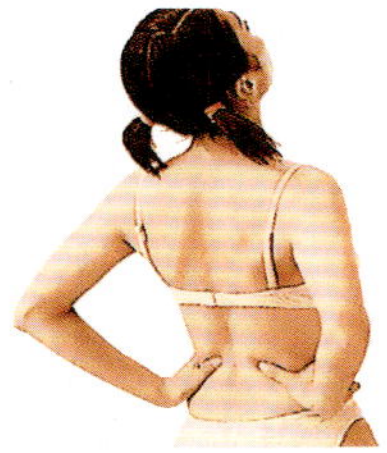

大肠俞 双手拇指同时按压同侧穴位。

Chapter 3:
Super Quick-acting Three-step Symptomatic Massage Manipulations

❶ Black Rim of Eyes

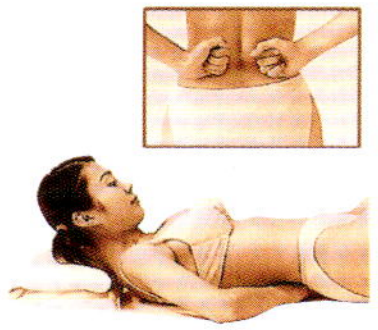

Shènshū(BL23) : Lie on the back, clench the fists, press against the acupoint with the protuberance of the fist, press the acupoint by weight.

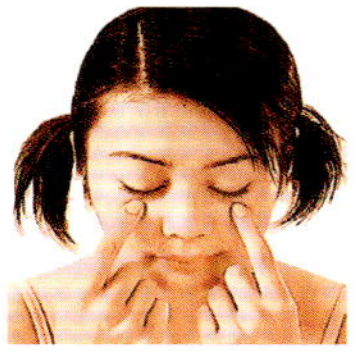

Sìbái(ST2) : Press the acupoints in each side with index finger of both hands at the same time.

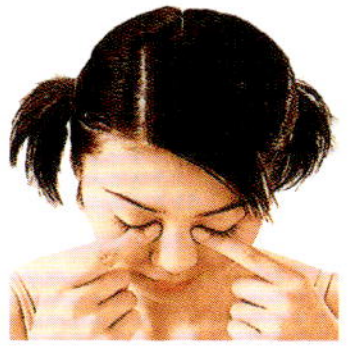

Jīngmíng(BL1) : Press the acupoints in each side with index finger of both hands at the same time.

❷ Anti-wrinkle and Wrinkle Prevention

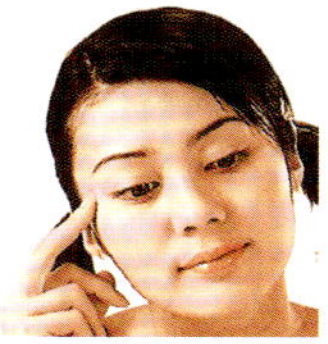

Tóngzǐliáo(GB1) : Press the acupoint with middle finger.

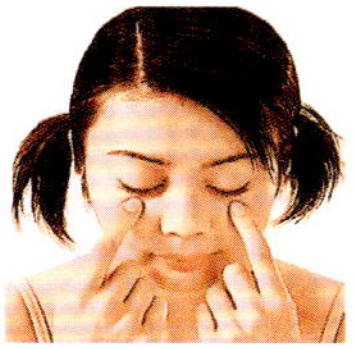

Sìbái(ST2) : Put the index finger on the acupoint in each side, close eyes and press the acupoints with the head forward.

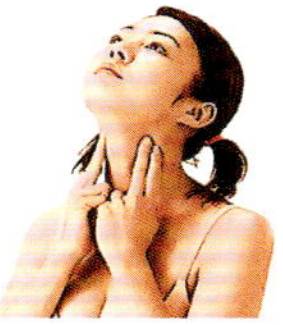

Rényíng(ST9) : Put the middle finger and index finger together and press the acupoint in each side, flat-pushing with the acupoint as the center with finger pulp.

❸ Whitening and Freckle Removal

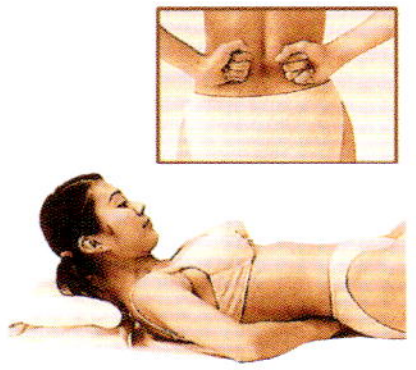

Shènshū(BL23) : Lie on the back, clench the fists, press against the acupoint with the protuberance of the fist, press the acupoint by weight.

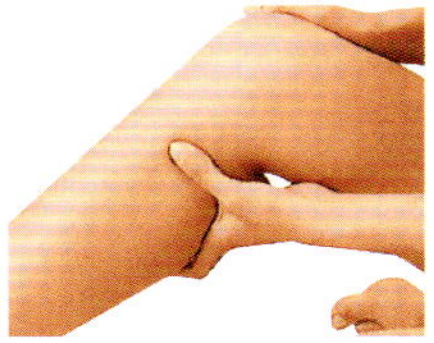

Yīnlíngquán(SP9) : One hand fix the knee, the thumb of the other hand press the acupoint directly.

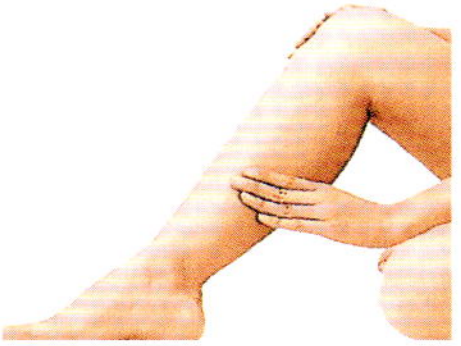

Sānyīnjiāo(SP6) : Use four fingers except the thumb to do flat-pushing from bottom up with the acupoint as the center.

❹ Hair Blackening and Beauty

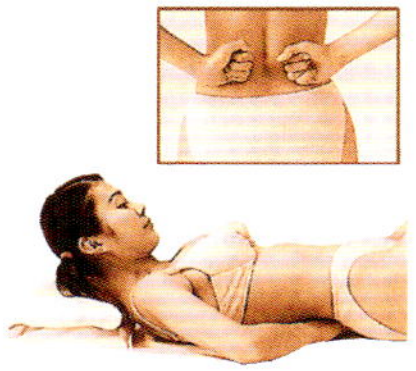

Shènshū(BL23) : Lie on the back, clench the fists, press against the acupoint with the protuberance of the fist, press the acupoint by weight.

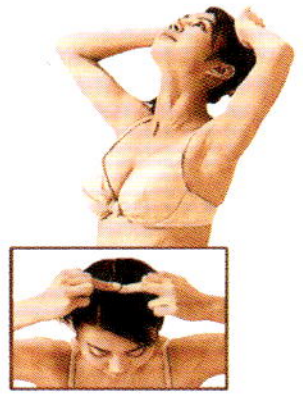

Bǎihuì(GV20) : Press the acupoint with middle fingers stacked.

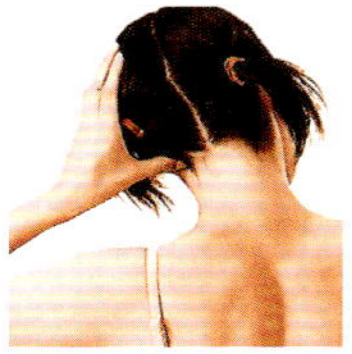

Fēngchí(GB20) : Press the acupoint by thumb on the same side.

❺ Weight Loss

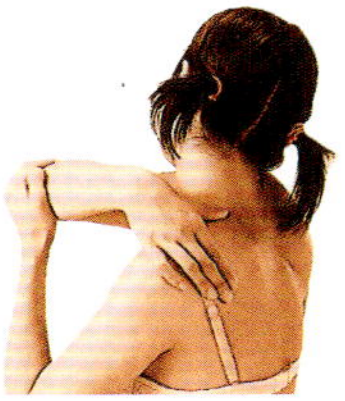

Jiānjǐng(GB21) : Press the acupoint in the other side by thumb.

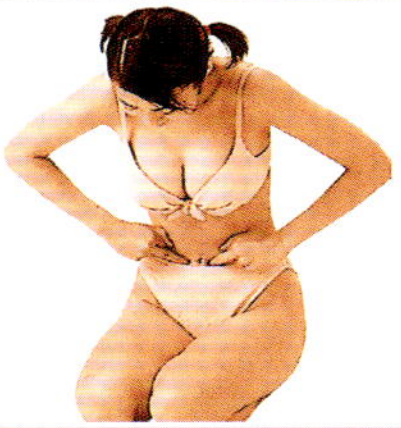

Tiānshū(ST25) : Press acupoint in each side with both middle fingers.

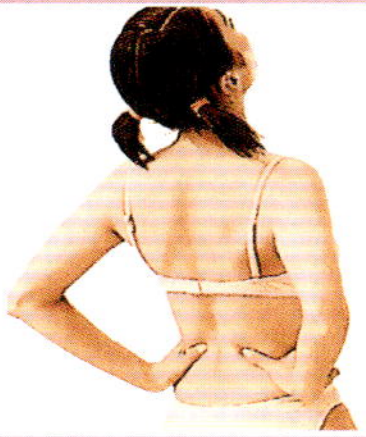

Dàchángshū(BL25) : Press acupoint in each side with both thumbs at the same time.

6 经前乳胀

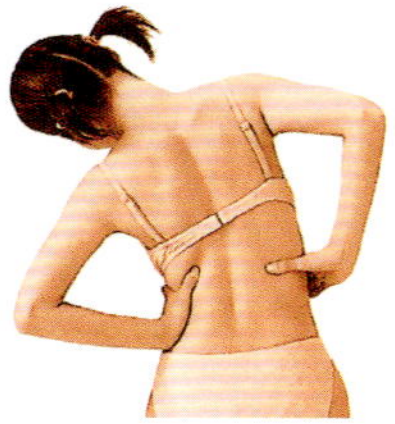

肝俞 两手拇指分别按同侧穴位。

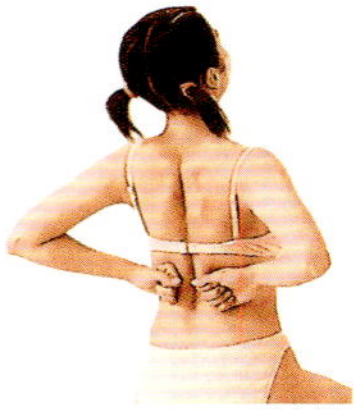

胃俞 双手握拳，用拳头突起的关节按穴位。

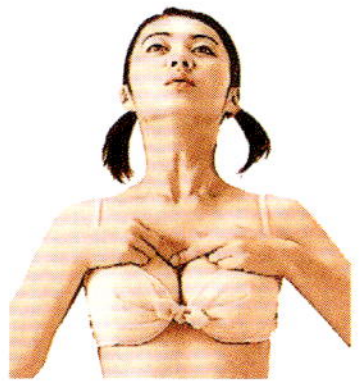

膻中 用中指按压穴位。

7 痛经、月经周期不规则

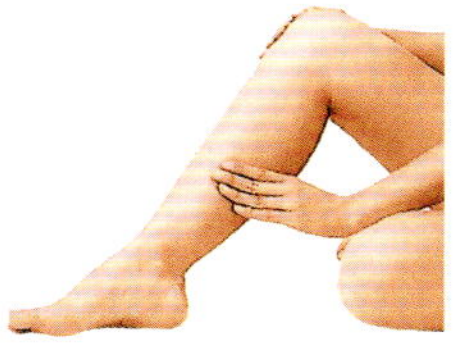

三阴交 用除拇指外的四指，以穴位为中心，从下向上平推。

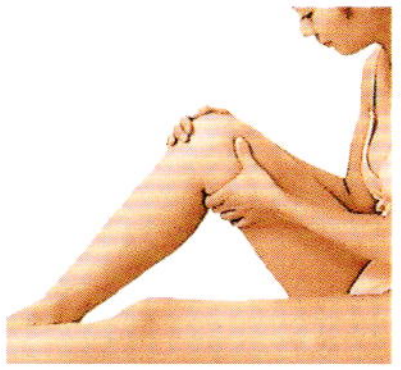

血海 拇指按穴位，做小范围的按揉。

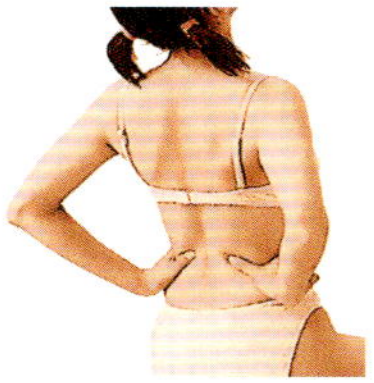

肾俞 两手拇指分别按同侧穴位。

8 月经量少或量多

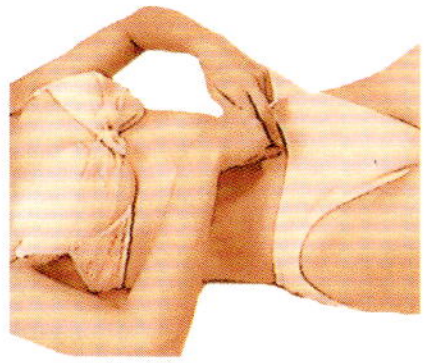

关元 仰卧、用双手中指叠放在一起按揉。

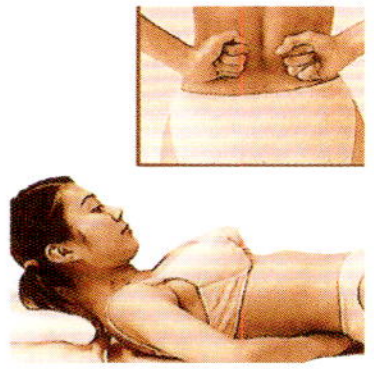

肾俞 仰卧，双手握拳，用拳头突出的关节顶住穴位，利用体重按压穴位。

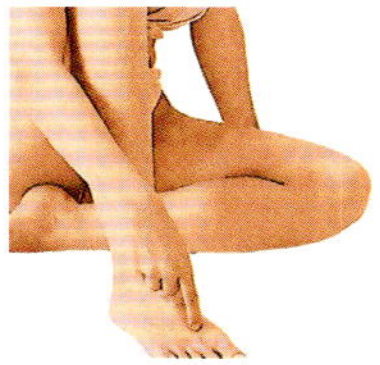

太冲 食指按揉穴位。

9 更年期综合征

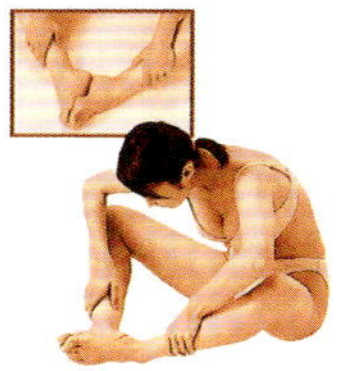

三阴交 两手拇指分别按压同侧穴位。

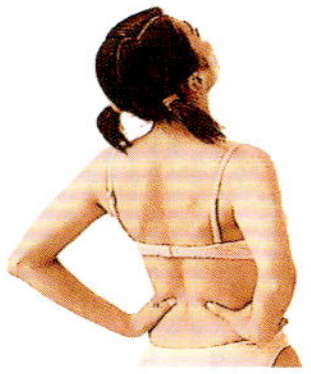

肾俞 两手拇指分别按同侧穴位。

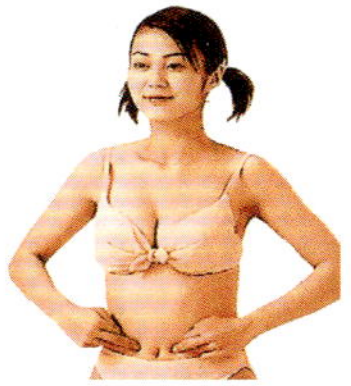

天枢 两手中指分别按同侧穴位。

10 贫血

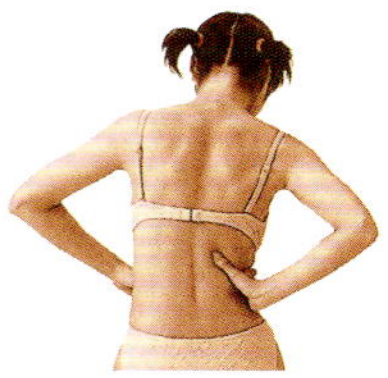

肝俞 用拇指按同侧穴位。

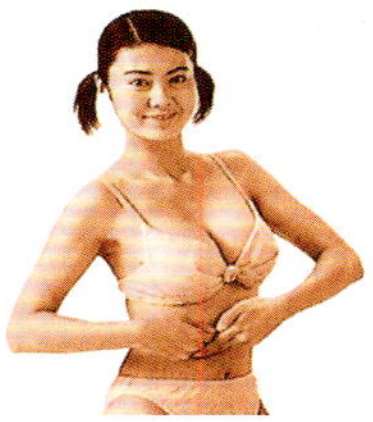

期门 两手中指叠放在穴位上按压。

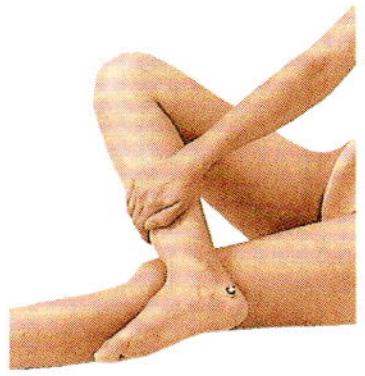

水泉 用艾炷灸，烧至有痛感为止。

11 腰膝寒冷

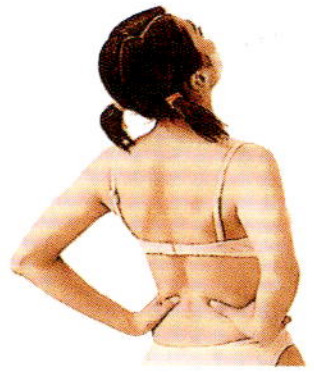

肾俞 两手中指同时按压同侧穴位。

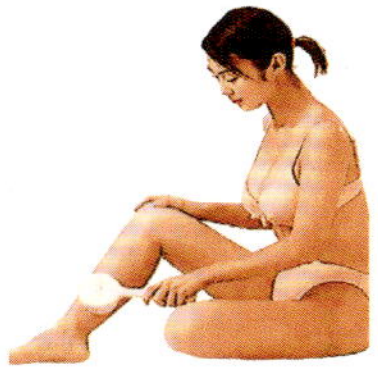

三阴交 用浴刷，以穴位为中心，从下向上在5~10厘米范围上下刷动。

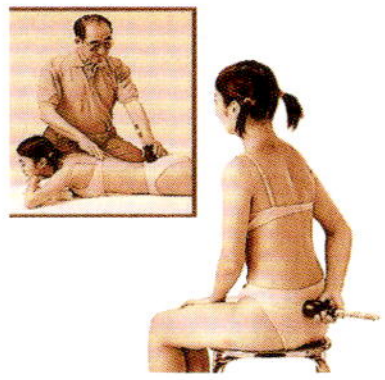

次髎 用温灸器温灸穴位10~20秒，做3~5次。

6 Breast Distention before Menstruation

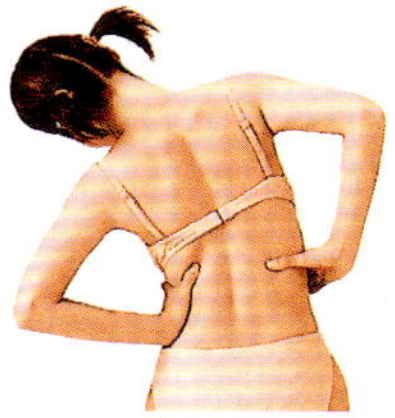

Gānshū(BL18) : Press acupoint in each side with both thumbs.

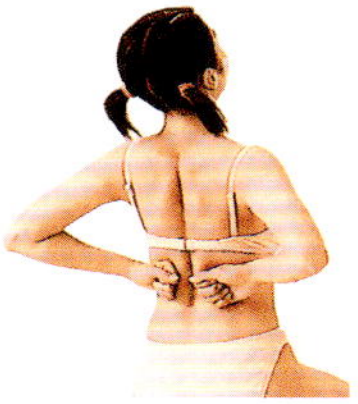

Wèishū(BL21) : Clench the fists, press against the acupoint with the protuberance of the fist.

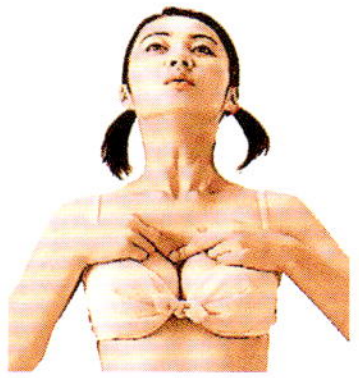

Dànzhōng(CV17) : Press the acupoint with middle fingers.

7 Dysmenorrhea and Irregular Menstruation

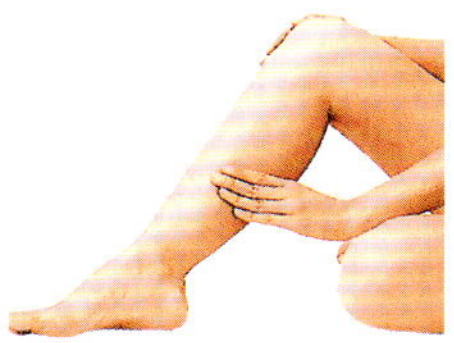

Sānyīnjiāo(SP6) : Use four fingers except the thumb to do flat-pushing from bottom up with the acupoint as the center.

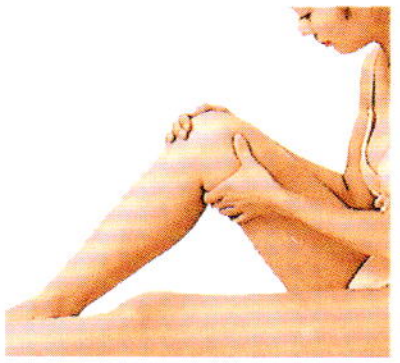

Xuèhǎi(SP10) : Press the acupoint by thumb and massage in small area.

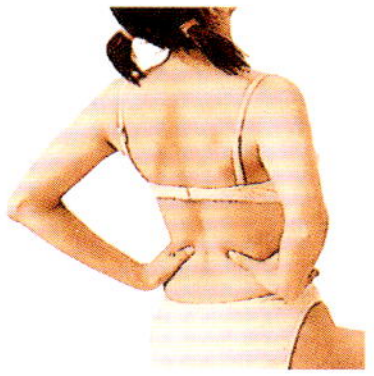

Shènshū(BL23) : Press the acupoint in each side with both thumbs.

8 Hypomenorrhea or Hypermenorrhea

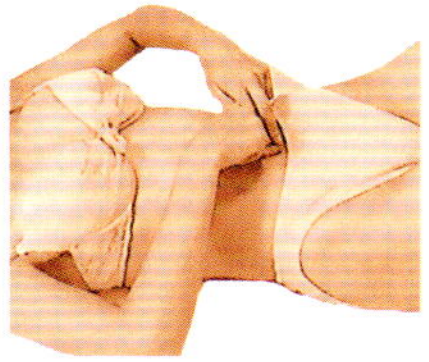

Guānyuán(CV4) : Lie on the back, press with both middle fingers stacked on the acupoint.

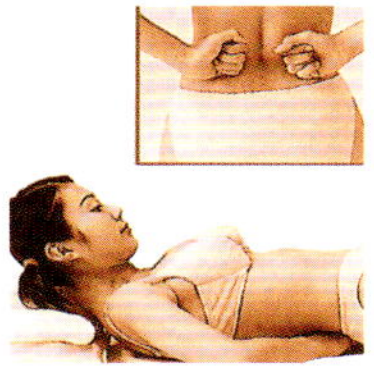

Shènshū(BL23) : Lie on the back, clench the fists, press against the acupoint with the protuberance of the fist, press the acupoints by weight.

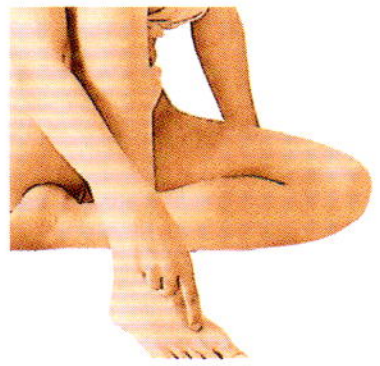

Tàichōng(LR3) : Press acupoint with index finger.

9 Climacteric Syndrome

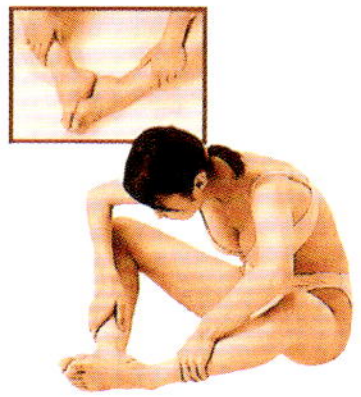

Sānyīnjiāo(SP6) : Press acupoint in each side with both thumbs.

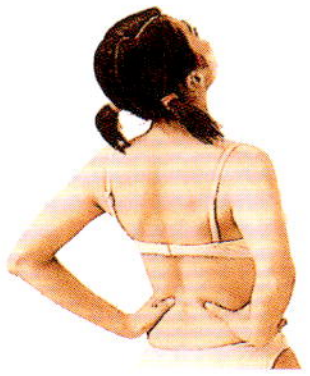

Shènshū(BL23) : Press acupoint in each side with both thumbs.

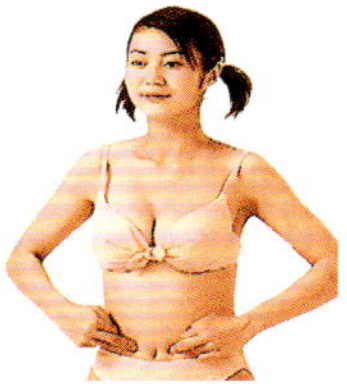

Tiānshū(ST25) : Press acupoint in each side with both middle fingers.

10 Anemia

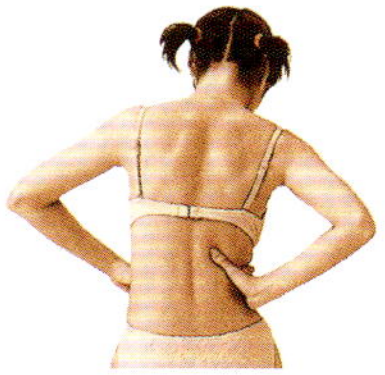

Gānshū(BL18) : Press acupoint by thumb on the same side.

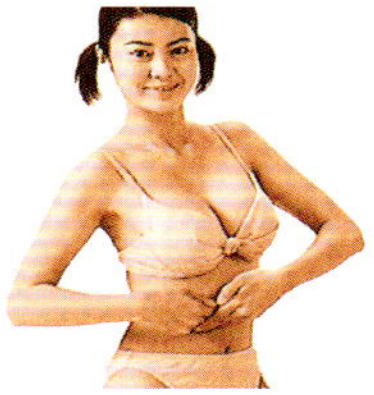

Qīmén(LR14) : Press acupoint with both middle fingers stacked.

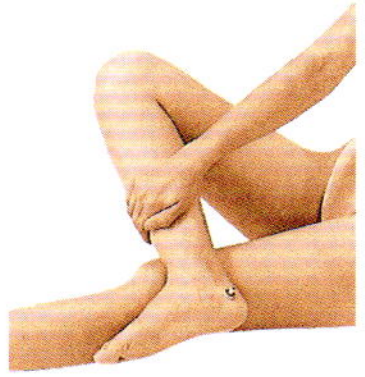

Shuǐquán(KI5) : Burning until there is pain by moxibustion with moxa cone.

11 Coldness in Waist and Knees

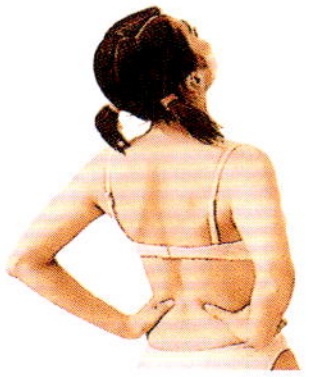

Shènshū(KI16) : Press acupoint in each side with both middle fingers at the same time.

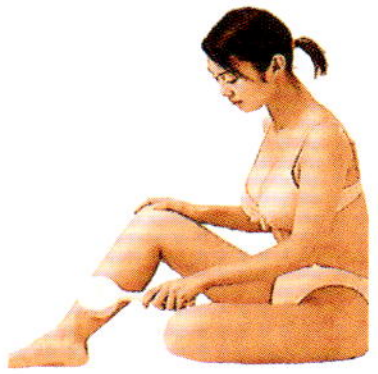

Sānyīnjiāo(SP6) : Brush from bottom to top within 5 to 10 centimeters with the acupoint as the center by brush.

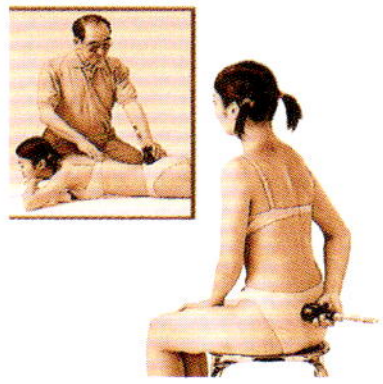

Cìliáo(BL32) : Warm the acupoint with moxa burner 10 to 20 seconds for 3 to 5 times.

12 妊娠反应

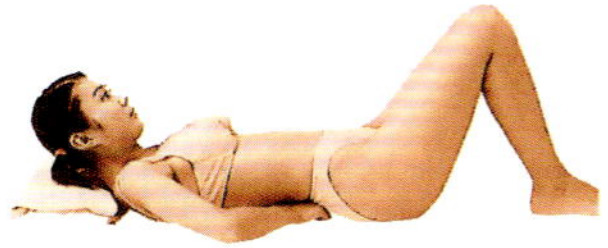

膈俞 仰卧，双手握拳，用拳头突出的关节顶住穴位，利用体重按压穴位。

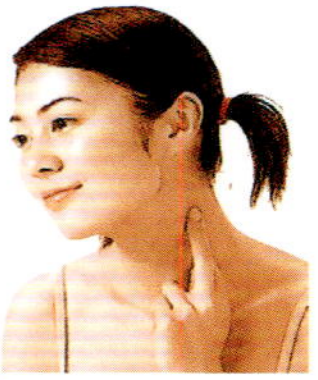

扶突 中指按揉同侧穴位。

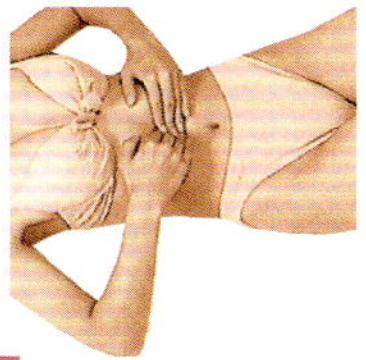

中脘 仰卧，除拇指外四指放在穴位上，做大范围按揉。

13 不孕症

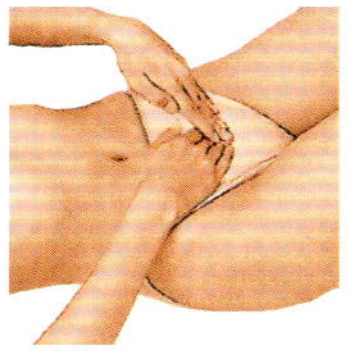

关元 仰卧，用除拇指以外的四指叠放在一起按揉。

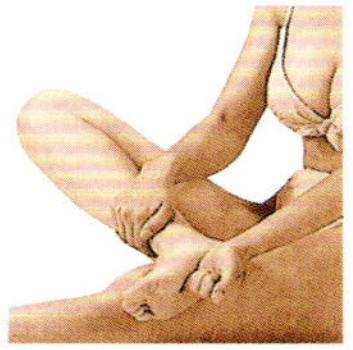

涌泉 握拳，以脉搏的节奏缓慢敲击以对侧穴位为中心的区域 100 次。

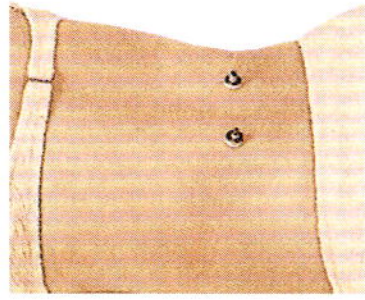

肾俞 在穴位上做艾炷灸，直至烧完。

14 习惯性流产

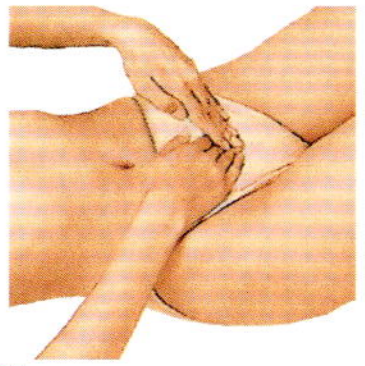

关元 仰卧，用除拇指以外的四指叠放在一起按揉。

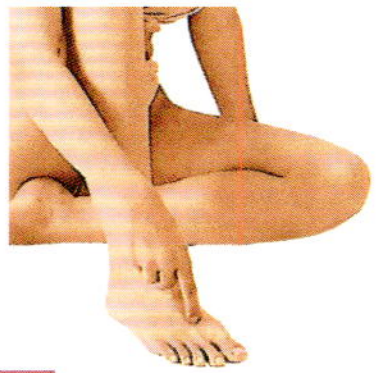

太冲 食指按揉穴位。

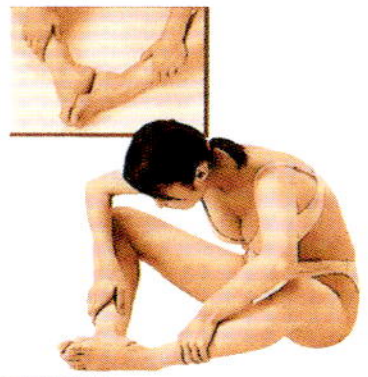

三阴交 两手拇指分别按压同侧穴位。

15 产后腰痛

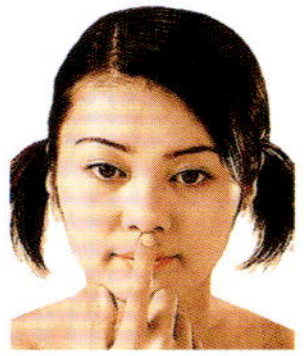

水沟 食指按揉穴位，注意不要用力过大。

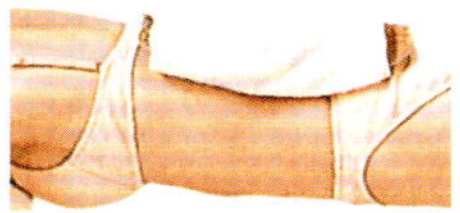

命门 用毛巾包裹住热水袋，平放在腰部进行热敷，每次 8~10 分钟。

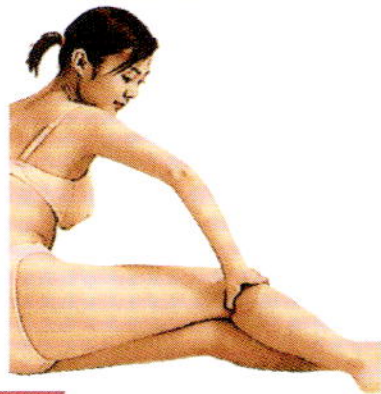

委中 用拇指按压穴位。

16 产后宫缩痛

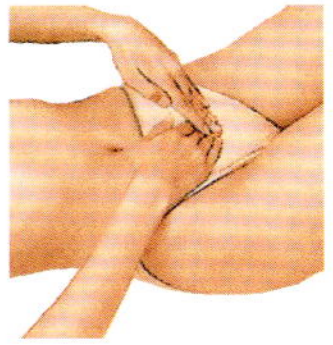

中极 用除拇指外的四指，以穴位为中心顺时针按揉。

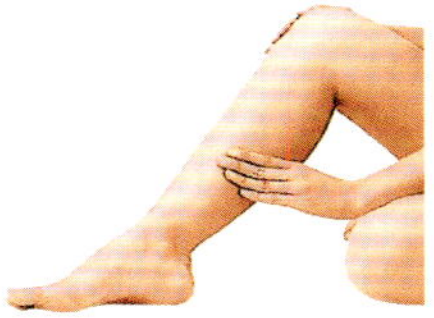

三阴交 用除拇指外的四指，以穴位为中心，从下向上平推。

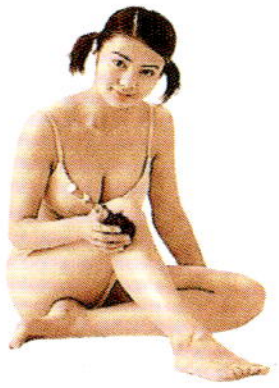

足三里 用带罩的温灸器，将艾条以适宜的温度接近穴位，艾灸 10~20 秒就拿开。

17 母乳不畅

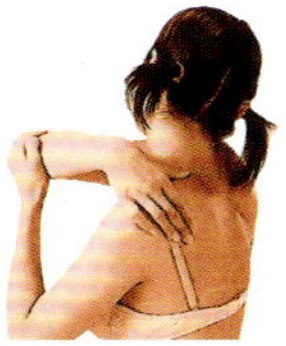

肩井 侧倾颈部的同时，用拇指按压对侧肩部穴位。

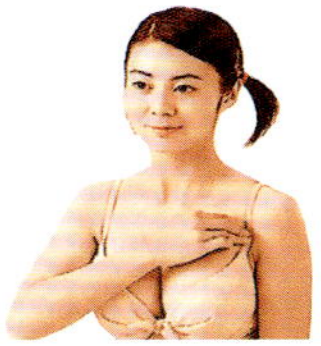

中府 用除拇指外的四指按对侧穴位，做环形按揉。

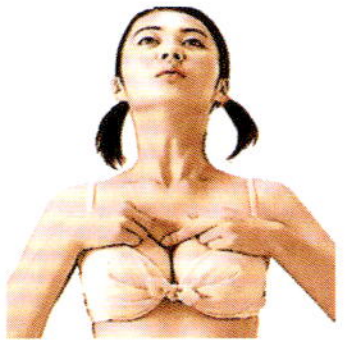

膻中 用中指按压穴位。

12 Pregnancy Reaction

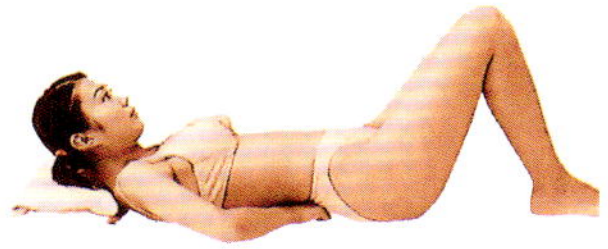
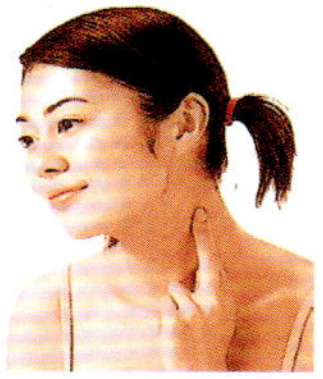
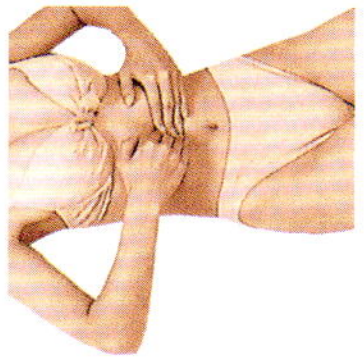

Géshū(BL17) : Lie on the back, clench the fists, press against the acupoint with the protuberance of the fists, press the acupoint by weight.

Fútū(LI18) : Press the acupoint in the same side with the middle finger.

Zhōngwǎn(CV12) : Lie on the back, put four fingers on the acupoint except the thumb and massage on a large area.

13 Sterility

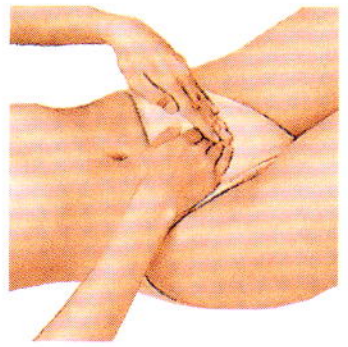
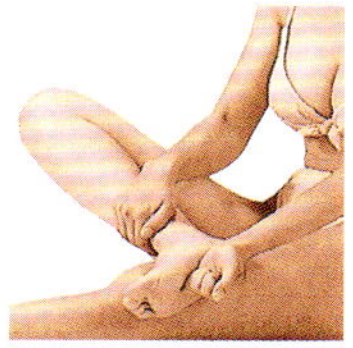
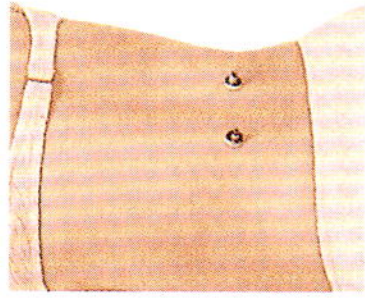

Guānyuán(CV4) : Lie on the back, massage with four fingers stacked except the thumbs.

Yǒngquán(KI1) : Clench the fists, knock slowly on the area with the acupoint on the other side as the center at the speed of pulse for 100 times.

Shènshū(BL23) : Do moxibustion with moxa cone till it burns down.

14 Habitual Abortion

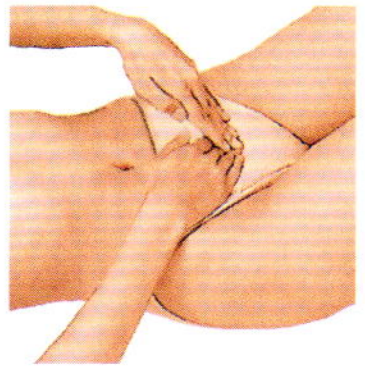
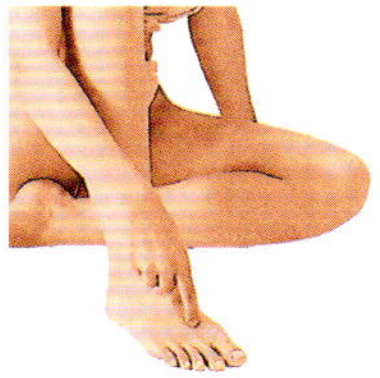
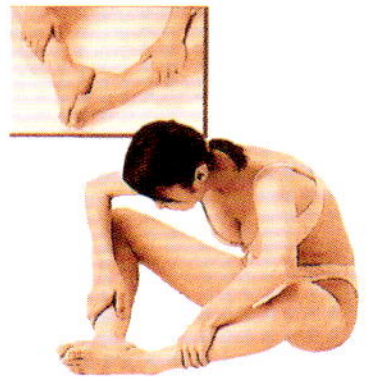

Guānyuán(CV4) : Lie on the back, use four fingers stacked except the thumbs to knead the acupoints.

Tàichōng(LR3) : Press the acupoint with index fingers.

Sānyīnjiāo(SP6) : Press acupoint in each side with both thumbs.

15 Postpartum Lumbago

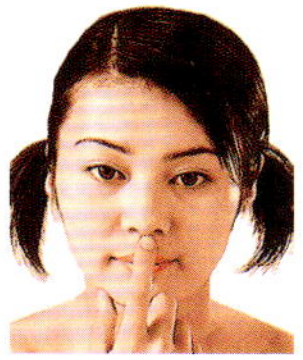
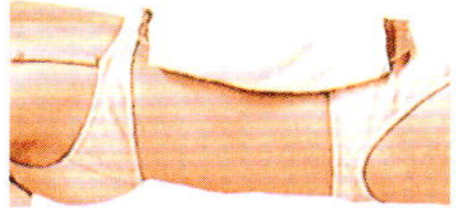
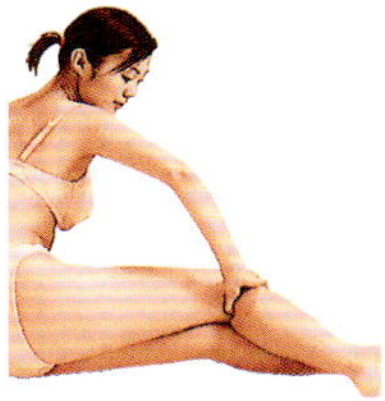

Shuǐgōu(GV26) : Press acupoint with index finger gently.

Mìngmén(GV4) : Wrap the hot water bag with a towel and put it on the waist for 8 to 10 minutes each time.

Wěizhōng(BL40) : Press the acupoint with thumb.

16 Postpartum Uterus Systole Pain

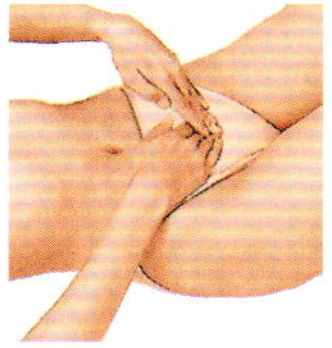
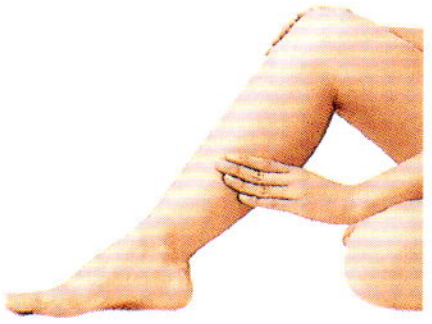
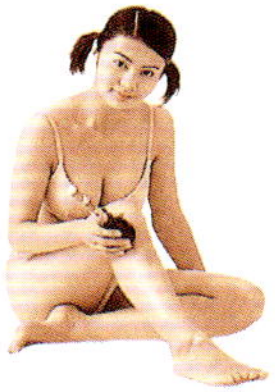

Zhōngjí(CV3) : Massage clockwise with the acupoint as the center with four fingers except the thumb.

Sānyīnjiāo(SP6) : Use four fingers except the thumb, do flat-pushing from bottom to top with the acupoint as the center.

Zúsānlǐ(ST36) : Use the moxa burner with cover to make the moxa stick near the acupoint with the appropriate temperature and move it away after 10 to 20 seconds.

17 Scanty Breast Milk

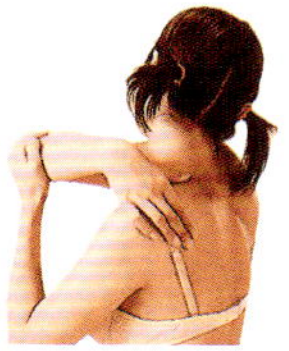
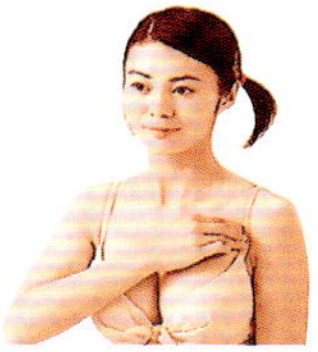
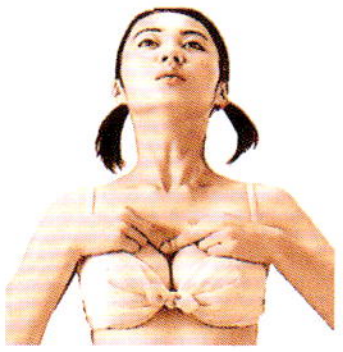

Jiānjǐng(GB21) : Press the acupoint on the shoulder with the thumb on the other side while heeling the neck.

Zhōngfǔ(LU1) : Use four fingers except the thumb to press the acupoint on the other side and knead in a circle.

Dànzhōng(CV17) : Press the acupoint with the middle finger.

18 慢性盆腔炎

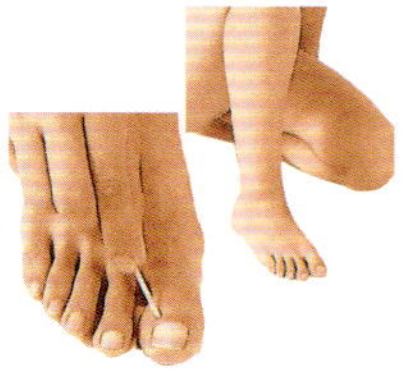

大敦 用牙签粗的一头向趾尖方向轻轻按压刺激穴位。

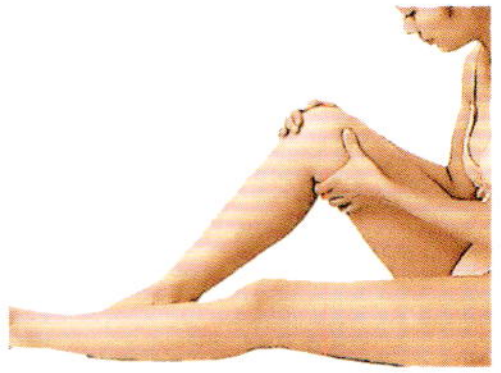

曲泉 屈膝，用拇指做小范围的环形按揉。

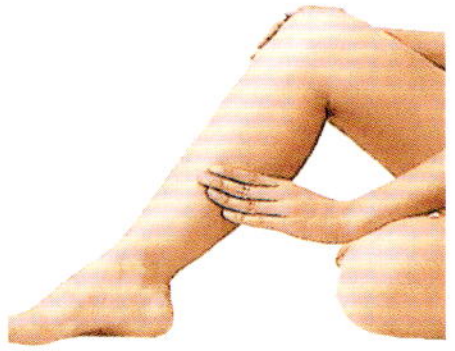

三阴交 用除拇指外的四指，以穴位为中心，从下向上平推。

19 女性复发性尿道炎

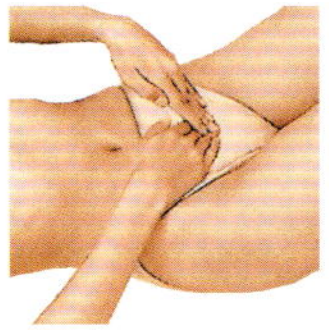

中极 用除拇指外的四指，以穴位为中心顺时针按揉。

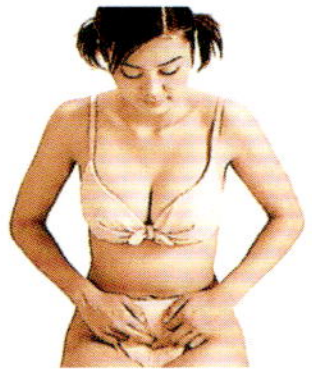

曲骨 用中指按压穴位。

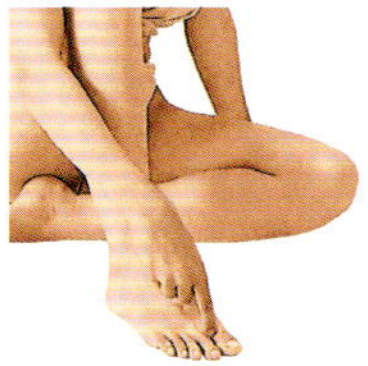

行间 用食指按压同侧穴位。

20 子宫脱垂

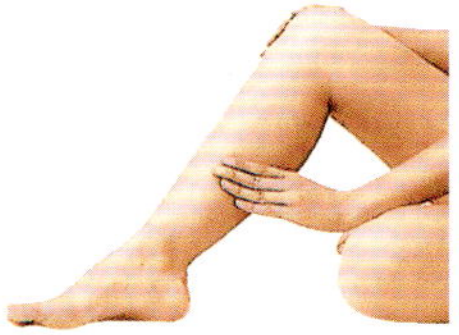

三阴交 用除拇指外的四指，以穴位为中心，从下向上平推。

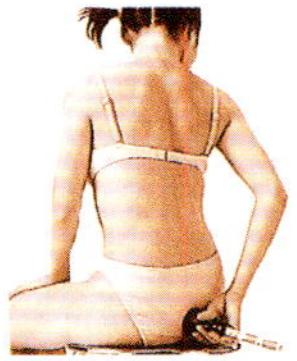

长强 把艾条装入带罩的温灸器中，放到穴位上做艾灸。

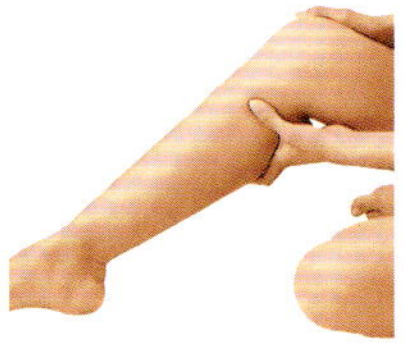

阴陵泉 屈膝，用对侧手拇指按压穴位。

21 子宫后位

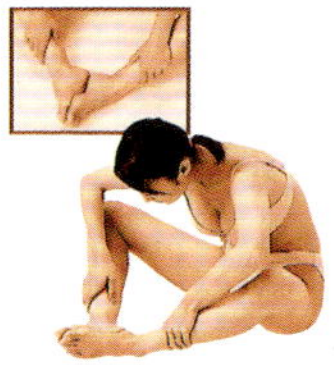

三阴交 用双手拇指同时按压同侧穴位。

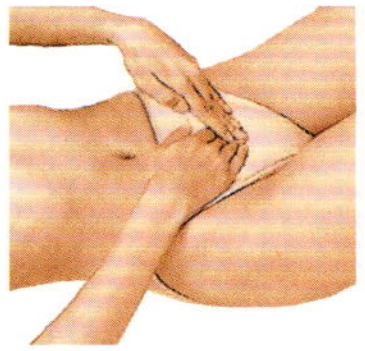

中极 用除拇指外的四指，以穴位为中心顺时针按揉。

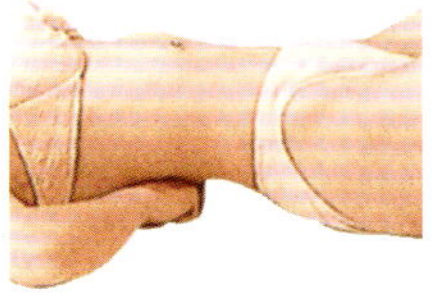

中脘 用艾炷灸至有痛感为止。

22 输卵管炎

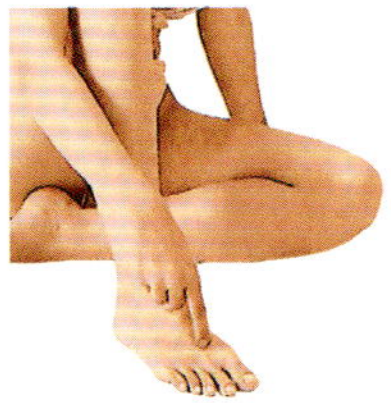

太冲 用食指按揉穴位。

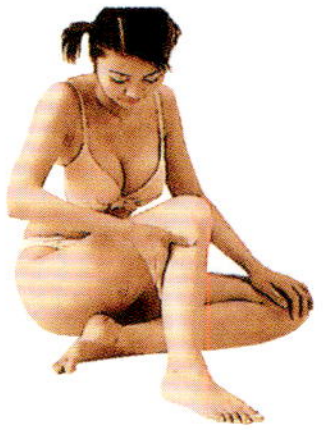

足三里 用拇指按压同侧穴位。

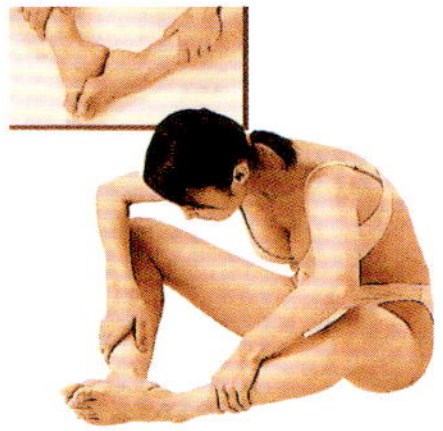

三阴交 用双手拇指同时按压同侧穴位。

23 颈椎劳损

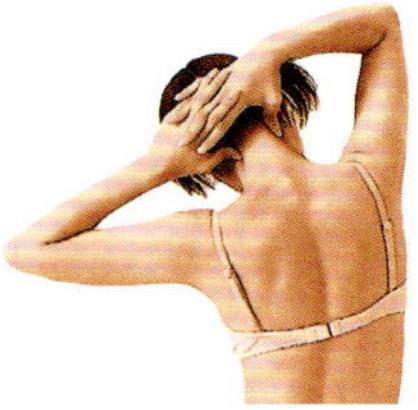

风池 用双手拇指同时按压同侧穴位。

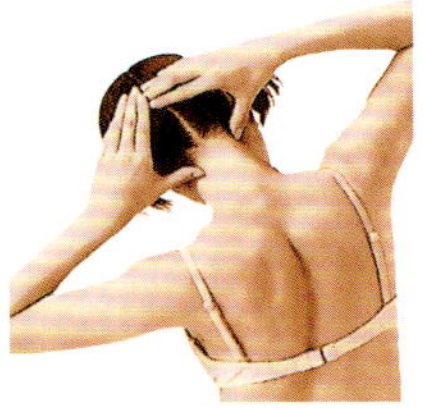

天柱 用双手拇指同时按压同侧穴位。

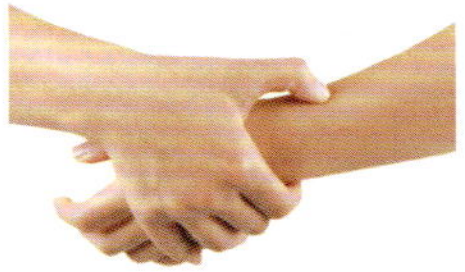

列缺 用拇指按压对侧穴位。

18 Chronic Pelvic Inflammatory Disease

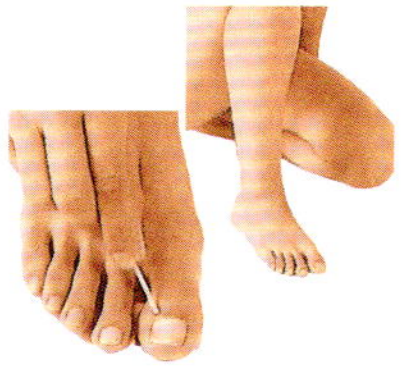

Dàdūn(LR1) : Gently press the acupoint with the thick part of the toothpick in the direction of the toetip.

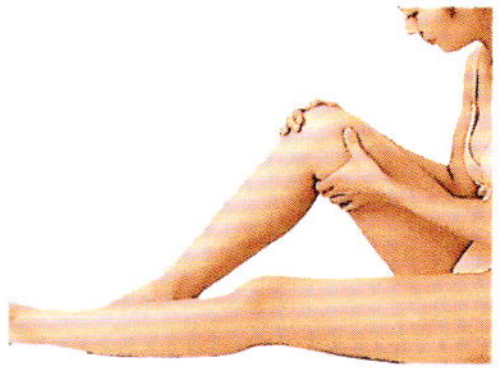

Qūquán(LR8) : Bend the knees, knead in a circle in small area with the thumb.

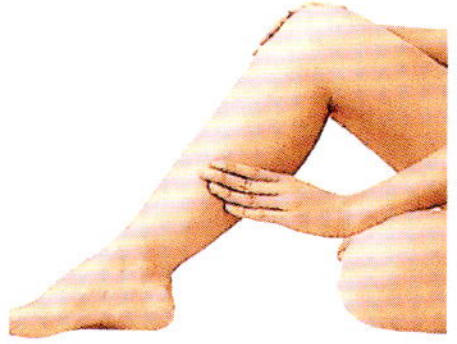

Sānyīnjiāo(SP6) : Use four fingers except the thumb to do flat-pushing from bottom to top with the acupoint as the center.

19 Female Recurrent Urethritis

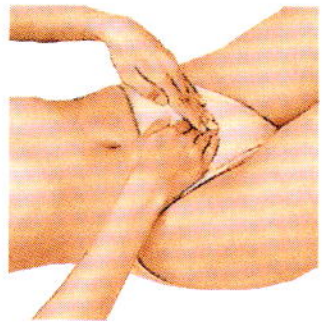

Zhōngjí(CV3) : Use four fingers except the thumb to knead clockwise with the acupoint as the center.

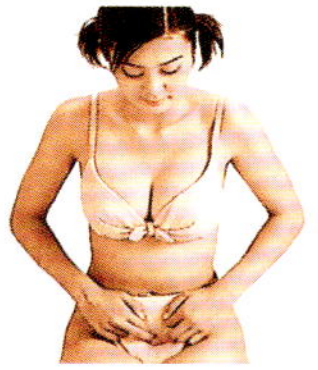

Qūgǔ(CV2) : Press the acupoint with the middle finger.

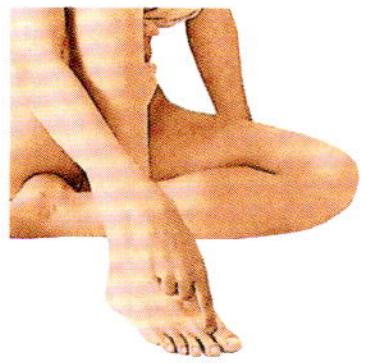

Xíngjiān(LR2) : Press the acupoint with the index finger on the same side.

20 Uterus prolapse

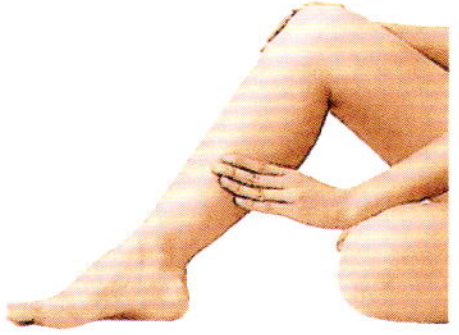

Sānyīnjiāo(SP6) : Use four fingers except the thumb to do flat-pushing from bottom to top with the acupoint as the center.

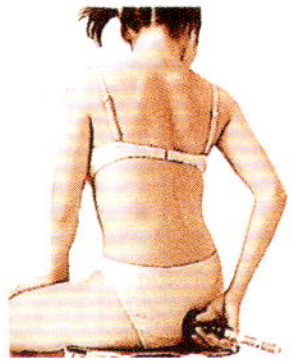

Chángqiáng(GV1) : Put the moxa stick in the moxa burner with cover and put it on the acupoint.

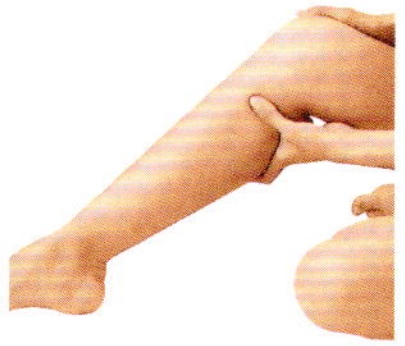

Yīnlíngquán(SP9) : Bend the knee, press the acupoint with the thumb on the other side.

21 Uterus Retroposition

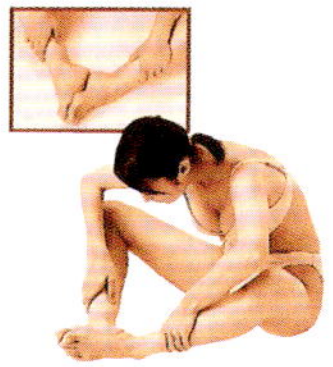

Sānyīnjiāo(SP6) : Press the acupoint with both thumbs on the same side at the same time.

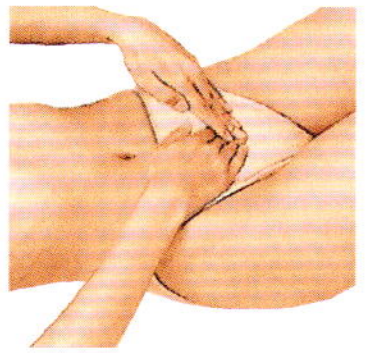

Zhōngjí(CV3): Use four fingers except the thumb, knead clockwise with the acupoint as the center.

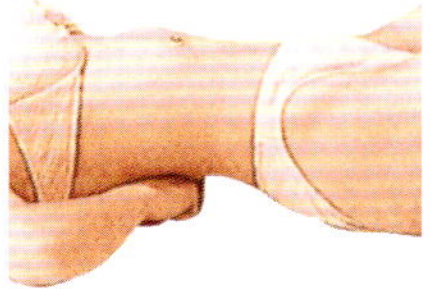

Zhōngwǎn(CV12) : Use the moxa cone till you feel a little bit pain.

22 Salpingitis

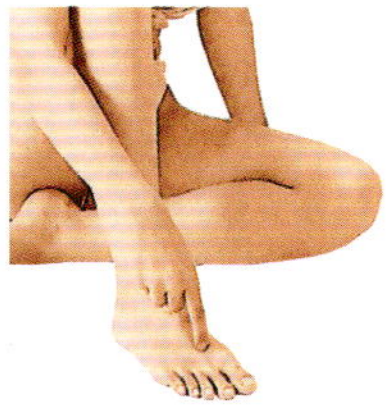

Tàichōng(LR3) : Knead the acupoint with the index finger.

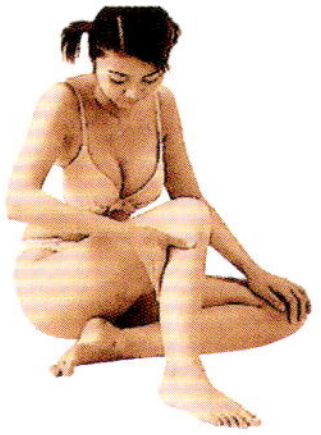

Zúsānlǐ(ST36) : Press the acupoint with the thumb on the same side.

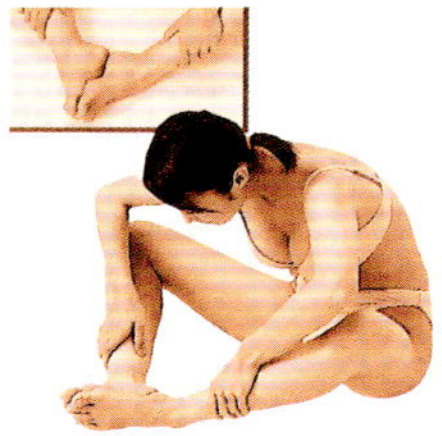

Sānyīnjiāo(SP6) : Press the acupoint with both thumbs on the same side at the same time.

23 Cervical Vertebra Strain

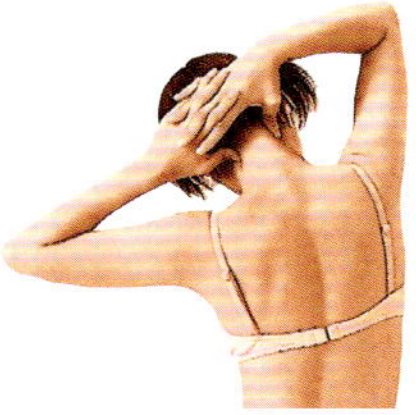

Fēngchí(GB20) : Press the acupoint with both thumbs on the same side at the same time.

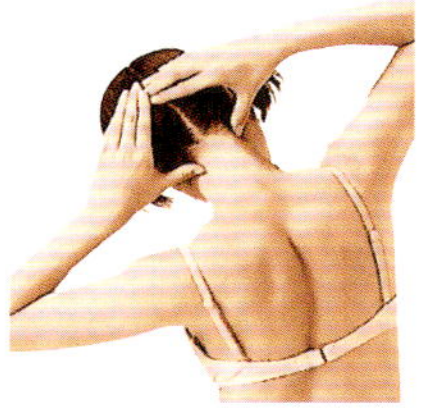

Tiānzhù(BL10) : Press the acupoint with both thumbs on the same side at the same time.

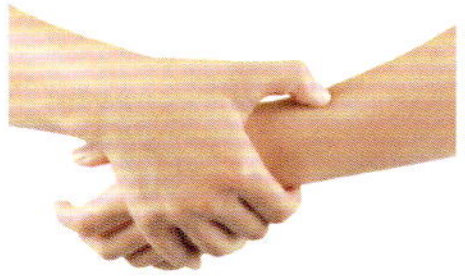

Lièquē(LU7) : Press the acupoint with the thumb on the other side.

24 落枕

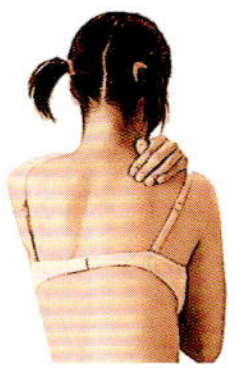

肺俞 用中指按揉对侧穴位。

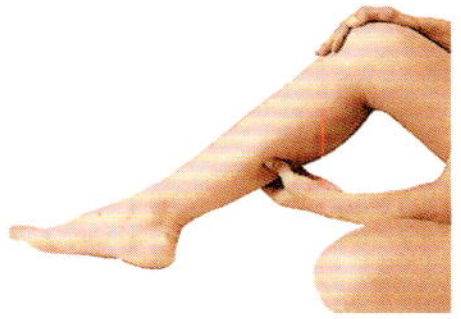

承筋 用拇指按压穴位，做大范围的环形按揉。

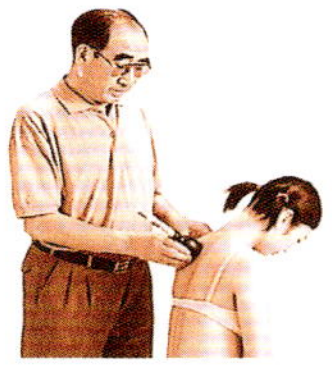

身柱 温灸器放到穴位上加热，感到烫就拿开，反复做。

25 肩周炎

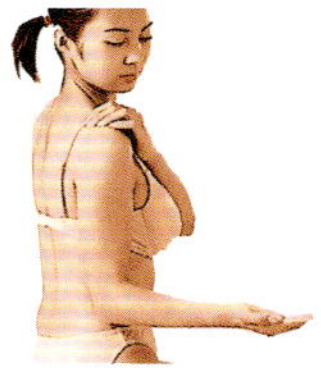

巨骨 用中指按揉对侧穴位。

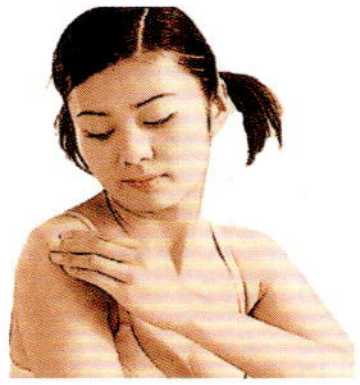

肩髃 用除拇指外的四指按对侧穴位，做大范围的环形按揉。

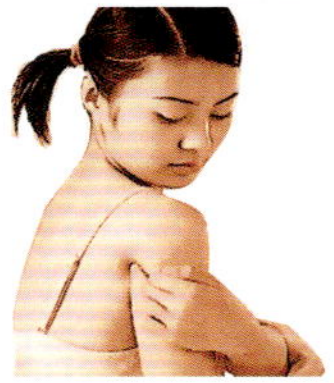

肩贞 用中指按摩对侧穴位，做小范围按揉。

26 腰背痛（骨质疏松）

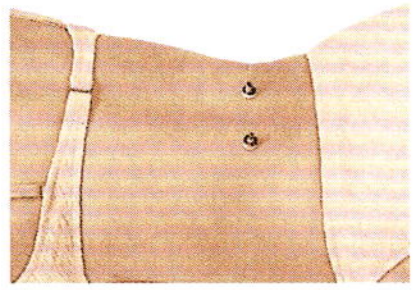

肾俞 在穴位上做艾炷，每次灸感到烫就拿掉，注意不要烫伤，连续做3~5次。

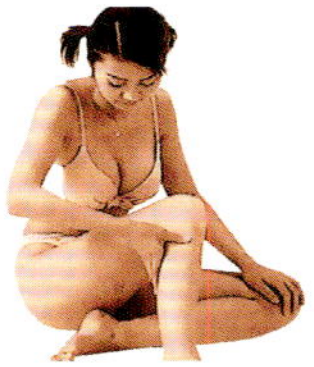

足三里 用拇指按压同侧穴位。

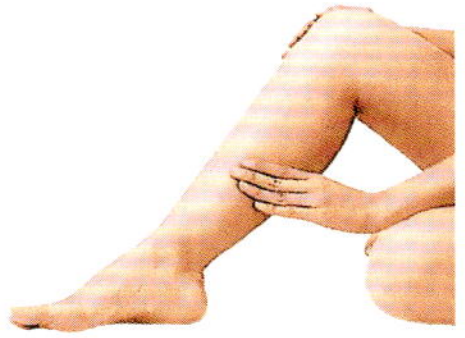

三阴交 用除拇指外的四指，以穴位为中心，从下向上平推。

27 失眠

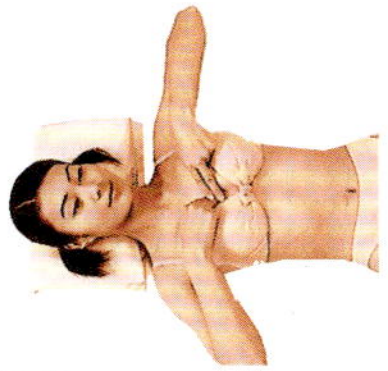

膻中 用中指按揉穴位。

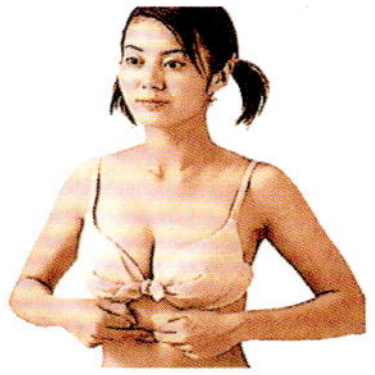

巨阙 用中指按揉穴位。

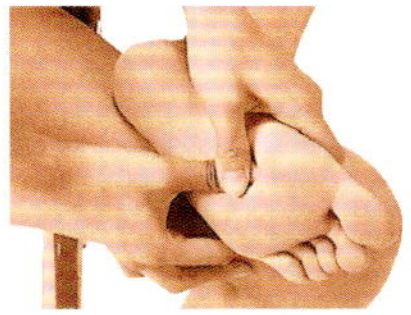

涌泉 拇指垂直按压穴位，做小范围按揉。

28 头痛、头重

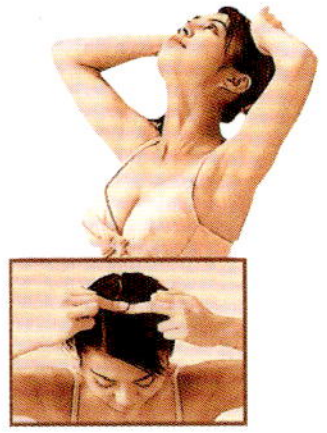

百会 两手中指叠放在穴位上按压。

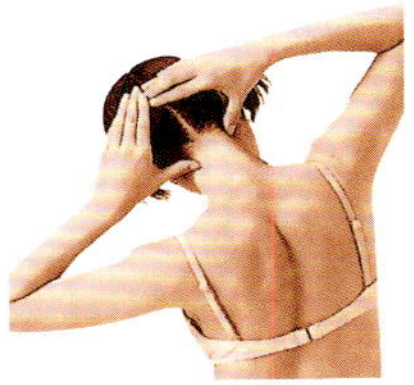

天柱 两拇指分别按同侧穴位，其余四指支撑头部。

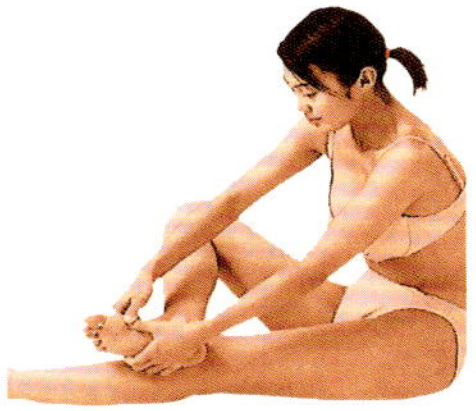

太白 两拇指叠放在穴位上按揉穴位。

29 头晕目眩

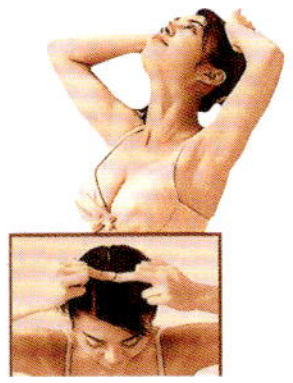

百会 用双手中指叠放在穴位上按压。

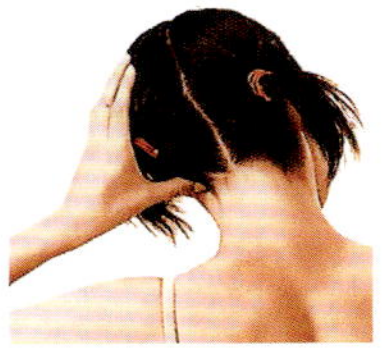

风池 用拇指按压同侧穴位。

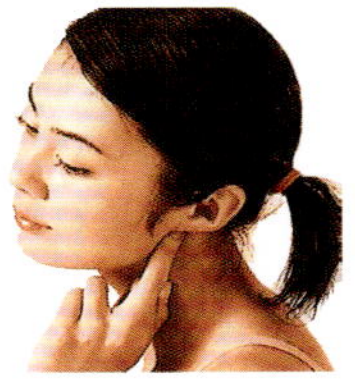

翳风 用中指按压同侧穴位。

24 Stiff Neck

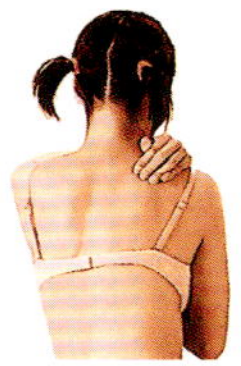

Fèishū(BL13) : Massage the acupoint with the middle finger on the other side.

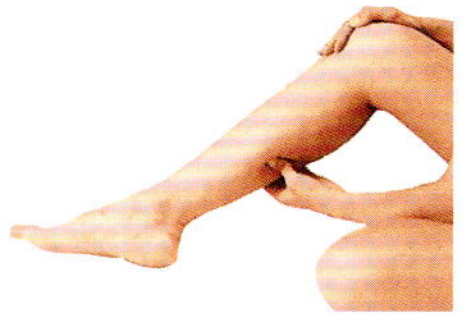

Chéngjīn(BL56) : Press the acupoint with the thumb and knead in a large area in a circle.

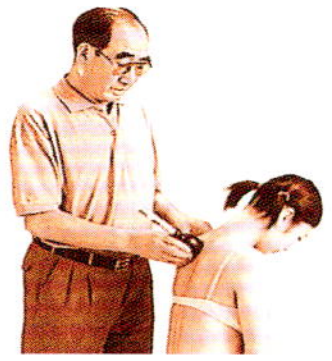

Shēnzhù(GV12) : Put the moxa burner on the acupoint and remove it when you feel hot, do it repeatedly.

25 Shoulder Periarthritis

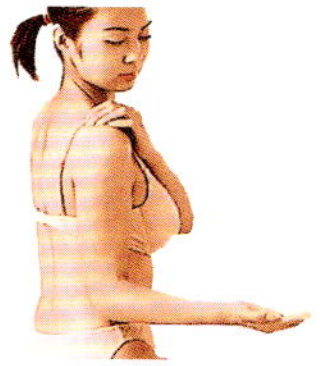

Jùgǔ(LI16) : Knead the acupoint with the middle finger on the other side.

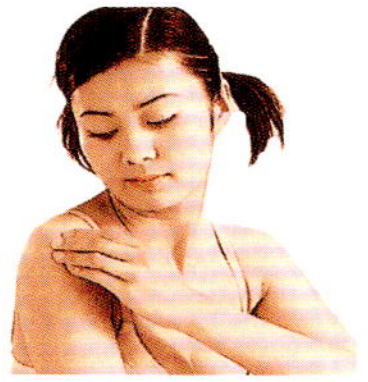

Jiānyú(LI15) : Use four fingers except the thumb to knead the acupoint in the other side and massage in a large area in a circle.

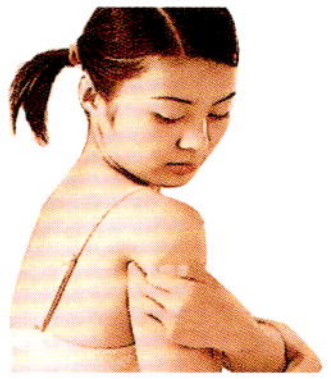

Jiānzhēn(SI9) : Use middle finger to massage the acupoint in the other side in a small area.

26 Lumbago and Back Pain (Osteoporosis)

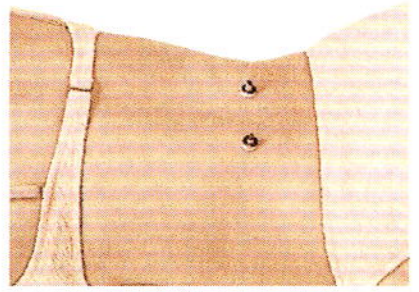

Shènshū(BL23) : Use moxa cone on the acupoint and remove it when you feel hot. Beware of empyrosis, do it for three to five times.

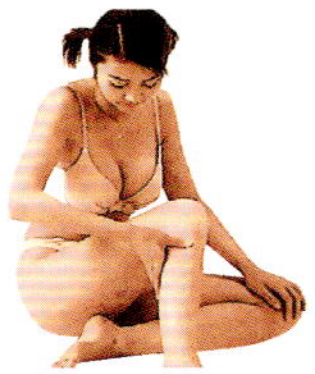

Zúsānlǐ(ST36) : Press the acupoint with thumb on the same side.

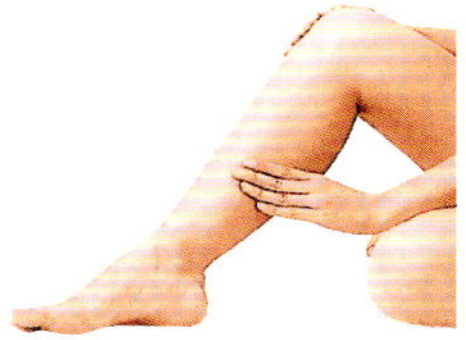

Sānyīnjiāo(SP6) : Use four fingers except the thumb to do flat-pushing from bottom with the acupoint as the center.

27 Insomnia

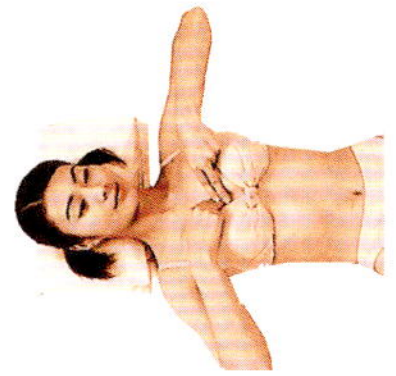

Dànzhōng(CV17) : Knead the acupoint with the middle finger.

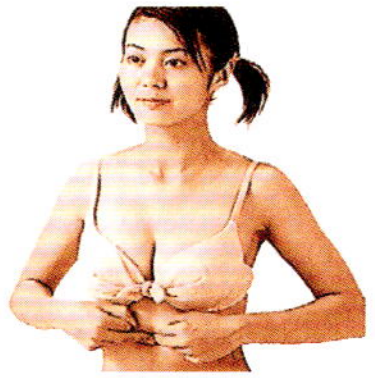

Jùquè(CV14) : Knead the acupoint with the middle finger.

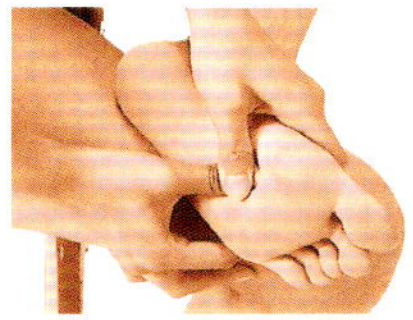

Yǒngquán(KI1) : Press the acupoint with the thumb vertically and massage in a small area.

28 Headache and Heavy Sensation of Head

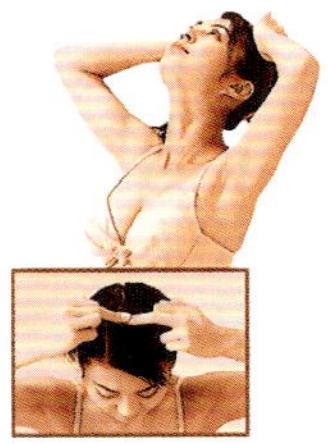

Bǎihuì(GV20): Press the acupoint with both middle fingers stacked.

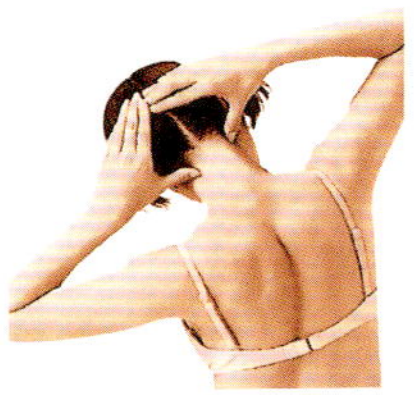

Tiānzhù(BL10) : Press the acupoint with the thumb on the same side and use the other four fingers to support the head.

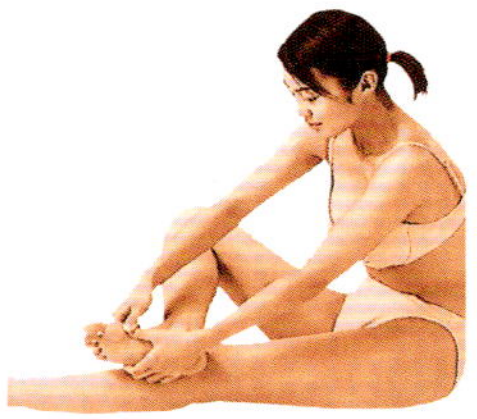

Tàibái(SP3): Press the acupoint with two thumbs stacked.

29 Dizziness

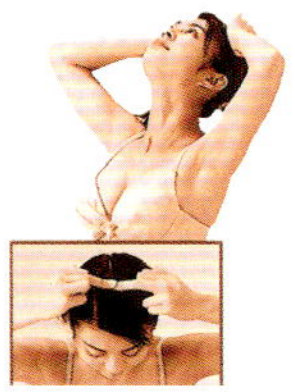

Bǎihuì(GV20) : Press the acupoint with both middle fingers stacked.

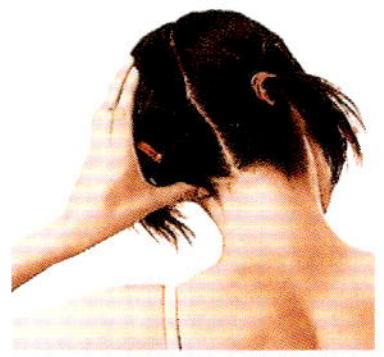

Fēngchí(GB20) : Press the acupoint with thumb on the same side.

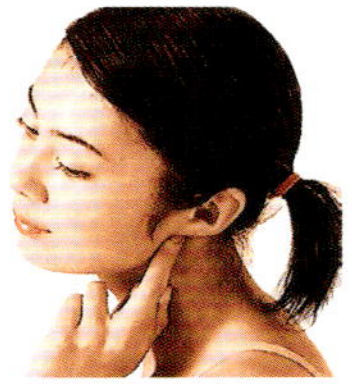

Yìfēng(TE17) : Press the acupoint with middle fingers on the same side.

30 体质虚弱

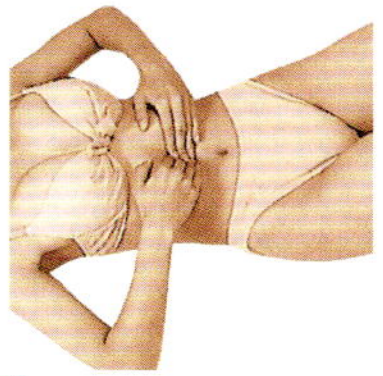
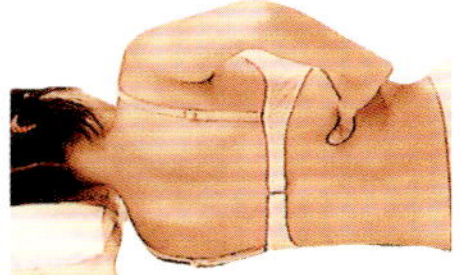
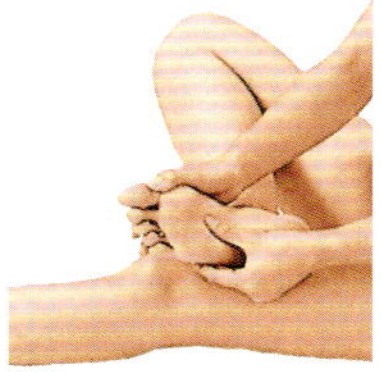

中脘 用除拇指外的四指小范围按揉穴位。

胃俞 侧卧，用上方手按压同侧穴位。

涌泉 一手固定足背，另一手拇指按压穴位，做小范围按揉。

31 牙痛

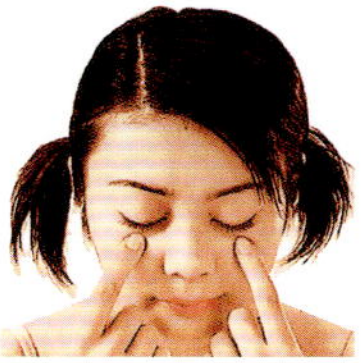
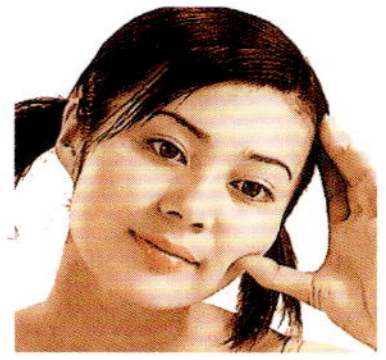
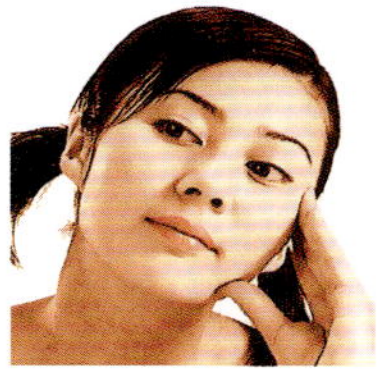

四白 双手食指同时按压同侧穴位。

下关 用拇指由下向上顶压穴位。

大迎 用拇指按压同侧穴位。

32 口臭

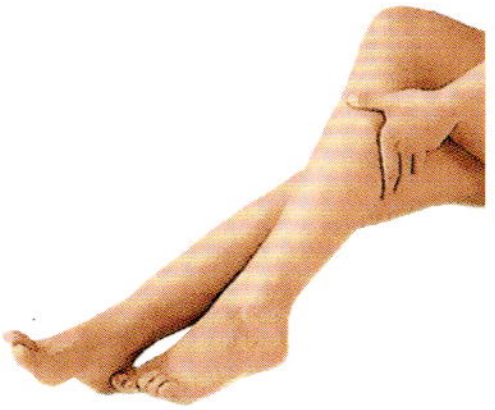
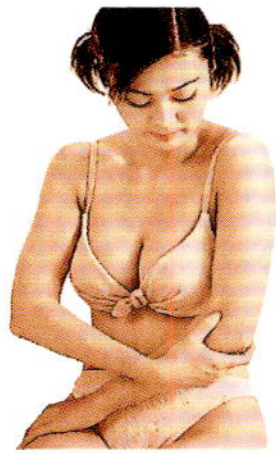
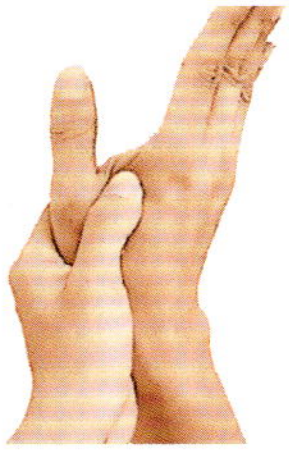

足三里 用拇指指腹按揉穴位。

曲池 拇指按揉对侧穴位。

合谷 从穴位处向食指侧用力按压。

33 慢性咽炎

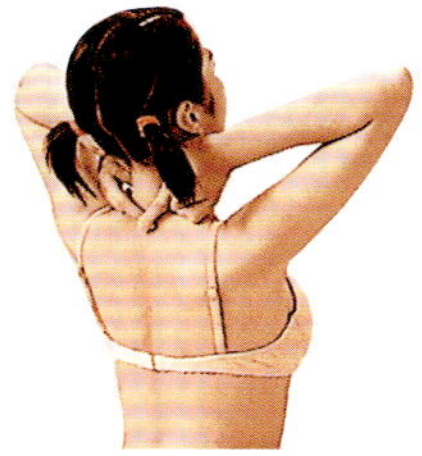
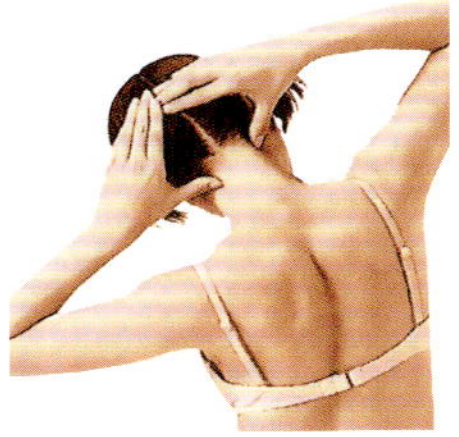
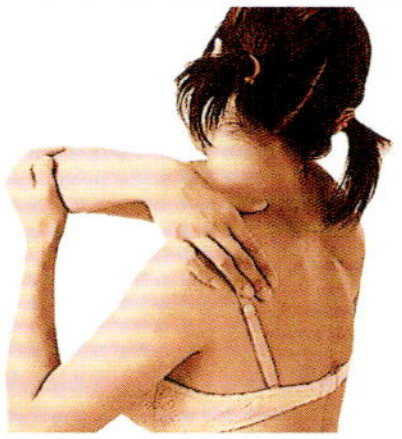

大椎 用两手中指叠放在穴位上按压。

天柱 两手拇指同时按压同侧穴位。

肩井 拇指按压对侧穴位。

34 面瘫（贝尔麻痹）

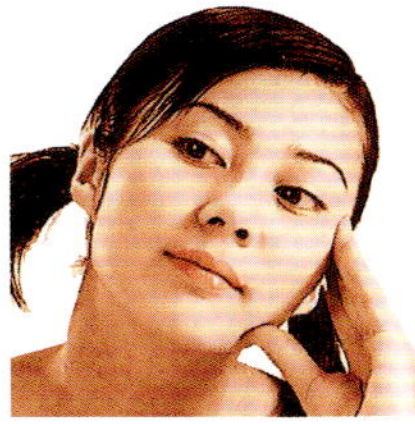
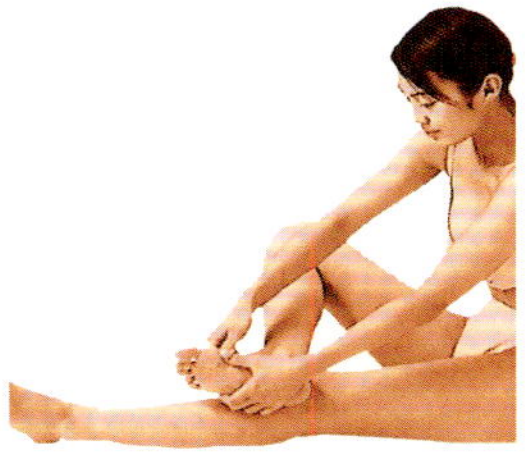
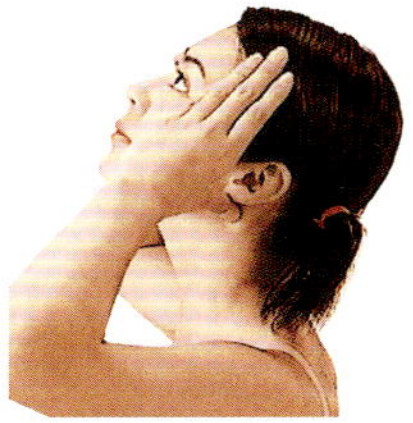

大迎 用拇指按压同侧穴位。

太白 用双手拇指叠放在穴位上按揉。

翳风 两手拇指同时按压同侧穴位。

35 便秘

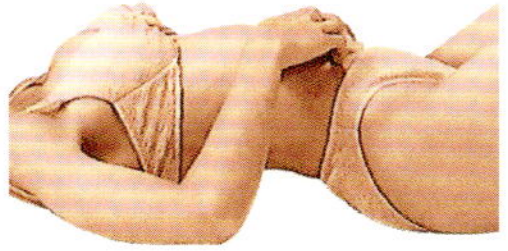
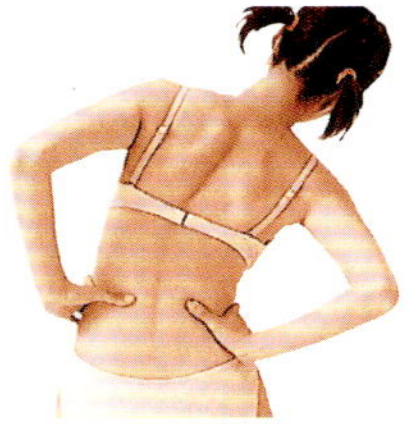
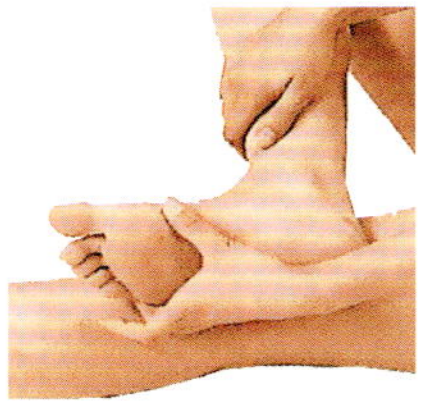

大巨 仰卧、屈膝。两手中指分别按同侧穴位。

大肠俞 两手拇指分别按同侧穴位。

太白 以穴位为中心，从足趾向脚踝方向缓慢地平推。

30 Weak Constitution

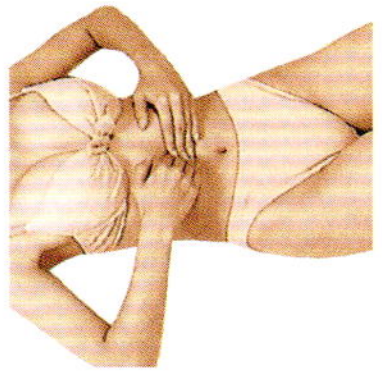

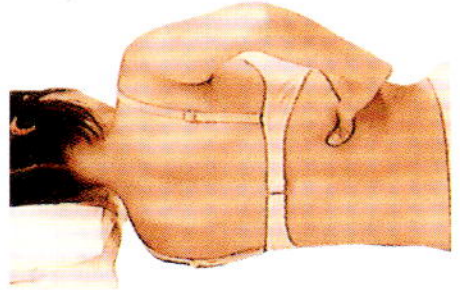

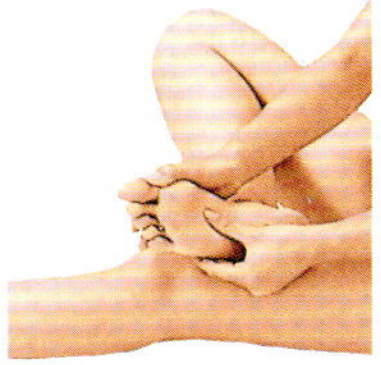

Zhōngwǎn(CV12) : Use four fingers except the thumb to knead the acupoint in a small area.

Wèishū(BL21) : Lie on the side and press the acupoint with the hand above the body.

Yǒngquán(KI1) : One hand holds the foot and the thumb of the other hand presses the acupoint and kneads in a small area.

31 Toothache

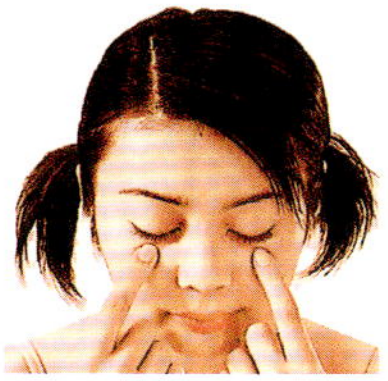

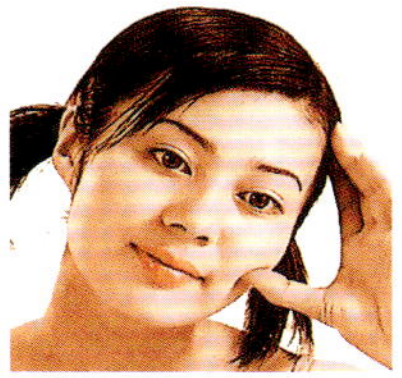

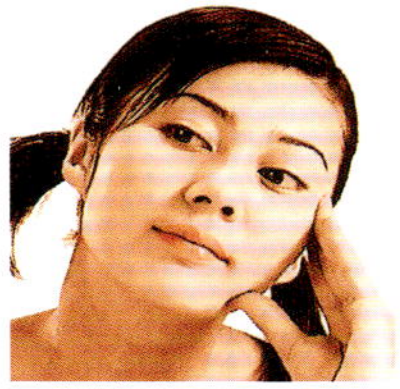

Sìbái(ST2) : Press acupoint in each side with index fingers on the same side at the same time.

Xiàguān(ST7) : Use the thumb to press against the acupoint from bottom to up.

Dàyíng(ST5) : Press the acupoint with thumb on the same side.

32 Halitosis

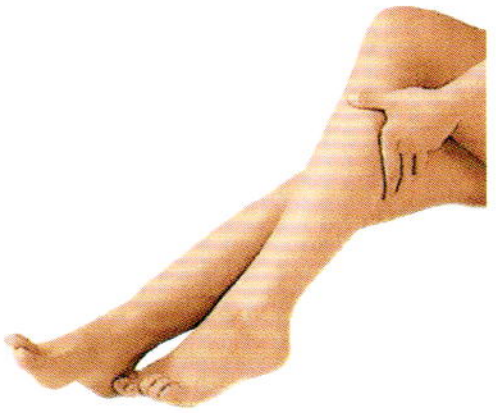

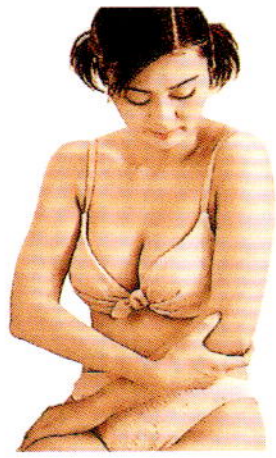

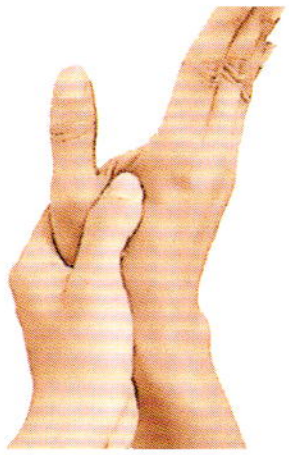

Zúsānlǐ(ST36) : Press acupoint with the finger palm of the thumb.

Qūchí(LI11) : Press and knead acupoint with thumb on the other side.

Hégǔ(LI4) : Press hard from the acupoint to the side of the index finger.

33 Chronic Pharyngitis

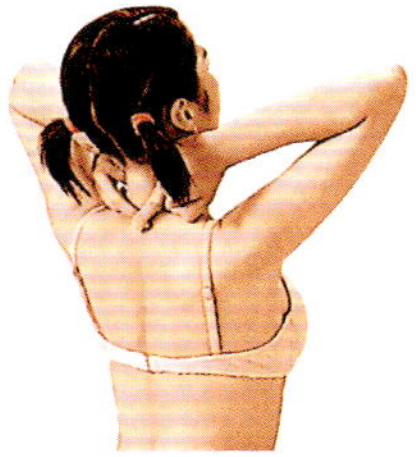

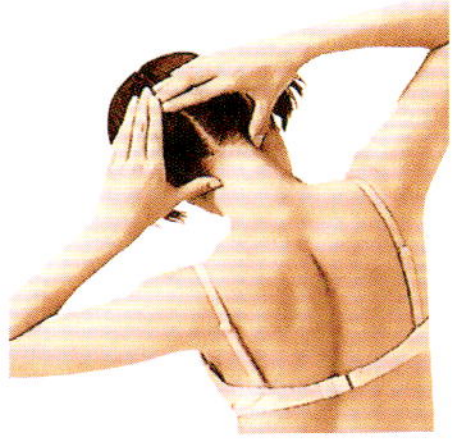

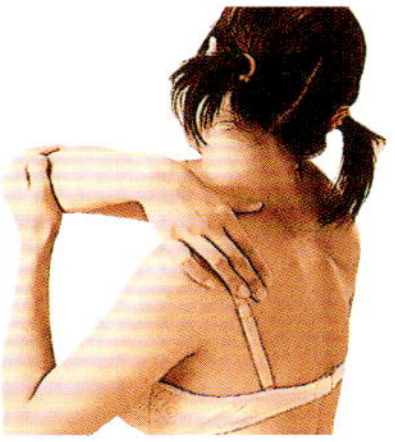

Dàzhuī(GV14) : Press with two middle fingers stacked on the acupoint.

Tiānzhù(BL10) : Press acupoint in each side with thumb on the same side at the same time.

Jiānjǐng(GB21) : Press acupoint with thumb on the other side.

34 Facial Paralysis (Bell's Palsy)

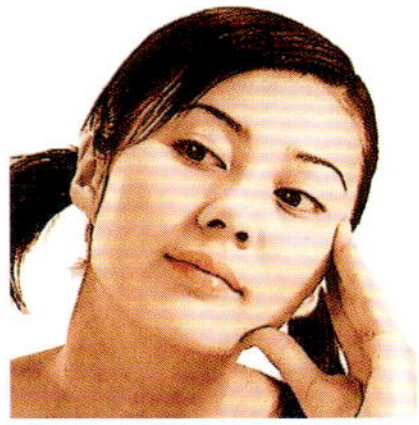

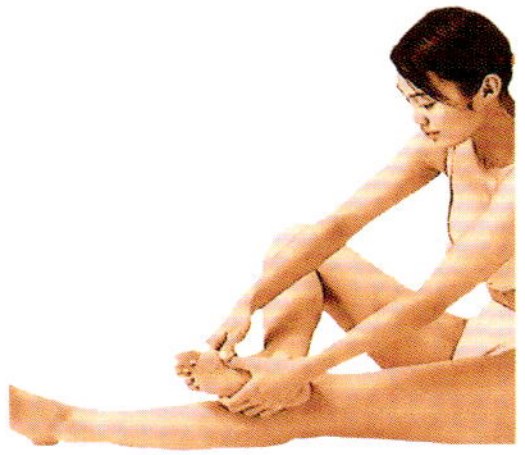

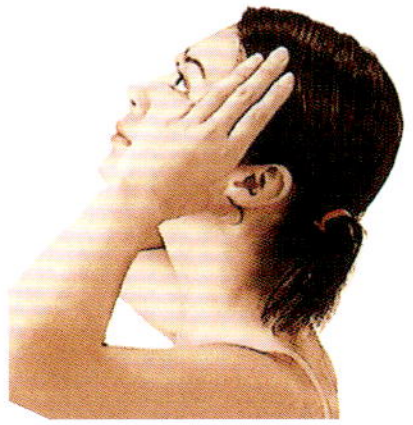

Dàyíng(ST5) : Press acupoint with thumbs on the same side.

Tàibái(SP3) : Massage with two thumbs stacked on the acupoint.

Yìfēng(TE17) : Press acupoint in each side with thumb on the same side at the same time.

35 Constipation

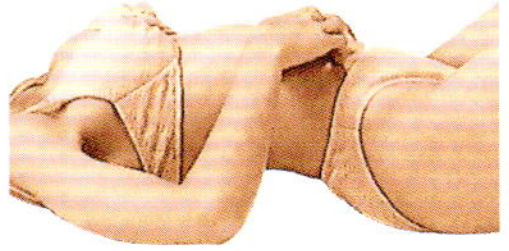

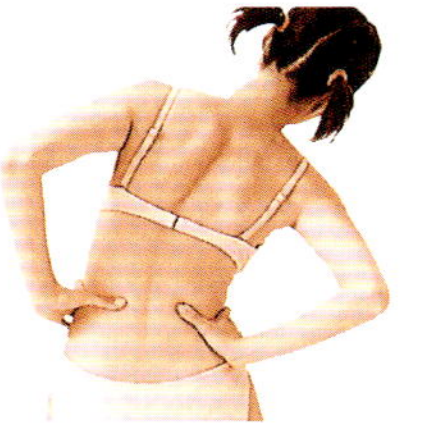

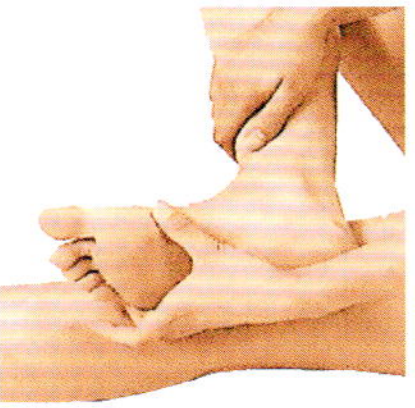

Dàjù(ST27) : Lie on the back, bend knees and press acupoint in each side with middle fingers on the same side.

Dàchángshū(BL25) : Press acupoint in each side with thumb on the same side.

Tàibái(SP3) : Do flat-pushing from the toe to the ankle with the acupoint as the center.

附录　经外奇穴图解

Appendix: Diagrams of Extra Points

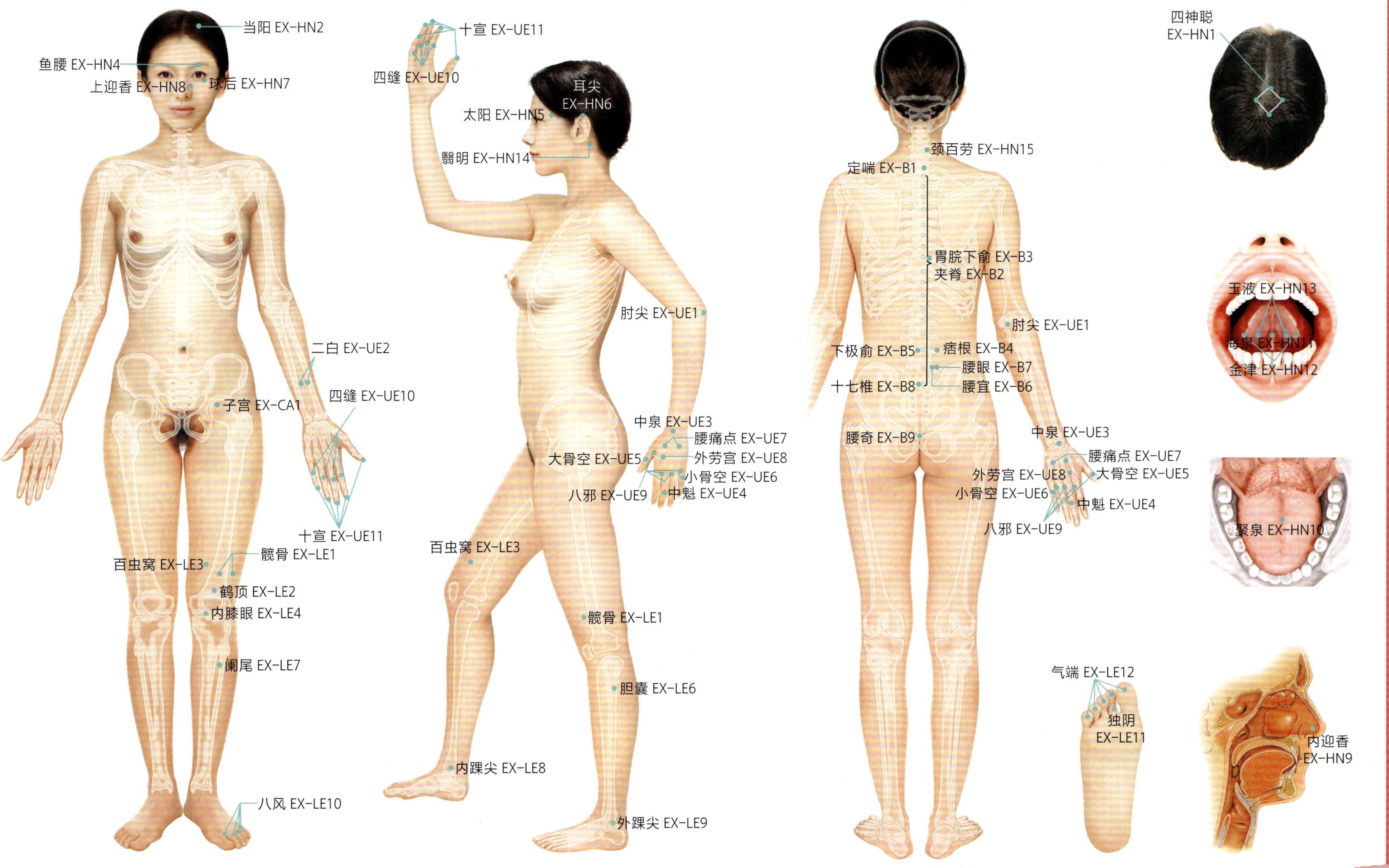

EX-HN	穴名	主 治
1	四神聪	头痛、眩晕、失眠、健忘、癫痫、痴呆
2	当阳	偏、正头痛，眩晕，目赤肿痛
4	鱼腰	目赤肿痛、目翳、眼睑下垂、眼睑痉挛、眉棱骨痛、高血压
5	太阳	头痛、目疾、牙痛、面痛、头晕、神经衰弱、假性近视
6	耳尖	目赤肿痛、目翳、睑腺炎、咽喉肿痛
7	球后	目疾
8	上迎香	鼻塞、鼻窦炎、目赤肿痛、迎风流泪、头痛
9	内迎香	鼻疾、目赤肿痛
10	聚泉	舌强、舌缓、食不知味、2 型糖尿病、气喘
11	海泉	舌体肿胀、舌缓不收、2 型糖尿病
12	金津	舌强不语、舌肿、口疮、呕吐、2 型糖尿病
13	玉液	舌强不语、舌肿、口疮、呕吐、2 型糖尿病
14	翳明	目疾、耳鸣、失眠、头痛
15	颈百劳	颈项强痛、咳嗽、气喘、潮热、盗汗

EX-HN	Acupoints	Indications
1	Sìshéncōng	Headache; dizziness; insomnia; forgetfulness; epilepsy; dementia
2	Dāngyáng	Migraine; headache; dizziness; redness and swelling of eyes
4	Yúyāo	Swelling and pain of eye; nephelium; blepharoptosis; blepharospasm; forehead pain, hypertension
5	Tàiyáng	Headache; eye diseases; toothache; facial pain; dizziness; neurasthenia; pseudo-myopia
6	Ěrjiān	Redness, swelling and pain of eye; nephelium; hordeolum; swollen sore throat
7	Qiúhòu	Eye diseases
8	Shàngyíngxiāng	Rhinobyon; nasosinusitis; swelling and pain of eye; epiphora induced by wind; headache
9	Nèiyíngxiāng	Nose diseases; redness, swelling and pain of eyes
10	Jùquán	Stiff tongue; slack tongue; inability to taste food; type 2 diabetes; asthma
11	Hǎiquán	Swelling of the tongue body; flaccid tongue; type 2 diabetes
12	Jīnjīn	Aphasia due to stiff tongue; paraglossa; aphtha; vomiting; type 2 diabetes
13	Yùyè	Aphasia due to stiff tongue; paraglossa; aphtha; vomiting; type 2 diabetes
14	Yìmíng	Eye diseases; tinnitus; insomnia; headache
15	Jìngbǎiláo	Neck pain; cough; asthma; tidal fever, night sweat

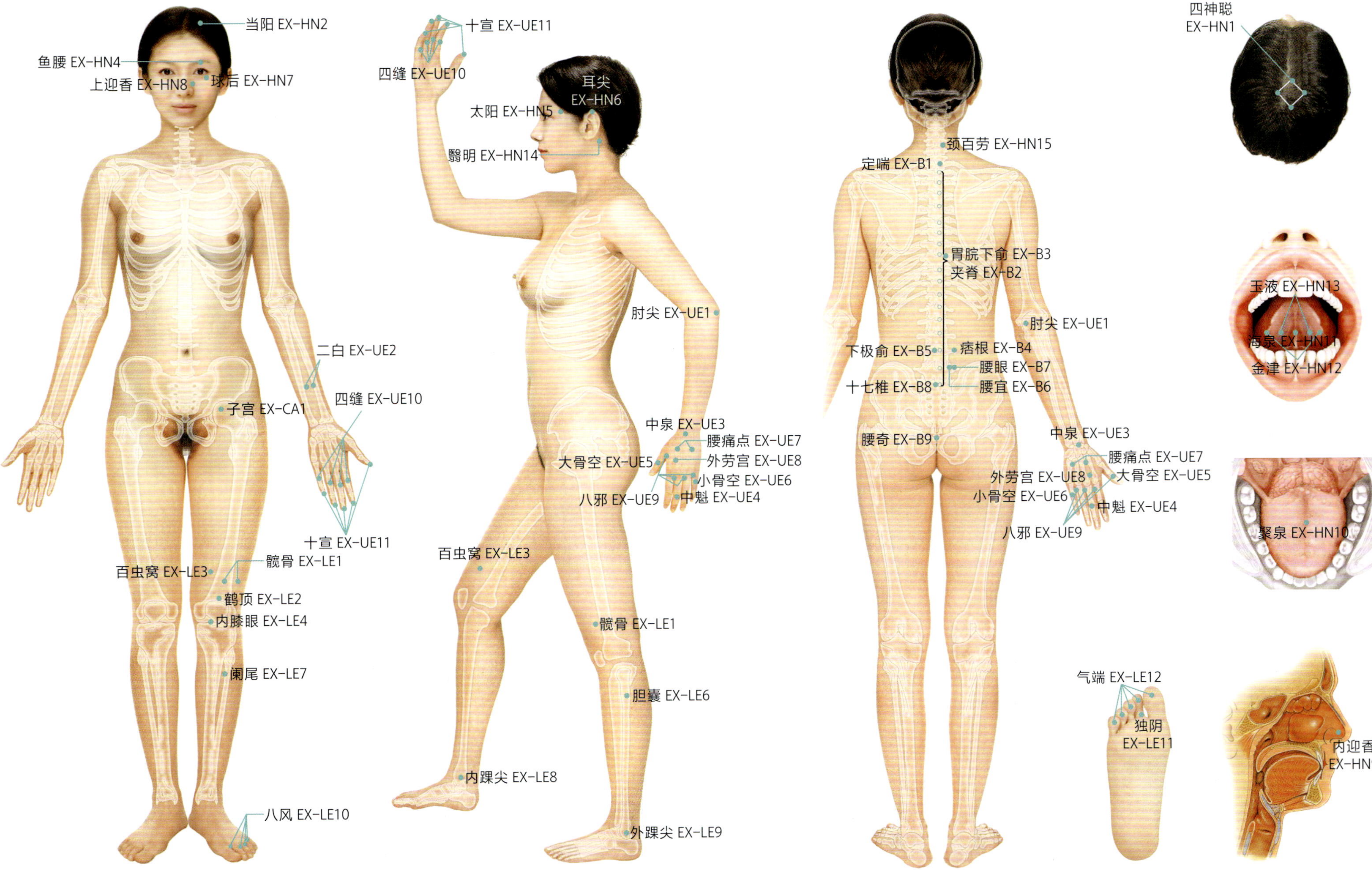
当阳 EX-HN2
鱼腰 EX-HN4
球后 EX-HN7
上迎香 EX-HN8
十宣 EX-UE11
四缝 EX-UE10
耳尖 EX-HN6
太阳 EX-HN5
翳明 EX-HN14
肘尖 EX-UE1
二白 EX-UE2
四缝 EX-UE10
子宫 EX-CA1
十宣 EX-UE11
百虫窝 EX-LE3
髋骨 EX-LE1
鹤顶 EX-LE2
内膝眼 EX-LE4
阑尾 EX-LE7
八风 EX-LE10
中泉 EX-UE3
腰痛点 EX-UE7
大骨空 EX-UE5
外劳宫 EX-UE8
小骨空 EX-UE6
八邪 EX-UE9
中魁 EX-UE4
百虫窝 EX-LE3
髋骨 EX-LE1
胆囊 EX-LE6
内踝尖 EX-LE8
外踝尖 EX-LE9
颈百劳 EX-HN15
定喘 EX-B1
胃脘下俞 EX-B3
夹脊 EX-B2
肘尖 EX-UE1
下极俞 EX-B5
痞根 EX-B4
腰眼 EX-B7
十七椎 EX-B8
腰宜 EX-B6
腰奇 EX-B9
中泉 EX-UE3
腰痛点 EX-UE7
外劳宫 EX-UE8
大骨空 EX-UE5
小骨空 EX-UE6
中魁 EX-UE4
八邪 EX-UE9
四神聪
EX-HN1
玉液 EX-HN13
海泉 EX-HN11
金津 EX-HN12
聚泉 EX-HN10
气端 EX-LE12
独阴
EX-LE11
内迎香
EX-HN9

EX-LE	穴名	主 治
1	髋骨	结核性关节炎、下肢痿痹
2	鹤顶	膝关节酸痛、腿足无力、结核性关节炎
3	百虫窝	皮肤瘙痒、风疹、湿疹、疮疡、蛔虫病
4	内膝眼	膝肿痛、膝骨性关节炎
6	胆囊	胆囊炎、胆石症、胆绞痛、胆道蛔虫症
7	阑尾	急、慢性阑尾炎
8	内踝尖	乳蛾、牙痛、小儿不语、霍乱转筋
9	外踝尖	十趾拘急、小腿外侧肌肉拘紧疼痛、牙痛、舌下血脉肿胀
10	八风	趾痛、足背肿痛、足趾麻木
11	独阴	胸胁痛、心绞痛、呕吐、胞衣不下、月经不调、疝气
12	气端	足趾麻木、足背红肿疼痛、卒中

EX-LE	Acupoints	Indications
1	Kuāngǔ	Tuberculous arthritis; lower limb paralysis
2	Hèdǐng	Soreness of knee joint; weakness of leg and foot; tuberculous arthritis
3	Bǎichóngwō	Skin itching; rubella; eczema; sores; ascariasis
4	Nèixīyǎn	Knee swelling and pain; knee osteoarthritis
6	Dǎnnáng	Cholecystitis; cholelithiasis; biliary colic; biliary ascariasis
7	Lánwěi	Acute and chronic appendicitis
8	Nèihuáijiān	Acute tonsillitis; toothache; aphasia of children; cholera cramps
9	Wàihuáijiān	Spasm of the ten toes; tighten pain of the lateral leg muscles; toothache; sublingual veins swelling
10	Bāfēng	Toe pain; swelling and pain of the dorsum of foot, numbness of the toes
11	Dúyīn	Chest pain; angina; vomiting; placenta retension; irregular menstruation; hernia
12	Qìduān	Numbness of the toes; swelling and pain in the dorsal foot; stroke

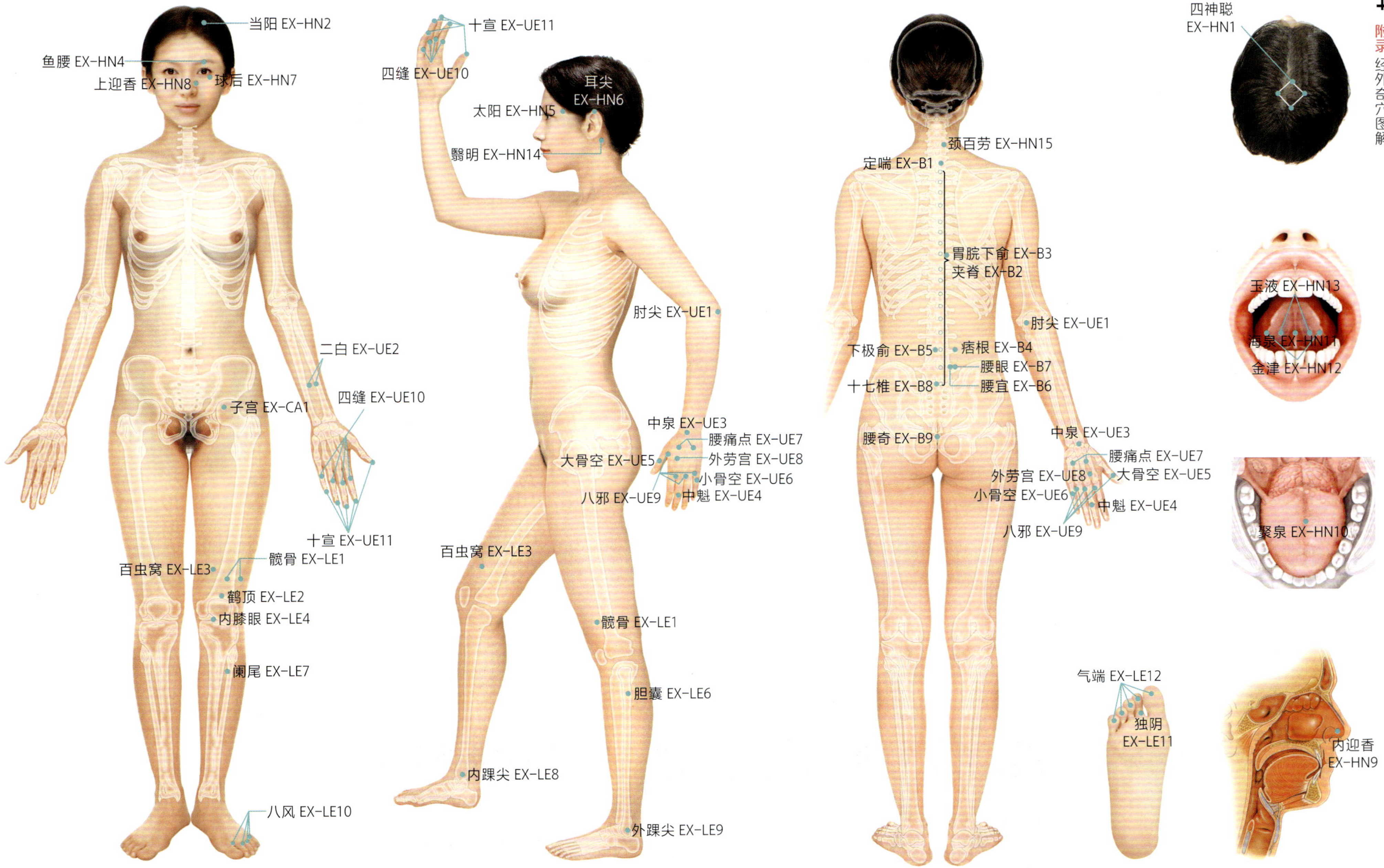
当阳 EX-HN2
鱼腰 EX-HN4
球后 EX-HN7
上迎香 EX-HN8
二白 EX-UE2
四缝 EX-UE10
子宫 EX-CA1
十宣 EX-UE11
髋骨 EX-LE1
百虫窝 EX-LE3
鹤顶 EX-LE2
内膝眼 EX-LE4
阑尾 EX-LE7
八风 EX-LE10
十宣 EX-UE11
四缝 EX-UE10
耳尖
EX-HN6
太阳 EX-HN5
翳明 EX-HN14
肘尖 EX-UE1
中泉 EX-UE3
腰痛点 EX-UE7
外劳宫 EX-UE8
大骨空 EX-UE5
小骨空 EX-UE6
八邪 EX-UE9
中魁 EX-UE4
百虫窝 EX-LE3
髋骨 EX-LE1
胆囊 EX-LE6
内踝尖 EX-LE8
外踝尖 EX-LE9
颈百劳 EX-HN15
定喘 EX-B1
胃脘下俞 EX-B3
夹脊 EX-B2
肘尖 EX-UE1
下极俞 EX-B5
痞根 EX-B4
腰眼 EX-B7
十七椎 EX-B8
腰宜 EX-B6
腰奇 EX-B9
中泉 EX-UE3
腰痛点 EX-UE7
外劳宫 EX-UE8
大骨空 EX-UE5
小骨空 EX-UE6
中魁 EX-UE4
八邪 EX-UE9
四神聪
EX-HN1
玉液 EX-HN13
海泉 EX-HN11
金津 EX-HN12
聚泉 EX-HN10
气端 EX-LE12
独阴
EX-LE11
内迎香
EX-HN9

EX-CA	穴名	主 治
1	子宫	子宫脱垂、不孕、痛经、崩漏、月经不调

续表

EX-B	穴名	主 治
1	定喘	哮喘、咳嗽、落枕、肩背痛、上肢疼痛不举
2	夹脊	①胸 1~5 夹脊：心肺、胸部及上肢疾病。②胸 6~12 夹脊：胃肠、脾、肝、胆疾病。③腰 1~5 夹脊：下肢疼痛，腰、骶、小腹部疾病
3	胃脘下俞	胃痛、腹痛、胸胁痛、2 型糖尿病、胰腺炎
4	痞根	腰痛、腹部肿块、癥瘕
5	下极俞	腰痛、小便不利、遗尿
6	腰宜	妇人血崩、腰痛、脊柱强直
7	腰眼	腰痛、尿频、月经不调、带下、坐骨神经痛
8	十七椎	腰骶痛、痛经、崩漏、月经不调、遗尿
9	腰奇	便秘、癫痫、失眠、头痛

EX-CA	Acupoints	Indications
1	Zǐgōng	Uterine prolapse; sterility; dysmenorrhea; metrorrhagia and metrostaxis; irregular menstruation

EX-B	Acupoints	Indications
1	Dìngchuǎn	Asthma; cough; stiff neck; shoulder and back pain; causalgia in upper limb
2	Jiájǐ	① Chest 1 to 5 Jiaji: cardiopulmonary, chest and upper extremity diseases. ② Chest 6~12 Jiaji: gastrointestinal, spleen, liver and gallbladder diseases. ③ Waist 1 to 5 Jiaji: lower limb pain, waist、sacral and abdominal diseases
3	Wèiwǎnxiàshū	Stomach pain; abdominal pain; chest pain; type 2 diabetes; pancreatitis
4	Pǐgēn	Lumbago; abdominal mass; mass
5	Xiàjíshū	Lumbago; difficult urination; enuresis
6	Yāoyí	Metrorrhagia; lumbago; spinal stiffness
7	Yāoyǎn	Lumbago; frequent urination; irregular menstruation; leukorrheal diseases; sciatica
8	Shíqīzhuī	Lumbosacral pain, dysmenorrhea; metrorrhagia and metrostaxis; irregular menstruation; enuresis
9	Yāoqí	Constipation; epilepsy; insomnia; headache

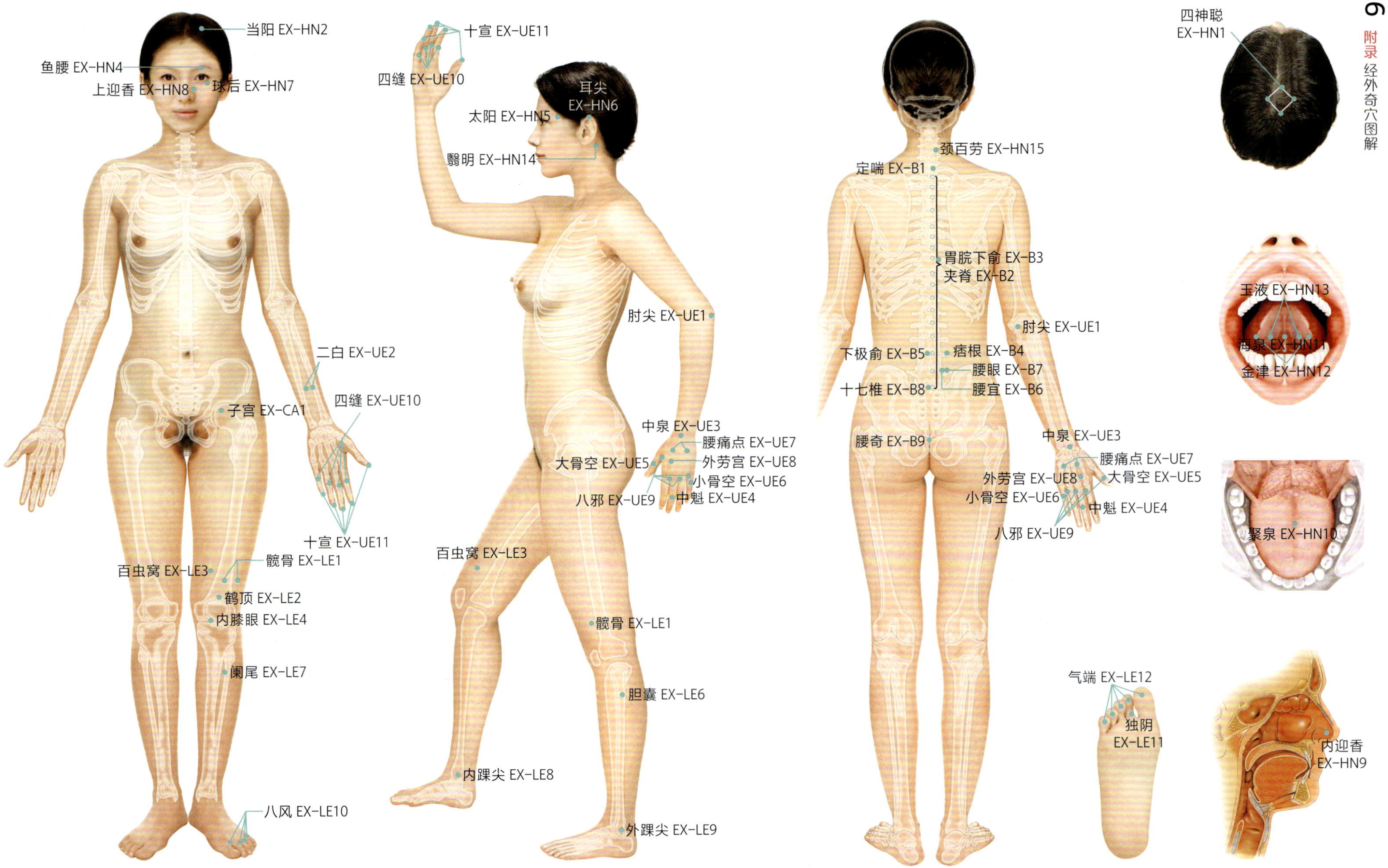
当阳 EX-HN2
鱼腰 EX-HN4
上迎香 EX-HN8
球后 EX-HN7
二白 EX-UE2
四缝 EX-UE10
子宫 EX-CA1
十宣 EX-UE11
百虫窝 EX-LE3
髋骨 EX-LE1
鹤顶 EX-LE2
内膝眼 EX-LE4
阑尾 EX-LE7
八风 EX-LE10
十宣 EX-UE11
四缝 EX-UE10
太阳 EX-HN5
耳尖
EX-HN6
翳明 EX-HN14
肘尖 EX-UE1
中泉 EX-UE3
腰痛点 EX-UE7
大骨空 EX-UE5
外劳宫 EX-UE8
小骨空 EX-UE6
八邪 EX-UE9
中魁 EX-UE4
百虫窝 EX-LE3
髋骨 EX-LE1
胆囊 EX-LE6
内踝尖 EX-LE8
外踝尖 EX-LE9
颈百劳 EX-HN15
定喘 EX-B1
胃脘下俞 EX-B3
夹脊 EX-B2
肘尖 EX-UE1
下极俞 EX-B5
痞根 EX-B4
腰眼 EX-B7
十七椎 EX-B8
腰宜 EX-B6
腰奇 EX-B9
中泉 EX-UE3
腰痛点 EX-UE7
外劳宫 EX-UE8
大骨空 EX-UE5
小骨空 EX-UE6
中魁 EX-UE4
八邪 EX-UE9
四神聪
EX-HN1
玉液 EX-HN13
海泉 EX-HN11
金津 EX-HN12
聚泉 EX-HN10
气端 EX-LE12
独阴
EX-LE11
内迎香
EX-HN9

续表

EX-UE	穴名	主 治
1	肘尖	痈疽、疔疮、颈淋巴结结核
2	二白	痔疮、脱肛、前臂痛、胸胁痛
3	中泉	胸胁胀满、咳嗽、气喘、心痛、胃脘疼痛、掌心发热
4	中魁	牙痛、鼻出血、反胃、呕吐
5	大骨空	目痛、目翳、吐泻、鼻出血
6	小骨空	目赤肿痛、目翳、咽喉肿痛
7	腰痛点	急性腰扭伤
8	外劳宫	落枕、手指麻木、手指屈伸不利
9	八邪	烦热、目痛、毒蛇咬伤、手背肿痛、手指麻木、小儿厌食
10	四缝	小儿疳积、百日咳
11	十宣	昏迷、高热、昏厥、中暑、癫痫、咽喉肿痛

EX-UE	Acupoints	Indications
1	Zhǒujiān	Ulcer; furunculosis; tuberculosis of cervical lymphnode
2	Èrbái	Hemorrhoids; prolapse of the anus; forearm pain; chest pain
3	Zhōngquán	Fullness of chest and hypochondrium; cough; asthma; heartache; epigastric pain; palm fever
4	Zhōngkuí	Toothache; nose bleeding; nausea; vomiting
5	Dàgǔkōng	Painful eyes; nephelium, diarrhea; nose bleeding
6	Xiǎogǔkōng	Swelling and pain of eye; nephelium; swollen sore throat
7	Yāotòngdiǎn	Acute lumbar sprain
8	Wàiláogōng	Stiff neck; numbness of the fingers; inhibited bending and stretching of hands
9	Bāxié	Dysphoria with smothery sensation; painful eyes; snake bites; pain on the dorsum of hand; numb fingers; anorexia in children
10	Sìfèng	Infantile malnutrition; whooping cough
11	Shíxuān	Coma; high fever; syncope; heat stroke; epilepsy; swollen sore throat

Three-Dimension

Colored Diagrams for

Meridians and Acupoints

（Chinese-English Edition）

三维经络穴位全彩图集

（中英对照版）

编　著　（按姓氏笔画排序）

老中医养生堂　刘嘉瑶
许博捷　杨丽雯
余骏腾　张金金
张晓雯　张淑巧
陈谷超　林　芳
段牡薇　贾荣曼
高玉伟　郭修兵
曹柏川　曹琳琰

Acupoints with Special Effects for Children

儿童特效穴位

编　著　（按姓氏笔画排序）

杨丽雯　余骏腾
张淑巧　林　芳
贾荣曼

海峡出版发行集团 | 福建科学技术出版社

THE STRAITS PUBLISHING & DISTRIBUTING GROUP | FUJIAN SCIENCE & TECHNOLOGY PUBLISHING HOUSE

目 录 CONTENTS

第二章　儿童特效穴位分部图解 20

Chapter 2: Diagrams for Acupoints with Specific Effects for Children in Different Divisions

第三章　儿童超速效对症按摩 118

Chapter 3: Super Quick-acting Pediatric Symptomatic Massage

本书特色与使用说明

1. 收录儿童全身特效穴位。这些特效穴位除了少数为经穴、奇穴外，多数为儿童按摩所特有的“特定穴”。

2. 本书结合 AR 技术展示十四经脉循行，可作为读者认识儿童经络的参考。读者通过扫描并关注“健康乐读汇”微信公众号，按提示下载客户端，扫描识别码即可观看。

3. 内容全面、直观，查找方便。以部位为纲，分部位展示儿童特效穴位和按摩方法。

4. 穴位应用不求人。收录 40 种儿童保健和常见病症的超速效按摩方法，简单、实用、疗效佳。

Features and Instructions

1. The book has included pediatric acupoints with specific effects in the whole body. Except for few meridian acupoints and extra points, most are "specific points" for children massage.

2. The book has demonstrated the circulation of the 14 meridians combining with AR technology as the reference for readers to understand meridians and collaterals of children. Readers may scan the QR code in back cover and register on WeChat public account of ***Happy Reading On Health.*** Download the client App under the instructions and you can read after scanning the identification code.

3. With comprehensive and straightforward contents, the book, convenient for search, demonstrates the acupoints with specific effects for children and massage manipulations in different divisions of the body.

4. Acupoints massage self-application: super quick-acting symptomatic massage manipulations for 40 common syndromes are included. It is simple and practical with well curative effect.

第一章　儿童十四经络穴位图解

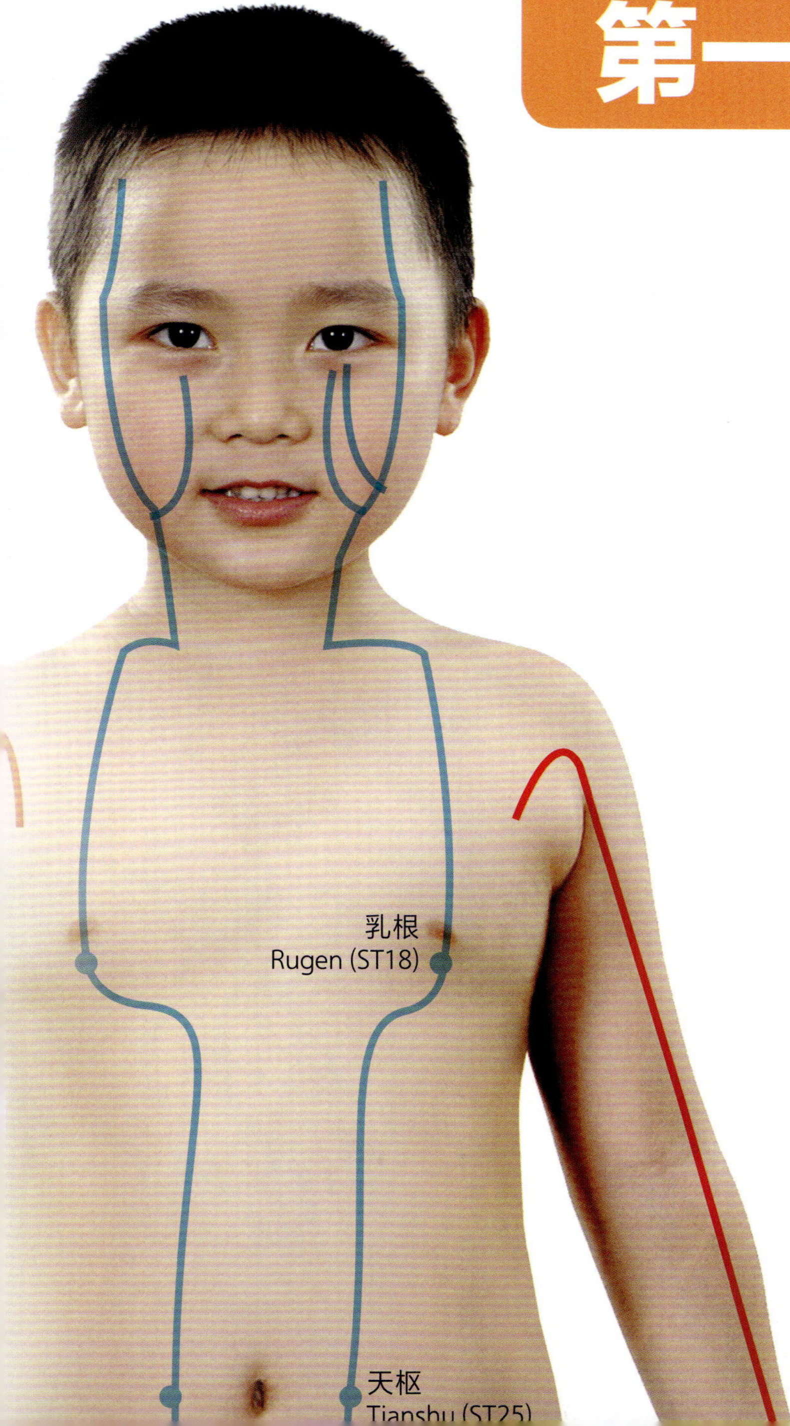

手太阴肺经

手太阴肺经：从胸部上外侧开始，经前臂的桡侧→手掌桡侧→拇指桡侧的少商穴为止。

足阳明胃经

足阳明胃经：从眼睛下方开始，经口角→下颌→耳前→额角；从颈部胸锁乳突肌的前缘开始，经锁骨下凹陷→胸部→前腹部→腹股沟→腿→足第 2 趾末节外侧为止。

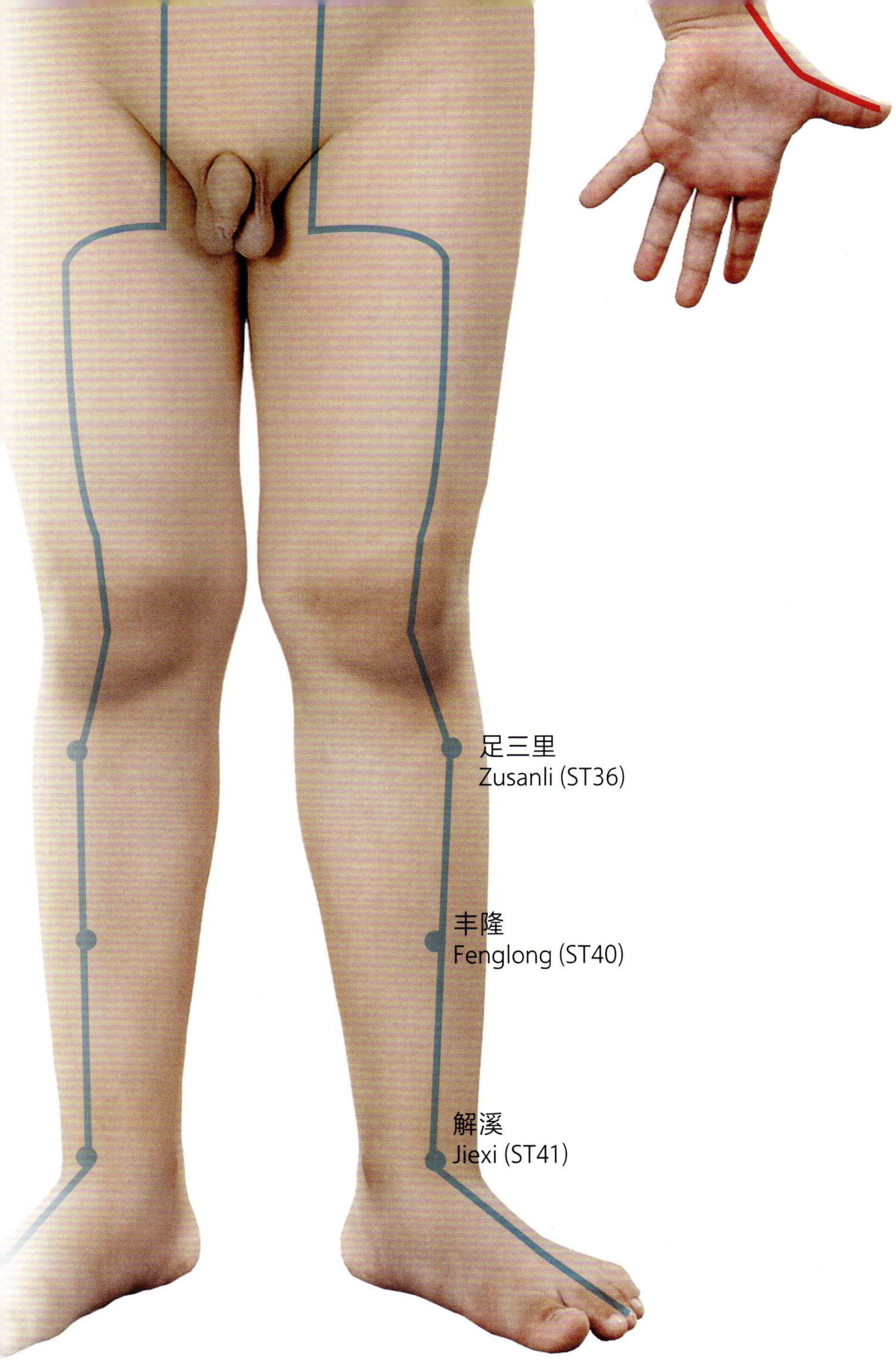

Chapter 1: Diagrams for Acupoints in 14 Meridians for Children

Lung Meridian of Hand-Taiyin, LU

Lung Meridian of Hand-Taiyin: starting from the superior lateral side of the chest, it passes through the radial side of the forearm → radial side of the palm and ends at Shaoshang (LU11) in the radial side of the thumb.

Stomach Meridian of Foot-Yangming, ST

Stomach Meridian of Foot-Yangming: starting below the eye, it passes through the corner of the mouth→ mandible→anterior part of the ear→ the corner of the forehead. Starting from the anterior border of the sternocleidomastoid in the neck, it passes through the infraclavicular depression→ chest→upper abdomen→ groin→leg→lateral side of the distal segment of the 2nd toe and ends at the toe.

手阳明大肠经

手阳明大肠经：从食指末端桡侧开始，经手臂→肩部→锁骨上窝→侧颈部→鼻翼旁为止。

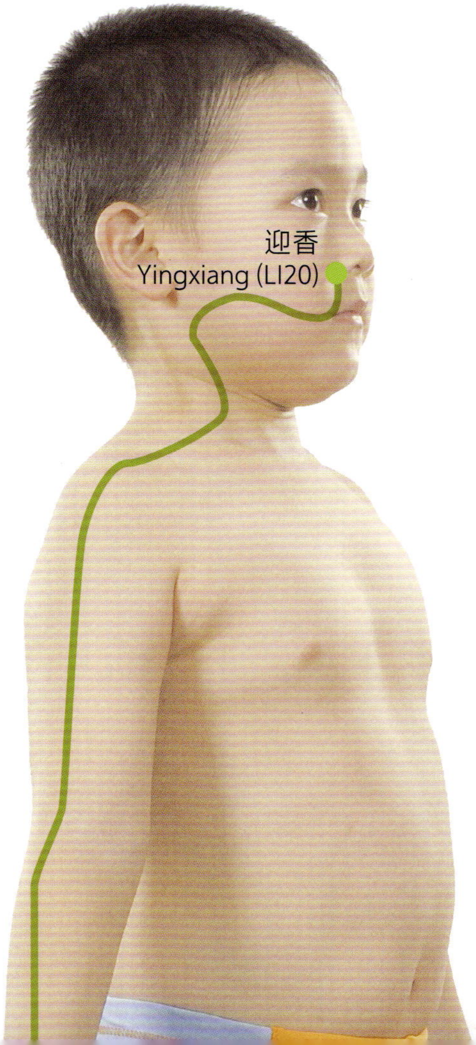

足太阴脾经

足太阴脾经：从踇趾内侧、趾甲根角旁开始，经腿→腹股沟→前腹部→胸部→腋下→侧胸壁第 7 肋间位置为止。

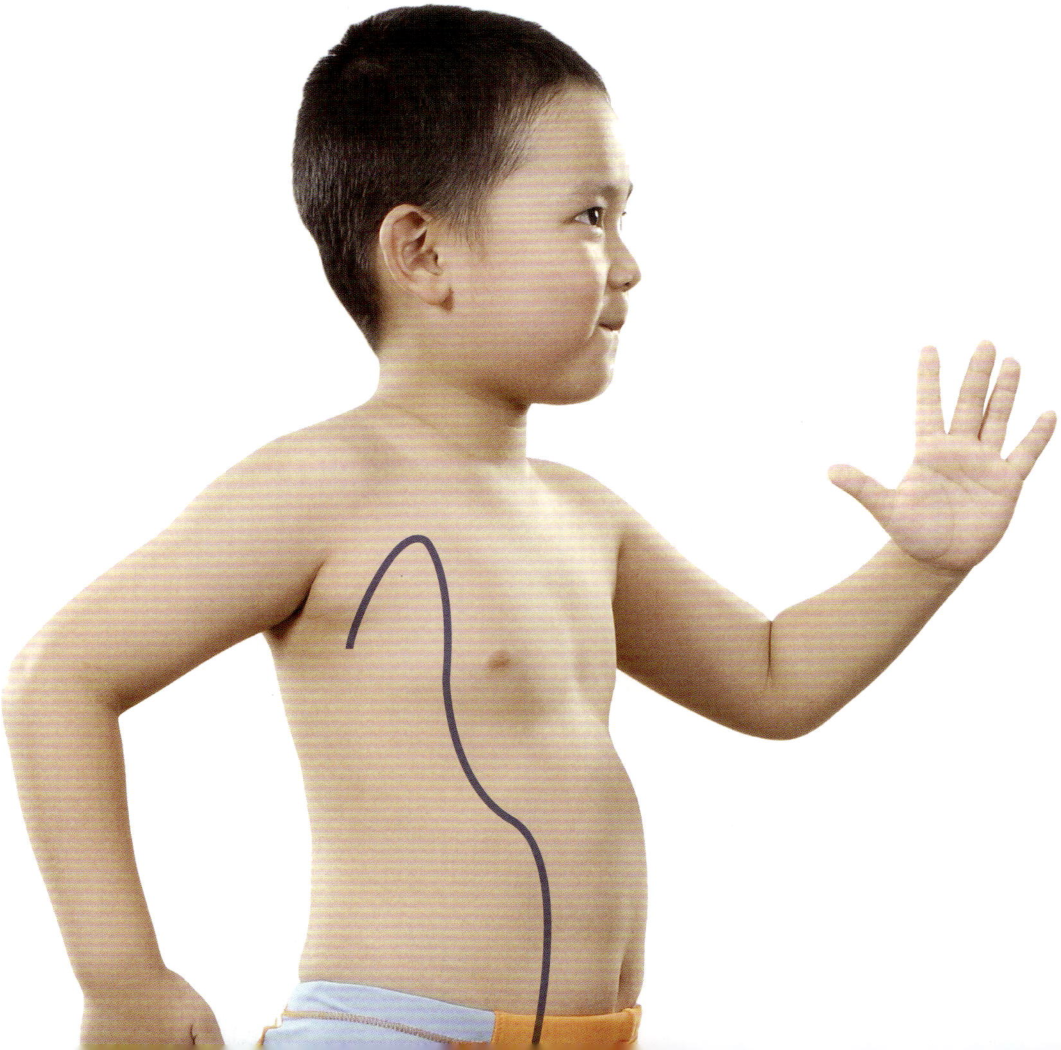

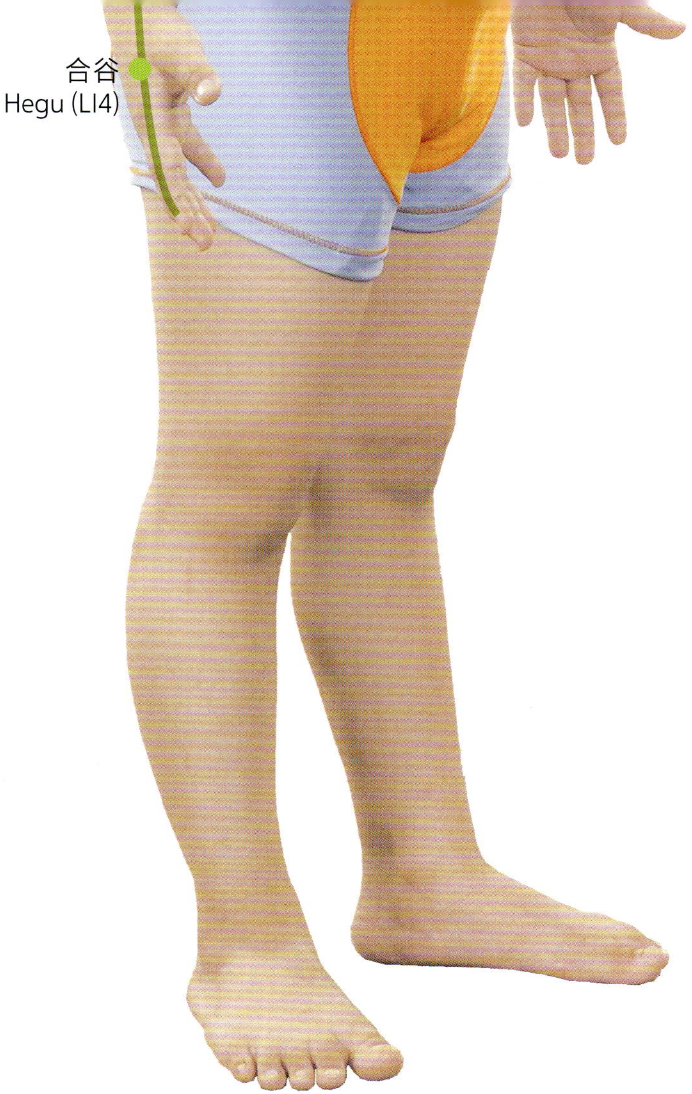

Large Intestine Meridian of Hand-Yangming, LI

Large Intestine Meridian of Hand-Yangming: starting from the distal radial side of the index finger, it passes through arm→shoulder→supraclavicular fossa→lateral side of the neck and ends at the lateral ala nasi.

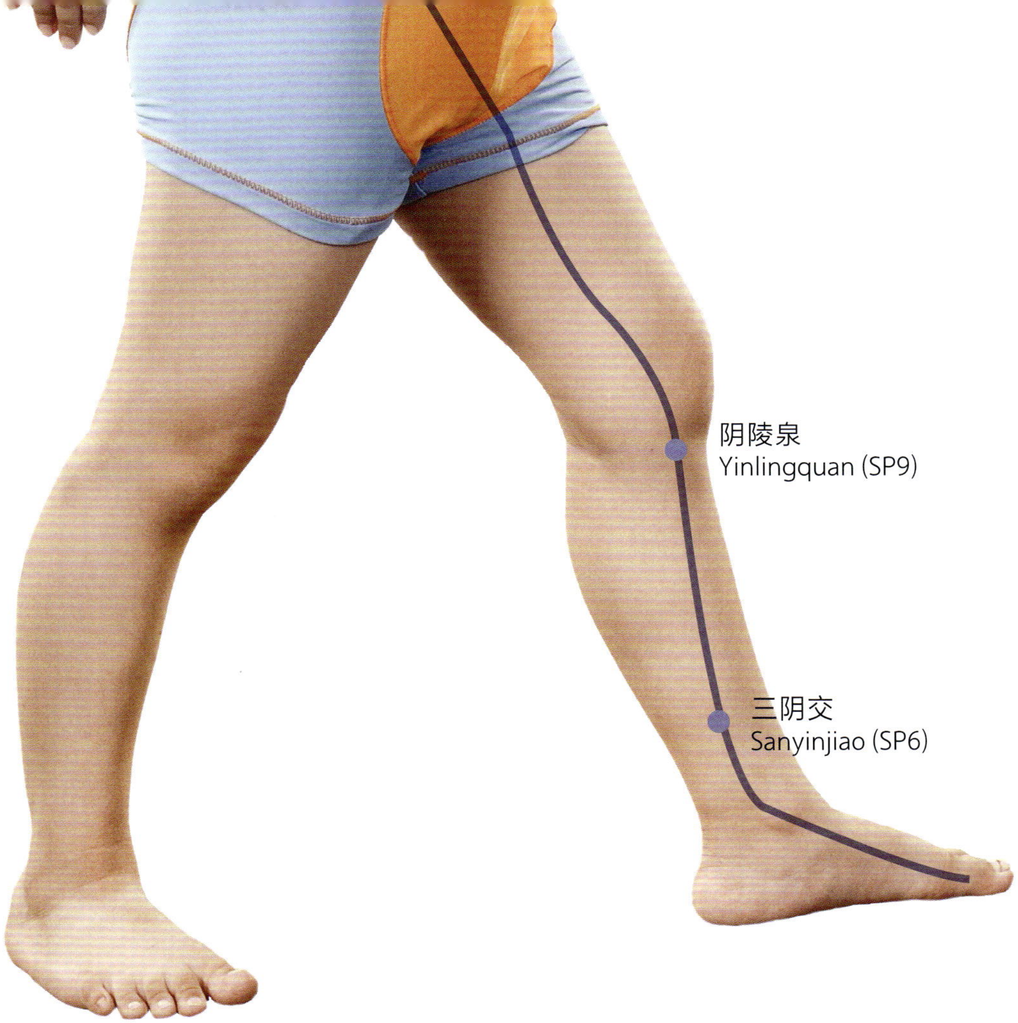

Spleen Meridian of Foot-Taiyin, SP

Spleen Meridian of Foot-Taiyin: starting from the inner side of the big toe at the nail root, it passes through the leg→ groin→ upper abdomen→ chest→ axilla and ends at the 7th intercostal space of the lateral thoracic wall.

手少阴心经

手少阴心经：起于心中，从腋下开始，经手臂→手腕→手掌→小指末节桡侧为止。

Heart Meridian of Hand-Shaoyin, HT

Heart Meridian of Hand-Shaoyin: starting from the heart, it flows from the axilla→ arm→ wrist→ palm and ends at the distal radial side of the little finger.

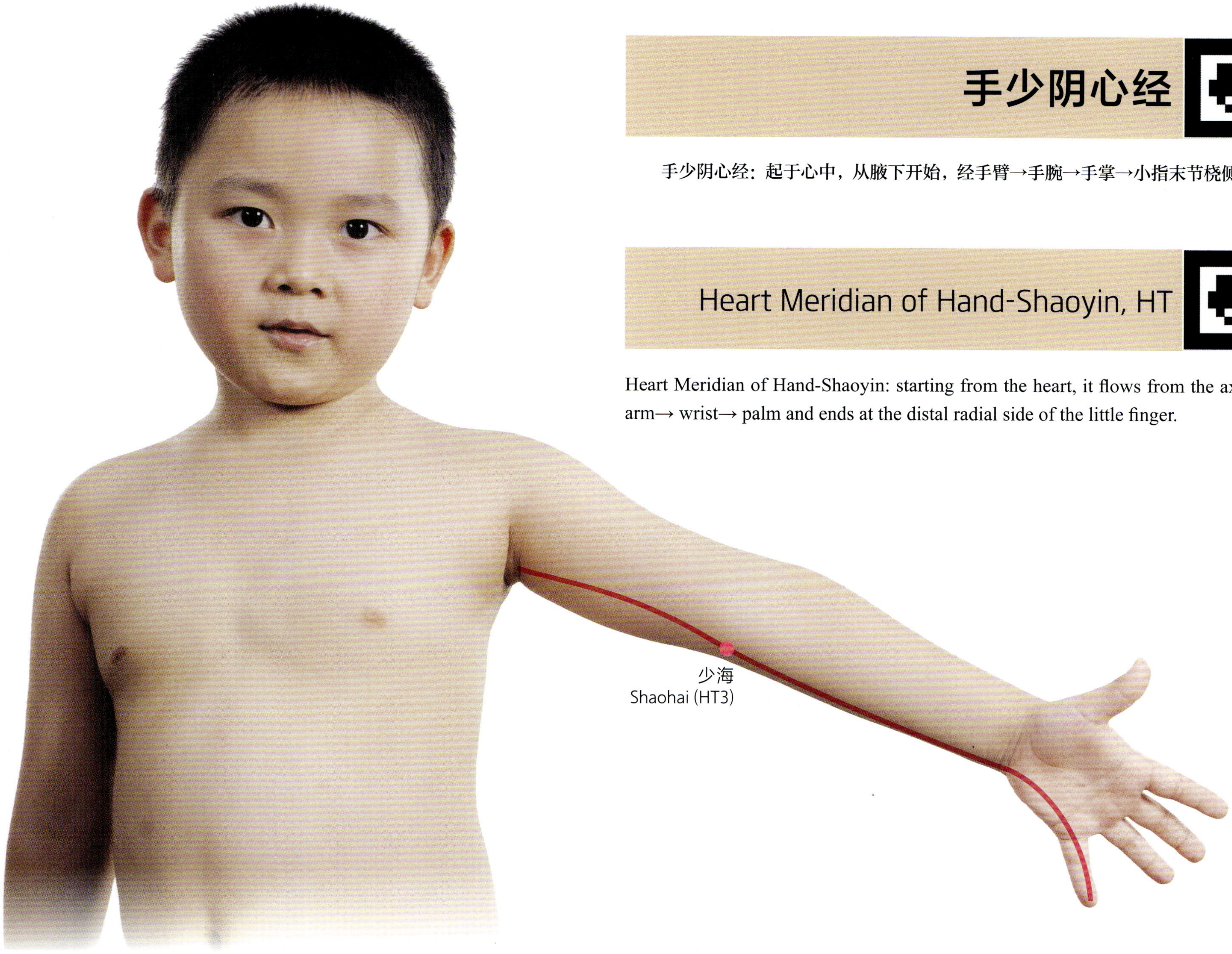

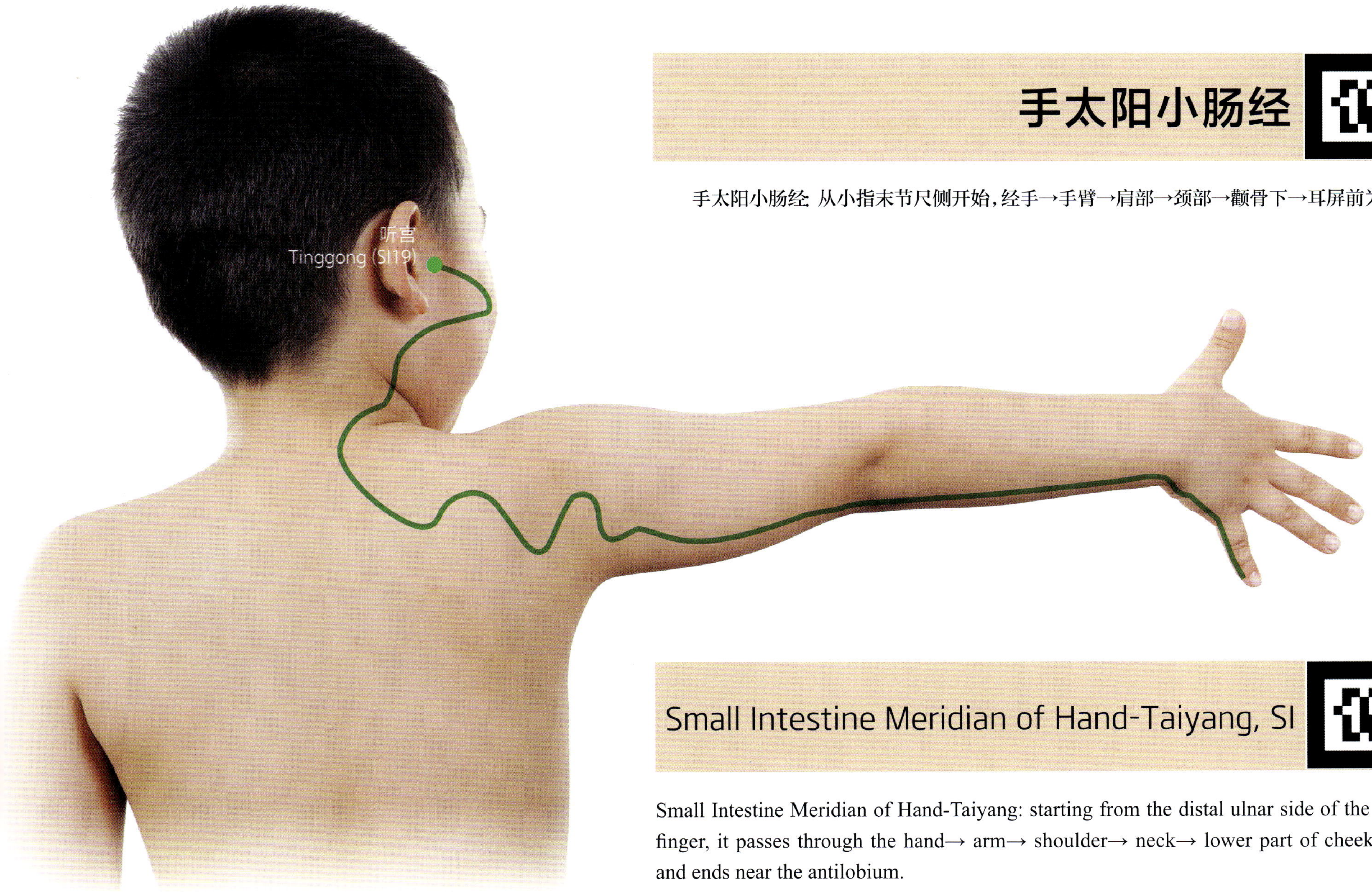

手太阳小肠经

手太阳小肠经：从小指末节尺侧开始，经手→手臂→肩部→颈部→颧骨下→耳屏前为止。

Small Intestine Meridian of Hand-Taiyang, SI

Small Intestine Meridian of Hand-Taiyang: starting from the distal ulnar side of the little finger, it passes through the hand→ arm→ shoulder→ neck→ lower part of cheekbone and ends near the antilobium.

足太阳膀胱经

足太阳膀胱经：从内眼角开始，经后头部→颈部→背部→腰→腿→足小趾末节外侧为止。

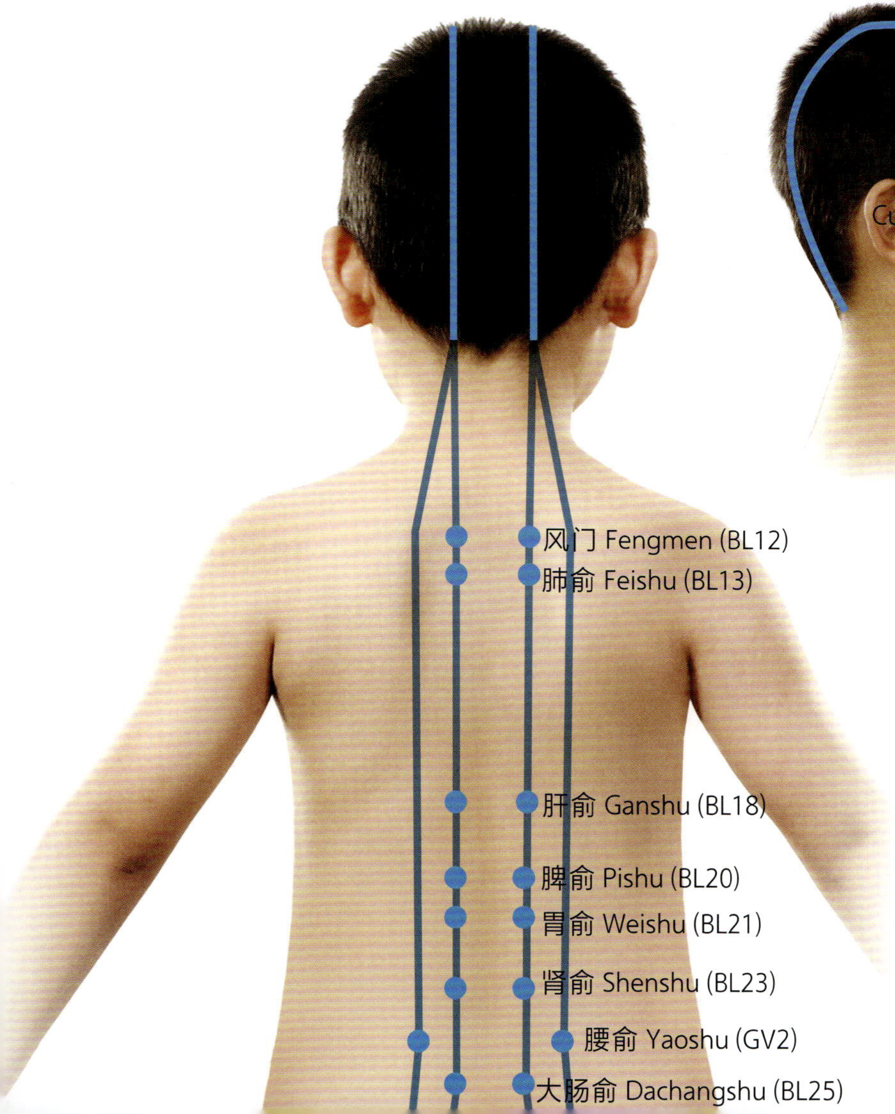

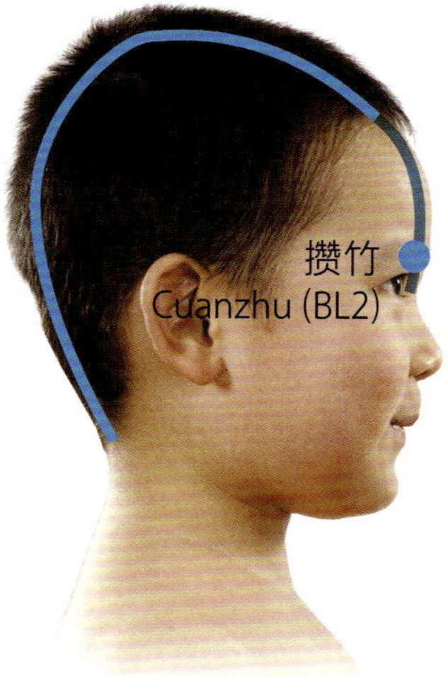

足少阴肾经

足少阴肾经：从足底开始，经腿→前腹部→胸部锁骨下缘为止。

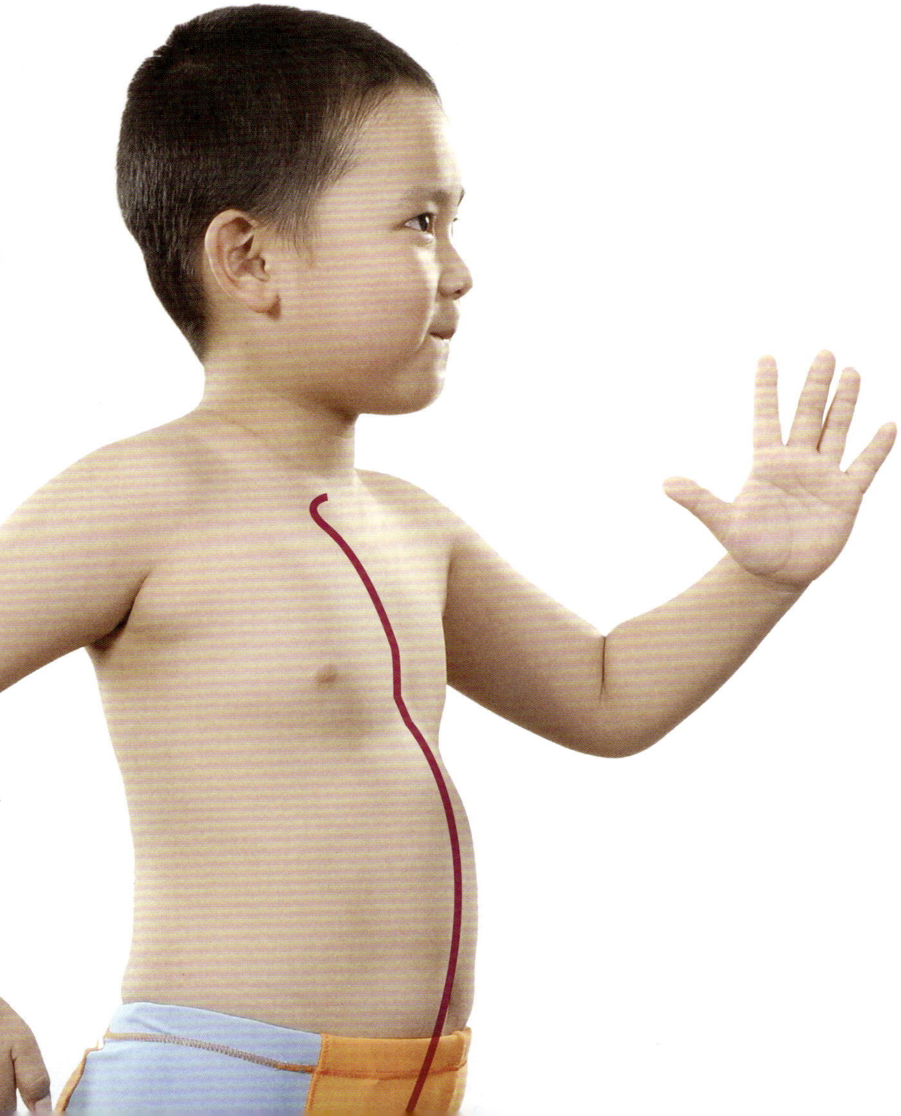

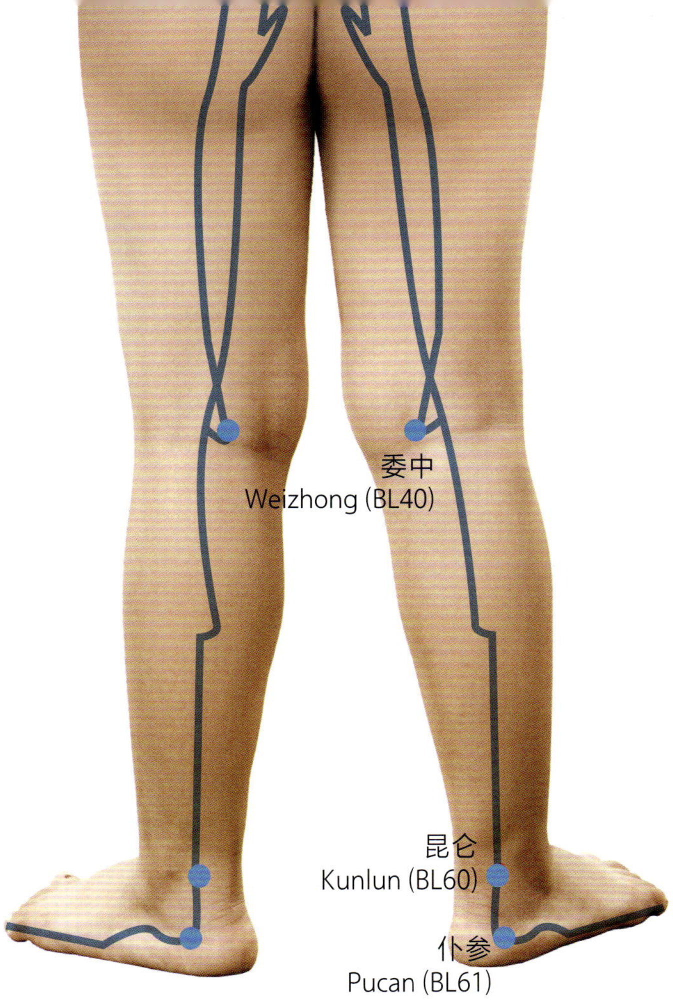

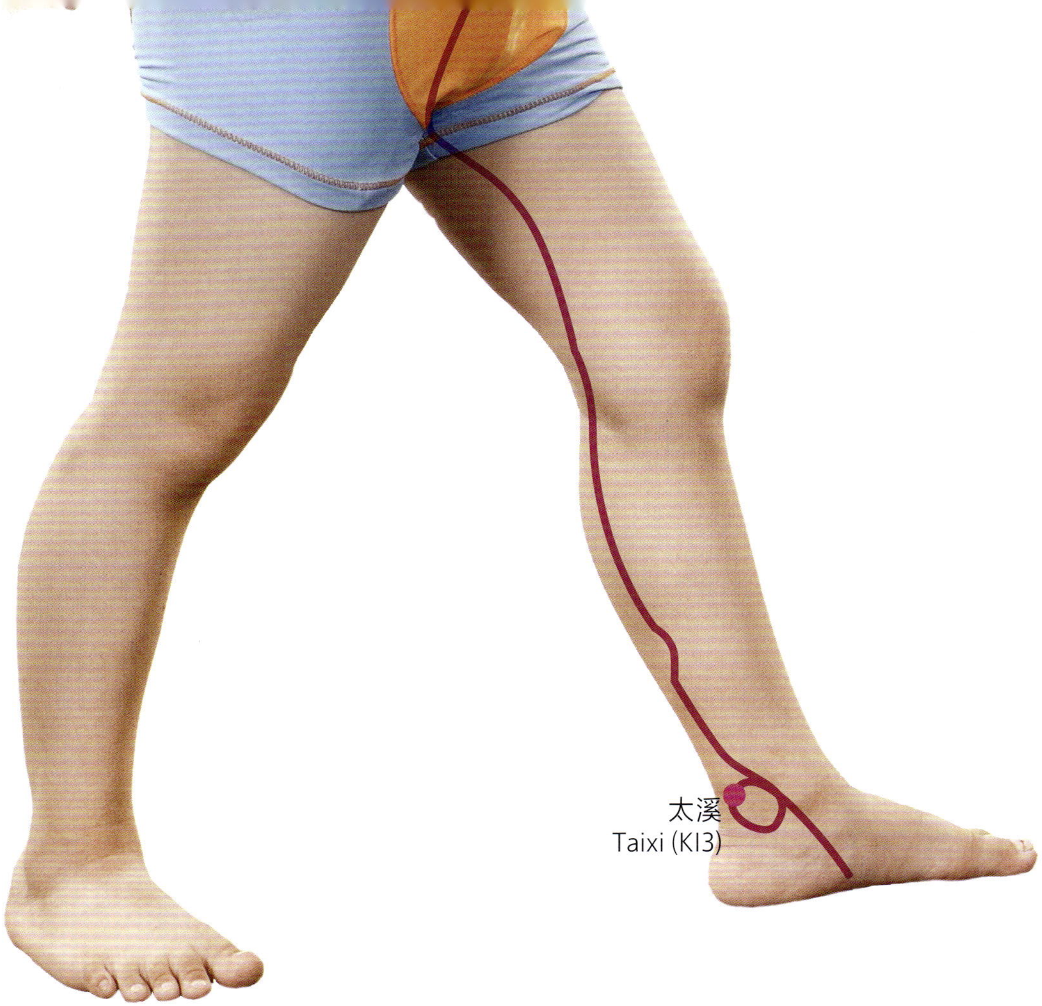

Bladder Meridian of Foot-Taiyang, BL

Bladder Meridian of Foot-Taiyang: starting from the inner canthus, it passes through the occiput→ neck→ back→ waist→ leg and ends at the distal lateral side of the little toe.

Kidney Meridian of Foot-Shaoyin, KI

Kidney Meridian of Foot-Shaoyin: starting from the planta pedis, it passes through the leg→the upper abdomen and ends at the inferior border of clavicle in the chest.

手厥阴心包经

手厥阴心包经：从胸部的乳头外侧开始，经手臂→手掌→手中指尖为止。

Pericardium Meridian of Hand-Jueyin, PC

Pericardium Meridian of Hand-Jueyin: starting from the lateral side of the nipple in the chest, it passes through the arm→ palm and ends at the middle fingertip.

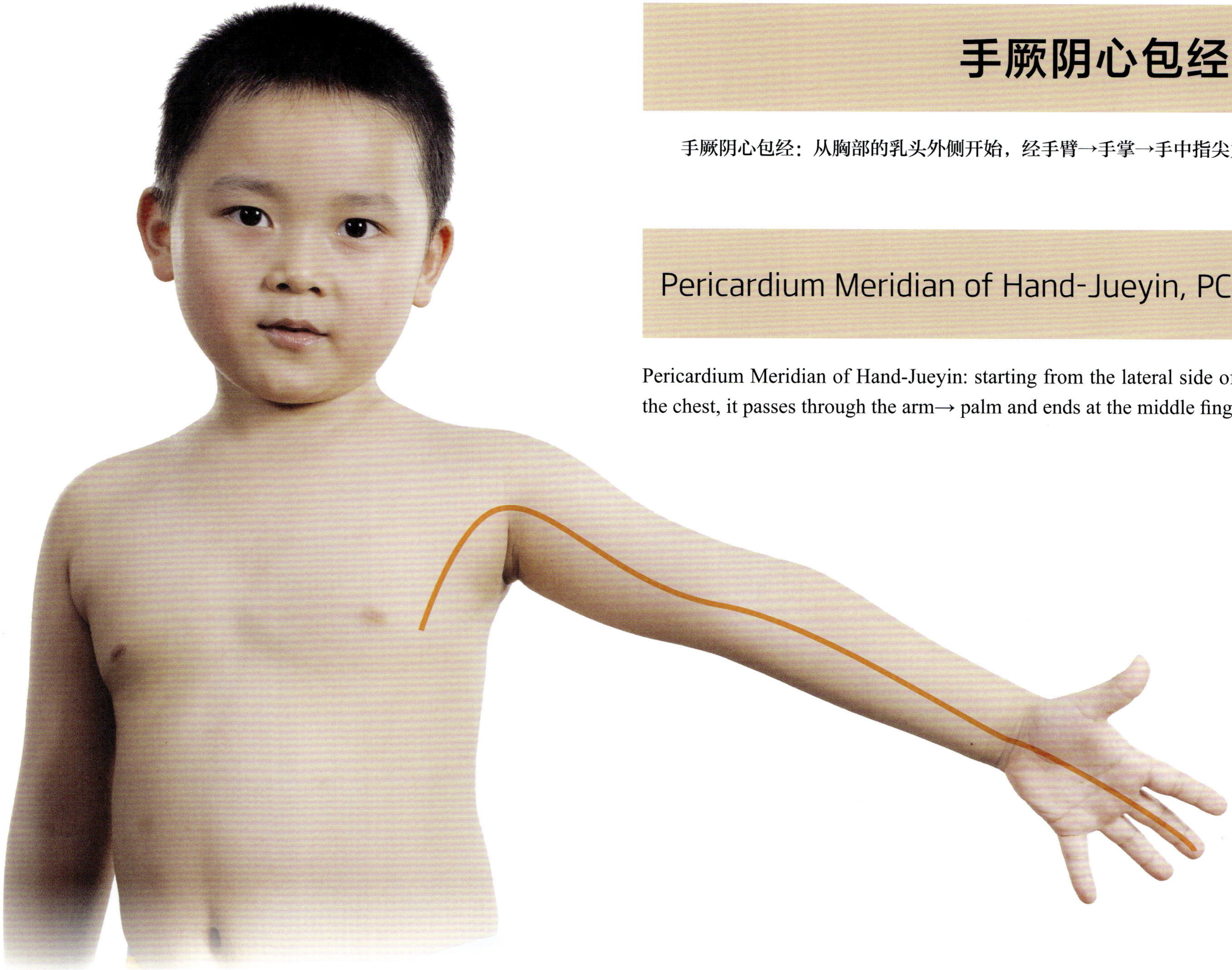

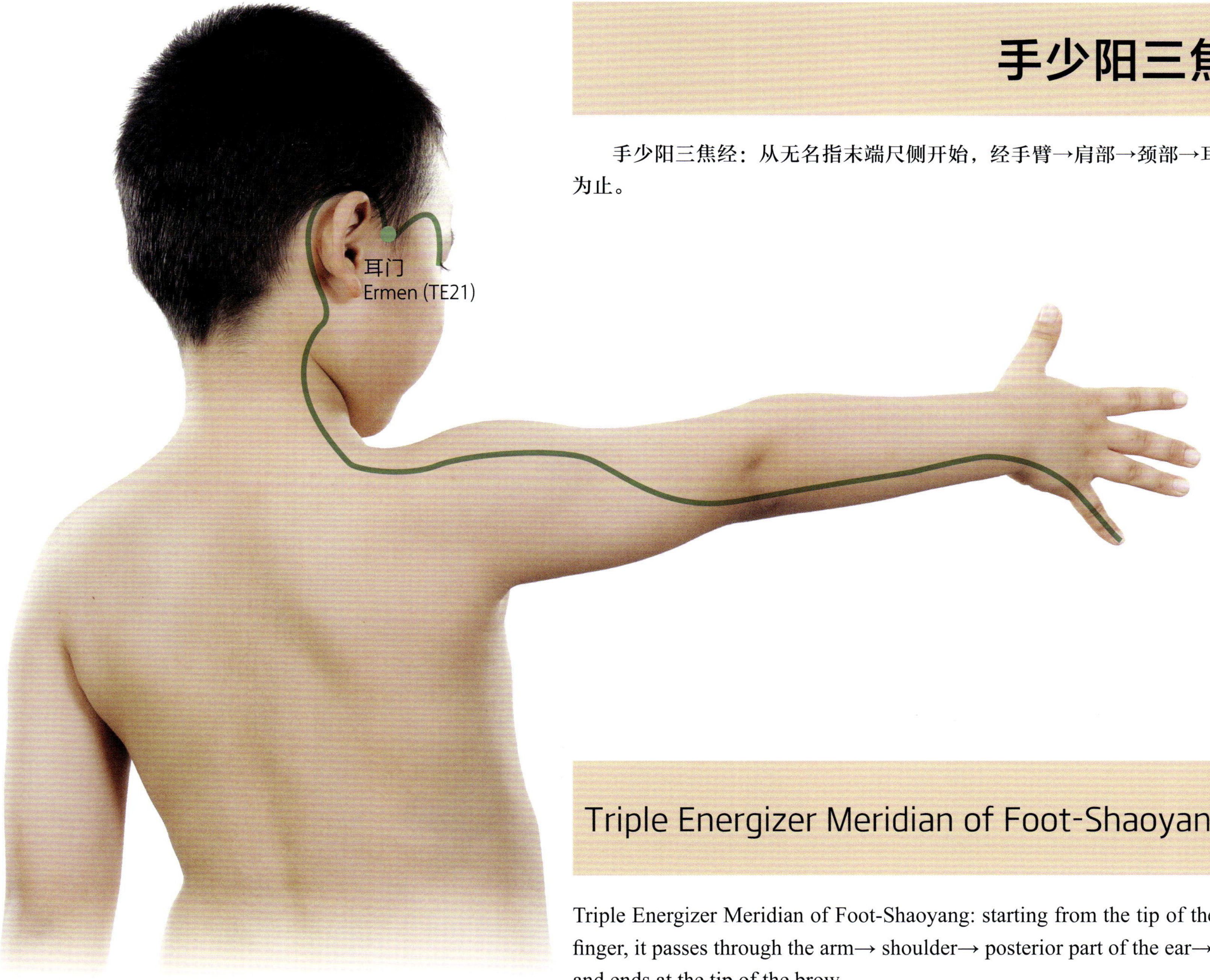

手少阳三焦经

手少阳三焦经：从无名指末端尺侧开始，经手臂→肩部→颈部→耳后→耳前→眉梢末端为止。

Triple Energizer Meridian of Foot-Shaoyang, TE

Triple Energizer Meridian of Foot-Shaoyang: starting from the tip of the ulnar side of the ring finger, it passes through the arm→ shoulder→ posterior part of the ear→anterior part of the ear and ends at the tip of the brow.

足少阳胆经

足少阳胆经：从外眼角开始，经耳周→颈部→肩部→上体侧面→腿→足第 4 趾末节外侧为止。

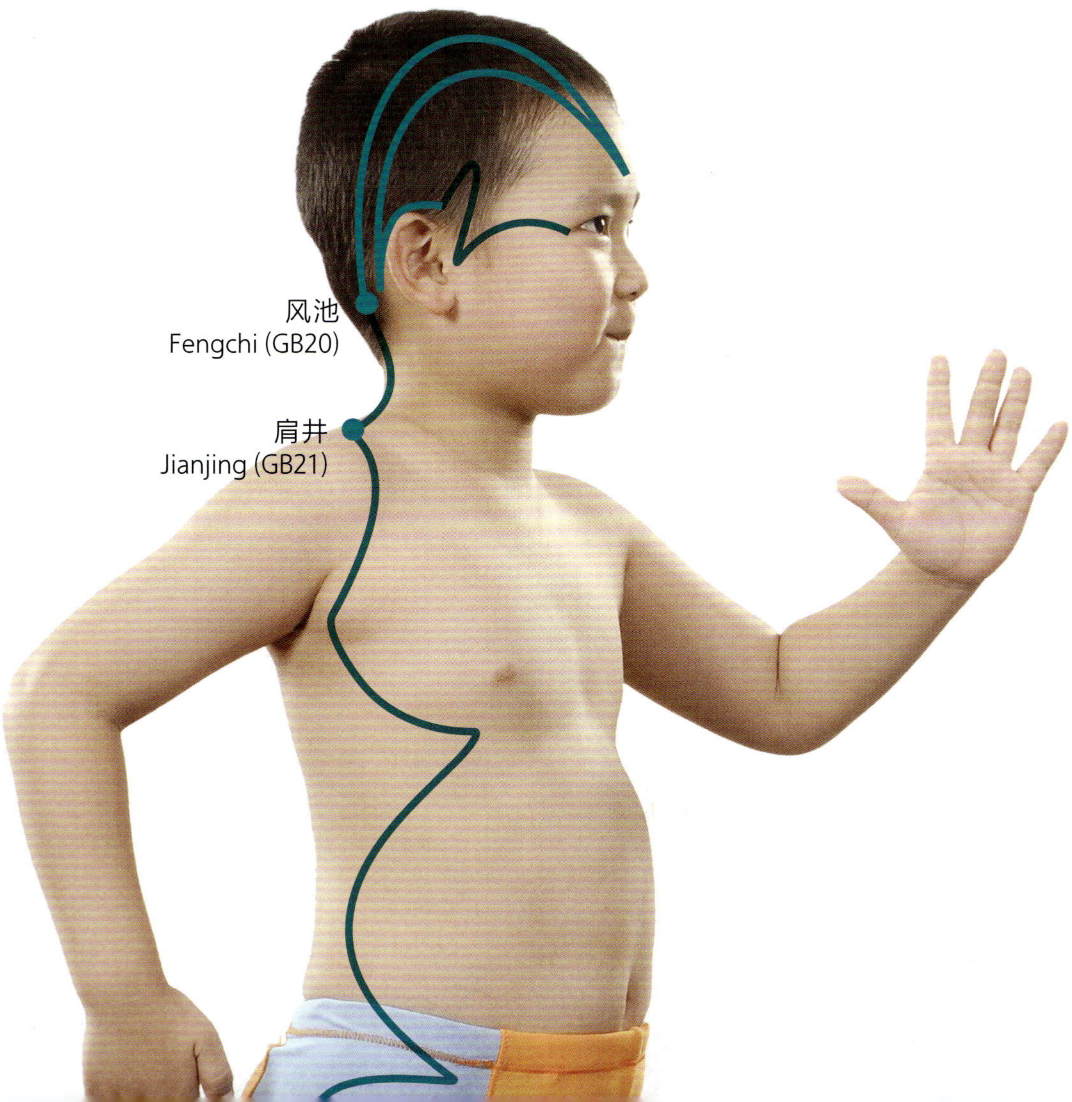

足厥阴肝经

足厥阴肝经：从踇趾末节外侧开始，经腿→腹部→乳头下第 6 肋间为止。

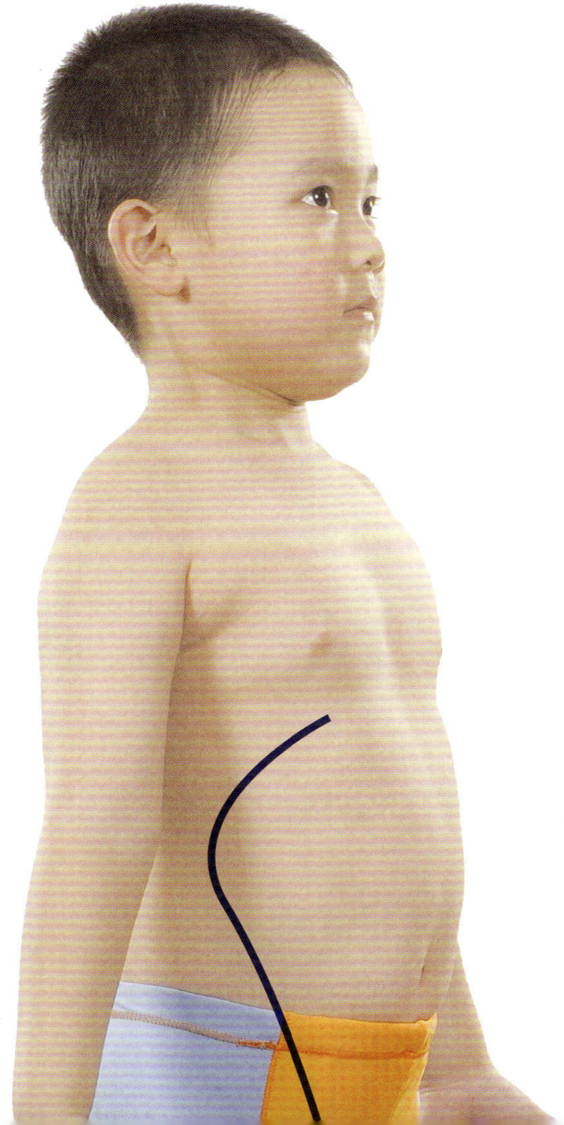

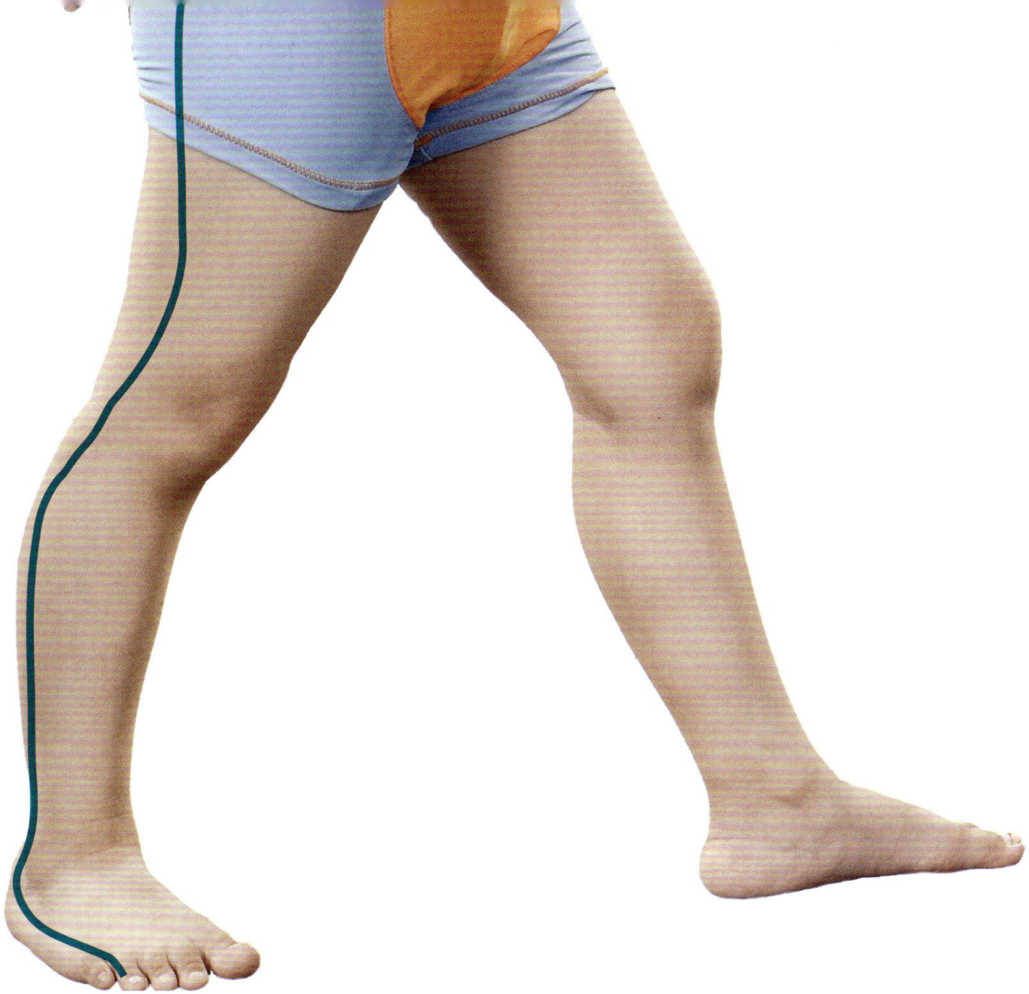

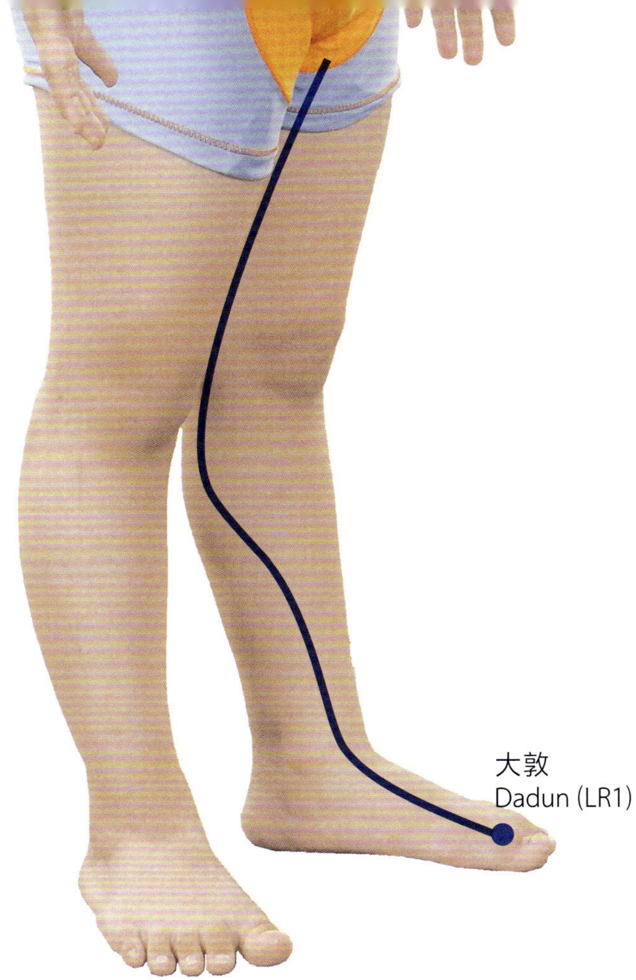

Gallbladder Meridian of Foot-Shaoyang, GB

Gallbladder Meridian of Foot-Shaoyang: starting from the outer canthus, it goes around the ear→ neck→ shoulder→ lateral side of the upper body→ leg and ends at the distal lateral side of the 4th toe.

Liver Meridian of Foot-Jueyin, LR

Liver Meridian of Foot-Jueyin: starting from the distal lateral side of the big toe, it passes through the leg→ abdomen and ends at the 6th intercostal space below the nipple.

督脉

督脉：从尾骨尖开始，沿背部正中线向上，经腰→背→后头部→头顶→鼻尖→上唇内上唇系带与齿龈连接处为止。

任脉

任脉：从会阴开始，沿体前正中向上，经腹部→胸部→面部颏唇沟的正中凹陷处为止。

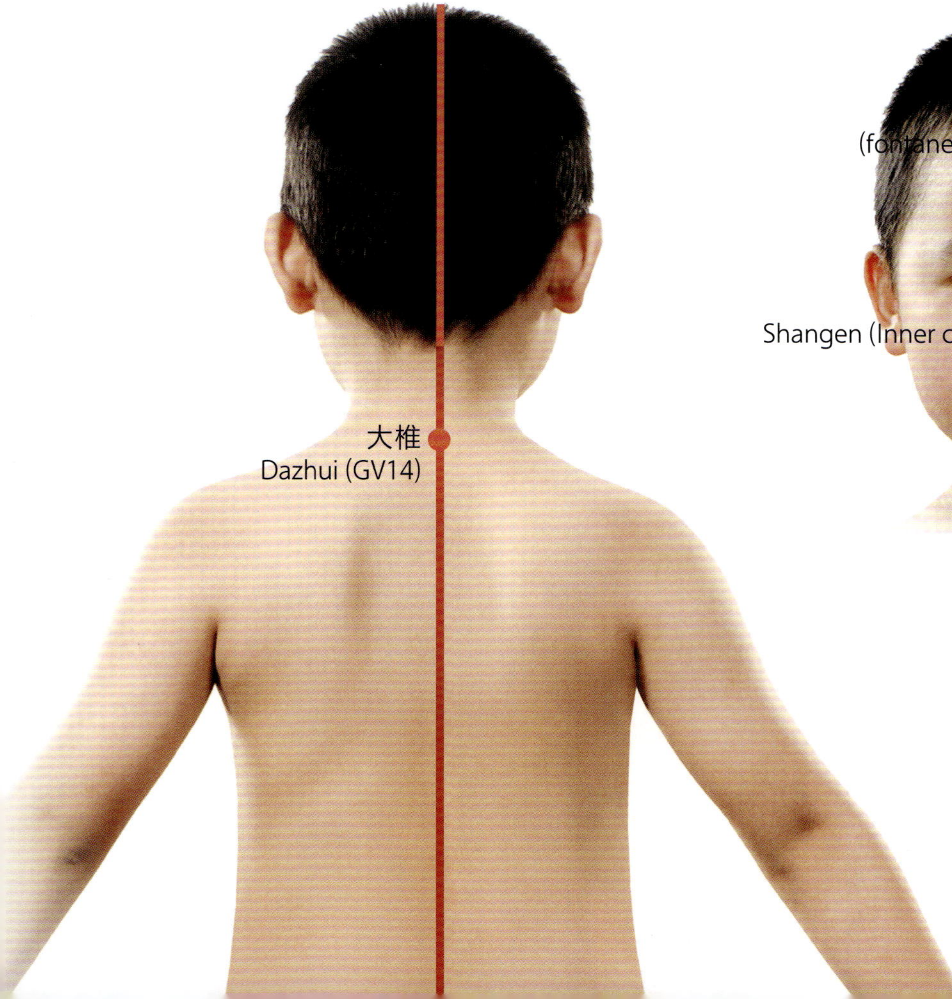

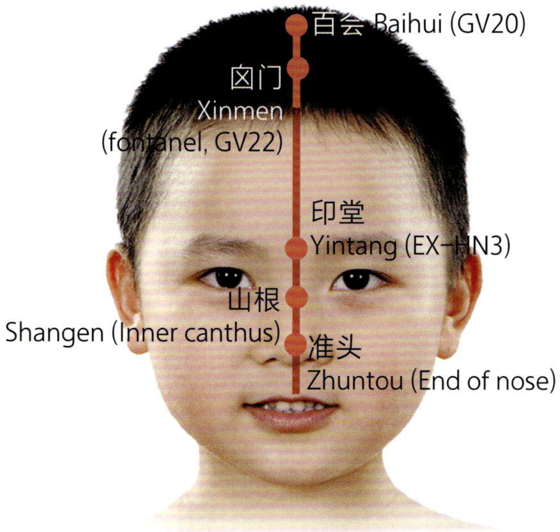

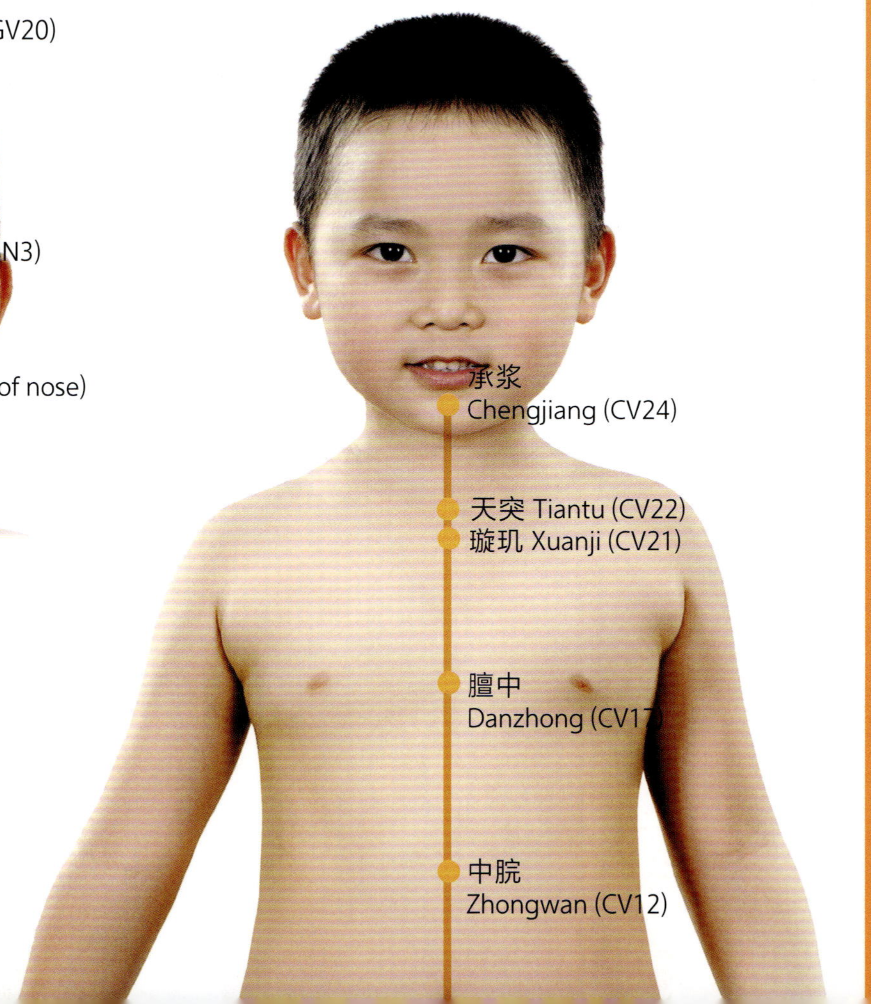

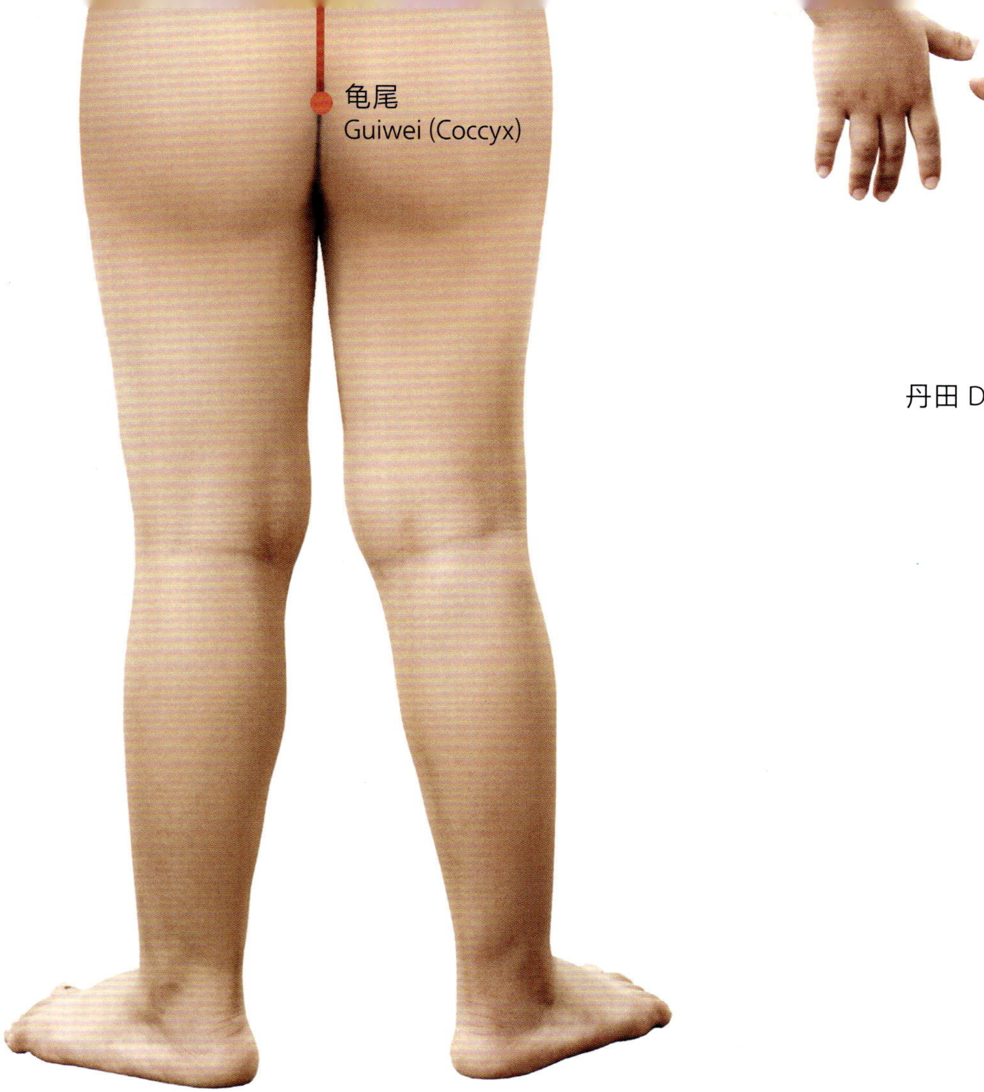

Governor Vessel Meridian, GV

Governor Vessel Meridian: starting from the coccygeal tip, it flows upward along the middle line of the back→waist→ back→ occiput→ the top of the head→ apex nasi and ends at the junction of upper labial frenum and gingival in the upper lip.

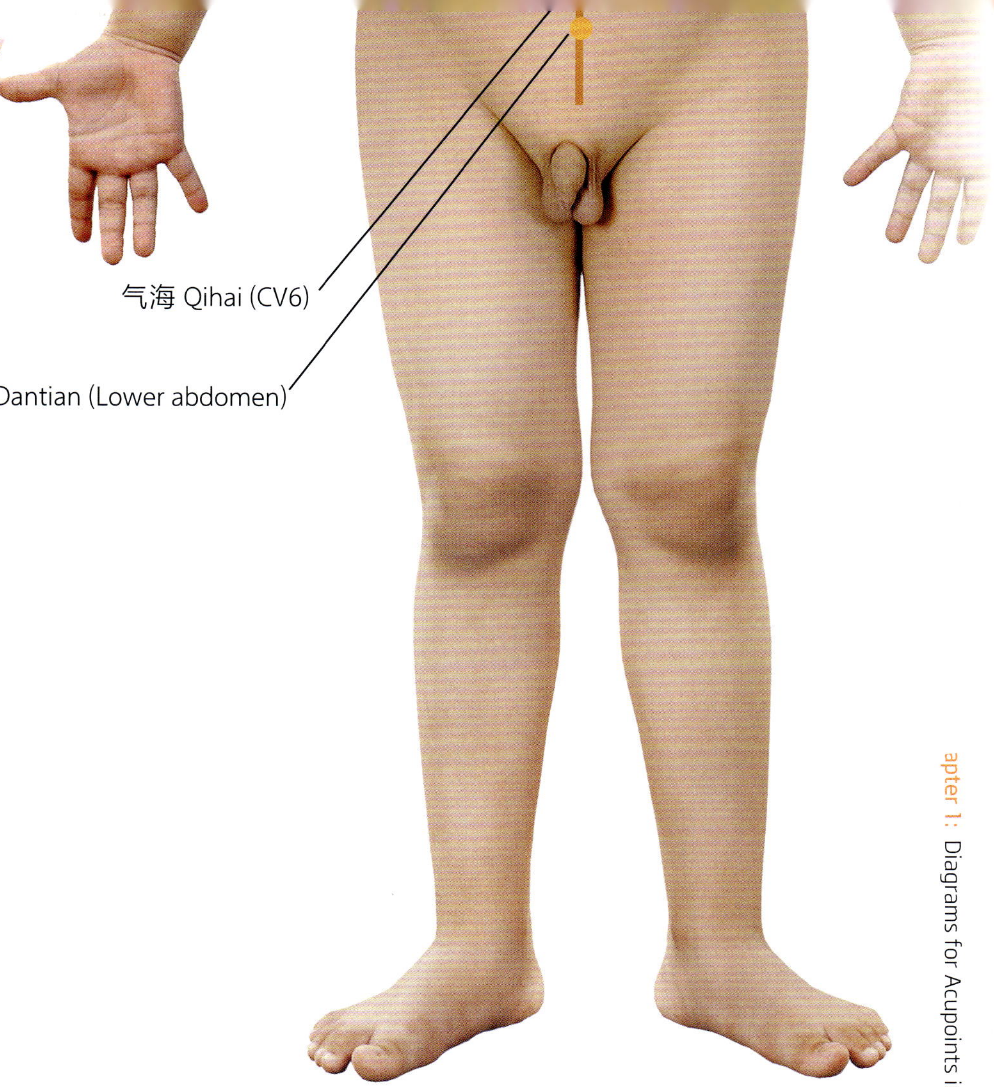

Conception Vessel Meridian, CV

Conception Vessel Meridian: starting from the perineum, it flows upward along the middle line of the front body→abdomen→ chest and ends at the middle depression of the mentolabial sulcus in the face.

第二章 儿童特效穴位分部图解

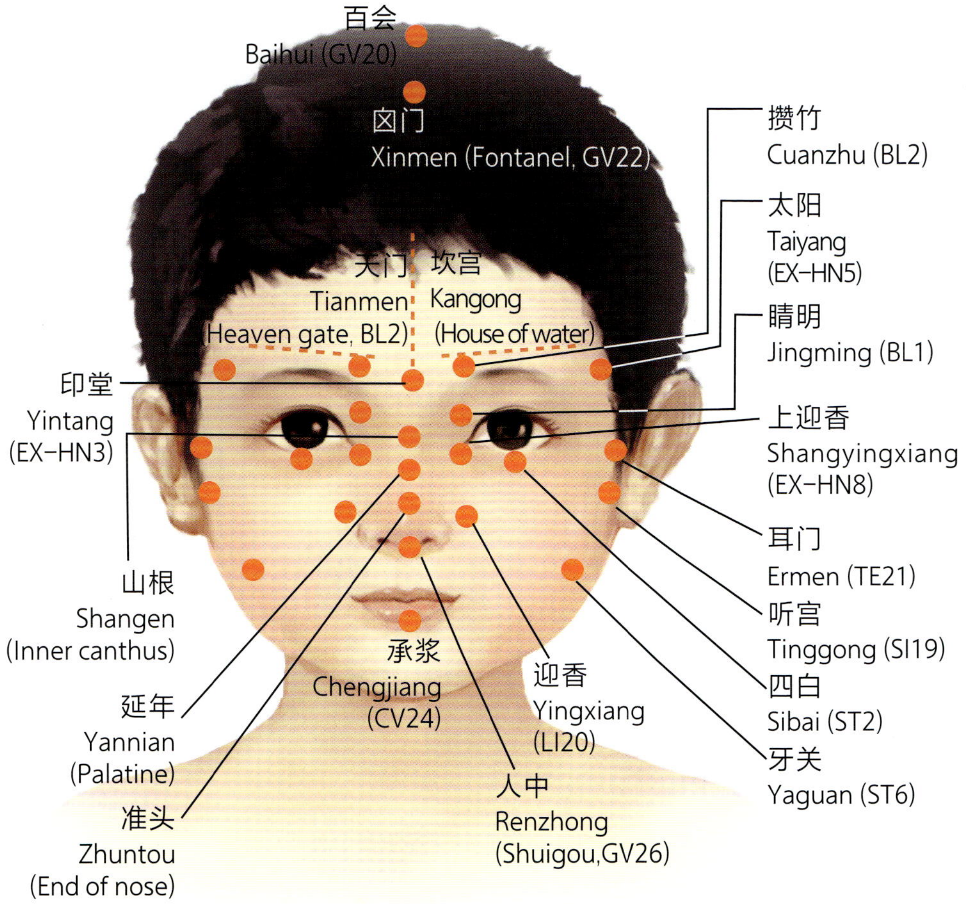

头面颈项部经典按摩手法

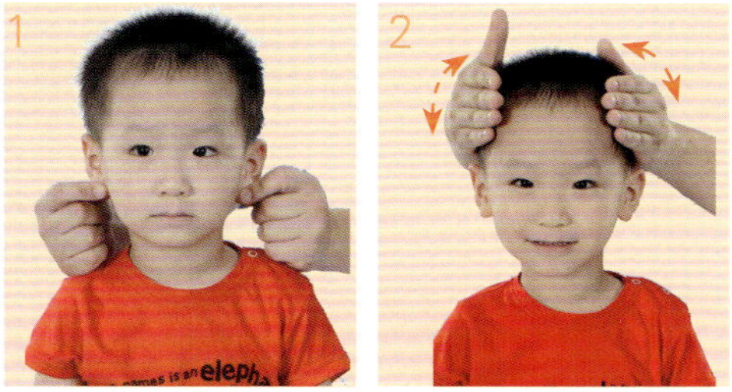

揉耳摇头

本法可以开关镇惊、调和气血。用于治疗惊风。

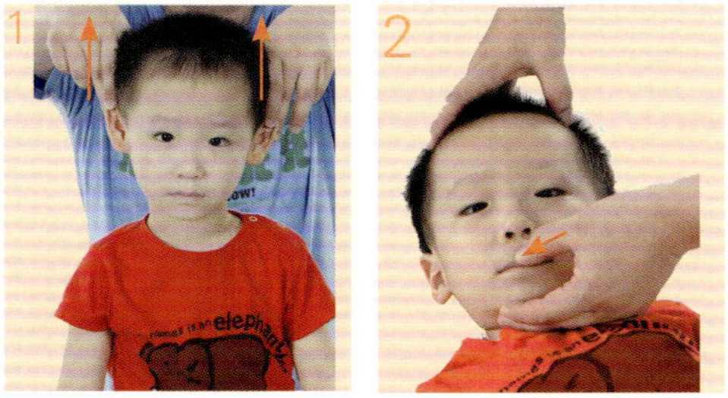

双凤展翅

本法可以祛风寒、温肺经、止咳化痰。用于外感风寒，咳嗽痰多等上呼吸道疾患。

Chapter 2: Diagrams for Acupoints with Specific Effects for Children in Different Divisions

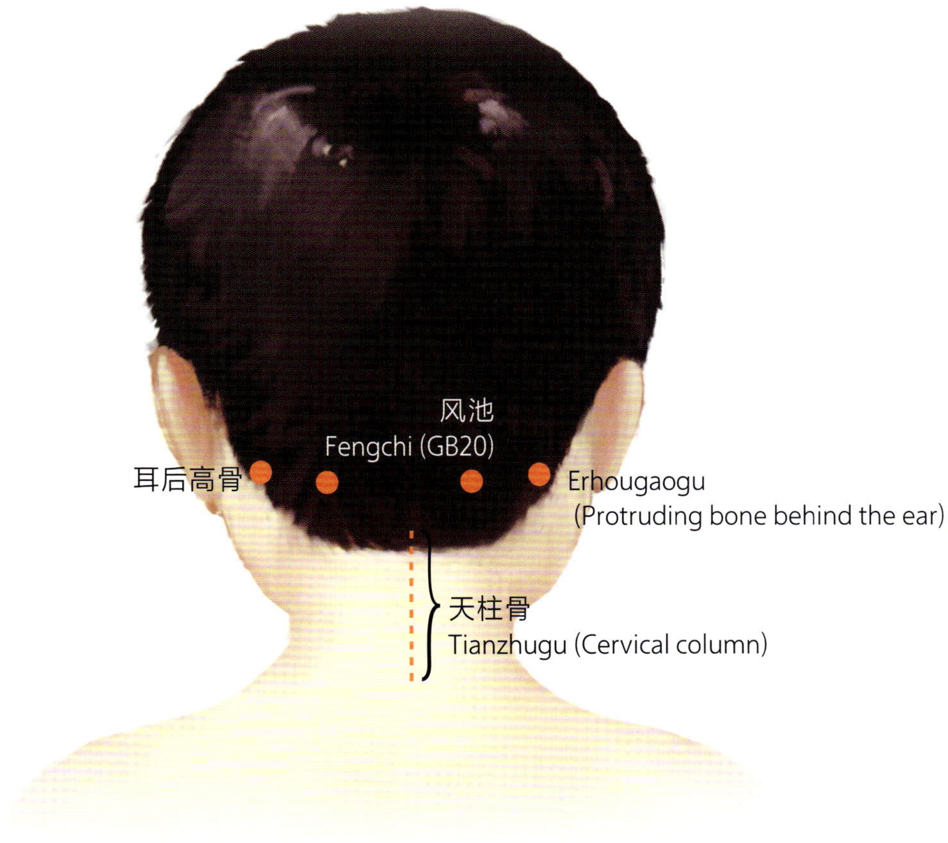

Classic Massage Manipulations in Head and Neck

Rou Er Yao Tou(Knead the ear and rotate the head)

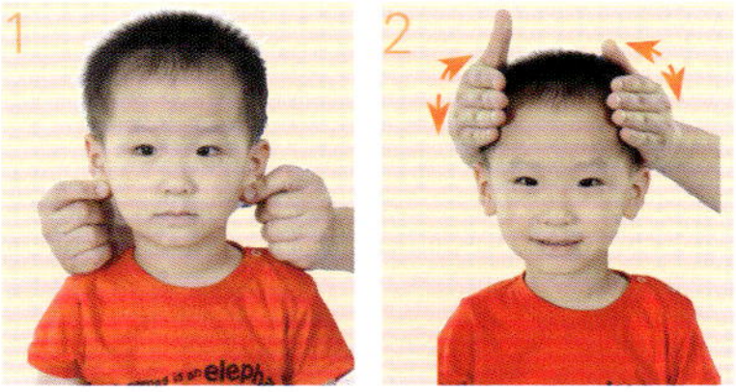

The manipulation can open the blockage and calm fright, and harmonize Qi and blood to treat infantile convulsion.

Shuang Feng Zhan Chi(Moving hands like the phoenix spreading wings)

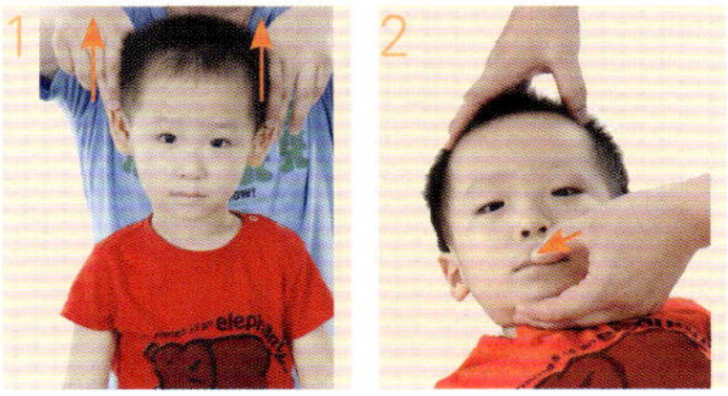

The manipulation can dispel wind-cold, warm the Lung Meridian, relieve cough and resolve phlegm. It can be applied in the diseases of upper respiratory tract such as the affection of exogenous wind-cold and cough with excessive phlegm.

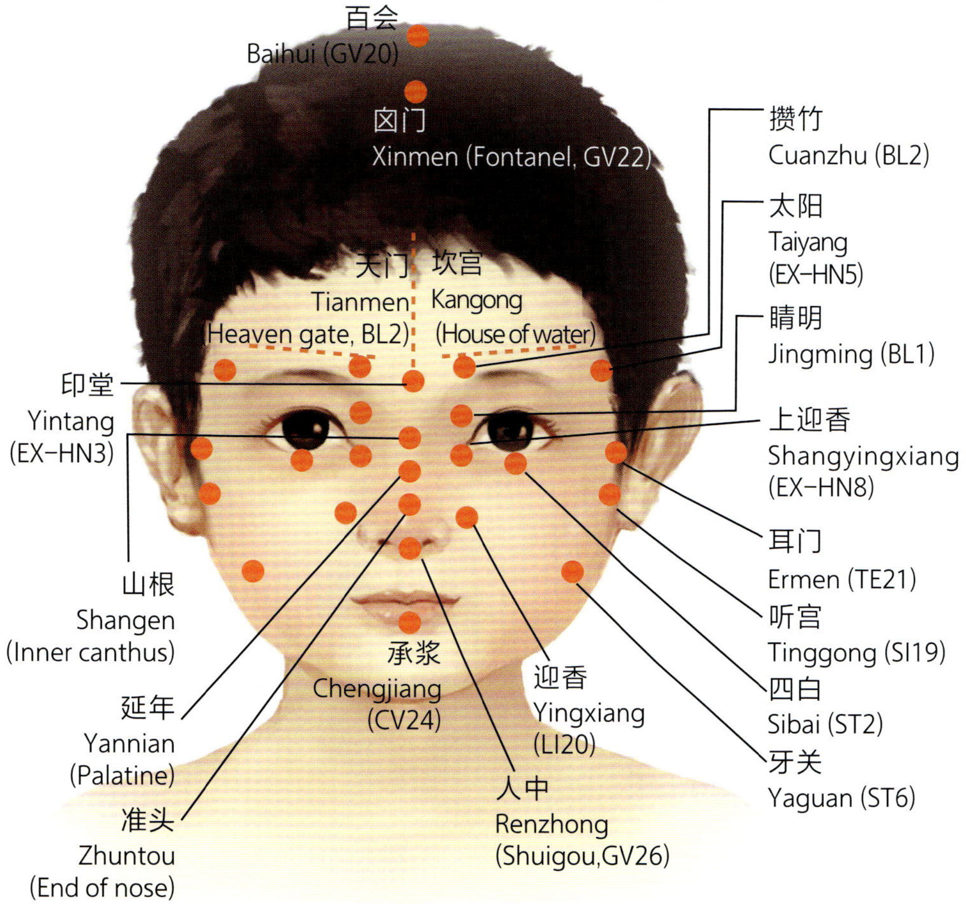
百会
Baihui (GV20)
囟门
Xinmen (Fontanel, GV22)
攒竹
Cuanzhu (BL2)
太阳
Taiyang
(EX-HN5)
睛明
Jingming (BL1)
天门
Tianmen
(Heaven gate, BL2)
坎宫
Kangong
(House of water)
印堂
Yintang
(EX-HN3)
上迎香
Shangyingxiang
(EX-HN8)
耳门
Ermen (TE21)
听宫
Tinggong (SI19)
四白
Sibai (ST2)
牙关
Yaguan (ST6)
山根
Shangen
(Inner canthus)
延年
Yannian
(Palatine)
准头
Zhuntou
(End of nose)
承浆
Chengjiang
(CV24)
迎香
Yingxiang
(LI20)
人中
Renzhong
(Shuigou,GV26)

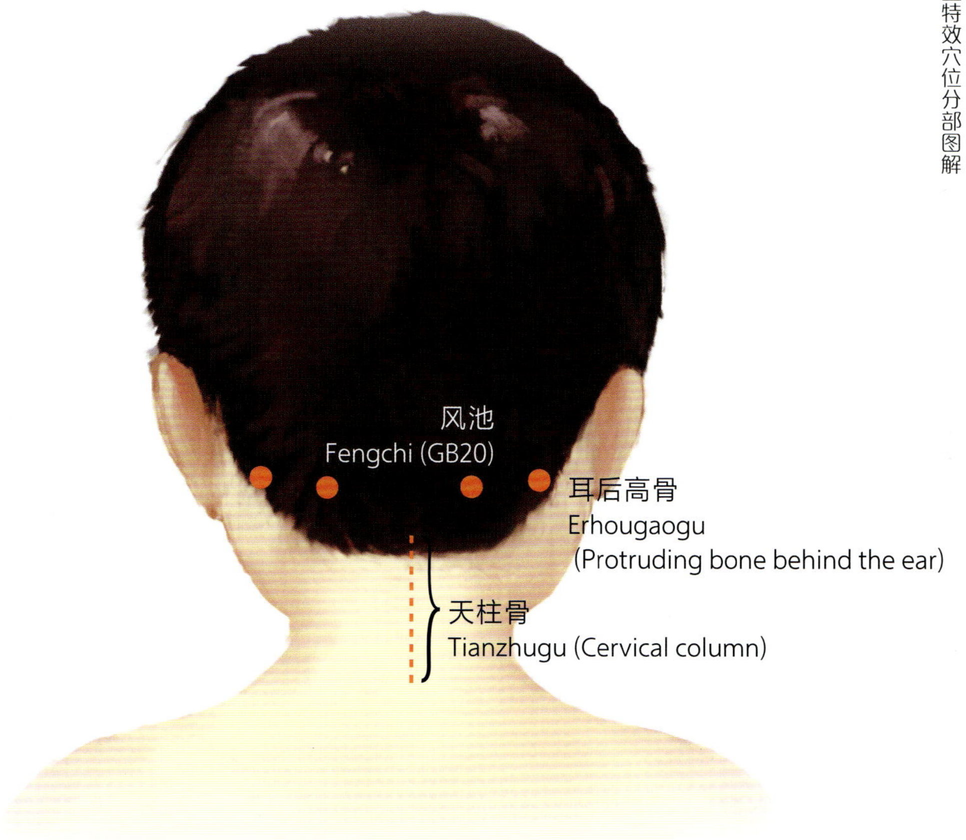
风池
Fengchi (GB20)
耳后高骨
Erhougaogu
(Protruding bone behind the ear)
天柱骨
Tianzhugu (Cervical column)

按摩方法速览
Quick Look of Massage Manipulations

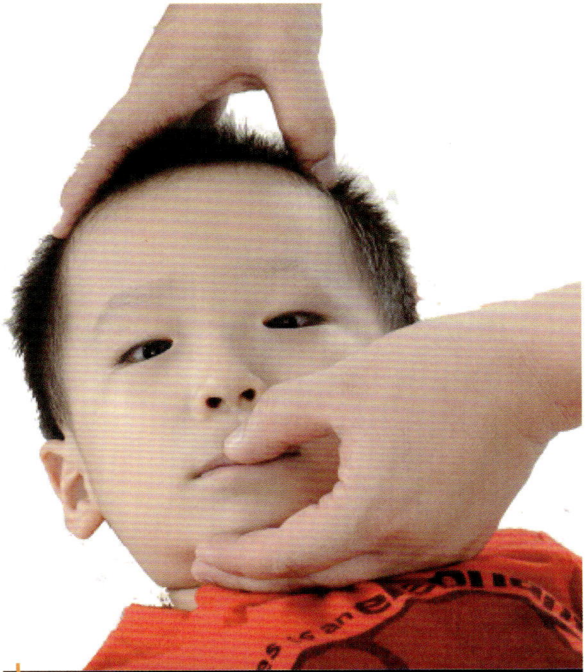

掐人中 Pinch Renzhong (Shuigou GV26)

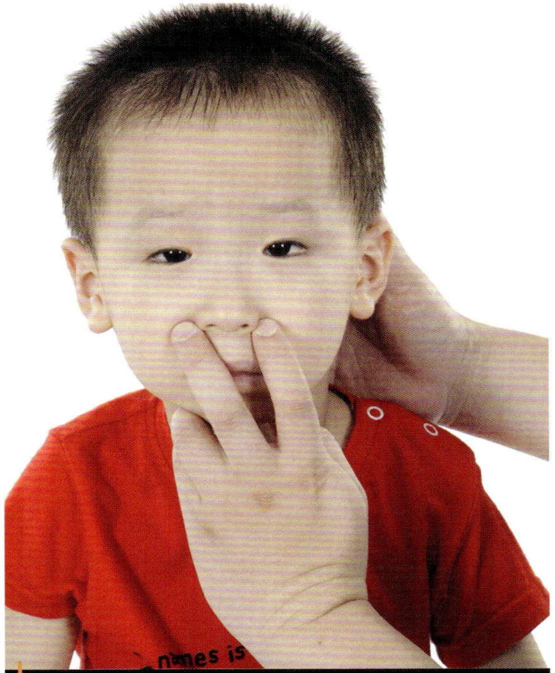

揉迎香 Knead Yingxiang (LI20)

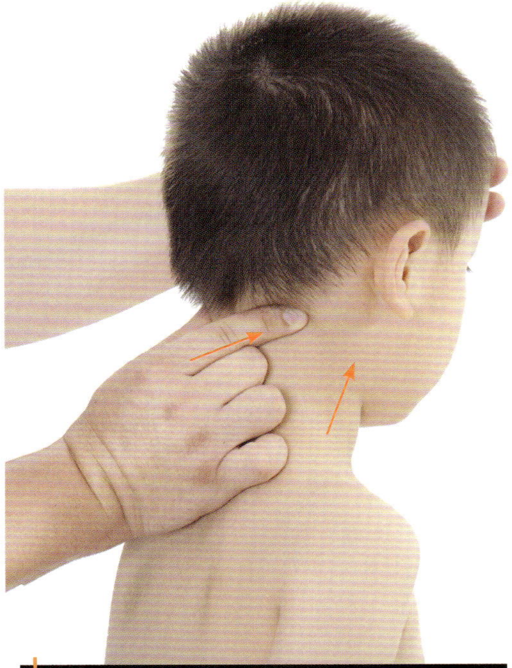

拿风池 Grasp Fengchi (GB20)

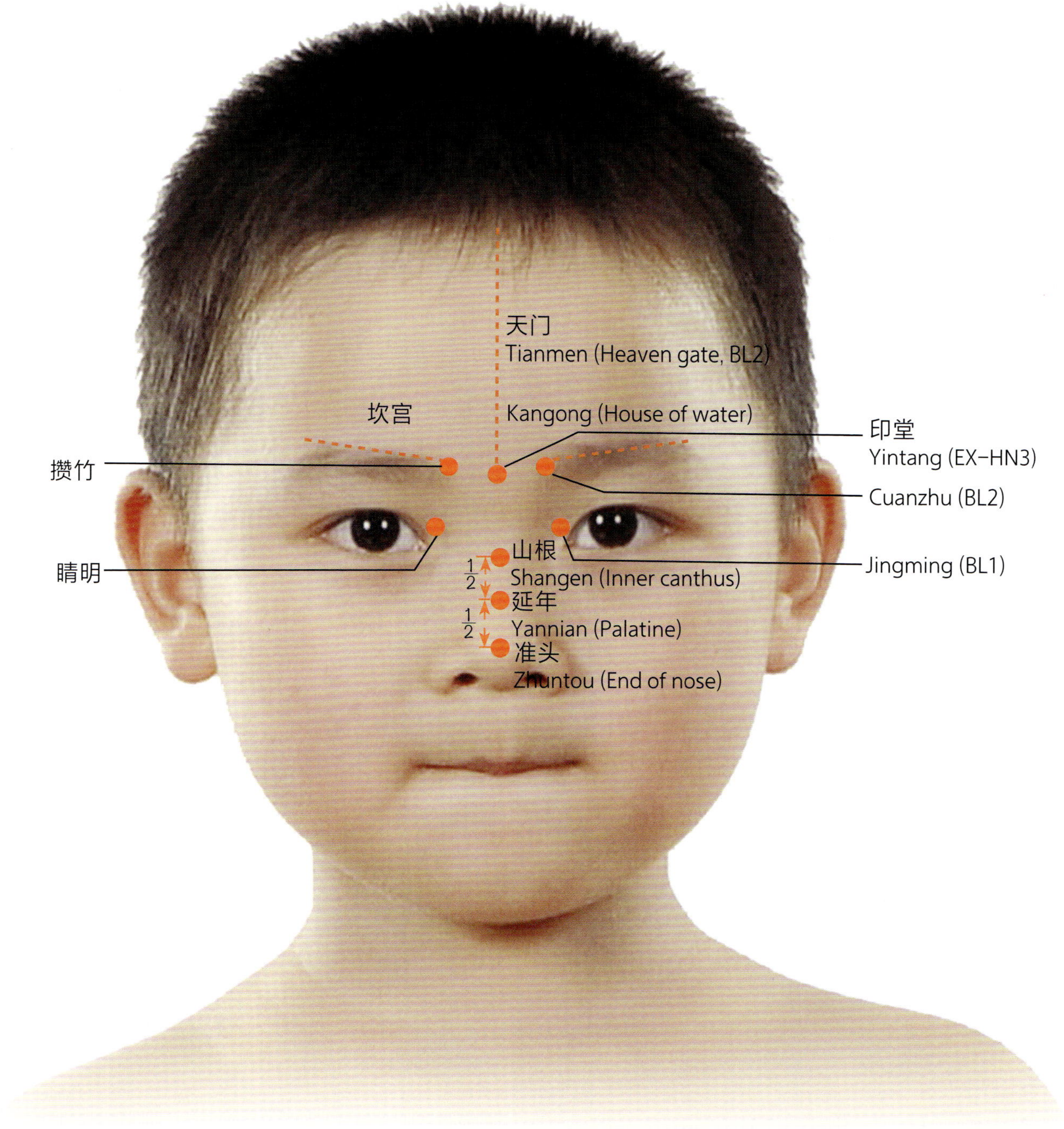
天门
Tianmen (Heaven gate, BL2)
坎宫
Kangong (House of water)
印堂
Yintang (EX-HN3)
攒竹
Cuanzhu (BL2)
睛明
Jingming (BL1)
山根
Shangen (Inner canthus)
1/2
延年
Yannian (Palatine)
1/2
准头
Zhuntou (End of nose)

穴 位	定 位	按摩方法	功效主治
天门	两眉中间至前发际成一直线	推法：从眉心向额上交替直推，称开天门，推 30~50 次	发汗解表，镇静安神，清脑止痛。主治发热、头痛、感冒、精神萎靡、惊恐不安
坎宫	自眉头起沿眉向眉梢成一横线	推法：用两拇指自眉心向眉梢分推 30~50 次	发汗解表，清脑明目，止头痛。主治感冒、发热、抽搐、癫痫、头痛、目赤痛
印堂	在额部，当两眉头之中间	掐法或揉法：用拇指指甲掐 3~5 次，或用指端揉，揉 20~30 次	醒脑安神，祛风通窍。主治感冒头痛、昏厥、抽搐、癫痫
攒竹	面部眉头凹陷中，眶上切迹处	揉法：用拇指指腹按揉 50~100 次	清热明目，祛风通络。主治感冒发热、头痛、精神萎靡、惊风

Acupoints	Location	Massage Manipulations	Efficacy and Indications
Tianmen (Heaven gate, BL2)	The line between the midpoint of the 2 eyebrows and the anterior hairline	Pushing manipulation: Push the point directly upward from the midpoint of the eyebrows to the forehead alternatively for 30 to 50 times, which is called Open Tianmen (Heaven gate, BL 2)	It can induce sweating to release exterior, tranquilize and calm mind, clear brain and relieve pain, mainly used for fever, headache, cold, low spirit and fear
Kangong (House of water)	The transverse line starting from the brow tip to the brow end	Pushing manipulation: Push Kangong (House of water)from the midpoint to the end of the eyebrow with the 2 thumbs for 30 to 50 times	It can induce sweating to release exterior, clear brain and improve vision, and relieve headache, mainly used for cold, fever, convulsion, epilepsy, headache and red eyes with pain
Yintang (EX-HN3)	In the frontal part, the midpoint of the 2 eyebrows	Pinching or Kneading Manipulation: Pinch the point for 3 to 5 times with the fingernail of the thumb, or knead the point for 20 to 30 times with the finger tip	It can restore consciousness and tranquilize mind, dispel wind and relieve stuffy orifices, mainly used for cold with headache, syncope, convulsion and epilepsy
Cuanzhu (BL2)	In the depression of the medial end of the eyebrow on the face, in the supraorbital notch	Kneading manipulation: Press-knead the point for 50 to 100 times with the finger pulp of the thumb	It can clear heat and improve vision, dispel wind and sooth collaterals, mainly used for cold, fever, headache, low spirit and infantile convulsion

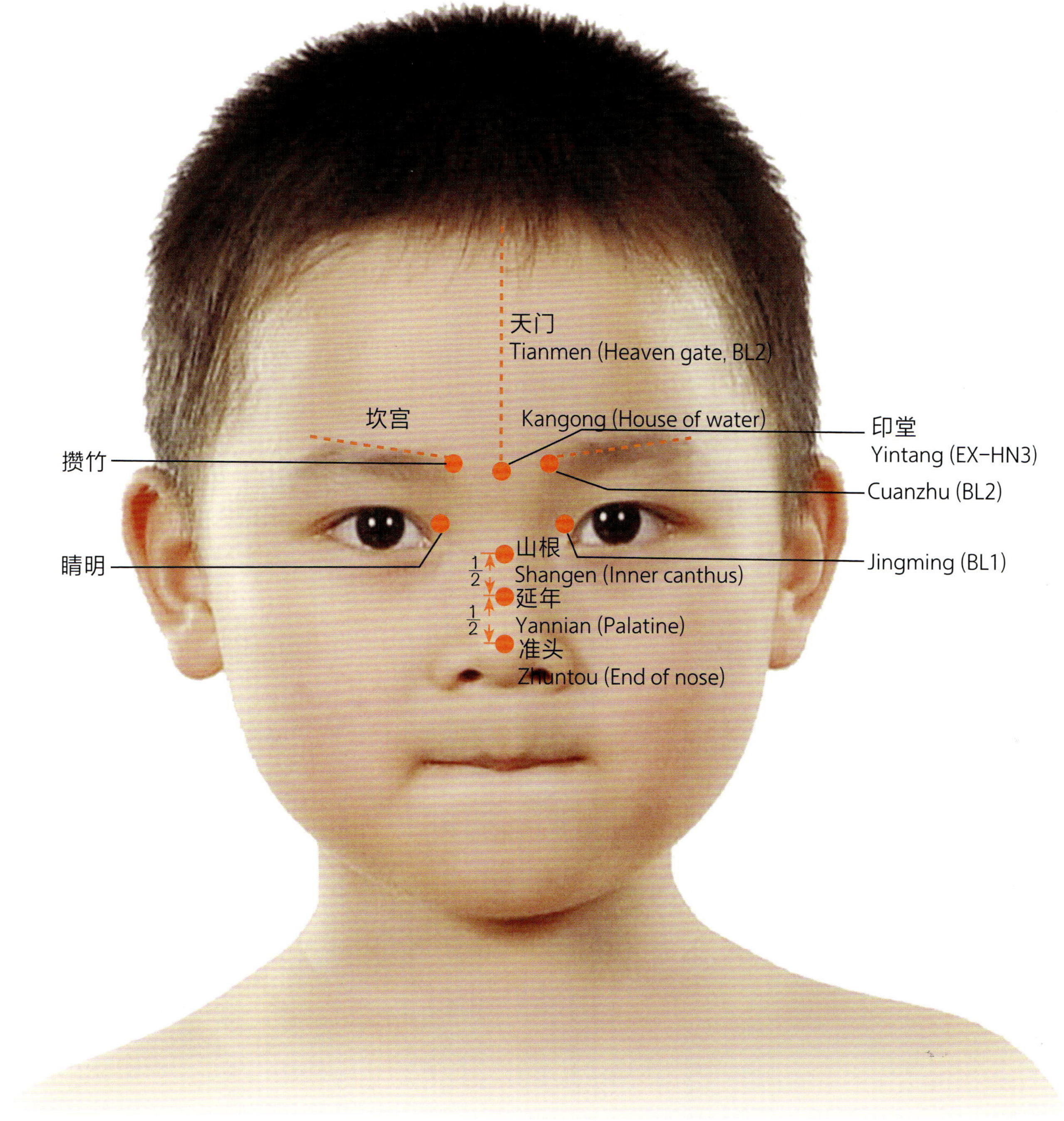
天门
Tianmen (Heaven gate, BL2)
坎宫
Kangong (House of water)
印堂
Yintang (EX-HN3)
攒竹
Cuanzhu (BL2)
睛明
Jingming (BL1)
山根
Shangen (Inner canthus)
延年
Yannian (Palatine)
准头
Zhuntou (End of nose)
1/2
1/2

续表

穴 位	定 位	按摩方法	功效主治
睛明	目内眦（内眼角）稍上方凹陷处	揉法：用拇指指腹按揉 50~100 次	祛风，清热，明目。主治目赤肿痛、近视、色盲、夜盲
山根	两目内眦（内眼角）之中点，鼻梁上低洼处	掐法：用拇指指甲掐 3~5 次	退热定惊，开关通窍，醒目安神。主治抽搐、癫痫、目赤痛
延年	鼻梁骨高耸处，山根穴与准头穴之间	掐法：用拇指指甲掐 3~5 次	开窍醒神，止抽搐。主治外感风寒、惊厥
准头	鼻尖中央	掐法或揉法：用拇指或食指指甲掐 3~5 次，继之以中指螺纹面揉 10~20 次	开窍醒神，健脾定喘，祛风清热。主治抽搐、癫痫、鼻塞不通

Continued

Acupoints	Location	Massage Manipulations	Efficacy and Indications
Jingming (BL1)	In the depression slightly above the Inner canthus	Kneading manipulation: Press-knead the point for 50 to 100 times with the finger pulp of the thumb	It can dispel wind, clear heat and improve vision, mainly used for red eyes with swelling and pain, nearsightedness, color blindness and nyctalopia
Shangen (Inner canthus)	The midpoint of the 2 inner canthus, in the low-lying area of the nasal bridge	Pinching manipulation: Pinch the point for 3 to 5 times with the fingernail of the thumb	It can bring down fever, relieve convulsion, open the blockage and relieve stuffy orifices, restore vision and tranquilize mind, mainly used for convulsion, epilepsy and red eyes with pain
Yannian (Palatine)	In the high area of the nasal bone, between Shangen (Inner canthus) and Zhuntou (End of nose) points	Pinching manipulation: Pinch the point for 3 to 5 times with fingernail of the thumb	It can open orifice, induce resuscitation and arrest convulsion, mainly used for affection of exogenous wind-cold and convulsion
Zhuntou (End of nose)	The middle of apex nasi	Pinching or kneading manipulation: Pinch the point for 3 to 5 times with fingernail of the thumb or index finger, and then knead the point for 10 to 20 times with the middle finger	It can open orifice, induce resuscitation, invigorate spleen, relieve dyspnea,dispel wind and clear heat, mainly used for convulsion, epilepsy and nasal congestion

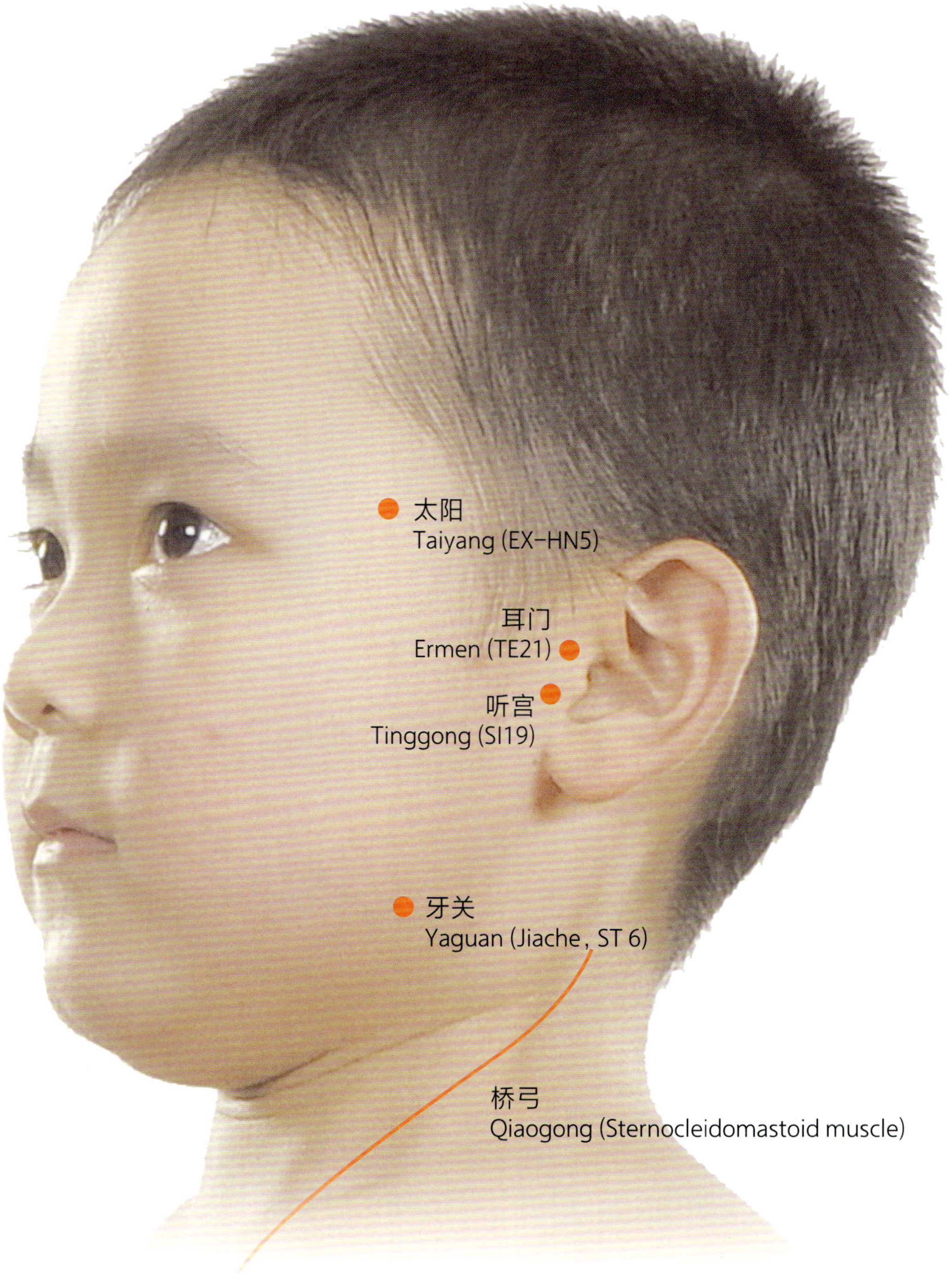
太阳
Taiyang (EX-HN5)
耳门
Ermen (TE21)
听宫
Tinggong (SI19)
牙关
Yaguan (Jiache, ST 6)
桥弓
Qiaogong (Sternocleidomastoid muscle)

穴 位	定 位	按摩方法	功效主治
太 阳	眉梢与目外眦（外眼角）之间，向后约 1 横指之凹陷处	揉法：用拇指或中指指端揉 30~50 次	疏风清热，开窍镇惊。主治感冒、发热、头痛、目赤肿痛、口眼㖞斜
耳 门	耳屏上切迹之前方，张口凹陷处	揉法：用食指或中指揉 30~50 次	镇惊开窍，聪耳，止牙痛。主治耳鸣、耳聋、抽搐、癫痫、牙痛、口眼㖞斜
听 宫	耳屏前，下颌骨髁状突的后方，张口时呈凹陷处	揉法：用食指或中指揉 30~50 次	聪耳开窍。主治耳鸣、耳聋、中耳炎、外耳道炎、失音症、聋哑

Acupoints	Location	Massage Manipulations	Efficacy and Indications
Taiyang (EX-HN5)	Between the brow tip and outer canthus, in the depression about one finger-breadth backward	Kneading manipulation: Knead the point for 30 to 50 times with the fingertip of the thumb or middle finger	It can disperse wind and clear heat, open orifice and calm fright, mainly used for cold, fever, headache, red eyes with swelling and pain and facial palsy
Ermen (TE21)	Near the supratragic notch, in the depression when open the mouth	Kneading manipulation: Knead the point for 30 to 50 times with index or middle finger	It can calm fright and open orifice, improve hearing and relieve toothache, mainly used for tinnitus, deafness, convulsion, epilepsy, toothache and facial palsy
Tinggong (SI19)	Near the tragus, posterior to the mandibular condyle, in the depression when open the mouth	Kneading manipulation: Knead the point for 30 to 50 times with index or middle finger	It can improve hearing and open orifice, mainly used for tinnitus, deafness, tympanitis, external otitis, aphonia and deafmutism

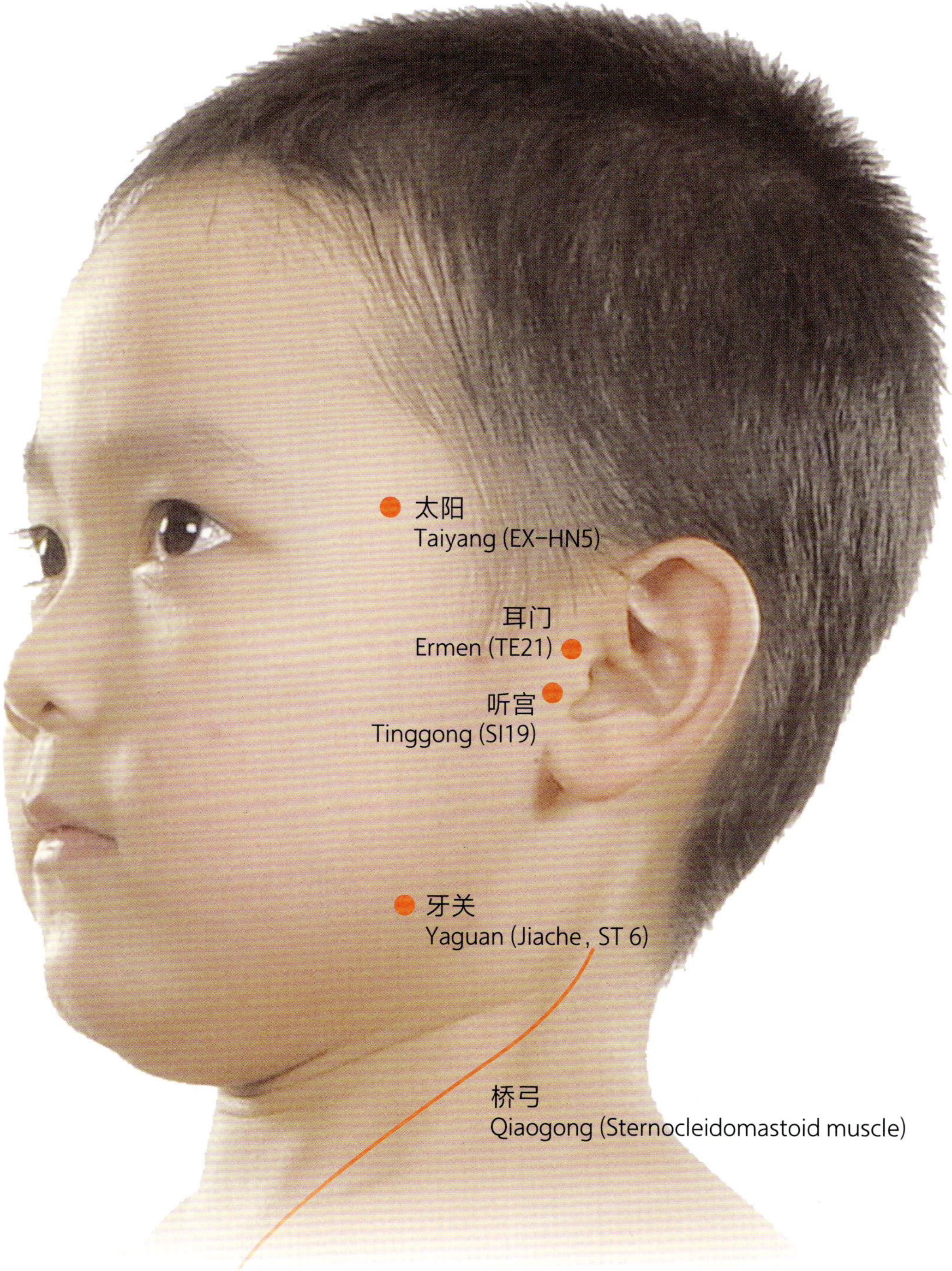
太阳
Taiyang (EX-HN5)
耳门
Ermen (TE21)
听宫
Tinggong (SI19)
牙关
Yaguan (Jiache，ST 6)
桥弓
Qiaogong (Sternocleidomastoid muscle)

续表

穴 位	定 位	按摩方法	功效主治
牙关	耳下 1 寸，下颌骨凹陷中	揉法或掐法：用拇指或中指按揉牙关穴 10~20 次，或用指端掐揉牙关穴 5~10 次	开窍，疏风，止痛。主治牙关紧闭、口眼㖞斜、颞颌关节痛、牙痛
桥弓	颈部两侧，沿胸锁乳突肌呈一直线	拿法或推法：用一手拇指、食指自上而下拿 3~5 次，或自上而下推 30~50 次。注意：手法轻重要适当，部位要准确，不可拿捏颈总动脉	舒筋活络，调和气血，平肝潜阳。主治先天性斜颈、抽搐、癫痫

Continued

Acupoints	Location	Massage Manipulations	Efficacy and Indications
Yaguan (Jiache, ST 6)	1 cun below the ear, in the depression of the mandible	Kneading or pinching manipulation: Press-knead Yaguan (Jiache, ST 6) with thumb or middle finger for 10 to 20 times, or pinch-knead Yaguan (Jiache, ST 6) with the fingertip for 5 to 10 times	It can open orifice, dispel wind and relieve pain, mainly used for jaw clenching, facial palsy, pain of temporomandibular joint and toothache
Qiaogong (Sternocleido mastoid muscle)	The straight line along the sternocleidomastoid in the both sides of the neck.	Grasping or pushing manipulation: Grasp the point for 3 to 5 times from top to bottom with the thumb and index finger, or push the point for 30 to 50 times from top to bottom. Notes: The manipulation shall be applied with appropriate strength, accurate location and the arteria carotis communis shall not be grapsed or pinched	It can relax sinew and activate collaterals, harmonize Qi and blood, pacify liver and subdue Yang, mainly used for congenital torticollis, convulsion and epilepsy

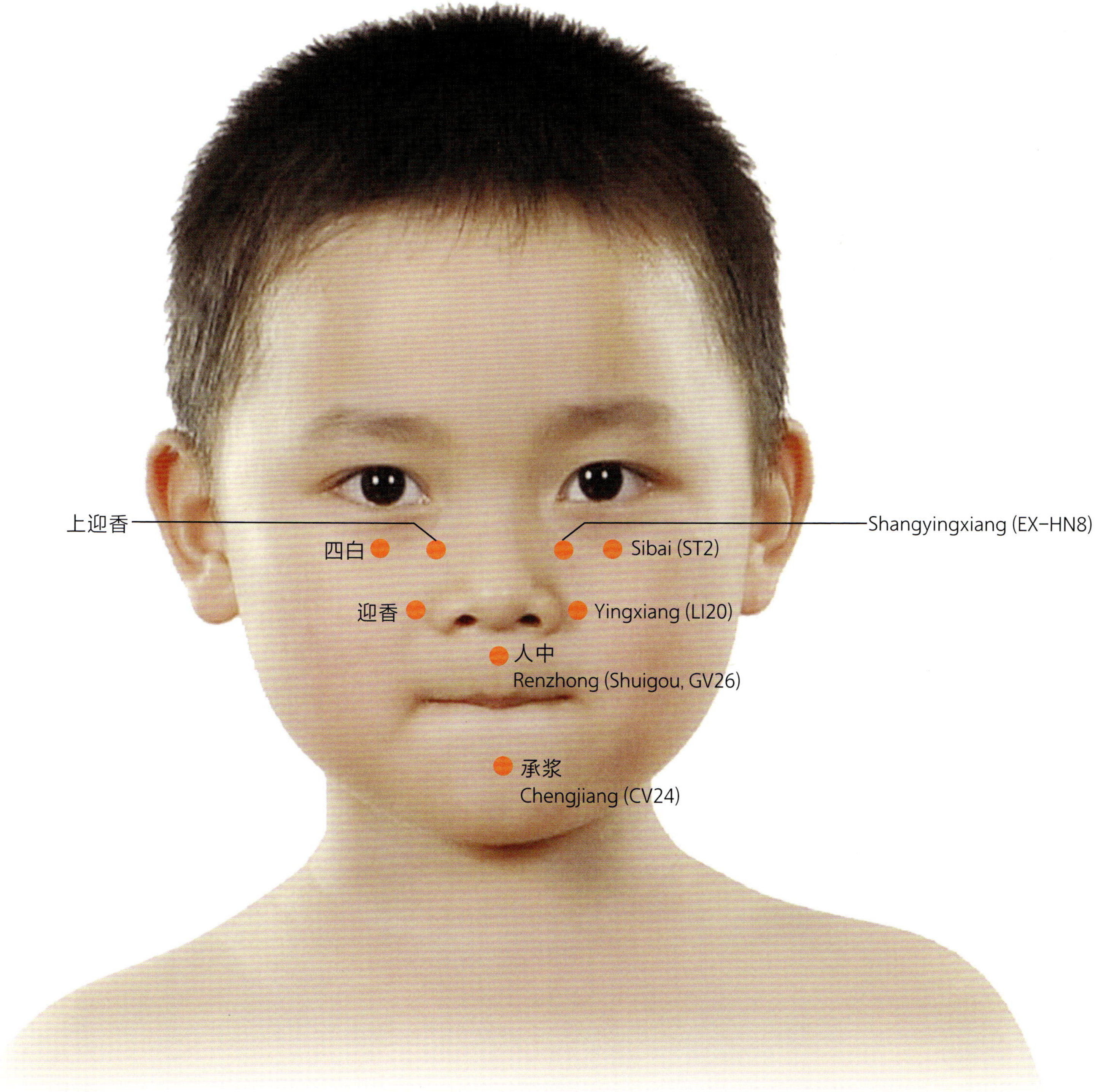
上迎香
Shangyingxiang (EX-HN8)
四白
Sibai (ST2)
迎香
Yingxiang (LI20)
人中
Renzhong (Shuigou, GV26)
承浆
Chengjiang (CV24)

穴 位	定 位	按摩方法	功效主治
上迎香	鼻翼软骨与鼻甲的交界处，近鼻唇沟上端处	揉法：用拇指指腹按揉 30~50 次	清利鼻窍，通络止痛。主治过敏性鼻炎、鼻窦炎、头痛
四白	瞳孔直下，眶下孔凹陷处	揉法：用拇指指腹按揉 30~50 次	祛风明目，通经活络。主治三叉神经痛、面神经麻痹、角膜炎、近视、青光眼、头痛、眩晕
迎香	鼻翼旁 0.5 寸，鼻唇沟中	揉法：用食指、中指两指或两拇指按揉两侧穴位，揉 50~100 次	疏散风热，通利鼻窍。主治鼻炎、鼻塞、口眼㖞斜

Acupoints	Location	Massage Manipulations	Efficacy and Indications
Shangyingxiang (EX-HN8)	In the junction of nasal alar cartilage and turbinalia near the upper edge of the nasolabial fold	Kneading manipulation: Press-knead the point for 30 to 50 times with the finger pulp of the thumb	It can clear nasal orifice, sooth collaterals and relieve pain, mainly used for allergic rhinitis, nasosinusitis and headache
Sibai (ST2)	Directly below the pupil, in the depression of the infraorbital foramen	Kneading manipulation: Press-knead the point for 30 to 50 times with the finger pulp of the thumb	It can dispel wind and improve vision, sooth meridians and activate collaterals, mainly used for trigeminal neuralgia, facial paralysis, keratitis, nearsightedness, glaucoma, headache and vertigo
Yingxiang (LI20)	0.5 cun lateral to the nasal ala, in the nasolabial fold	Kneading manipulation: Press-knead the point in both sides for 50 to 100 times with index and middle fingers or the 2 thumbs	It can disperse wind-heat and Relieving Stuffy Nose, mainly used for rhinitis, nasal congestion and facial palsy

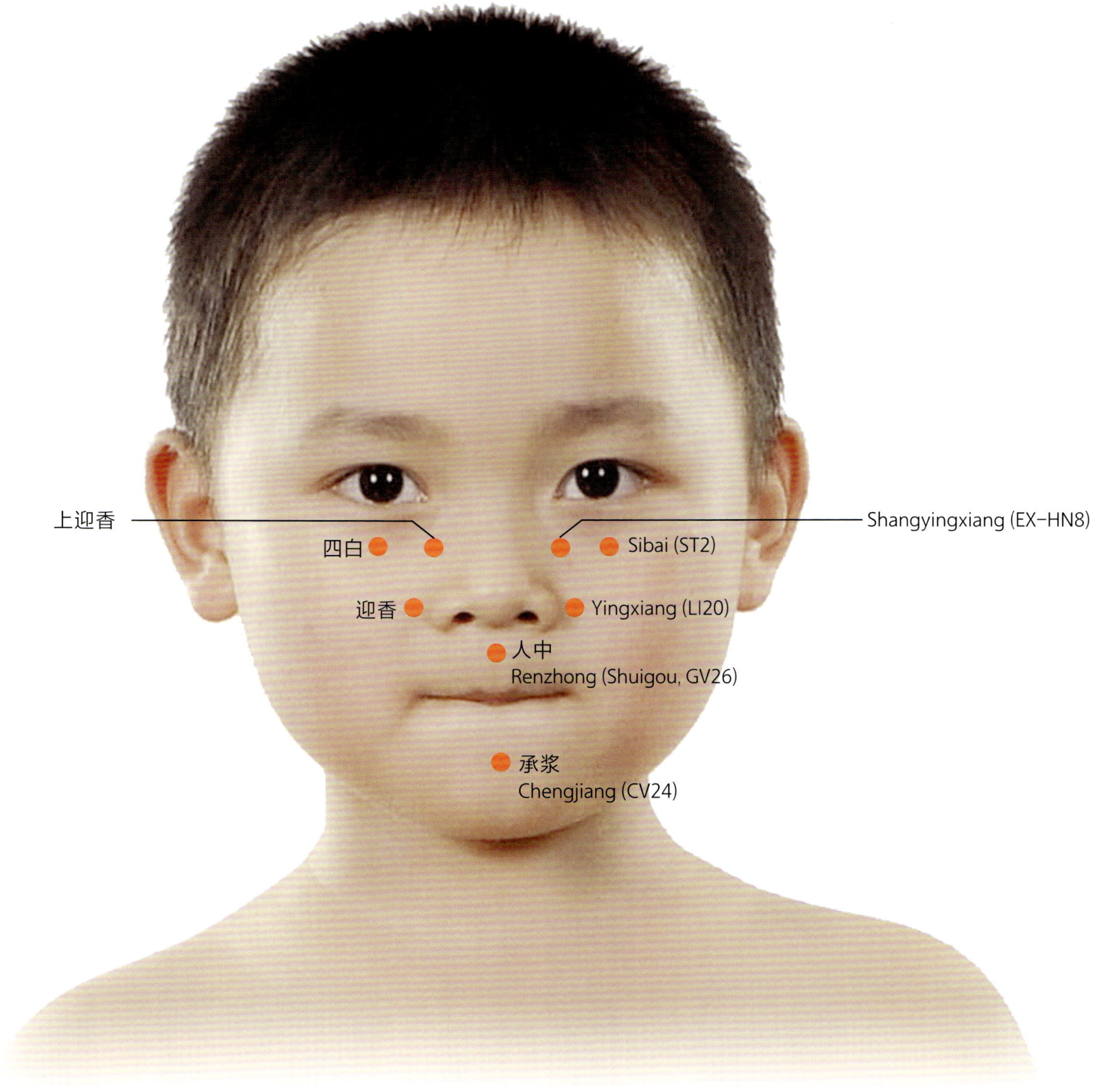
上迎香
Shangyingxiang (EX-HN8)
四白
Sibai (ST2)
迎香
Yingxiang (LI20)
人中
Renzhong (Shuigou, GV26)
承浆
Chengjiang (CV24)

续表

穴 位	定 位	按摩方法	功效主治
人 中	面部人中沟的上 1/3 与中 1/3 交界处	掐法：用拇指指甲掐 5 次	开窍醒神。主治抽搐、癫痫、昏厥
承 浆	颏唇沟的正中凹陷处	掐法：用食指或拇指指甲掐 3~5 次	祛风，开窍，醒神。主治抽搐、癫痫、口眼㖞斜
百 会	在头部，当前发际正中直上 5 寸，或两耳尖连线的中点处	按法或揉法：用拇指按 30~50 次，或用拇指揉 100~200 次。注意：囟门未闭者不宜按摩	安神镇惊，升阳举陷，止头痛。主治头痛、脱肛、久泄、癫痫、抽搐

Continued

Acupoints	Location	Massage Manipulations	Efficacy and Indications
Renzhong (Shuigou, GV26)	At the junction of the upper 1/3 and middle 1/3 of the philtrum in the face	Pinching manipulation: Pinch the point for 5 times with the fingernail of the thumb	It can open orifice and induce resuscitation, mainly used for convulsion, epilepsy and syncope
Chengjiang (CV24)	In the depression of the middle of the mentolabial sulcus	Pinching manipulation: Pinch the point for 3 to 5 times with the fingernail of the index finger or thumb	It can dispel wind, open orifice and induce resuscitation, mainly used for convulsion, epilepsy and facial palsy
Baihui (GV20)	On the head, 5 cun directly above the middle of the anterior hairline, or the midpoint of the line between tips of the 2 ears	Pressing or kneading manipulation: Press the point for 30 to 50 times with the thumb, or knead the point for 100 to 200 times with the thumb. Note: It is not suitable to massage for those with open fontanel	It can tranquilize mind and calm fright, elevate Yang and collapse, and relieve headache, mainly used for headache, prolapse of rectum, chronic diarrhea, epilepsy and convulsion

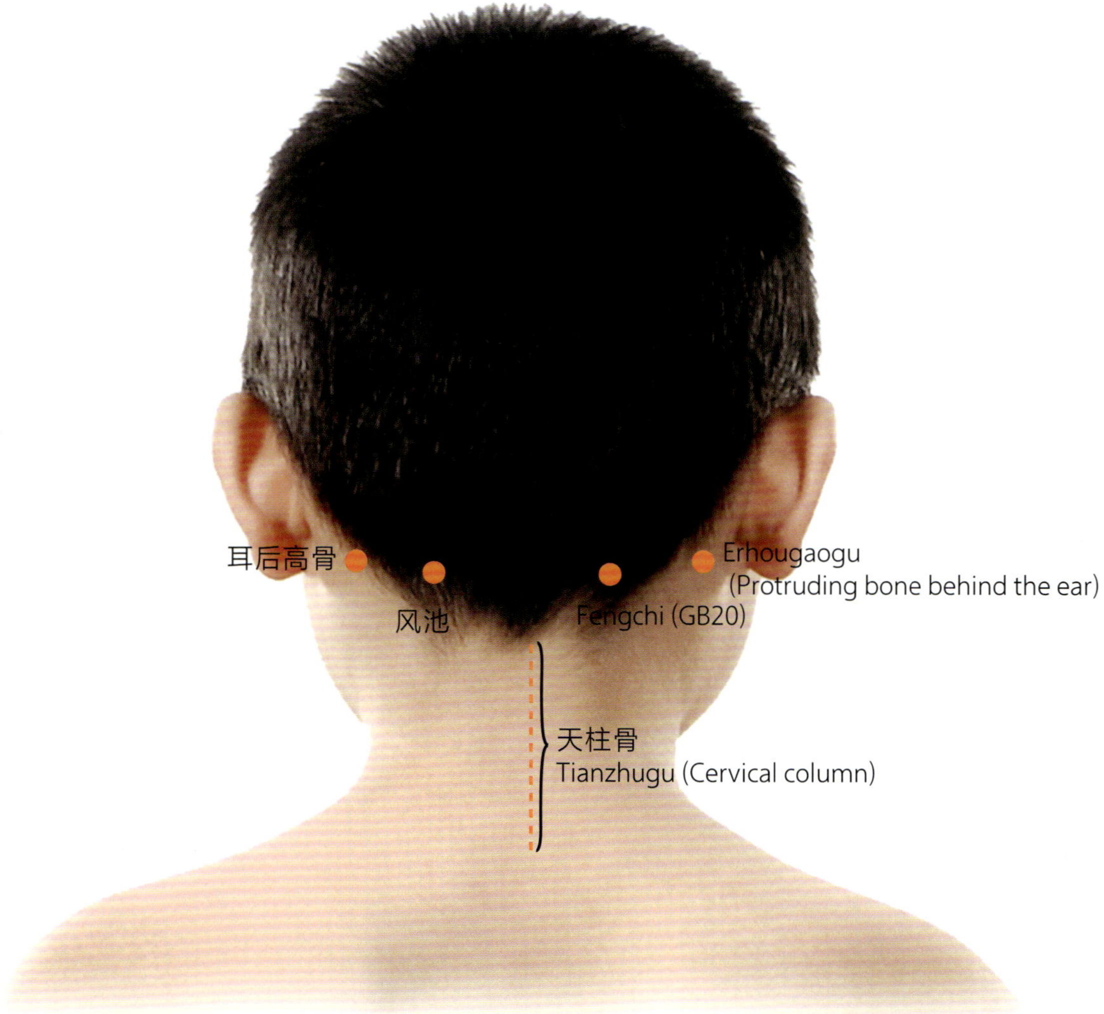
耳后高骨
风池
Erhougaogu
(Protruding bone behind the ear)
Fengchi (GB20)
天柱骨
Tianzhugu (Cervical column)

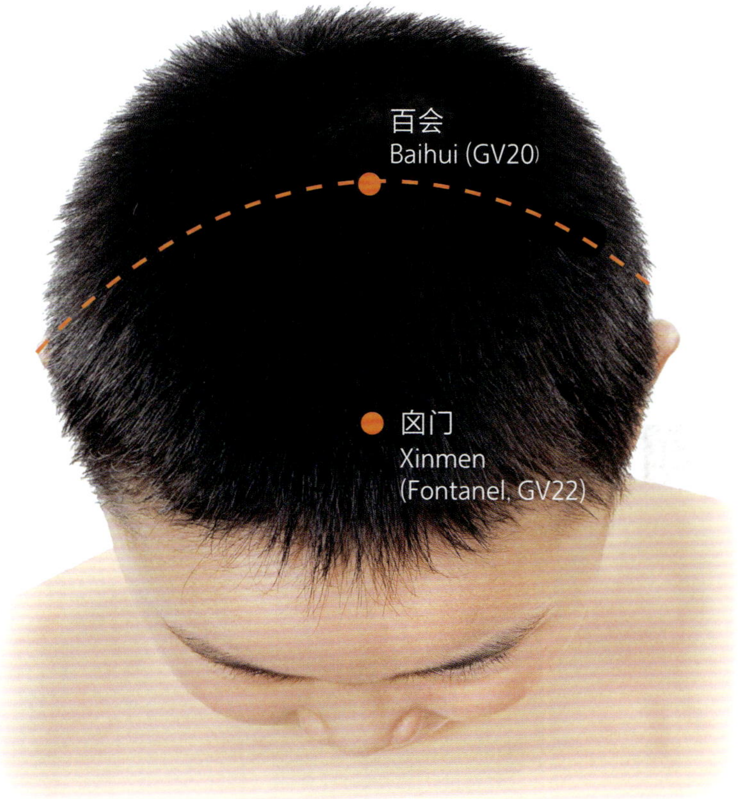
百会
Baihui (GV20)
囟门
Xinmen
(Fontanel, GV22)

穴 位	定 位	按摩方法	功效主治
囟门	前发际正中直上 2 寸，百会前骨之凹陷中	揉法或推法：用拇指腹面轻揉，或用拇指腹面自前发际向该穴反复推 50~100 次。注意：囟门未闭者不宜按摩	镇惊，醒神，通窍。主治抽搐、癫痫、头痛、鼻塞、鼻出血
耳后高骨	耳后入发际高骨下凹陷中	揉法：用中指指端揉 30~50 次	疏风解表，安神除烦。主治头痛、抽搐、癫痫、烦躁不安

Acupoints	Location	Massage Manipulations	Efficacy and Indications
Xinmen (Fontanel, GV22)	2 cun directly above the midpoint of the anterior hairline, in the depression of the prehallus of Baihui (GV20)	Kneading or pushing manipulation: Knead the point slightly with the finger pulp of the thumb, or push repeatedly from anterior hairline to Xinmen (Fontanel, GV22) with the finger pulp of the thumb for 50 to 100 times. Note: It is not suitable to massage for those with open fontanel	It can calm fright, induce resuscitation and relieve stuffy orifices, mainly used for convulsion, epilepsy, headache, nasal congestion and nasal bleeding
Erhougaogu (Protruding bone behind the ear)	In the depression below the Erhougaogu (Protruding bone behind the ear)entering the hairline	Kneading manipulation: Knead the point for 30 to 50 times with the tip of middle finger	It can disperse wind, release the exterior, tranquilize mind and relieve dysphoria, mainly used for headache, convulsion, epilepsy and dysphoria

续表

穴 位	定 位	按摩方法	功效主治
风 池	颈后枕骨下大筋外侧凹陷中	拿法或揉法：用拇指、食指指端按揉 30~50 次，或用拇指、食指指端拿 3~5 次	平肝息风，祛风解毒，通利官窍。主治头痛、感冒、发热、颈项强痛
天 柱 骨	颈后发际正中至大椎穴成一直线	推法：用拇指或食指、中指两指指腹自上而下直推 100~500 次	降逆止呕，祛风散寒。主治呕吐、恶心、颈项强痛、发热、抽搐、癫痫

Continued

Acupoints	Location	Massage Manipulations	Efficacy and Indications
Fengchi (GB20)	In the depression of the lateral side the large tendon below the occipital bone below the neck	Grasping or pushing manipulation: Press-knead the point with tips of the thumb and index finger for 30 to 50 times, or grasp the point for 3 to 5 times with tips of the thumb and index finger	It can pacify liver and extinguish wind, dispel wind remove toxin, and relieve organs and stuffy orifices, mainly used for headache, cold, fever and painful and stiff neck
Tianzhugu (Cervical column)	The straight line between the midpoint of the posterior hairline behind the neck and Dazhui (GV 14)	Pushing manipulation: Push the point directly from top to bottom with finger pulps of the thumb, or index and middle fingers for 100 to 500 times	It can descend adverse Qi to relieve hiccup, dispel wind and dissipate cold, mainly used for vomiting, nausea, painful and stiff neck, fever, convulsion and epilepsy

按摩方法详解
Detailed Diagram of Massage Manipulations

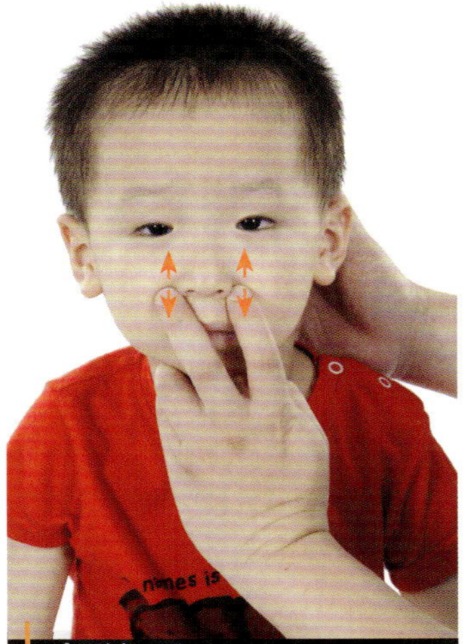

揉迎香

按摩者用食指、中指两指指端按揉之。操作 20~30 次。

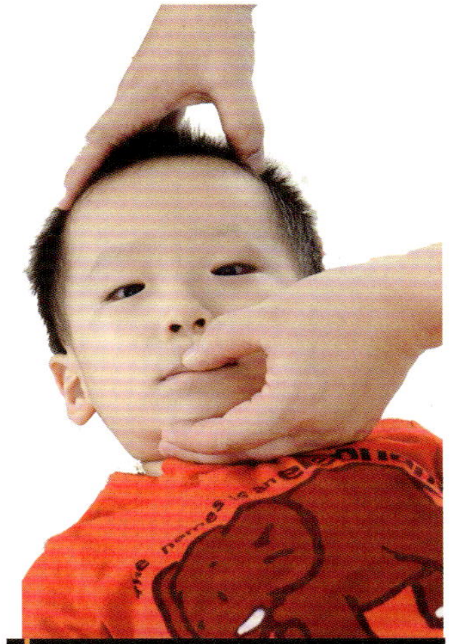

掐人中

拇指指甲掐，一般 5 次。

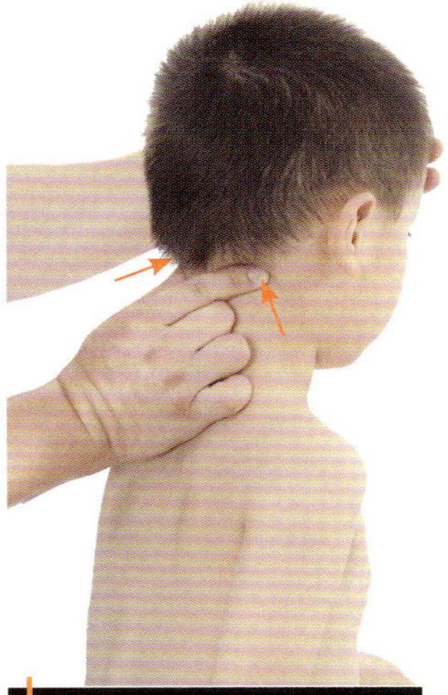

拿风池

按摩者位于小儿身后，以两手之四指扶住小儿头侧，用拇指拿之。一般拿3~5次。

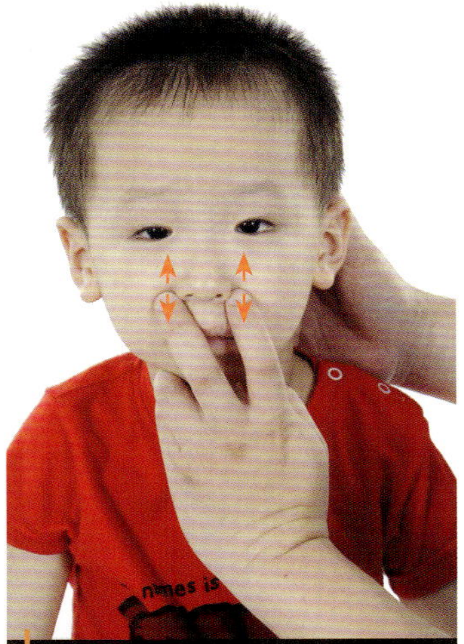

Knead Yingxiang (LI20)

Press-knead Ying xiang (LI20) with the finger tips of the index and middle fingers for 20 to 30 times.

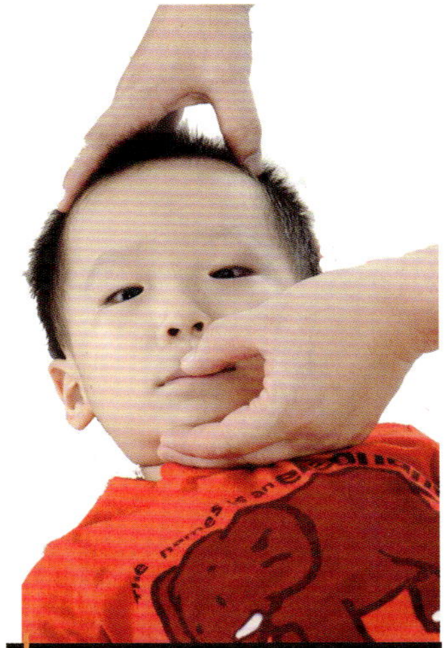

Pinch Renzhong (Shuigou, GV26)

Pinch with the fingernail of the thumb for generally 5 times.

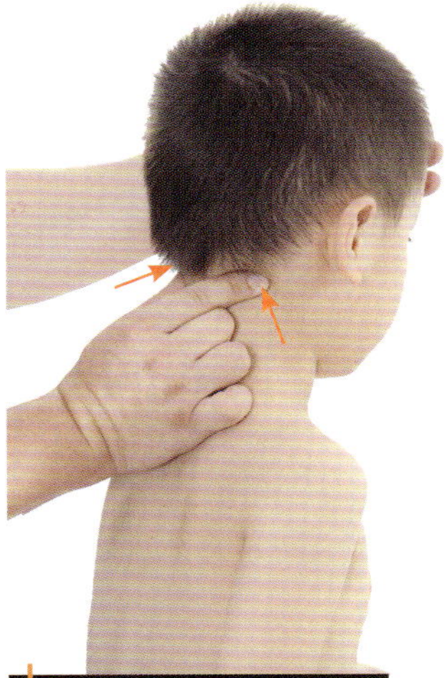

Grasp Fengchi (GB20)

Stand behind the child.Hold the head of the child with index, middle, ring and little fingers of the 2 hands and grasp Fengchi (GB20) with the thumbs for 3 to 5 times generally.

胸腹部穴位及按摩手法

Acupoints and Massage Manipulations in Chest and Abdomen

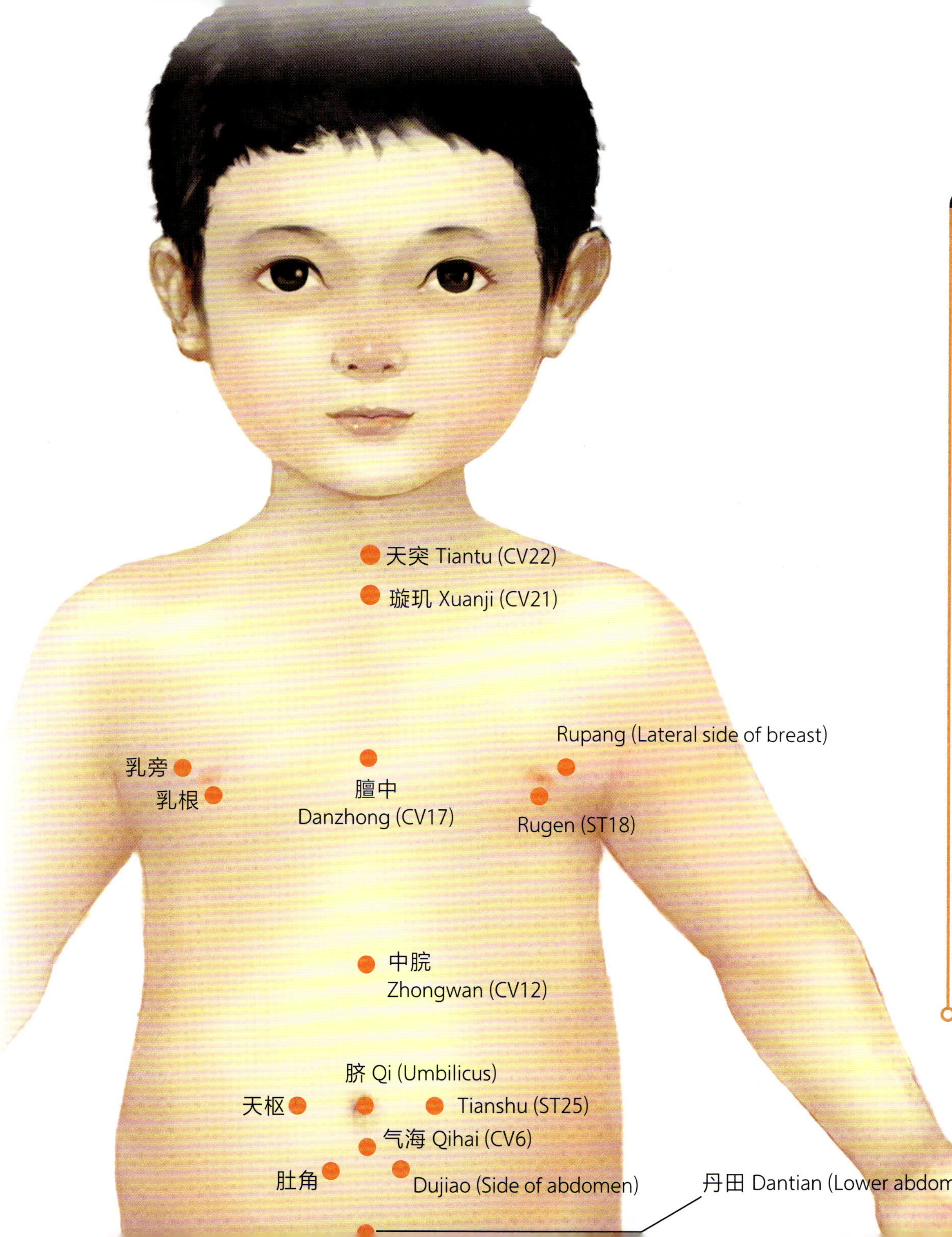

胸腹部经典按摩手法

开璇玑

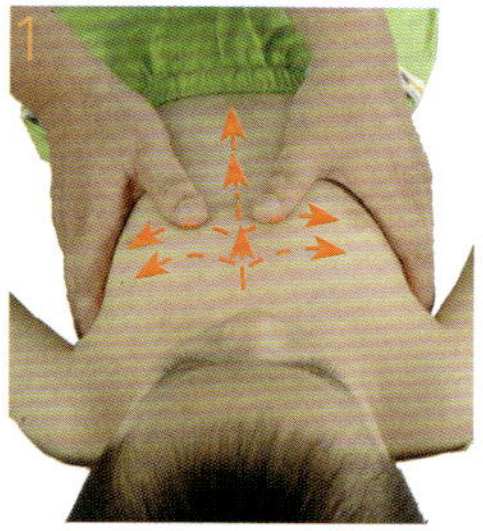

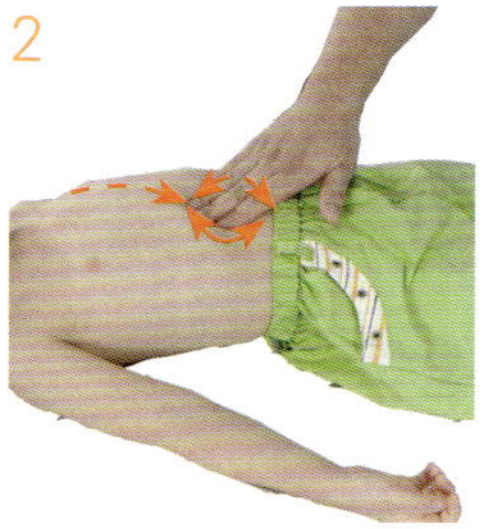

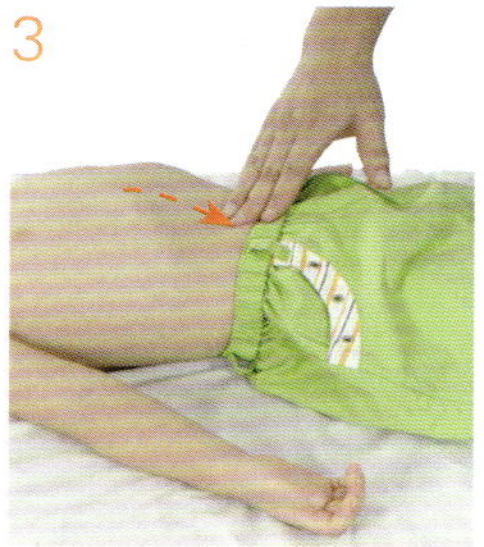

本法具有宽胸理气，健脾和胃的功效。主治胸闷咳喘、痰鸣气急、恶心呕吐、腹痛腹泻、便秘等症。

按弦搓摩

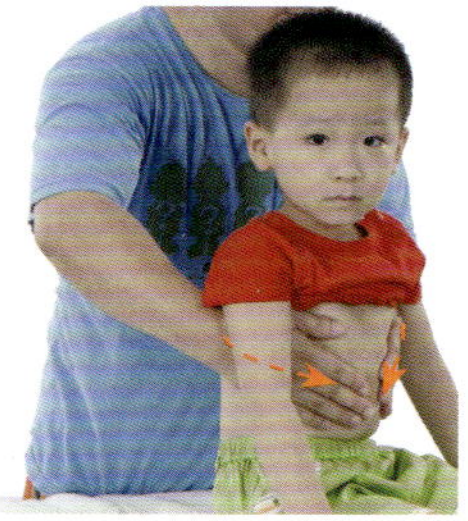

本法主要用于胸闷、气机不利、咳喘气急、痰喘不利等。

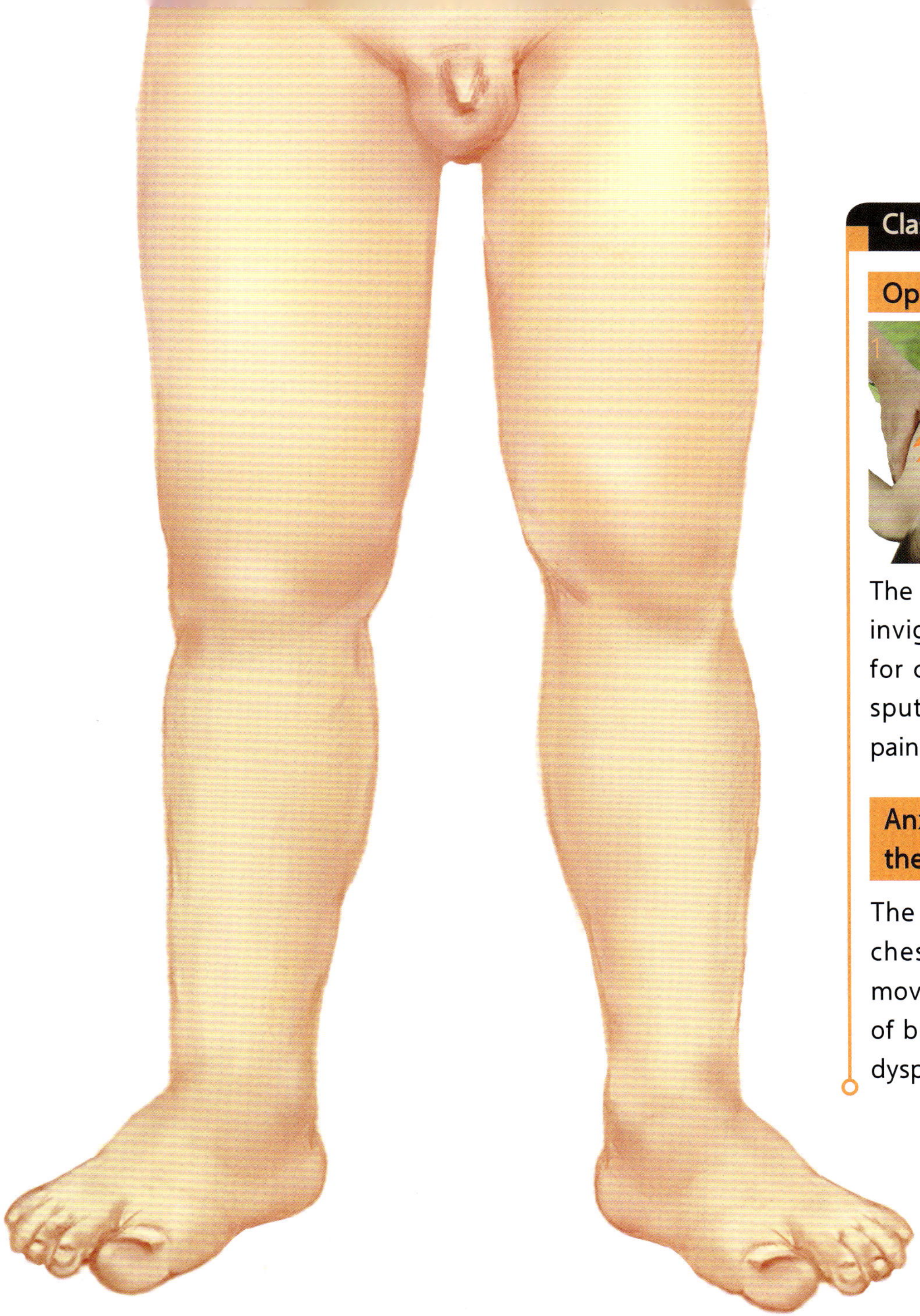

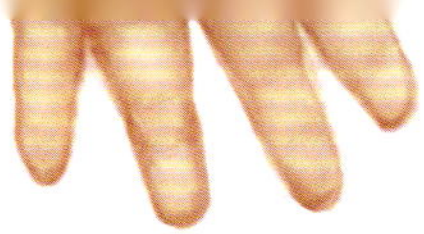

Classic Massage Manipulations in Chest and Abdomen

Open Xuanji (CV21)

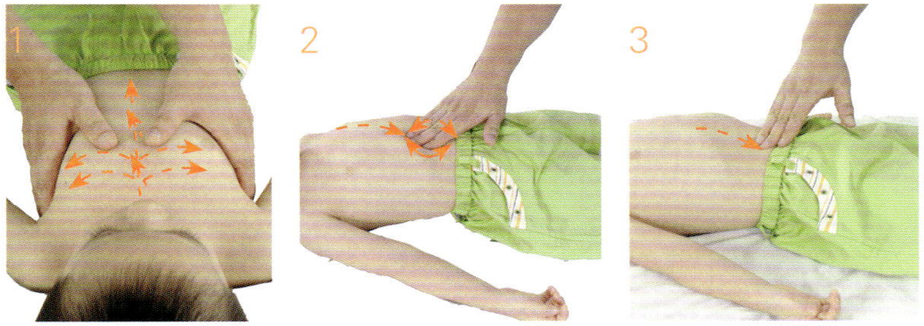

The manipulation can smooth the chest and regulate Qi, invigorate spleen and harmonize stomach, mainly used for chest stuffiness, cough and asthma, gurgling with sputum, short of breath, nausea, vomiting, abdominal pain, diarrhea, constipation and other symptoms.

Anxian Cuomo (Twisting and Rubbing like Plucking the String)

The manipulation is mainly used for chest stuffiness, disturbance of Qi movement, cough and asthma, short of breath, disturbance of phlegmatic dyspnea and so on.

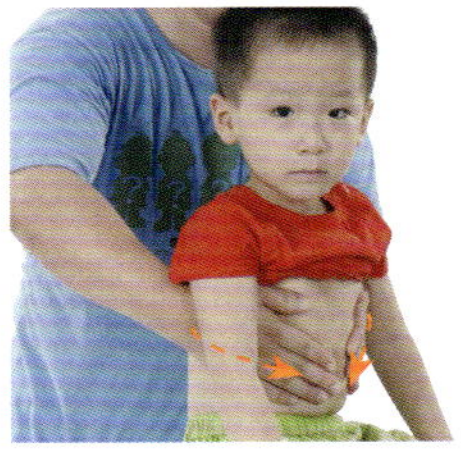

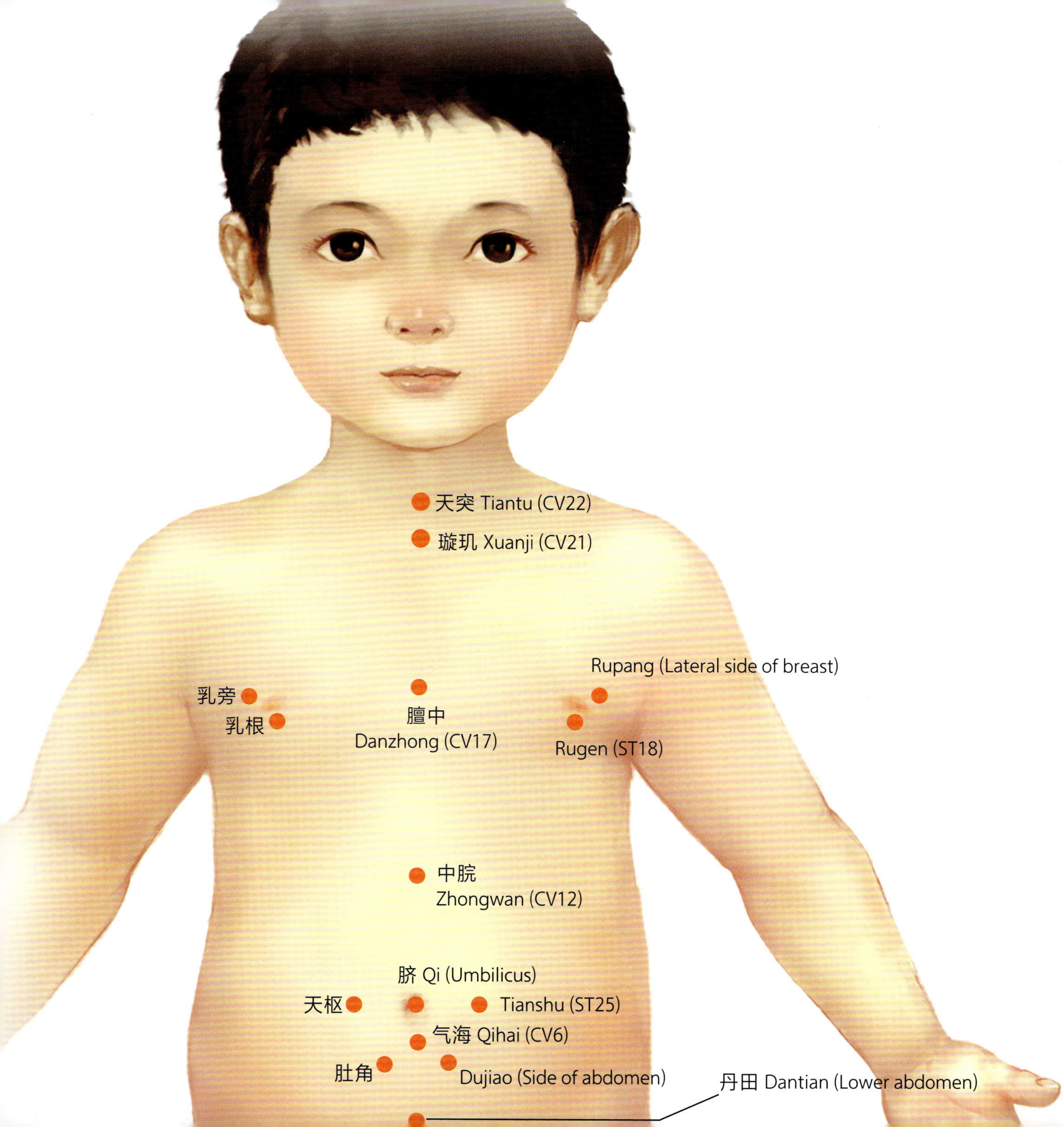

按摩方法速览
Quick Look of Massage Manipulations

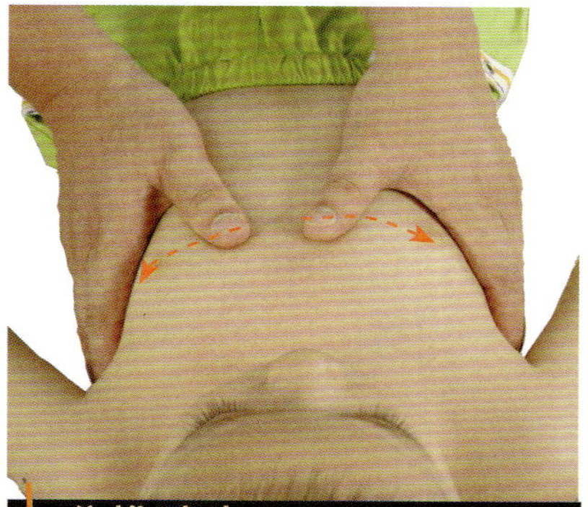

分推膻中 Part-Push Manipulation of Danzhong (CV17)

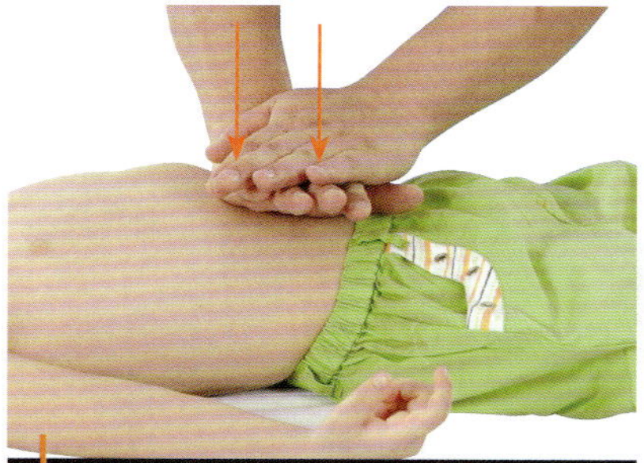

按中脘 Press Zhongwan (CV12)

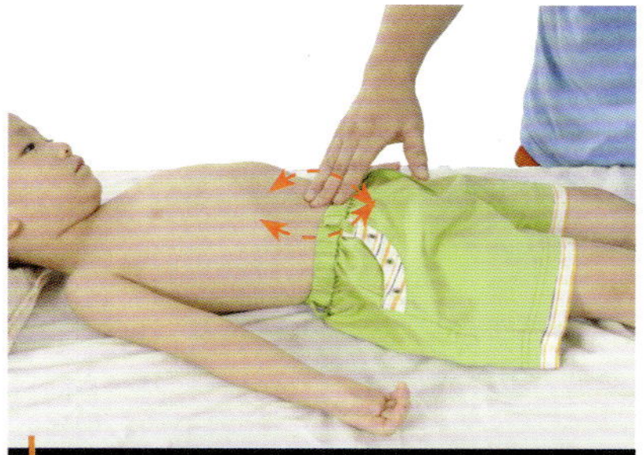

揉脐 Knead Qi (Umbilicus)

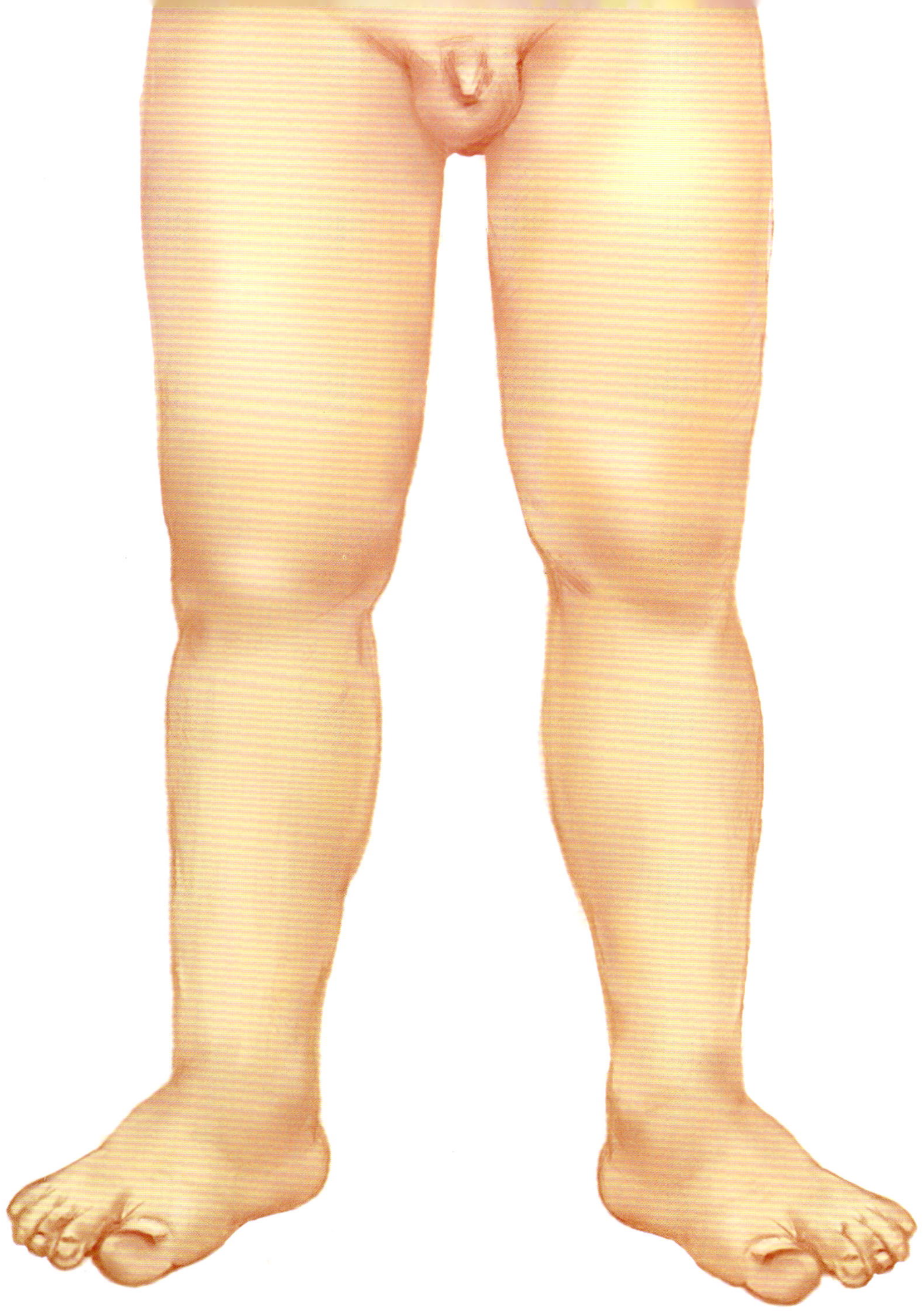

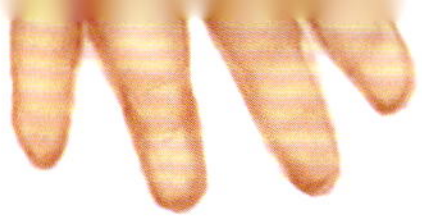

按摩方法速览
Quick Look of Massage Manipulations

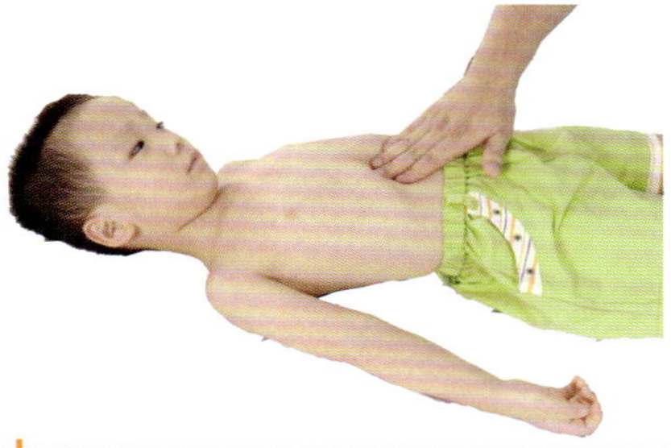

揉中脘 Knead Zhongwan (CV12)

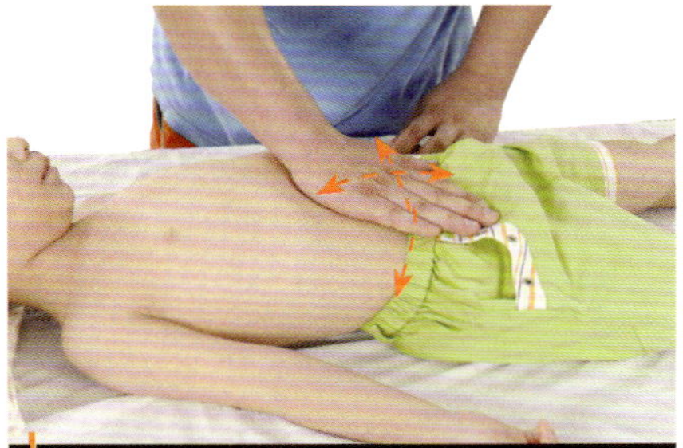

摩腹 Rub Fu (Abdomen)

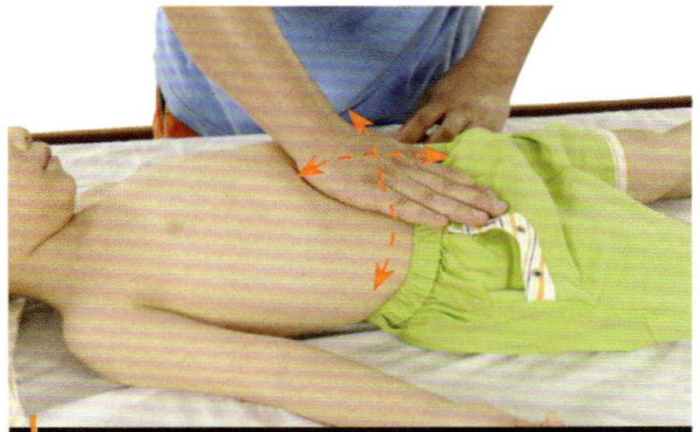

摩脐 Rub Qi (Umbilicus)

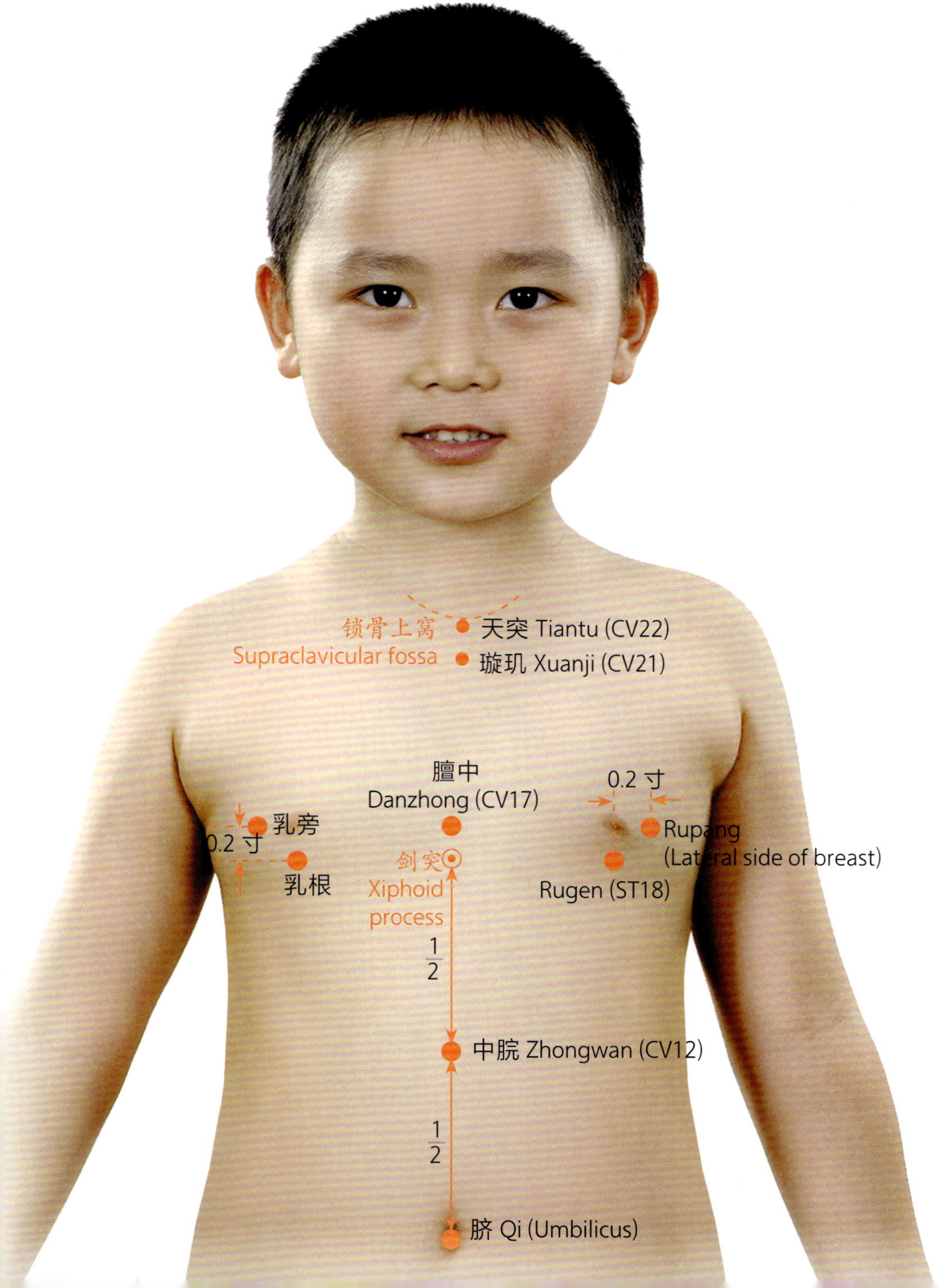

穴 位	定 位	按摩方法	功效主治
天突	颈部前正中线上，胸骨上窝中央	揉法：用中指指端按揉 30 次	理气化痰，降逆平喘，止呕。主治咳嗽、哮喘、呕吐
璇玑	胸部前正中线上，天突穴下 1 寸	揉法：用中指指端揉 100~300 次	利咽止痛，平喘，开胸利气。主治咳嗽气喘、咽喉肿痛
膻中	胸部前正中线上两乳头连线的中点	摩法、揉法或推法：用手掌面或食指、中指、无名指螺纹面作顺时针或逆时针方向环形移动摩擦 5 分钟，或用中指指端揉 100~300 次，或用两拇指桡侧自膻中向两旁分推至乳头，或以食指、中指自膻中向下推至剑突各 100~300 次	宽胸理气，止咳化痰。主治咳嗽、气喘、呕吐
乳旁	乳头外旁开 0.2 寸	揉法：常用食指、中指指端分别对准乳根、乳旁，同时按揉 30~50 次	宽胸理气，化痰止咳。主治胸闷、咳嗽、痰鸣、呕吐

Acupoints	Location	Massage Manipulations	Efficacy and Indications
Tiantu (CV22)	On the anterior midline of the neck, in the middle of suprasternal fossa	Kneading manipulation: Press-knead the point with the tip of middle finger for 30 times	It can regulate Qi and resolve phlegm, descend counterflow of Qi and relieve dyspnea and arrest vomiting, mainly used for cough, asthma and vomiting
Xuanji (CV21)	On the anterior midline of the chest, 1 cun below Tiantu (CV22)	Kneading manipulation: Knead the point with the tip of middle finger for 100 to 300 times	It can relieve sore throat and pain, relieve dyspnea, smooth the chest and promote circulation of Qi, mainly used for cough, asthma and sore throat.
Danzhong (CV17)	On the anterior midline of the chest, at the midpoint of the line between the 2 nipples	Rubbing, kneading or pushing manipulation: Rub the point in a circle clockwise or anticlockwise with the palm or index, middle and ring fingers for 5 minutes, or knead the point with the tip of middle finger for 100 to 300 times, or implement parting-pushing manipulation from Danzhong (CV17) to nipples with the radial side of the 2 thumbs for 100 to 300 times, or push downward from Danzhong (CV17) to xiphoid process with index and middle finger for 100 to 300 times	It can smooth the chest and regulate Qi, relieve cough and resolve phlegm, mainly used for cough, asthma and vomiting
Rupang (Lateral side of breast)	0.2 cun lateral to the nipple	Kneading manipulation: Press-knead Rugen (ST18) and Rupang (Lateral side of breast) with tips of index and middle fingers simultaneously for 30 to 50 times.	It can smooth the chest and regulate Qi, resolve phlegm and relieve cough, mainly used for chest stuffiness, cough, gurgling with sputum and vomiting

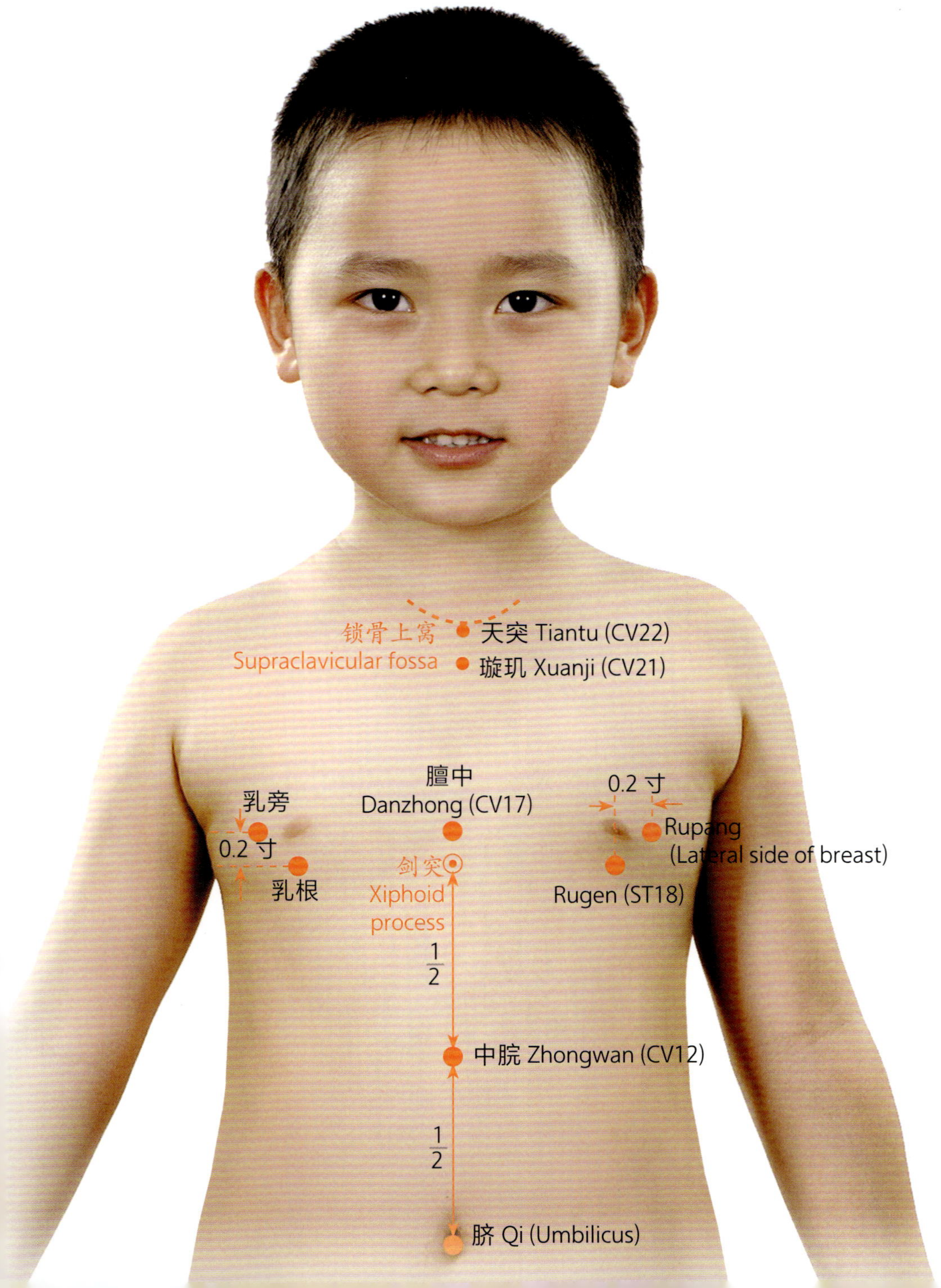

续表

穴位	定位	按摩方法	功效主治
乳根	胸部当乳头直下，乳房根部，第 5 肋间隙处	揉法：常用食指、中指指端分别对准乳根、乳旁，同时按揉 30~50 次	宣肺理气，止咳化痰。主治咳嗽、气喘
中脘	上腹部，前正中线上，脐上 4 寸	揉法、摩法或推法：用指端或掌根按揉 100~300 次，或用掌心或四指摩 5 分钟，或自喉下向下推至中脘 100~300 次	健脾和胃，消食和中。主治胃痛、腹胀、呕吐、呃逆(打嗝)、泄泻(腹泻)、黄疸、脾胃虚弱
脐	肚脐	揉法或摩法：用中指指端或掌根揉 100~300 次，或用食指、中指、无名指或掌心摩脐 5 分钟	温阳散寒，补益气血，和胃健脾，消食导滞。主治腹胀、腹痛、食积、便秘、肠鸣、吐泻

Continued

Acupoints	Location	Massage Manipulations	Efficacy and Indications
Rugen (ST18)	Direct below the nipples in the chest, in the root of the nipples, at the 5th intercostal space	Kneading manipulation: Press-knead Rupang (Lateral side of breast) and Rugen (ST 18) with tips of index and middle fingers simultaneously for 30 to 50 times.	It can ventilate lung and regulate Qi, relieve cough and resolve phlegm, mainly used for cough and asthma
Zhongwan (CV12)	In the epigastrium, on the anterior midline, 4 cun above the umbilicus	Kneading, rubbing or pushing manipulation: Press-knead the point with the fingertips or root of palm for 100 to 300 times, or rub the point for 5 minutes with the palm or 4 fingers, or push downward from the inferior throat to Zhongwan (CV12) for 100 to 300 times	It can invigorate spleen and harmonize stomach, promote digestion and harmonize the middle, mainly used for stomachache, abdominal distension, vomiting, hiccup, diarrhea, jaundice and spleen-stomach weakness
Qi (Umbilicus)	At the umbilicus	Kneading or rubbing manipulation: Knead the point with the tip of middle finger of root of palm for 100 to 300 times, or rub the umbilicus with index, middle and ring fingers or palm for 5 minutes	It can warm Yang and dissipate cold, tonify and replenish Qi and blood, invigorate spleen and harmonize stomach, promote digestion and remove food stagnation, mainly used for abdominal distension, abdominal pain, food accumulation, constipation, borborygmus, vomiting and diarrhea

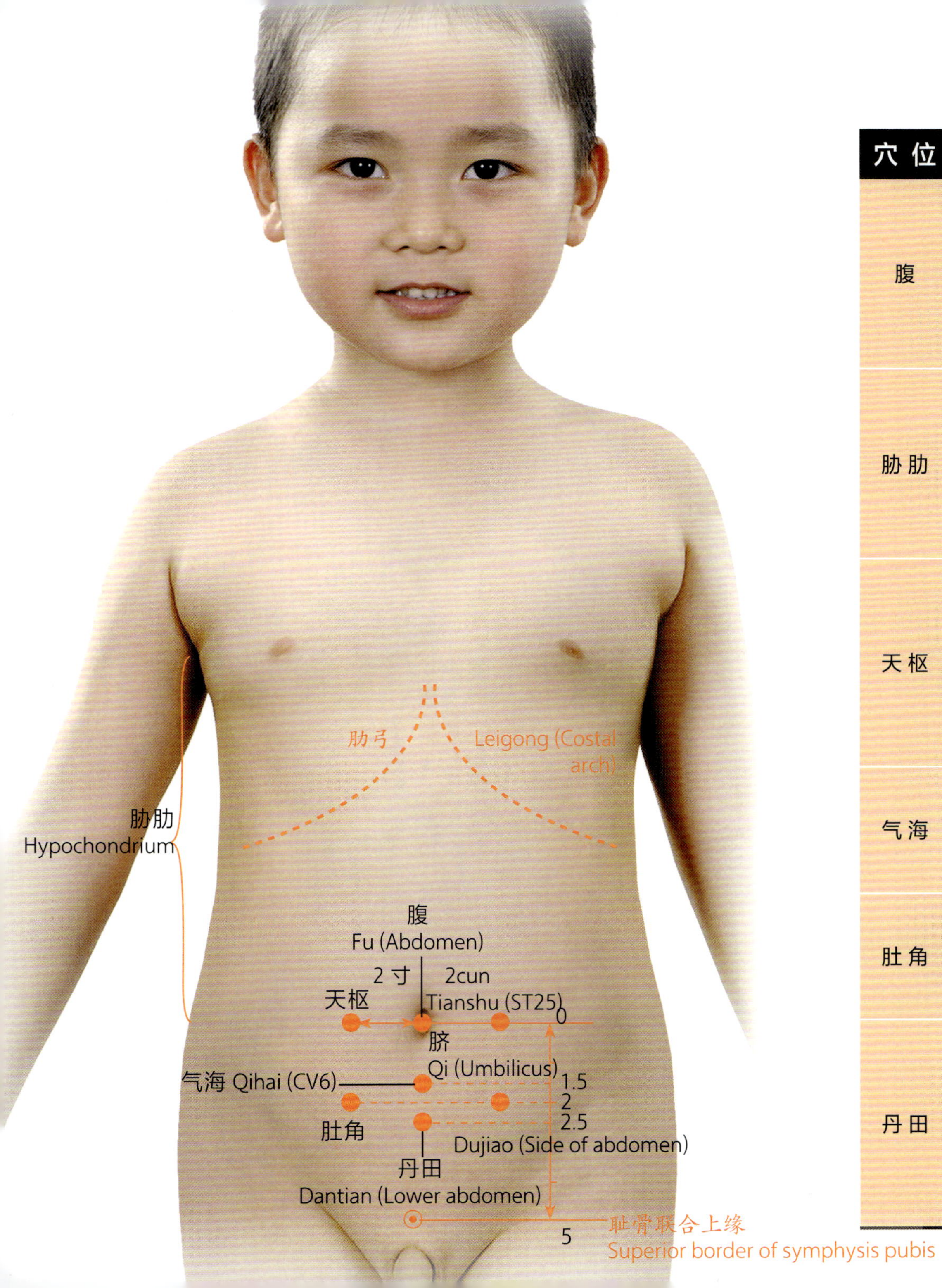

穴位	定位	按摩方法	功效主治
腹	腹部	摩法或推法：用掌心或四指指面摩 5 分钟，或以两拇指指腹沿肋弓角边缘向两旁分推（称分推腹阴阳）200~300 次	消食导滞，理气和胃。主治腹痛、腹胀、呕吐、泄泻（腹泻）、便秘、消化不良
胁肋	自腋下两胁至天枢处	搓法：用双手掌自两胁腋下至天枢搓摩 50~100 次	顺气化痰，除胸闷，开积聚。主治胁痛、胸闷、疳积（营养不良）、气急痰喘、肝脾肿大
天枢	腹中部，距脐中 2 寸	揉法：以食指、中指两指分别揉 50~100 次	疏调大肠，理气消滞。主治腹胀肠鸣、绕脐腹痛、泄泻（腹泻）、便秘、痢疾
气海	脐下 1.5 寸	揉法或按法：用拇指或中指或掌根揉 50~100 次，或用拇指或中指指端点按 1 分钟	调气，补元气。主治腹痛、腹胀、泄泻（腹泻）、便秘、遗尿（尿床）
肚角	脐下 2 寸，前正中线旁开 2 寸	按法或拿法：用拇指、食指、中指三指作拿法，或用中指指端按，各 3~5 次	止腹痛，消腹胀。主治腹胀、腹痛、泻痢
丹田	脐下 2 寸与 3 寸之间	揉法或摩法：用食指、中指、无名指三指揉 30~50 次，或用食指、中指、无名指三指摩 5 分钟	培肾固本，温补下元，分清泌浊。主治少腹痛、遗尿（尿床）、脱肛、小便赤少

Acupoints	Location	Massage Manipulation	Efficacy and Indications
Fu (Abdomen)	At the abdomen	Rubbing or pushing manipulation: Rub abdomen with the palm or 4 fingers except the thumb for 5 minutes, or push abdomen with the finger pulps of the 2 thumbs to both sides along the border of angulus infrasternalis (also called Parting-Pushing Manipulation of Yin-Yang)for 200 to 300 times	It can promote digestion and remove food stagnation, regulate Qi and harmonize stomach, mainly used for abdominal pain, abdominal distension, vomiting, diarrhea, constipation and dyspepsia
Hypochondrium	From costal regions below the axilla to Tianshu (ST25)	Twisting manipulation: Twist and rub hypochondrium from the costal regions below the axilla to Tianshu (ST25) for 50 to 100 times with the 2 palms	It can move Qi and resolve phlegm, remove chest stuffiness and relieve abdominal mass, mainly used for costalgia, chest stuffiness, malnutrition, short of breath with phlegmatic asthma and hepatosplenomegaly
Tianshu (ST25)	In the middle of abdomen, 2 cun lateral to the umbilicus	Kneading manipulation: Knead the point for respective 50 to 100 times with index and middle fingers	It can disperse and regulate large intestine, regulate Qi and remove stagnation, mainly used for abdominal distension, borborygmus, or abdominal pain around the umbilical region, diarrhea, constipation and dysentery
Qihai (CV6)	1.5 cun below the umbilicus	Kneading or pressing manipulation: Knead the point for 50 to 100 times with the thumb or middle finger or root of palm, or digital-press the tip of the thumb or middle finger for 1 minute	It can regulate Qi and tonify original Qi, mainly used for abdominal pain and abdominal distension, diarrhea, constipation and enuresis
Dujiao (Side of abdomen)	2 cun below the umbilicus, 2 cun lateral to the anterior midline	Pressing or grasping manipulation: Grasp the point with the thumb, index and middle fingers, or press the point with the tip of middle finger for respective 3 to 5 times	It can relieve abdominal pain and remove abdominal distension, mainly used for abdominal distension, abdominal pain and diarrhea and dysentery
Dantian (Lower abdomen)	Between 2 cun and 3 cun below the umbilicus	Kneading or rubbing manipulation: Knead the point with the index, middle and ring fingers for 30 to 50 times, or rub the point with the index, middle and ring fingers for 5 minutes	It can bank up kidney and consolidate root, warm and tonify kidney Qi, and separate clear and turbid, mainly used for lower abdominal pain, enuresis, prolapse of rectum and little red urine

按摩方法详解
Detailed Diagram of Massage Manipulations

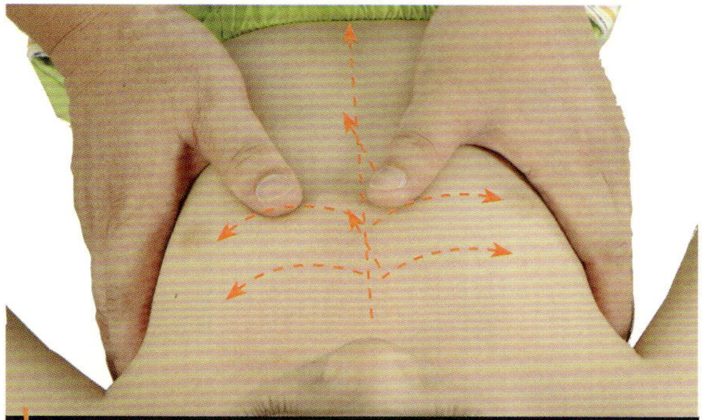

开璇玑

按摩者两拇指由小儿璇玑开始，顺着肋间隙向两旁分推；再由鸠尾向下直推至神阙；然后顺时针摩腹或在脐两旁推拿；最后从脐中向下推至小腹。

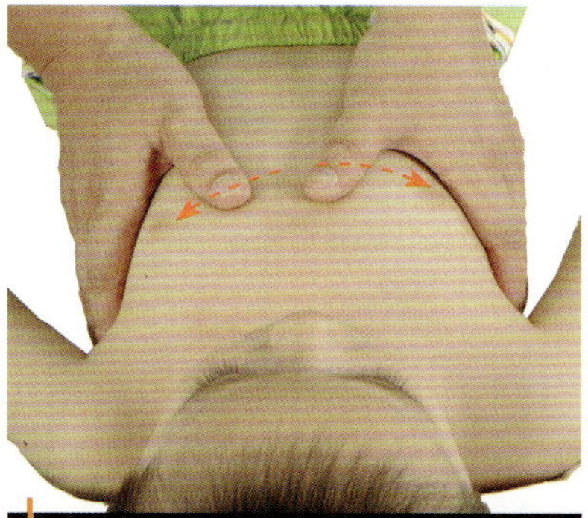

分推膻中

拇指自穴中向两旁分推至乳头。推 100~300 次。

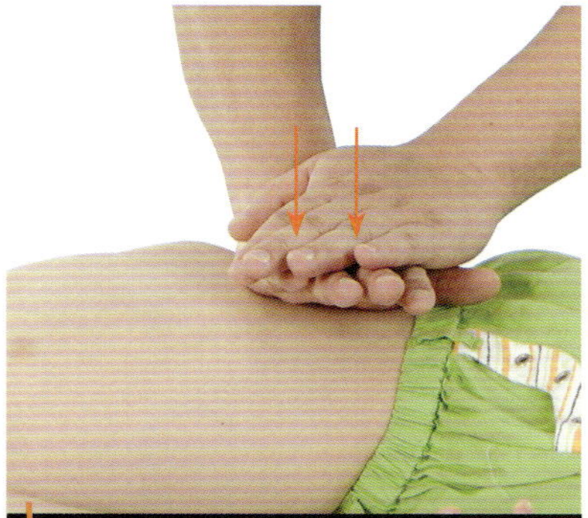

按中脘

用指端或掌根按揉。一般揉 100~300 次。

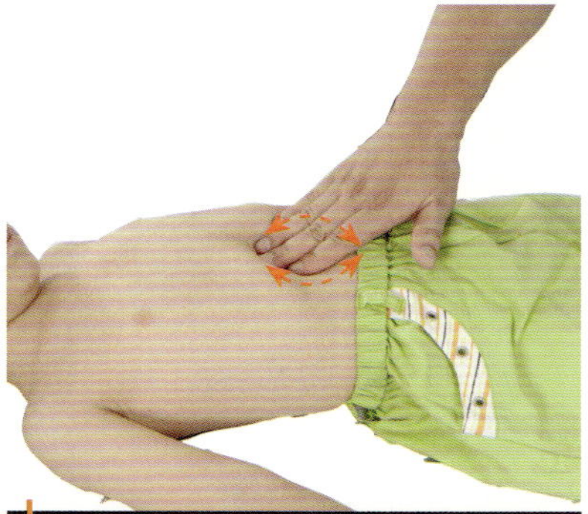

揉中脘

用指端或掌根按揉。一般揉 100~300 次。

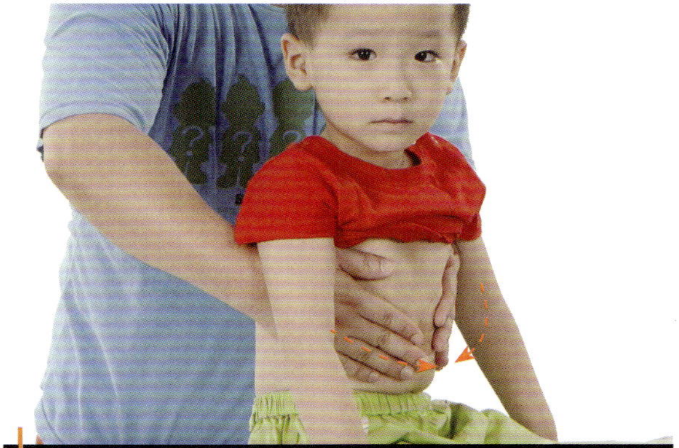

按弦搓摩

两手掌面着力，轻贴在小儿两侧胁肋部，对称性地搓摩至肚角处，手法自上而下，不可逆之。以 50~500 次为宜。

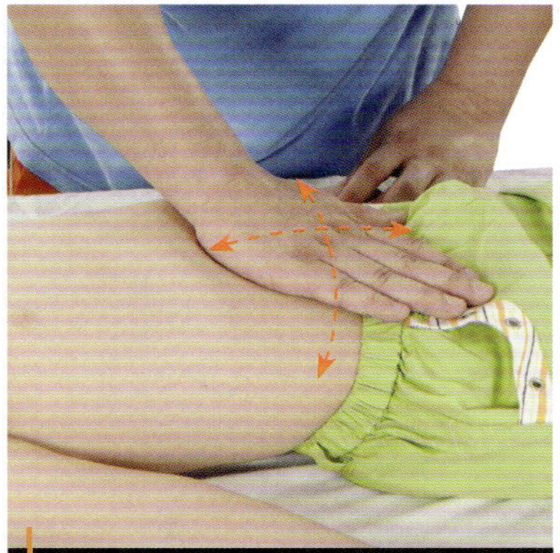

摩腹

小儿仰卧，按摩者以全掌或食指、中指、无名指三指指面摩上腹部。摩 3~5 分钟。

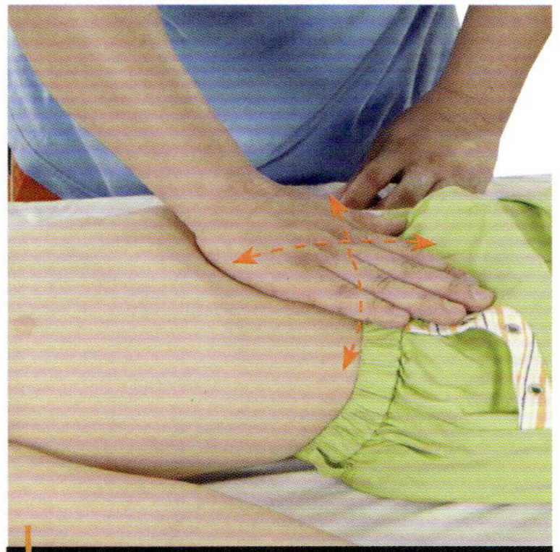

摩脐

用指端或掌根摩。揉脐摩 3~5 分钟。

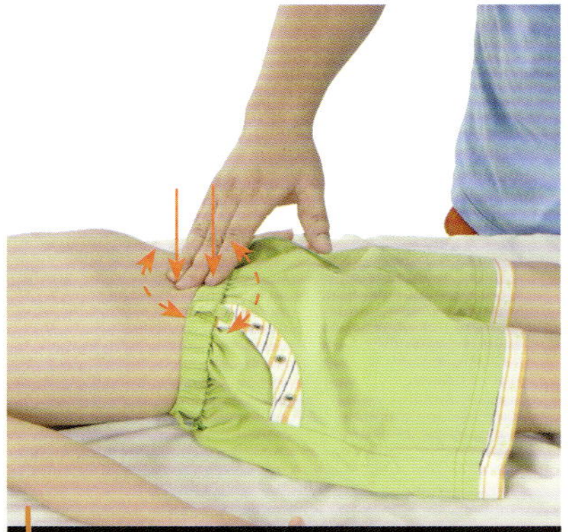

揉脐

用指端按揉。一般揉 100~300 次。

按摩方法详解
Detailed Diagram of Massage Manipulations

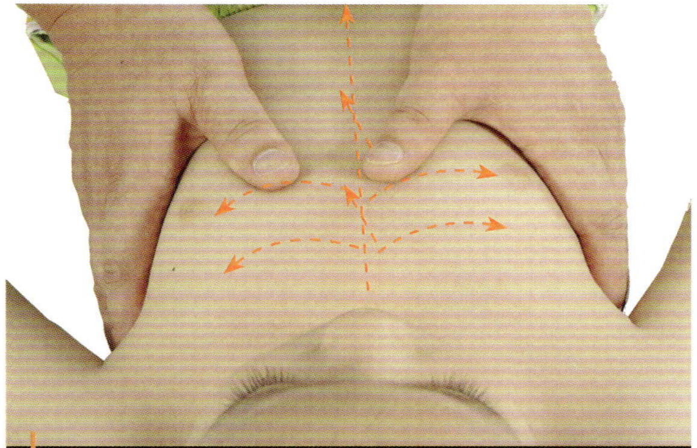

Open Xuanji (CV21)

Push from Xuanji (CV21) of the child along the intercostal spaces to the both sides with the 2 thumbs. Then push directly from Jiuwei (CV15) downward to Shenque (CV8). Afterwards, rub abdomen clockwise or carry out massage in both sides of umbilicus and finally push from the middle of umbilicus to lower abdomen.

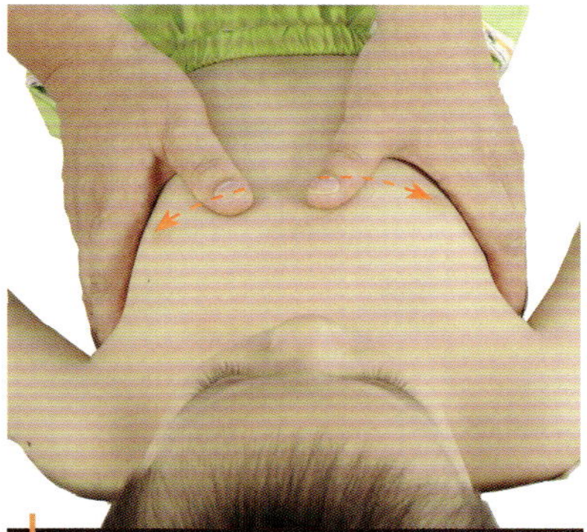

Part-Push Manipulation of Danzhong (CV17)

Push Danzhong (CV17) to the nipples in both sides with the thumbs for 100 to 300 times.

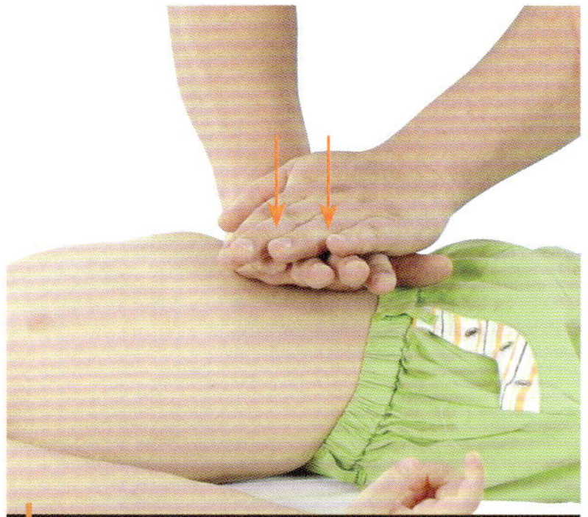

Press Zhongwan (CV12)

Press-knead the point with the fingertip or root of palm for 100 to 300 times generally.

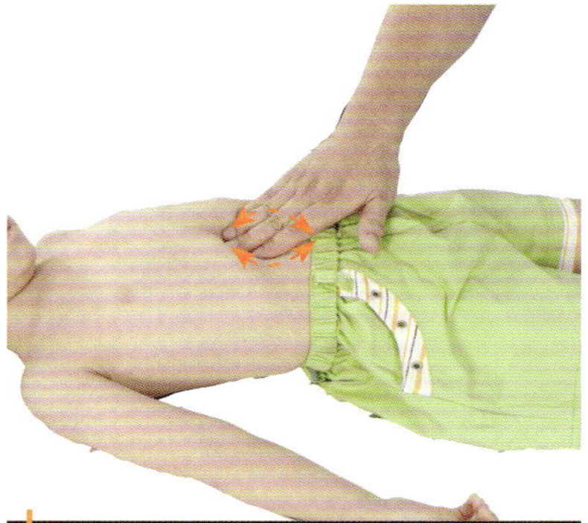

Knead Zhongwan (CV12)

Press-knead the point with the fingertip or root of palm for 100 to 300 times generally.

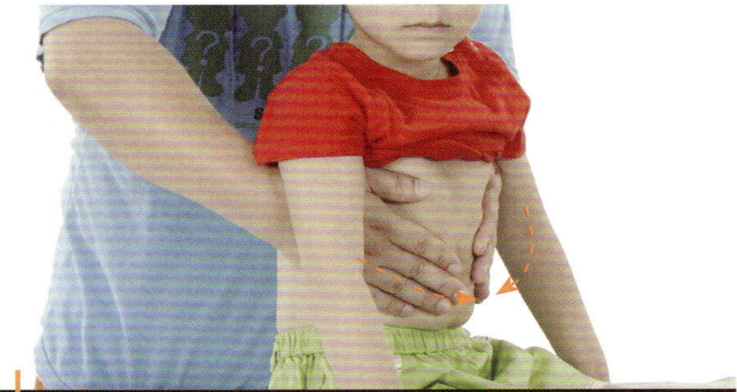

Anxian Cuomo (Twisting and Rubbing like Plucking the String)

Exert efforts with the 2 palms, and slightly put them to the both sides of the hypochondrium. Rub and twist it symmetrically to the location of Dujiao (Side of abdomen) with the manipulation from top to bottom irreversibly for appropriately 50 to 500 times.

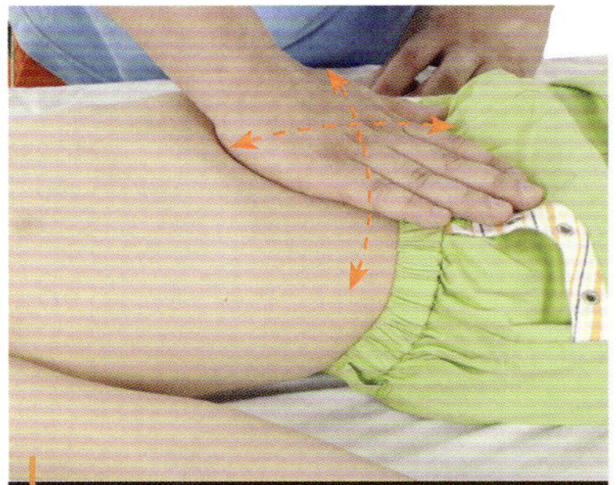

Rub Fu (Abdomen)

Let the child lie in supine position. Rub the upper abdomen with the whole palm or facies digitales of the index, middle and ring fingers for 3 to 5 minutes.

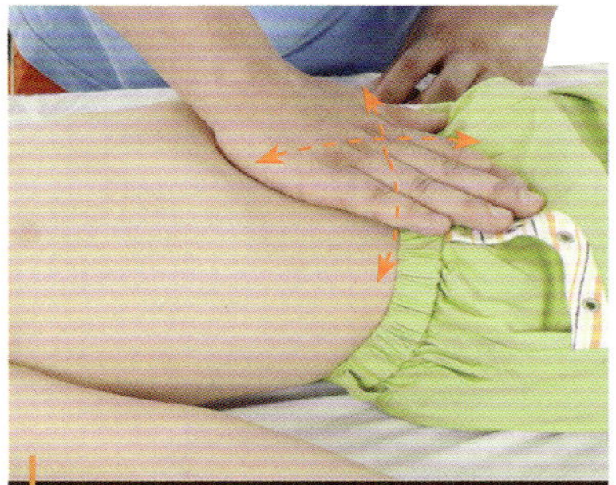

Rub Qi (Umbilicus)

Rub umbilicus with the fingertip or root of palm. Knead umbilicus for 3 to 5 minutes.

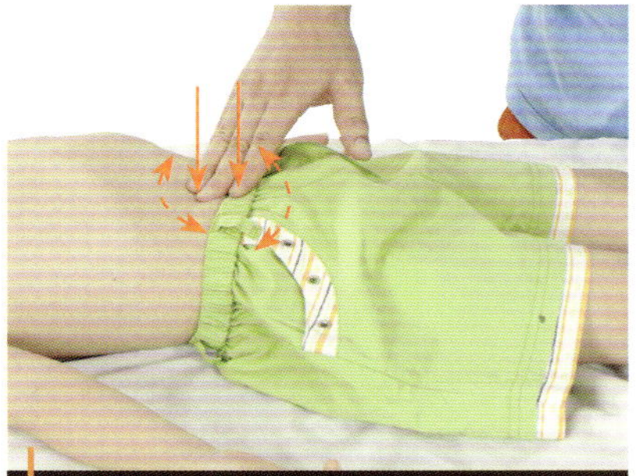

Knead Umbilicus

Press and knead umbilicus with the fingertip for generally 100 to 300 times.

背部穴位及按摩手法
Acupoints and Massage Manipulations in Back

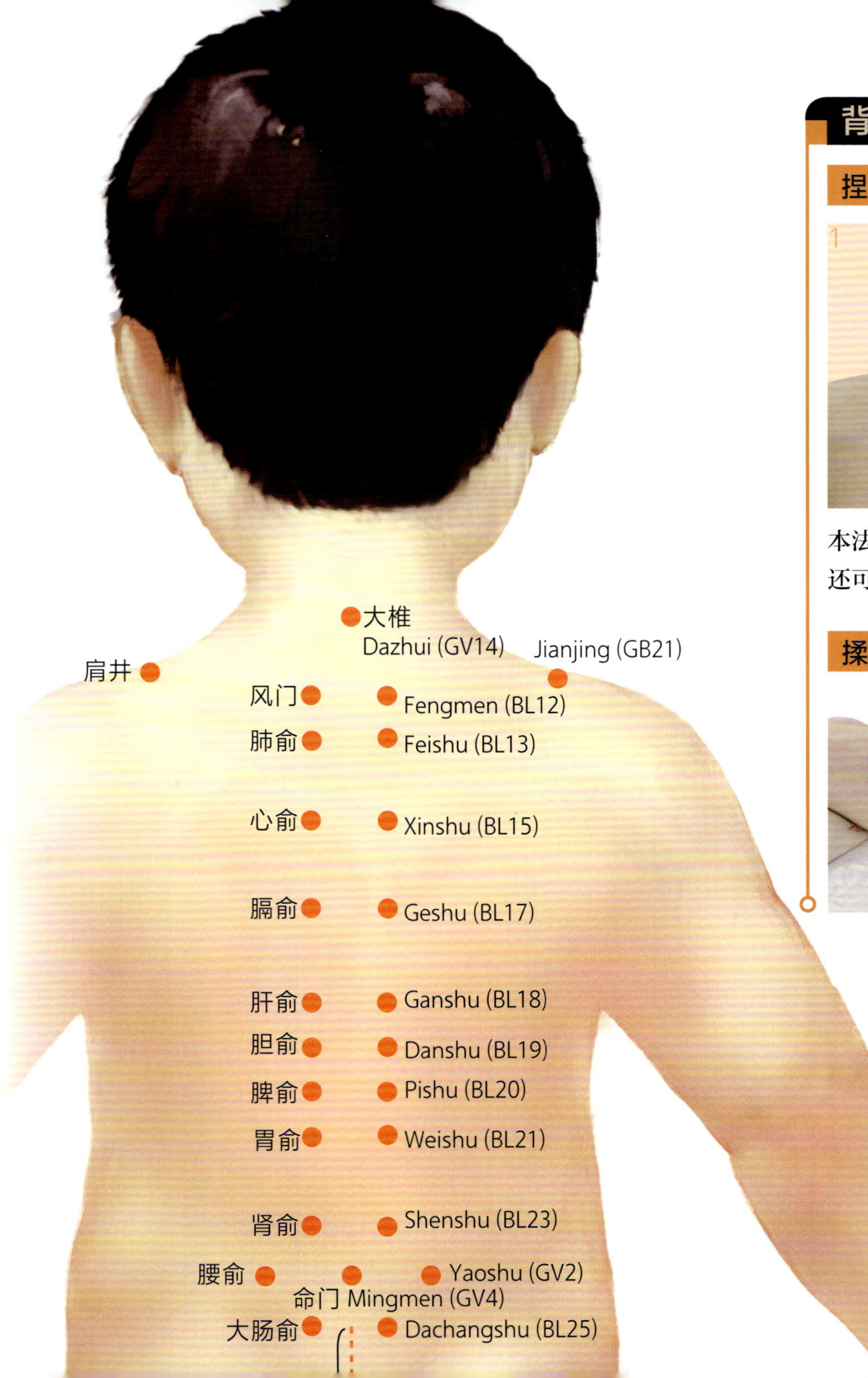

背部经典按摩手法

捏脊

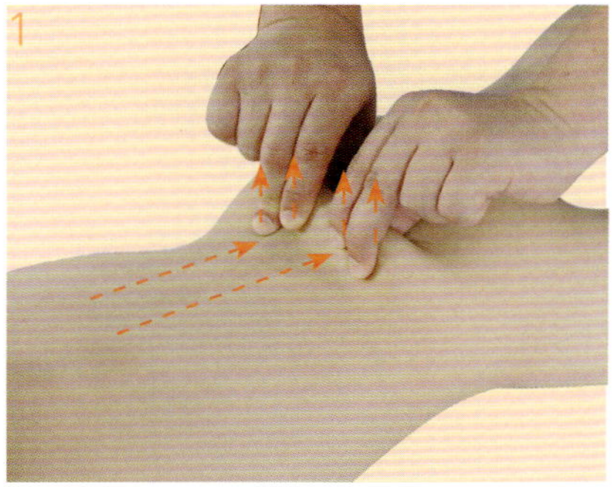

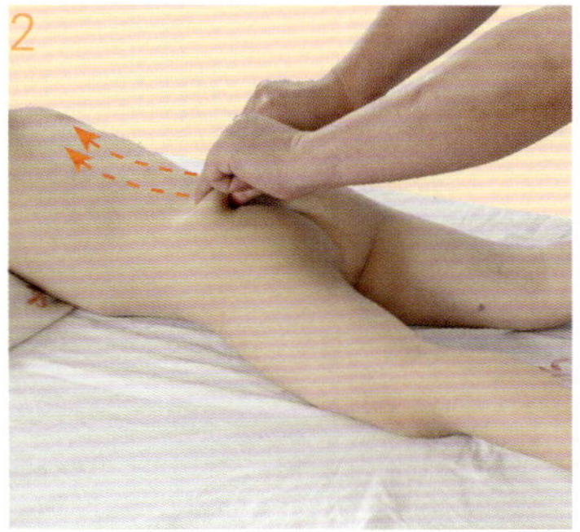

本法是治疗小儿消化不良、厌食、腹泻等消化道疾病的有效手法，还可用于小儿保健，增强抵抗力。

揉龟尾并推七节骨

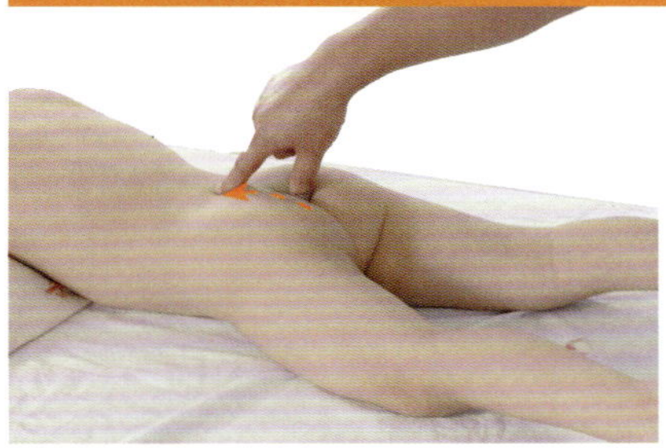

本法有通便止泻、调节大肠功能的作用。

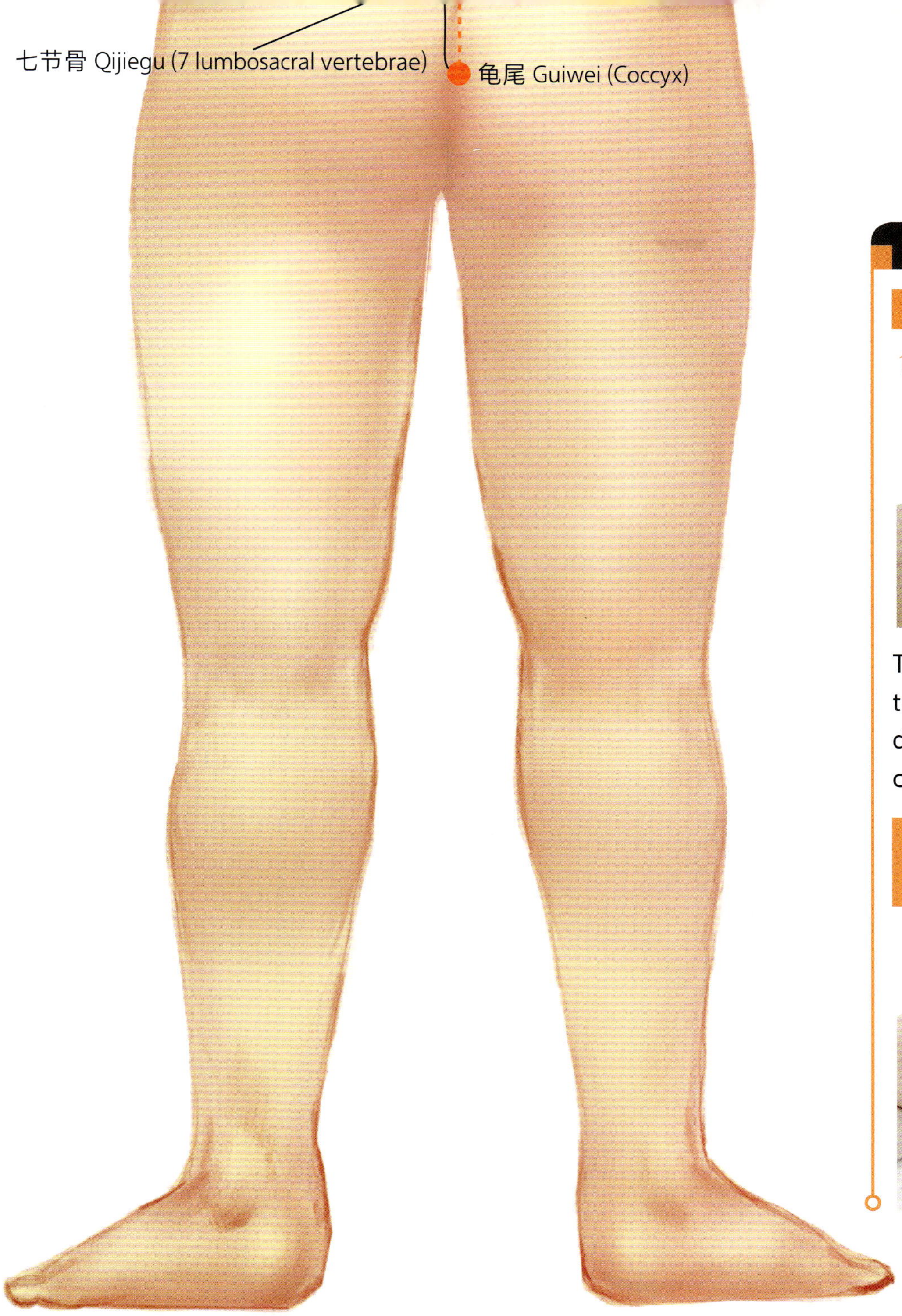

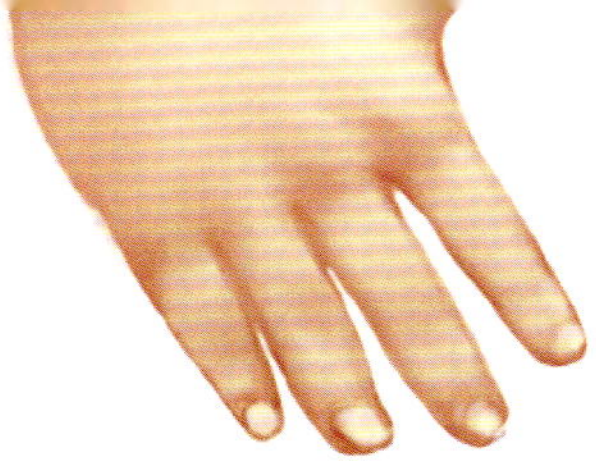

Classic Massage Manipulations in Back

Pinch Spine

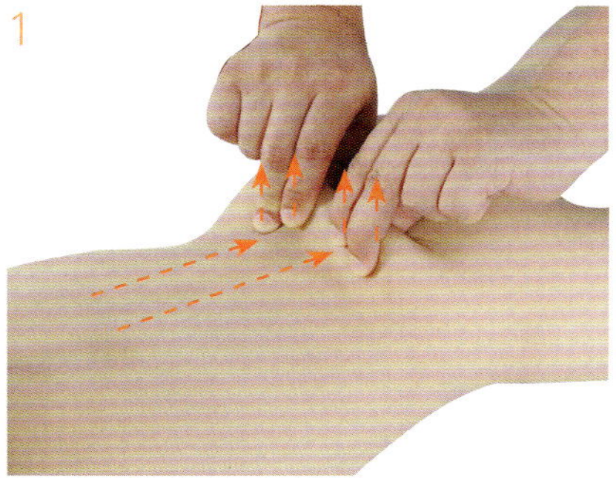

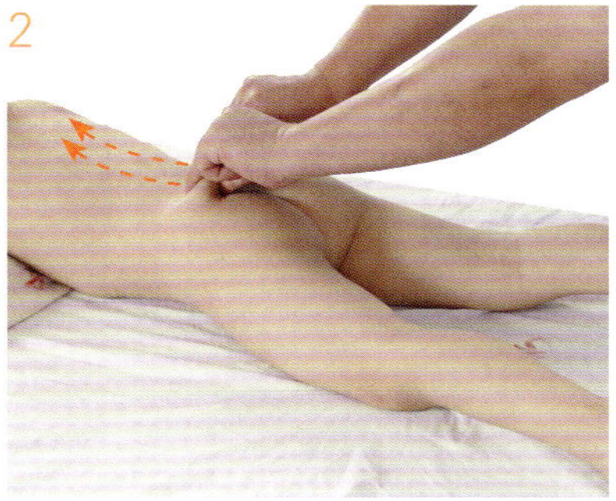

The manipulation is an effective technique used for digestive tract diseases of children such as dyspepsia, anorexia and diarrhea. It can also protect health and enhance resistance of children.

Knead Guiwei (Coccyx) and Push Qijiegu (7 lumbosacral vertebrae)

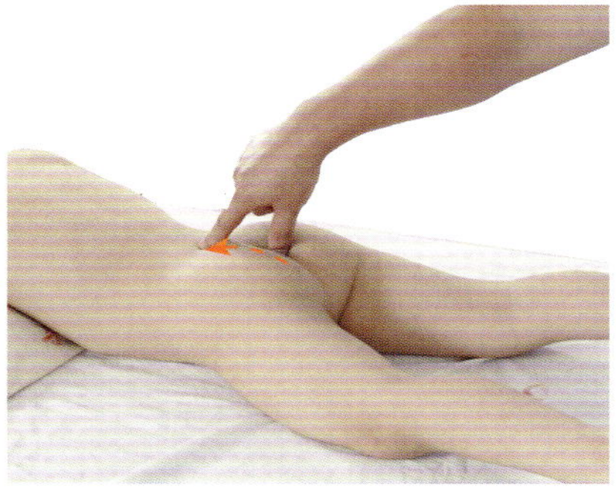

The manipulation has effects of purgation, relieving diarrhea and regulating functions of large intestine.

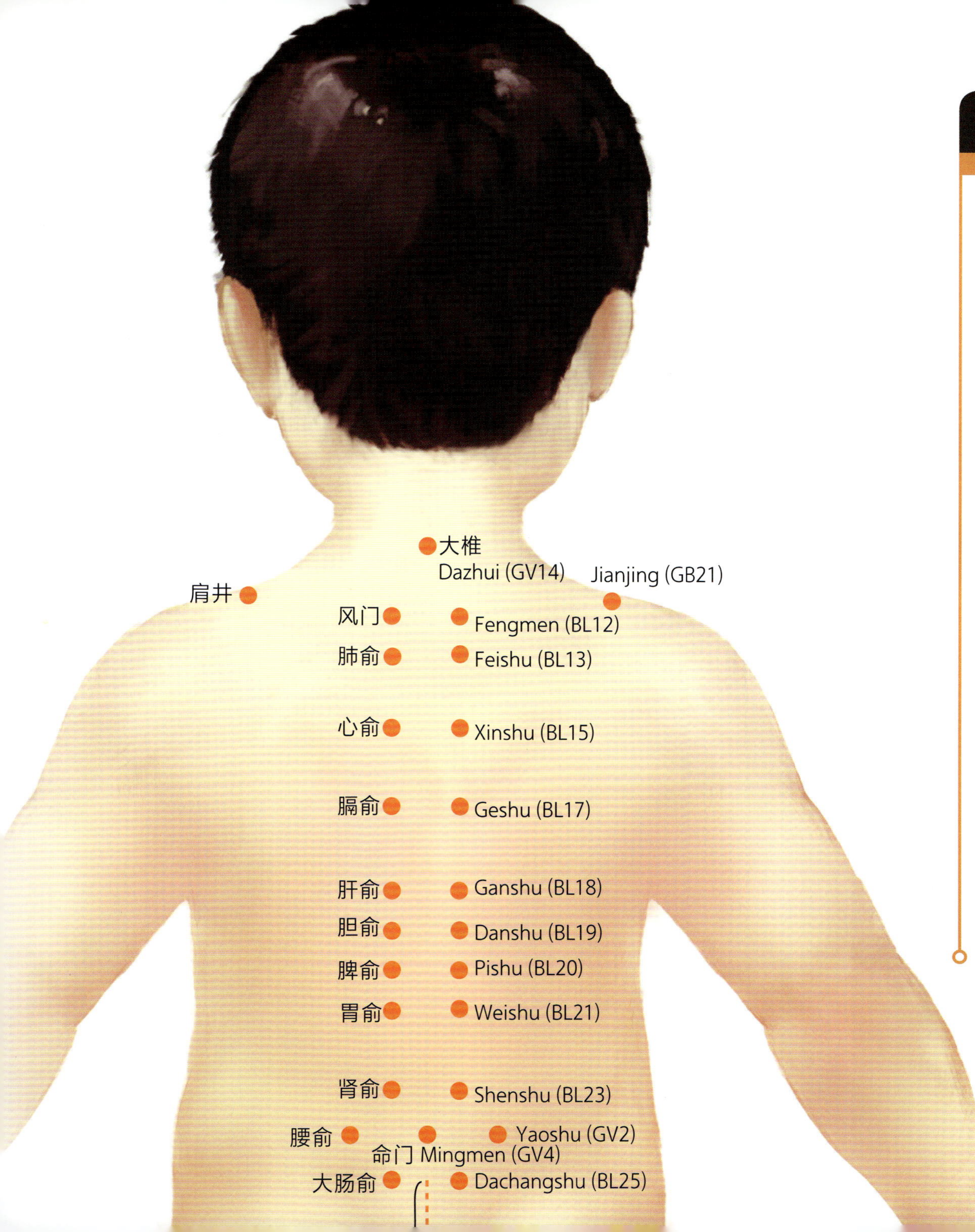

按摩方法速览
Quick Look of Massage Manipulations

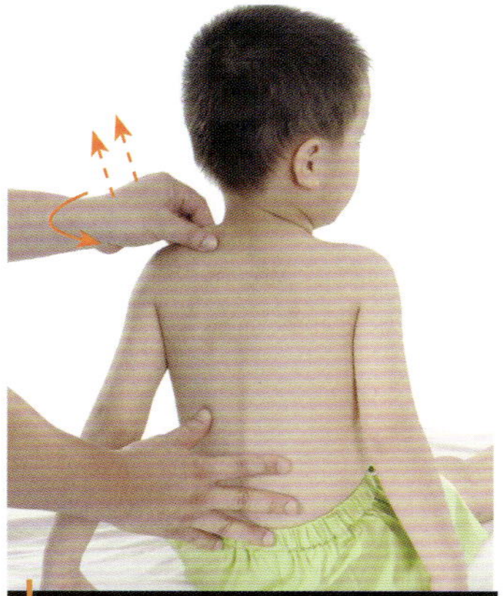

拿肩井 Grasp Jianjing (GB21)

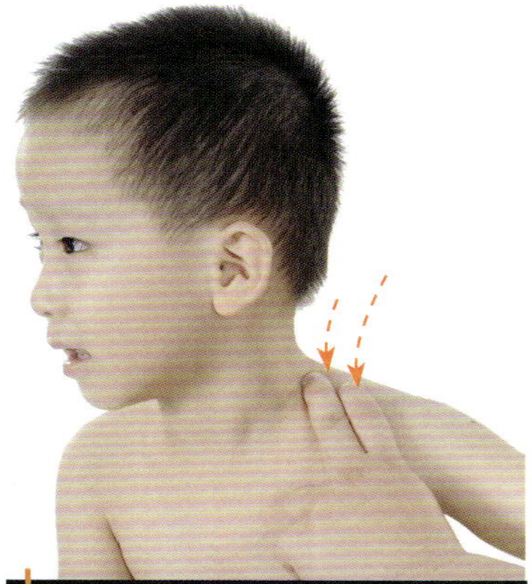

按肩井 Press ianjing (GB21)

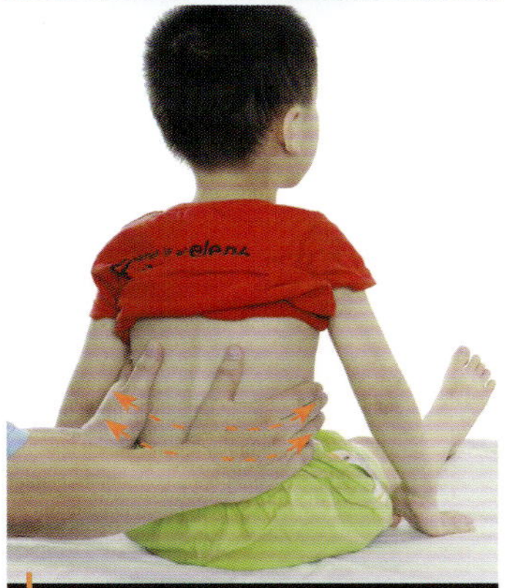

搓肾俞 Twist Shenshu (BL23)

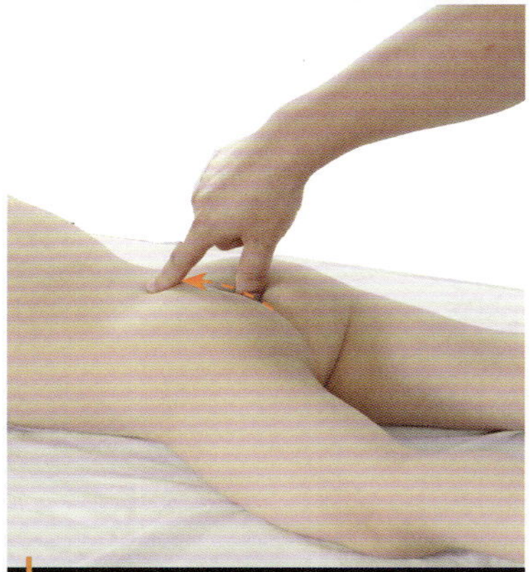

推七节骨 Push Qijiegu (7 lumbosacral vertebrae)

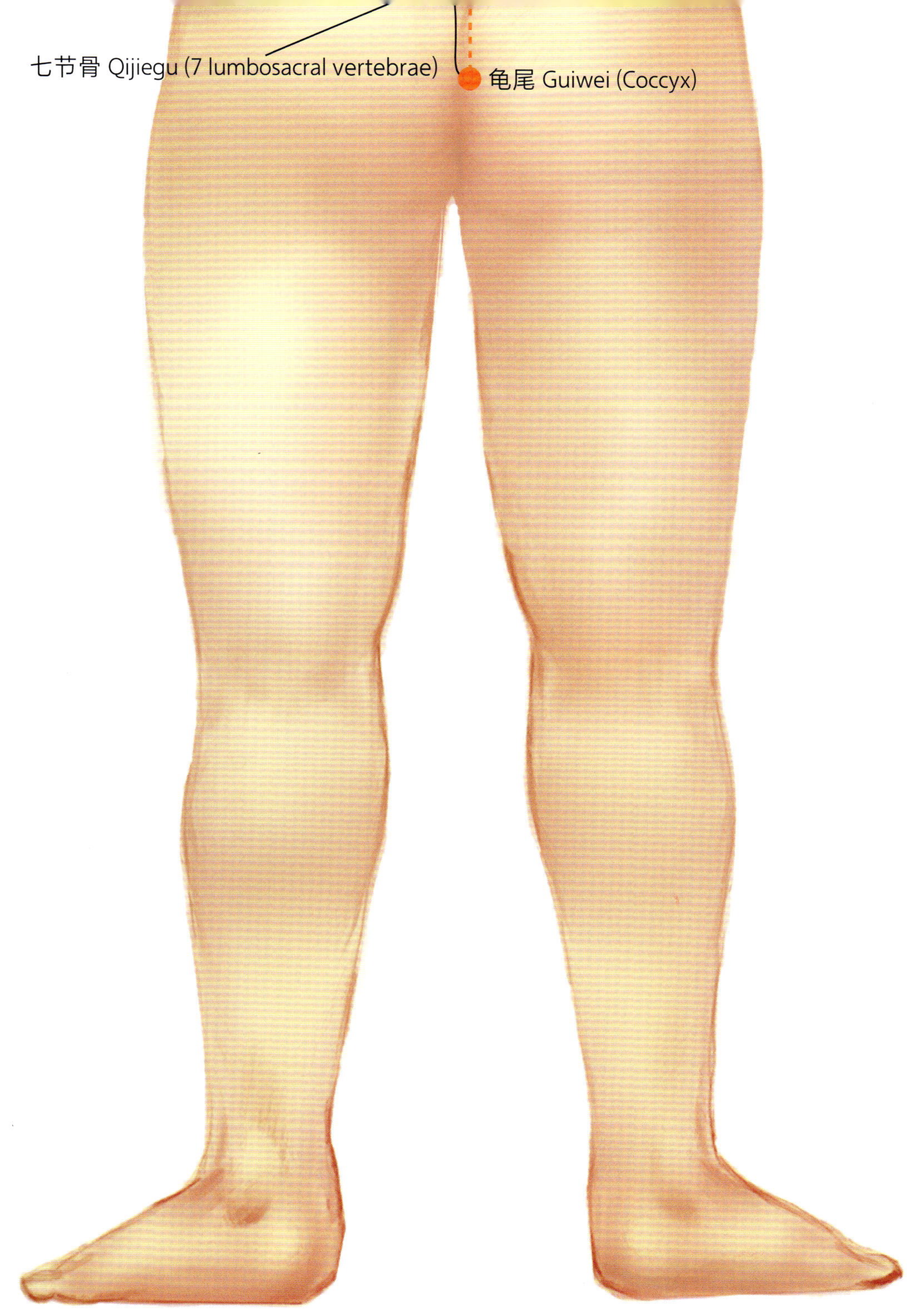

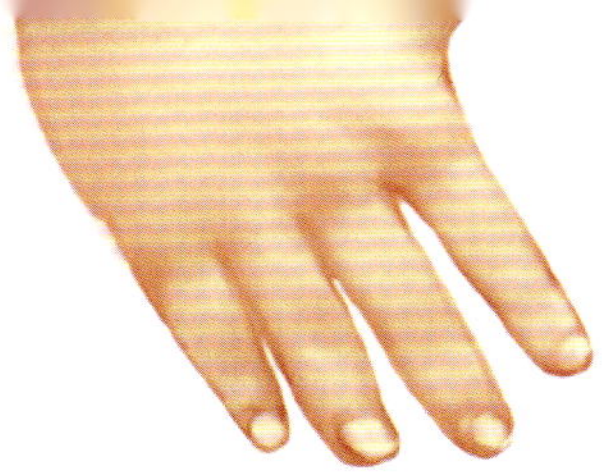

按摩方法速览
Quick Look of Massage Manipulations

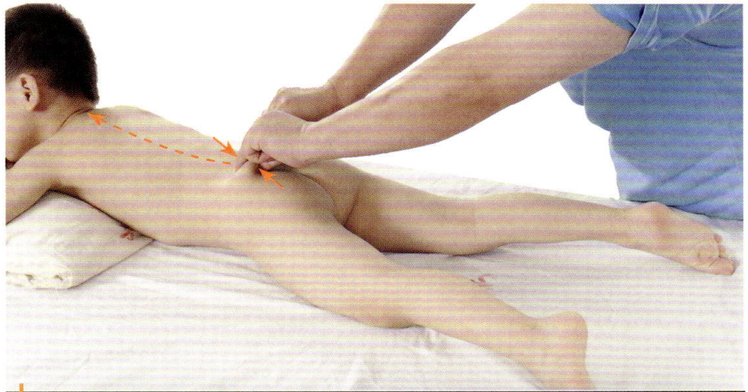

捏脊 Pinch Spine

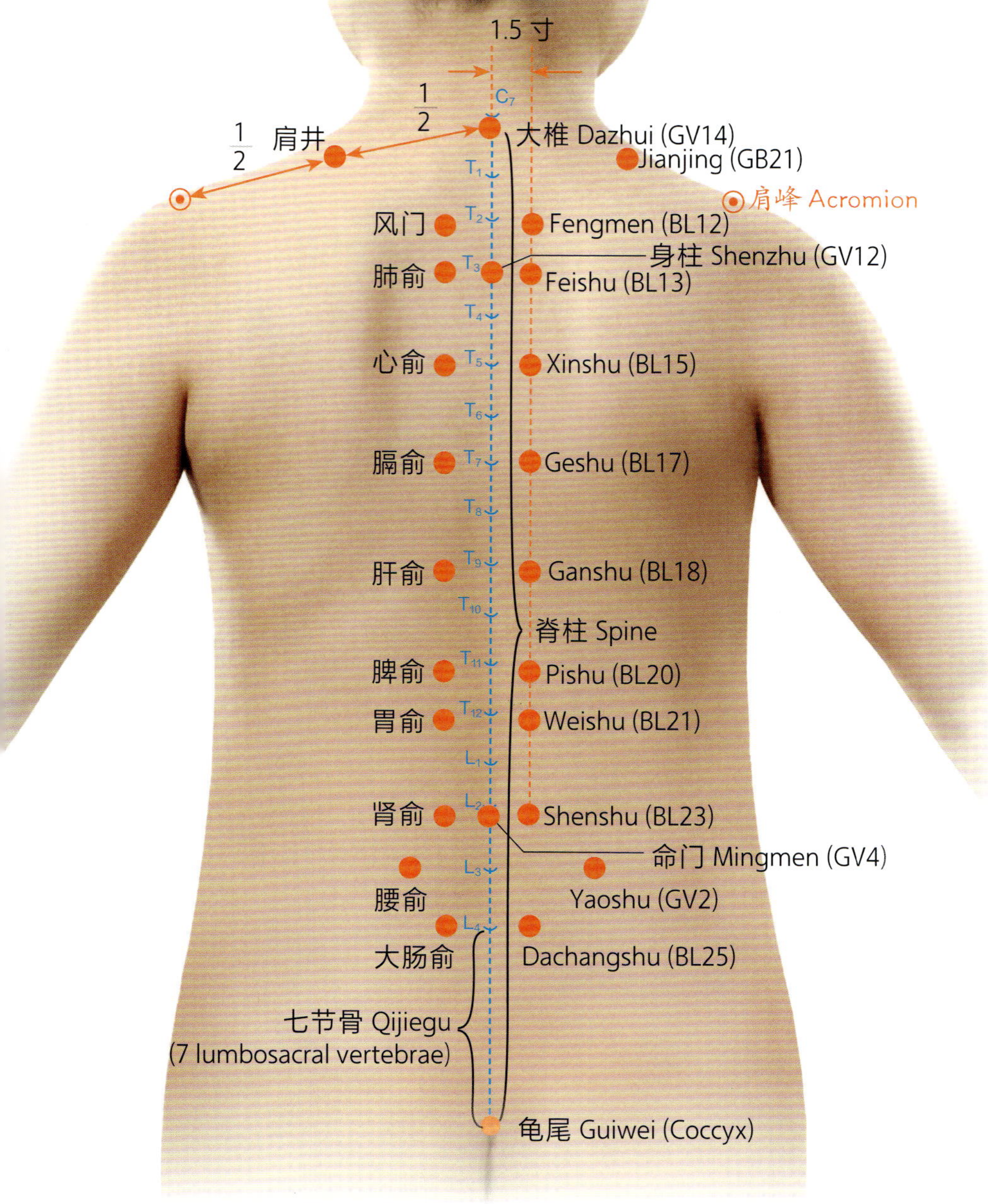

C: 颈椎棘突 Spinous process of cervical vertebra
T: 胸椎棘突 Spinous process of thoracic vertebra
L: 腰椎棘突 Spinous process of lumbar vertebra

穴位	定位	按摩方法	功效主治
大椎	第 7 颈椎棘突下	揉法或捏法：以右手中指指端揉 30~50 次，或用两手食指、中指屈曲挤捏至局部皮肤充血潮红	疏风解表，通经活络。主治感冒、发热、咳嗽、抽搐、癫痫
肩井	大椎与肩峰连线中点	拿法或按法：以拇指、食指对称用力提拿 3~5 次，或用拇指指端按 1 分钟	发汗解表，宣通气血。主治感冒、抽搐、癫痫、上肢活动不利、颈项疼痛
风门	第 2 胸椎棘突下旁开 1.5 寸	揉法：以两手食指、中指指端揉 50 次	止咳平喘，解表通络。主治感冒、咳嗽、痰喘
身柱	第 3 胸椎棘突下凹陷中	揉法：以两手食指、中指指端揉 50 次	宣肺清热，宁神镇咳。主治腰脊强痛、小儿急惊风、支气管哮喘
肺俞	第 3 胸椎棘突下，旁开 1.5 寸	揉法或推法：以食指、中指指端或两拇指指端揉 50~100 次，或两拇指指端分别自肩胛骨内缘由上向下分推 100~200 次	调肺气，补虚损，止咳嗽。主治咳嗽、气喘、盗汗、感冒、发热
心俞	第 5 胸椎棘突下，旁开 1.5 寸	揉法：以食指、中指指端或两拇指指端揉 50~100 次	宽胸理气，通络安神。主治心房纤颤、心动过速、癫痫、胃出血、食道狭窄、背部软组织损伤

Acupoints	Location	Massage Manipulations	Efficacy and Indications
Dazhui (GV14)	Below the spinous process of the 7th cervical vertebra	Kneading or pinching manipulation: Knead the point with the tip of middle finger of the right hand for 30 to 50 times, or pinch the point with the bending index and middle fingers of the 2 hands until the local skin shows hyperemia and flush	It can disperse wind and release exterior, sooth meridians and activate collaterals, mainly used for cold, fever, cough, convulsion and epilepsy
Jianjing (GB21)	At the midpoint of the line joining Dazhui (GV14) and the acromion	Grasping or pressing manipulation: Exert strength symmetrically with the thumb and index finger to lift and grasp the point for 3 to 5 times, or press the point with the fingertip of the thumb for 1 minute	It can induce sweating to release exterior and promote Qi and blood, mainly used for cold, convulsion, epilepsy, impaired physical activity of upper limb and pain of neck
Fengmen (BL12)	1.5 cun lateral to the depression below the spinous process of the 2nd thoracic vertebra	Kneading manipulation: Knead the point with tips of index and middle fingers of the 2 hands for 50 times	It can relieve cough and dyspnea, release exterior and sooth collaterals, mainly used for cold, cough, phlegmatic dyspnea
Shenzhu (GV12)	In the depression below the spinous process of the 3rd thoracic vertebra	Kneading manipulation: Knead the point with tips of index and middle fingers of the 2 hands for 50 times	It can ventilate lung and clear heat, calm mind and tranquilize cough, mainly used for painful and stiff waist and backbone, acute infantile convulsion and bronchial asthma
Feishu (BL13)	1.5 cun lateral to the depression below the spinous process of the 3rd thoracic vertebra	Kneading or pushing manipulation: Knead the point with tips of index and middle fingers or the fingertips of the 2 thumbs for 50 to 100 times, or push from top to bottom starting from the interior border of scapula with fingertips of the 2 thumbs for 100 to 200 times	It can regulate lung Qi, tonify deficiency and relieve cough, mainly used for cough, asthma, night sweat, cold and fever.
Xinshu (BL15)	1.5 cun lateral to the depression below the spinous process of the 5th thoracic vertebra	Kneading manipulation: Knead the point with tips of index and middle fingers or the fingertips of the 2 thumbs for 50 to 100 times	It can smooth the chest and regulate Qi, sooth collaterals and tranquilize mind, mainly used for atrial fibrillation, tachycardia, epilepsy, stomach bleeding, esophageal stenosis and soft tissue injury of back

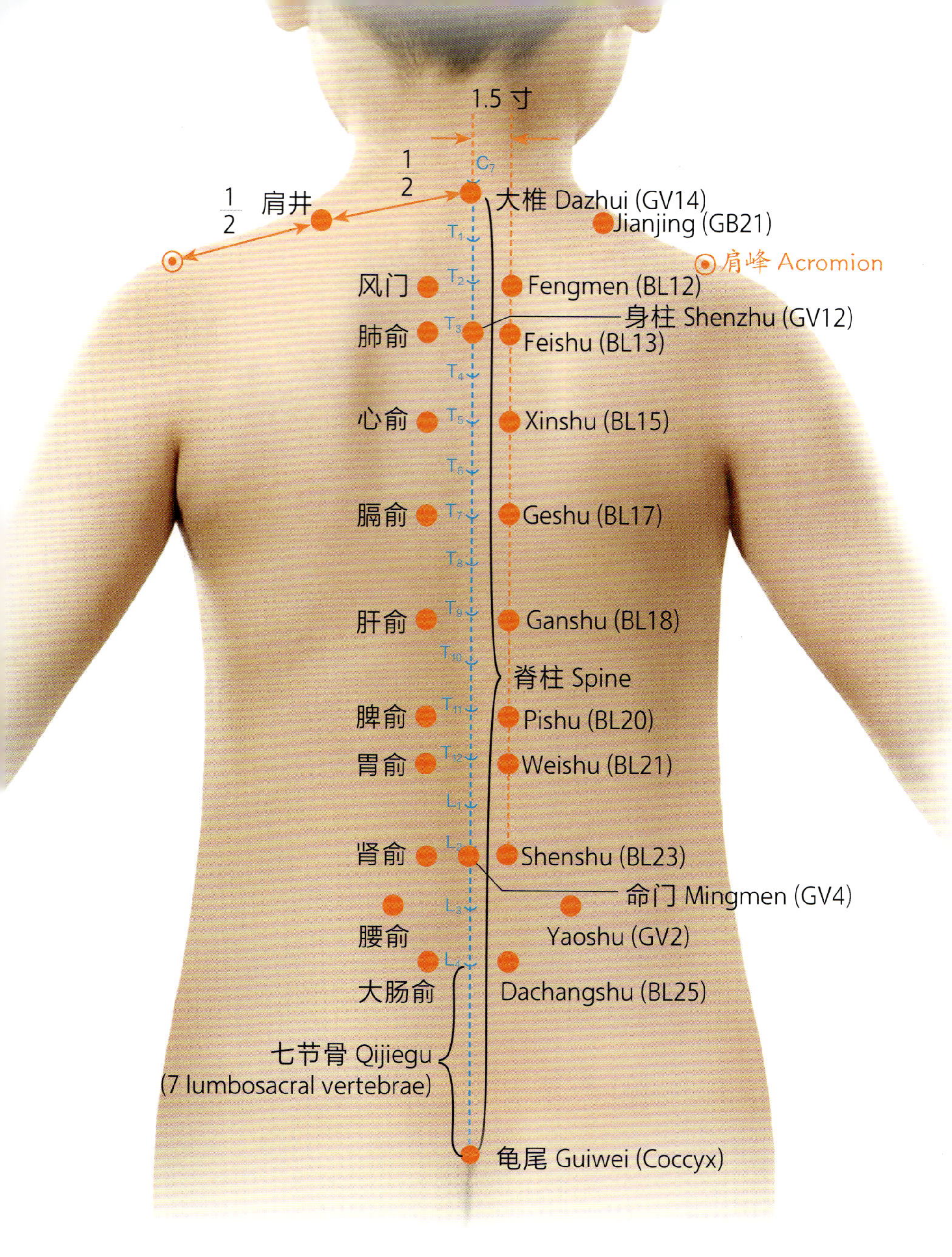

续表

穴 位	定 位	按摩方法	功效主治
膈 俞	第 7 胸椎棘突下，旁开 1.5 寸	揉法：以食指、中指指端或两拇指指端揉 50~100 次	理气宽胸，活血通脉。主治神经性呕吐、淋巴结结核、小儿营养不良、荨麻疹、哮喘、支气管炎
肝 俞	第 9 胸椎棘突下，旁开 1.5 寸	揉法：用两手拇指指端揉 50~100 次	疏肝利胆，理气明目。主治黄疸、眩晕、目赤、胁痛、脊背痛
脊 柱	大椎直下至尾骨端长强穴成一直线	推法或捏法：用食指、中指两指指面在背部自上向下直推 50~100 次，或用捏脊法自下而上捏提 3~5 遍	调和阴阳，补益气血，培补元气，强健脾胃，清热退热。主治发热、感冒、腹泻、腹痛、恶心、呕吐、疳积（营养不良）、便秘、抽搐、癫痫、夜啼、脱肛、遗尿（尿床）等
脾 俞	第 11 胸椎棘突下，旁开 1.5 寸	揉法：以食指、中指指端或两拇指指端揉 50~100 次	健脾胃，助运化，祛水湿。主治厌食、腹胀、呕吐、泄泻（腹泻）、便血、黄疸、胁痛、水肿
胃 俞	第 12 胸椎棘突下，旁开 1.5 寸	揉法：以食指、中指指端或两拇指指端揉 50~100 次	健脾和胃。主治胃脘痛、胸胁痛、腹胀、呕吐、肠鸣、完谷不化（消化不良，大便里含有未消化的食物）
肾 俞	第 2 腰椎棘突下，旁开 1.5 寸	揉法：以食指、中指指端或两拇指指端揉 50~100 次	滋阴壮阳，补益肾气。主治腰膝酸痛、遗尿（尿床）、小便频数、水肿

Acupoints	Location	Massage Manipulations	Efficacy and Indications
Geshu (BL17)	1.5 cun lateral to the depression below the spinous process of the 7th thoracic vertebra	Kneading manipulation: Knead the point with tips of index and middle fingers or the fingertips of the 2 thumbs for 50 to 100 times	It can regulate Qi and sooth the chest, activate blood and dredge vessels, mainly used for nervous vomiting, lymphatic tuberculosis, infantile malnutrition, urticaria, asthma and bronchitis
Ganshu (BL18)	1.5 cun lateral to the depression below the spinous process of the 9th thoracic vertebra	Kneading manipulation: Knead the point with the fingertips of the 2 thumbs for 50 to 100 times	It can sooth liver and promote bile secretion, regulate Qi and improve vision, mainly used for jaundice, vertigo, red eye, hypochondriac and back pain
Spine	The line between Dazhui (GV14) downward to Changqiang (GV1) at the end of coccygeal bone	Pushing or pinching manipulation: Push directly the back from top to bottom with the facies digitales of index and middle fingers for 50 to 100 times, or pinch and lift the back from top to bottom with spine pinching manipulation for 3 to 5 times.	It can harmonize Yin and Yang, tonify and replenish Qi and blood, bank up and tonify original Qi, invigorate spleen and stomach, clear heat and bring down a fever, mainly used for fever, cold, diarrhea, abdominal pain, nausea, vomiting, infantile malnutrition with accumulation, constipation, convulsion, epilepsy, night crying, prolapse of rectum and enuresis and so on
Pishu (BL20)	1.5 cun lateral to the depression below the spinous process of the 11th thoracic vertebra	Kneading manipulation: Knead the point with tips of index and middle fingers or fingertips of the 2 thumbs for 50 to 100 times	It can invigorate spleen and stomach to promote transportation and transformation and remove dampness, mainly used for anorexia, abdominal distension, vomiting, diarrhea, bloody stool, jaundice, hypochondriac pain and edema
Weishu (BL21)	1.5 cun lateral to the depression below the spinous process of the 12th thoracic vertebra	Kneading manipulation: Knead the point with tips of index and middle fingers or fingertips of the 2 thumbs for 50 to 100 times	It can invigorate spleen and harmonize stomach, mainly used for stomach, pain of chest and hypochondrium, abdominal distension, vomiting, borborygmus and undigested food in stool
Shenshu (BL23)	1.5 cun lateral to the depression below the spinous process of the 2nd lumbar vertebra	Kneading manipulation: Knead the point with tips of index and middle fingers or fingertips of the 2 thumbs for 50 to 100 times	It can nourish Yin and tonify Yang, and tonify and replenish kidney Qi, mainly used for aching pain of waist and knees, enuresis, frequent urination and edema

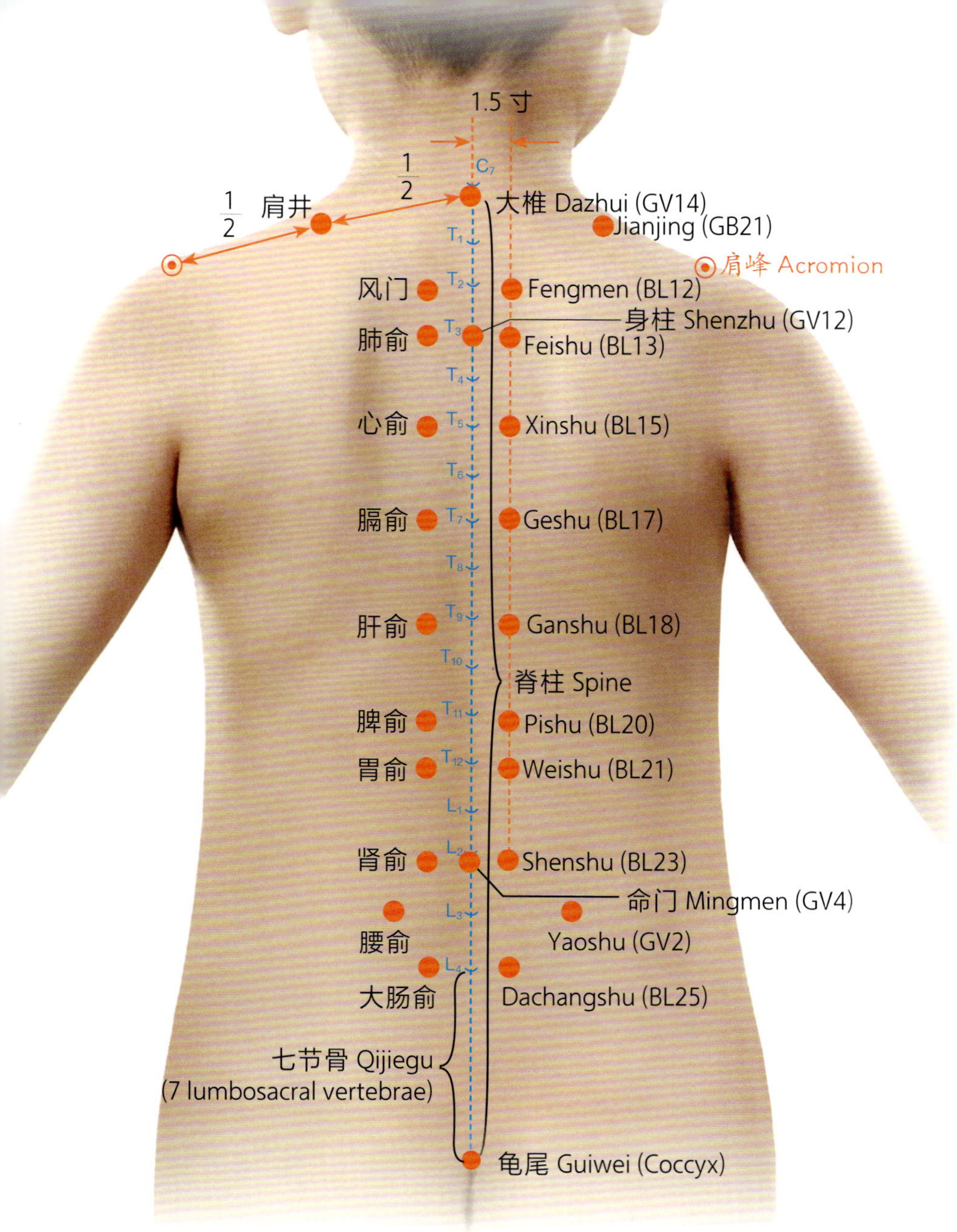

C: 颈椎棘突 Spinous process of cervical vertebra
T: 胸椎棘突 Spinous process of thoracic vertebra
L: 腰椎棘突 Spinous process of lumbar vertebra

续表

穴 位	定 位	按摩方法	功效主治
命门	第 2 腰椎棘突下凹陷中	揉法：以食指、中指指端或两拇指指端揉 50~100 次	补肾壮阳。主治遗尿、汗不出、小儿惊风
大肠俞	第 4 腰椎棘突下，旁开 1.5 寸	揉法：用两手拇指指端揉 50~100 次	通便，止痛。主治腹痛、腹胀、肠鸣、泄泻（腹泻）、便秘
腰俞	第 3 腰椎棘突下，旁开 3 寸	揉法：用两拇指或食指、中指指端揉 50~100 次	通经活络。主治腰痛、泄泻（腹泻）
七节骨	第 4 腰椎至尾骨端成一直线	推法：用拇指桡侧面或食指、中指螺纹面，自下向上或自上向下直推 100~500 次。分别称为推上七节骨和推下七节骨	温阳止泻，益气通便。主治泄泻（腹泻）、便秘、腹胀、脱肛
龟尾	尾椎骨端	揉法：用拇指或中指指端揉 100~300 次	止泻，通便。主治泄泻（腹泻）、痢疾、便秘、脱肛、遗尿（尿床）

Continued

Acupoints	Location	Massage Manipulations	Efficacy and Indications
Mingmen (GV4)	In the depression below the spinous process of the 2nd lumbar vertebra	Kneading manipulation: Knead the point with tips of index and middle fingers or fingertips of the 2 thumbs for 50 to 100 times	It can tonify kidney Yang, mainly used for enuresis, anhidrosis and infantile convulsion
Dachangshu (BL25)	1.5 cun lateral to the depression below the spinous process of the 4th lumbar vertebra	Kneading manipulation: Knead the point with the fingertips of the 2 thumbs for 50 to 100 times	It can relieve constipation and pain, mainly used for abdominal pain and abdominal distension, borborygmus, diarrhea and constipation
Yaoshu (GV2)	3 cun lateral to the depression below the spinous process of the 3th lumbar vertebra	Kneading manipulation: Knead the point with fingertips of the 2 thumbs or tips of index and middle fingers for 50 to 100 times	It can sooth meridians and activate collaterals, mainly used for lumbago and diarrhea
Qijiegu (7 lumbosacral vertebrae)	The line between the 4th lumbar vertebra and the end of coccygeal bone	Pushing manipulation: Push directly Qijiegu (7 lumbosacral vertebrae) with the radial side of the thumb or index and middle fingers for 100 to 500 times from bottom to top or from top to bottom, which is called Push Upper Qijiegu (7 lumbosacral vertebrae) and Push Lower Qijiegu (7 lumbosacral vertebrae) respectively	It can warm Yang and relieve diarrhea, replenish Qi and relieve constipation, mainly used for diarrhea, constipation, abdominal distension and prolapse of rectum
Guiwei (Coccyx)	At the end of coccygeal vertebra	Kneading manipulation: Knead the point with fingertips of the thumb or middle finger for 100 to 300 times	It can relieve diarrhea and constipation, mainly used for diarrhea, dysentery, constipation, prolapse of rectum and enuresis

按摩方法详解
Detailed Diagram of Massage Manipulations

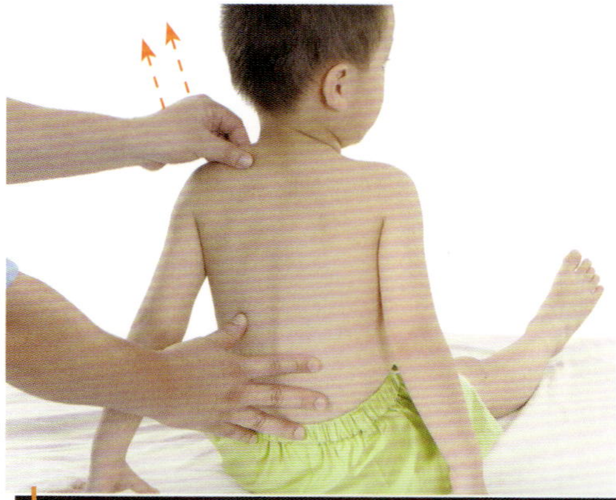

拿肩井

用拇指与食指、中指两指对称用力提拿本穴。拿 3~5 次。

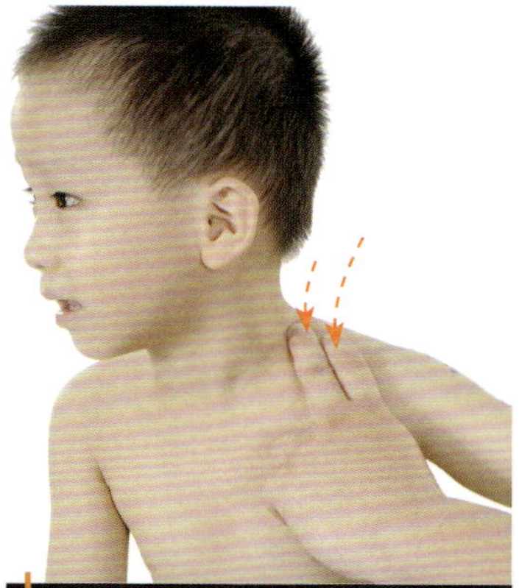

按肩井

用指端按穴位，按 0.5~1 分钟。本法是诸法推毕的结束手法，又称为总收法。

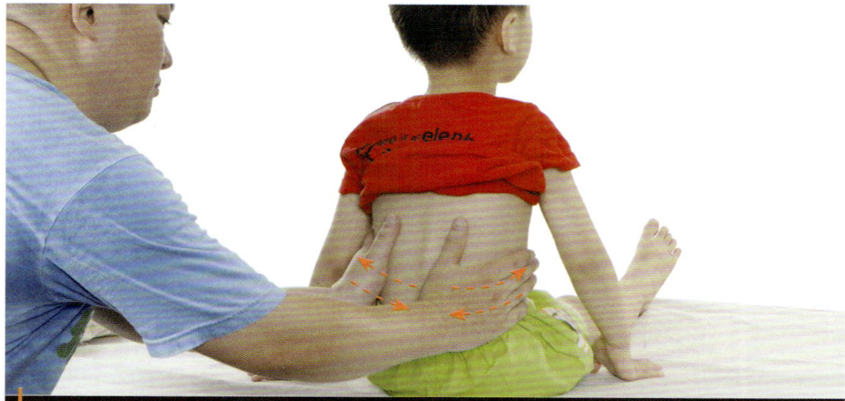

搓肾俞

双手掌挟住肾俞处，交替用力向相反方向来回搓动，同时上下往返移动。

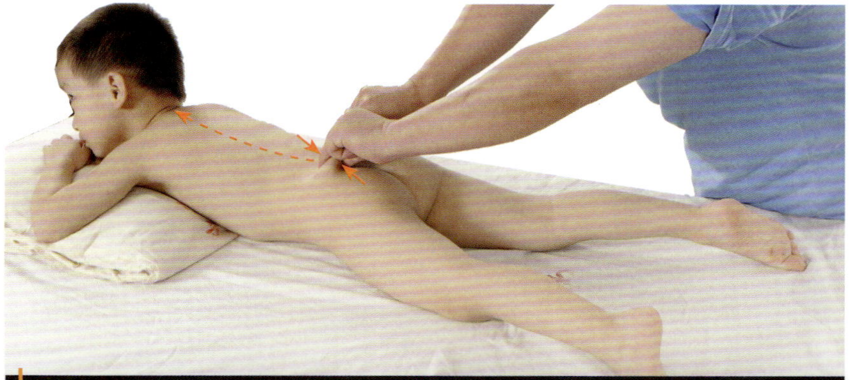

捏脊

小儿俯卧，按摩者用双手拇指、食指自小儿腰骶部开始把皮肤捏起，自下而上捏提至大椎穴处。一般捏 3~5 遍，以脊柱两侧皮肤微有潮红为有效。

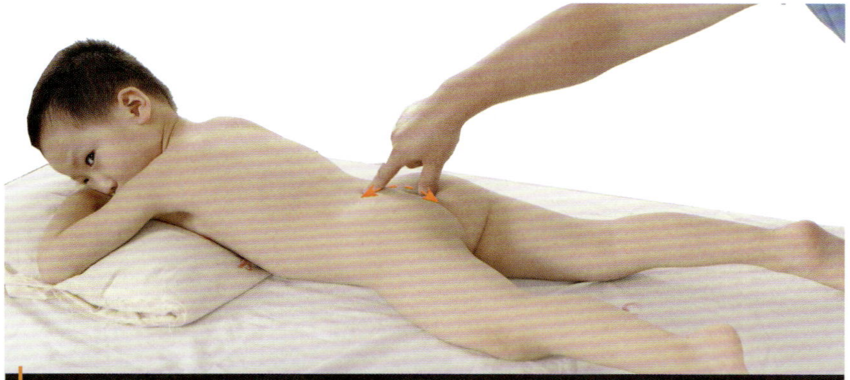

推七节骨

用拇指面或食指、中指两指面自下向上或自上向下作直推。推 100~500 次。

按摩方法详解
Detailed Diagram of Massage Manipulations

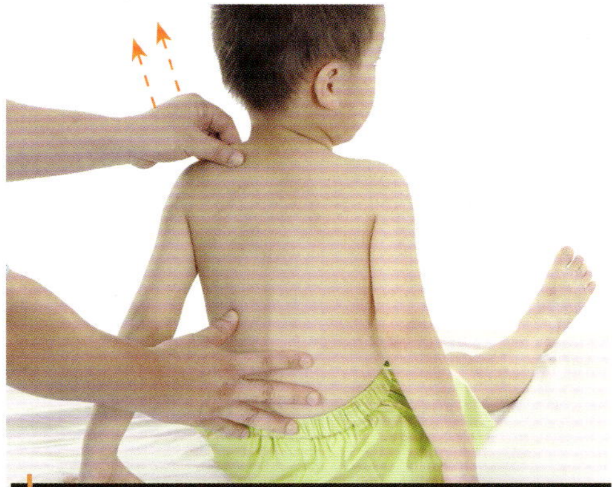

Grasp Jianjing (GB21)

Exert strength symmetrically with the thumb and index, middle fingers to lift and grasp the point for 3 to 5 times.

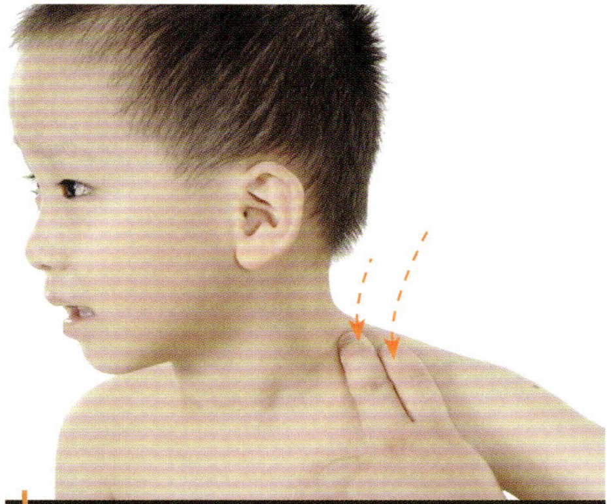

Press Jianjing (GB21)

Press the point with the fingertips for 0.5 to 1 minutes. The manipulation is the last ending technique for all manipulations, which is also called Completing Technique.

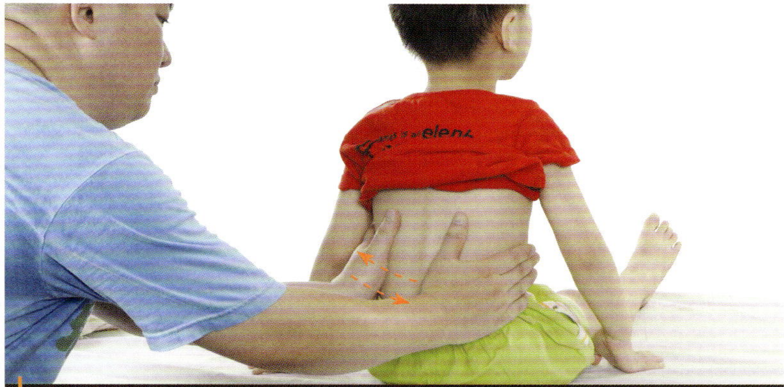

Twist Shenshu (BL23)

Hold the region of Shenshu (BL23) with the 2 palms. Exert strength to twist back and forth alternatively in opposite direction and move the palm up and down at the same time.

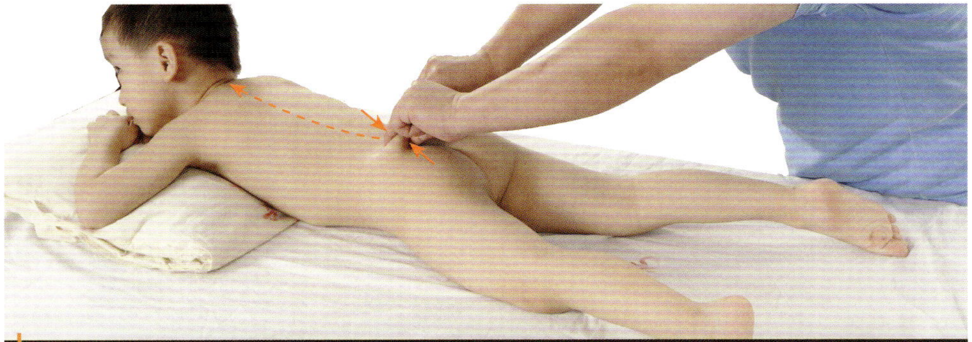

Pinch spine

Let the child lie in prone position. Pinch the skin from bottom to top with the thumbs and index fingers of the 2 hands starting from the lumbosacral region to Dazhui (GV14) for 3 to 5 times generally until the bilateral skin around spine turns slightly flush.

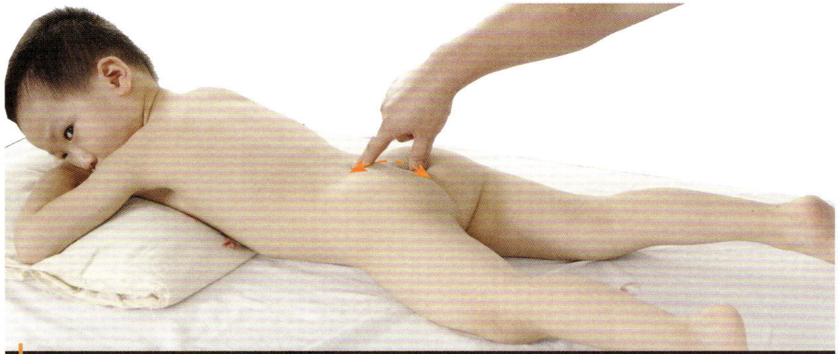

Push Qijiegu (7 lumbosacral vertebrae)

Push directly Qijiegu (7 lumbosacral vertebrae) from bottom to top or from top to bottom with the facial digitales of the thumb or index and middle fingers for 100 to 500 times.

上肢穴位及按摩手法
Acupoints and Massage Manipulations in Upper Limbs

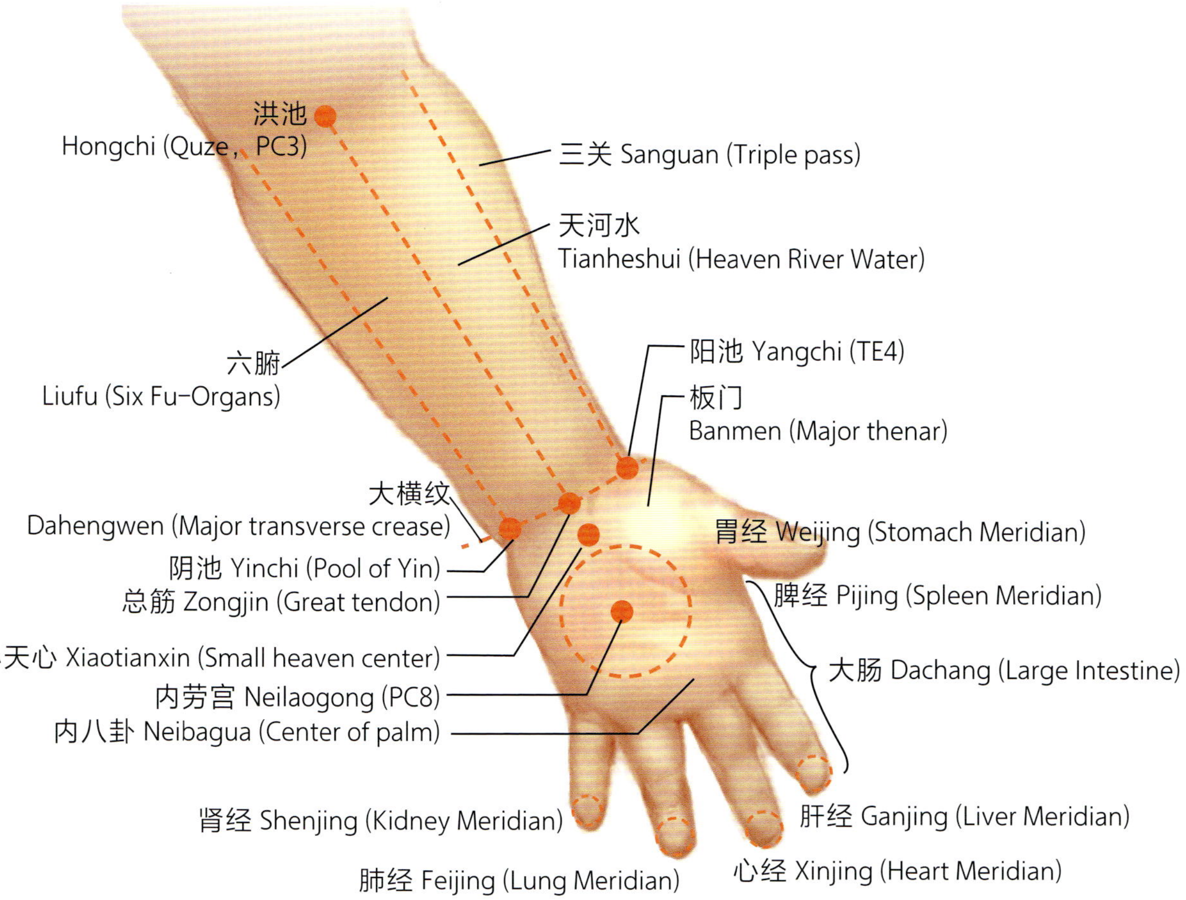

上肢部经典按摩手法

运水入土

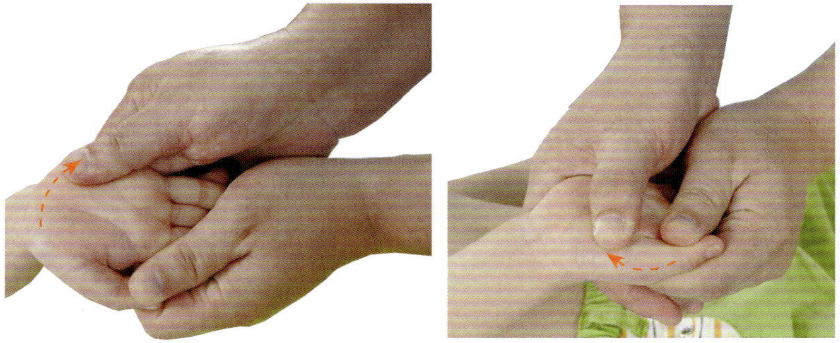

本法有健脾、润燥、通便的作用。

打马过天河

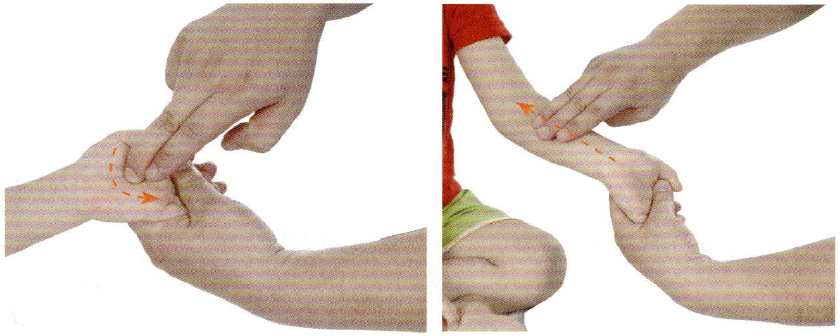

本法可以清火退热，用于治疗一切热病发热。

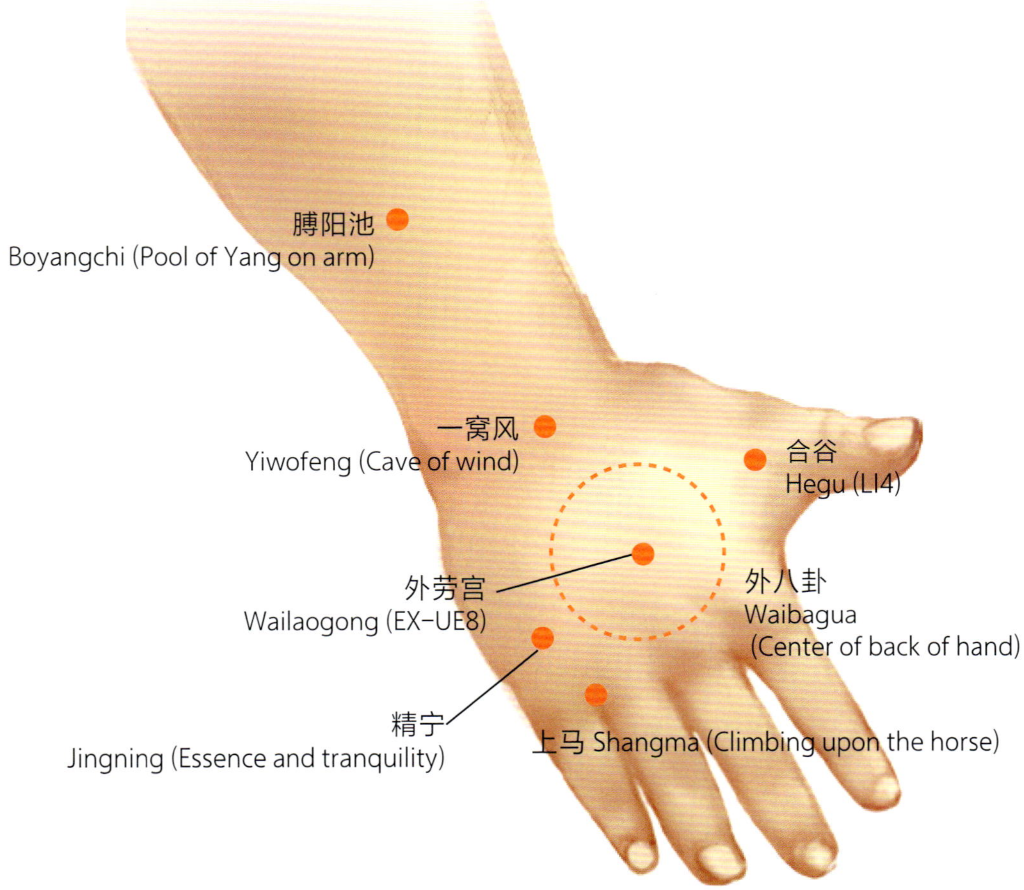

Classic Massage Manipulations in Upper Limbs

Yunshui Rutu (Transforming Water into Earth)

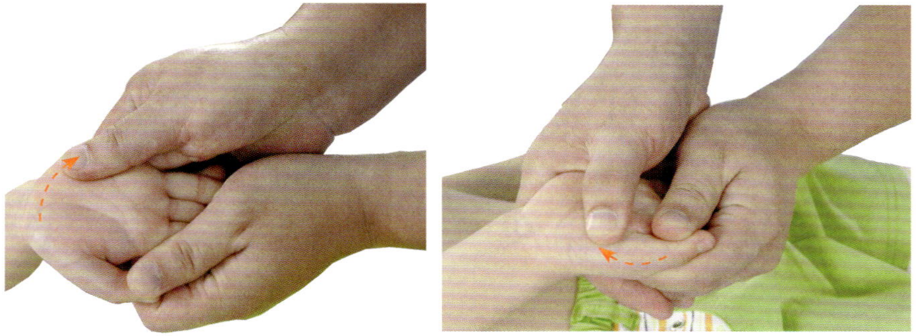

The manipulation can invigorate spleen, moisten dry and relieve constipation.

Dama Guotianhe (Beating the Horse to Cross Heaven River)

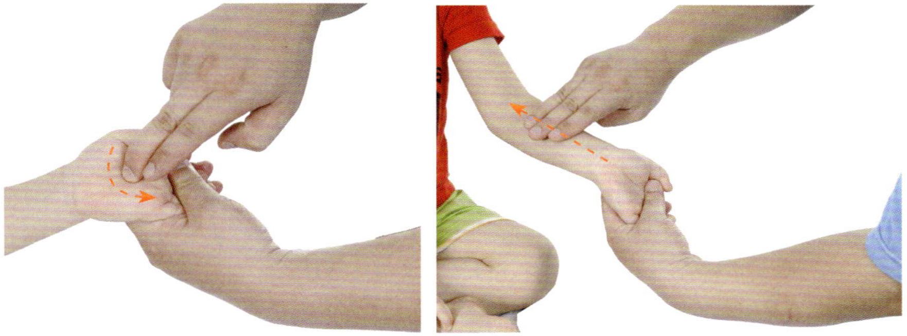

The manipulation can clear fire and bring down a fever to treat fever in all kinds of febrile diseases.

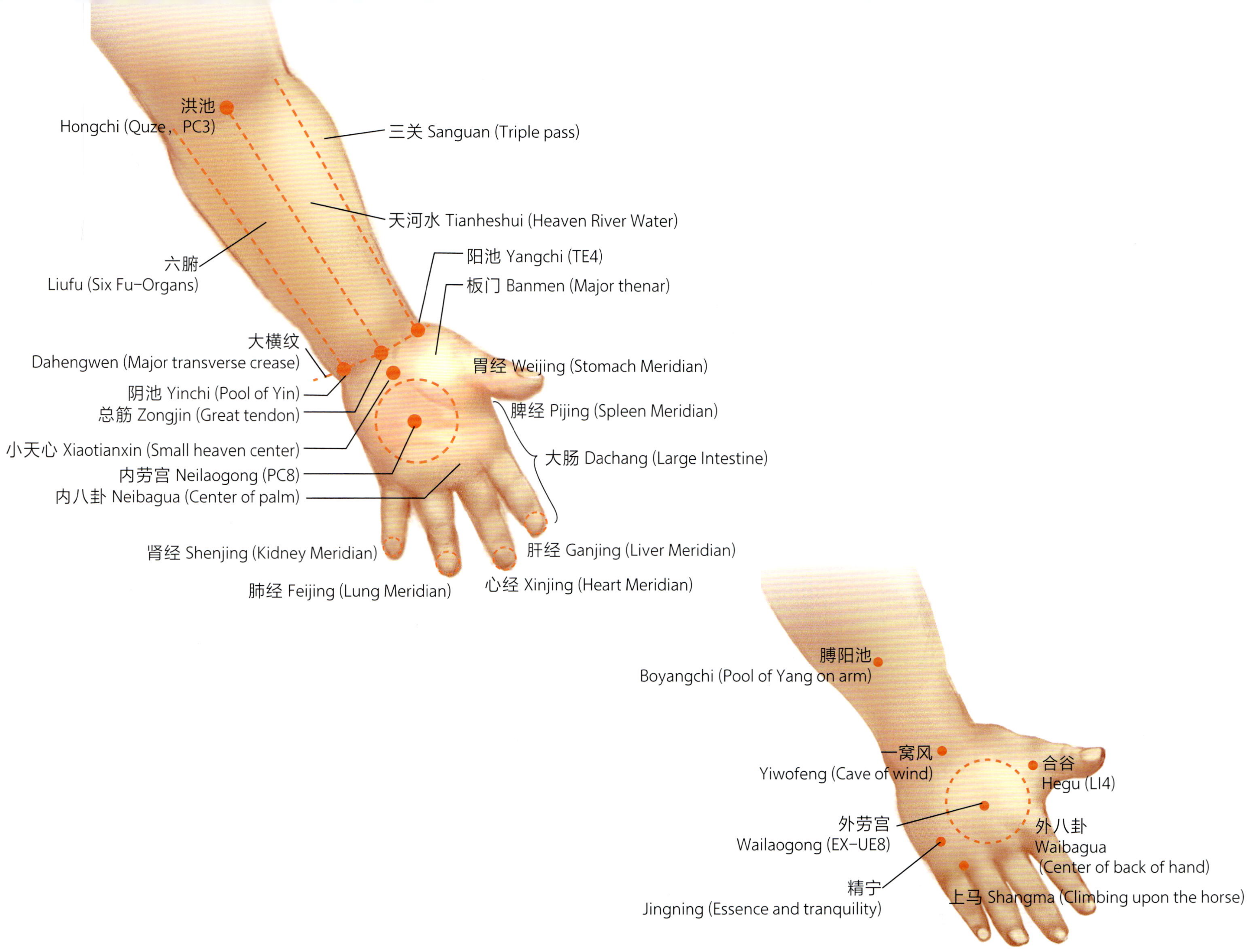
洪池
Hongchi (Quze，PC3)
三关 Sanguan (Triple pass)
天河水 Tianheshui (Heaven River Water)
六腑
Liufu (Six Fu-Organs)
阳池 Yangchi (TE4)
板门 Banmen (Major thenar)
大横纹
Dahengwen (Major transverse crease)
胃经 Weijing (Stomach Meridian)
阴池 Yinchi (Pool of Yin)
总筋 Zongjin (Great tendon)
脾经 Pijing (Spleen Meridian)
小天心 Xiaotianxin (Small heaven center)
大肠 Dachang (Large Intestine)
内劳宫 Neilaogong (PC8)
内八卦 Neibagua (Center of palm)
肾经 Shenjing (Kidney Meridian)
肝经 Ganjing (Liver Meridian)
肺经 Feijing (Lung Meridian)
心经 Xinjing (Heart Meridian)
膊阳池
Boyangchi (Pool of Yang on arm)
一窝风
Yiwofeng (Cave of wind)
合谷
Hegu (LI4)
外劳宫
Wailaogong (EX-UE8)
外八卦
Waibagua
(Center of back of hand)
精宁
Jingning (Essence and tranquility)
上马 Shangma (Climbing upon the horse)

按摩方法速览
Quick Look of Massage Manipulations

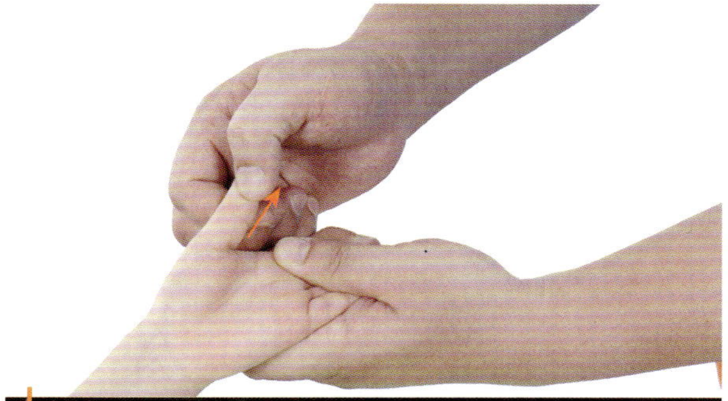

推胃经 Push Weijing (Stomach Meridian)

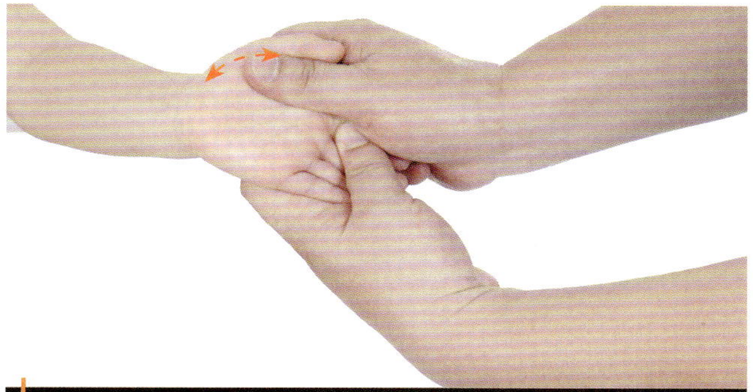

推板门 Push Banmen (Major thenar)

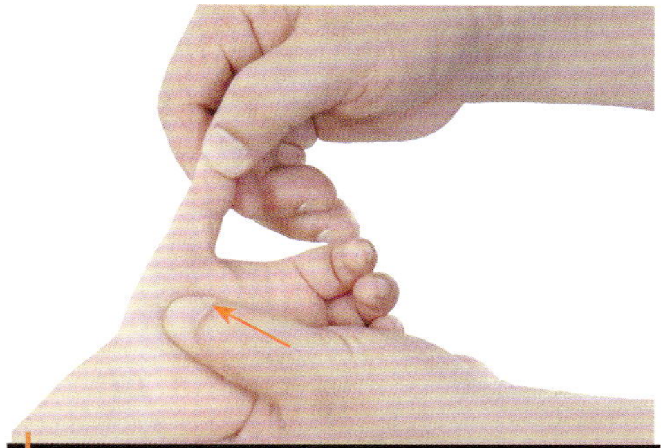

掐脾经 Pinch Pijing (Spleen Meridian)

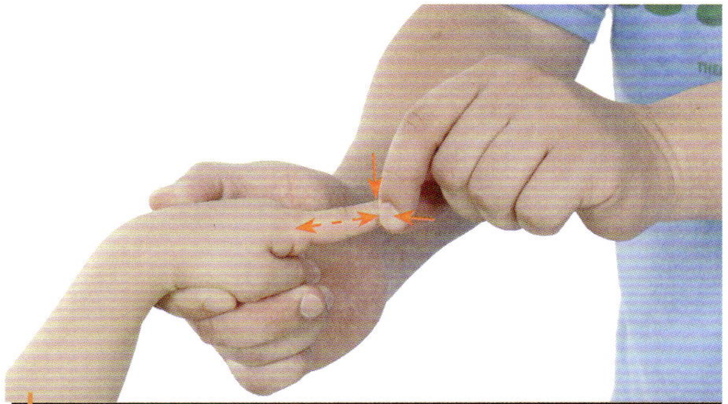

捻大肠 Twirl Dachang (Large Intestine)

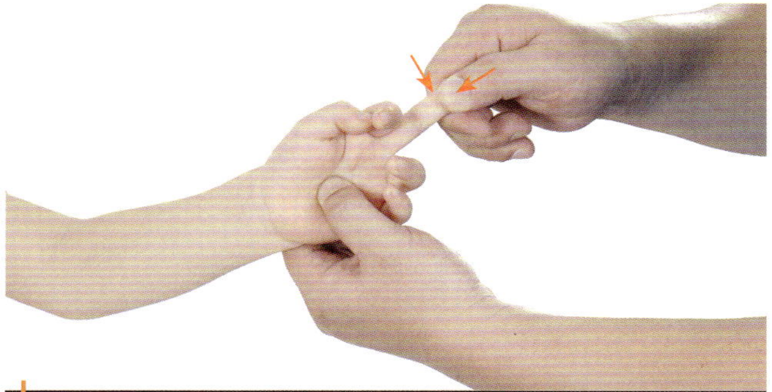

掐心经 Pinch Xinjing (Heart Meridian)

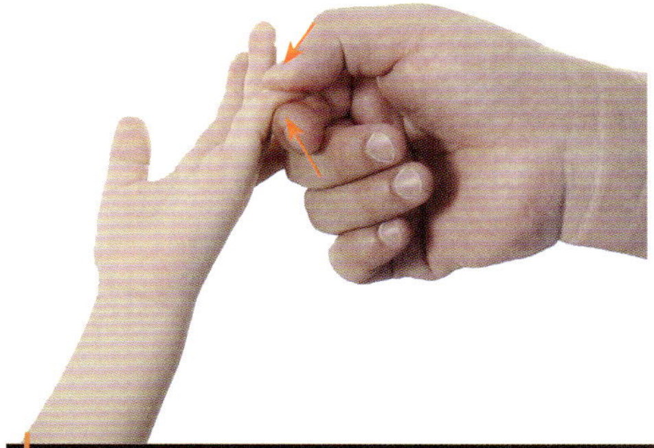

捏肾经 Pinch Shenjing (Kidney Meridian)

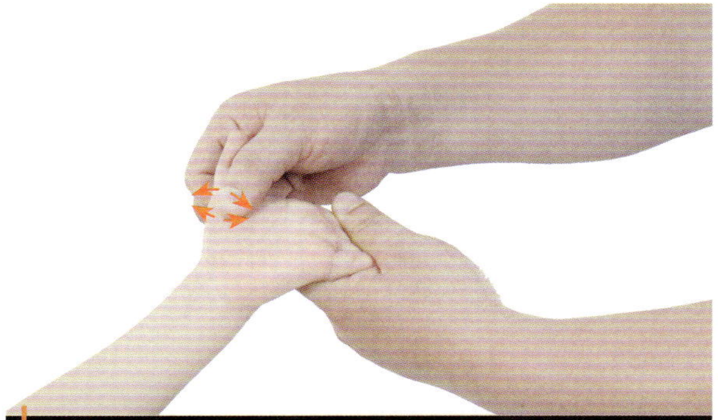

揉板门 Knead Banmen (Major thenar)

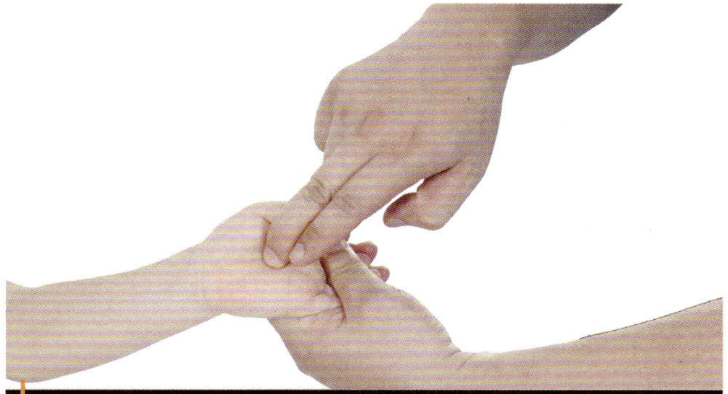

运内劳宫 Circularly push Neilaogong (PC8)

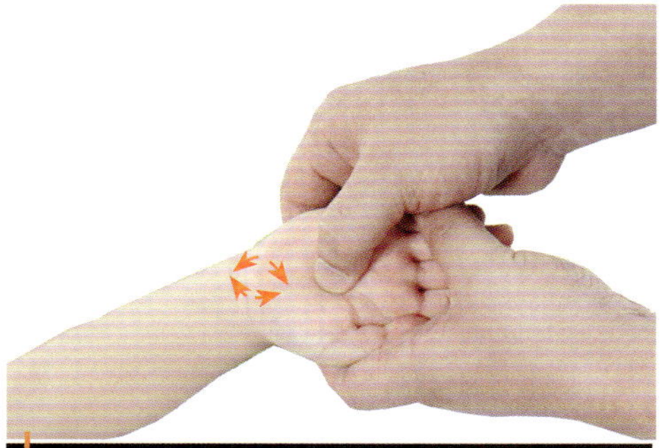

揉内劳宫 Knead Neilaogong (PC8)

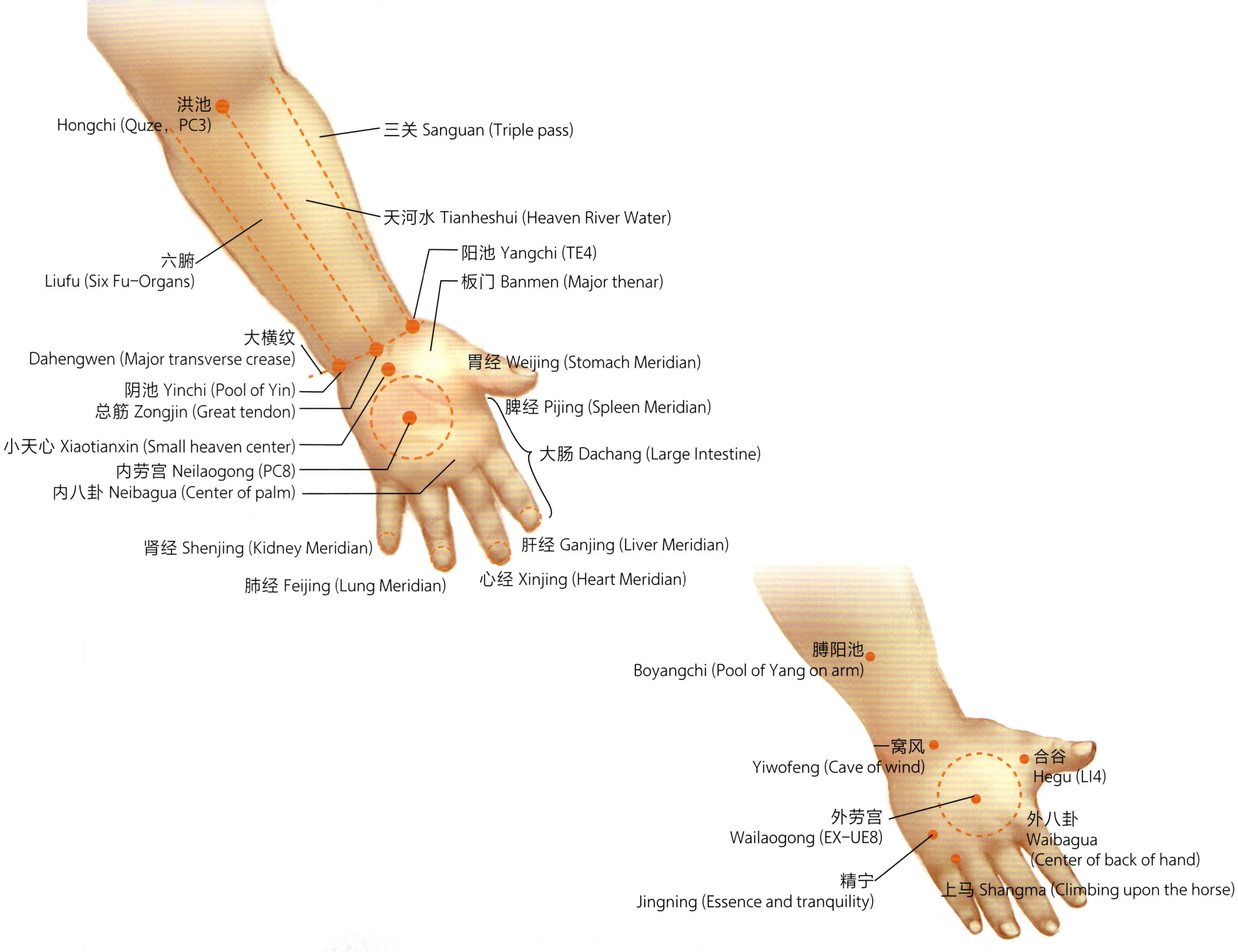
洪池
Hongchi (Quze，PC3)
三关 Sanguan (Triple pass)
天河水 Tianheshui (Heaven River Water)
六腑
Liufu (Six Fu-Organs)
阳池 Yangchi (TE4)
板门 Banmen (Major thenar)
大横纹
Dahengwen (Major transverse crease)
胃经 Weijing (Stomach Meridian)
阴池 Yinchi (Pool of Yin)
总筋 Zongjin (Great tendon)
脾经 Pijing (Spleen Meridian)
小天心 Xiaotianxin (Small heaven center)
大肠 Dachang (Large Intestine)
内劳宫 Neilaogong (PC8)
内八卦 Neibagua (Center of palm)
肾经 Shenjing (Kidney Meridian)
肝经 Ganjing (Liver Meridian)
肺经 Feijing (Lung Meridian)
心经 Xinjing (Heart Meridian)
膊阳池
Boyangchi (Pool of Yang on arm)
一窝风
Yiwofeng (Cave of wind)
合谷
Hegu (LI4)
外劳宫
Wailaogong (EX-UE8)
外八卦
Waibagua
(Center of back of hand)
精宁
Jingning (Essence and tranquility)
上马 Shangma (Climbing upon the horse)

按摩方法速览
Quick Look of Massage Manipulations

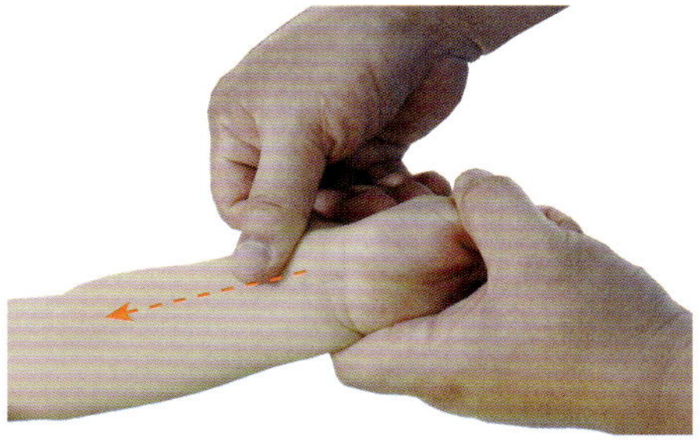
推上三关 Push Upper Sanguan (Triple pass)

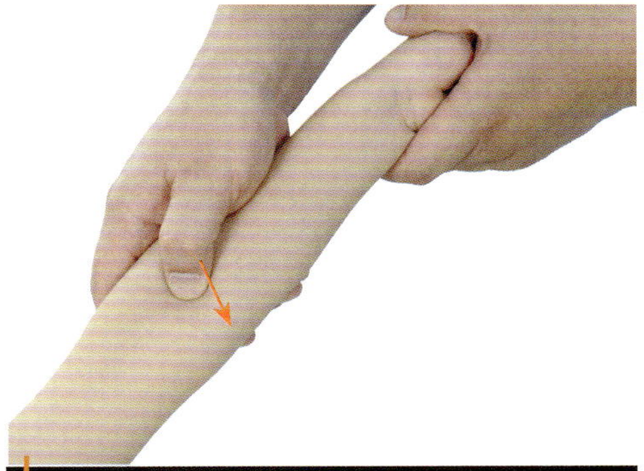
掐洪池 Pinch Hongchi (Quze，PC3)

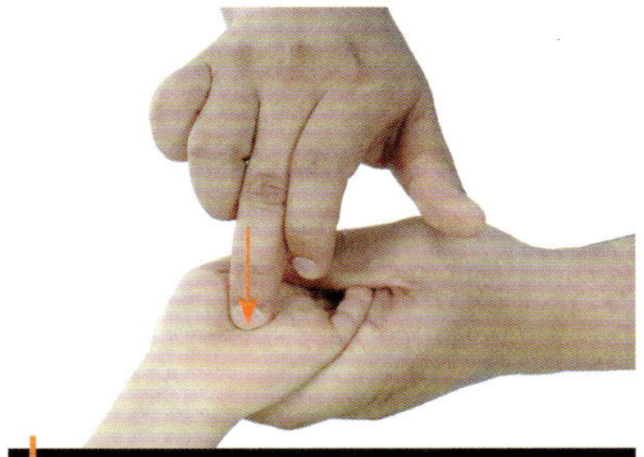
捣小天心 Pound Xiaotianxin (Small heaven center)

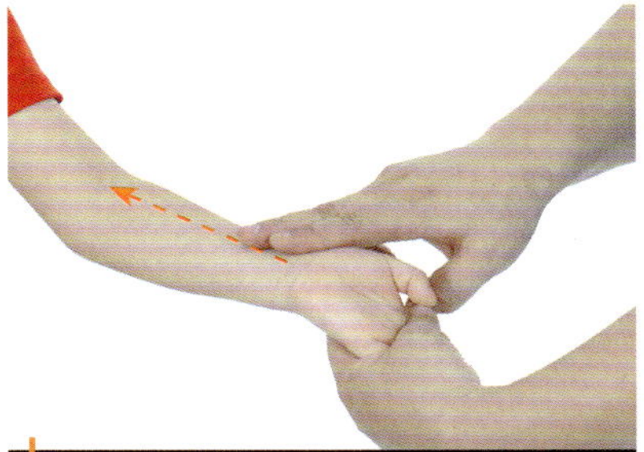
打马过天河 Dama Guotianhe (Beating the Horse to Cross Heaven River)

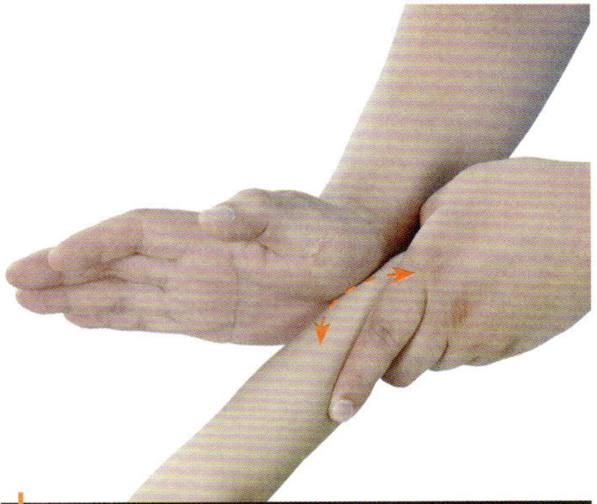
揉一窝风 Knead Yiwofeng (Cave of wind)

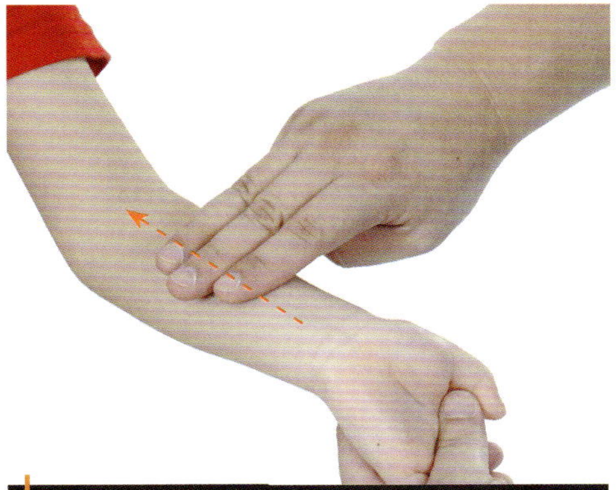
推天河水 Push Tianheshui (Heaven river water)

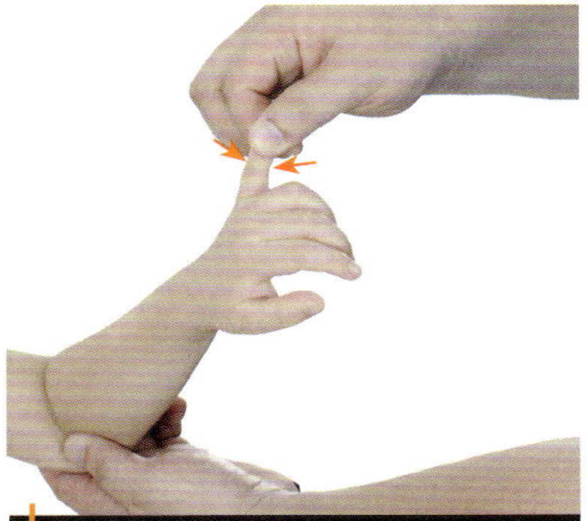
揉五指节 Knead Wuzhijie (Interphalangeal joints of 5 fingers)

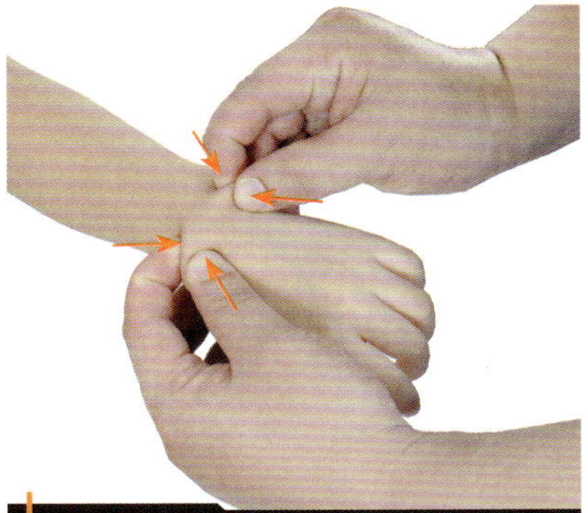
提捏螺蛳骨 Lift-Pinch Luosigu (Bilateral protrusion of wrist)

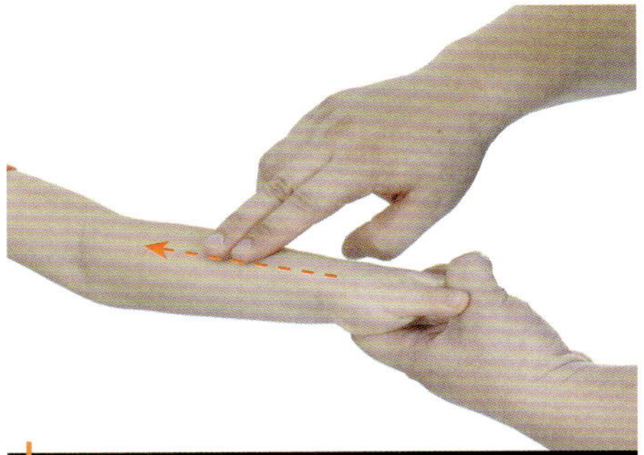
推上三关 Push Upper Sanguan (Triple pass)

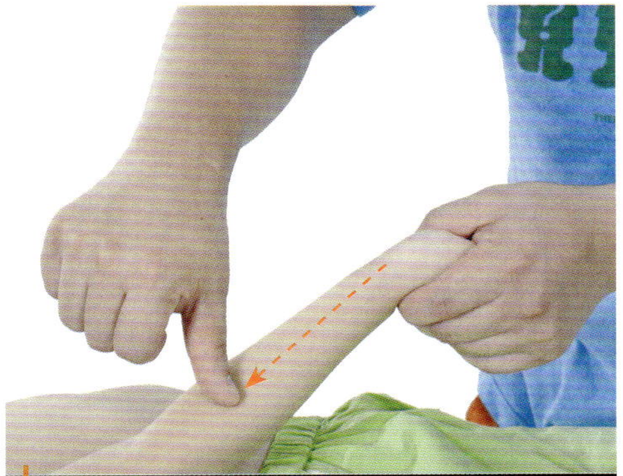
刮三关 Scrape Sanguan (Triple pass)

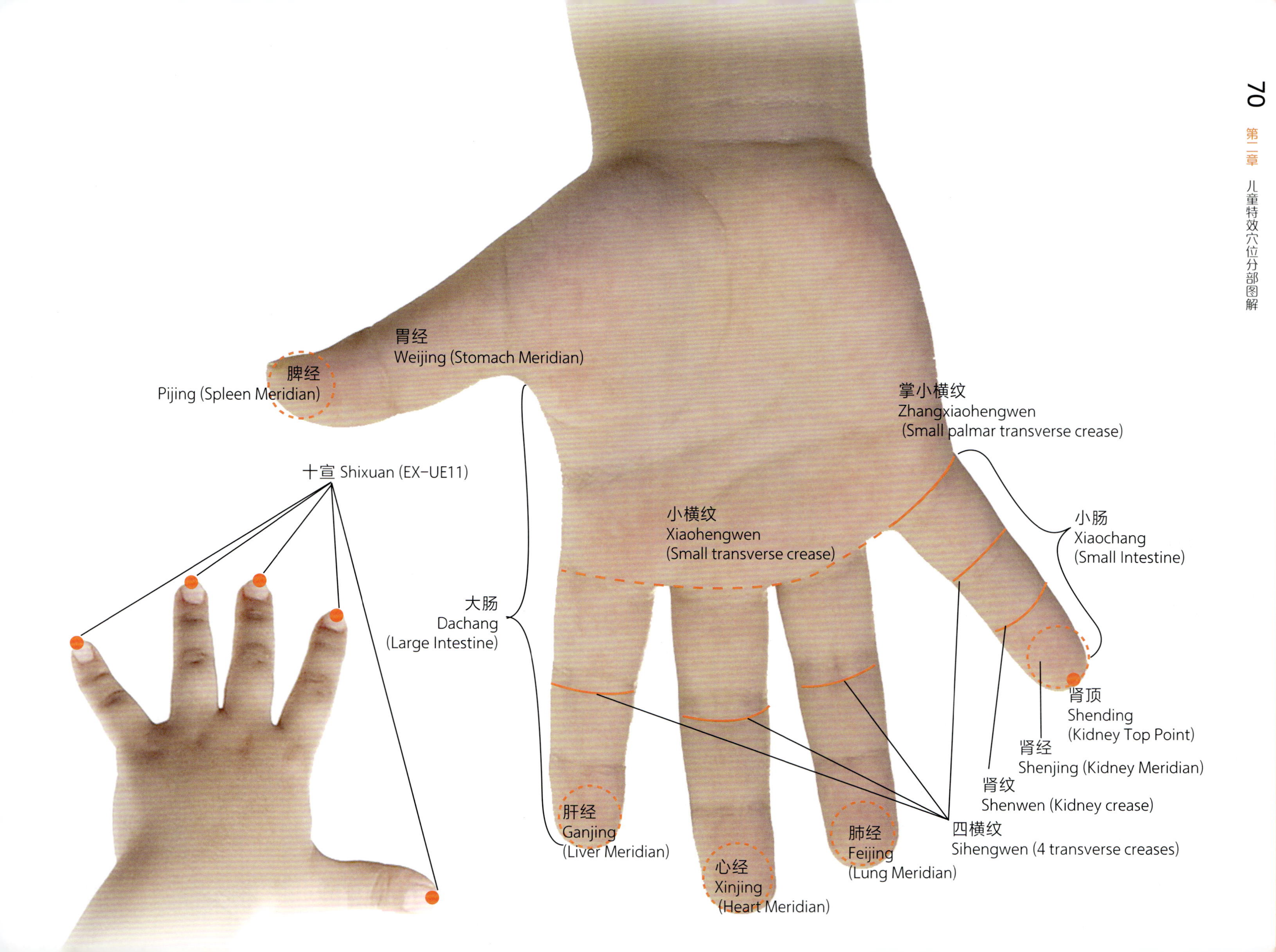
胃经
Weijing (Stomach Meridian)
脾经
Pijing (Spleen Meridian)
掌小横纹
Zhangxiaohengwen
(Small palmar transverse crease)
十宣 Shixuan (EX-UE11)
小横纹
Xiaohengwen
(Small transverse crease)
小肠
Xiaochang
(Small Intestine)
大肠
Dachang
(Large Intestine)
肾顶
Shending
(Kidney Top Point)
肾经
Shenjing (Kidney Meridian)
肾纹
Shenwen (Kidney crease)
四横纹
Sihengwen (4 transverse creases)
肝经
Ganjing
(Liver Meridian)
肺经
Feijing
(Lung Meridian)
心经
Xinjing
(Heart Meridian)

穴 位	定 位	按摩方法	功效主治
胃 经	拇指掌面近掌端第 1 节，或大鱼际桡侧赤白肉际处	直推法：自指根（指横纹）向掌根（掌指横纹）方向直推 100~500 次，称补胃经；反之为清胃经	补胃经，可健脾和胃，消食化积；清胃经，可降逆止呕，泻胃火，清中焦湿热。主治烦渴善饥、食欲不振、呕恶、嗳气（打嗝）、吐血、鼻出血
脾 经	拇指末节螺纹面或拇指桡侧缘	直推法：将儿童拇指微屈，从拇指桡侧边缘向指根方向直推，称补脾经；由指根向指端方向直推，称清脾经；自指尖到指根来回直推为平补平泻，称清补脾经。一般脾经多用补法，直推 100~500 次	补脾经，可健脾和胃，补益气血；清脾经，可清利湿热，消积导滞，化痰止呕。主治伤食（饮食不当，损伤脾胃）、腹泻、便秘、呕吐、痢疾、食欲不振、黄疸、精神萎靡

Acupoints	Location	Massage Manipulations	Efficacy and Indications
Weijing (Stomach Meridian)	The palm of the 1st distal knuckle of the thumb, or the dorso-ventral boundary of the hand in the radial side of the great thenar	Direct-pushing manipulation: Push Weijing (Stomach Meridian) directly from the finger root (transverse striation of fingers) to the root of palm (metacarpophalangeal crease) for 100 to 500 times, named tonifying Weijing (Stomach Meridian), while pushing in the opposite direction is clearing Weijing (Stomach Meridian)	The manipulation of tonifying Weijing (Stomach Meridian) can invigorate spleen and harmonize stomach, promote digestion and resolve food stagnation. The manipulation of clearing Weijing (Stomach Meridian) can descend adverse Qi and arrest vomiting, purge stomach fire and clear dampness-heat of middle energizer. It is mainly used for polydipsia and hyperorexia, poor appetite, vomiting and nausea, hiccup, hematemesis and nasal bleeding
Pijing (Spleen Meridian)	The distal segment of the thumb or the radial border of the thumb	Direct-pushing manipulation: Bend the thumb of the child slightly. Push Pijing (Spleen Meridian) directly from the radial border to the root of the thumb, named tonifying Pijing (Spleen Meridian), while pushing from the root to tip of the thumb is clearing Pijing (Spleen Meridian). The manipulation of pushing directly back and forth from the tip to root of the thumb is neutral reinforcement and reduction, named moistening and tonifying Pijing (Spleen Meridian).Pijing (Spleen Meridian) is generally suitable for tonifying. Push Pijing (Spleen Meridian) directly for 100 to 500 times	The manipulation of tonifying Pijing (Spleen Meridian) can invigorate spleen and harmonize stomach, tonify and replenish Qi and blood. The manipulation of clearing Pijing (Spleen Meridian) can clear dampness-heat, resolve accumulation and remove food stagnation, resolve phlegm and arrest vomiting. It is mainly used for dyspepsia (Spleen and stomach are injured by improper diet), diarrhea, constipation, vomiting, dysentery, poor appetite, jaundice and low spirit

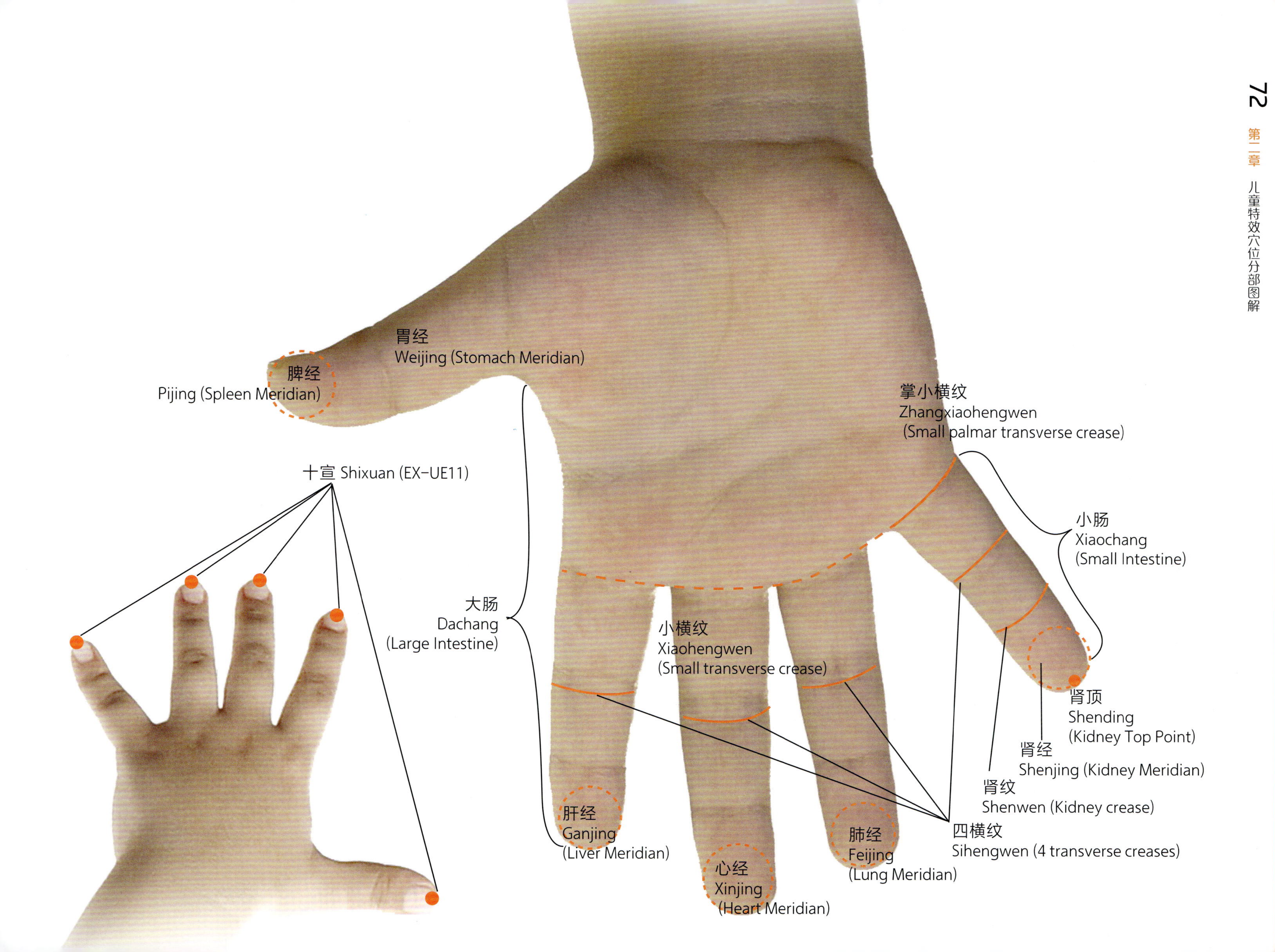
胃经
Weijing (Stomach Meridian)
脾经
Pijing (Spleen Meridian)
掌小横纹
Zhangxiaohengwen
(Small palmar transverse crease)
十宣 Shixuan (EX-UE11)
小肠
Xiaochang
(Small Intestine)
大肠
Dachang
(Large Intestine)
小横纹
Xiaohengwen
(Small transverse crease)
肾顶
Shending
(Kidney Top Point)
肾经
Shenjing (Kidney Meridian)
肾纹
Shenwen (Kidney crease)
四横纹
Sihengwen (4 transverse creases)
肝经
Ganjing
(Liver Meridian)
肺经
Feijing
(Lung Meridian)
心经
Xinjing
(Heart Meridian)

续表

穴 位	定 位	按摩方法	功效主治
肝经	食指末端螺纹面	直推法：从食指掌面末节指纹向食指尖方向直推为清，称清肝经，反之为补肝经。一般肝经宜清不宜补，直推 100~500 次	平肝泻火，解郁除烦，和气生血。主治烦躁不安、五心烦热、口苦咽干、头痛、头晕、目赤、抽搐、癫痫
心经	中指末节螺纹面	直推法：自中指掌面末节指纹向指尖方向直推为清，称清心经，反之为补心经。一般心经宜清不宜补，直推 100~500 次	清心经可清心火；补心经可补气血、养心安神。主治高热神昏、五心烦热、口舌生疮、小便赤涩、心烦不安

Continued

Acupoints	Location	Massage Manipulations	Efficacy and Indications
Ganjing (Liver Meridian)	The tip of index finger	Direct-pushing manipulation: Push Ganjing (Liver Meridian) directly from the distal segment to the tip of index finger, which is clearing method, named clearing Ganjing (Liver Meridian), while pushing in the opposite direction is tonifying Ganjing (Liver Meridian). Ganjing (Liver Meridian) is generally suitable for clearing instead of tonifying. Push Ganjing (Liver Meridian) directly for 100 to 500 times	It can pacify liver and purge fire, resolve depression and relieve dysphoria, harmonize Qi and generate blood, mainly used for restlessness, vexing heat in chest, palms and soles, bitter taste in mouth and dry throat, headache, vertigo, red eye, convulsion and epilepsy
Xinjing (Heart Meridian)	The distal segment of middle finger	Direct-pushing manipulation: Push Xinjing (Heart Meridian) directly from the distal segment to the tip of middle finger, which is clearing method, named clearing Xinjing (Heart Meridian), while pushing in the opposite direction is tonifying Xinjing (Heart Meridian). Xinjing (Heart Meridian) is generally suitable for clearing instead of tonifying. Push Xinjing (Heart Meridian) directly for 100 to 500 times	The manipulation of clearing Xinjing (Heart Meridian) can clear heart fire, while the manipulation of tonifying Xinjing (Heart Meridian) can tonify Qi and blood, nourish heart and tranquilize mind. It is mainly used for hyperpyrexia and unconsciousness, vexing heat in chest, palms and soles, sore in the mouth, difficult and red urination, vexation and restlessness

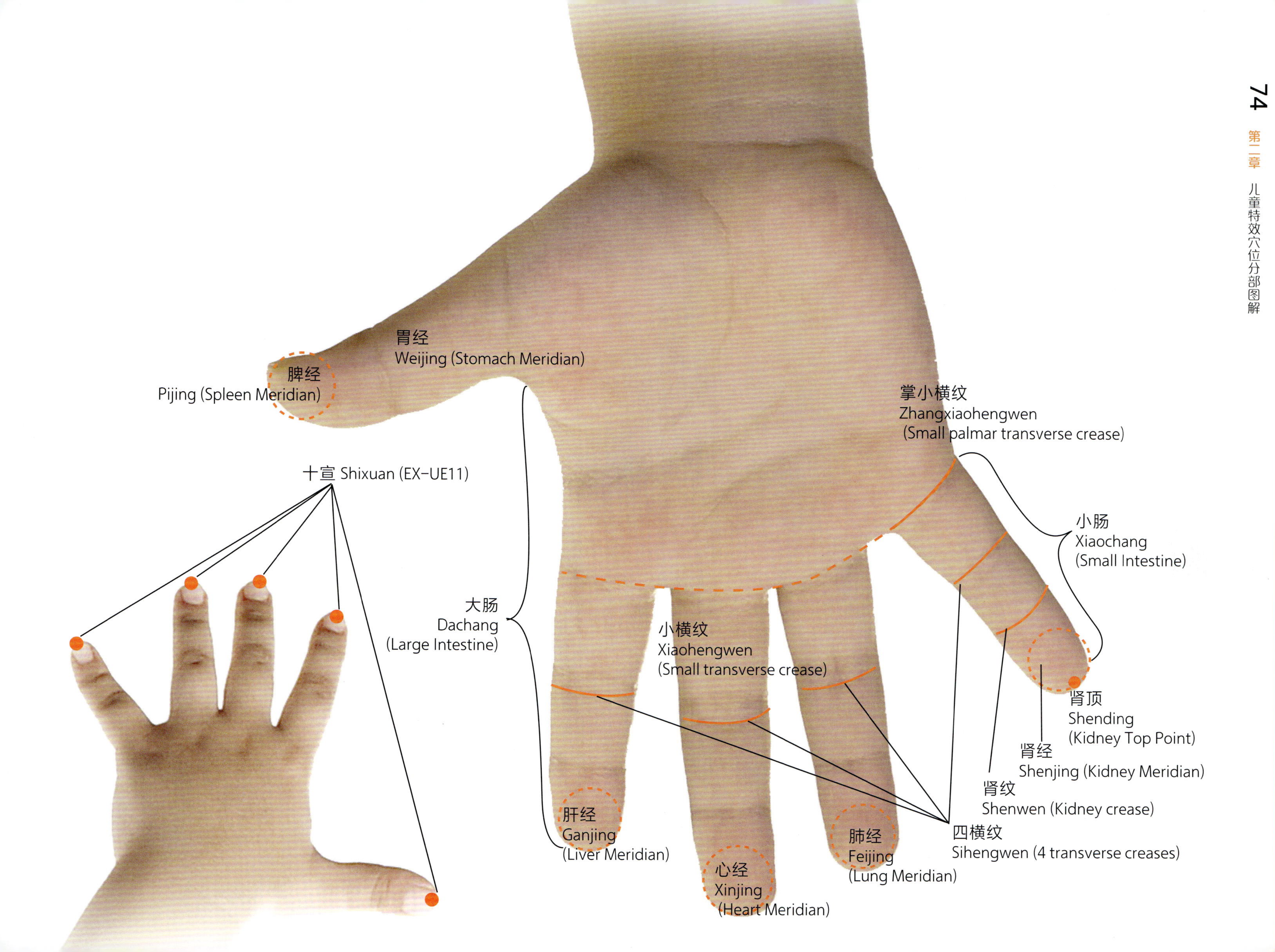
胃经
Weijing (Stomach Meridian)
脾经
Pijing (Spleen Meridian)
掌小横纹
Zhangxiaohengwen
(Small palmar transverse crease)
十宣 Shixuan (EX-UE11)
小肠
Xiaochang
(Small Intestine)
大肠
Dachang
(Large Intestine)
小横纹
Xiaohengwen
(Small transverse crease)
肾顶
Shending
(Kidney Top Point)
肾经
Shenjing (Kidney Meridian)
肾纹
Shenwen (Kidney crease)
四横纹
Sihengwen (4 transverse creases)
肝经
Ganjing
(Liver Meridian)
心经
Xinjing
(Heart Meridian)
肺经
Feijing
(Lung Meridian)

续表

穴 位	定 位	按摩方法	功效主治
肺 经	无名指末节螺纹面	直推法：自无名指掌面末节指纹向指尖方向直推为清，称清肺经，反之为补肺经。直推 100~500 次	补肺经可补益肺气；清肺经可清泻肺热，止咳化痰。主治感冒、发热、咳嗽、气喘、胸闷、脱肛、虚汗怕冷
肾 经	小指末节螺纹面，或小指尖至掌根尺侧边缘成一直线	直推法：从指根向指尖方向直推为补，称补肾经，反之为清肾经。直推 100~500 次	补肾经可温补下元，滋肾壮阳；清肾经可清热利尿。主治肾虚腹泻、遗尿（尿床）、虚喘、先天不足、久病体虚、膀胱湿热之小便赤涩
肾 顶	小指顶端处	揉法：用拇指或中指指端按揉 100~500 次	固表止汗，收敛元气。主治盗汗、自汗、解颅（儿童囟门应合不合）

Continued

Acupoints	Location	Massage Manipulations	Efficacy and Indications
Feijing (Lung Meridian)	The distal segment of ring finger	Direct-pushing manipulation: Push Feijing (Lung Meridian) directly from the distal segment to the tip of ring finger, which is clearing method, named clearing Feijing (Lung Meridian), while pushing in the opposite direction is tonifying Feijing (Lung Meridian). Push Feijing (Lung Meridian) directly for 100 to 500 times	The manipulation of tonifying Feijing (Lung Meridian) can tonify and replenish lung Qi. The manipulation of clearing Feijing (Lung Meridian) can clear and purge lung heat, relieve cough and resolve phlegm. It is mainly used for cold, fever, cough, asthma, chest stuffiness, prolapse of rectum, abnormal sweating due to general debility and fear of cold
Shenjing (Kidney Meridian)	The distal segment of little finger, or the line between the tip of little finger to the ulnar border of root of palm	Direct-pushing manipulation: Push Shenjing (Kidney Meridian) directly from the root to tip of fingers, which is tonifying method, named tonifying Shenjing (Kidney Meridian), while pushing in the opposite direction is clearing Shenjing (Kidney Meridian). Push Shenjing (Kidney Meridian) directly for 100 to 500 times.	The manipulation of tonifying Shenjing (Kidney Meridian) can warm and tonify kidney Qi, nourish kidney Yin and tonify kidney Yang. The manipulation of clearing Shenjing (Kidney Meridian) can clear heat and induce urination. It is mainly used for diarrhea caused by kidney deficiency, enuresis, deficient dyspnea, innate deficiency, physical weakness due to enduring diseases, and red and difficult urination due to dampness-heat of bladde
Shending (Tip of little finger)	The tip of little finger	Kneading manipulation: Press-knead the point with the fingertip of the thumb or middle finger for 100 to 500 times	It can consolidate exterior and stop sweating, and astringe original Qi, mainly used for night seat, spontaneous sweating and ununited skull (The fontanel of the child should have been closed)

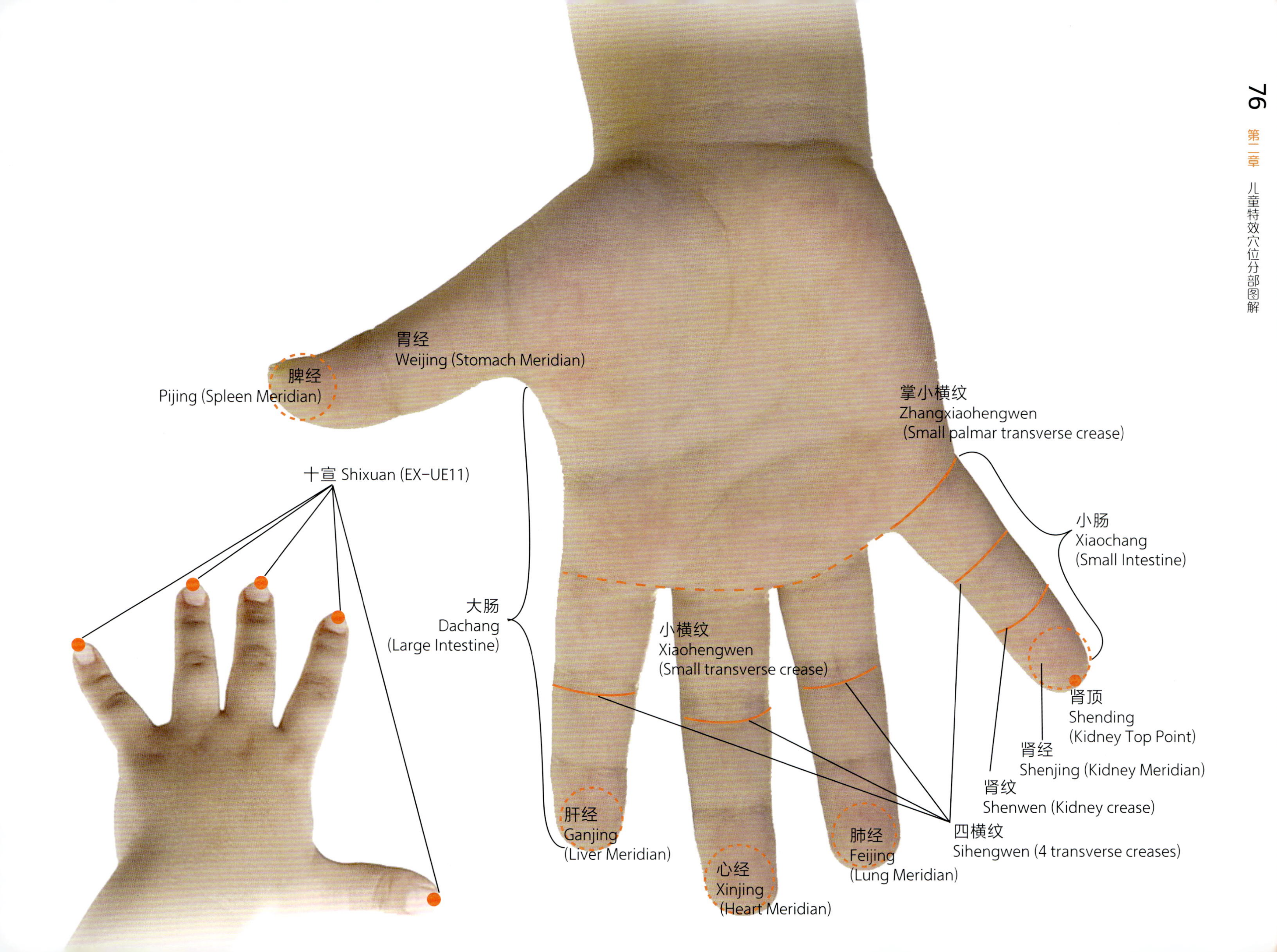
胃经
Weijing (Stomach Meridian)
脾经
Pijing (Spleen Meridian)
十宣 Shixuan (EX-UE11)
掌小横纹
Zhangxiaohengwen
(Small palmar transverse crease)
小肠
Xiaochang
(Small Intestine)
大肠
Dachang
(Large Intestine)
小横纹
Xiaohengwen
(Small transverse crease)
肾顶
Shending
(Kidney Top Point)
肾经
Shenjing (Kidney Meridian)
肾纹
Shenwen (Kidney crease)
四横纹
Sihengwen (4 transverse creases)
肝经
Ganjing
(Liver Meridian)
心经
Xinjing
(Heart Meridian)
肺经
Feijing
(Lung Meridian)

续表

穴 位	定 位	按摩方法	功效主治
肾 纹	手掌面，小指第 2 指间关节横纹处	揉法：用拇指端或中指端按揉 100~500 次	祛风明目，清热散结。主治高热、目赤肿痛、鹅口疮
大 肠	食指桡侧缘，自食指尖至虎口成一直线	直推法：从食指尖向虎口直推为补，称补大肠，反之称清大肠。直推 100~300 次	补大肠可固肠止泻；清大肠可清利大肠湿热，消导积滞。主治泄泻（腹泻）、痢疾、便秘、脱肛、腹痛
小 肠	小指尺侧边缘，自指尖到指根成一直线	推法：从指尖向指根方向直推为补，称补小肠，反之为清小肠。直推 100~300 次	分清泌浊，清热利尿。主治水泻（泻下稀水，如水下注）、遗尿（尿床）、小便赤涩、尿闭、口舌糜烂

Continued

Acupoints	Location	Massage Manipulations	Efficacy and Indications
Shenwen (Kidney crease)	In the palm surface, the transverse striation of the 2nd interphalangeal joint of the little finger	Kneading manipulation: Press-knead the point with the fingertip of the thumb or middle finger for 100 to 500 times	It can dispel wind and improve vision, clear heat and dissipate mass, mainly used for hyperpyrexia, red eye with swollen pain and thrush
Dachang (Large Intestine)	In the radial border of index finger, the line between the tip of index finger to Hukou (the part between the thumb and the index finger).	Direct-pushing manipulation: Push Dachang (Large Intestine) directly from the tip of index finger to Hukou (the part between the thumb and the index finger), which is tonifying method, named tonifying Dachang (Large Intestine), while pushing in the opposite direction is clearing Dachang (Large Intestine). Push directly for 100 to 300 times	The manipulation of tonifying Dachang (Large Intestine) can astringe intestines and relieve diarrhea. The manipulation of clearing Dachang (Large Intestine) can clear dampness-heat of large intestine, resolve accumulation and remove food stagnation. It is mainly used for diarrhea, dysentery, constipation, prolapse of rectum and abdominal pain
Xiaochang (Small Intestine)	In the ulnar border of little finger, the line between the fingertip to the root of finger	Pushing manipulation: Push Xiaochang (Small Intestine) directly from the tip to root of fingers, which is tonifying method, named tonifying Xiaochang (Small Intestine), while pushing in the opposite direction is clearing Xiaochang (Small Intestine). Push Xiaochang (Small Intestine) directly for 100 to 300 times	It can distinguish clear and turbid, clear heat and induce urination, mainly used for watery diarrhea (The stool is like water), enuresis, red and difficult urination, anuresis and erosion of mucous membrane in the oral cavity

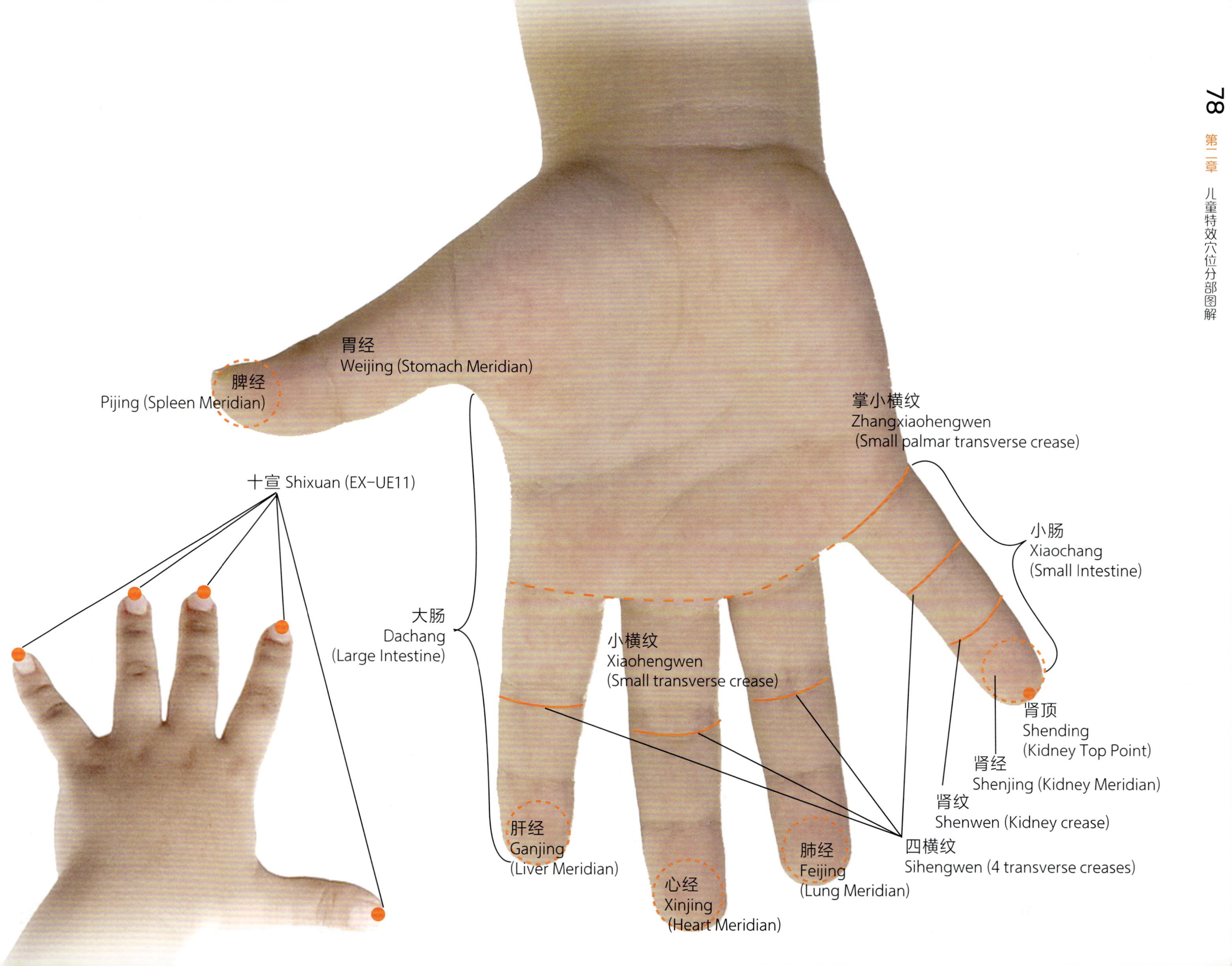
胃经
Weijing (Stomach Meridian)
脾经
Pijing (Spleen Meridian)
掌小横纹
Zhangxiaohengwen
(Small palmar transverse crease)
十宣 Shixuan (EX-UE11)
小肠
Xiaochang
(Small Intestine)
大肠
Dachang
(Large Intestine)
小横纹
Xiaohengwen
(Small transverse crease)
肾顶
Shending
(Kidney Top Point)
肾经
Shenjing (Kidney Meridian)
肾纹
Shenwen (Kidney crease)
肝经
Ganjing
(Liver Meridian)
肺经
Feijing
(Lung Meridian)
四横纹
Sihengwen (4 transverse creases)
心经
Xinjing
(Heart Meridian)

续表

穴位	定位	按摩方法	功效主治
四横纹	手掌面，食指、中指、无名指、小指的第1指间关节横纹处	掐法或推法：用拇指指甲依次掐揉3~5次，或四指并拢从食指横纹处向小指横纹处推100~300次	调和气血，消肿散结，退热除烦。主治腹胀痛、消化不良、抽搐、癫痫、疳积（营养不良）
小横纹	手掌面，食指、中指、无名指、小指掌指关节横纹处	掐法或推法：用拇指指甲依次掐3~5次，或以拇指指侧推100~300次	清热除烦，消肿散结。主治口疮、唇裂、烦躁、腹胀
掌小横纹	手掌面，小指根下，尺侧掌纹头	揉法：用拇指或中指指端按揉100~500次	清热化痰，开胸散结。主治口舌生疮、痰热喘咳、百日咳、肺炎、流涎
十宣	手背十指尖端，距指甲游离缘0.1寸，左右各5穴，共10穴	掐法：用拇指指甲掐之，每穴各掐5次	清热，醒神，开窍。主治昏迷、中暑、高热、抽搐、癫痫

Continued

Acupoints	Location	Massage Manipulations	Efficacy and Indications
Sihengwen (4 transverse creases)	In the palm surface, the transverse striation of the 1st interphalangeal joint of index, middle, ring and little fingers	Pinching or pushing manipulation: Pinch-knead the points with fingernail of the thumb for 3 to 5 times successively, or push the points from the transverse striation of index finger to the little finger with 4 fingers closing together for 100 to 300 times	It can harmonize Qi and blood, reduce swelling and dissipate mass, bring down a fever and relieve dysphoria, mainly used for abdominal distension and pain, dyspepsia, convulsion, epilepsy and infantile malnutrition with accumulation
Xiaohengwen (Small transverse crease)	In the palm surface, the transverse striation of the metacarpophalangeal joint of index, middle, ring and little fingers	Pinching or pushing manipulation: Pinch the points with fingernail of the thumb for 3 to 5 times successively, or push the points with the side of the thumb for 100 to 300 times	It can clear heat and relieve dysphoria, reduce swelling and dissipate mass, mainly used for aphtha, cleft lip, vexation and abdominal distension
Zhangxiaohengwen (Small palmar transverse crease)	On the palm surface, below the root of little finger, in the ulnar side of the palmprint	Kneading manipulation: Press-knead the point with the fingertip of the thumb or middle finger for 100 to 500 times	It can clear heat and resolve phlegm, smooth the chest and dissipate mass, mainly used for sore in the mouth, phlegm-heat, asthma and cough, whooping cough, pneumonia and drooling
Shixuan (EX-HN 11)	The tips of 10 fingers on the dorsum of hand, 0.1 cun lateral to the free margin of nails. There are 5 points in each hand for total 10 points	Pinching manipulation: Pinch the points with fingernail of the thumb for 5 times in every point	It can clear heat, induce resuscitation and open orifice, mainly used for unconsciousness, heat stroke, hyperpyrexia, convulsion and epilepsy

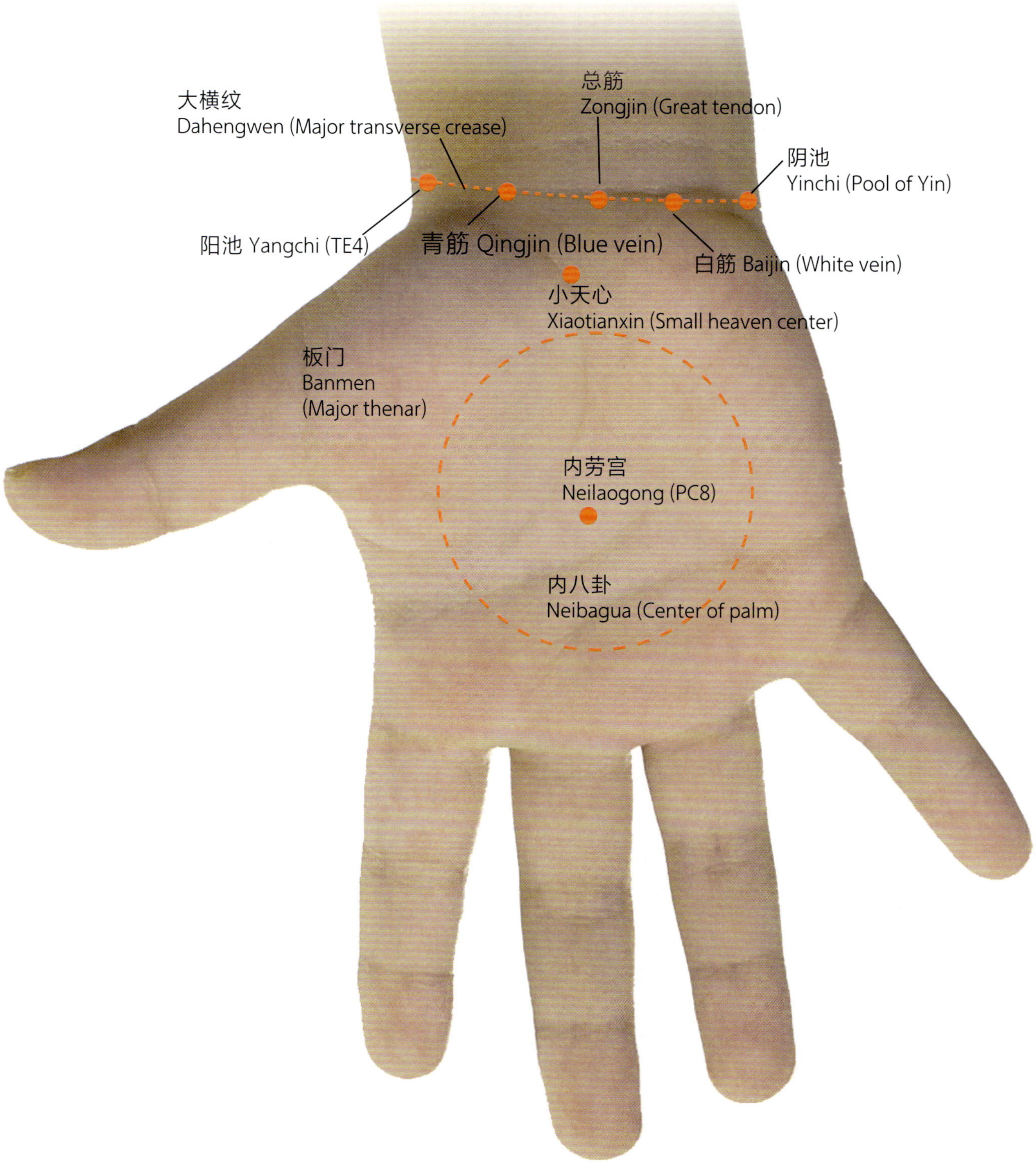
大横纹
Dahengwen (Major transverse crease)
总筋
Zongjin (Great tendon)
阴池
Yinchi (Pool of Yin)
阳池 Yangchi (TE4)
青筋 Qingjin (Blue vein)
白筋 Baijin (White vein)
小天心
Xiaotianxin (Small heaven center)
板门
Banmen
(Major thenar)
内劳宫
Neilaogong (PC8)
内八卦
Neibagua (Center of palm)

穴位	定位	按摩方法	功效主治
大横纹	仰掌，掌后横纹。近拇指端称阳池，近小指端称阴池	分推或合推：用双手拇指自掌后横纹中点（总筋）向两侧分推，称分阴阳；自两旁向总筋处合推，称合阴阳。各推 30~50 次	平衡阴阳，调和气血，祛痰散结，行滞消食。主治腹泻、腹胀、痢疾、寒热往来（发热与恶寒交替出现）、呕吐、食积、烦躁不安、痰结咳嗽
总筋	掌后腕横纹中点	揉法或掐法：用拇指或中指按揉 100~300 次，或用拇指指甲掐 3~5 次	通调气机，清热止痉。主治癫痫、抽搐、夜啼、口舌生疮
青筋	总筋与阳池连线之中点	掐法或揉法：用拇指指甲掐 3~5 次，或用拇指指端揉 30~50 次	清心明目。主治目赤、视物模糊
白筋	总筋与阴池连线之中点	掐法或揉法：用拇指指甲掐 3~5 次，或用拇指指端揉 30~50 次	顺气化痰，开胸利膈。主治胸闷、痰喘

Acupoints	Location	Massage Manipulations	Efficacy and Indications
Dahengwen (Major transverse crease)	At the transverse crease of wrist with the palm upward, the point near the side of the thumb is Yangchi (TE4), while the point near the side of the little finger is Yinchi (Pool of Yin).	Parting-pushing or meeting-pushing manipulation: Push from the midpoint of the transverse crease of wrist ［Zongjin (Great tendon)］ to both sides with the 2 thumbs, named Yin and Yang Seperation, while the meet-pushing manipulation from both sides to Zongjin (Great tendon) is called Meet Yin and Yang. The 2 manipulations are repeated for respective 30 to 50 times	It can balance Yin and Yang, harmonize Qi and blood, dispel phlegm and dissipate mass, move stagnation and promote digestion, mainly used for diarrhea, abdominal distension, dysentery, alternating chills and fever (Fever and chills occur alternatively), vomiting, food stagnation, vexation and restlessness and phlegmatic cough
Zongjin (Great tendon)	The midpoint of the transverse crease of wrist	Kneading or pinching manipulation: Press-knead Zongjin (Great tendon) with the thumb or middle finger for 100 to 300 times, or pinch Zongjin (Great tendon) with the fingernail of the thumb for 3 to 5 times	It can regulate Qi movement, clear heat and stop convulsion, mainly used for epilepsy, convulsion, night crying and sore in the mouth
Qingjin (Blue vein)	The midpoint of the line between Zongjin (Great tendon) and Yangchi (TE4)	Pinching or kneading manipulation: Pinch Qingjin with the fingernail of the thumb for 3 to 5 times, or knead Qingjin (Blue vein) with the fingertip of the thumb for 30 to 50 times	It can clear heart and improve vision, mainly used for red eye and blurred vision
Baijin (White vein)	The midpoint of the line between Zongjin (Great tendon) and Yinchi (Pool of Yin)	Pinching or kneading manipulation: Pinch Qingjin (Blue vein) with the fingernail of the thumb for 3 to 5 times, or knead Qingjin (Blue vein) with the fingertip of the thumb for 30 to 50 times.	It can guide Qi downward, resolve phlegm, sooth the chest and disinhibit diaphragm, mainly used for chest stuffiness and phlegmatic dyspnea

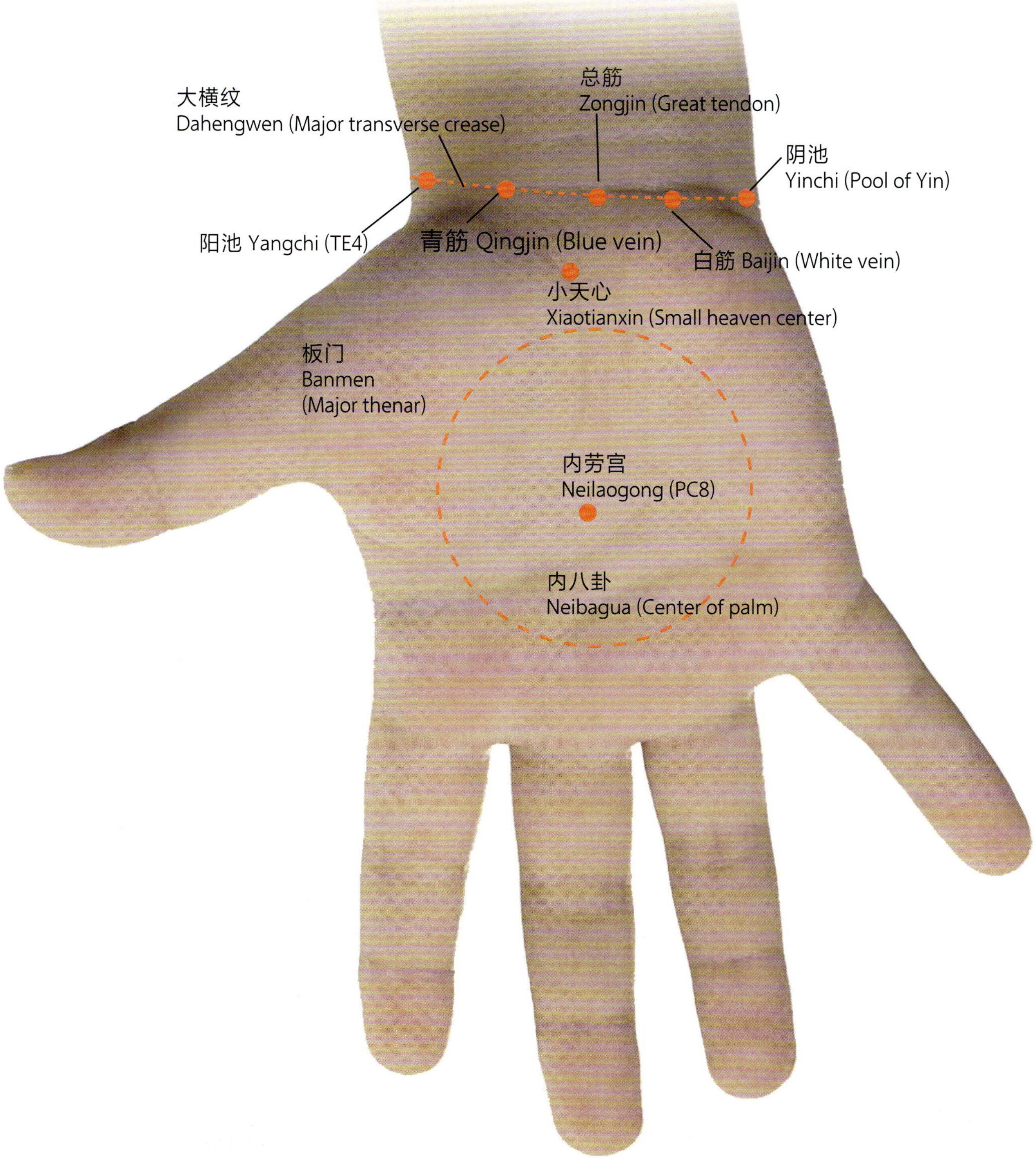
大横纹
Dahengwen (Major transverse crease)
总筋
Zongjin (Great tendon)
阴池
Yinchi (Pool of Yin)
阳池 Yangchi (TE4)
青筋 Qingjin (Blue vein)
白筋 Baijin (White vein)
小天心
Xiaotianxin (Small heaven center)
板门
Banmen
(Major thenar)
内劳宫
Neilaogong (PC8)
内八卦
Neibagua (Center of palm)

续表

穴位	定位	按摩方法	功效主治
小天心	手掌面大小鱼际交接处凹陷中	揉法、掐法或捣法：用中指指端揉 100~300 次，或用拇指指甲掐 5~20 次，或用中指指尖或屈曲的指间关节捣 5~20 次	清热，镇惊，利尿，明目。主治烦躁不安、夜啼、癫痫、抽搐、目赤痛、小便赤涩
板门	手掌大鱼际平面	揉法或推法：用拇指、食指指端或指腹揉，或自拇指指根推向腕横纹（可止泻），亦可由腕横纹推向拇指指根（可止呕），各推 100~300 次	健脾和胃，消食化滞，止呕吐，除腹胀。主治食欲不振、食积、腹胀、呕吐、腹泻、嗳气（打嗝）
内劳宫	手掌心中，握拳时中指与无名指之间处	揉法或运法：用中指指端揉 100~300 次，或用中指指端自小指指根经掌小横纹、小天心运至内劳宫，10~30 次	发汗，清心火，补气除烦。主治发热、口疮、齿龈糜烂、虚烦内热

Continued

Acupoints	Location	Massage Manipulations	Efficacy and Indications
Xiaotianxin (Small heaven center)	In the depression of the joint of the greater thenar and hypothenar in the surface of palm	Kneading, pinching or pounding manipulation: Knead Xiaotianxin (Small heaven center) with the tip of middle finger for 100 to 300 times, or pinch Xiaotianxin (Small heaven center) with the fingernail of the thumb for 5 to 20 times, or pound Xiaotianxin (Small heaven center) with the tip of middle finger or the bending interphalangeal joint for 5 to 20 times	It can clear heat, calm fright, induce urination and improve vision, mainly used for vexation and restlessness, night crying, epilepsy, convulsion, red and painful eye, and red and difficult urination
Banmen (Major thenar)	The plane of the great thenar of the palm	Kneading or pushing manipulation: Knead Banmen (Major thenar) with the tips or finger pulps of the thumb and index finger, or push from the root of the thumb to the transverse crease of wrist (which can relieve diarrhea), or push from transverse crease of wrist to the root of the thumb (which can arrest vomiting). The manipulations are repeated for respective 100 to 300 times	It can invigorate spleen and harmonize stomach, promote digestion and resolve food stagnation, stop vomiting and remove abdominal distension, mainly used for poor appetite, food stagnation, abdominal distension, vomiting, diarrhea and hiccup
Neilaogong (PC8)	In the middle of the palm, between the middle and ring fingers when clench fist	Kneading or transporting manipulation: Knead the point with the tip of middle finger for 100 to 300 times, or transport from the root of little finger to Neilaogong (PC8) through Zhangxiaohengwen (Small palmar transverse crease) and Xiaotianxin (Small heaven center) with the tip of middle finger for 10 to 30 times	It can induce sweating, clear heart fire, tonify Qi and relieve dysphoria, mainly used for fever, aphtha, gingival erosion, deficient dysphoria and internal thermal

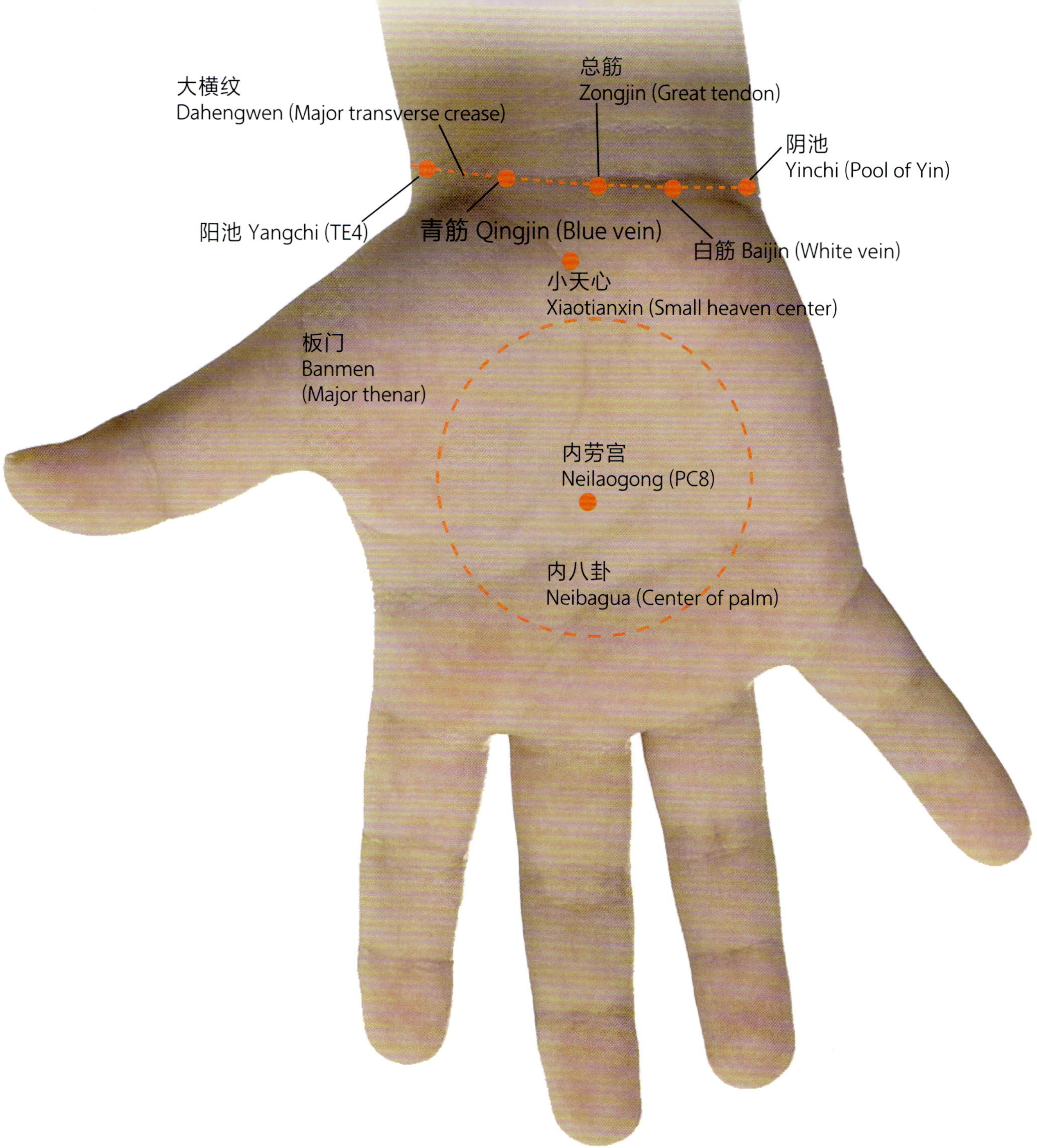
大横纹
Dahengwen (Major transverse crease)
总筋
Zongjin (Great tendon)
阴池
Yinchi (Pool of Yin)
阳池 Yangchi (TE4)
青筋 Qingjin (Blue vein)
白筋 Baijin (White vein)
小天心
Xiaotianxin (Small heaven center)
板门
Banmen
(Major thenar)
内劳宫
Neilaogong (PC8)
内八卦
Neibagua (Center of palm)

续表

穴 位	定 位	按摩方法	功效主治
内八卦	手掌面，以手心为圆心，以圆心至中指根横纹约 2/3 处为半径作圆周	运法：用拇指或食指、中指作顺时针方向掐运 100~300 次	宽胸利膈，理气化痰，行滞消食。主治气喘、胸闷、心烦、咳嗽、呕吐、腹胀、腹泻

Continued

Acupoints	Location	Massage Manipulations	Efficacy and Indications
Neibagua (Center of palm)	In the surface of the palm, the circle with the center of the palm as the center of the circle, and the 2/3 of the length of the line between the center of the circle and the transverse crease of the root of middle finger as the radius	Circularly pushing manipulation: Pinch-transport Neibagua (Center of palm) with the thumb, or index and middle fingers clockwise for 100 to 300 times	It can smooth the chest and disinhibit diaphragm, regulate Qi and resolve phlegm, move stagnation and promote digestion, mainly used for dyspnea, chest stuffiness, dysphoria, cough, vomiting, abdominal distension and diarrhea

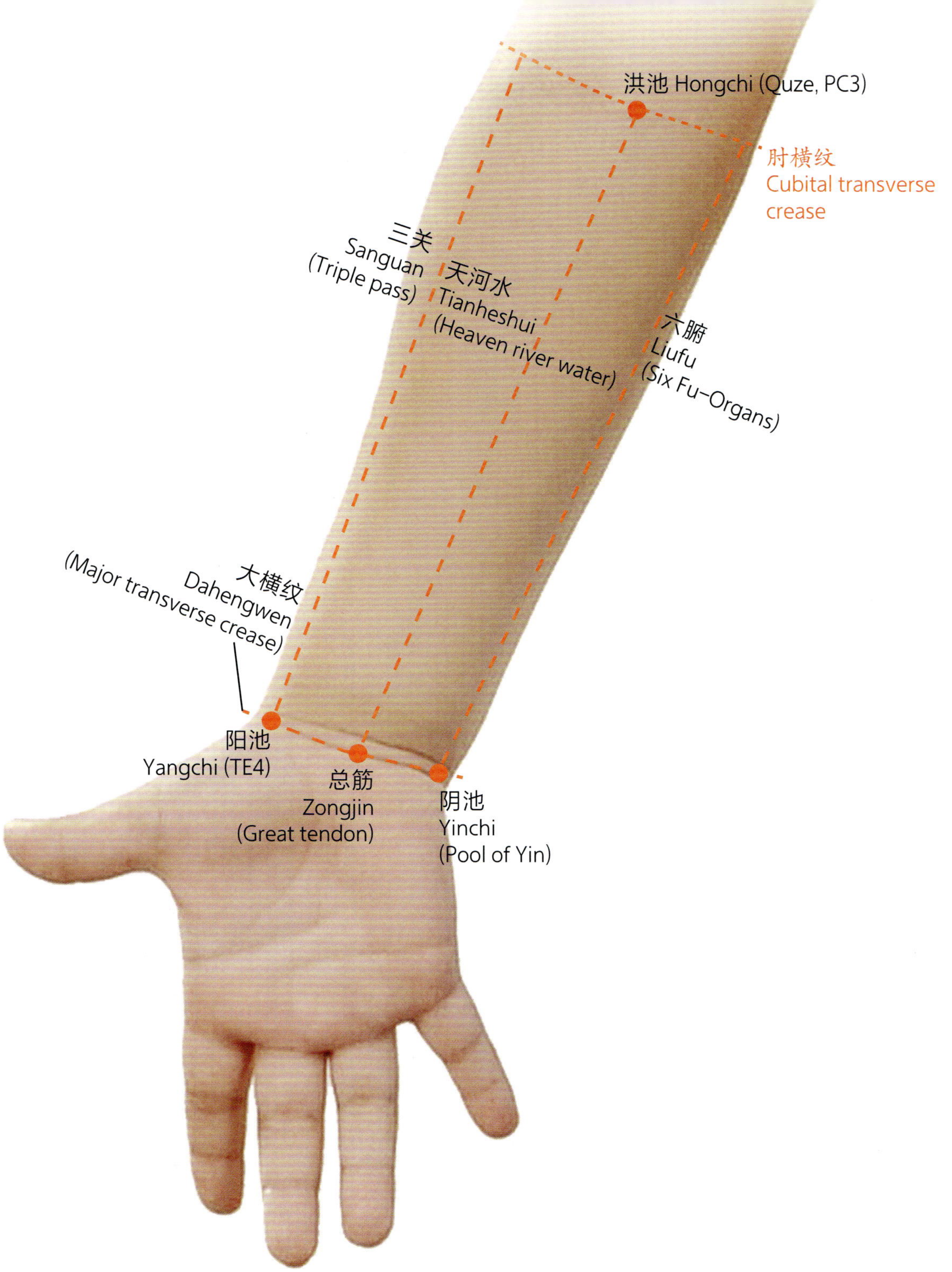
洪池 Hongchi (Quze, PC3)
肘横纹
Cubital transverse
crease
三关
Sanguan
(Triple pass)
天河水
Tianheshui
(Heaven river water)
六腑
Liufu
(Six Fu-Organs)
大横纹
Dahengwen
(Major transverse crease)
阳池
Yangchi (TE4)
总筋
Zongjin
(Great tendon)
阴池
Yinchi
(Pool of Yin)

穴 位	定 位	按摩方法	功效主治
洪 池	肘横纹中，肱二头肌腱（肘部可摸到的一条大筋）的内（尺）侧	揉法、拿法或掐法：以拇指按揉 30~50 次，或用拇指和其他四指相对用力拿 3~5 次，或用拇指指甲掐 3~5 次	清心火，定惊镇静。主治肘臂痛、惊风（抽搐神昏）
天 河 水	前臂掌侧正中，自腕横纹中点至肘横纹中点（即总筋至洪池）成一直线	直推法：用食指、中指两指指腹面自腕横纹推至肘横纹，称清天河水；或用食指、中指沾水自总筋处，一起一落弹打，如弹琴状，直至洪池，同时一面用口吹气随之，称打马过天河。各 100~300 次	清热解表，泻心火，除烦躁，化燥痰。主治外感发热、高热、烦躁不安、口渴、抽搐、癫痫

Acupoints	Location	Massage Manipulations	Efficacy and Indications
Hongchi (Quze, PC3)	In the cubital transverse crease, the inner(ulnar) side of the biceps (the big tendon which can be touched in the elbow)	Kneading, grasping or pinching manipulation: Press-knead the point with the thumb for 30 to 50 times, or exert strength relatively with the thumb and another four fingers to grasp the point for 3 to 5 times, or pinch the point with the fingernail of the thumb for 3 to 5 times	It can clear heart fire, calm fright and tranquilize mind, mainly used for pain of elbow and arms and infantile convulsion (convulsion and unconsciousness)
Tianheshui (Heaven river water)	In the middle of the palm-side of the forearm, the line between the midpoint of the transverse crease of wrist and the midpoint of the cubital transverse crease [(the line between Zongjin (Great tendon) and Hongchi (Quze, PC3)].	Direct-pushing manipulation: Push from the transverse crease of wrist to cubital transverse crease with the finger pulps of index and middle fingers, named Clear Tianheshui (Heaven river water); or flick-strike from Zongjin (Great tendon) to Hongchi (Quze, PC3) with the index and middle fingers dipping water like playing piano and blow gas with mouth at the same time, named Dama Guo tianhe. The manipulations are repeated for respective 100 to 300 times	It can clear heat and release exterior, purge heart fire, relieve vexation and resolve dry-phlegm, mainly used for external-contraction fever, hyperpyrexia, vexation and restlessness, thirst, convulsion and epilepsy

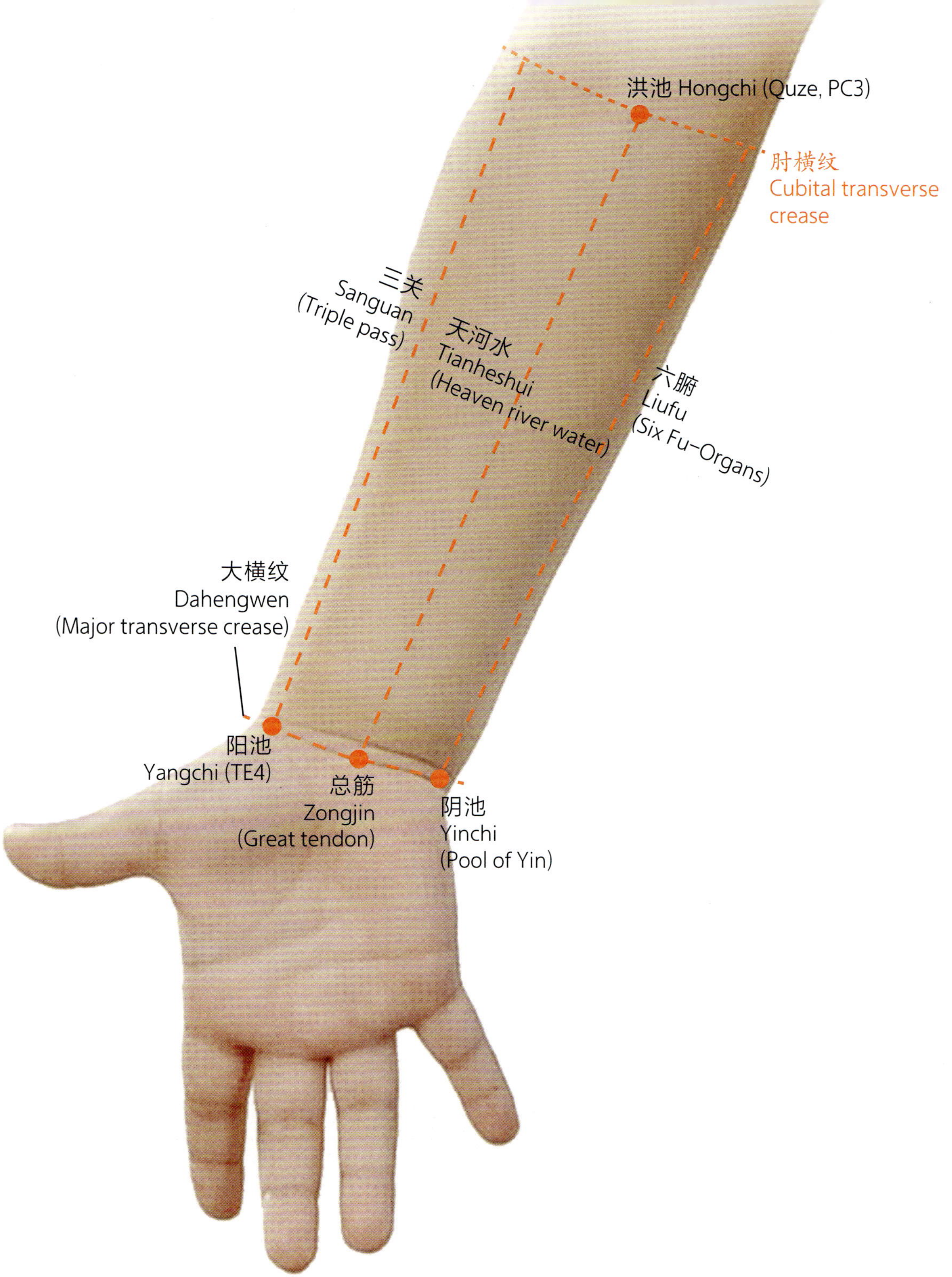
洪池 Hongchi (Quze, PC3)
肘横纹
Cubital transverse crease
三关
Sanguan
(Triple pass)
天河水
Tianheshui
(Heaven river water)
六腑
Liufu
(Six Fu-Organs)
大横纹
Dahengwen
(Major transverse crease)
阳池
Yangchi (TE4)
总筋
Zongjin
(Great tendon)
阴池
Yinchi
(Pool of Yin)

续表

穴 位	定 位	按摩方法	功效主治
六 腑	前臂尺侧，从肘横纹至腕横纹成一直线	直推法：用拇指指面或食指、中指螺纹面自肘向腕直推 100~300 次，称退六腑，为大凉之法。注意：若儿童平素大便溏薄（稀软），脾虚腹泻则慎用本法	清热，解毒，凉血。主治高热、烦渴、抽搐、癫痫、鹅口疮、咽喉肿痛、热痢、大便干燥
三 关	前臂桡侧，腕横纹至肘横纹成一直线	直推法：食指、中指两指并拢，用指腹面自腕横纹或拇指桡侧直推至肘横纹 100~300 次。此为大热之法	温阳散寒，益气活血，培补元气，发汗解表。主治气血虚弱、阳虚肢冷、腹痛、泄泻（腹泻）、风寒感冒、疹出不透

Continued

Acupoints	Location	Massage Manipulations	Efficacy and Indications
Liufu (Six Fu-Organs)	In the ulnar side of the forearm, the line between the cubital transverse crease and the transverse crease of wrist	Direct-pushing manipulation: Push directly from elbow to wrist with the facies digitales of the thumb or index and middle fingers for 100 to 300 times, named Reducing Liufu (Six Fu Organs), a great cooling method. Note: If the child usually has loose stool, the manipulation shall be used with caution for the diarrhea due to spleen deficiency	It can clear heat, remove toxin and cool blood, mainly used for hyperpyrexia, vexation, convulsion, epilepsy, thrush, swollen sore throat, heat dysentery and dry stool
Sanguan (Triple pass)	In the radial side of the forearm, the line between the transverse crease of wrist and the cubital transverse crease	Direct-pushing manipulation: Push directly from the transverse crease of wrist or the radial side of the thumb to cubital transverse crease with the finger pulps of the closing index and middle fingers for 100 to 300 times. It is the great heating method.	It can warm Yang and dissipate cold, replenish Qi and activate blood, bank up and tonify original Qi and induce sweating to release exterior, mainly used for deficient Qi and blood, cold limb due to Yang deficiency, abdominal pain, diarrhea, cold due to wind-cold and incomplete appearance of rashes

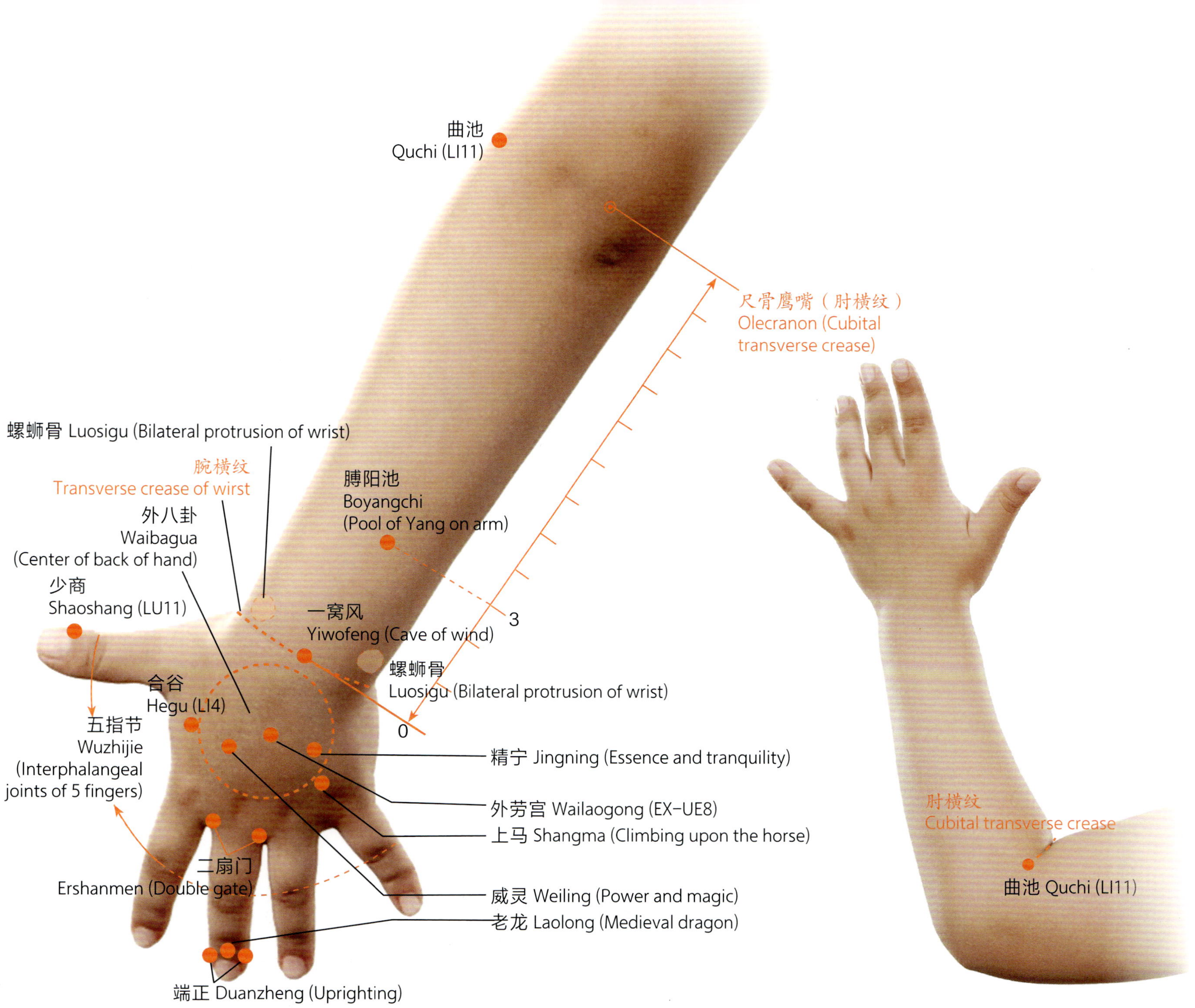
曲池
Quchi (LI11)
尺骨鹰嘴（肘横纹）
Olecranon (Cubital transverse crease)
螺蛳骨 Luosigu (Bilateral protrusion of wrist)
腕横纹
Transverse crease of wirst
膊阳池
Boyangchi
(Pool of Yang on arm)
外八卦
Waibagua
(Center of back of hand)
少商
Shaoshang (LU11)
一窝风
Yiwofeng (Cave of wind)
3
螺蛳骨
Luosigu (Bilateral protrusion of wrist)
合谷
Hegu (LI4)
0
五指节
Wuzhijie
(Interphalangeal joints of 5 fingers)
精宁 Jingning (Essence and tranquility)
外劳宫 Wailaogong (EX-UE8)
上马 Shangma (Climbing upon the horse)
二扇门
Ershanmen (Double gate)
威灵 Weiling (Power and magic)
老龙 Laolong (Medieval dragon)
端正 Duanzheng (Uprighting)
肘横纹
Cubital transverse crease
曲池 Quchi (LI11)

穴 位	定 位	按摩方法	功效主治
曲 池	肘横纹外侧端凹陷中	揉法：用拇指或中指指端按揉 100~200 次	发汗解表，开窍通络。主治发热、咽喉肿痛、齿痛、瘾疹、吐泻
膊 阳 池	手背，一窝风后 3 寸处	掐法或揉法：用拇指指甲掐或指端揉，各 50~100 次	通大便，利小便，止头痛。主治大便秘结、小便赤涩、感冒头痛
螺 蛳 骨	腕部两侧骨突起处，即尺、桡骨茎突处	捏法：用食指、拇指提捏该处皮肤 10~20 次	健脾镇惊，退热。主治消化不良、惊悸、腱鞘炎
少 商	在手拇指末节桡侧，距指甲角 0.1 寸	掐法：以拇指指甲掐 5~10 次	清热散风，利咽止痛，开窍醒神。主治咽喉肿痛、发热、鼻出血、昏迷

Acupoints	Location	Massage Manipulations	Efficacy and Indications
Quchi (LI11)	In the depression of the lateral side of the cubital transverse crease	Kneading manipulation: Press-knead the point with the fingertip of the thumb or middle finger for 100 to 200 times	It can induce sweating to release exterior, open orifice and sooth collaterals, mainly used for fever, swollen sore throat, toothache, urticaria, vomiting and diarrhea
Boyangchi (Pool of Yang on arm)	On the dorsum of hand, 3 cun behind Yiwofeng (Cave of wind)	Pinching or kneading manipulation: Pinch the point with the nail of the thumb or knead the point with fingertip of the thumb for respective 50 to 100 times	It can relieve constipation, promote urination and relieve headache, mainly used for constipation, red and difficult urination, cold and headache
Luosigu (Bilateral protrusion of wrist)	At the prominence of the bones in both sides of wrist, namely at the styloid process of radius and ulna	Pinching manipulation: Pinch the local skin with the thumb and index finger for 10 to 20 times	It can invigorate spleen, calm fright and reduce fever, mainly used for dyspepsia, palpitation due to fright and tenosynovitis
Shaoshang (LU11)	In the radial side of the thumb tip, 0.1 cun lateral and posterior to the corner of the fingernail	Pinching manipulation: Pinch the point with the nail of the thumb for 5 to 10 times	It can clear heat and disperse wind, relieve sore throat, open orifice and induce resuscitation, mainly used for sore throat, fever, nasal bleeding and coma

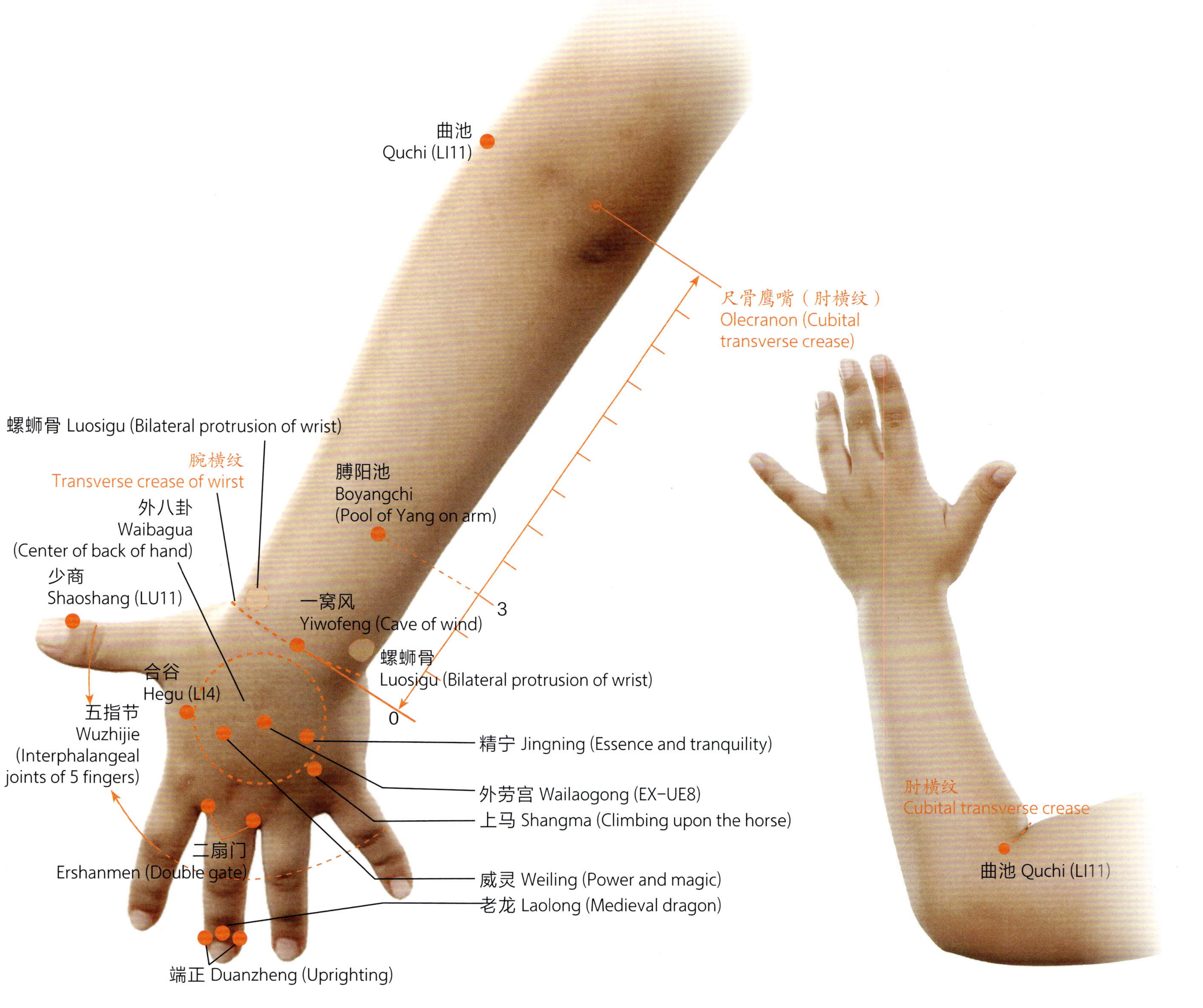
曲池
Quchi (LI11)
尺骨鹰嘴（肘横纹）
Olecranon (Cubital transverse crease)
螺蛳骨 Luosigu (Bilateral protrusion of wrist)
腕横纹
Transverse crease of wirst
腫阳池
Boyangchi
(Pool of Yang on arm)
外八卦
Waibagua
(Center of back of hand)
少商
Shaoshang (LU11)
一窝风
Yiwofeng (Cave of wind)
3
螺蛳骨
Luosigu (Bilateral protrusion of wrist)
合谷
Hegu (LI4)
0
五指节
Wuzhijie
(Interphalangeal joints of 5 fingers)
精宁 Jingning (Essence and tranquility)
外劳宫 Wailaogong (EX-UE8)
上马 Shangma (Climbing upon the horse)
二扇门
Ershanmen (Double gate)
威灵 Weiling (Power and magic)
老龙 Laolong (Medieval dragon)
端正 Duanzheng (Uprighting)
肘横纹
Cubital transverse crease
曲池 Quchi (LI11)

续表

穴 位	定 位	按摩方法	功效主治
一窝风	手背腕横纹正中凹陷处	揉法：用拇指或中指指端揉 100~300 次	通经络，温中行气，止痹痛，利关节。主治关节痹痛、腹痛肠鸣、伤风感冒
合谷	在手背第 1、2 掌骨间，当第 2 掌骨桡侧的中点处	掐法和揉法：用拇指指甲掐 5 次，继而用拇指指腹揉 50~100 次	开闭，泻热，镇惊止痛。主治头痛、齿痛、鼻出血、感冒、腹痛、便秘
威灵	手背外劳宫穴旁，第 2、3 掌骨间	掐法：用拇指指甲掐 3~5 次	醒神，开窍，镇惊。主治抽搐、癫痫、头痛、昏迷不醒
精宁	手背外劳宫旁，第 4、5 掌骨间	掐法：用拇指指甲掐 5~10 次。注意：体虚者慎用本法	行气，破结，化痰。主治疳积（营养不良）、痰喘、干呕

Continued

Acupoints	Location	Massage Manipulations	Efficacy and Indications
Yiwofeng (Cave of wind)	In the depression of the middle of transverse crease of wrist on the dorsum of hand	Kneading manipulation: Knead the point with the fingertip of the thumb or middle finger for 100 to 300 times	It can sooth meridians and collaterals, warm the middle and move Qi, relieve pain and promote articular motion, mainly used for arthralgia, abdominal pain, borborygmus and cold
Hegu (LI4)	Between the 1st and 2nd metacarpal bones on the dorsum of hand, at the midpoint of the radial side of the 2nd metacarpal bone	Pinching and kneading manipulation: Pinch the point with the nail of the thumb for 5 times, then knead the point with the finger pulp of the thumb for 50 to 100 times	It can open orifices, purge heat, calm fright and relieve pain, mainly used for headache, toothache, nasal bleeding, cold, abdominal pain and constipation
Weiling (Power and magic)	Lateral to Wailaogong (EX-UE8) on the dorsum of hand, between the 2nd and the 3rd metacarpal bones.	Pinching manipulation: Pinch the point with the nail of the thumb for 3 to 5 times	It can induce resuscitation, open orifice and calm fright, mainly used for convulsion, epilepsy, headache and unconsciousness
Jingning (Essence and tranquility)	Lateral to Wailaogong (EX-UE8) on the dorsum of hand, between the 4th and 5th metacarpal bones	Pinching manipulation: Pinch the point with the nail of the thumb for 5 to 10 times. Note: Those with physical weakness shall apply the manipulation with caution	It can move Qi, remove stagnation and phlegm, mainly used for infantile malnutrition with accumulation, phlegmatic dyspnea and retching

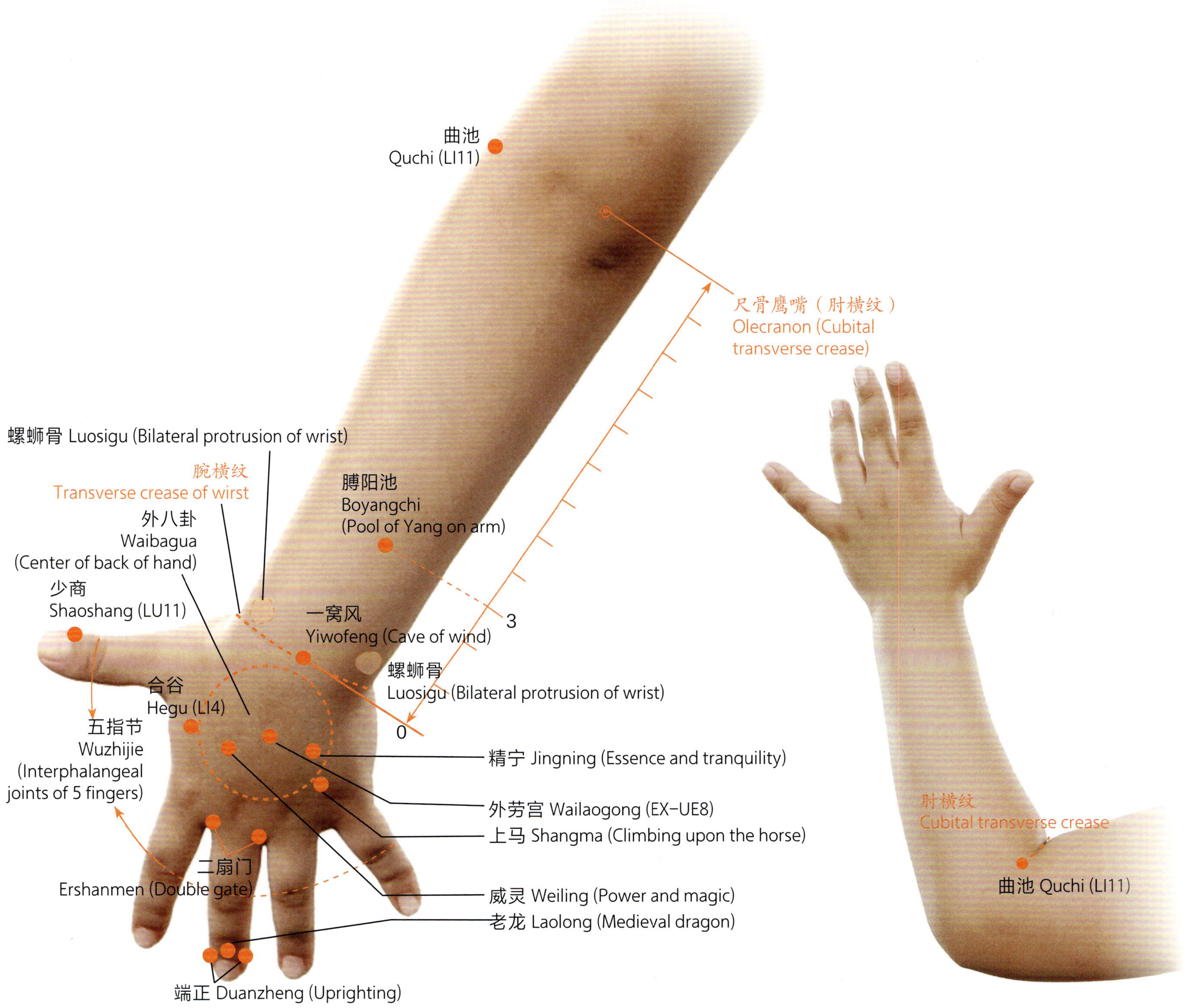
曲池
Quchi (LI11)
尺骨鹰嘴（肘横纹）
Olecranon (Cubital transverse crease)
螺蛳骨 Luosigu (Bilateral protrusion of wrist)
腕横纹
Transverse crease of wirst
膊阳池
Boyangchi
(Pool of Yang on arm)
外八卦
Waibagua
(Center of back of hand)
少商
Shaoshang (LU11)
一窝风
Yiwofeng (Cave of wind)
3
螺蛳骨
Luosigu (Bilateral protrusion of wrist)
合谷
Hegu (LI4)
0
五指节
Wuzhijie
(Interphalangeal joints of 5 fingers)
精宁 Jingning (Essence and tranquility)
外劳宫 Wailaogong (EX-UE8)
上马 Shangma (Climbing upon the horse)
二扇门
Ershanmen (Double gate)
威灵 Weiling (Power and magic)
老龙 Laolong (Medieval dragon)
端正 Duanzheng (Uprighting)
肘横纹
Cubital transverse crease
曲池 Quchi (LI11)

续表

穴位	定位	按摩方法	功效主治
外劳宫	手掌中，与内劳宫相对	揉法或掐法：用食指、中指指端揉 100~300 次，或用指尖掐 3~5 次	发汗解表，温阳散寒，升阳举陷。主治风寒感冒、腹痛腹胀、肠鸣腹泻、痢疾、脱肛、遗尿（尿床）、疝气
上马	手背无名指、小指掌指关节间的后陷中	揉法或掐法：用拇指指端揉 100~500 次，或用拇指指端掐 3~5 次	滋阴补肾，顺气散结，利水通淋。主治小便赤涩、消化不良、腹痛、体虚、喘咳、脱肛、遗尿（尿床）
二扇门	手掌背中指根本节（中指掌指关节前方）两侧凹陷处	掐法或揉法：用拇指指甲掐 3~5 次，或用拇指侧面按揉 100~500 次	发汗解表，退热平喘。主治癫痫、抽搐、身热无汗、感冒

Continued

Acupoints	Location	Massage Manipulations	Efficacy and Indications
Wailaogong (EX-UE8)	In the palm, the opposite of Neilaogong (PC8)	Kneading or pinching manipulation: Knead the point with tips of index and middle fingers for 100 to 300 times, or pinch the point with fingertips for 3 to 5 times	It can induce sweating to release exterior, warm Yang and dissipate cold, elevate Yang and raise the drooping, mainly used for cold due to wind-cold, abdominal pain and distension, borborygmus, diarrhea, dysentery, prolapse of rectum, enuresis and hernia
Shangma (Climbing upon the horse)	In the posterior depression between metacarpophalangeal joints of ring and little fingers on the dorsum of hand	Kneading or pinching manipulation: Knead the point with the fingertip of the thumb for 100 to 500 times, or pinch the point with the fingertip of the thumb for 3 to 5 times	It can nourish Yin and tonify kidney, guide Qi downward and dissipate mass, promote urination and relieve stranguria, mainly used for red and difficult urination, dyspepsia, abdominal pain, physical weakness, phlegmatic dyspnea, prolapse of rectum and enuresis
Ershanmen (Double gate)	In the depression of both sides of the root of middle finge (near the metacarpophalangeal joint of the middle finger) on the dorsum of hand	Pinching or kneading manipulation: Pinch the point with the nail of the thumb for 3 to 5 times, or press-knead the point with the lateral thumb for 100 to 500 times.	It can induce sweating to release exterior, reduce fever and relieve asthma, mainly used for epilepsy, convulsion, fever without sweating and cold

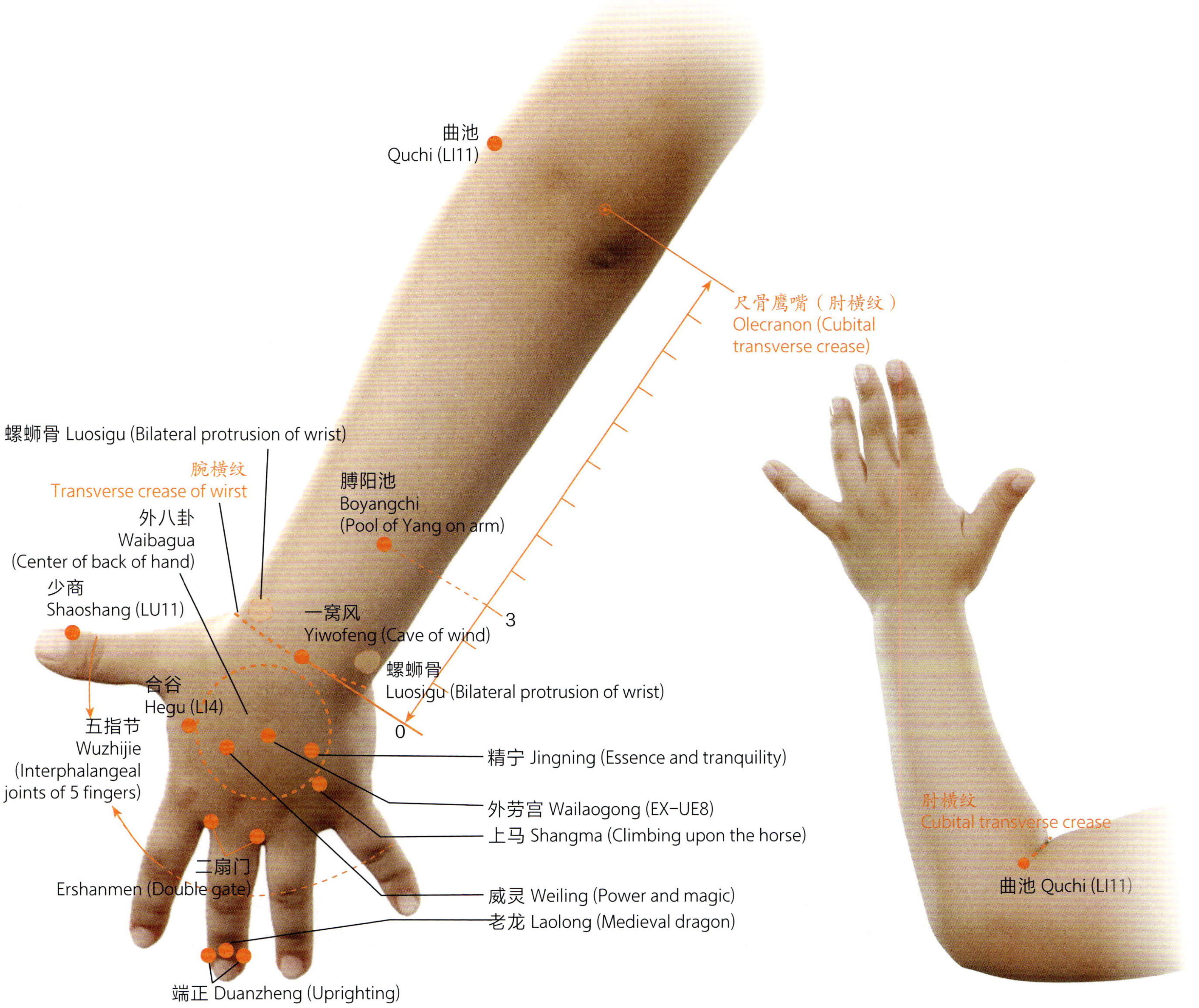
曲池
Quchi (LI11)
尺骨鹰嘴（肘横纹）
Olecranon (Cubital transverse crease)
螺蛳骨 Luosigu (Bilateral protrusion of wrist)
腕横纹
Transverse crease of wirst
膊阳池
Boyangchi
(Pool of Yang on arm)
外八卦
Waibagua
(Center of back of hand)
少商
Shaoshang (LU11)
一窝风
Yiwofeng (Cave of wind)
3
螺蛳骨
Luosigu (Bilateral protrusion of wrist)
合谷
Hegu (LI4)
0
五指节
Wuzhijie
(Interphalangeal joints of 5 fingers)
精宁 Jingning (Essence and tranquility)
外劳宫 Wailaogong (EX-UE8)
上马 Shangma (Climbing upon the horse)
二扇门
Ershanmen (Double gate)
威灵 Weiling (Power and magic)
老龙 Laolong (Medieval dragon)
端正 Duanzheng (Uprighting)
肘横纹
Cubital transverse crease
曲池 Quchi (LI11)

续表

穴 位	定 位	按摩方法	功效主治
五指节	掌背 5 指第 1 指间关节	掐法或揉法：用拇指指甲依次掐 3~5 次，或用拇指指端揉搓 30~50 次	安神镇惊，祛风痰，开关窍。主治抽搐、癫痫、惊恐不安、吐涎、咳嗽
老龙	中指指甲后一分处	掐法和揉法：先用拇指指甲掐 3~5 次，继而揉之	退热，开窍醒神。主治抽搐、癫痫、高热、昏迷不醒
端正	中指甲根两侧赤白肉际处。桡侧称左端正，尺侧称右端正	掐法和揉法：用拇指指甲掐 5 次，或用拇指螺纹面揉 50 次	左端正升阳止泻；右端正降逆止呕，止血。主治呕吐、泄泻（腹泻）、痢疾、鼻出血、抽搐、癫痫

Continued

Acupoints	Location	Massage Manipulations	Efficacy and Indications
Wuzhijie (Interphalangeal joints of 5 fingers)	The 1st interphalangeal joint of the 5 fingers on the dorsum of hand	Pinching or kneading manipulation: Pinch the points successively with the nail of the thumb for 3 to 5 times, or knead-twist the points with the fingertip of the thumb for 30 to 50 times	It can tranquilize mind and calm fright, dispel wind-phlegm and open orifices, mainly used for convulsion, epilepsy, panic, drooling and cough
Laolong (Medieval dragon)	1 fen posterior to the nail of middle finger	Pinching and kneading manipulation: Pinch the point firstly with the nail of the thumb for 3 to 5 times, and then knead the point	It can reduce fever, open orifice and induce resuscitation, mainly used for convulsion, epilepsy, hyperpyrexia and unconsciousness
Duanzheng (Uprighting)	At the dorso-ventral boundary of both sides of the root of middle finger. The one in the radial side is called Left Duanzheng (Uprighting), while the one in the ulnar side is Right Duanzheng (Uprighting)	Pinching and kneading manipulation: Pinch the point with the nail of the thumb for 5 times, or knead the point with the thumb for 50 times	The Left Duanzheng (Uprighting) can elevate Yang to relieve diarrhea, while the Right Duanzheng (Uprighting) can descend adverse Qi, arrest vomiting and stop bleeding, mainly used for vomiting, diarrhea, dysentery, nasal bleeding, convulsion and epilepsy

按摩方法详解
Detailed Diagram of Massage Manipulations

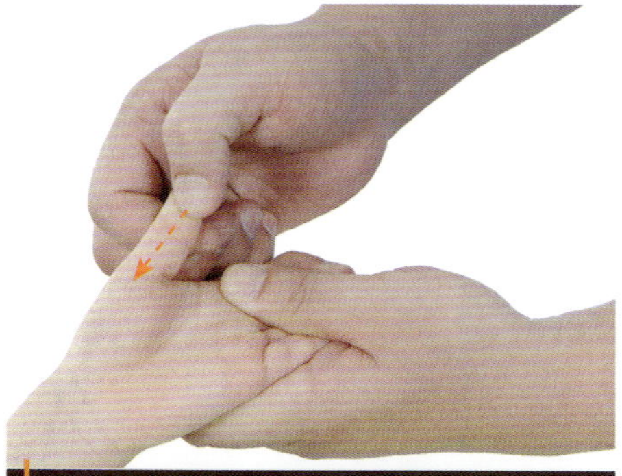

清胃经

旋推拇指掌面第 1 节，从指根向指尖方向为补胃经，从指尖向指根方向直推称为清胃经。一般推 100~300 次。

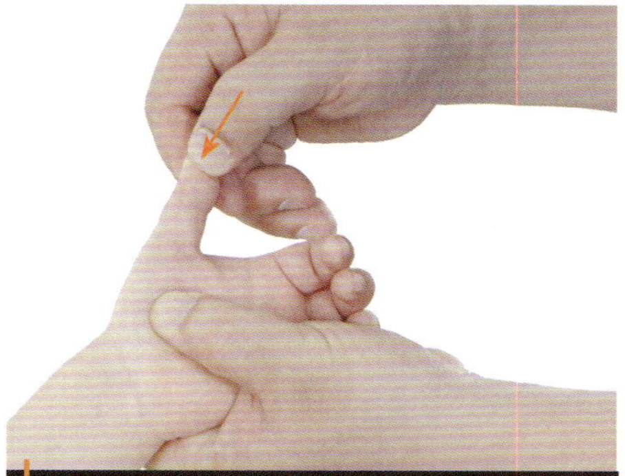

掐脾经

用拇指指甲掐之。一般掐3~5次。

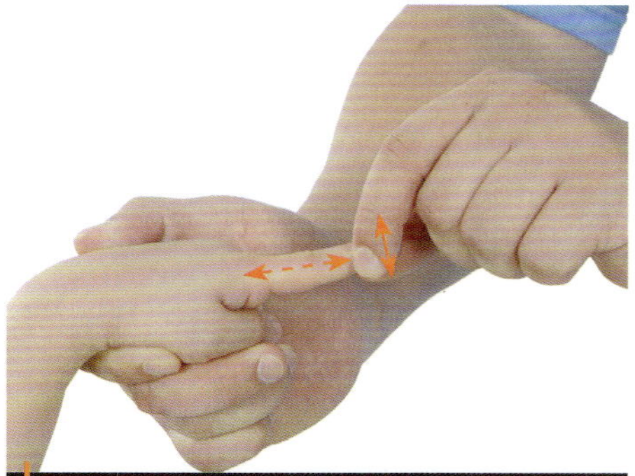

捻大肠

用拇指和食指螺纹面挟住小儿的食指两侧，快速捻搓的同时，沿大肠做往返移动。一般操作 0.5~1 分钟。

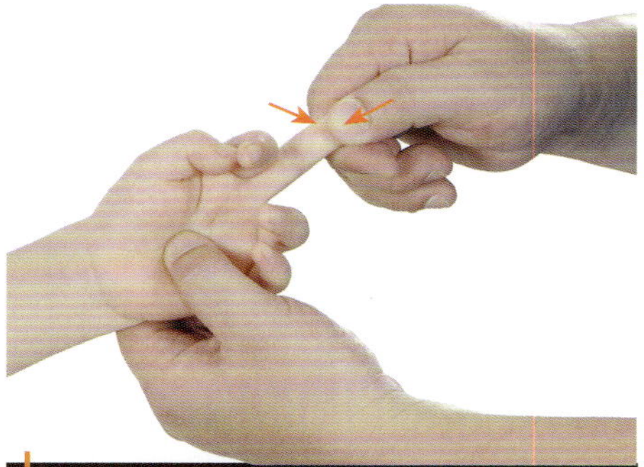

掐心经

用拇指指甲掐之。一般掐 3~5 次。

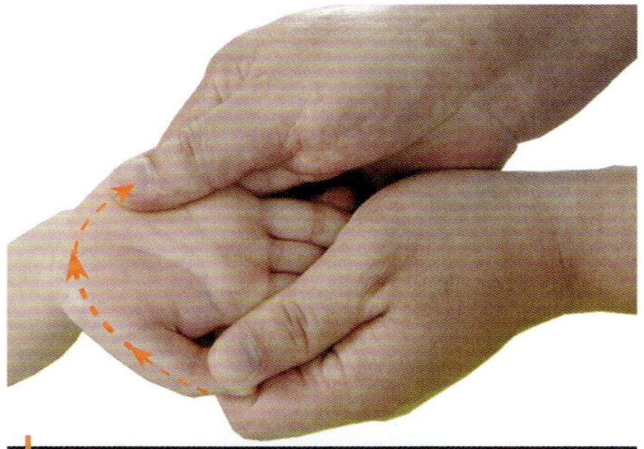

运土入水

自小儿拇指脾经穴起，沿手掌跟部、尺侧部至小指肾经穴。以 50~100 次为宜。

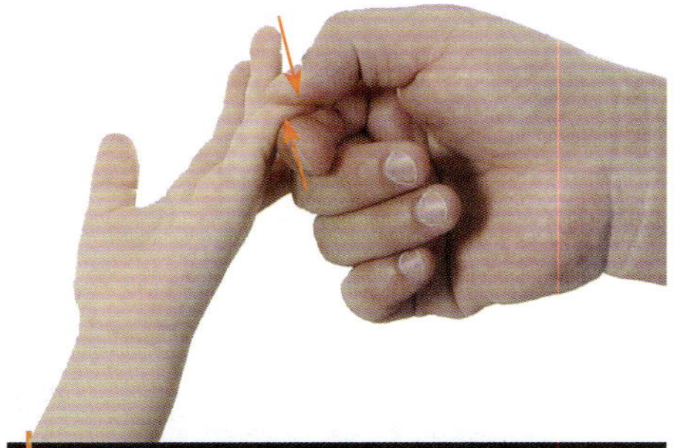

捏肾经

一般捏 100~300 次。

按摩方法详解
Detailed Diagram of Massage Manipulations

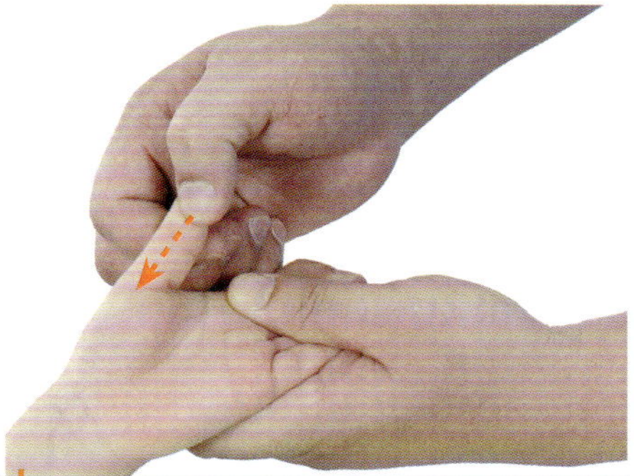

Clear Weijing (Stomach Meridian)

Rotate and push the distal phalange of thumb from the thumb root to the tip, which is called tonifying Weijing (Stomach Meridian), while push in the opposite direction from tip to bottom of the thumb is clearing Weijing (Stomach Meridian). The pushing manipulation is generally repeated for 100 to 300 times.

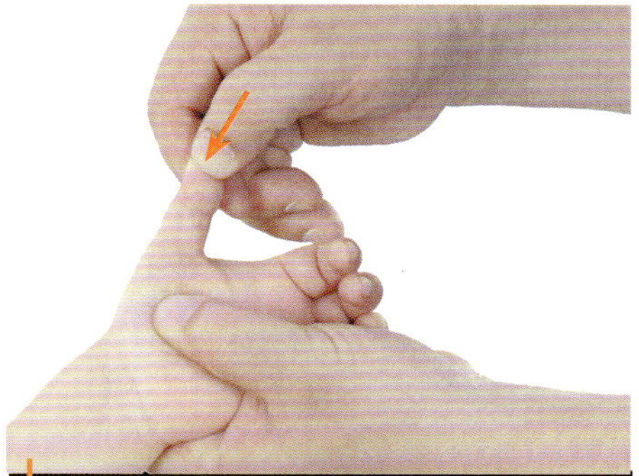

Pinch Pijing (Spleen Meridian)

Pinch Pijing with the fingernail of the thumb for generally 3 to 5 times.

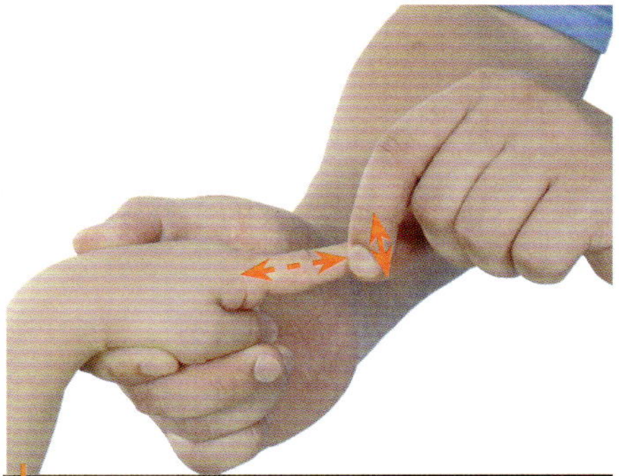

Twirl Dachang (Large Intestine)

Hold the both sides of the index finger of the child with the thumb and index finger for quick twirling and twisting. At the same time, move Dachang (Large Intestine) back and forth for generally 0.5 to 1 minutes.

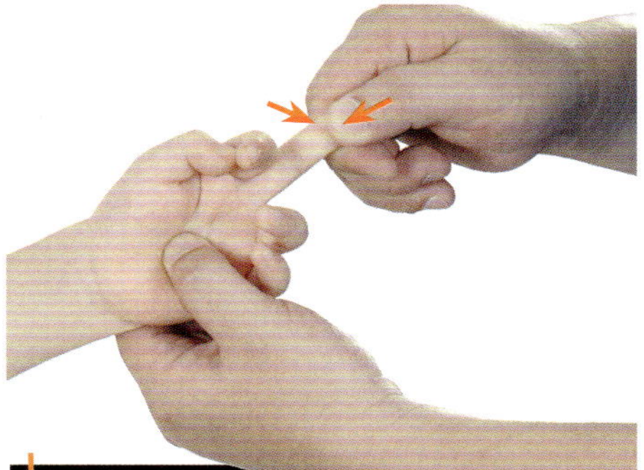

Pinch Xinjing (Heart Meridian)

Pinch Xinjing (Heart Meridian) with the fingernail of the thumb for generally 3 to 5 times.

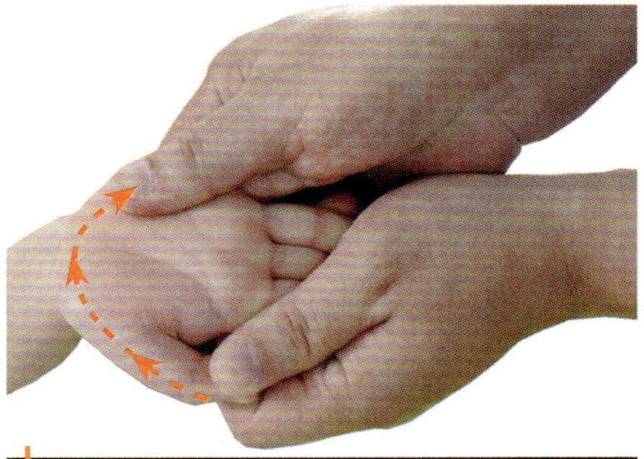

Yuntu Rushui (Transforming Earth into Water)

Start from Pijing (Spleen Meridian) of the thumb of the child to Shenjing (Kidney Meridian) in the little finger along the root of palm and the ulnar side of the palm for appropriately 50 to 100 times.

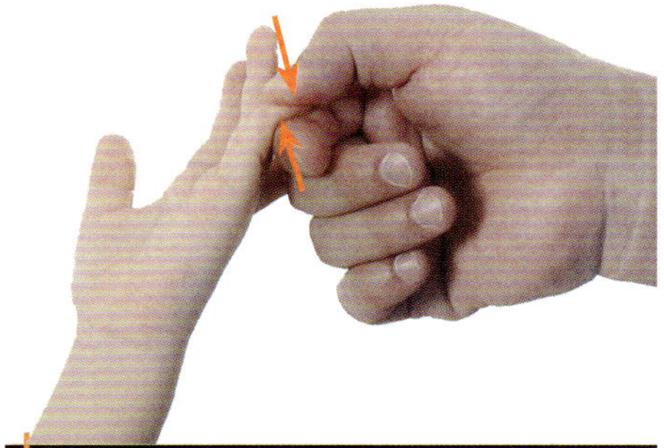

Pinch Shenjing (Kidney Meridian)

Pinch Shenjing (Kidney Meridian) for generally 100 to 300 times.

按摩方法详解
Detailed Diagram of Massage Manipulations

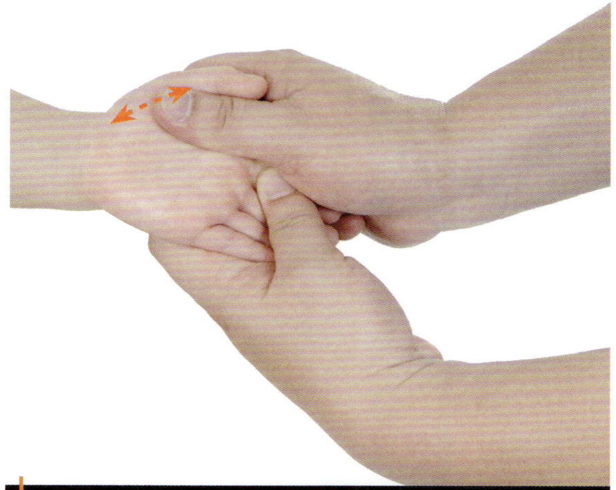

推板门

自拇指指根推向腕横纹，称板门推向横纹；反之，称为横纹推向板门。一般推 100~300 次。

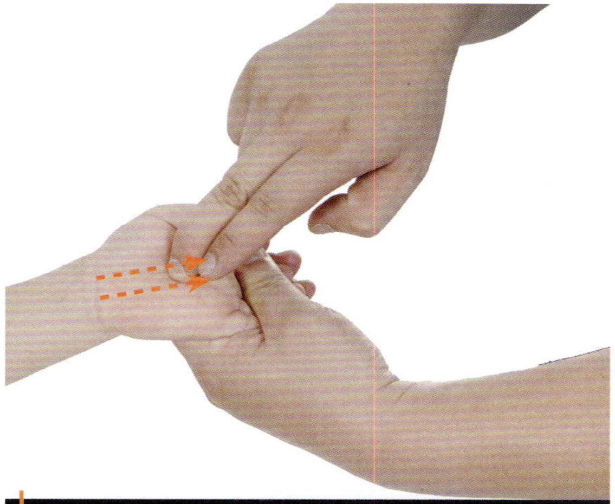

运内劳宫

用中指指端，经掌横纹、小天心掐运至内劳宫。

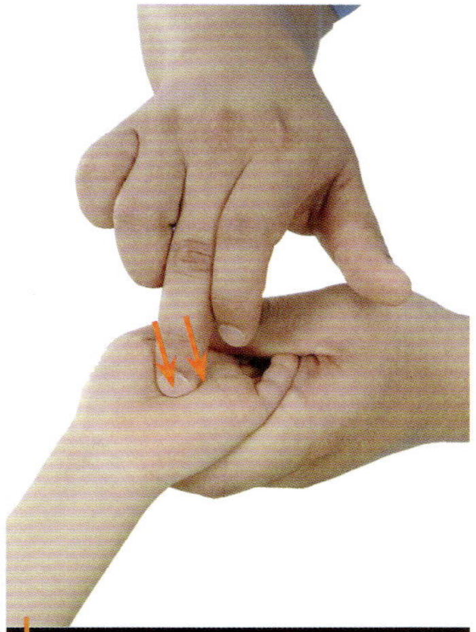

捣小天心

用中指指尖或屈曲的指间关节捣。捣 5~20 次。

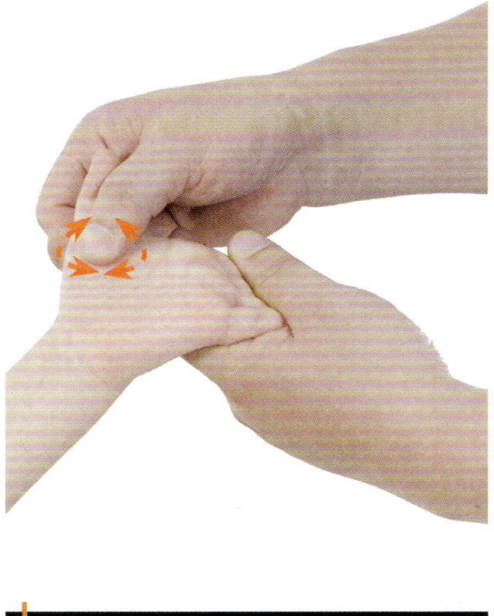

揉板门

指端揉大鱼际。一般揉 100~300 次。

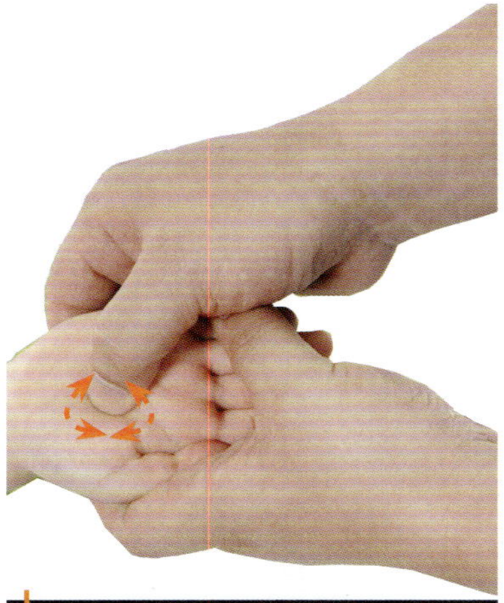

揉内劳宫

用指端揉，一般揉 100~300 次。

按摩方法详解
Detailed Diagram of Massage Manipulations

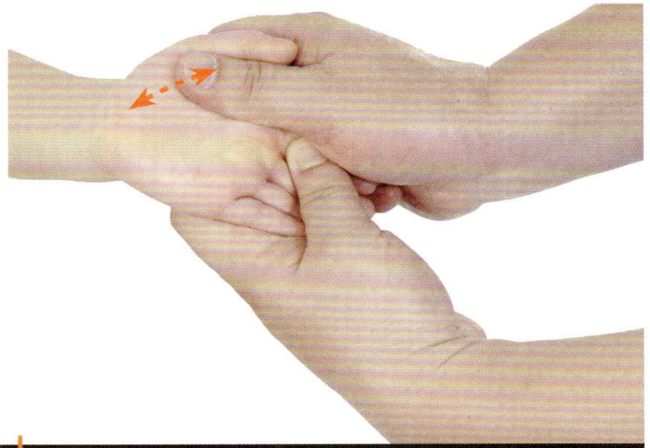
Push Banmen (Major thenar)

Pushing the point from the root of the thumb to the wrist crease is named Banmen (Major thenar)to Transverse Crease Push, while pushing in the opposite direction is called Transverse Crease to Banmen (Major thenar)Push. It is usually repeated for 100 to 300 times.

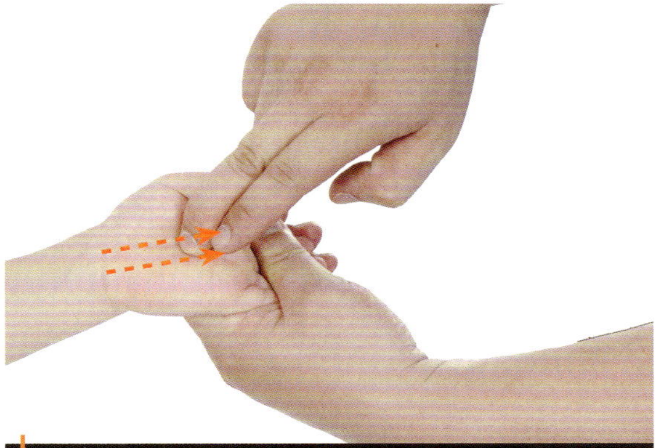
Circularly push Neilaogong (PC8)

Pinch and transport to Neilaogong (PC8) through Zhanghengwen and Xiaotianxin (Small heaven center) with the tip of middle finger.

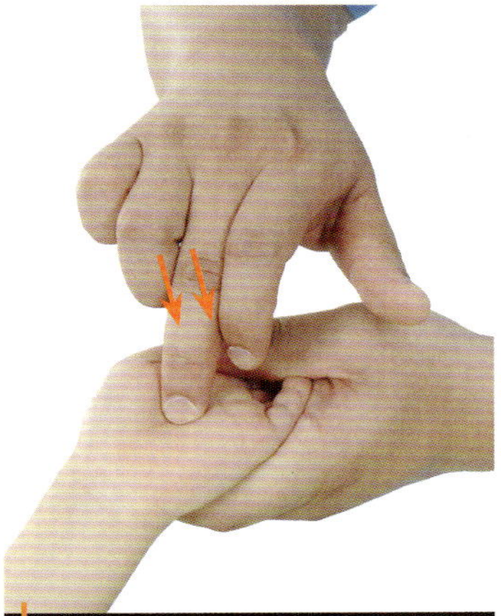
Pound Xiaotianxin (Small heaven center)

Pound Xiaotian xin (Small heaven center) with the tip of middle finger or the bending interphalangeal joint for 5 to 20 times.

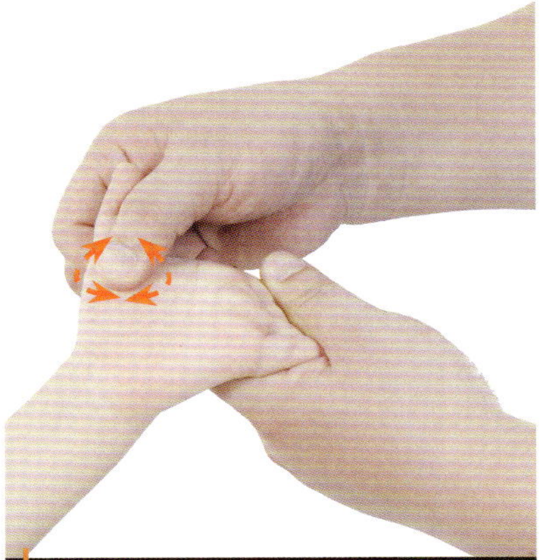
Knead Banmen (Major thenar)

Knead the greater thenar with the fingertips for generally 100 to 300 times.

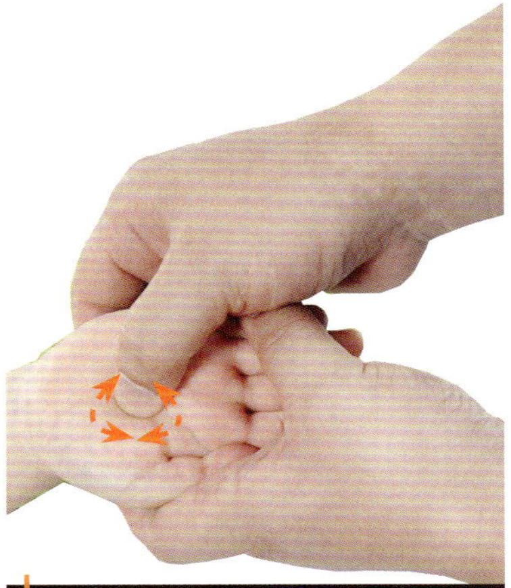
Knead Neilaogong (PC8)

Knead the point with the fingertip for generally 100 to 300 times.

按摩方法详解
Detailed Diagram of Massage Manipulations

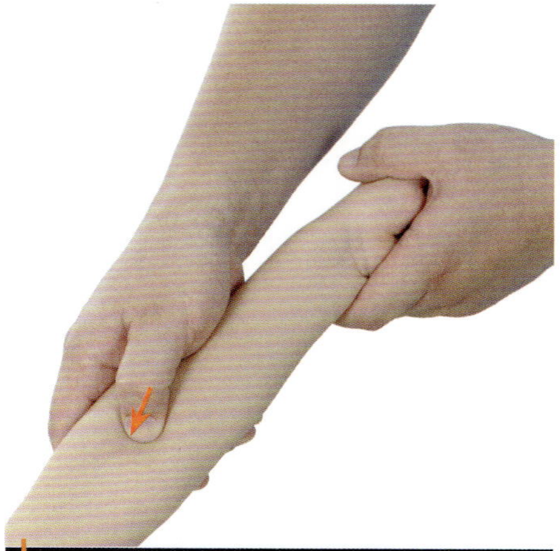

掐洪池

按摩者一手握住小儿之手，另一手拇指指甲掐该穴。一般 3~5 次。

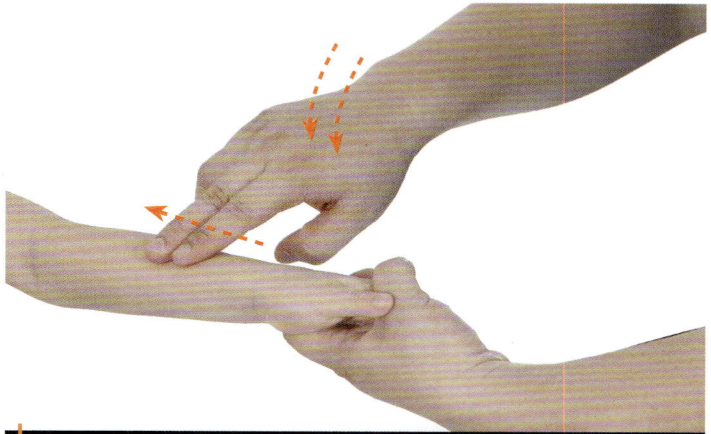

推上三关

用拇指指面或食指、中指指面自腕横纹向上推至肘横纹。推 100~300 次。

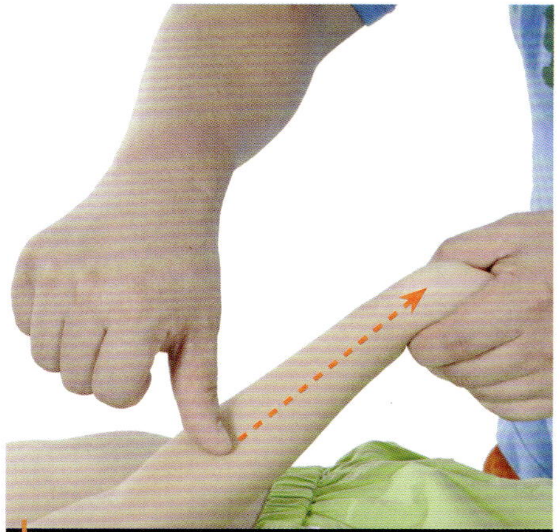

刮三关

用拇指桡侧缘，蘸清水、药水等润滑剂后，沿穴位做单方向的快速刮动。

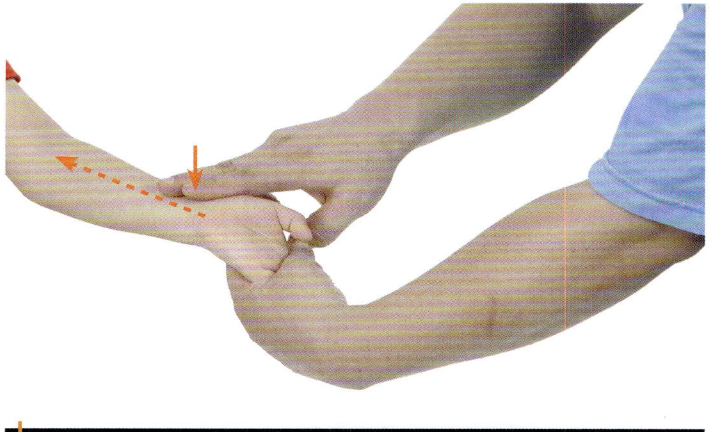

打马过天河

用一手捏住小儿四指，将掌心向上，用另一手的中指指面运内劳宫后，再用食指、中指、无名指三指由总筋起沿天河水打至洪池穴，或用食指、中指沿天河水弹击至肘弯处。弹击 20~30 遍。

按摩方法详解
Detailed Diagram of Massage Manipulations

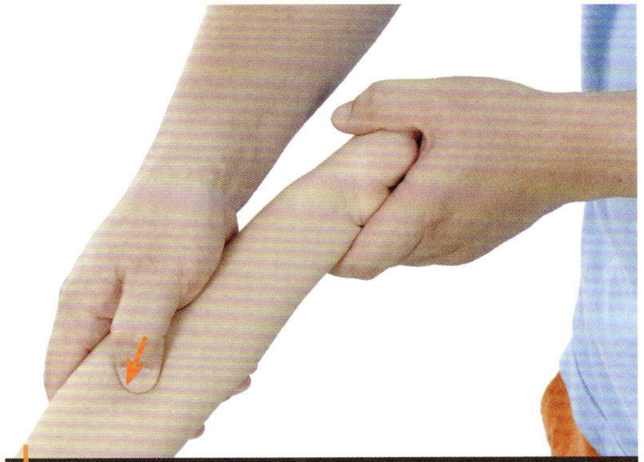

Pinch Hongchi (Quze, PC3)

Hold 1 hand of the child, and pinch the point with the fingernail of the thumb of the other hand for generally 3 to 5 times.

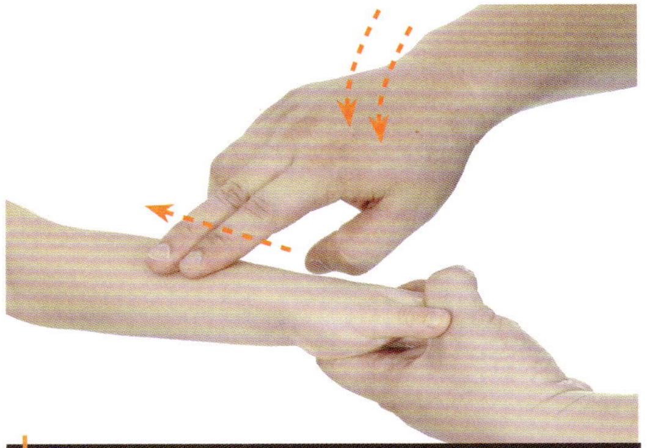

Push Upper Sanguan (Triple pass)

Push from the transverse crease of wrist upward to the cubital transverse crease with the facies digitales of the thumb or index and middle fingers for 100 to 300 times

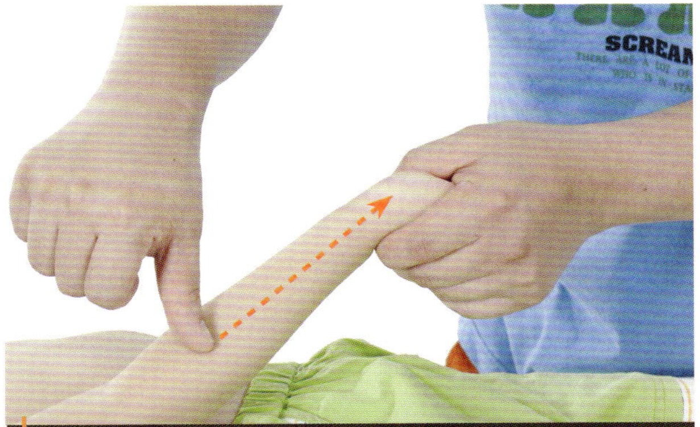

Scrape Sanguan (Triple pass)

Scrape quickly along the point in a single direction with the radial border of the thumb after dipping lubricating agent such as rinsing and liquid medicine

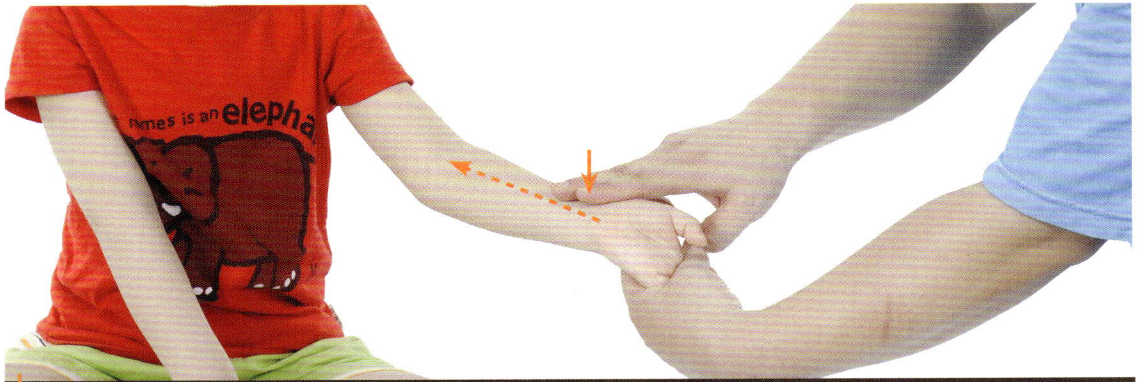

Dama Guotianhe (Beating the Horse to Cross Heaven River)

Pinch 4 fingers (index, middle, ring and little fingers) of the child with the palm upward. Circularly push Neilaogong (PC8) with the facies digitales of middle finger of the other hand. Then flap from Zongjin (Great tendon) to Hongchi Quze, (PC3) along the Tianheshui (Heaven river water) with the index, middle and ring fingers, or flick-strike along the Tianheshui (Heaven river water) to the elbow bend with the index and middle fingers for 20 to 30 times.

按摩方法详解
Detailed Diagram of Massage Manipulations

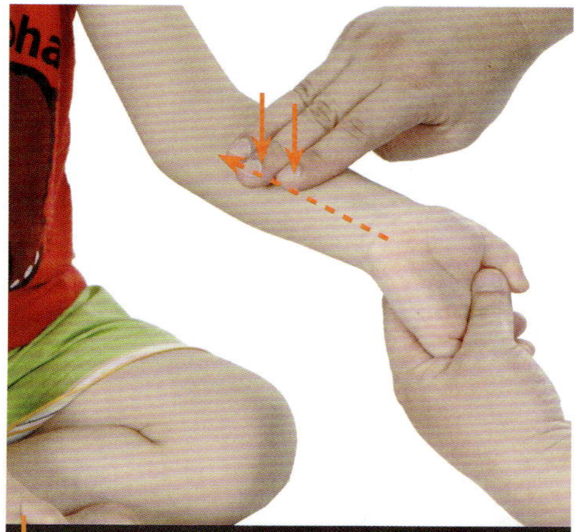

推天河水

用食指、中指、无名指三指由总筋起沿天河水打至洪池穴。以20~30次为宜。

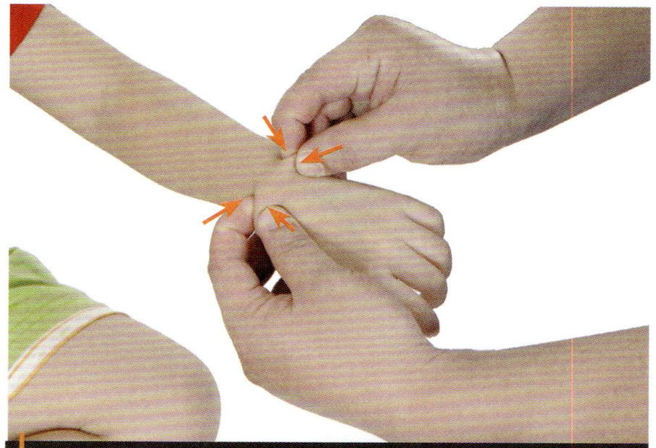

提捏螺蛳骨

用拇指、食指两指提捏该处皮肤10~20次。

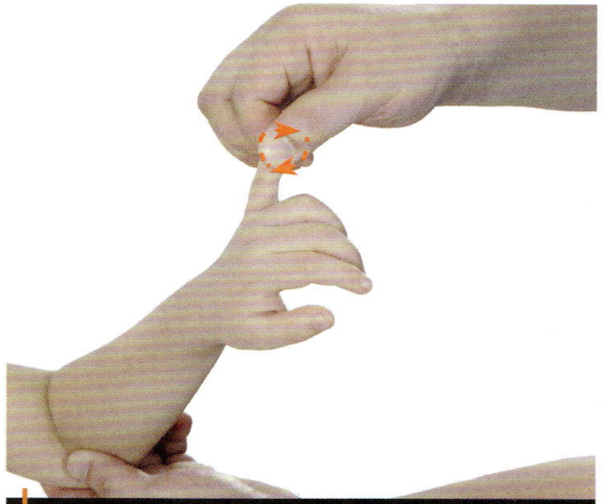

揉五指节

用拇指、食指揉搓。揉30~50次。

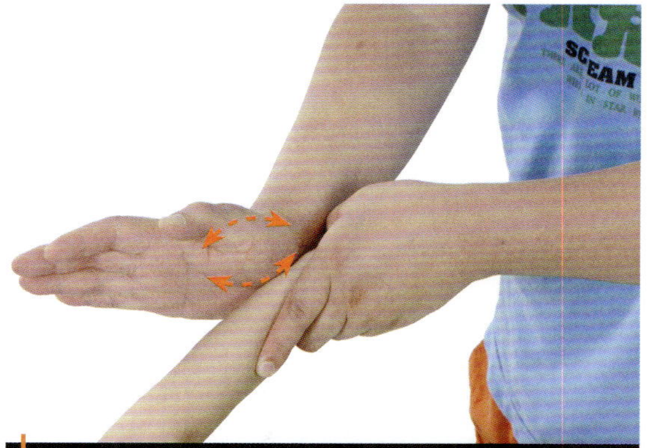

揉一窝风

以指端或掌根揉100~300次。

按摩方法详解
Detailed Diagram of Massage Manipulations

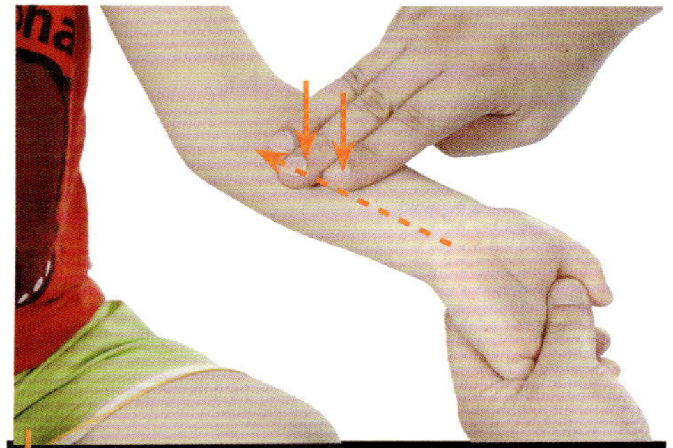

Push Tianheshui (Heaven river water)

Flap from Zongjin (Great tendon) to Hongchi (Quze, PC3) along the Tianheshui (Heaven river water) with the index, middle and ring fingers for appropriately 20 to 30 times.

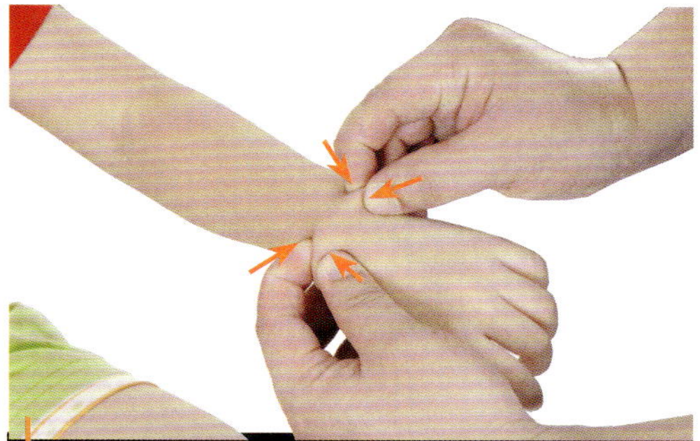

Lift-Pinch Luosigu (Bilateral protrusion of wrist)

Lift-pinch the local skin with the thumb and index finger for 10 to 20 times.

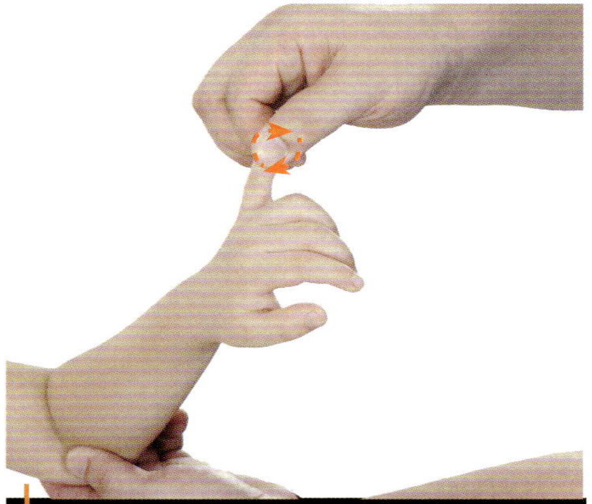

Knead Wuzhijie (Interphalangeal joints of 5 fingers)

Knead and twist Wuzhijie (Interphalangeal joints of 5 fingers) with the thumb and index finger for 30 to 50 times.

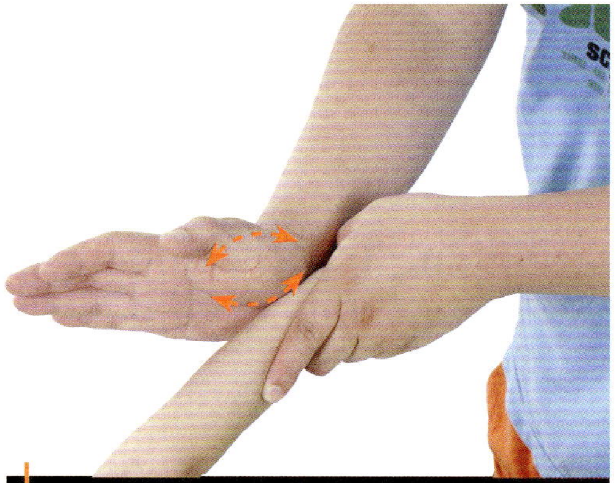

Knead Yiwofeng (Cave of wind)

Knead Yiwofeng (Cave of wind) with the fingertip or the root of palm for 100 to 300 times.

下肢穴位及按摩手法
Acupoints and Massage Manipulations in Lower Limbs

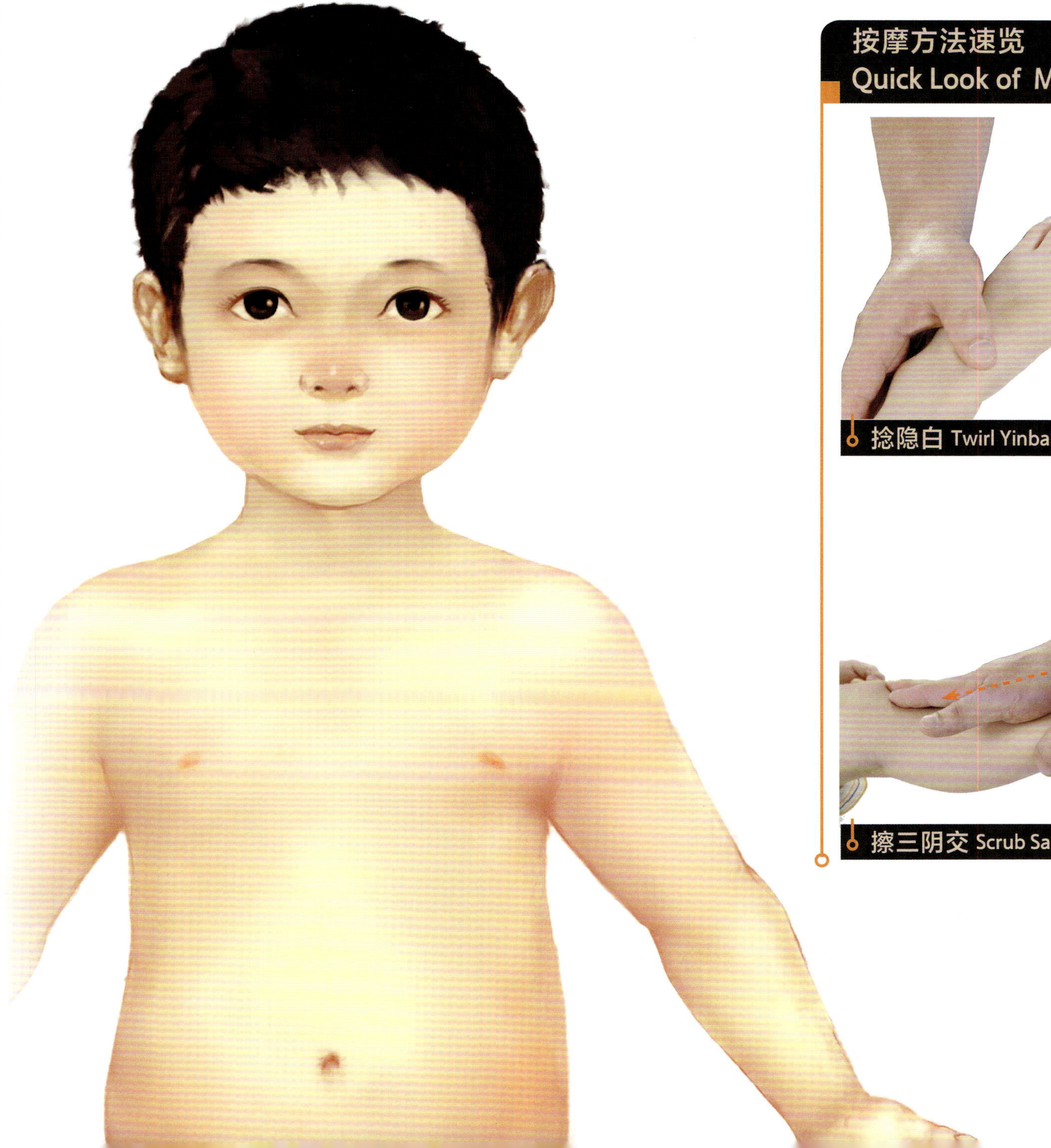

按摩方法速览
Quick Look of Massage Manipulations

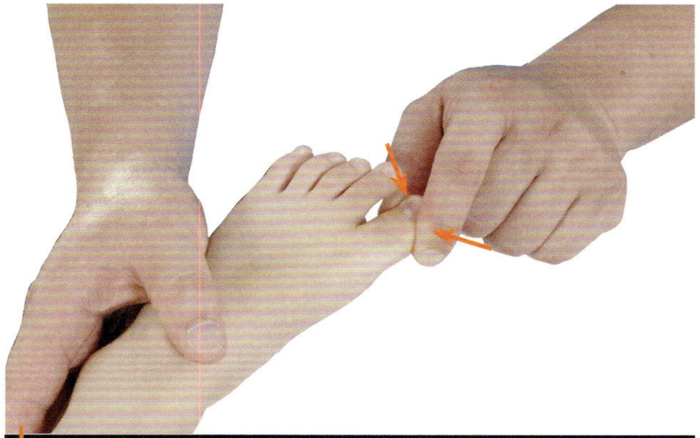

捻隐白 Twirl Yinbai (SP1)

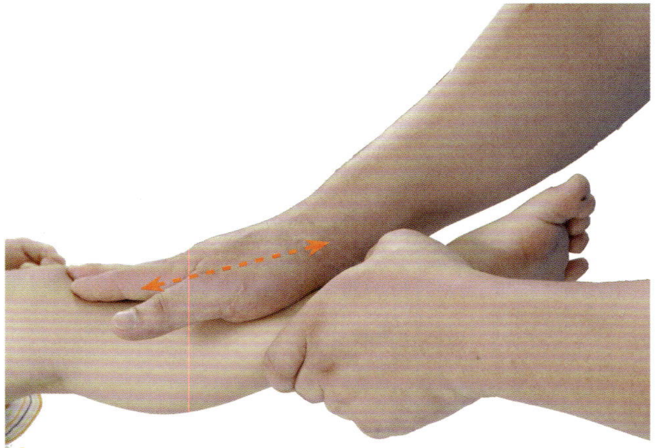

擦三阴交 Scrub Sanyinjiao (SP6)

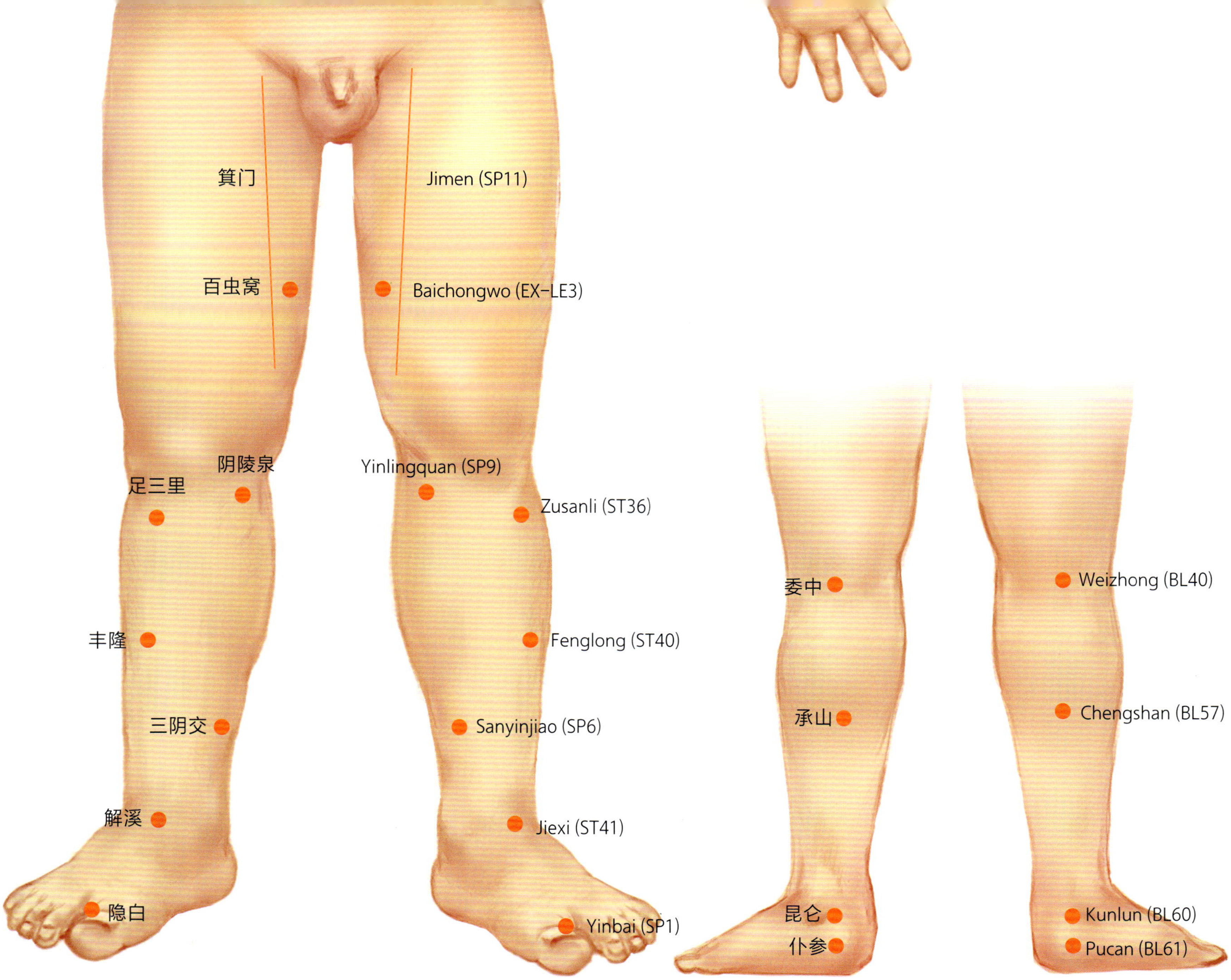
箕门
Jimen (SP11)
百虫窝
Baichongwo (EX-LE3)
阴陵泉
足三里
Yinlingquan (SP9)
Zusanli (ST36)
丰隆
Fenglong (ST40)
三阴交
Sanyinjiao (SP6)
解溪
Jiexi (ST41)
隐白
Yinbai (SP1)
委中
Weizhong (BL40)
承山
Chengshan (BL57)
昆仑
仆参
Kunlun (BL60)
Pucan (BL61)

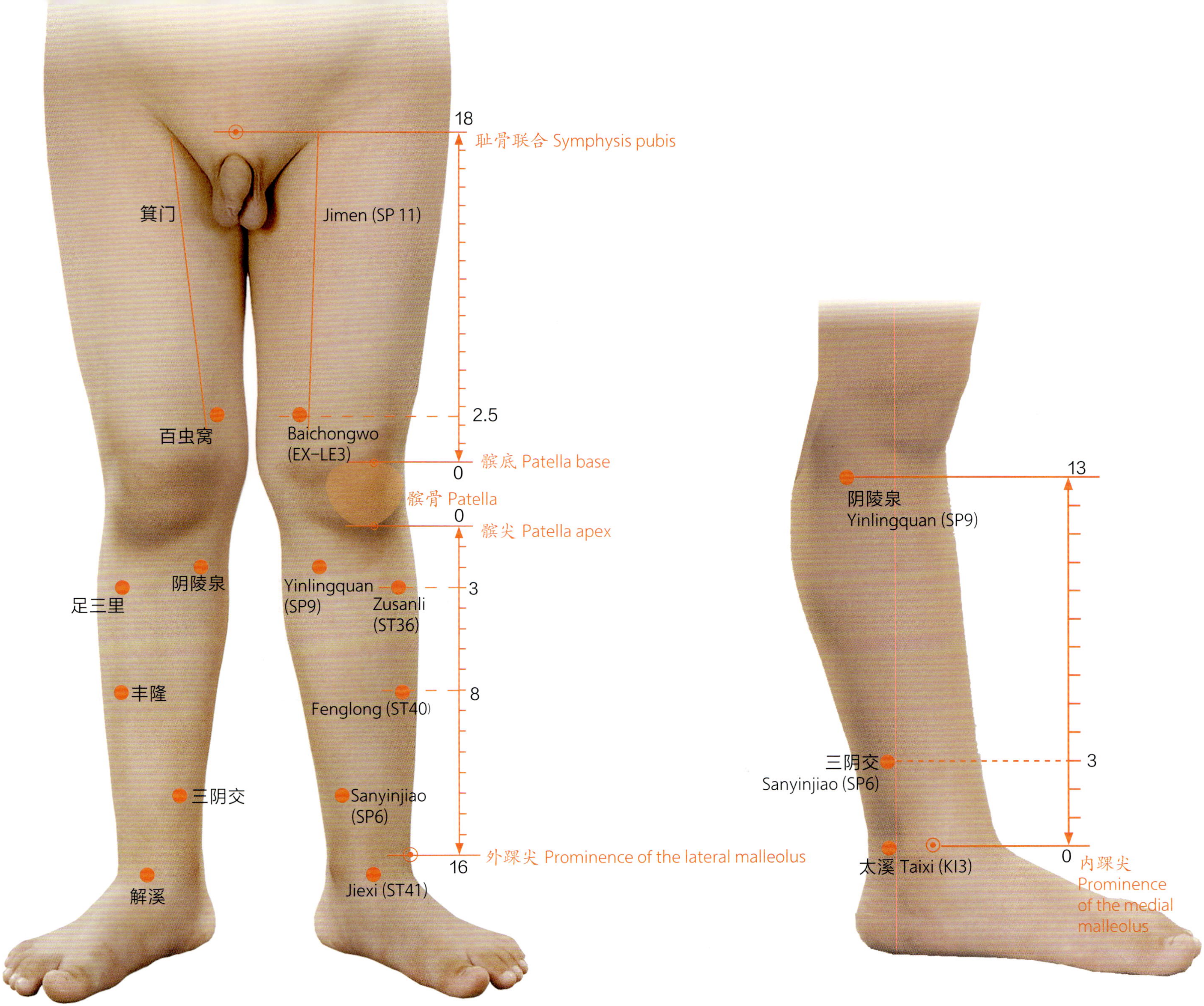
18
耻骨联合 Symphysis pubis
箕门
Jimen (SP 11)
2.5
百虫窝
Baichongwo
(EX-LE3)
髌底 Patella base
0
髌骨 Patella
0
髌尖 Patella apex
阴陵泉
足三里
Yinlingquan
(SP9)
3
Zusanli
(ST36)
丰隆
8
Fenglong (ST40)
三阴交
Sanyinjiao
(SP6)
外踝尖 Prominence of the lateral malleolus
16
解溪
Jiexi (ST41)
13
阴陵泉
Yinlingquan (SP9)
三阴交
Sanyinjiao (SP6)
3
太溪 Taixi (KI3)
0
内踝尖
Prominence
of the medial
malleolus

穴 位	定 位	按摩方法	功效主治
箕门	大腿内侧，从膝盖上缘至腹股沟成一直线	推法：用食指、中指指腹面，从膝盖内侧上缘直上，推至腹股沟根部 100~300 次	利尿，清热，通小便。主治小便赤涩、尿闭（小便不通）、尿潴留
百虫窝	膝上内侧肌肉丰厚处	拿法或揉法：用拇指和食指、中指两指指腹拿 3~5 次，或以拇指或中指指端揉 30~50 次	通经络，止抽搐。主治下肢瘫痪、抽搐、癫痫、昏迷
阴陵泉	小腿内侧，胫骨内侧髁后下方凹陷处	揉法：用食指或拇指指腹揉 50~100 次	健脾利湿。主治腹胀、泄泻（腹泻）、小便不利或失禁、黄疸

Acupoints	Location	Massage Manipulation	Efficacy and Indications
Jimen (SP11)	In the medial side of the thigh, the line from the interior border of the knee to groin	Pushing manipulation: Push directly from the interior border of the medial side of the knee to the root of groin with the finger pulps of index and middle fingers for 100 to 300 times	It has diuretic effect, and the effects of clearing heat and inducing urination,mainly used for red and difficult urination, anuresis and urine retention
Baichongwo (EX-LE3)	At the thick muscular part above the medial side of the knee	Grasping or kneading manipulation: Grasp the point with the finger pulps of the thumb and index and middle fingers for 3 to 5 times, or knead the point with the fingertip of the thumb or middle finger for 30 to 50 times	It cansooth meridians and collaterals, and stop convulsion, mainly used for lower limb paralysis, convulsion, epilepsy and coma
Yinlingquan (SP9)	In the medial leg, the posterior inferior depression of the medial condyle of tibia	Kneading manipulation: Knead the point with the finger pulp of the index finger or the thumb for 50 to 100 times	It can invigorate spleen and eliminate dampness, mainly used for abdominal distension, diarrhea, difficult urination or urinary incontinence and jaundice

续表

穴位	定位	按摩方法	功效主治
足三里	小腿前外侧，犊鼻下 3 寸，距胫骨前缘 1 横指（中指）	揉法：以拇指指端按揉 50~100 次	健脾和胃，调中理气，导滞通络。主治胃痛、腹胀、呕吐、泄泻（腹泻）、消化不良、疳积（营养不良）、便秘、水肿、下肢疾患。此穴可强身防病，为儿童保健要穴
丰隆	在小腿前外侧，当外踝尖上 8 寸，距胫骨前缘 2 横指（中指）	揉法：以拇指指端按揉 50~100 次	和胃，化痰，通便。主治痰多、咳嗽、哮喘、便秘、下肢疼痛
三阴交	小腿内侧，足内踝尖上 3 寸，胫骨内侧缘后方	揉法：以拇指指端按揉 50~100 次	通血脉，活经络，健脾胃，助运化，疏下焦。主治惊风（抽搐神昏）、腹胀肠鸣、泄泻（腹泻）、遗尿（尿床）、小便不利、瘾疹（风疹、荨麻疹）
解溪	踝关节前横纹中点，两筋之间凹陷处	揉法或掐法：用拇指指端揉 50~100 次，或用拇指指甲掐 3~5 次	镇惊止搐，止吐泻。主治惊风（抽搐神昏）、头痛、踝关节屈伸不利、吐泻

Continued

Acupoints	Location	Massage Manipulation	Efficacy and Indications
Zusanli (ST36)	In the anterior lateral side of the leg, 3 cun below Dubi (ST35), and 1 finger-breadth (fingers) lateral to the anterior border of the tibia	Kneading manipulation: Press-knead the point with the fingertip of the thumb for 50 to 100 times	It can invigorate spleen and harmonize stomach, regulate middle Qi, remove stagnation and sooth collaterals, mainly used for stomachache, abdominal distension, vomiting, diarrhea, dyspepsia, infantile malnutrition with accumulation, constipation, edema and diseases of lower limb. The point can strengthen body to prevent diseases as an important point of children for healthcare
Fenglong (ST40)	In the anterior lateral side of the leg, 8 cun above the prominence of the lateral malleolus, and 2 middle finger below the anterior border of the tibia	Kneading manipulation: Press-knead the point with the tip of the thumb for 50 to 100 times	It can harmonize stomach, resolve phlegm and relieve constipation, mainly used for excessive phlegm, cough, asthma, constipation and pain of lower limb
Sanyinjiao (SP6)	In the medial leg, 3 cun above the prominence of the medial malleolus of foot, behind the medial border of the tibia	Kneading manipulation: Press-knead the point with the fingertip of the thumb for 50 to 100 times	It can promote blood circulation, activate meridians and collaterals, invigorate spleen and stomach to promote transportation and transformation, and dredge lower energizer, mainly used for infantile convulsion (convulsion and unconsciousness), abdominal distension, borborygmus, diarrhea, enuresis, difficult urination and urticaria (rubella and nettle-rash)
Jiexi (ST41)	At the midpoint of the anterior transverse crease of the ankle joint, in the depression between the 2 tendons	Kneading or pinching manipulation: Knead the point with the fingertip of the thumb for 50 to 100 times, or pinch the point with the nail of the thumb for 3 to 5 times	It can calm fright and stop convulsion, and relieve vomiting and diarrhea, mainly used for infantile convulsion (convulsion and unconsciousness), headache, difficult extension and flexion of ankle, vomiting and diarrhea

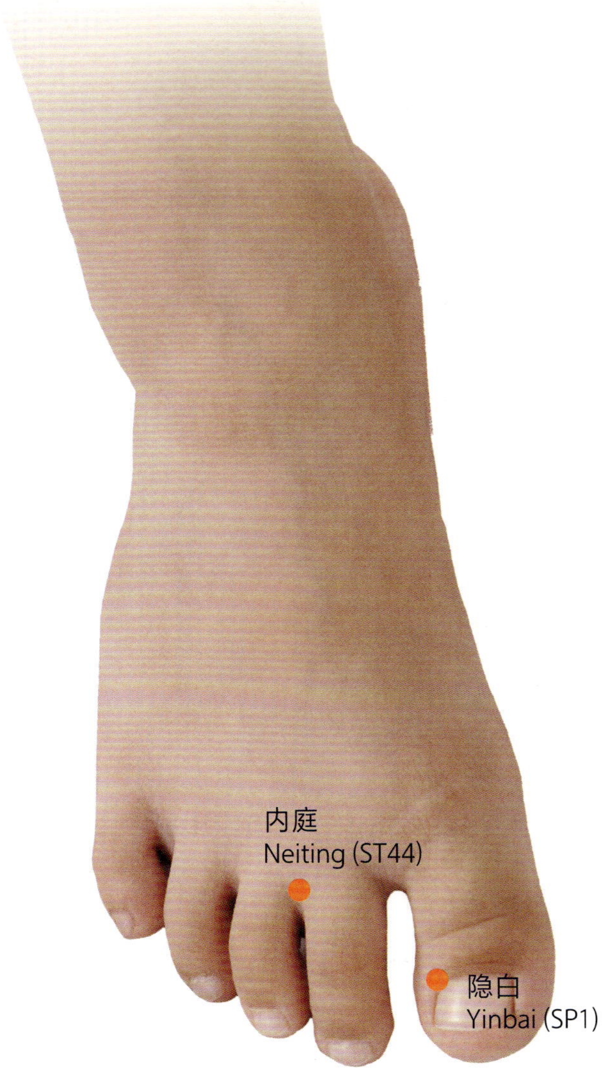
内庭
Neiting (ST44)
隐白
Yinbai (SP1)

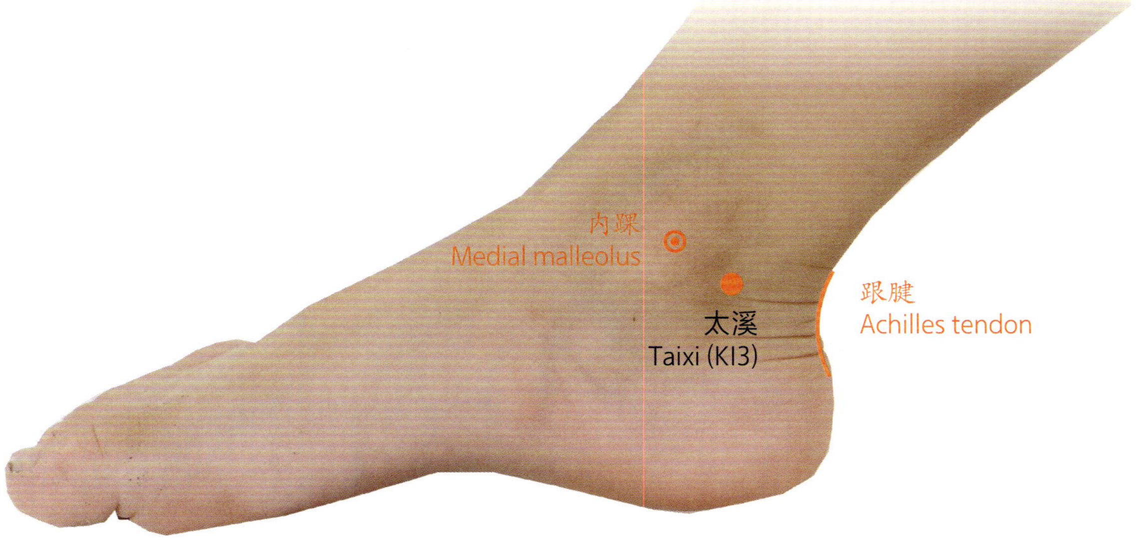
内踝
Medial malleolus
太溪
Taixi (KI3)
跟腱
Achilles tendon

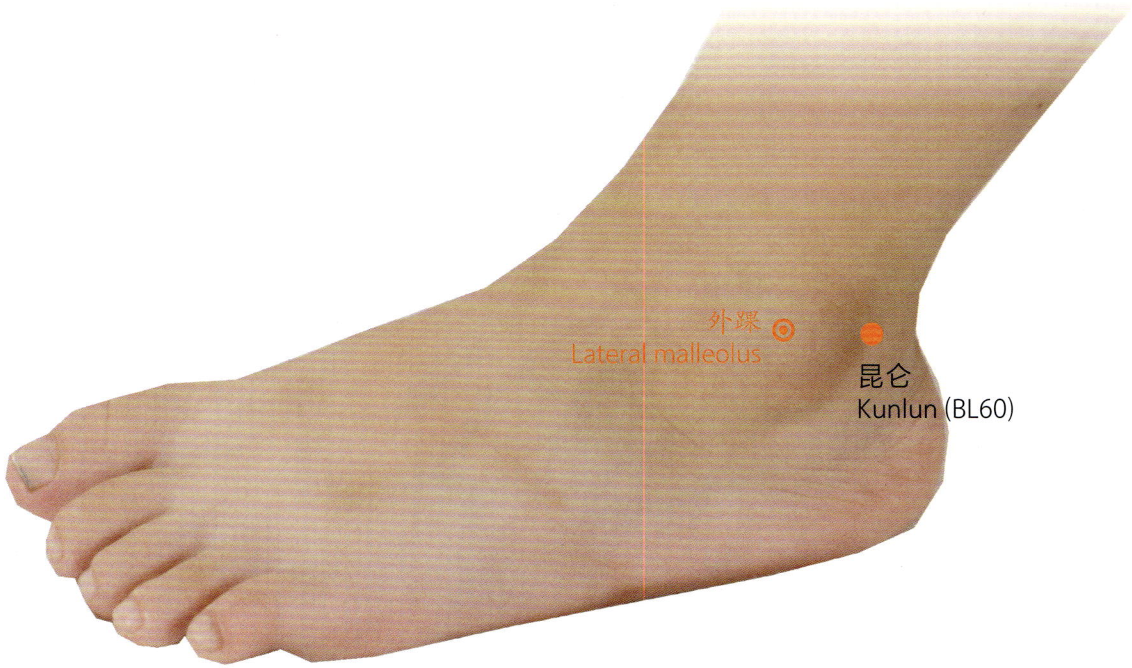
外踝
Lateral malleolus
昆仑
Kunlun (BL60)

穴位	定位	按摩方法	功效主治
太溪	足内踝尖与跟腱之间的凹陷处	揉法：用食指指端揉 50~100 次	滋阴益肾，壮阳强腰。主治肾炎、遗尿、支气管炎、哮喘、口腔炎、耳鸣、足跟痛、膈肌痉挛
内庭	足背，第 2、3 趾间，趾蹼缘后方赤白肉际处	揉法：用食指指端揉 50~100 次	清胃泻火，理气止痛。主治三叉神经痛、牙痛、齿龈炎、扁桃体炎、胃痉挛、急慢性肠炎
隐白	足大趾末节内侧，距趾甲角 0.1 寸	揉法：用食指指端揉 50~100 次	调经统血，健脾回阳。主治牙龈出血、鼻出血、小儿惊风、消化道出血、急性胃肠炎、尿血

Acupoints	Location	Massage Manipulations	Efficacy and Indications
Taixi (KI3)	In the depression between the prominence of the medial malleolus of foot and achilles tendon	Kneading manipulation: Knead the point with the tip of index finger for 50 to 100 times	It can nourish Yin and replenish kidney, strengthen Yang and waist, mainly used for nephritis, enuresis, bronchitis, asthma, stomatitis, tinnitus, painful heel and spasm of diaphragm
Neiting (ST44)	On the dorsum of foot, between the 2nd and the 3rd toes, at the dorsal-ventral boundary of the posterior toe line	Kneading manipulation: Knead the point with the tip of index finger for 50 to 100 times	It can clear and purge stomach fire, regulate Qi and relieve pain, mainly used for trigeminal neuralgia, toothache, gingivitis, tonsillitis, gastrospasm and acute and chronic enteritis
Yinbai (SP1)	In the medial side of the tip of the big toe, 0.1 cun lateral to the corner of the toenail	Kneading manipulation: Knead the point with the tip of index finger for 50 to 100 times	It can regulate meridians and control blood, invigorate spleen and restore Yang, mainly used for gingival bleeding, nasal bleeding, infantile convulsion, gastrointestinal bleeding, acute gastroenteritis and hematuria

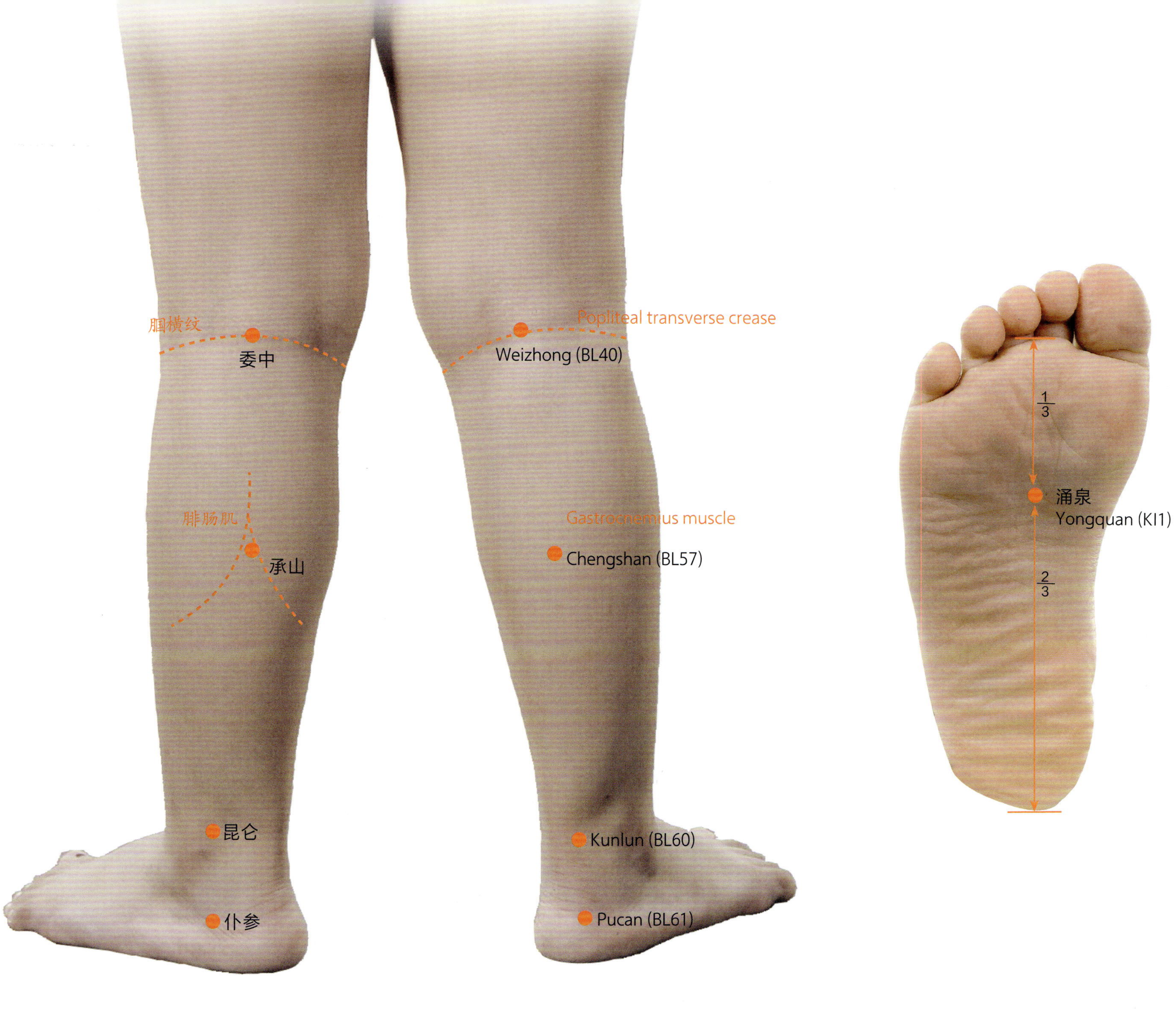
腘横纹
委中
Popliteal transverse crease
Weizhong (BL40)
腓肠肌
承山
Gastrocnemius muscle
Chengshan (BL57)
昆仑
Kunlun (BL60)
仆参
Pucan (BL61)
1/3
涌泉
Yongquan (KI1)
2/3

续表

穴位	定位	按摩方法	功效主治
委中	腘窝中，腘横纹的中央凹陷中	拿法：以拇指和其他手指相对用力拿 3~5 次	镇惊，舒筋，通络。主治惊风（神昏抽搐）、中暑、腹痛、吐泻、腰腿痛、下肢瘫痪
承山	小腿后面正中、腓肠肌腹下陷中	拿法或直推法：以拇指、食指、中指指端相对用力拿 3~5 次，或以食指、中指两指直推 100~500 次	通经络，止抽搐，止腹泻，通大便。主治便秘、腹泻、腿痛、瘫痪、抽筋
昆仑	外踝尖与跟腱的中点凹陷中	拿法或掐法：以拇指、食指两指相对用力拿 3~5 次，或以拇指掐 3~5 次	镇惊定痫。主治头痛、抽搐、癫痫、腰痛、足内翻、足跟痛

Continued

Acupoints	Location	Massage Manipulations	Efficacy and Indications
Weizhong (BL40)	Inside the popliteal fossa, in the depression of the middle of the popliteal transverse crease	Grasping manipulation: Exert proper strength with the thumb and other fingers to grasp the point for 3 to 5 times	It can calm fright, relax sinew and sooth collaterals, mainly used for infantile convulsion (unconsciousness and convulsion), heat stroke, abdominal pain, vomiting and diarrhea, pain of waist and leg, and paralysis of lower limb
Chengshan (BL57)	In the middle of the back of leg, in the depression below the muscle belly of gastrocnemius muscle	Grasping or direct-pushing manipulation: Exert proper strength with tips of the thumb, index and middle fingers to grasp the point for 3 to 5 times, or carry out direct-pushing manipulation with the index and middle fingers for 100 to 500 times	It can sooth meridians and collaterals, stop convulsion, relieve diarrhea and constipation, mainly used for constipation, diarrhea, painful leg, paralysis and cramp
Kunlun (BL60)	In the depression of the midpoint of the line between the prominence of lateral malleolus and achilles tendon	Grasping or pinching manipulation: Exert proper strength with the thumb and index finger to grasp the point for 3 to 5 times, or pinch the point with the thumb for 3 to 5 times	It can calm fright and stabilize epilepsy, mainly used for headache, convulsion, epilepsy, lumbago, strephenopodia and heel pain

续表

穴位	定位	按摩方法	功效主治
仆参	足跟外踝后下凹陷中	拿法或掐法：用拇指、食指、中指指端相对用力拿 3~5 次，或用拇指掐 3~5 次	镇惊，复苏。主治腰痛、脚跟痛、昏迷
涌泉	屈足趾，脚掌心前正中凹陷中	推法或揉法：用拇指螺纹面向足趾方向推，或用拇指指端揉，各 50~100 次	引火归原，退虚热，止吐泻。主治发热、五心烦热、呕吐、腹泻

Continued

Acupoints	Location	Massage Manipulations	Efficacy and Indications
Pucan (BL61)	In the depression of posterior inferior to the lateral malleolus of the heel	Grasping or pinching manipulation: Exert proper strength with tips of the thumb, index and middle fingers for 3 to 5 times, or pinch the point with the thumb for 3 to 5 times	It can calm fright and induce resuscitation, mainly used for lumbago, heel pain and coma
Yongquan (KI1)	Bend the toes, in the depression of the anterior median sole	Pushing or kneading manipulation: Push the point toward the toe with the thumb, or knead the point with the fingertip of the thumb for respective 50 to 100 times	It can return fire to its origin, reduce deficiency-heat and relieve vomiting and diarrhea, mainly used for fever, vexing heat in chest, palms and soles, vomiting and diarrhea

按摩方法详解
Detailed Diagram of Massage Manipulations

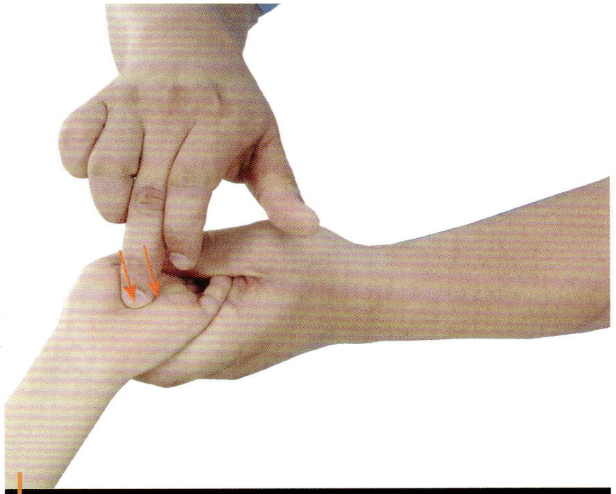

擦三阴交

以手指、掌、大鱼际、小鱼际放在该处皮肤上，做直线往返运动。擦100~200次。

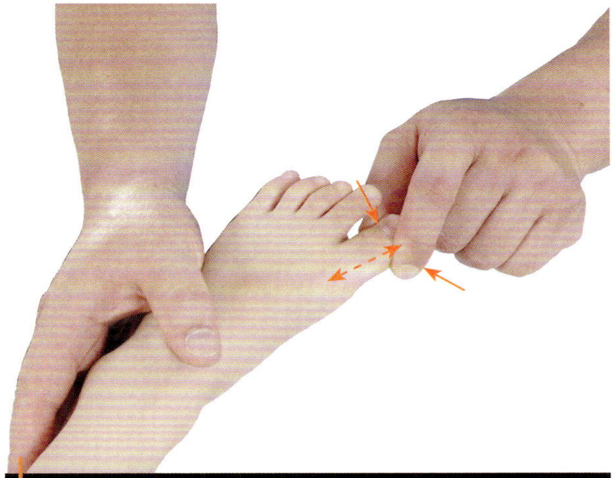

捻隐白

用拇指和食指捏住小儿足部大指，做对称、来回快速捻搓。一般捻搓0.5~1分钟。

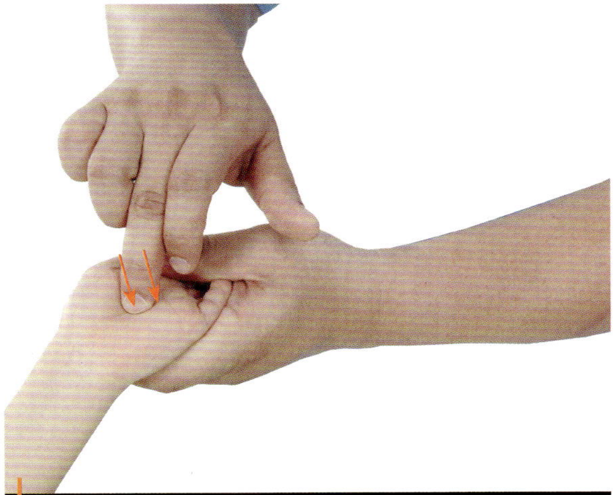

Scrub Sanyinjiao (SP6)

Put the fingers, palm, great thenar and hypothenar to the local skin. Move back and forth in a line and scrub for 100 to 200 times.

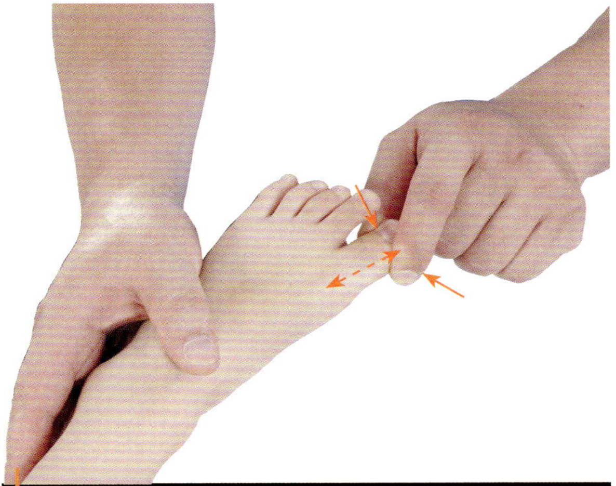

Twirl Yinbai (SP1)

Pinch the big toe of children with the thumb and index finger. Carry out quick twirling and twisting movement symmetrically back and forth for generally 0.5 to 1 minutes.

第三章 儿童超速效对症按摩

1 感冒

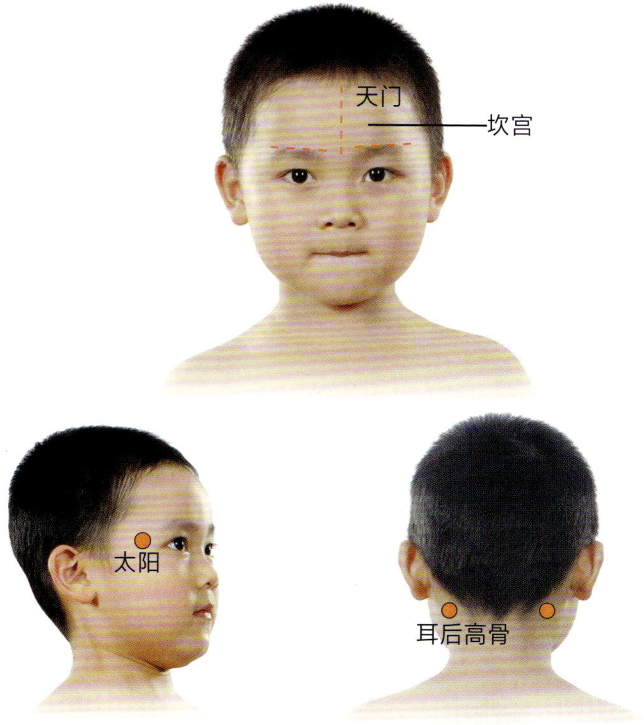

经典配穴

天门：两眉中至前发际呈一直线。

坎宫：从眉头起沿眉向眉梢呈一横线。

太阳：眉梢与眼外角连线的中点。

耳后高骨：耳后高骨后下凹陷中。

按摩操作

开天门：两拇指自下而上地交替直推，推30次。

推坎宫：亦称分阴阳，两拇指自眉头向眉梢分推，推30次。

揉太阳：用拇指或食指指腹揉，两侧各揉30次。

揉耳后高骨：用拇指或食指指腹揉，两侧各揉30次。

2 发热

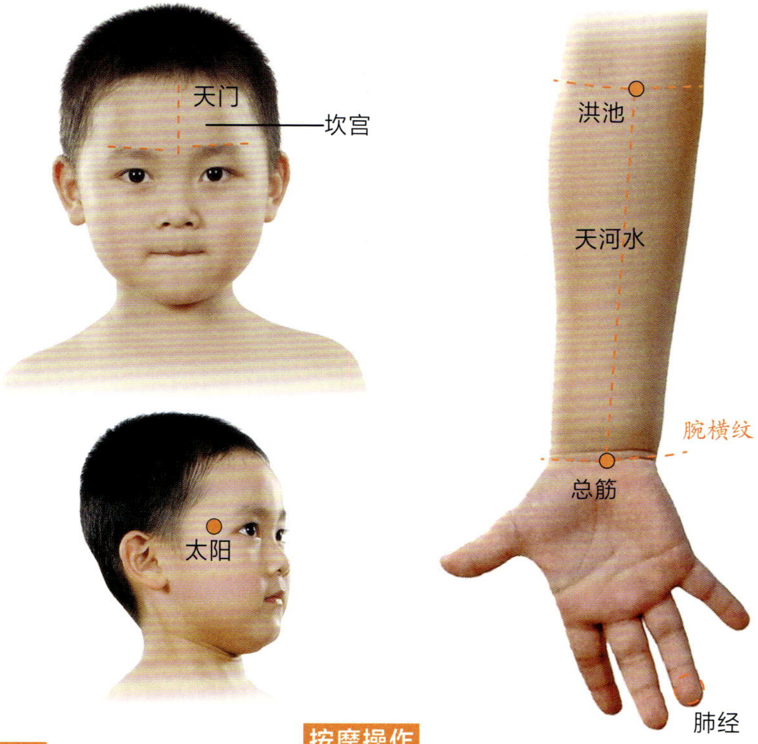

经典配穴

天门：两眉中至前发际呈一直线。

坎宫：从眉头起沿眉向眉梢呈一横线。

太阳：眉梢与眼外角连线的中点。

肺经：无名指末节指腹。

天河水：前臂掌侧正中，自腕横纹中点至肘横纹中点呈一直线。

按摩操作

开天门：两拇指自下而上地交替直推，推50次。

推坎宫：亦称分阴阳，两拇指自眉头向眉梢分推，推50次。

揉太阳：用拇指或食指指腹揉，两侧各揉50次。

清肺经：从无名指掌面末节指纹处向指尖方向推。

清天河水：用食指、中指两指自腕横纹向上推至肘横纹处，推300次。

Chapter 3:
Super Quick-acting Pediatric Symptomatic Massage

1 Cold

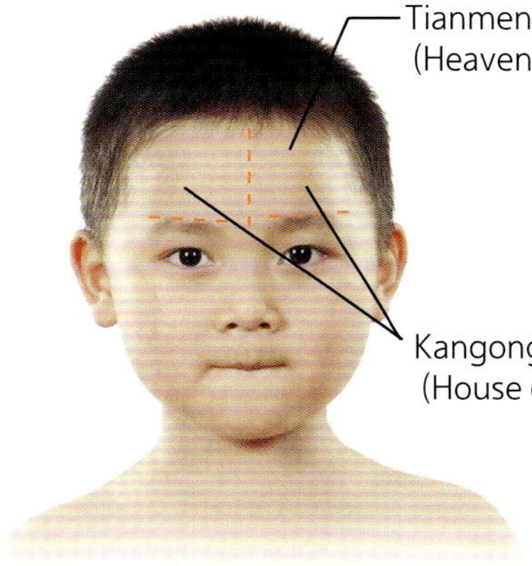

Classic Acupoints Matching

Tianmen (Heaven gate, BL2): The line between the midpoint of the 2 eyebrows and the anterior hairline.
Kangong (House of water): The transverse line starting from the brow tip to the brow end along the brow.
Taiyang (EX-HN5): The midpoint of the line between the brow tip to the outer canthus.
Erhougaogu (Protruding bone behind the ear): In the depression of the posterior inferior protruding bone behind the ear.

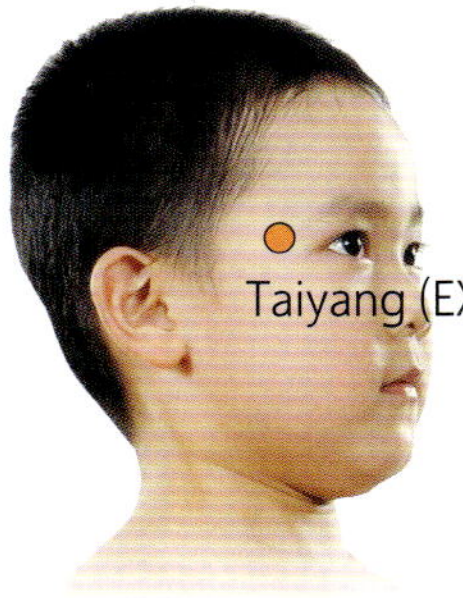

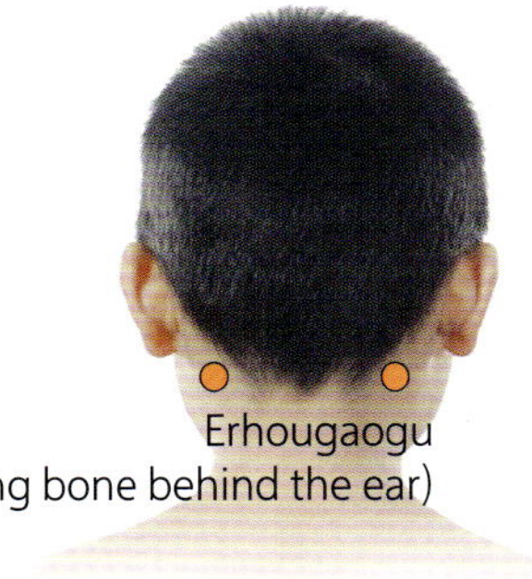

Massage Manipulations

Open Tianmen (Heaven gate, BL2): Push directly and alternatively from bottom to top with the 2 thumbs for 30 times.
Push Kangong (House of water): Push from the brow tip to the brow end with the 2 thumbs for each side for 30 times, also called Yin and Yang seperation.
Knead Taiyang (EX-HN5): Knead the point with the finger pulp of the thumb or index finger for respective 30 times in both sides of the head.
Knead Erhougaogu (Protruding bone behind the ear): Knead the point with the finger pulp of the thumb or index finger for respective 30 times in both sides of the head.

2 Fever

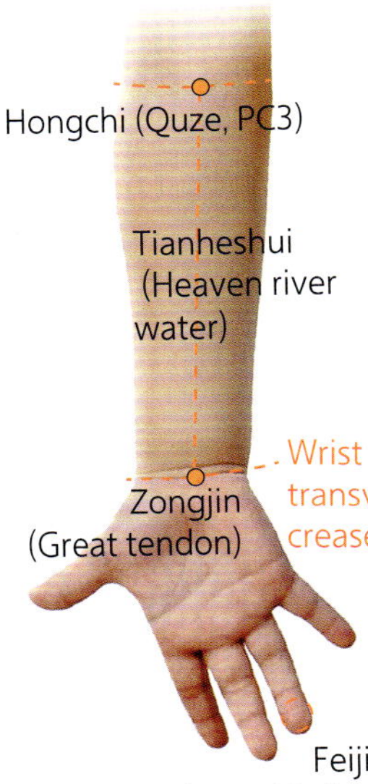

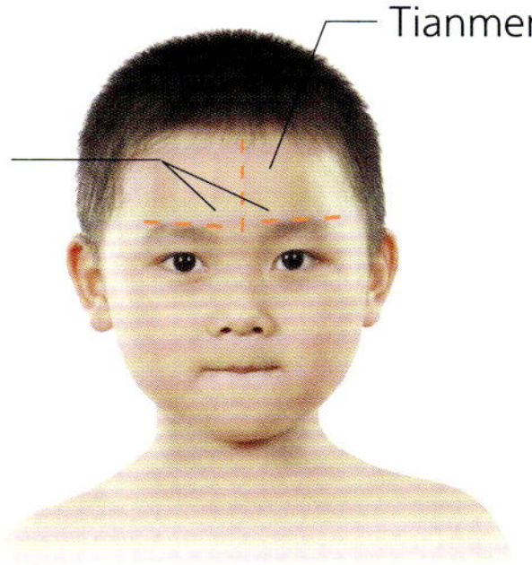

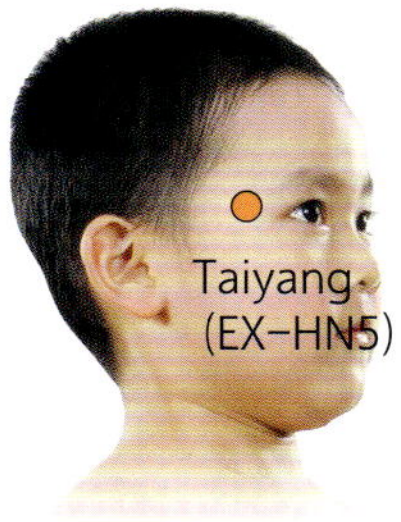

Classic Acupoints Matching

Tianmen (Heaven gate, BL2): The line between the midpoint of the 2 eyebrows and the anterior hairline.
Kangong (House of water): The transverse line starting from the brow tip to the brow end.
Taiyang (EX-HN5): The midpoint of the line between the brow tip to the outer canthus.
Feijing (Lung Meridian): The finger pulp of the distal segment of ring finger.
Tianheshui (Heaven river water): In the middle of the palm-side of the forearm, the line between the midpoint of the transverse crease of wrist and the midpoint of the cubital transverse crease.

Massage Manipulations

Open Tianmen (Heaven gate, BL2): Push directly and alternatively from bottom to top with the 2 thumbs for 50 times.
Push Kangong (House of water): Push from the tip to end of the eyebrow with the 2 thumbs for 50 times, also called Yin and Yang separation.
Knead Taiyang (EX-HN5): Knead the point with the finger pulp of the thumb or index finger for respective 50 times in both sides of the head.
Clear Feijing (Lung Meridian): Push from the fingerprint of the distal segment of ring finger in the palm-side to the tip of ring finger.
Clear Tianheshui (Heaven river water): Push upward from the transverse crease of wrist to the cubital transverse crease with the index and middle fingers for 300 times.

3 惊风

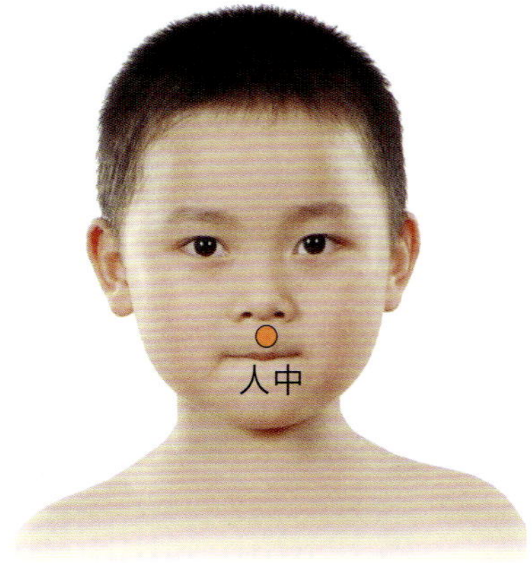

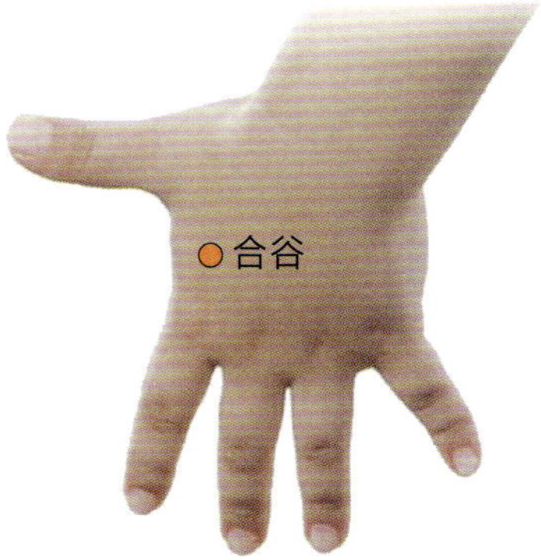

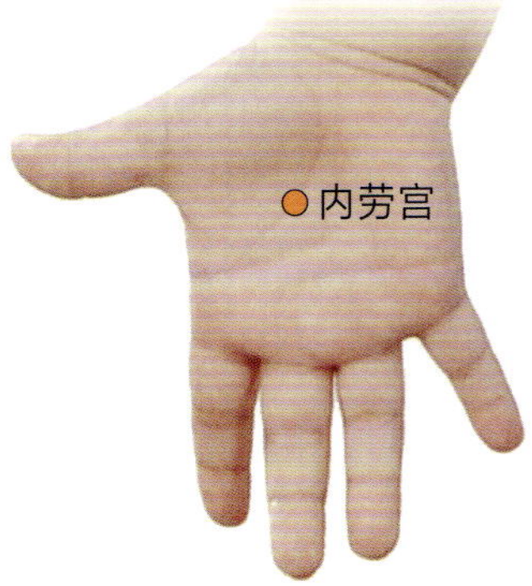

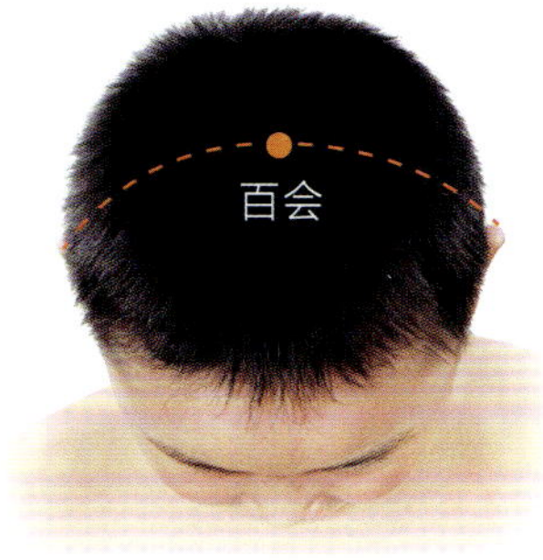

经典配穴

人中：人中沟上1/3与下2/3交界处。
内劳宫：掌心，握拳时中指、无名指指端中点所在处。
百会：头顶正中线与两耳尖连线的交叉点。
合谷：手背第1、2掌骨之间，约平第2掌骨中点处。

按摩操作

掐人中：用拇指指甲掐，掐50次。
揉内劳宫：用中指指端揉，揉150次。
按压百会：用拇指指腹按压，按100次。
揉合谷：用拇指指腹揉，揉100次。

4 咳嗽

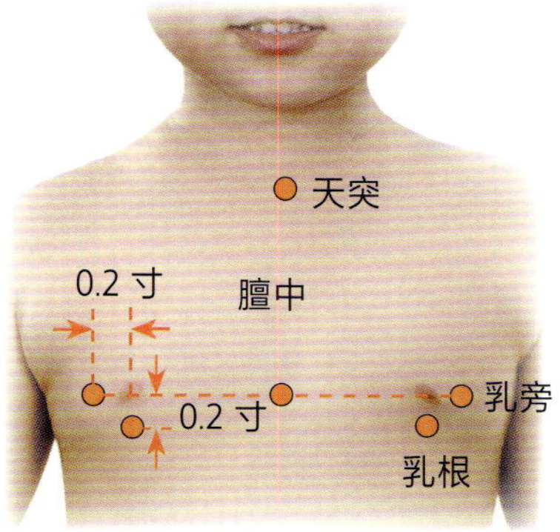

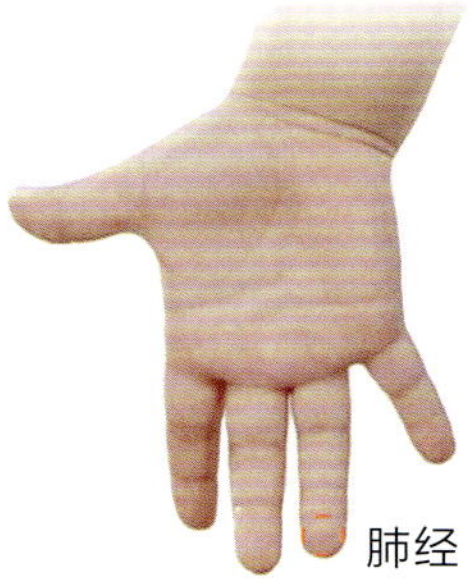

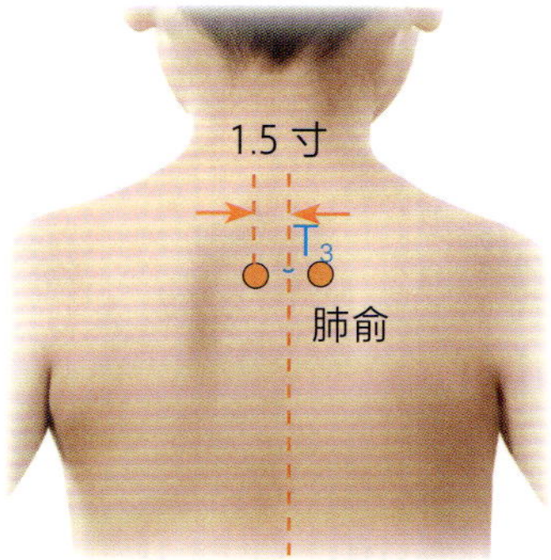

经典配穴

肺经：无名指末节指腹。
天突：胸骨上窝正中。
膻中：两乳头连线的中点。
乳旁：乳头外旁开0.2寸。
乳根：第5肋间隙，乳头直下0.2寸。
肺俞：第3胸椎棘突下，旁开1.5寸处。

按摩操作

清肺经：从无名指掌面末节指纹向指尖方向推，推100次。
按天突：用食指指腹按压，按压5分钟。
推膻中：用食指、中指两指自胸骨切迹向下推至剑突，推150次。
揉乳旁：用两手食指指腹揉，揉20次。
揉乳根：用两手食指指腹揉，揉20次。
揉肺俞：用两手拇指或食指指腹揉，以透热为度。

3 Infantile Convulsion

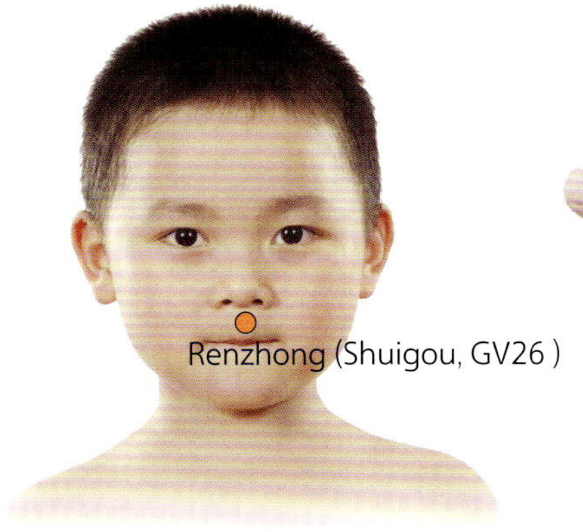

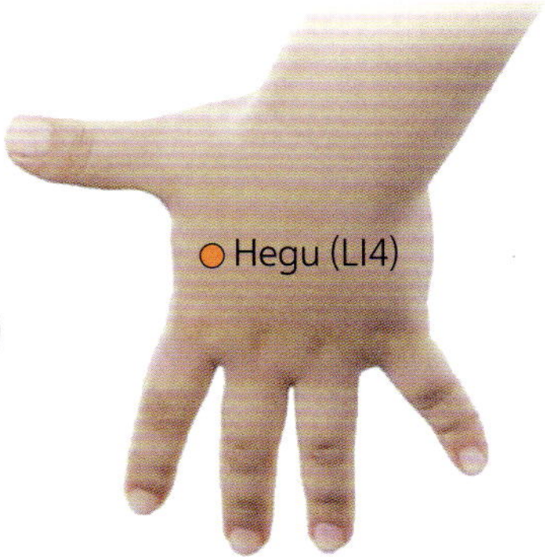

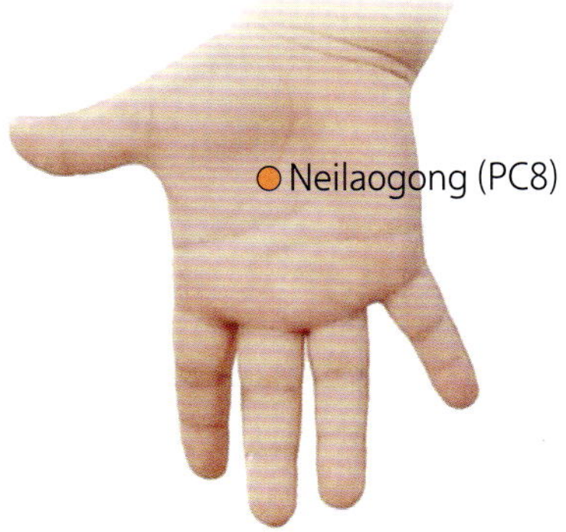

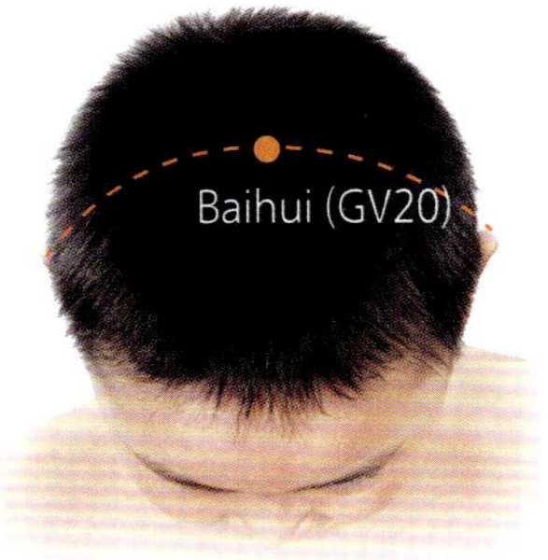

Classic Acupoints Matching

Renzhong (Shuigou GV26): At the junction of the upper 1/3 and lower 2/3 of the philtrum.
Neilaogong (PC8): In the center of the palm, at the midpoint of the tip of middle and ring fingers when clench fist.
Baihui (GV20): The crossing point of the midline of the vertex and the line of the 2ears tips.
Hegu (LI4): Between the 1st and the 2nd metacarpal bones on the dorsum of hand, at around the midpoint of the radial side of the 2nd metacarpal bone.

Massage Manipulations

Pinch Renzhong (Shuigou GV26): Pinch the point with the nail of the thumb for 50 times.
Knead Neilaogong (PC8): Knead the point with the tip of middle finger for 150 times.
Press Baihui (GV20): Press the point with the finger pulp of the thumb for 100 times.
Knead Hegu (LI4): Knead the point with the finger pulp of the thumb for 100 times.

4 Cough

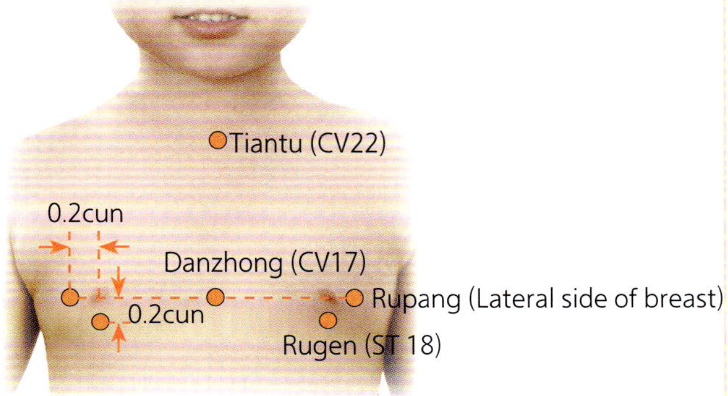

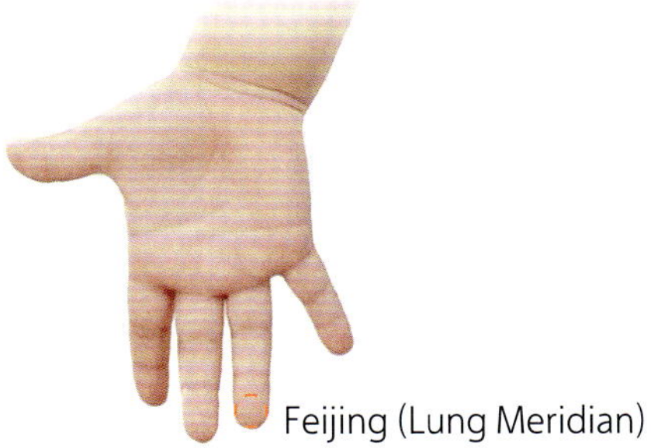

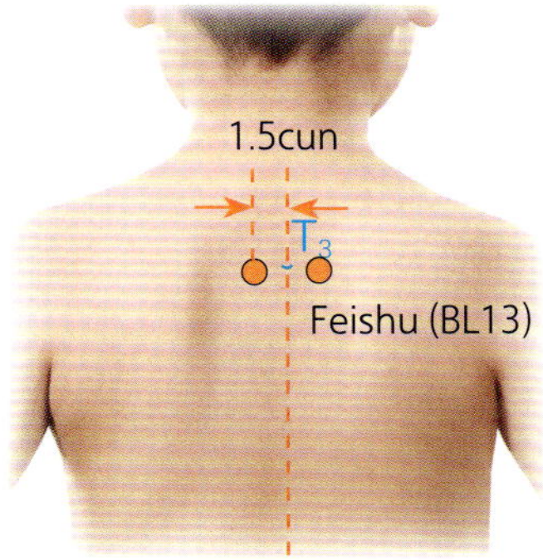

Classic Acupoints Matching

Feijing (Lung Meridian): The finger pulp of the distal segment of ring finger.
Tiantu (CV22): In the middle of suprasternal fossa.
Danzhong (CV17): At the midpoint of the line of the 2 nipples.
Rupang (Lateral side of breast): 0.2 cun lateral to the nipple.
Rugen (ST18): In the 5th intercostal space,directly below the nipples.
Feishu (BL13): 1.5 cun lateral to the depression below the spinous process of the 3rd thoracic vertebra.

Massage Manipulations

Clear Feijing (Lung Meridian): Push from the fingerprint of the distal segment of ring finger to the fingertip for 100 times.
Press Tiantu (CV22): Press the point with the finger pulp of the index finger for 5 minutes.
Push Danzhong (CV17): Push downward from the sterna notch to xiphoid process with the index and middle fingers for 150 times.
Knead Rupang (Lateral side of breast): Knead the point with the finger pulps of the index fingers of the 2 hands for 20 times.
Knead Rugen (ST18): Knead the point with the finger pulps of the index fingers of the 2 hands for 20 times.
Knead Feishu (BL13): Knead the point with the finger pulps of the thumbs or index fingers of the 2 hands until local skin feels warm.

5 扁桃体炎

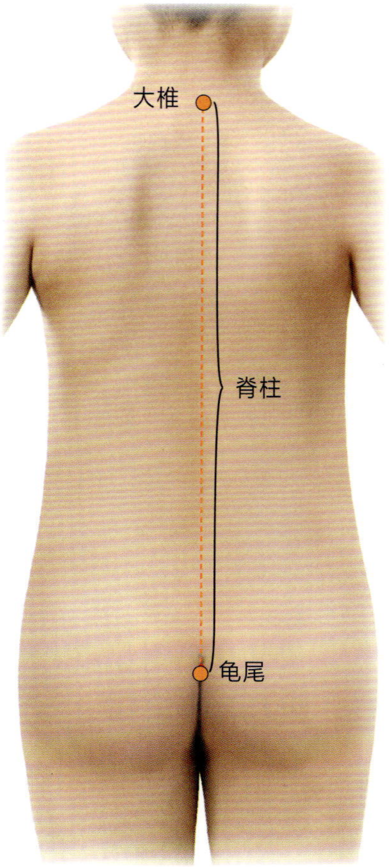

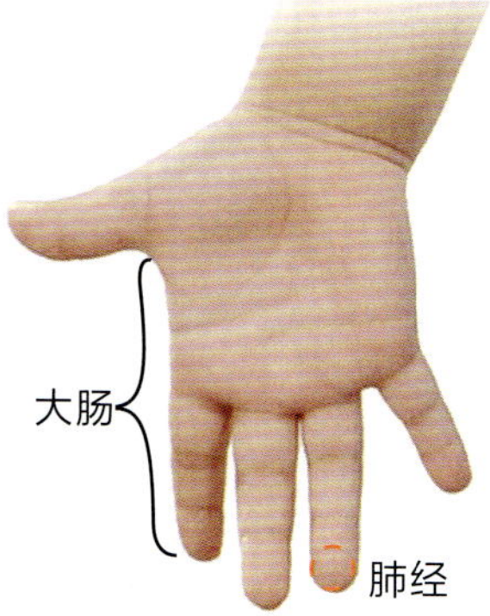

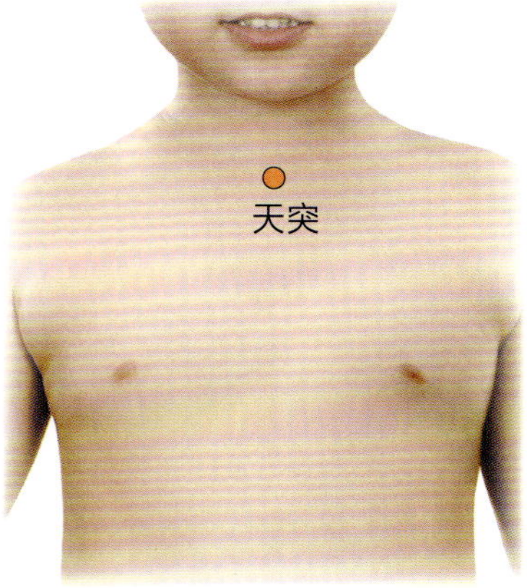

经典配穴

肺经：无名指末节指腹。
大肠：食指桡侧边缘，自指尖至虎口呈一直线。
天突：胸骨上窝正中。
脊柱：大椎至尾骨端呈一直线。

按摩操作

清肺经：从无名指掌面末节指纹向指尖方向推，推 200 次。
清大肠经：由虎口向指尖方向推，推 100 次。
揉天突：用食指指腹揉，揉 200 次。
捏脊：小儿俯卧，按摩者用双手拇指、食指自小儿腰骶部开始把皮肤捏起，自下而上捏提至大椎穴处。一般捏 3~5 遍，以脊柱两侧皮肤微有潮红为有效。

6 哮喘

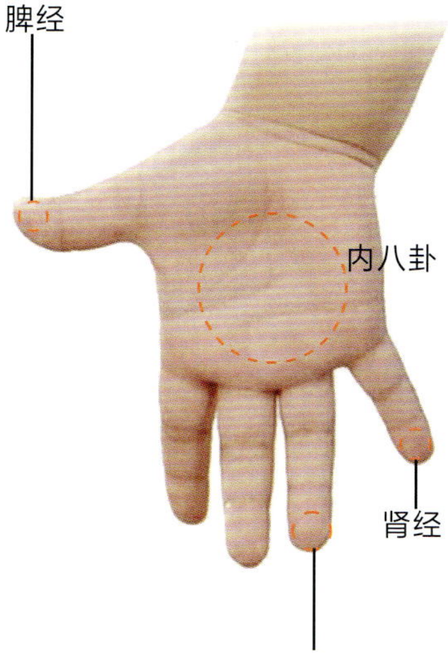

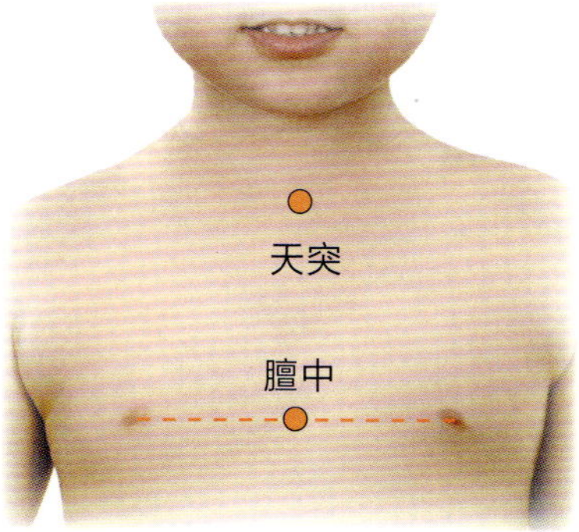

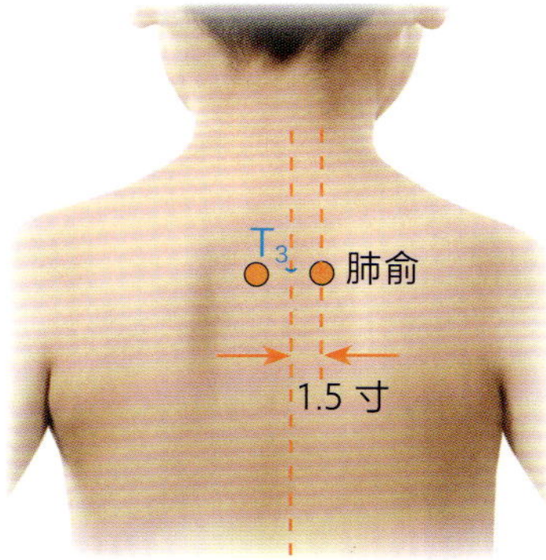

经典配穴

肺经：无名指末节指腹。
脾经：拇指末节指腹。
肾经：小指末节指腹。
内八卦：以掌心为圆心，从掌心到中指根横纹长度的 2/3 为半径所作圆周。
天突：胸骨上窝正中。
膻中：两乳头连线的中点。
肺俞：第 3 胸椎棘突下，旁开 1.5 寸处。

按摩操作

清肺经：从无名指掌面末节指纹向指尖方向推，推 200 次。
补脾经：从拇指指尖缘向指根方向直推，推 100 次。
补肾经：旋推或自指根直推至指尖，推 300 次。
运内八卦：用拇指甲沿顺时针方向掐运，运 200 次。
揉天突：用食指指腹揉，揉 50 次。
揉膻中：用食指指腹按揉，揉 50 次。
揉肺俞：用两手拇指或食指指腹揉，揉 50 次。

5 Tonsillitis

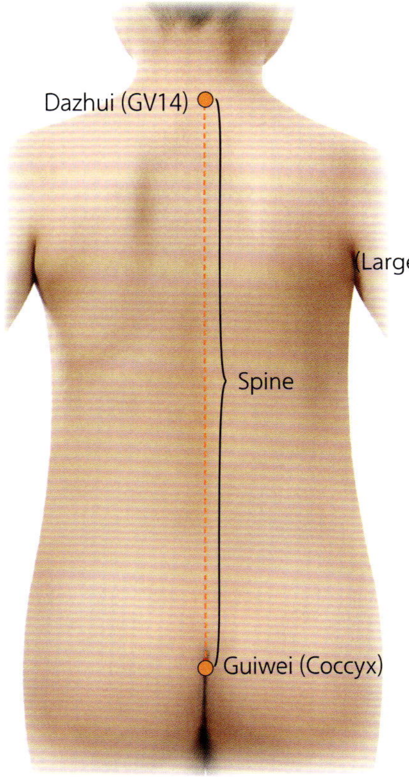

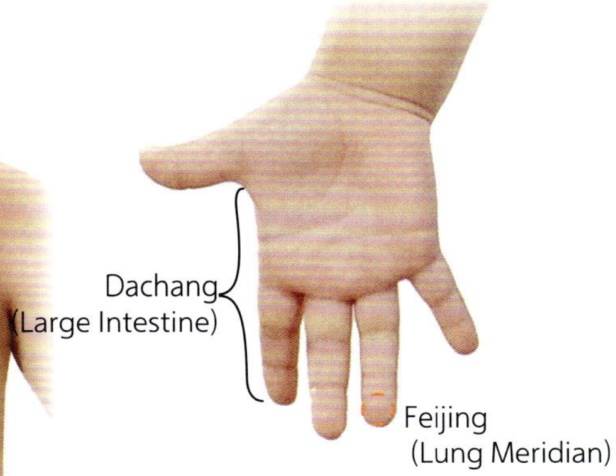

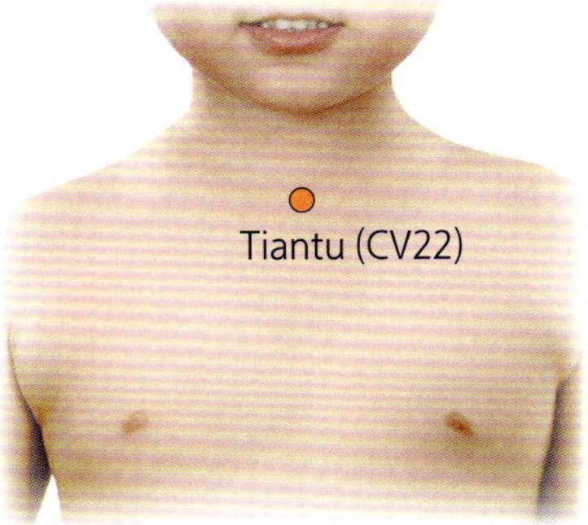

Classic Acupoints Matching

Feijing (Lung Meridian): The finger pulp of the distal segment of ring finger.
Dachang (Large Intestine): In the radial border of index finger, the line between the tip of index finger to Hukou (the part between the thumb and the index finger).
Tiantu (CV22): In the middle of suprasternal fossa.
Spine: The line between Dazhui (GV14) and the end of coccygeal bone.

Massage Manipulations

Clear Feijing (Lung Meridian): Push from the fingerprint of the distal segment of ring finger to the fingertip for 200 times.
Clear Dachangjing (Large Intestine Meridian): Push from Hukou(the part between the thumb and the index finger) to the fingertip for 100 times.
Knead Tiantu (CV22): Knead the point with the finger pulp of the index finger for 200 times.
Pinch Spine: Let the child lie in prone position. Pinch the skin from bottom to top with the thumb and index finger of 2 hands starting from the lumbosacral region to Dazhui (GV14) for generally 3 to 5 times until the skin in both sides of spine shows slightly flush.

6 Asthma

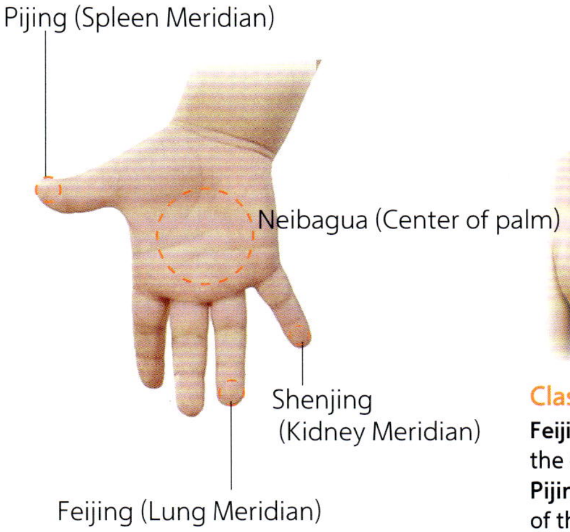

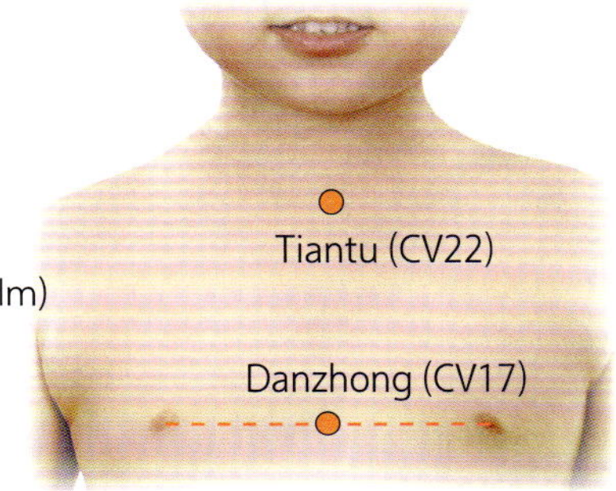

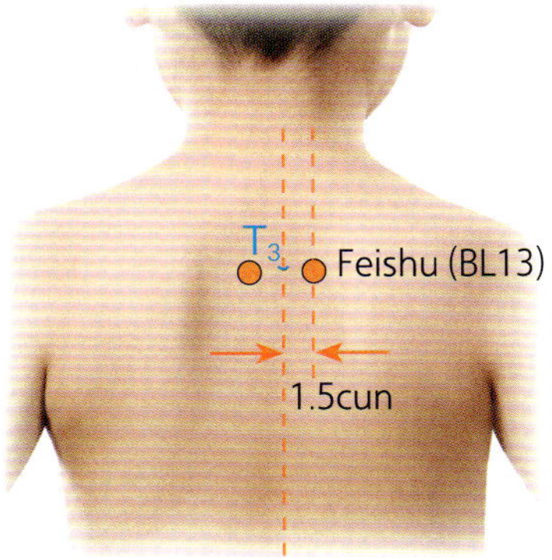

Classic Acupoints Matching

Feijing (Lung Meridian): The finger pulp of the distal segment of ring finger.
Pijing (Spleen Meridian): The finger pulp of the distal segment of the thumb.
Shenjing (Kidney Meridian): The finger pulp of the distal segment of little finger.
Neibagua (Center of palm): The circle with the center of the palm as the center of the circle, and the 2/3 of the length of the line between the center of the circle and the transverse crease of the root of middle finger as the radius.
Tiantu (CV22): In the middle of suprasternal fossa.
Danzhong (CV17): At the midpoint of the line of the 2 nipples.
Feishu (BL13): 1.5 cun lateral to the depression below the spinous process of the 3rd thoracic vertebra.

Massage Manipulations

Clear Feijing (Lung Meridian): Push from the fingerprint of the distal segment of ring finger to the fingertip for 200 times.
Tonify Pijing (Spleen Meridian): Push directly from the fingertip to the root of the thumb for 100 times.
Tonify Shenjing (Kidney Meridian): Rotate-push or push directly from the root to the tip of the finger for 300 times.
Circularly push Neibagua (Center of palm): Pinch-transport the point with the thumb nail clockwise for 200 times.
Knead Tiantu (CV22): Knead the point with the finger pulp of the index finger for 50 times.
Knead Danzhong (CV17): Press-knead the point with the finger pulp of the index finger for 50 times.
Knead Feishu (BL13): Knead the point with the finger pulps of the thumbs or index fingers of the 2 hands for 50 times.

7 过敏性鼻炎

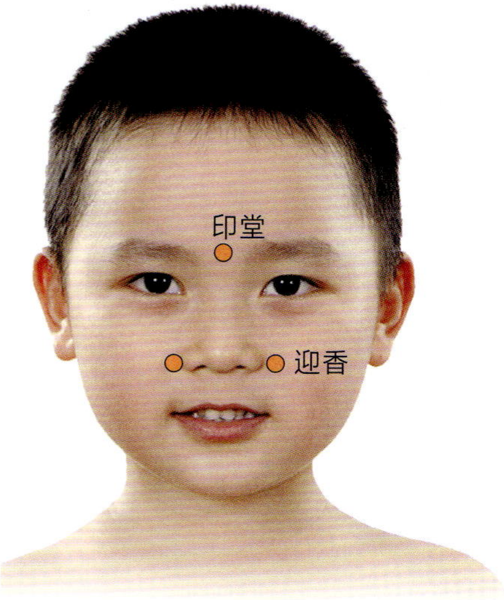

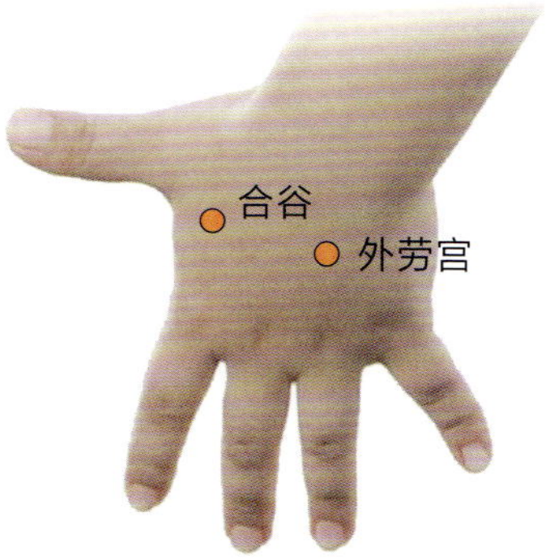

经典配穴

迎香：鼻翼旁0.5寸，鼻唇沟中。
印堂：两眉内侧端连线的中点处。
合谷：手背第1、2掌骨之间，约平第2掌骨中点处。
外劳宫：手背中央，与内劳宫相对。

按摩操作

按揉迎香：用食指、中指两指或两拇指指端按揉，揉200次。
推擦印堂：用拇指指端自眉心向上推至天庭，推100次。
掐揉合谷：用拇指指甲掐揉，掐揉100次。
揉外劳宫：用食指或者中指指端揉，揉100次。另外，可用拇指或食指搓擦两侧鼻翼100次，以局部产生温热感为度。

8 打嗝（呃逆）

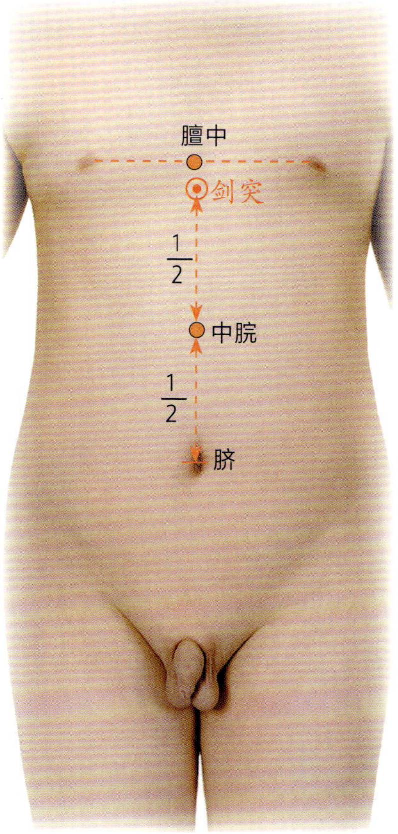

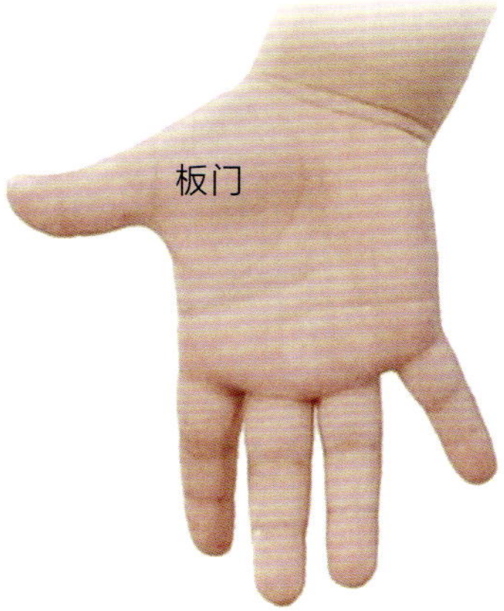

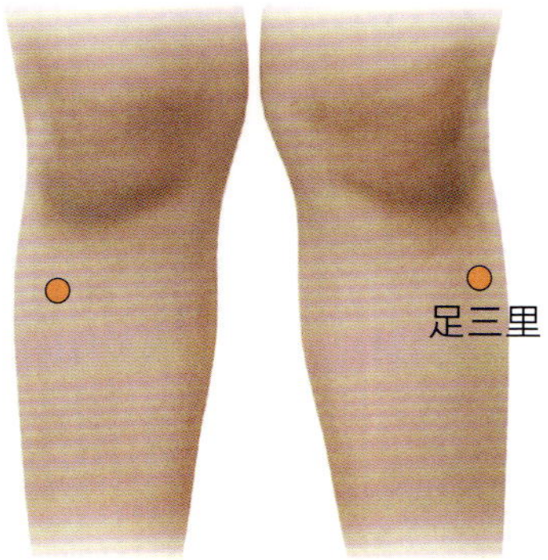

经典配穴

板门：手掌大鱼际处。
足三里：膝盖外侧凹陷直下3寸，胫骨旁1寸处。
膻中：两乳头连线的中点。
中脘：肚脐直上4寸处。

按摩操作

揉板门：用指端揉大鱼际，揉100次。
按揉足三里：以拇指指端按揉，揉100次。
揉膻中：用食指指腹按揉，揉100次。
揉中脘：用掌根按揉，揉50次。

7 Allergic Rhinitis

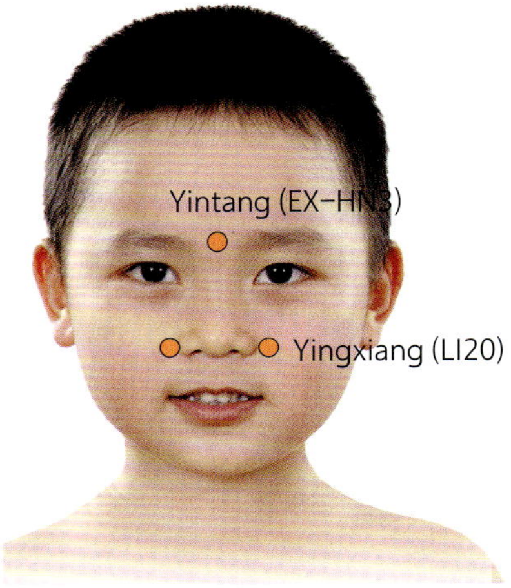

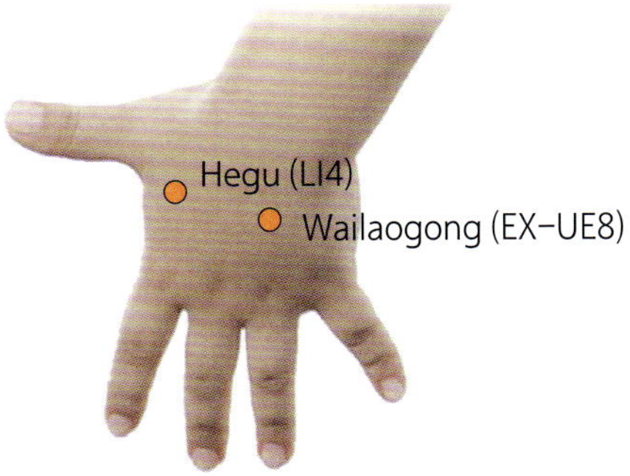

Classic Acupoints Matching

Yingxiang (LI20): 0.5 cun lateral to the nasal ala, in the nasolabial fold.
Yintang (EX-HN3): At the midpoint of the line between the medial side of the 2 eyebrows.
Hegu (LI4): Between the 1st and 2nd metacarpal bones on the dorsum of hand, at around the midpoint of the 2nd metacarpal bone.
Wailaogong (EX-UE8): In the center of the dorsum of hand, the opposite of Neilaogong (PC 8).

Massage Manipulations

Press-knead Yingxiang (LI20): Press-knead the point with tips of index and middle fingers or the fingertips of the 2 thumbs for 200 times.
Push-scrub Yintang (EX-HN3): Push upward from the middle of eyebrow to Tianting (BL 2) the middle of forehead with the fingertip of the thumb for 100 times.
Pinch-knead Hegu (LI4): Pinch-knead the point with the nail of the thumb for 100 times.
Knead Wailaogong (EX-UE8): Knead the point with the tip of index or middle finger for 100 times.
Besides, twist-scrub the both sides of nasal ala with the thumb or index finger for 100 times until the local skin feels warm.

8 Hiccup

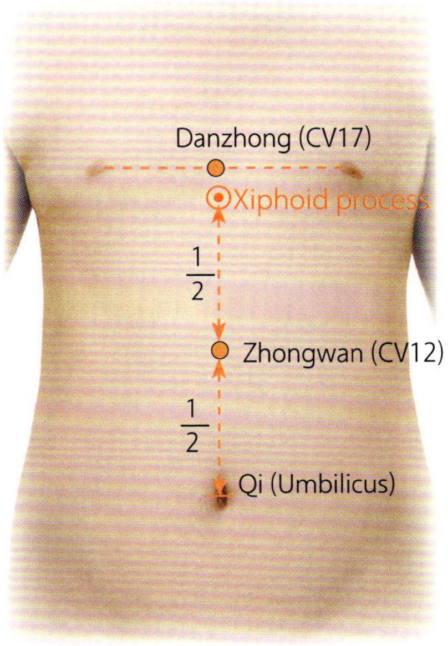

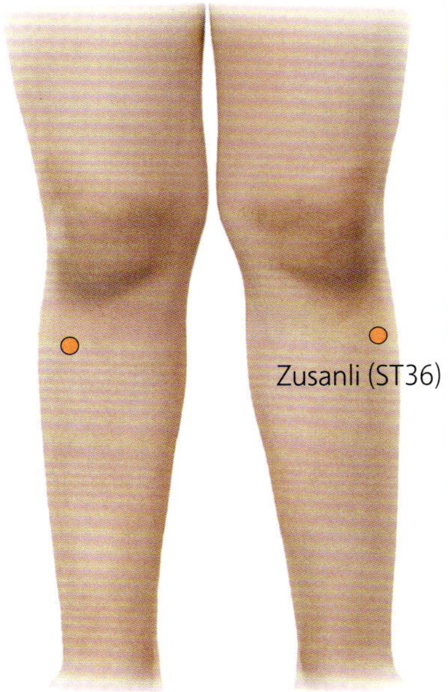

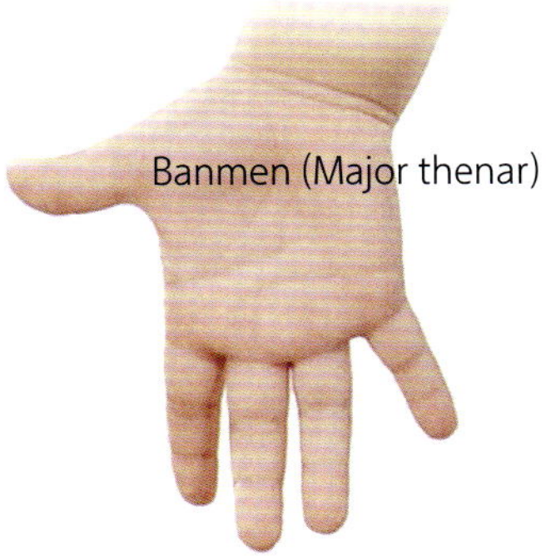

Classic Acupoints Matching

Banmen (Major thenar): At the great thenar of the palm.
Zusanli (ST36): 3 cun directly below the depression of the lateral side of the knee, 1 cun lateral to the tibia.
Danzhong (CV17): At the midpoint of the line between the 2 nipples.
Zhongwan (CV12): 4 cun directly above the umbilicus.

Massage Manipulations

Knead Banmen (Major thenar): Knead the great thenar with fingertips for 100 times.
Press-knead Zusanli (ST36): Press-knead the point with the fingertip of the thumb for 100 times.
Knead Danzhong (CV17): Press-knead the point with the finger pulp of the index finger for 100 times.
Knead Zhongwan (CV12): Press-knead the point with the root of palm for 50 times.

9 呕吐

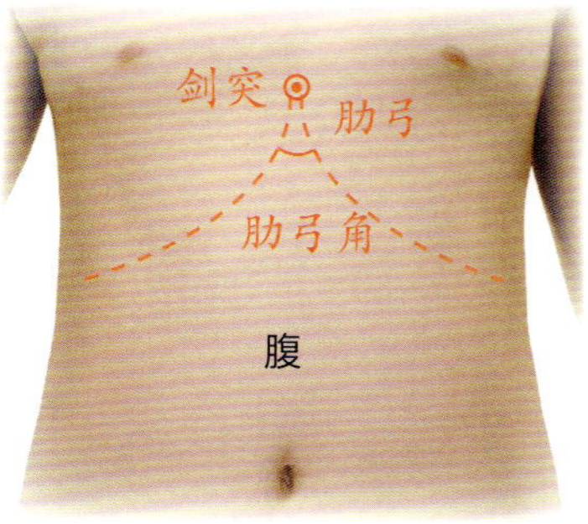

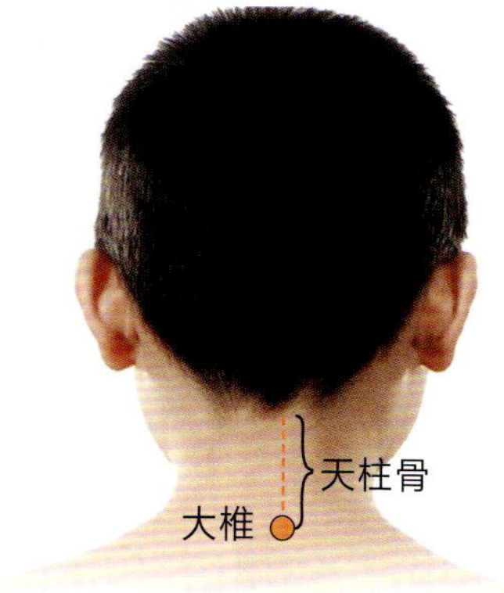

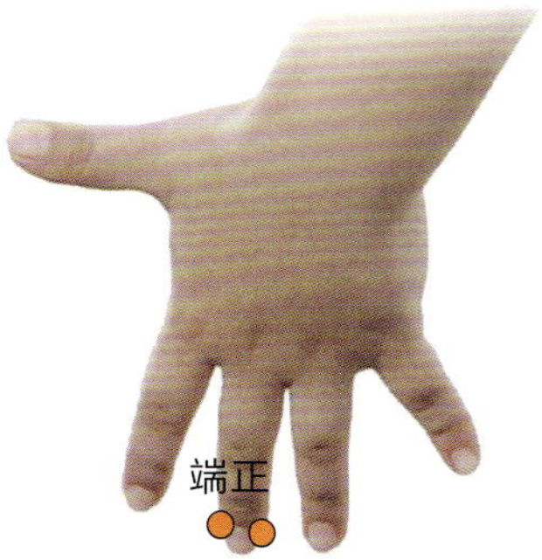

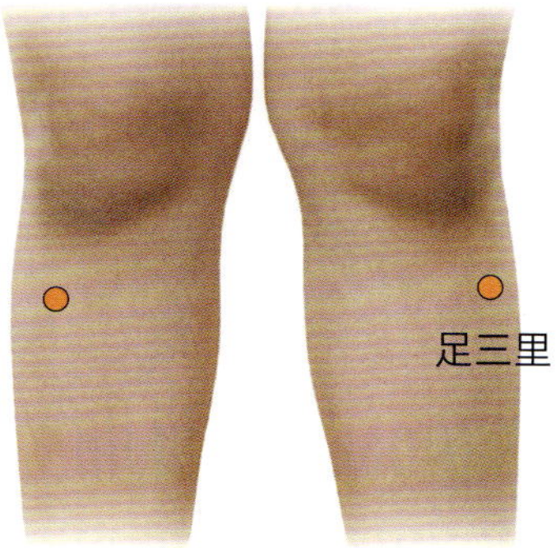

经典配穴

天柱骨：颈后发际正中至大椎穴呈一直线。

端正：中指甲根两侧赤白肉际处。桡侧称左端正，尺侧称右端正。

足三里：膝盖外侧凹陷直下3寸，胫骨旁1寸处。

腹：肋弓以下，肚脐以上。

按摩操作

推天柱骨：用拇指或食指自上向下直推，推100次。

掐揉端正：用拇指指甲掐5次，然后用拇指指腹揉50次。

按揉足三里：用拇指指端按揉，揉100次。

分推腹阴阳：用两拇指指腹沿肋弓角边缘向两旁分推，分推300次。

10 腹胀

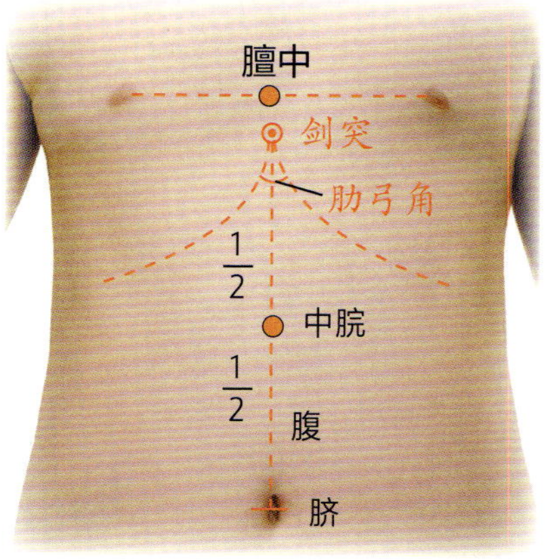

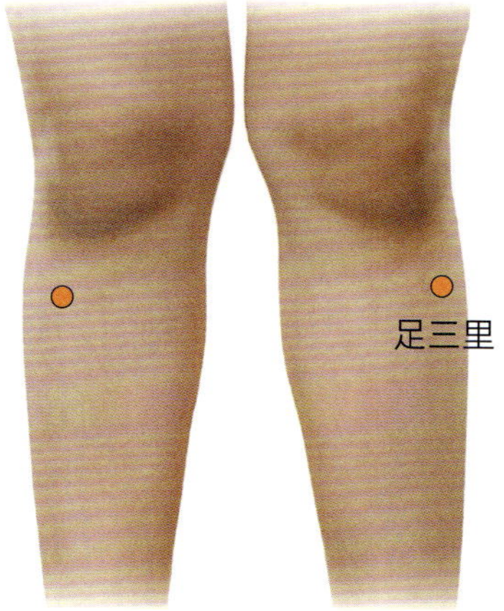

经典配穴

膻中：两乳头连线的中点。

腹：肋弓以下，肚脐以上。

中脘：肚脐直上4寸处。

足三里：膝盖外侧凹陷直下3寸，胫骨旁1寸处。

按摩操作

揉膻中：用食指指腹按揉，揉50次。

分推腹阴阳：用两拇指指腹沿肋弓角边缘向两旁分推，分推30次。

摩中脘：用掌心或四指摩，摩100次。

按揉足三里：用拇指指端按揉，揉50次。

9 Vomiting

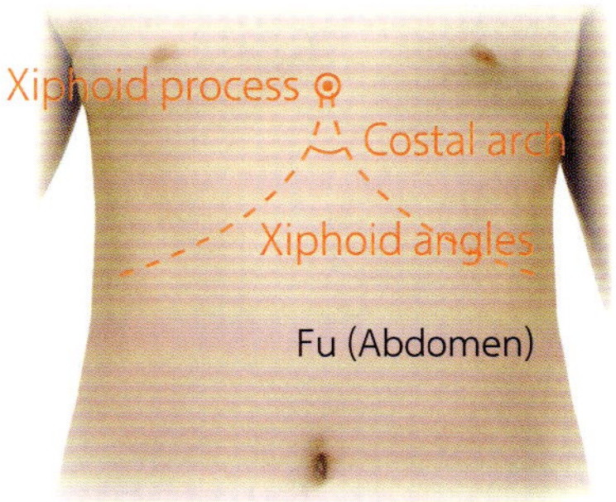

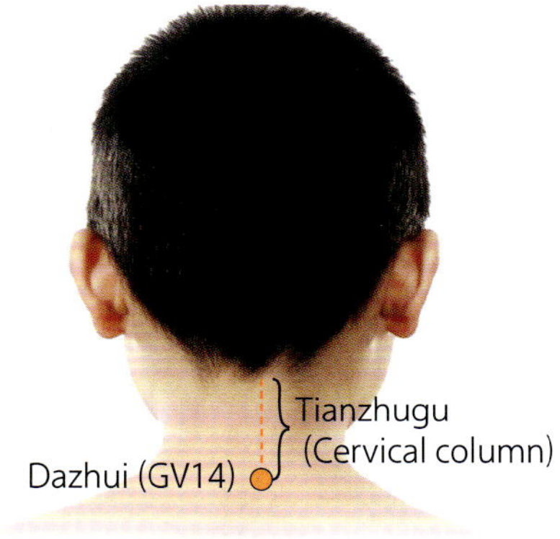

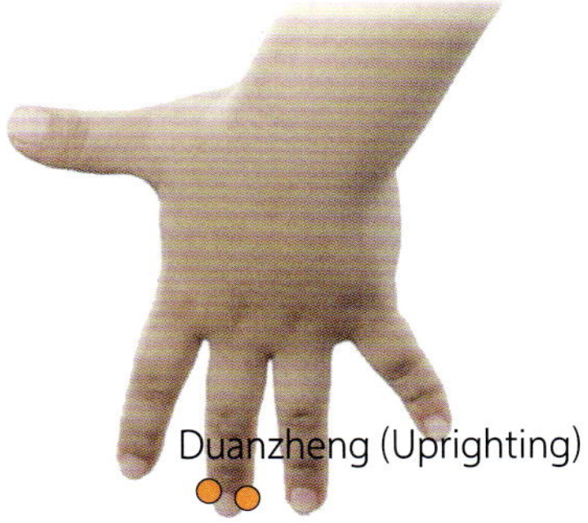

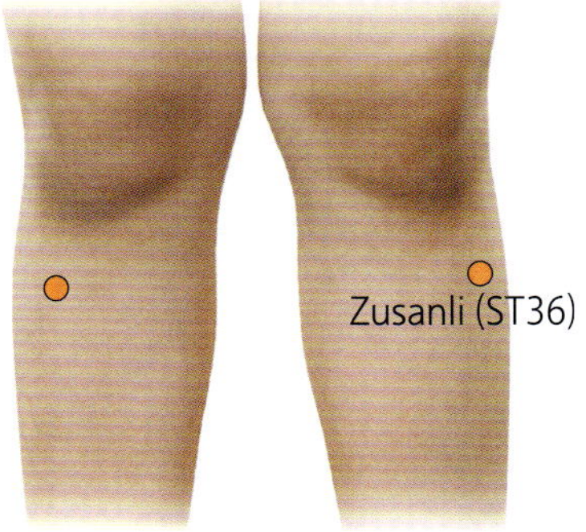

Classic Acupoints Matching

Tianzhugu (Cervical column): The straight line between the midpoint of the posterior hairline behind the neck and Dazhui (GV14).

Duanzheng (Uprighting): At the dorso-ventral boundary of both sides of the root of middle finger. The one in the radial side is called Left Duanzheng (Uprighting), while the one in the ulnar side is Right Duanzheng (Uprighting).

Zusanli (ST36): 3 cun directly below the depression of the lateral side of the knee, and 1 cun lateral to the tibia.

Fu (Abdomen): Below the costal arch, above the umbilicus.

Massage Manipulations

Push Tianzhugu (Cervical column): Push directly from top to bottom with the thumb or index finger for 100 times.

Pinch-knead Duanzheng (Uprighting): Pinch the point with the nail of the thumb for 5 times, and then knead the point with the finger pulp of the thumb for 50 times.

Press-knead Zusanli (ST36): Press-knead the point with the fingertip of the thumb for 100 times.

Part-push Yin and Yang of abdomen: Push along the border of xiphoid angles to both sides with the finger pulps of the 2 thumbs for 300 times respectively.

10 Abdominal Distension

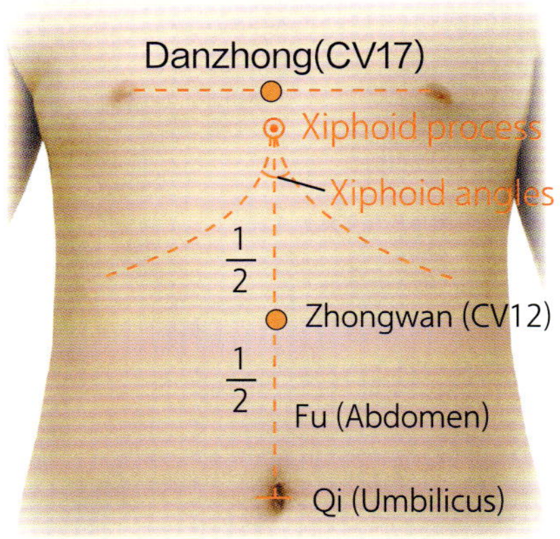

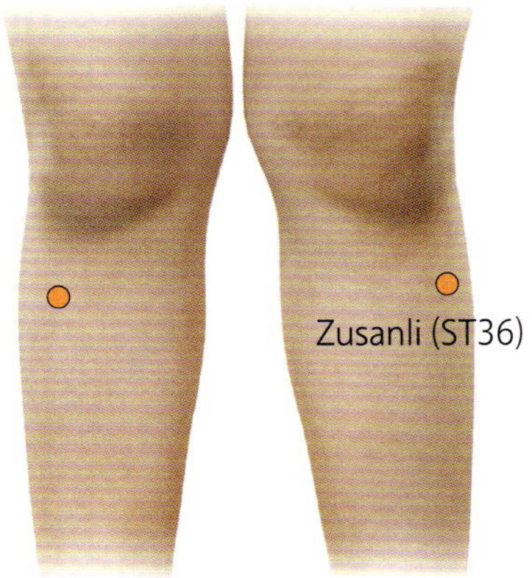

Classic Acupoints Matching

Danzhong (CV17): At the midpoint of the line between the 2 nipples.

Abdomen: Below the costal arch, above the umbilicus.

Zhongwan (CV12): 4 cun directly above the umbilicus.

Zusanli (ST36): 3 cun directly below the depression of the lateral side of the knee, 1 cun lateral to the tibia.

Massage Manipulations

Knead Danzhong (CV17): Press-knead the point with the finger pulp of the index finger for 50 times.

Part-push Yin and Yang of abdomen: Push along the border of xiphoid angles to both sides with the finger pulps of the 2 thumbs for 30 times.

Rub Zhongwan (CV12): Rub the point with the palm or the 4 fingers (index, middle, ring and little fingers) for 100 times.

Press-knead Zusanli (ST36): Press-knead the point with the fingertip of the thumb for 50 times.

11 腹痛

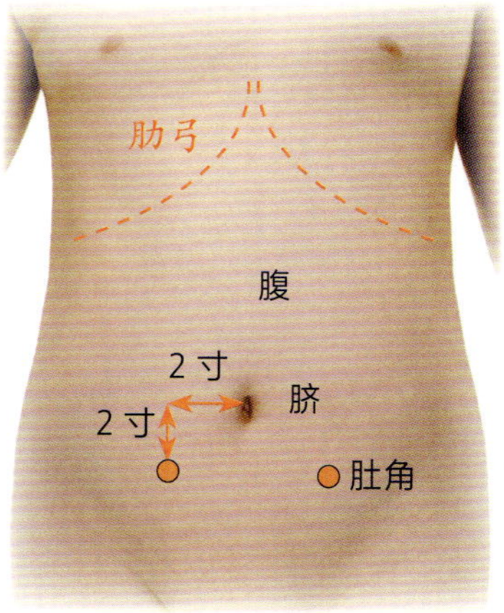

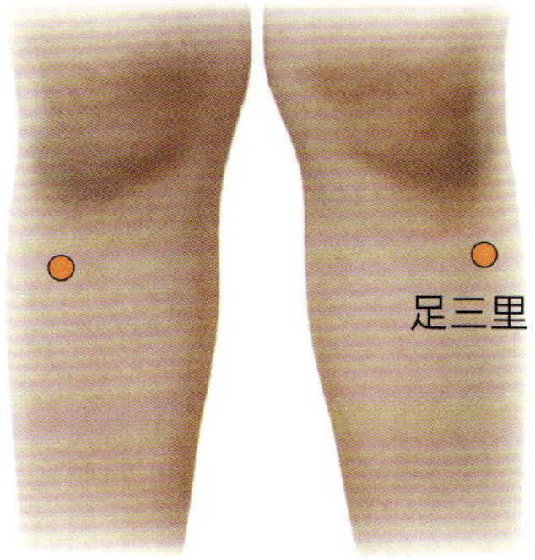

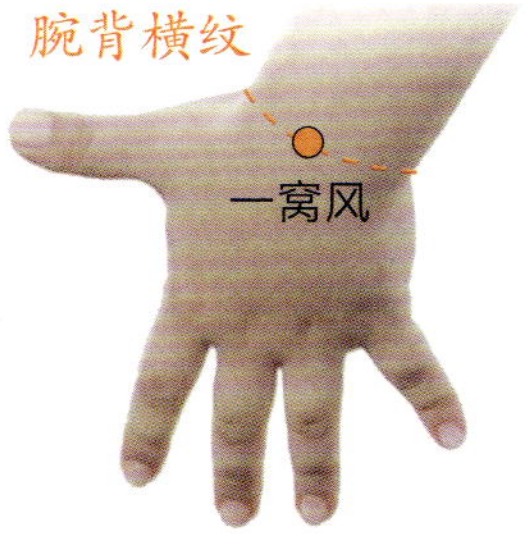

经典配穴

一窝风：手背腕横纹正中凹陷处。

足三里：膝盖外侧凹陷直下 3 寸，胫骨旁 1 寸处。

肚角：脐下 2 寸，旁开 2 寸两大筋上。

腹：肋弓以下，肚脐以上。

按摩操作

揉一窝风：用拇指或中指指端揉，揉 200 次。

揉足三里：用拇指指端按揉，揉 100 次。

拿肚角：小儿取仰卧位，按摩者用拇指、食指、中指三指向深处拿，拿 3 次。

摩腹：小儿仰卧，按摩者以全掌或食指、中指、无名指指腹摩上腹部，摩 3 分钟。

12 腹泻（泄泻）

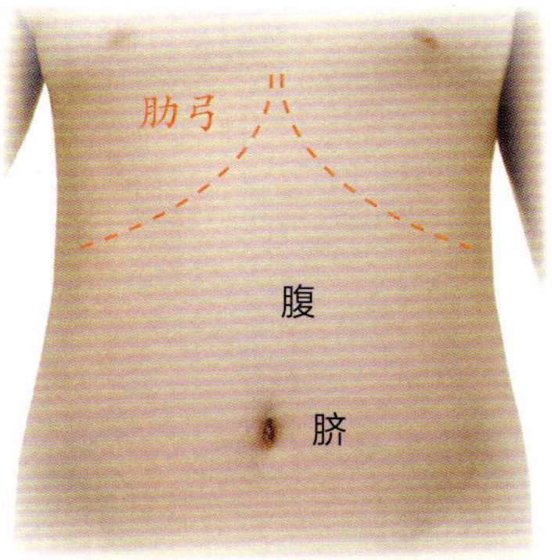

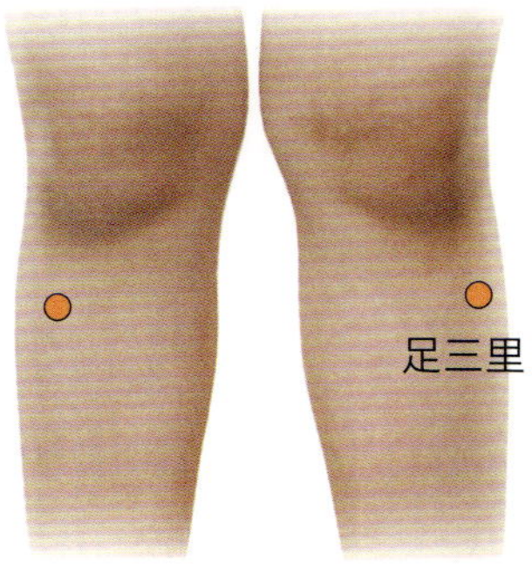

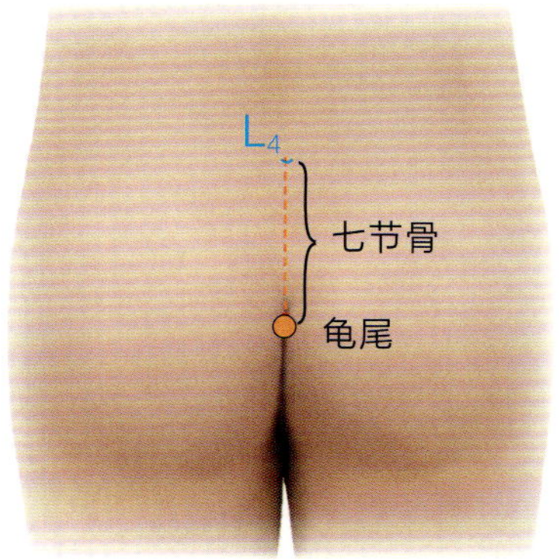

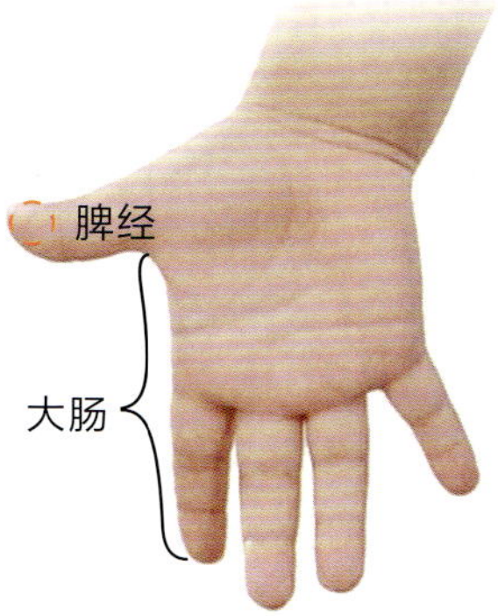

经典配穴

脾经：拇指末节指腹。

大肠：食指桡侧指尖至指根。

足三里：膝盖外侧凹陷直下 3 寸，胫骨旁 1 寸处。

腹：肋弓以下，肚脐以上。

脐：肚脐所在位置。

龟尾：尾椎骨处。

七节骨：第 4 腰椎至尾椎骨端呈一直线。

按摩操作

补脾经：从拇指指尖向指根方向直推，推 100 次。

补大肠：从食指指尖推向桡侧指根，推 100 次。

揉足三里：用拇指指端按揉，揉 100 次。

摩腹：小儿仰卧，按摩者以全掌或食指、中指、无名指指腹摩上腹部，摩 5 分钟。

揉脐：用掌根揉，揉 3 分钟。

揉龟尾：用拇指或中指指端揉，揉 100 次。

推上七节骨：用拇指指腹或食指、中指两指指腹自下而上作直推，推 100 次。

11 Abdominal Pain

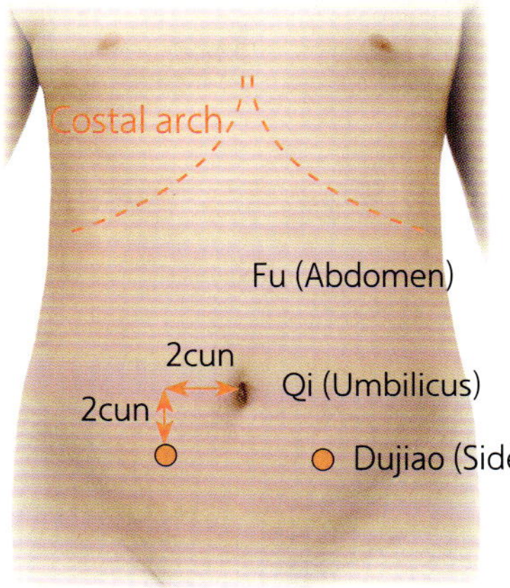

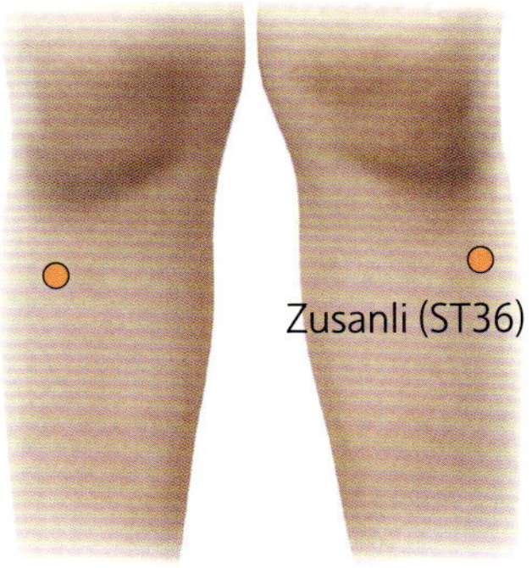

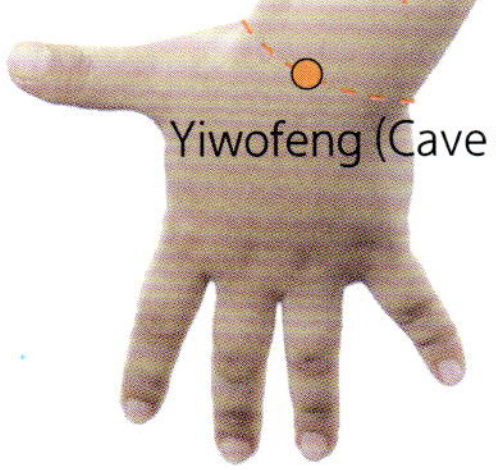

Classic Acupoints Matching

Yiwofeng (Cave of wind): In the depression of the middle of transverse crease of wrist on the dorsum of hand.

Zusanli (ST36): 3 cun directly below the depression of the lateral side of the knee, 1 cun lateral to the tibia.

Dujiao (Side of abdomen): 2 cun below the umbilicus, 2 cun lateral to the 2 great tendons.

Fu (Abdomen): Below the costal arch, above the umbilicus.

Massage Manipulations

Knead Yiwofeng (Cave of wind): Knead the point with the fingertip of the thumb or middle finger for 200 times.

Knead Zusanli (ST36): Press-knead the point with the fingertip of the thumb for 100 times.

Grasp Dujiao (Side of abdomen): Let the child lie in supine position. Grasp Dujiao (Side of abdomen) deeply with the thumb, index and middle fingers for 3 times.

Rub Fu (Abdomen): Let the child lie in supine position. Rub the upper abdomen with the whole palm or the finger pulp of index, middle and ring fingers for 3 minutes.

12 Diarrhea

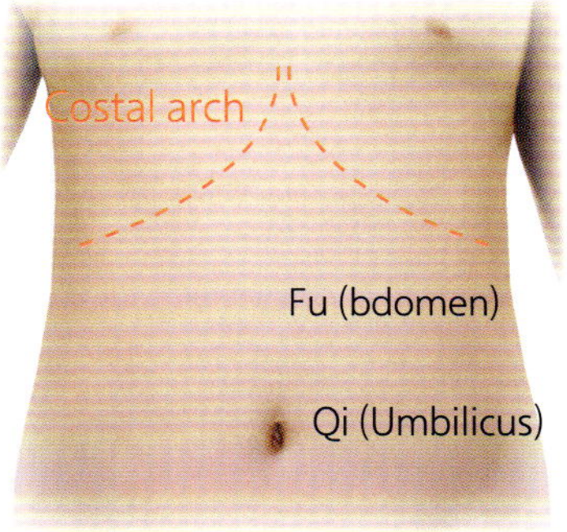

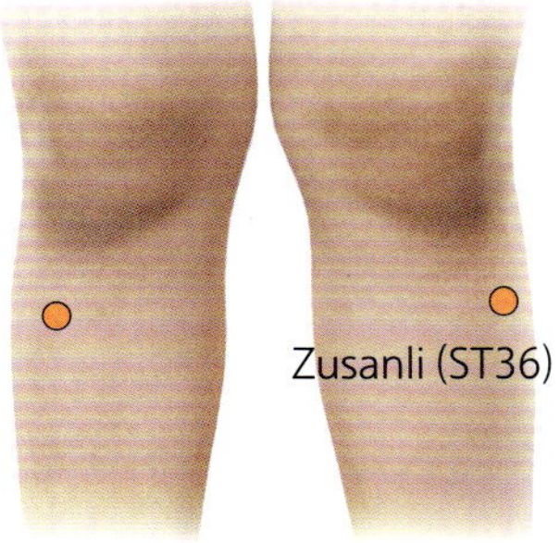

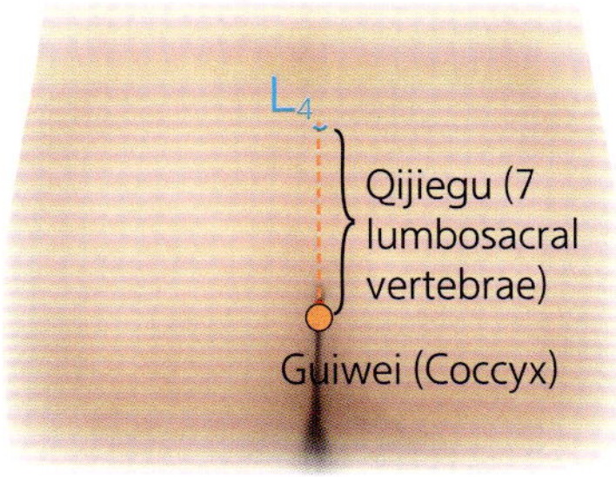

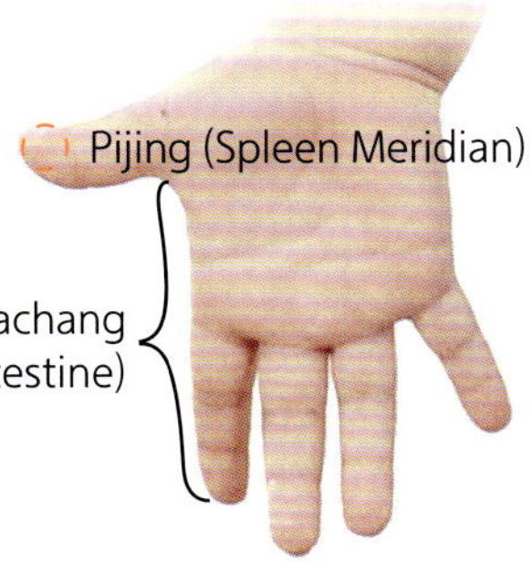

Classic Acupoints Matching

Pijing (Spleen Meridian): The finger pulp of the distal segment of thumb.

Dachang (Large Intestine): The tip to root of the radial side of the index finger.

Zusanli (ST36): 3 cun directly below the depression of the lateral side of the knee, 1 cun lateral to the tibia.

Fu (Abdomen): Below the costal arch, above the umbilicus.

Qi (Umbilicus): At the location of umbilicus.

Guiwei (Coccyx): At the coccygeal vertebra.

Qijiegu (7 lumbosacral vertebrae): The line between the 4th lumbar vertebra and the end of coccygeal vertebra.

Massage Manipulations

Tonify Pijing (Spleen Meridian): Push directly Pijing (Spleen Meridian) from the tip to the root of the thumb for 100 times.

Tonify Dachang (Large Intestine): Push from the tip of index finger to the root in the radial side for 100 times.

Knead Zusanli (ST36): Press-knead the point with the fingertip of the thumb for 100 times.

Rub Fu (Abdomen): Let the child lie in supine position. Rub the upper abdomen with the whole palm or the finger pulp of index, middle and ring fingers for 5 minutes.

Knead Qi (Umbilicus): Knead Qi (Umbilicus) with the root of palm for 3 minutes.

Knead Guiwei (Coccyx): Knead the point with the fingertip of thumb or middle finger for 100 times.

Push Upper Qijiegu (7 lumbrosacral vertebrae): Push directly from bottom to top with the finger pulp of the thumb or the finger pulps of index and middle fingers for 100 times.

13 便秘

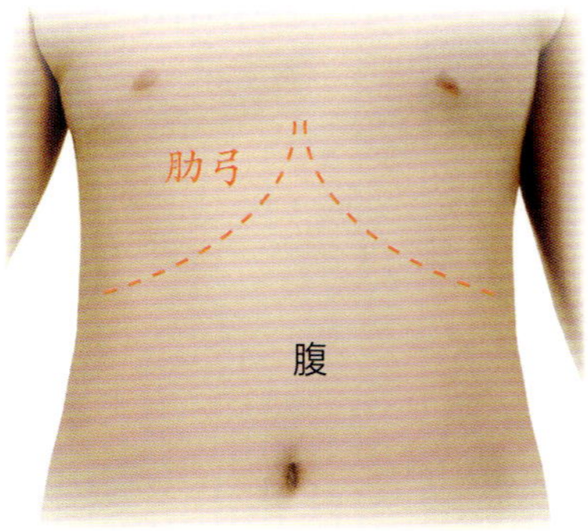

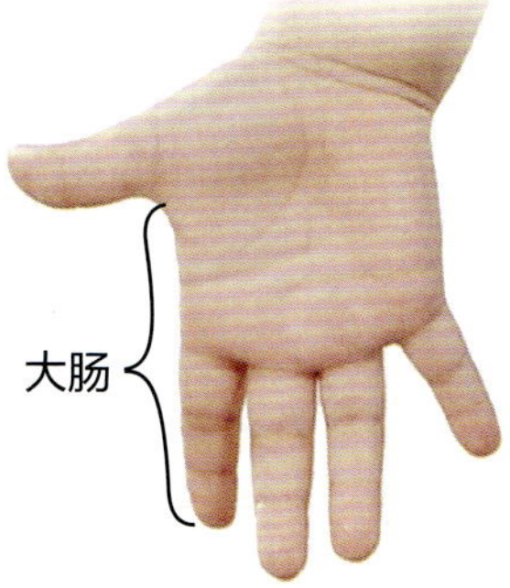

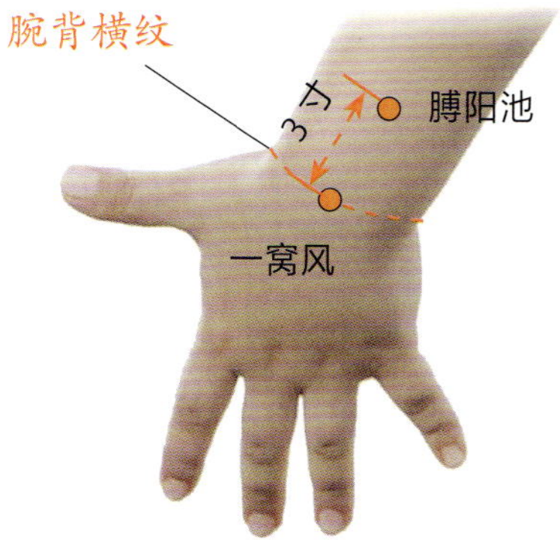

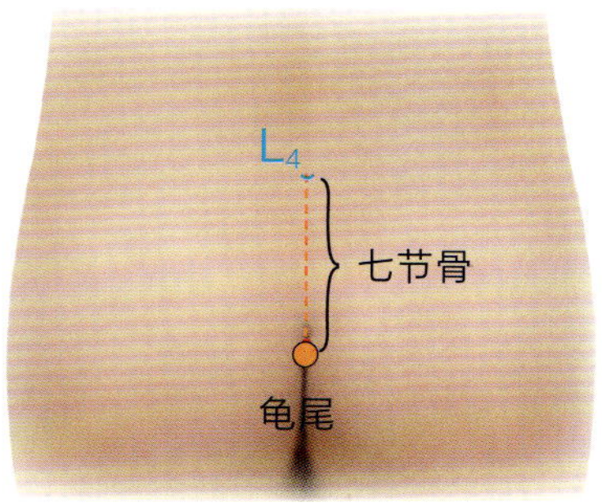

经典配穴

大肠：食指桡侧边缘，自指尖至虎口呈一直线。

膊阳池：在手背，一窝风后3寸处。

腹：肋弓以下，肚脐以上。

龟尾：尾椎骨处。

七节骨：第4腰椎至尾椎骨端呈一直线。

按摩操作

清大肠：从食指桡侧指根推向指尖，推100次。

按揉膊阳池：用指端按揉，揉50次。

摩腹：小儿仰卧，按摩者以全掌或食指、中指、无名指指腹摩上腹部，摩5分钟。

揉龟尾：用拇指或中指指端揉，揉100次。

推下七节骨：用拇指指腹或食指、中指两指指腹自上而下作直推，推100次。

14 厌食症

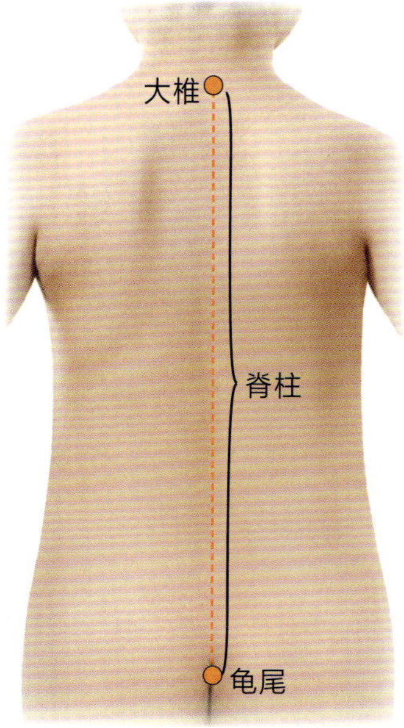

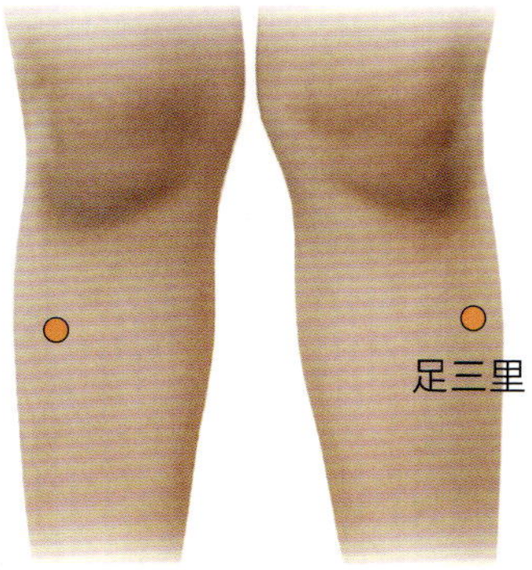

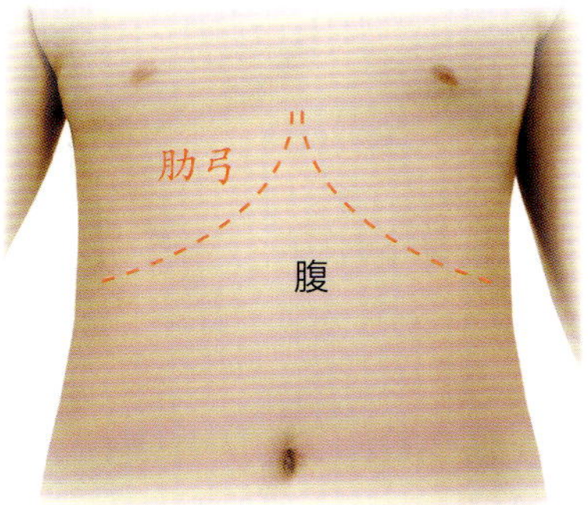

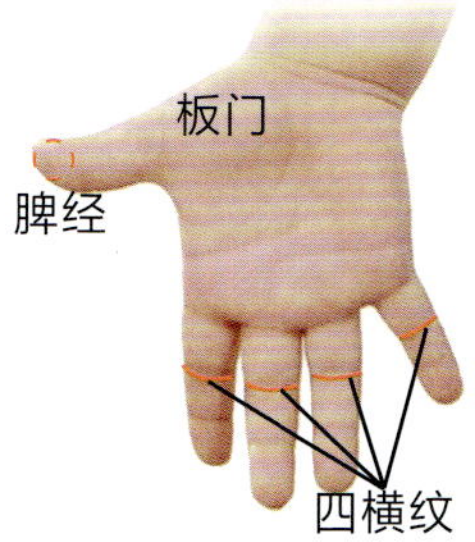

经典配穴

脾经：拇指末节指腹。

板门：手掌大鱼际处。

四横纹：掌面食指至小指，第2指间关节横纹处。

足三里：膝盖外侧凹陷直下3寸，胫骨旁1寸处。

腹：肋弓以下，肚脐以上。

脊柱：大椎至尾骨端呈一直线。

按摩操作

补脾经：从拇指指尖向指根方向直推，推300次。

揉板门：用指端揉大鱼际，揉100次。

推四横纹：小儿四指并拢，自小儿食指中节横纹推向小指中节横纹，推50次。

按揉足三里：用拇指指腹按揉，揉100次。

摩腹：小儿仰卧，按摩者以全掌或食指、中指、无名指指腹摩上腹部，摩100次。

捏脊：小儿俯卧，按摩者用双手拇指、食指自小儿腰骶部开始把皮肤捏起，自下而上捏提至大椎穴处。捏5遍，至脊柱两侧皮肤微有潮红。

13 Constipation

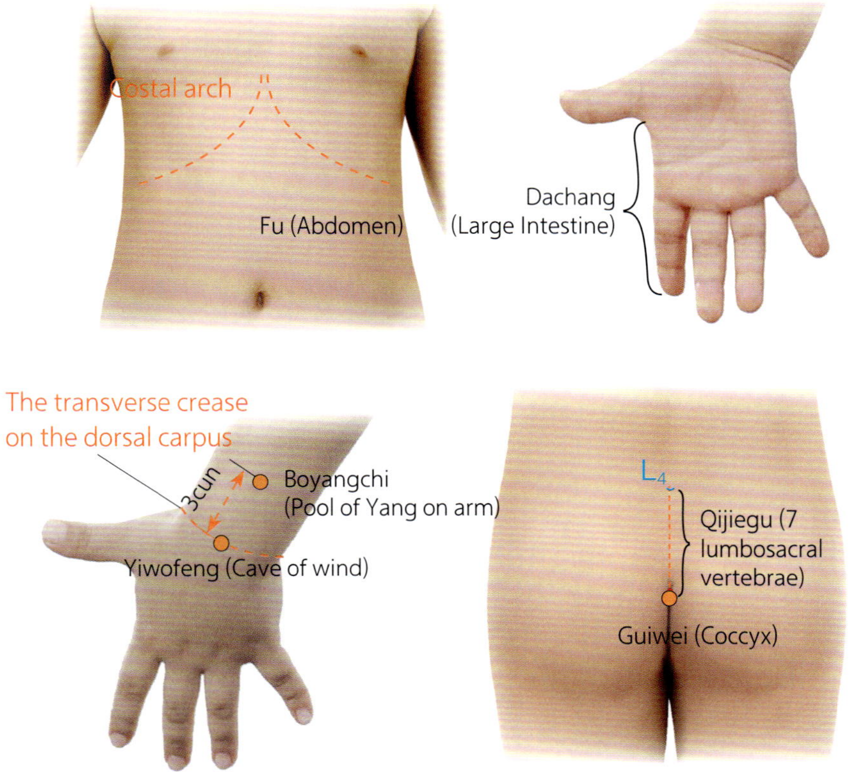

Classic Acupoints Matching

Dachang (Large Intestine): In the radial border of index finger, the line between the fingertip to Hukou (the part between the thumb and the index finger).
Boyangchi (Pool of Yang on arm): On the dorsum of hand, 3 cun behind Yiwofeng (Cave of wind).
Fu (Abdomen): Below the costal arch, above the umbilicus.
Guiwei (Coccyx): At the coccygeal vertebrae.
Qijiegu (7 lumbosacral vertebrae): The line between the 4th lumbar vertebra and the end of coccygeal vertebra.

Massage Manipulations

Clear Dachang (Large Intestine): Push from the root to tip of the radial side of index finger for 100 times.
Press-knead Boyangchi (Pool of Yang on arm): Press-knead Boyangchi (Pool of Yang on arm) with the fingertip for 50 times.
Rub Fu (Abdomen): Let the child lie in supine position. Rub the upper abdomen with the whole palm or the finger pulp of index, middle and ring fingers for 5 minutes.
Knead Guiwei (Coccyx): Knead the point with the fingertip of the thumb or middle finger for 100 times.
Push lower Qijiegu (7 lumbosacral vertebrae): Push directly from top to bottom with the finger pulp of the thumb or finger pulp of index and middle fingers for 100 times.

14 Anorexia

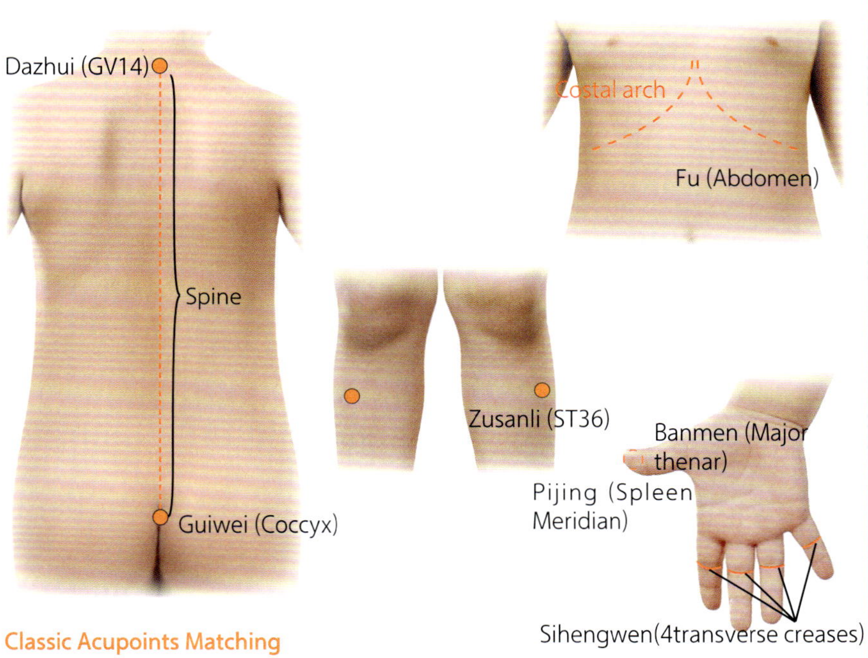

Classic Acupoints Matching

Pijing (Spleen Meridian): The finger pulp of the distal segment of the thumb.
Banmen (Major thenar): At the great thenar of the palm.
Sihengwen (4 transverse creases): At the transverse striation of the 2nd interphalangeal joint of index, middle, ring and little fingers in the palm surface.
Zusanli (ST36): 3 cun directly below the depression of the lateral side of the knee, 1 cun lateral to the tibia.
Fu (Abdomen): Below the costal arch, above the umbilicus.
Spine: The line between Dazhui (GV14) and the end of coccygeal bone.

Massage Manipulations

Tonify Pijing (Spleen Meridian): Push directly Pijing (Spleen Meridian) from fingertip to the root of the thumb for 300 times.
Knead Banmen (Major thenar): Knead the greater thenar with the fingertip for 100 times.
Push Sihengwen (4 transverse creases): Let the child close 4 fingers. Push from the transverse crease of the median segment of index finger to the transverse crease of the median segment of little finger of the child for 50 times.
Press-knead Zusanli (ST36): Press-knead the point with the finger pulp of the thumb for 100 times.
Rub Fu(Abdomen): Let the child lie in supine position. Rub the upper abdomen with the whole palm or the finger pulp of index, middle and ring fingers for 100 times.
Pinch Spine: Let the child lie in prone position. Pinch the skin from bottom to top with the thumb and index finger of 2 hands starting from the lumbosacral region to Dazhui (GV14) for generally 5 times until the skin in both sides of spine shows slightly flush.

15 中耳炎

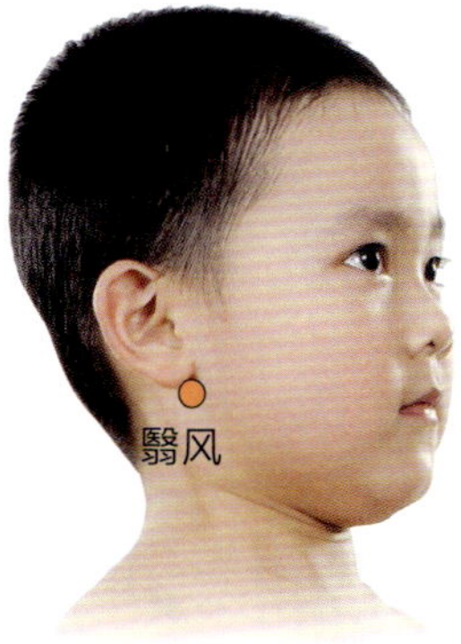

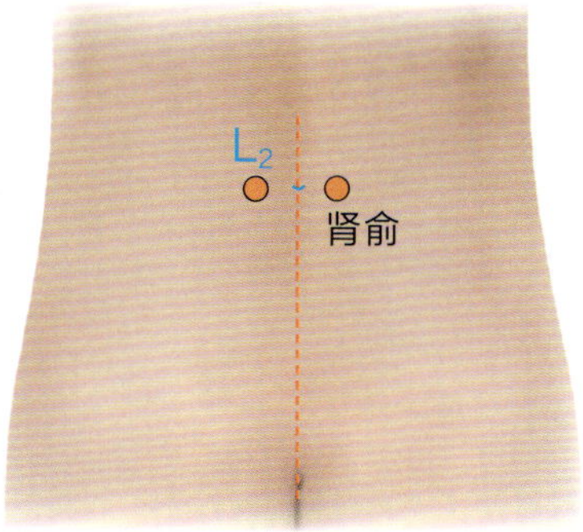

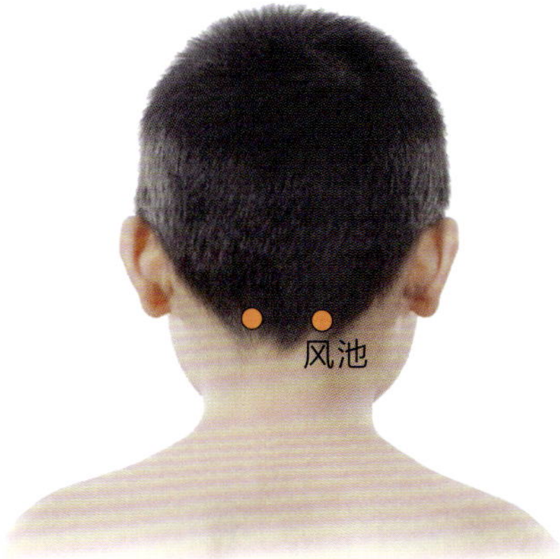

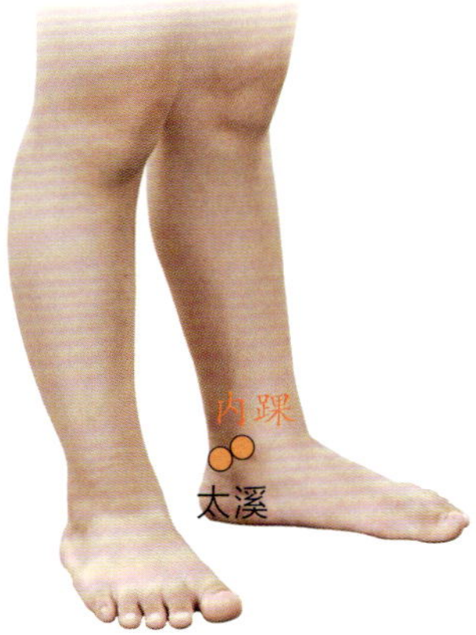

经典配穴

翳风：耳垂后，当乳突与下颌骨之间凹陷处。

太溪：足内踝尖与跟腱之间的凹陷处。

风池：颈后枕骨下大筋外侧凹陷中。

肾俞：第 2 腰椎棘突下，旁开 1.5 寸。

按摩操作

按翳风：用指端按，按 100 次。

按揉太溪：用食指指端按揉双侧穴位，按揉 150 次。

揉风池：用食指指端揉，揉 100 次。

揉肾俞：用两拇指指端揉两侧穴位，揉 100 次。

16 鼻出血

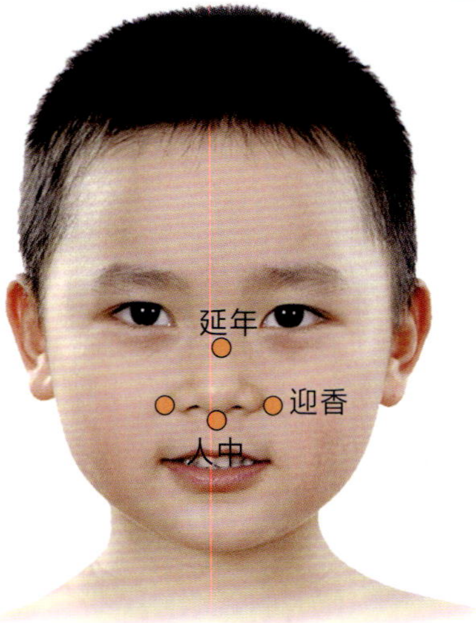

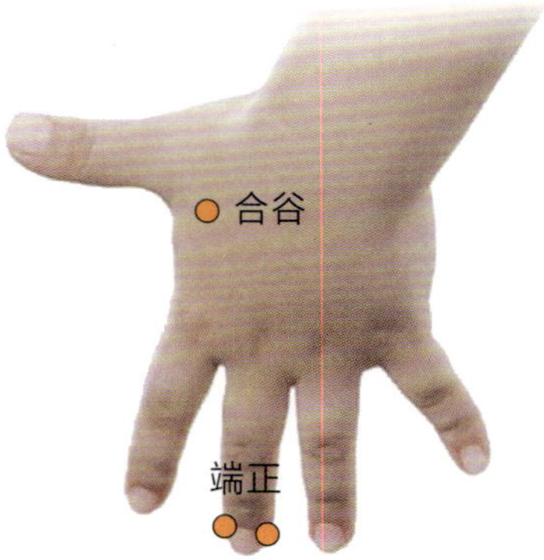

经典配穴

端正：中指甲根两侧赤白肉际处。桡侧称左端正，尺侧称右端正。

人中：人中沟上 1/3 与下 2/3 交界处。

延年：位于鼻梁骨高耸处，在山根穴与准头穴之间。

迎香：鼻翼旁 0.5 寸，鼻唇沟中。

合谷：手背第 1、2 掌骨之间，约平第 2 掌骨中点处。

按摩操作

掐端正：用拇指指甲掐，掐 10 次。

掐人中：用拇指指甲掐，掐 5 次。

掐延年：用拇指指甲掐，掐 5 次。

按揉迎香：用食指、中指两指或两拇指指端按揉两侧穴位，揉 50 次。

揉合谷：用拇指指腹揉，揉 30 次。

15 Tympanitis

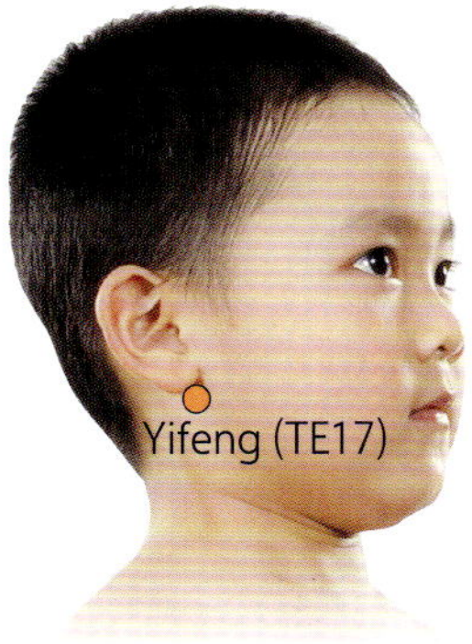

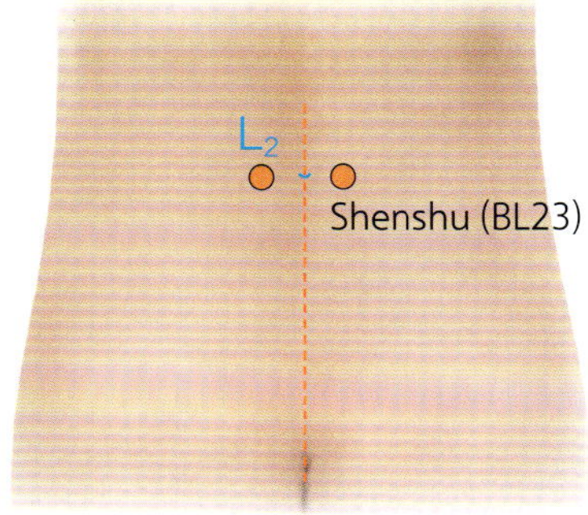

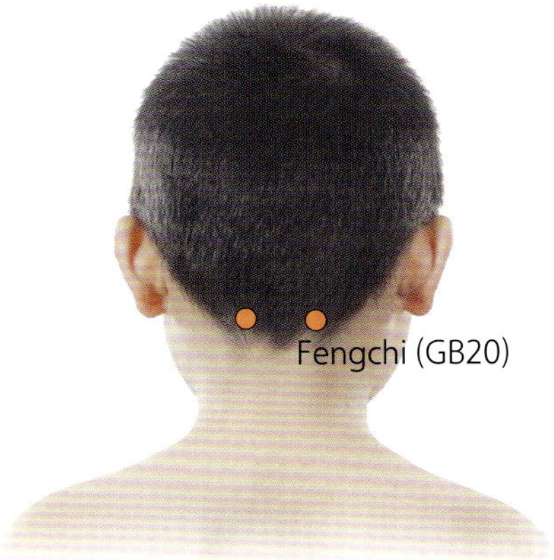

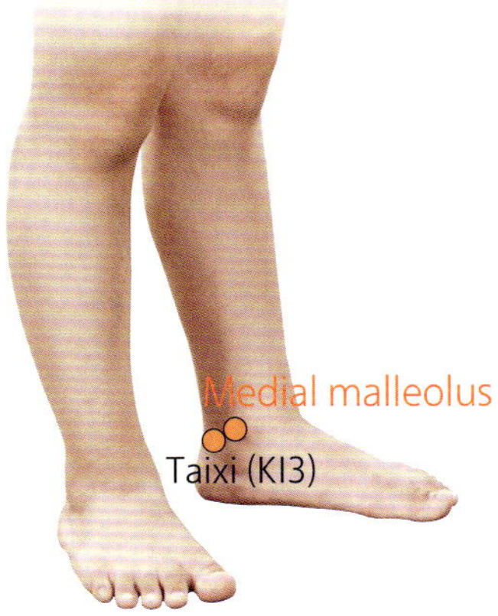

Classic Acupoints Matching

Yifeng (TE17): Behind the earlobe, in the depression between mastoid process and mandible.
Taixi (KI3): In the depression between the prominence of the medial malleolus of foot and achilles tendon.
Fengchi (GB20): In the depression of the lateral side of the great tendon below the occipital bone behind the neck.
Shenshu (BL23): 1.5 cun lateral to the depression below the spinous process of 2nd lumbar vertebra.

Massage Manipulations

Press Yifeng (TE17): Press the point with the fingertip for 100 times.
Press-knead Taixi (KI3): Press-knead the point in both sides with the tip of index finger for 150 times.
Knead Fengchi (GB20): Knead the point with the tip of index finger for 100 times.
Knead Shenshu (BL23): Knead the point in both sides with the fingertips of the 2 thumbs for 100 times.

16 Nasal Bleeding

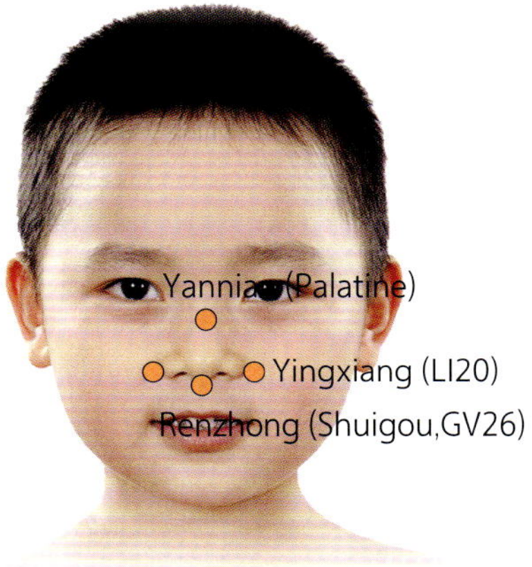

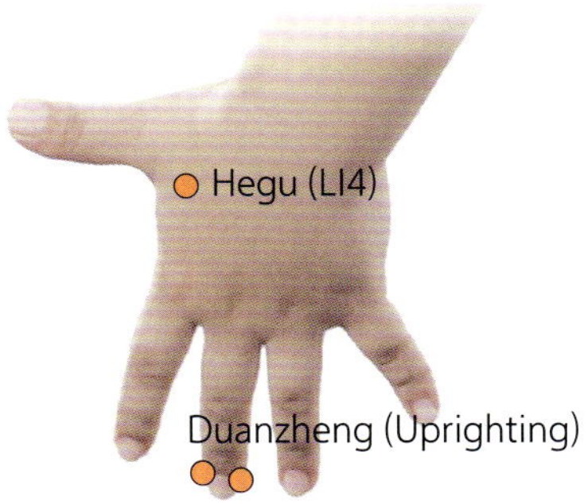

Classic Acupoints Matching

Duanzheng (Uprighting): At the dorso-ventral boundary of both sides of the root of middle fingernail. The one in the radial side is called Left Duanzheng (Uprighting), while the one in the ulnar side is Right Duanzheng (Uprighting).
Renzhong (Shuigou,GV26): At the junction of the upper 1/3 and lower 2/3 of the philtrum.
Yannian (Palatine): In the high area of the nasal bone, between Shangen (Inner canthus) and Zhuntou (End of nose) points.
Yingxiang (LI20): 0.5 cun lateral to the nasal ala, in the nasolabial fold.
Hegu (LI4): Between the 1st and 2nd metacarpal bones on the dorsum of hand, at around the midpoint of the radial side of the 2nd metacarpal bone.

Massage Manipulations

Pinch Duanzheng (Uprighting): Pinch the point with the nail of thumb for 10 times.
Pinch Renzhong (Shuigou,GV26): Pinch the point with the nail of the thumb for 5 times.
Pinch Yannian (Palatine): Pinch the point with the nail of the thumb for 5 times.
Press-knead Yingxiang (LI20): Press-knead the point in both sides with tips of index and middle fingers or the fingertips of the 2 thumbs for 50 times.
Knead Hegu (LI4): Knead the point with the finger pulp of the thumb for 30 times.

17 牙痛

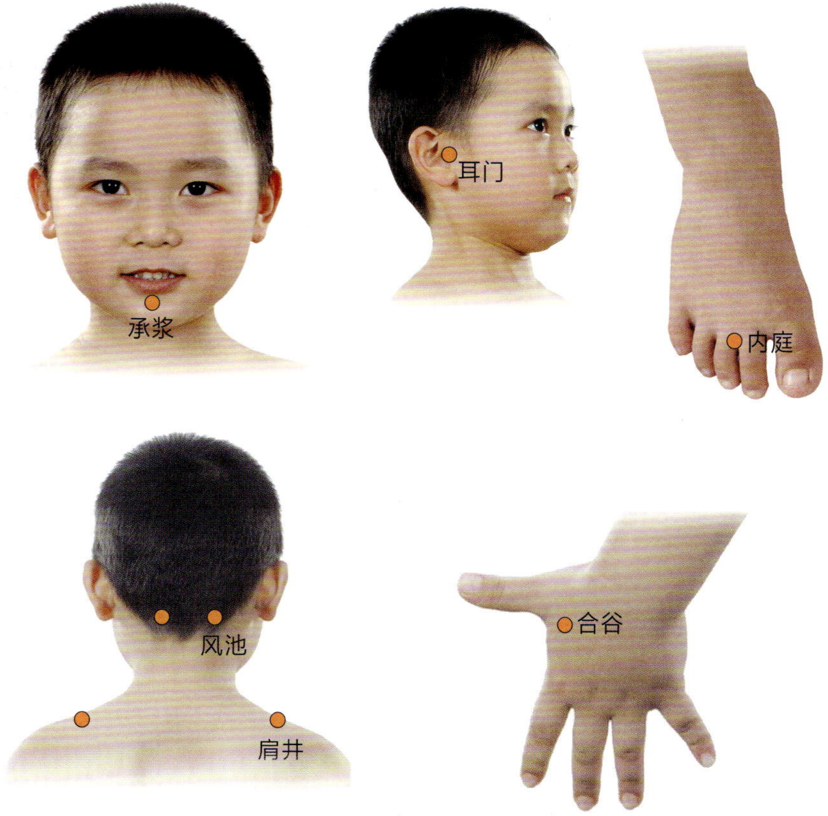

经典配穴

承浆：颏唇沟的正中凹陷处。

耳门：耳屏上切迹之前方，张口凹陷处。

风池：颈后枕骨下大筋外侧凹陷中。

合谷：手背第 1、2 掌骨之间，约平第 2 掌骨中点处。

内庭：足背，第 2、3 趾间，趾蹼缘后方赤白肉际处。

肩井：大椎与肩峰最高点连线的中点处。

按摩操作

点揉承浆：用食指指端揉，揉 200 次。

揉耳门：用食指指端揉，揉 200 次。

揉风池：用食指指端揉，揉 200 次。

按揉合谷：用拇指指腹揉，揉 100 次。

揉内庭穴：用食指指端揉，揉 100 次。

提拿肩井：小儿取坐位，按摩者用拇指与食指、中指两指对称用力提拿本穴，提拿 5 次。

18 口疮

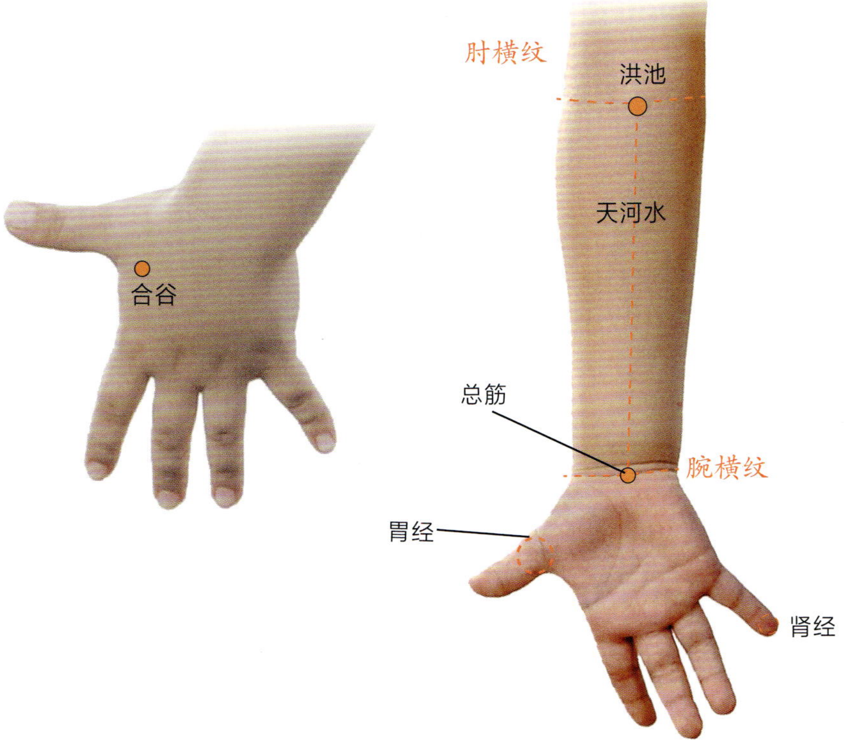

经典配穴

胃经：拇指掌面近掌端第 1 节处，或大鱼际外侧，赤白肉际处。

天河水：前臂掌侧正中，自腕横纹中点至肘横纹中点（即总筋至洪池）呈一直线。

肾经：小指末节指腹。

合谷：在手背，第 1、2 掌骨间，第 2 掌骨桡侧的中点处。

按摩操作

清胃经：自掌根（掌指横纹）向指根（指横纹）方向直推 200 次。

清天河水：用食指、中指两指自腕横纹向上推至肘横纹处，推 200 次。

补肾经：以指尖推向指根方向，推 300 次。

揉合谷：用拇指指腹揉，揉 3 分钟。

17 Toothache

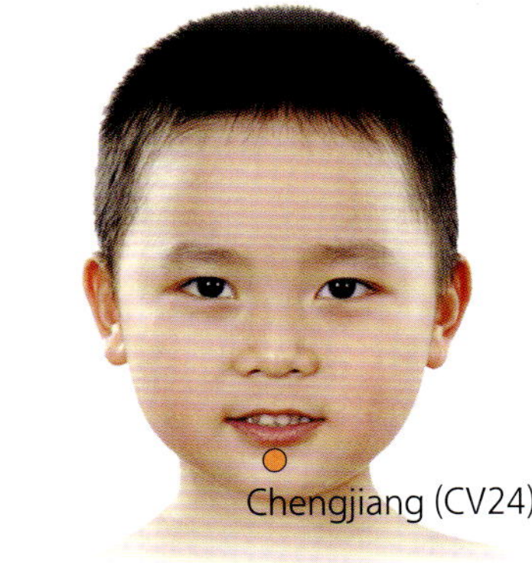

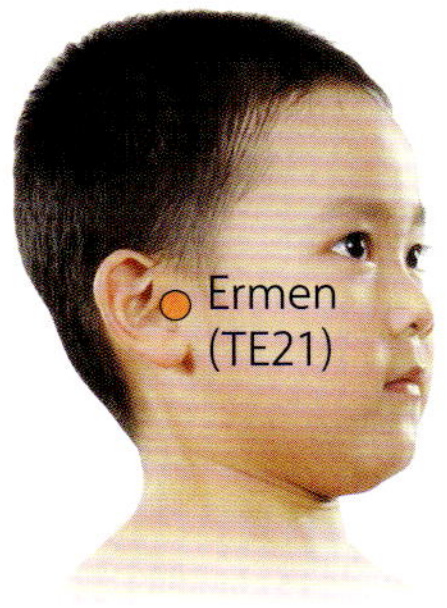

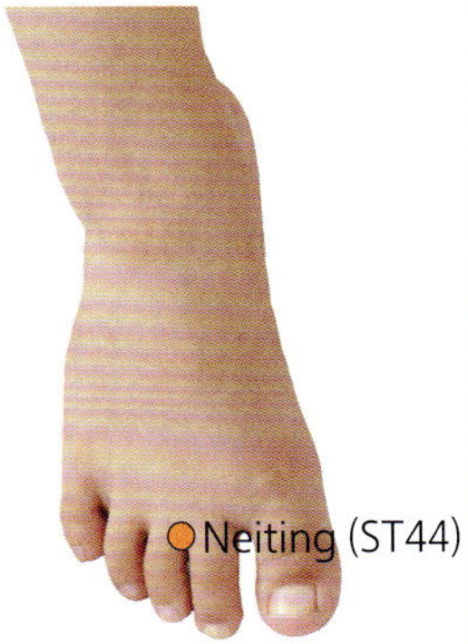

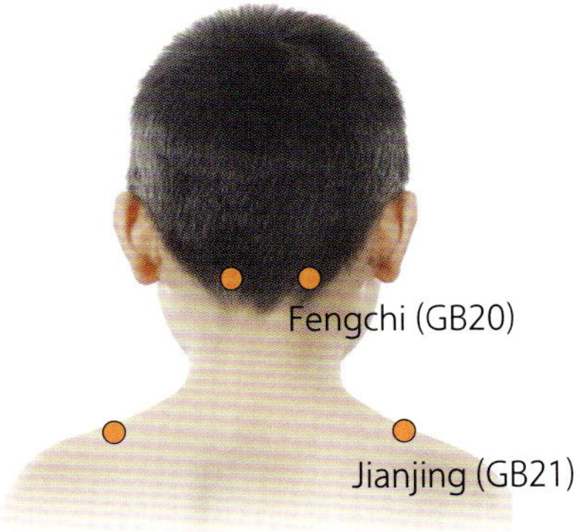

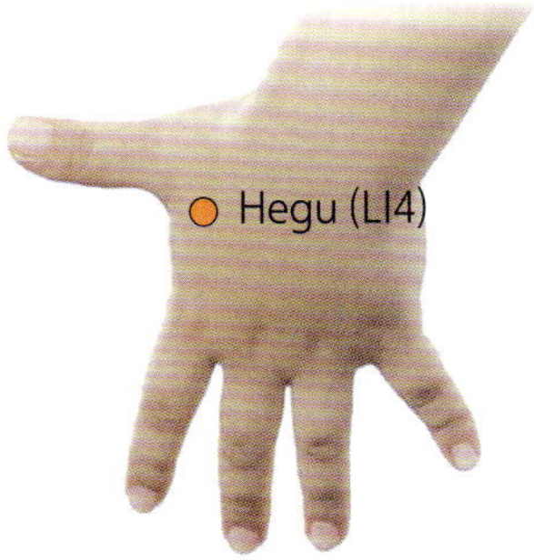

Classic Acupoints Matching

Chengjiang (CV24): In the depression of the middle of the mentolabial sulcus.

Ermen (TE21): In the depression of the anterior supratragic notch when open the mouth.

Fengchi (GB20): In the depression of the lateral side of the great tendon below the occipital bone behind the neck.

Hegu (LI4): Between the 1st and the 2nd metacarpal bones on the dorsum of hand, at around the midpoint of the radial side of the 2nd metacarpal bone.

Neiting (ST44): On the dorsum of foot, between the 2nd and the 3rd toes, at the dorsal-ventral boundary of the toe.

Jianjing (GB21): The midpoint of the line between Dazhui (GV14) to the peak of acromion.

Massage Manipulations

Point and knead Chengjiang (CV24): Knead the point with the tip of index finger for 200 times.

Knead Ermen (TE21): Knead the point with the tip of index finger for 200 times.

Knead Fengchi (GB20): Knead the point with the tip of index finger for 200 times.

Press-knead Hegu (LI4): Knead the point with the finger pulp of the thumb for 100 times.

Knead Neiting (ST44): Knead the point with the tip of index finger for 100 times.

Lift-grasp Jianjing (GB21): Let the child take a sitting position. Exert strength symmetrically with the thumb and index and middle fingers to lift and grasp the point for 5 times.

18 Aphtha

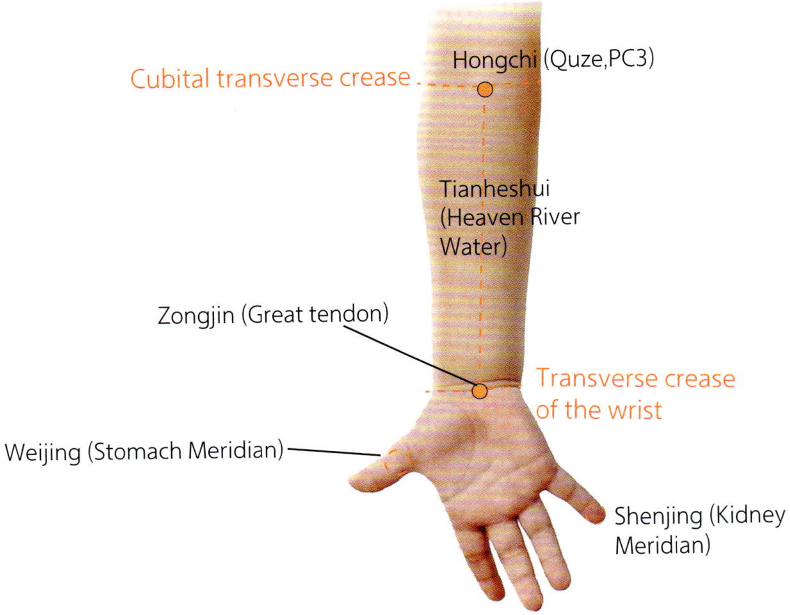

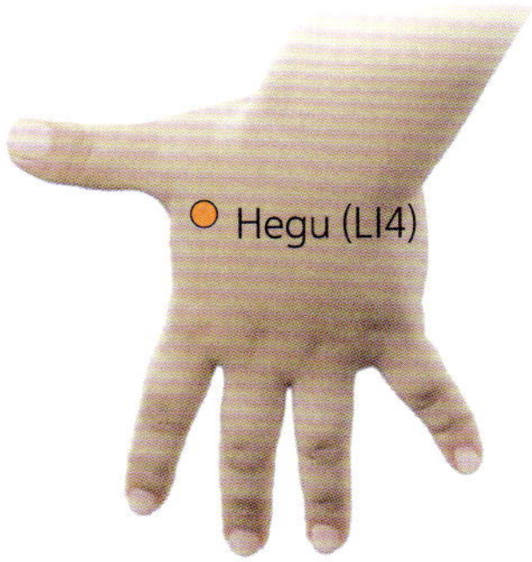

Classic Acupoints Matching

Weijing (Stomach Meridian): The palm of the 1st distal knuckle of the thumb, or the dorso-ventral boundary of the lateral side of the great thenar.

Tianheshui (Heaven River Water): In the middle of the palm-side of the forearm, the line between the midpoint of the transverse crease of wrist and the midpoint of the cubital transverse crease [the line between Zongjin (Great tendon) and Hongchi (Quze, PC 3)] .

Shenjing (Kidney Meridian): The finger pulp of the distal segment of little finger.

Hegu (LI4): Between the 1st and the 2nd metacarpal bones on the dorsum of hand, at the midpoint of the radial side of the 2nd metacarpal bone.

Massage Manipulations

Clear Weijing (Stomach Meridian): Push directly from the root of palm (metacarpophalangeal transverse crease) to the root of finger (finger crease) for 200 times.

Clear Tianheshui (Heaven River Water): Push upward from the transverse crease of wrist to the cubital transverse crease with the index and middle fingers for 200 times.

Tonify Shenjing (Kidney Meridian): Push from the tip to the root of the finger for 300 times.

Knead Hegu (LI4): Knead the point with the finger pulp of the thumb for 3 minutes.

19 水痘

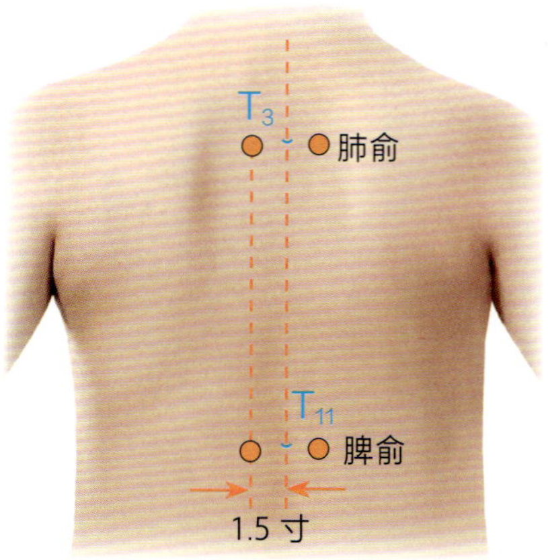

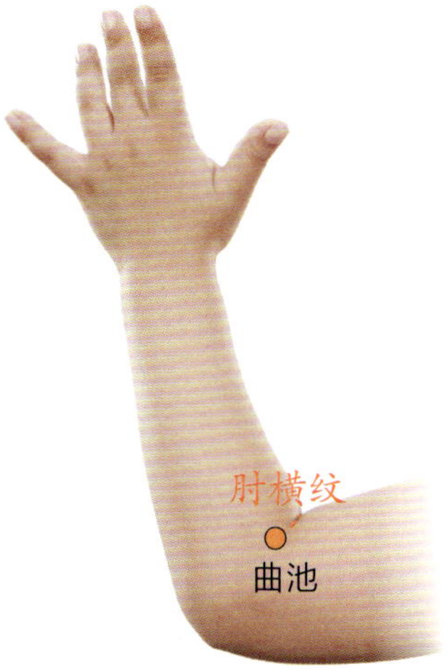

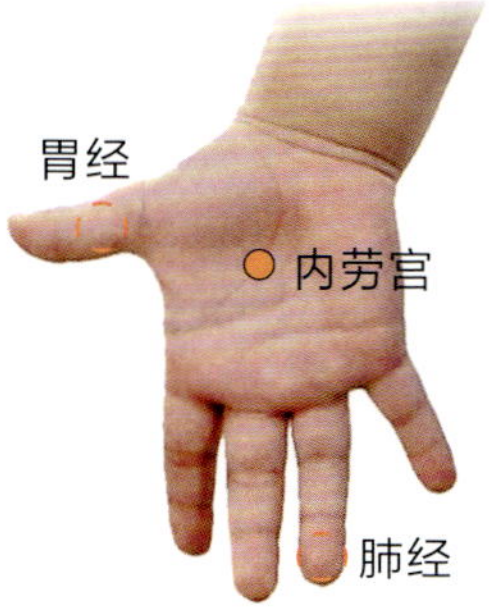

经典配穴

肺经：无名指末节指腹。

胃经：拇指掌面近掌端第 1 节处，或大鱼际外侧，赤白肉际处。

内劳宫：掌心，握拳时中指、无名指指端中点所在处。

曲池：在肘横纹外侧端凹陷中。

脾俞：第 11 胸椎棘突下，旁开 1.5 寸处。

肺俞：第 3 胸椎棘突下，旁开 1.5 寸处。

按摩操作

清肺经：从无名指末节指纹向指尖方向推，推 200 次。

清胃经：自掌根（掌指横纹）向指根（指横纹）方向直推 200 次。

揉内劳宫：用中指指端揉，揉 30 次。

按揉曲池：用拇指或中指指端揉，揉 50 次。

按揉脾俞：用两手拇指指腹或一手的食指和中指指端按揉，按揉 100 次。

揉肺俞：用两手拇指或食指指腹揉，揉 100 次。

20 麻疹

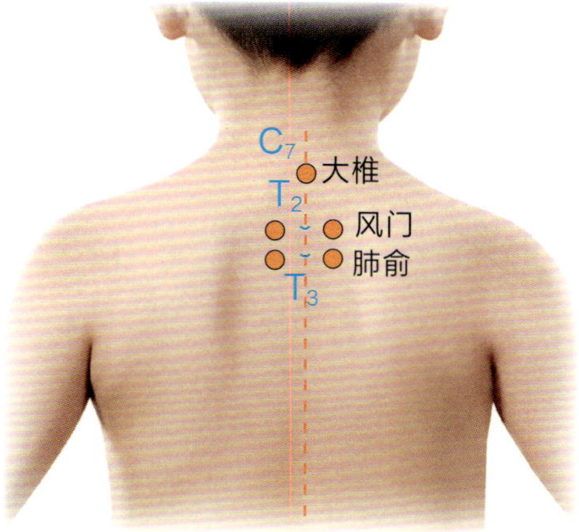

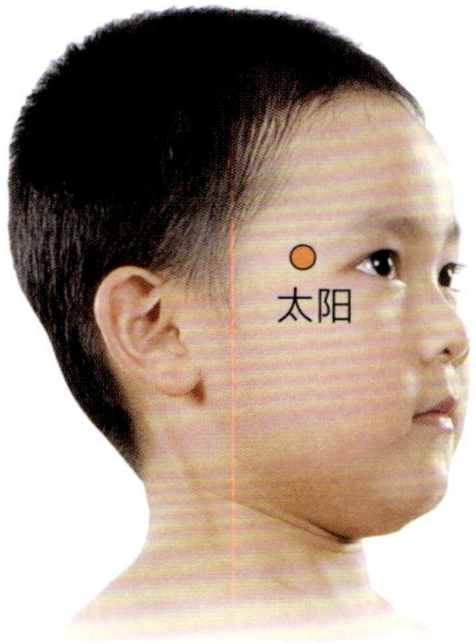

经典配穴

太阳：眉梢与眼外角连线的中点。

风门：第 2 胸椎棘突下旁开 1.5 寸处。

肺俞：第 3 胸椎棘突下，旁开 1.5 寸处。

大椎：第 7 颈椎棘突下。

按摩操作

揉太阳：用拇指或食指指腹揉，两侧各揉 50 次。

擦风门：用掌根擦两侧穴位，以透热为度。

按揉肺俞：用两手拇指或食指指腹揉，揉 100 次。

揉大椎：用中指指端揉，揉 100 次。

另外，从上向下分推两旁肩胛骨内侧缘 100 次。

19 Varicella

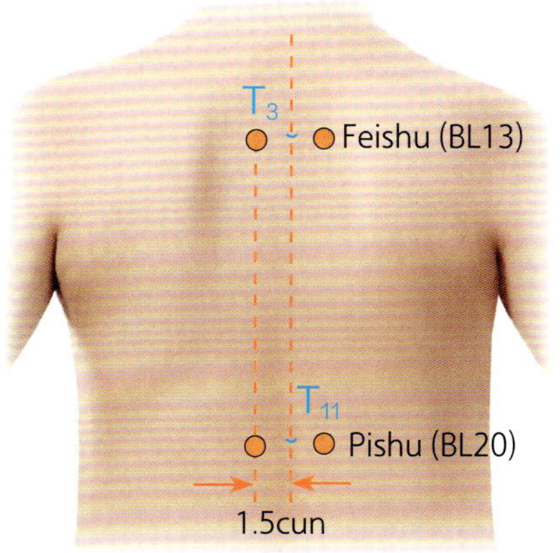

Classic Acupoints Matching

Feijing (Lung Meridian): The finger pulp of the distal segment of ring finger.
Weijing (Stomach Meridian): The palm of the 1st distal knuckle of the thumb, or the dorso-ventral boundary of the lateral side of the great thenar.
Neilaogong (PC8): In the center of the palm, at the midpoint of the tip of middle and ring fingers when clench fist.
Quchi (LI11): In the depression of the lateral side of cubital transverse crease.
Pishu (BL20): 1.5 cun lateral to the depression below the spinous process of the 11th thoracic vertebra.
Feishu (BL13): 1.5 cun lateral to the depression below the spinous process of the 3rd thoracic vertebra.

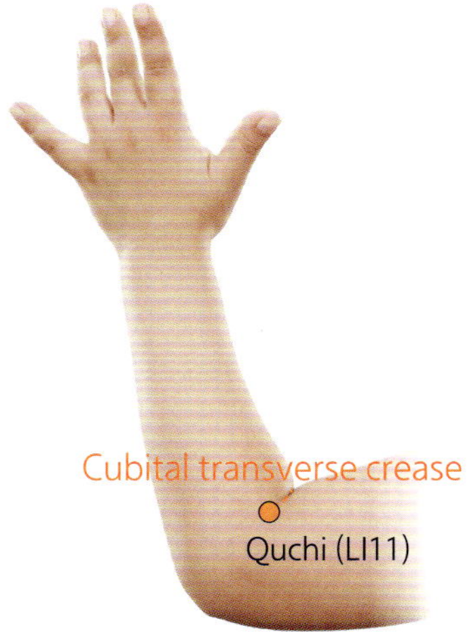

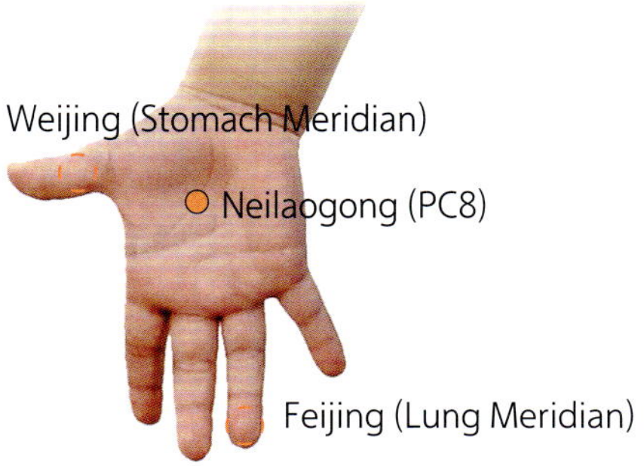

Massage Manipulations

Clear Feijing (Lung Meridian): Push from the fingerprint of the distal segment of ring finger to the fingertip for 200 times.
Clear Weijing (Stomach Meridian): Push directly from the root of palm (metacarpophalangeal crease) to the root of finger (finger crease) for 200 times.
Knead Neilaogong (PC8): Knead the point with the tip of middle finger for 30 times.
Press-knead Quchi (LI11): Knead the point with the fingertip of the thumb or middle finger for 50 times.
Press-knead Pishu (BL20): Press-knead the point with the finger pulps of the 2 thumbs or tips of index and middle fingers of 1 hand for 100 times.
Knead Feishu (BL13): Knead the point with the finger pulps of the thumbs or index fingers of the 2 hands for 100 times.

20 Measles

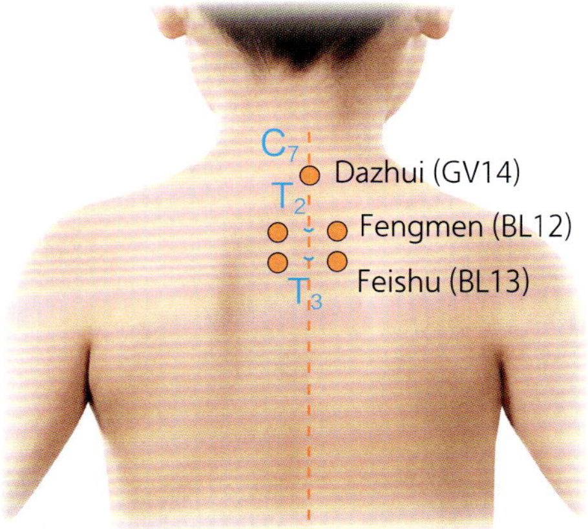

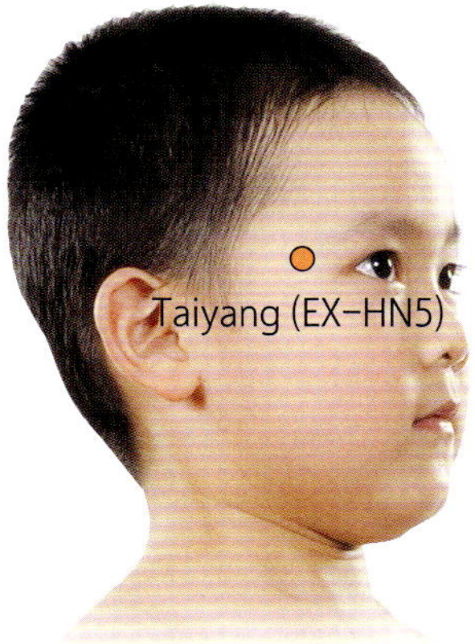

Classic Acupoints Matching

Taiyang (EX-HN5): The midpoint of the line between the brow tip to the outer canthus.
Fengmen (BL12): 1.5 cun lateral to the depression below the spinous process of the 2nd thoracic vertebra.
Feishu (BL13): 1.5 cun lateral to the depression below the spinous process of the 3rd thoracic vertebra.
Dazhui (GV14): Below the spinous process of the 7th cervical vertebra.

Massage Manipulations

Knead Taiyang (EX-HN5): Knead the point with the finger pulp of the thumb or index finger for respective 50 times in both sides.
Scrub Fengmen (BL12): Scrub the point in both sides with the root of palm until the skin feels warm.
Press-knead Feishu (BL13): Knead the point with the finger pulps of the thumbs or index fingers of the 2 hands for 100 times.
Knead Dazhui (GV14): Knead the point with the tip of middle finger for 100 times.
Besides, push the medial border of scapula from top to bottom for 100 times.

21 湿疹

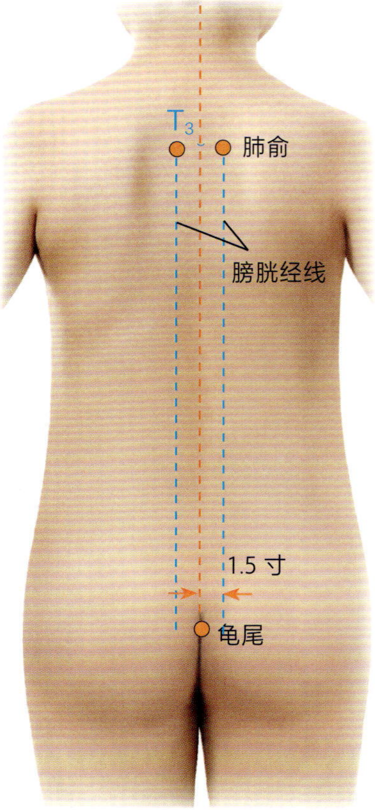

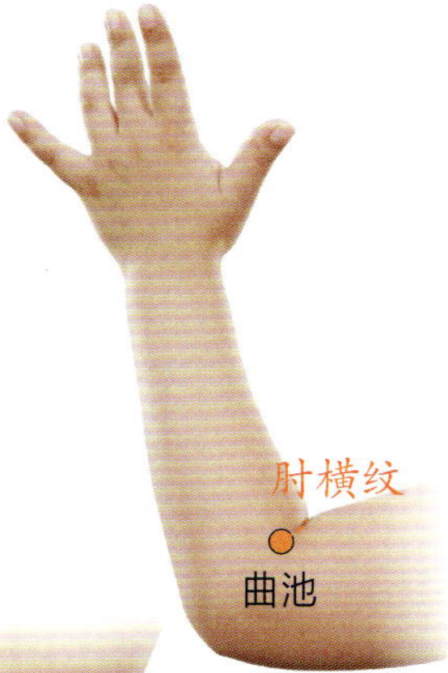

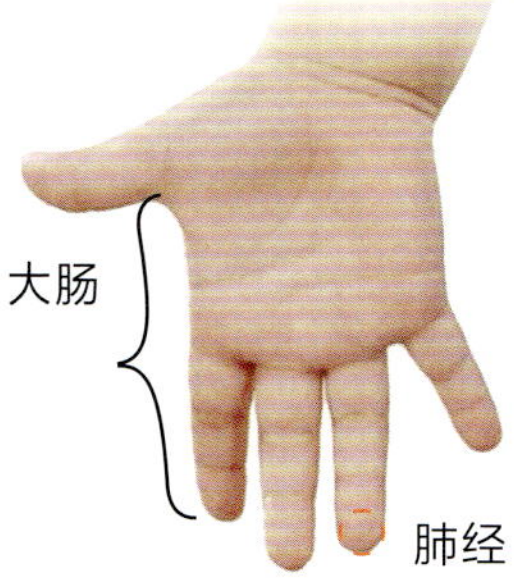

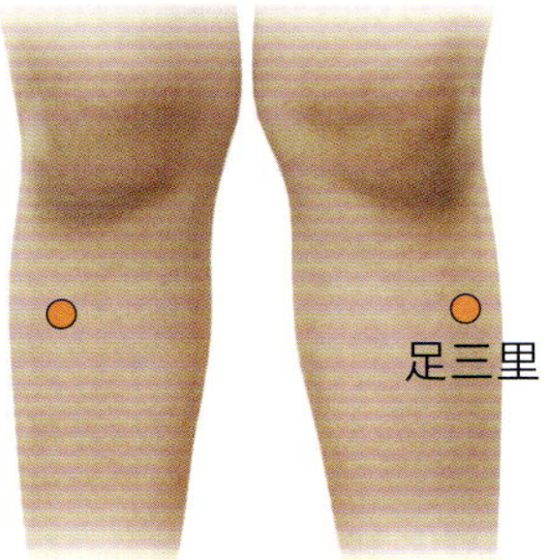

经典配穴

肺经： 无名指末节指腹。

大肠： 食指桡侧边缘，自指尖至虎口呈一直线。

曲池： 在肘横纹外侧端凹陷中。

足三里： 膝盖外侧凹陷直下3寸，胫骨旁1寸处。

膀胱经线： 脊柱旁开 1.5 寸，自肺俞开始至尾骨端止。

按摩操作

清肺经： 从无名指末节指纹向指尖方向推，推 300 次。

清大肠经： 从食指桡侧指根推向指尖，推 100 次。

按揉曲池： 用拇指或者中指指端揉，揉 100 次。

按揉足三里： 用拇指指腹揉，揉 100 次。

按揉背部膀胱经线： 用食指、中指两指自上而下揉，操作 30 次。

22 荨麻疹

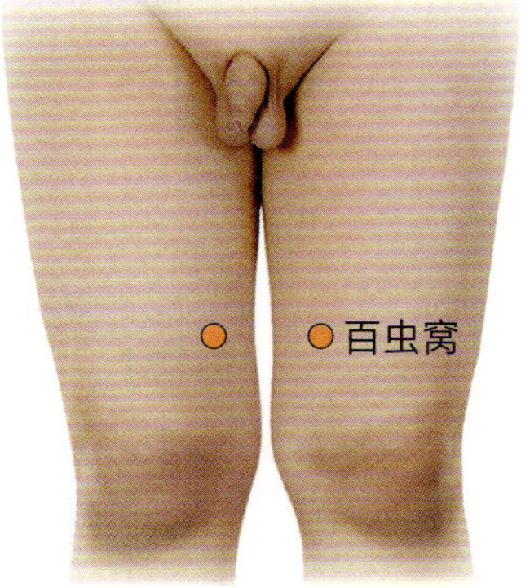

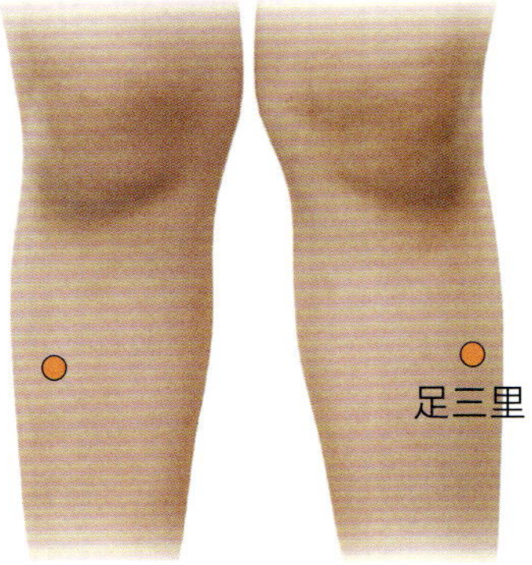

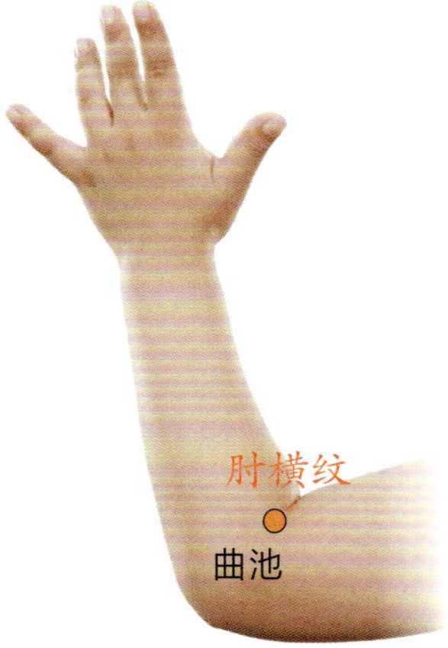

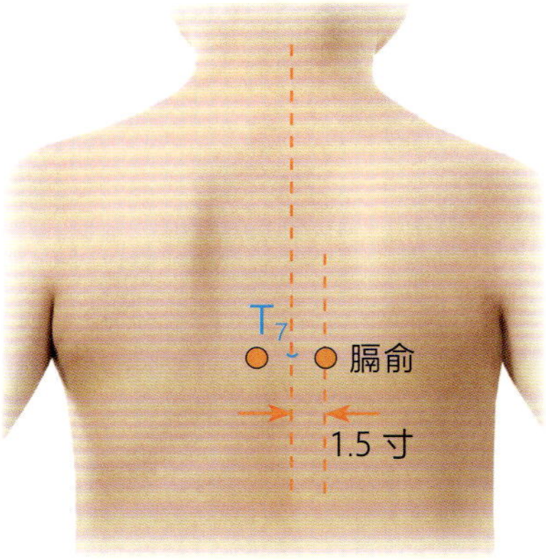

经典配穴

百虫窝： 膝上内侧肌肉丰厚处。

足三里： 膝盖外侧凹陷直下 3 寸，胫骨旁 1 寸处。

膈俞： 第 7 胸椎棘突下，旁开 1.5 寸处。

曲池： 在肘横纹外侧端凹陷中。

按摩操作

捏拿百虫窝： 用拇指和食指、中指两指指腹捏拿，两侧各拿 5 次。

按揉足三里： 用拇指指腹揉，两侧各揉 50 次。

按揉膈俞： 用指端按揉，按揉 10 次。

按揉曲池： 用拇指或者中指指端揉，两侧各揉 100 次。

21 Eczema

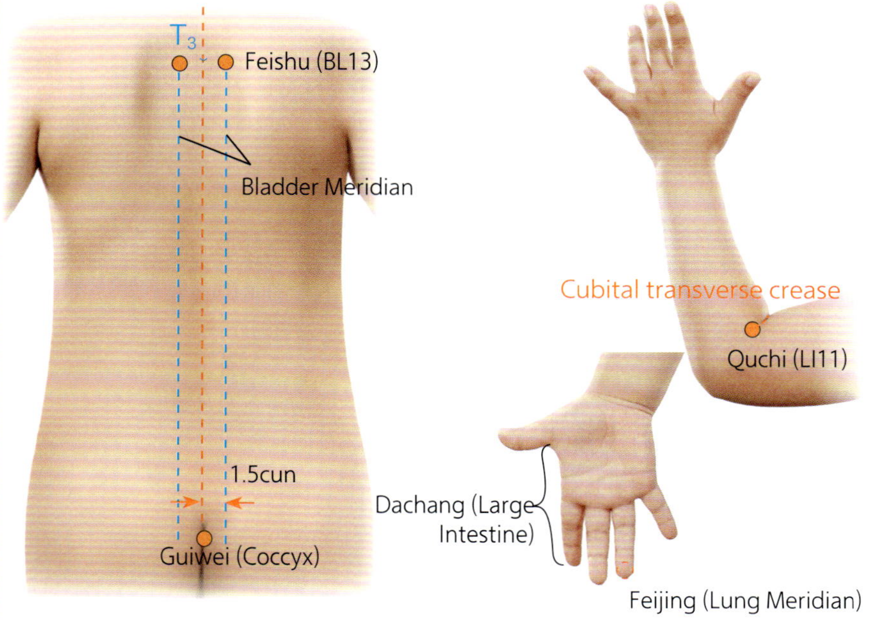

Classic Acupoints Matching

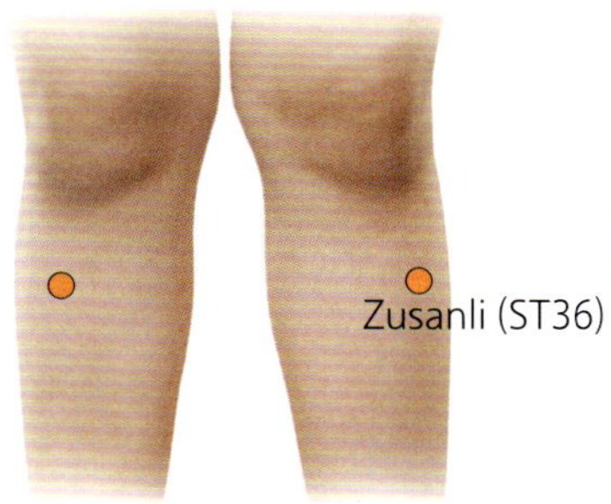

Feijing (Lung Meridian): The finger pulp of the distal segment of ring finger.
Dachang (Large Intestine): In the radial border of index finger, the line between the tip of index finger to Hukou (the part between the thumb and index finger).
Quchi (LI11): In the depression of the lateral side of the cubital transverse crease.
Zusanli (ST36): 3 cun directly below the depression of the lateral side of the knee, 1 cun lateral to the tibia.
Bladder Meridian: 1.5 cun lateral to the spine, starting from Feishu (BL13) and end at the coccygeal bone.

Massage Manipulations

Clear Feijing (Lung Meridian): Push from the fingerprint of the distal segment of ring finger to the fingertip for 300 times.
Clear Dachangjing (Large Intestine Meridian): Push from the root to the tip of the radial side of index finger for 100 times.
Press-knead Quchi (LI11): Knead the point with the tip of the thumb or middle finger for 100 times.
Press-knead Zusanli (ST36): Press-knead the point with the finger pulp of the thumb for 100 times.
Press-knead the Bladder Meridian in the back: Knead the meridian from top to bottom with index and middle fingers for 30 times.

22 Urticaria

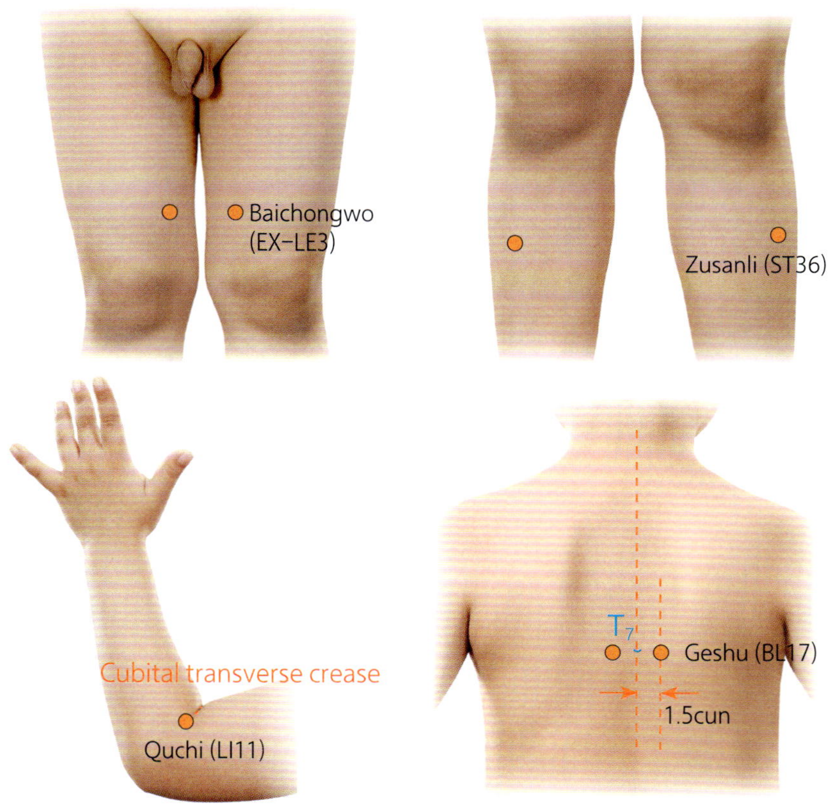

Classic Acupoints Matching

Baichongwo (EX-LE3): At the thick muscular part above the medial side of the knee.
Zusanli (ST36): 3 cun directly below the depression of the lateral side of the knee, 1 cun lateral to the tibia.
Geshu (BL17): 1.5 cun lateral to the depression below the spinous process of the 7th thoracic vertebra.
Quchi (LI11): In the depression of the lateral side of the cubital transverse crease.

Massage Manipulations

Pinch-grasp Baichongwo (EX-LE3): Pinch and grasp the point with the thumb and the finger pulps of index and middle fingers for respective 5 times in both sides.
Press-knead Zusanli (ST36): Press-knead the point with the fingertip of the thumb for respective 50 times in both sides.
Press-knead Geshu (BL17): Press-knead the point with the fingertip for 10 times.
Press-knead Quchi (LI11): Knead the point with the tip of the thumb or middle finger for respective 100 times in both sides.

23 暑热证（夏季热）

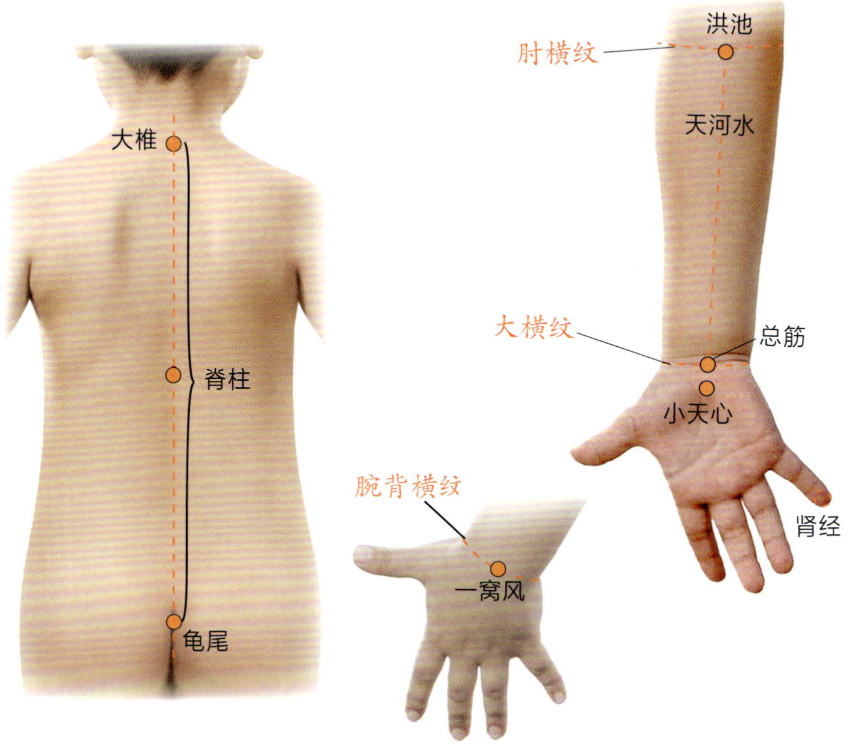

经典配穴

小天心：大小鱼际交接处凹陷中。

一窝风：手背腕横纹正中凹陷处。

肾经：小指末节指腹。

天河水：前臂掌侧正中，自腕横纹中点至肘横纹中点呈一直线。

大横纹：仰掌，掌后横纹，近拇指端称阳池，近小指端称阴池。

脊柱：大椎至尾骨端呈一直线。

按摩操作

揉小天心：用拇指指腹揉，揉 100 次。

揉一窝风：用拇指或中指指端揉，揉 200 次。

补肾经：旋推或自指根直推至指尖，推300 次。

清天河水：用食指、中指两指自腕横纹向上推至肘横纹处，推 300 次。

分阴阳：由小儿腕掌部中点向两侧分推，推 300 次。

捏脊：小儿俯卧，按摩者用双手拇指、食指自小儿腰骶部开始把皮肤捏起，自下而上捏提至大椎穴处。捏 3~5 遍，以脊柱两侧皮肤微有潮红为有效。

24 痄腮（流行性腮腺炎）

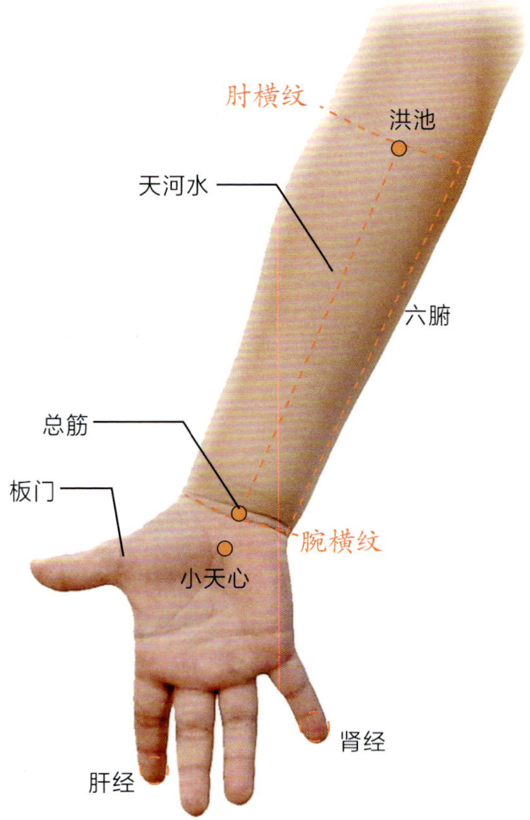

经典配穴

天河水：前臂掌侧正中，自腕横纹中点至肘横纹中点呈一直线。

肾经：小指末节指腹。

六腑：前臂尺侧，从肘横纹至腕横纹呈一直线。

肝经：食指末节指腹。

板门：手掌大鱼际处。

小天心：大小鱼际交接处凹陷中。

按摩操作

清天河水：用食指、中指两指自腕横纹向上推至肘横纹处，推 200 次。

补肾经：旋推或自指根直推至指尖，推 100 次。

退六腑：用拇指指面或食指、中指指面自肘横纹向腕横纹直推，推 300 次。

清肝经：以指根向指尖方向推，推 100 次。

揉板门：用指端揉大鱼际，揉 100 次。

揉小天心：用拇指指腹揉，揉 300 次。

23 Summer Fever

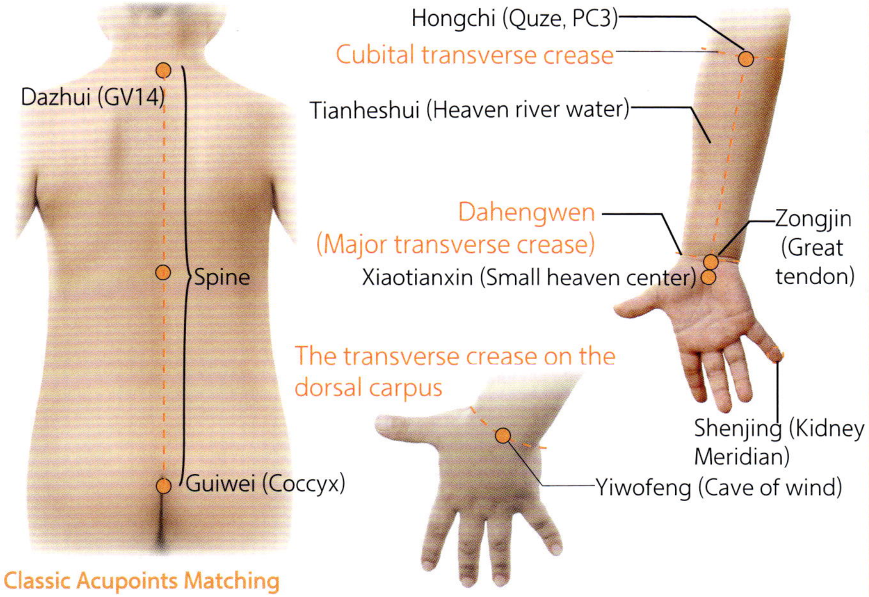

Classic Acupoints Matching

Xiaotianxin (Small heaven center): In the depression of the junction of the great thenar and hypothenar.
Yiwofeng (Cave of wind): In the depression of the middle of transverse crease on the dorsal carpus.
Shenjing (Kidney Meridian): The finger pulp of the distal segment of little finger.
Tianheshui (Heaven River Water): In the middle of the palm-side of the forearm, the line between the midpoint of the transverse crease of wrist and the midpoint of the cubital transverse crease.
Dahengwen (Major transverse crease): At the wrist transverse crease with the palm upward, the point near the side of the thumb is Yangchi (TE4), while the point near the side of the little finger is Yinchi (Pool of Yin).
Spine: The straight line between Dazhui (GV14) to the end of coccygeal bone.

Massage Manipulations

Knead Xiaotianxin (Small heaven center): Knead the point with the finger pulp of the thumb for 100 times.
Knead Yiwofeng (Cave of wind): Knead the point with the tip of the thumb or middle finger for 200 times.
Tonify Shenjing (Kidney Meridian): Rotate-push or push directly from the root to the tip of the finger for 300 times.
Clear Tianheshui (Heaven river water): Push upward from the transverse crease of wrist to the cubital transverse crease with the index and middle fingers for 300 times.
Part Yin and Yang: Push from the middle of the wrist palmar of the child to both sides for 300 times.
Pinch Spine: Let the child lie in prone position. Pinch the skin from bottom to top with the thumb and index finger of 2 hands starting from the lumbosacral region to Dazhui (GV14) for generally 3 to 5 times until the skin in both sides of spine shows slightly flush as an effective manipulation.

24 Mumps

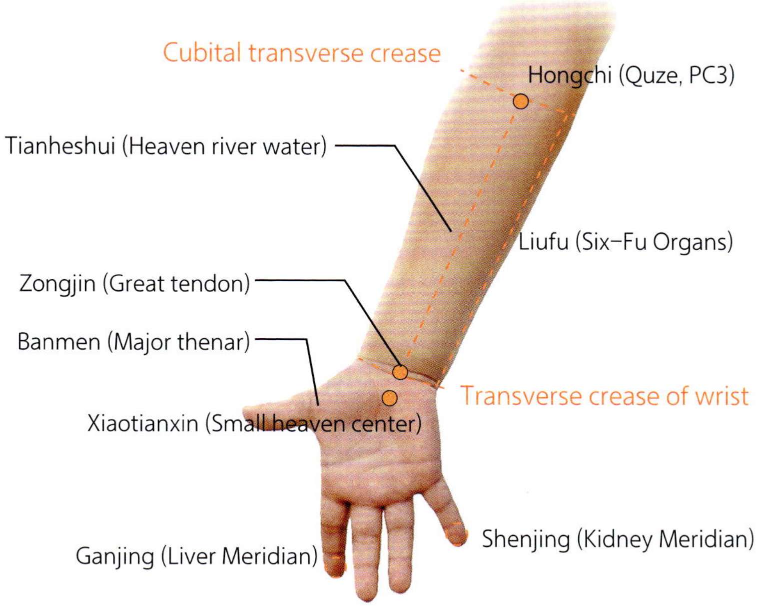

Classic Acupoints Matching

Tianheshui (Heaven River Water): In the middle of the palm-side of the forearm, the line between the midpoint of the transverse crease of wrist and the midpoint of the cubital transverse crease.
Shenjing (Kidney Meridian): The finger pulp of the distal segment of little finger.
Liufu (Six-Fu Organs): In the ulnar side of the forearm, the line between the cubital transverse crease to the wrist crease.
Ganjing (Liver Meridian): The finger pulp of the distal segment of index finger.
Banmen (Major thenar): At the great thenar of the palm.
Xiaotianxin (Small heaven center): In the depression of the junction of the great thenar and hypothenar.

Massage Manipulations

Clear Tianheshui (Heaven River Water): Push upward from the wrist crease to the cubital transverse crease with the index and middle fingers for 200 times.
Tonify Shenjing (Kidney Meridian): Rotate-push or push directly from the root to the tip of the finger for 100 times.
Relieve Liufu (Six-Fu Organs): Push directly from the cubital transverse crease to the wrist crease with the facies digitales of the thumb or the facies digitales of index and middle fingers for 300 times.
Clear Ganjing (Liver Meridian): Push from the root to the tip of the finger for 100 times.
Knead Banmen (Major thenar): Knead the great thenar with the fingertip for 100 times.
Knead Xiaotianxin (Small heaven center): Knead the point with the finger pulp of the thumb for 300 times.

25 肌性斜颈

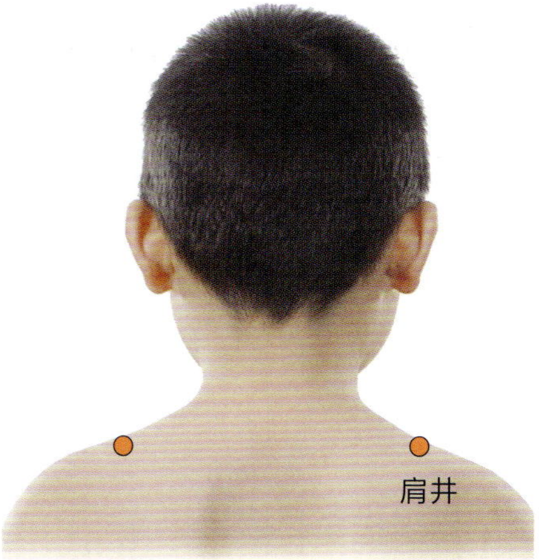

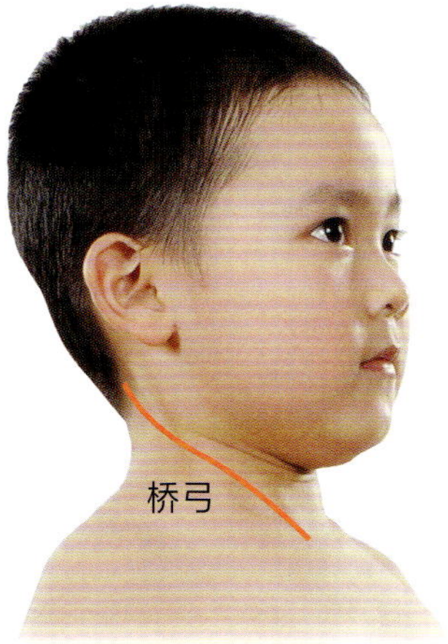

经典配穴

桥弓：在颈部两侧，沿胸锁乳突肌呈一直线。

肩井：大椎与肩峰最高点连线的中点处。

按摩操作

拿桥弓：用一手拇指、食指自上而下拿，操作5分钟。拿桥弓时手法轻重要适当，部位要准确，不可捏拿颈总动脉。

拿肩井：小儿取坐位，按摩者一手扶住小儿有肿块的一侧肩部，另一手按住头顶，使小儿头慢慢向无肿块的一侧倾斜，用拇指与食指、中指两指对称用力轻拿肩井3～5分钟，反复操作5～7次。（注意：手法宜由轻到重，幅度由小到大，不可超出生理范围。）

26 踝关节扭伤

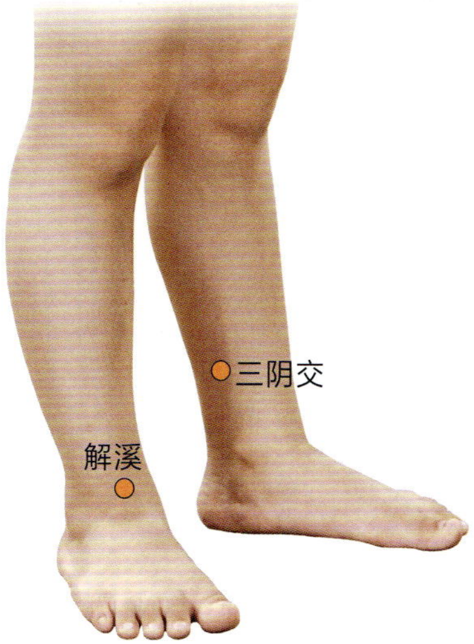

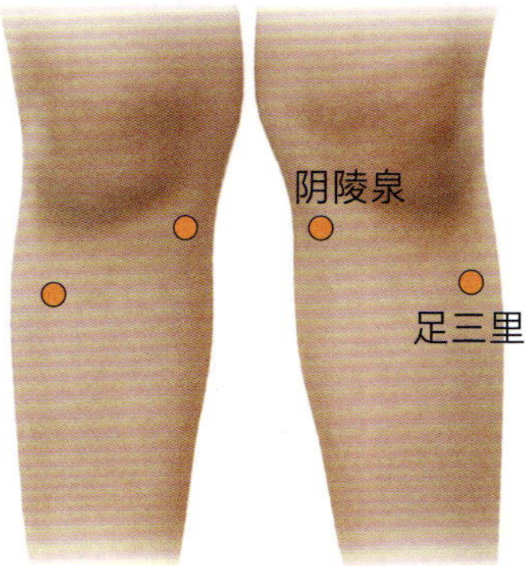

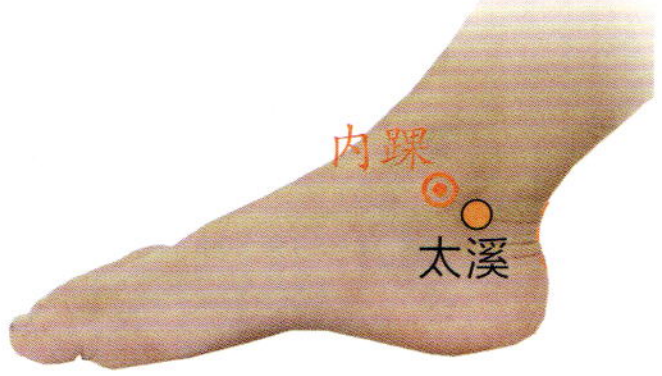

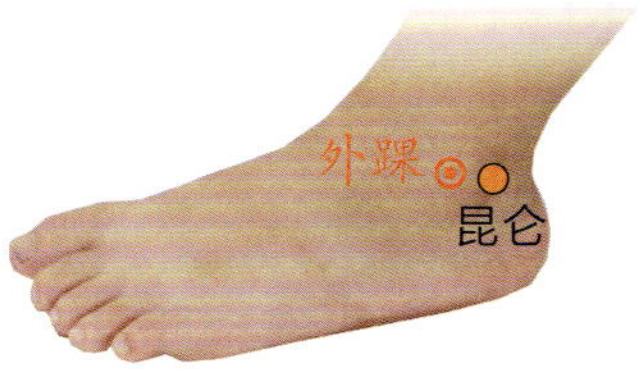

经典配穴

阴陵泉：小腿内侧，胫骨内侧髁后下方凹陷处。

足三里：膝盖外侧凹陷直下3寸，胫骨旁1寸处。

三阴交：小腿内侧，足内踝尖上3寸，胫骨内侧缘后方。

昆仑：外踝尖与跟腱的中点凹陷处。

太溪：足内踝尖与跟腱之间的凹陷处。

解溪：踝关节前横纹中点，两筋之间凹陷处。

按摩操作

按揉阴陵泉：用食指或拇指指腹揉，按揉50次。

按揉足三里：用拇指指端按揉，按揉50次。

按揉三阴交：用拇指指端按揉，按揉50次。

按揉昆仑：用指端按揉，揉30次。

按揉太溪：用指端按揉，揉30次。

掐解溪：用拇指指甲掐，掐5次。

25 Muscular Torticollis

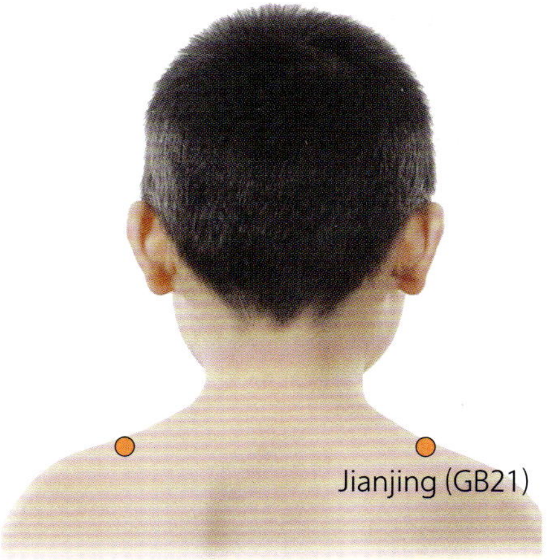

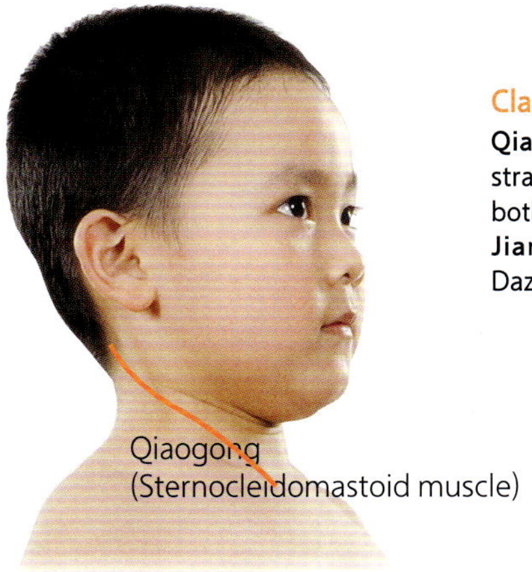

Classic Acupoints Matching

Qiaogong (Sternocleidomastoid muscle): The straight line along the sternocleidomastoid in the both sides of the neck.
Jianjing: The midpoint of the line between Dazhui (GV14) and the peak of acromion.

Massage Manipulations

Grasp Qiaogong (Sternocleidomastoid muscle): Grasp Qiaogong (Sternocleidomastoid muscle) from top to bottom with the thumb and index finger of one hand for 5 minutes. The grasping technique should be repeated with appropriate strength and exact location. The arteria carotis communis shall not be pinched or grasped.
Grasp Jianjing (GB21): Let the child take a sitting position. Hold the shoulder with a lump with one hand. Press the vertex with the other hand to let the head of the child lean on the side without the lump gradually. Exert strength symmetrically with the thumb, index and middle fingers to lift Jianjing (GB21) gently for 3 to 5 minutes. The manipulation is repeated repeatedly for 5 to 7 times. (Note: The technique shall be repeated from light to heavy strength, from small to big range without exceeding physiological range.)

26 Ankle Sprain

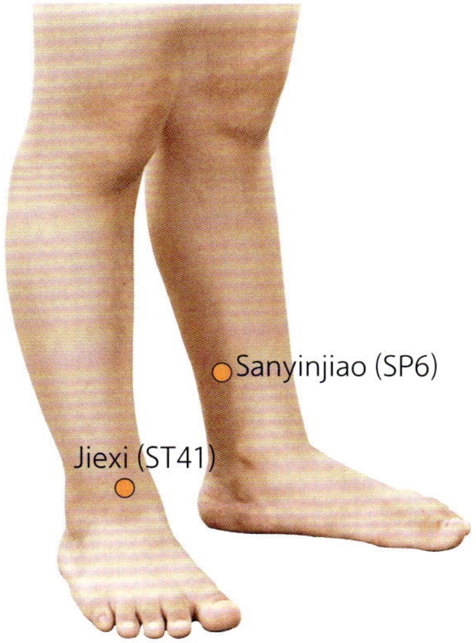

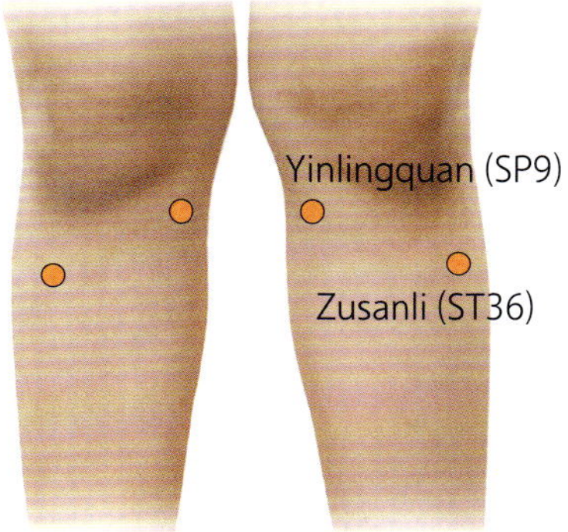

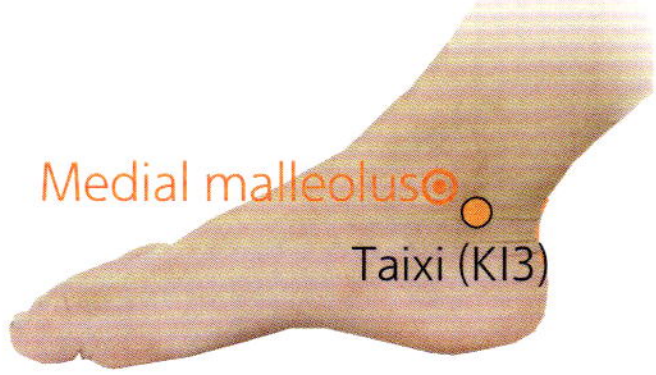

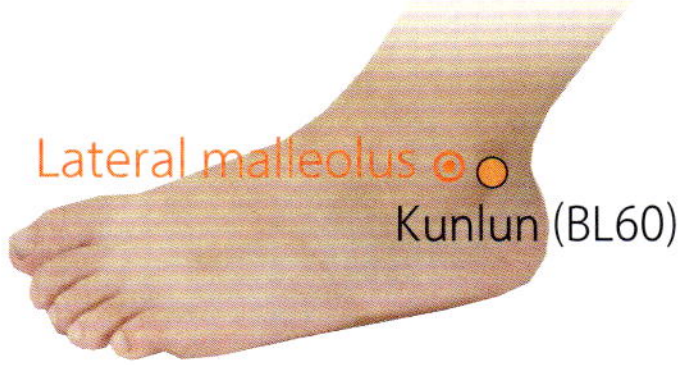

Classic Acupoints Matching

Yinlingquan (SP9): In the inner side of the leg, in the depression posterior inferior to the medial condyle of the tibia.
Zusanli (ST36): 3 cun directly below the depression of the lateral side of the knee, 1 cun lateral to the tibia.
Sanyinjiao (SP6): In the inner side of the leg, 3 cun above the prominence of the medial malleolus, posterior to the medial border of the tibia.
Kunlun (BL60): In the depression of the midpoint of line between the prominence of the lateral malleolus and achilles tendon.
Taixi (KI3): In the depression between the prominence of the medial malleolus and achilles tendons.
Jiexi (ST41): At the midpoint of the anterior crease of ankle joint, in the depression between the 2 tendons.

Massage Manipulations

Press-knead Yinlingquan (SP9): Knead the point with the finger pulp of the index finger or the thumb for 50 times.
Press-knead Zusanli (ST36): Press-knead the point with the fingertip of the thumb for 50 times.
Press-knead Sanyinjiao (SP6): Press-knead the point with the fingertip of the thumb for 50 times.
Press-knead Kunlun (BL60): Press-knead the point with the fingertip for 30 times.
Press-knead Taixi (KI3): Press-knead the point with the fingertip for 30 times.
Pinch Jiexi (ST41): Pinch the point with the nail of the thumb for 5 times.

27 多动症（注意缺陷障碍）

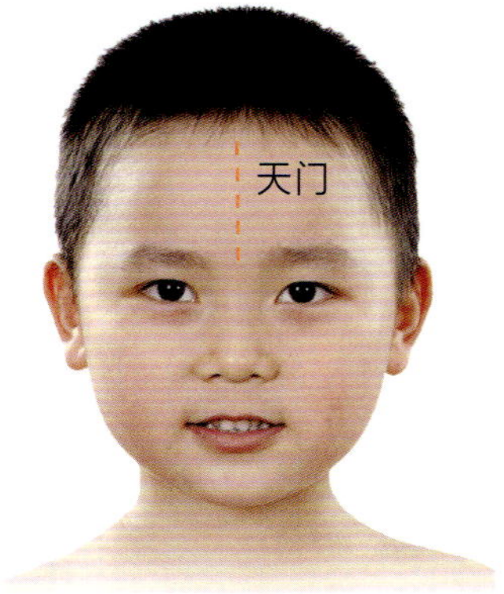

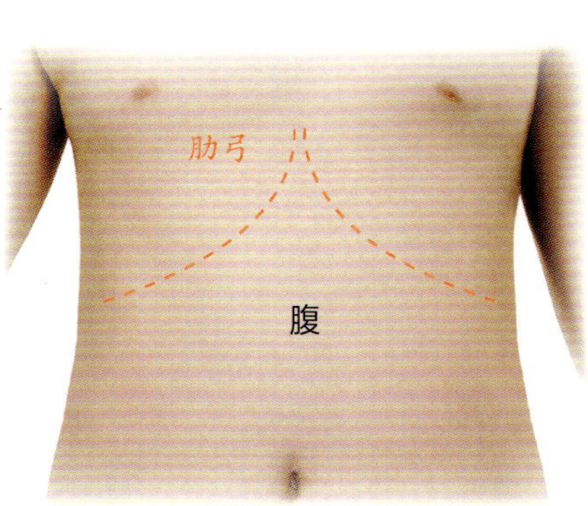

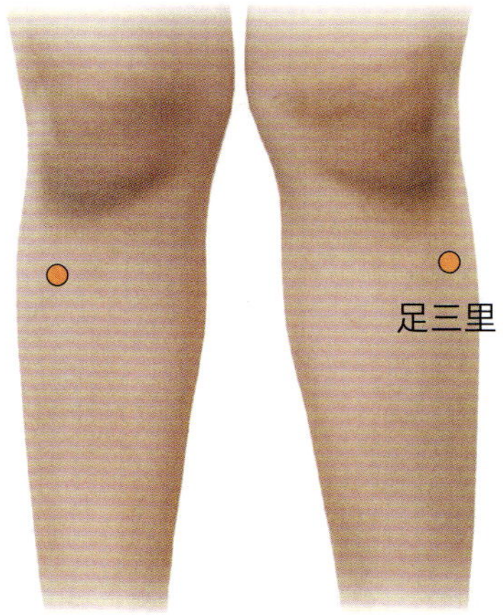

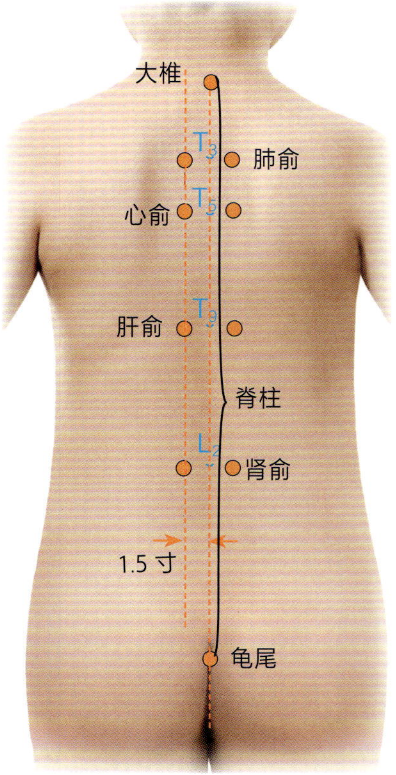

经典配穴

天门：两眉中至前发际呈一直线。

足三里：膝盖外侧凹陷直下 3 寸，胫骨旁 1 寸处。

腹：肋弓以下，肚脐以上。

肺俞：第 3 胸椎棘突下，旁开 1.5 寸处。

心俞：第 5 胸椎棘突下，旁开 1.5 寸处。

肝俞：第 9 胸椎棘突下，旁开 1.5 寸处。

肾俞：第 2 腰椎棘突下，旁开 1.5 寸处。

脊柱：大椎穴至尾骨端呈一直线。

按摩操作

开天门：两拇指自下而上地交替直推，推 100 次。

按揉足三里：用拇指指端按揉，按揉 5 分钟。

摩腹：小儿仰卧，按摩者以全掌或食指、中指、无名指指腹摩上腹部，按顺时针、逆时针方向摩腹各 100 次。

揉肺俞：用两手拇指或食指指腹揉，揉 50 次。

揉心俞：用两手拇指或食指指腹揉，揉 50 次。

揉肝俞：用两手拇指或食指指腹揉，揉 50 次。

揉肾俞：用两拇指端揉两侧穴位，揉 50 次。

捏脊：小儿俯卧，按摩者用双手拇指、食指自小儿腰骶部开始把皮肤捏起，自下而上捏提至大椎穴处，捏 5 遍，以脊柱两侧皮肤微有潮红为有效。

27 Attention Deficit Hyperactivity Disorder (ADHD)

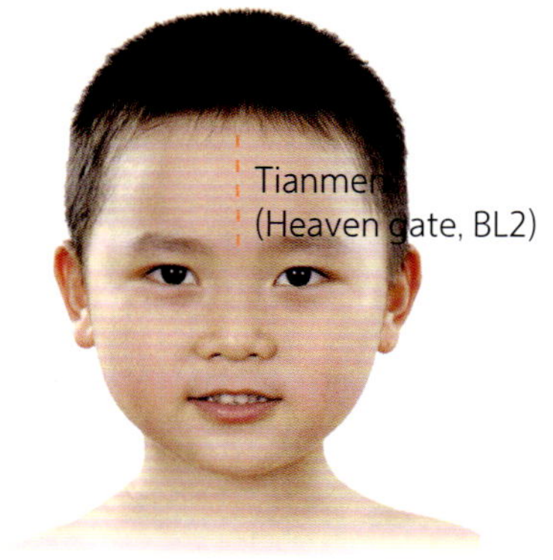

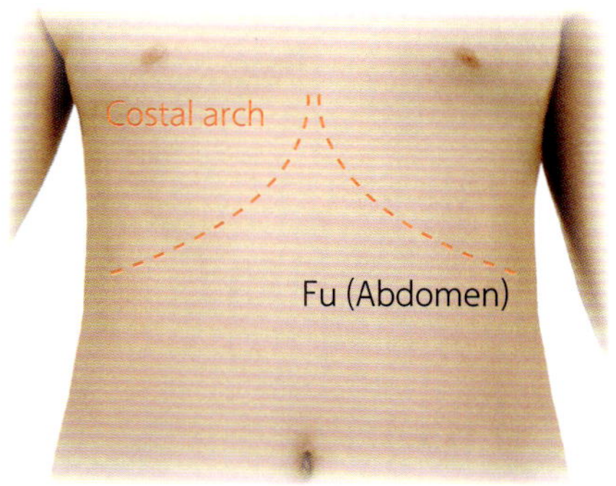

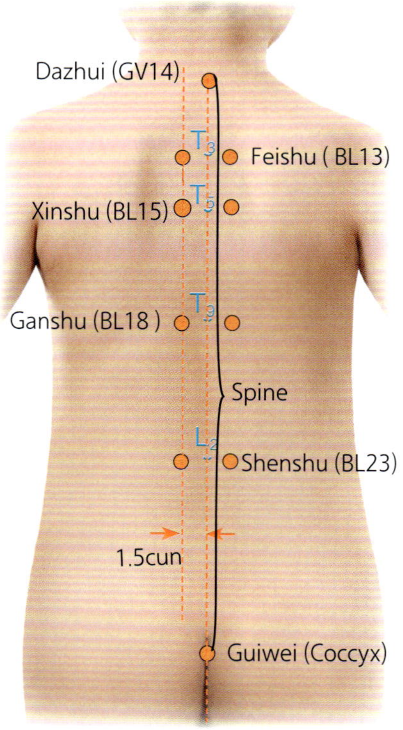

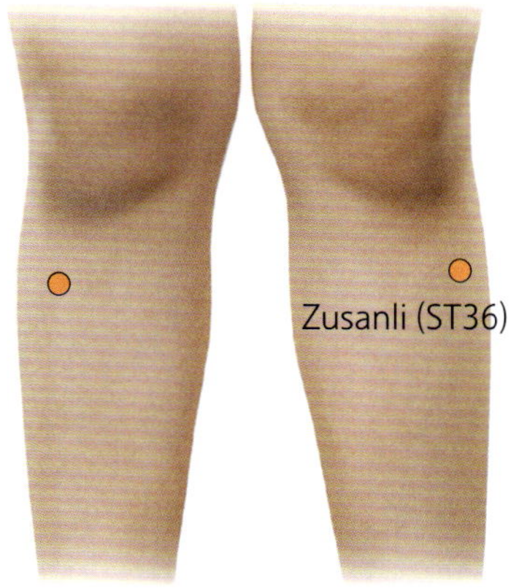

Classic Acupoints Matching

Tianmen (Heaven gate, BL2): The line between the midpoint of the 2 eyebrows and the anterior hairline.
Zusanli (ST36): 3 cun directly below the depression of the lateral side of the knee, 1 cun lateral to the tibia.
Fu (Abdomen): Below the costal arch, above the umbilicus.
Feishu (BL13): 1.5 cun lateral to the depression below the spinous process of the 3rd thoracic vertebra.
Xinshu (BL15): 1.5 cun lateral to the depression below the spinous process of the 5th thoracic vertebra.
Ganshu (BL18): 1.5 cun lateral to the depression below the spinous process of the 9th thoracic vertebra.
Shenshu (BL23): 1.5 cun lateral to the depression below the spinous process of the 2nd lumbar vertebra.
Spine: The straight line between Dazhui (GV14) to the end of coccygeal bone.

Massage Manipulations

Open Tianmen (Heaven gate, BL2): Push directly and alternatively from bottom to top with the 2 thumbs for 100 times.
Press-knead Zusanli (ST36): Press-knead the point with the fingertip of the thumb for 5 minutes.
Rub Fu (Abdomen): Let the child lie in supine position. Rub the upper abdomen with the whole palm or the finger pulp of index, middle and ring fingers for respective 100 times in the clockwise and anticlockwise direction.
Knead Feishu (BL13): Knead the point with the finger pulps of the thumbs or index fingers of the 2 hands for 50 times.
Knead Xinshu (BL15): Knead the point with the finger pulps of the thumbs or index fingers of the 2 hands for 50 times.
Knead Ganshu (BL18): Knead the point with the finger pulps of the thumbs or index fingers of the 2 hands for 50 times.
Knead Shenshu (BL23): Knead the point in both sides with the fingertips of the 2 thumbs for 50 times.
Pinch Spine: Let the child lie in prone position. Pinch the skin from bottom to top with the thumb and index finger of 2 hands starting from the lumbosacral region to Dazhui (GV14) for generally 5 times until the skin in both sides of spine shows slightly flush as an effective manipulation.

28 流口水（流涎）

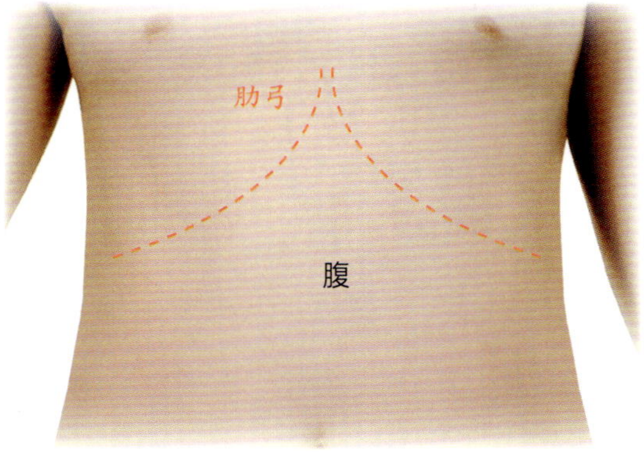

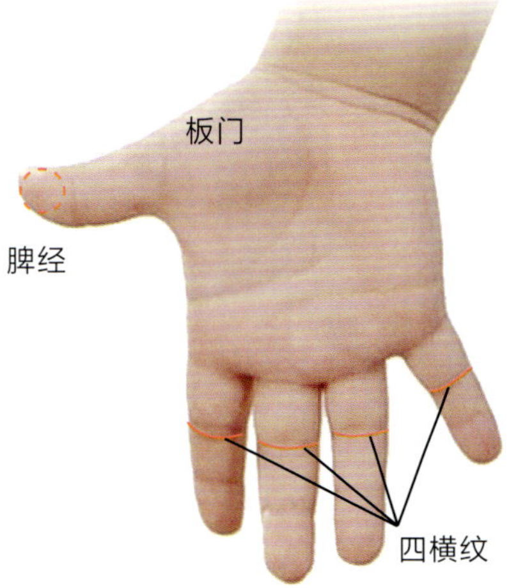

经典配穴

脾经：拇指末节指腹。
板门：手掌大鱼际处。
四横纹：掌面食指至小指，第 2 指间关节横纹处。
腹：肋弓以下，肚脐以上。

按摩操作

补脾经：从拇指指尖向指根方向直推，推 200 次。
揉板门：用指端揉大鱼际，揉 300 次。
掐揉四横纹：用拇指指甲依次掐揉，掐揉 100 次。
摩腹：小儿仰卧，按摩者以全掌或食指、中指、无名指指腹摩上腹部，摩 5 分钟。

29 夜啼

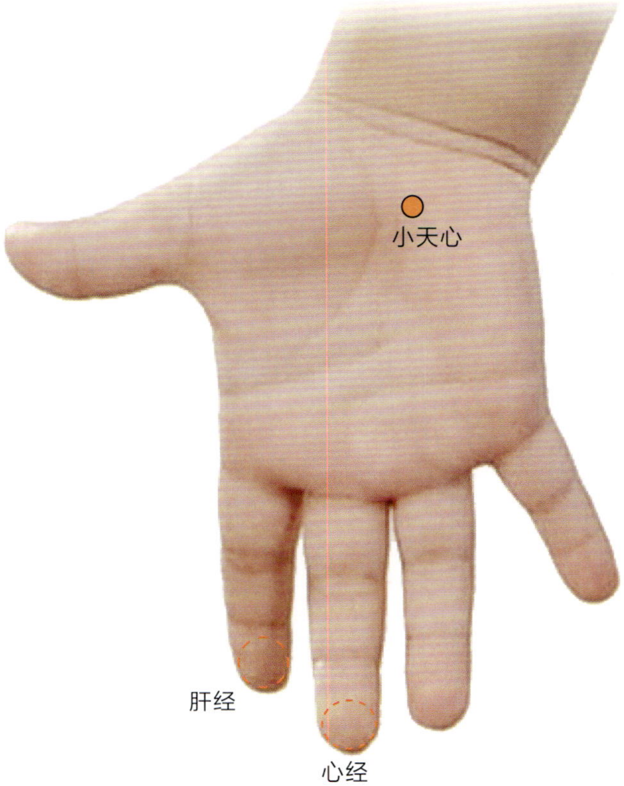

经典配穴

肝经：食指末节指腹。
心经：中指末节指腹。
小天心：大小鱼际交接处凹陷处。

按摩操作

清肝经：以指根向指尖方向推，推 100 次。
清心经：以指根向指尖方向推，推 100 次。
揉小天心：用拇指指腹揉，揉 5 次。

28 Drooling

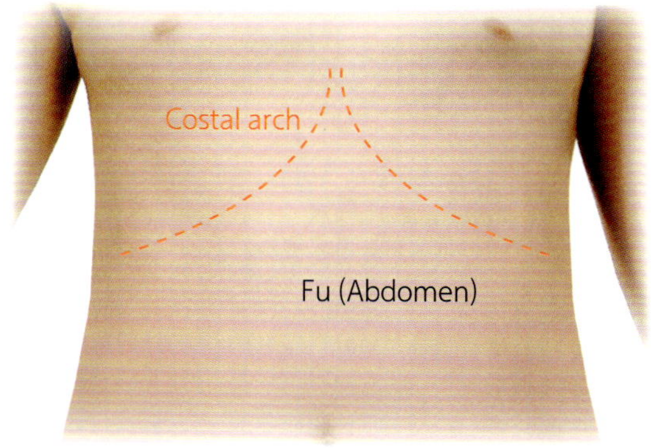

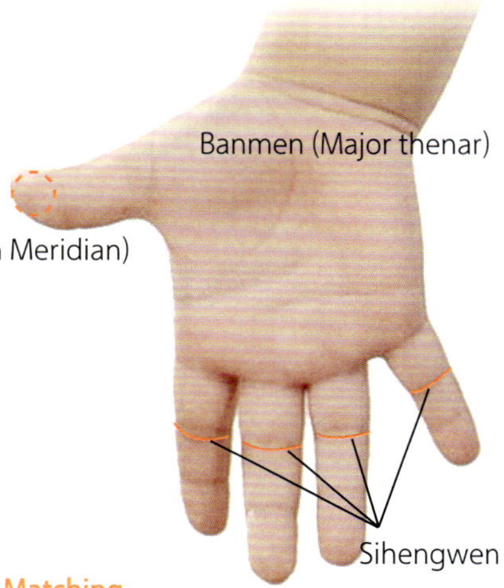

Classic Acupoints Matching

Pijing (Spleen Meridian): The finger pulp of the distal segment of thumb.
Banmen (Major thenar): At the great thenar of the palm.
Sihengwen (4 transverse creases): The transverse crease of the 2nd interphalangeal joint of the palm of the index, middle, ring and little fingers.
Fu (Abdomen): Below the costal arch, above the umbilicus.

Massage Manipulations

Tonify Pijing (Spleen Meridian): Push directly Pijing (Spleen Meridian) from the tip to the root of the thumb for 200 times.
Knead Banmen (Major thenar): Knead the great thenar with the fingertip for 300 times.
Pinch–knead Sihengwen (4 transverse creases): Pinch and knead the points successively with the nail of the thumb for 100 times.
Rub Fu (Abdomen): Let the child lie in supine position. Rub the upper abdomen with the whole palm or the finger pulp of index, middle and ring fingers for 5 minutes.

29 Night Crying

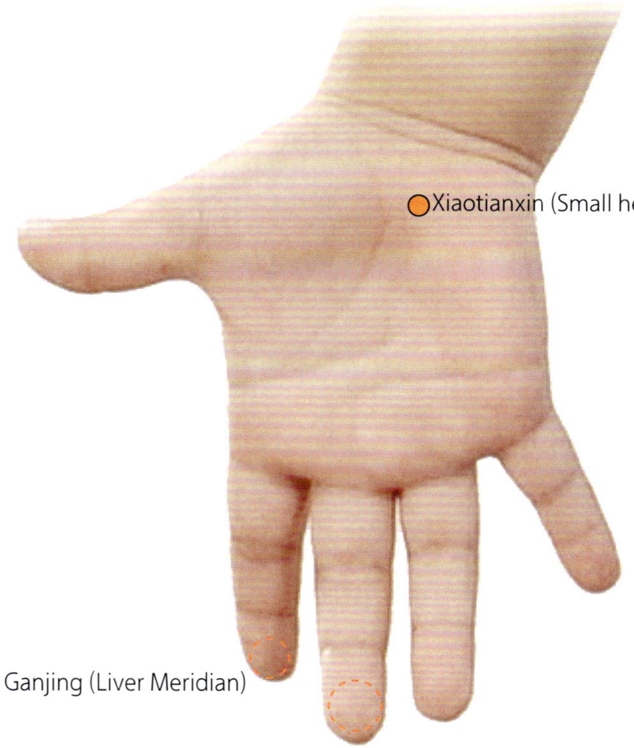

Classic Acupoints Matching

Ganjing (Liver Meridian): The finger pulp of the distal segment of the index finger.
Xinjing (Heart Meridian): The finger pulp of the distal segment of the middle finger.
Xiaotianxin (Small heaven center): In the depression of the junction of the great thenar and the hypothenar.

Massage Manipulations

Clear Ganjing (Liver Meridian): Push from the root to the tip of the finger for 100 times.
Clear Xinjing (Heart Meridian): Push from the root to the tip of the finger for 100 times.
Knead Xiaotianxin (Small heaven center): Knead the point with the finger pulp of the thumb for 5 times.

30 尿床（遗尿）

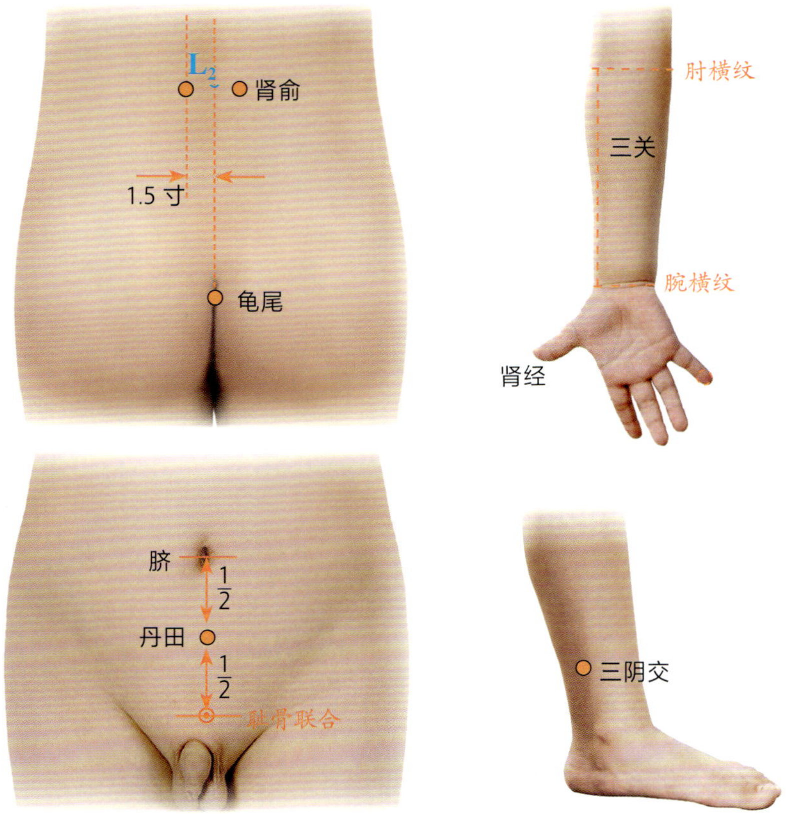

经典配穴

肾经： 小指末节指腹。

三关： 前臂桡侧，腕横纹至肘横纹呈一直线。

三阴交： 小腿内侧，足内踝尖上 3 寸，胫骨内侧缘后方。

丹田： 脐下 2 寸与 3 寸之间。

肾俞： 第 2 腰椎棘突下，旁开 1.5 寸处。

龟尾： 尾椎骨处。

按摩操作

补肾经： 旋推或自指根直推至指尖，推 200 次。

推三关： 食指、中指两指并拢，用指腹面自腕横纹或拇指桡侧直推至肘横纹，两侧各推 200 次。

按揉三阴交： 用拇指指端按揉，按揉 100 次。

揉丹田： 用食指、中指、无名指三指揉，揉 100 次。

揉肾俞： 用两拇指指端揉两侧穴位，揉 100 次。

揉龟尾： 用拇指或中指指端揉，揉 100 次。

31 近视

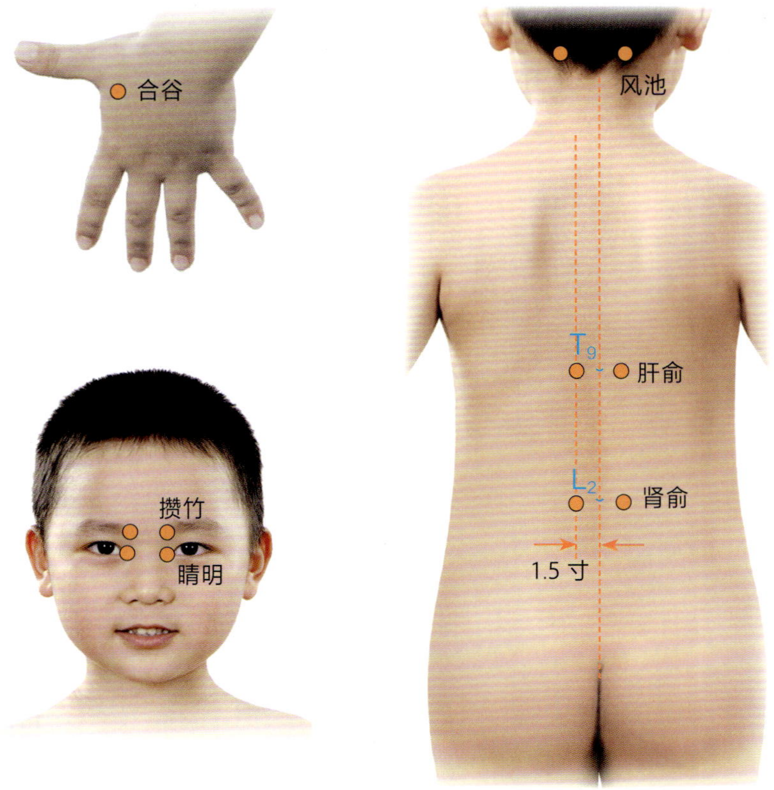

经典配穴

睛明： 目内眦内上方框内侧壁凹陷中。

攒竹： 眉毛内侧边缘凹陷处。

合谷： 手背第 1、2 掌骨之间，约平第 2 掌骨中点处。

风池： 颈后枕骨下大筋外侧凹陷中。

肾俞： 第 2 腰椎棘突下，旁开 1.5 寸处。

肝俞： 第 9 胸椎棘突下，旁开 1.5 寸处。

按摩操作

按揉睛明： 用食指指腹按揉，按揉 100 次。

按揉攒竹： 用拇指或食指指腹按揉，按揉 100 次。

按揉合谷： 用拇指指腹按揉，按揉 100 次。

揉风池： 按摩者站在小儿身后，以一手扶小儿头顶，另一手的拇指和其余四指相对用力，揉 100 次。

揉肾俞： 用两拇指指端揉两侧穴位，揉 30 次。

揉肝俞： 用两拇指指端揉两侧穴位，揉 30 次。

30 Enuresis

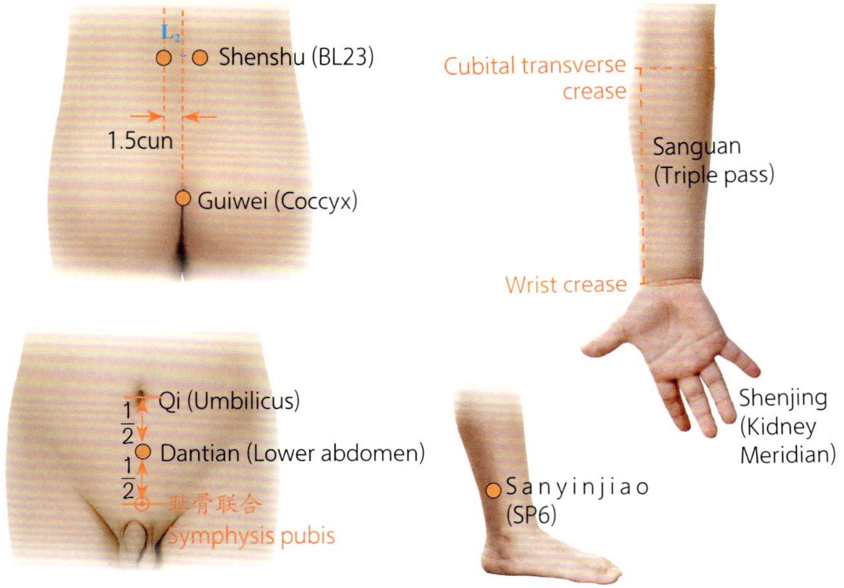

Classic Acupoints Matching

Shenjing (Kidney Meridian): The finger pulp of the distal segment of little finger.

Sanguan (Triple pass): In the radial side of the forearm, the line between wrist crease and cubital transverse crease.

Sanyinjiao (SP6): In the inner side of the leg, 3 cun above the prominence of the medial malleolus, behind the medial border of the tibia.

Dantian (Lower abdomen): Between 2 cun and 3 cun below the umbilicus.

Shenshu (BL23): 1.5 cun lateral to the depression below the spinous process of the 2nd lumbar vertebra.

Guiwei (Coccyx): At the coccygeal vertebra.

Massage Manipulations

Tonify Shenjing (Kidney Meridian): Rotate-push or push directly from the root to the tip of the finger for 200 times.

Push Sanguan (Triple pass): Close the index and middle fingers. Push directly from the wrist crease or the radial side of the thumb to the cubital transverse crease with the finger pulp for 200 times respectively.

Press-knead Sanyinjiao (SP6): Press-knead the point with the fingertip of the thumb for 100 times.

Knead Dantian (Lower abdomen): Knead the point with the index, middle and ring fingers for 100 times.

Knead Shenshu (BL23): Knead the point in both sides with the fingertips of the 2 thumbs for 100 times.

Knead Guiwei (Coccyx): Knead the point with the fingertip of the thumb or middle finger for 100 times.

31 Myopia

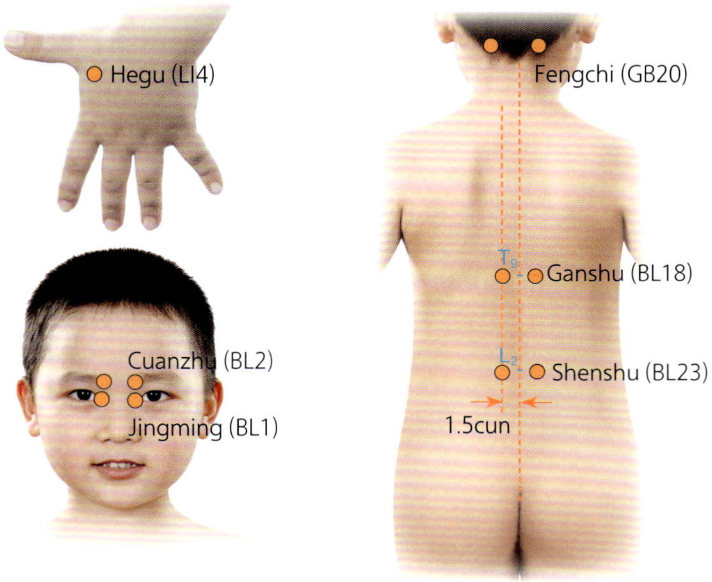

Classic Acupoints Matching

Jingming (BL1): In the depression of the medial wall of the medial superior inner canthus.

Cuanzhu (BL2): In the depression of the medial border of the eyebrow.

Hegu (LI4): Between the 1st and 2nd metacarpal bones on the dorsum of hand, at around the midpoint of the radial side of the 2nd metacarpal bone.

Fengchi (GB20): In the depression of the lateral side of the great tendon below the occipital bone behind the neck.

Shenshu (BL23): 1.5 cun lateral to the depression below the spinous process of the 2nd lumbar vertebra.

Ganshu (BL18): 1.5 cun lateral to the depression below the spinous process of the 9th thoracic vertebra.

Massage Manipulations

Press-knead Jingming (BL1): Press-knead the point with the finger pulp of the index finger for 100 times.

Press-knead Cuanzhu (BL2): Press-knead the point with the finger pulp of the thumb or index finger for 100 times.

Press-knead Hegu (LI4): Press-knead the point with the finger pulp of the thumb for 100 times.

Knead Fengchi (GB20): Stand behind the child. Hold the vertex of the child with 1 hand. Exert strength symmetrically with the thumb and other 4 fingers of the other hand to knead the point for 100 times.

Knead Shenshu (BL23): Knead the point in both sides with the fingertips of the 2 thumbs for 30 times.

Knead Ganshu (BL18): Knead the point in both sides with the fingertips of the 2 thumbs for 30 times.

32 自汗、盗汗

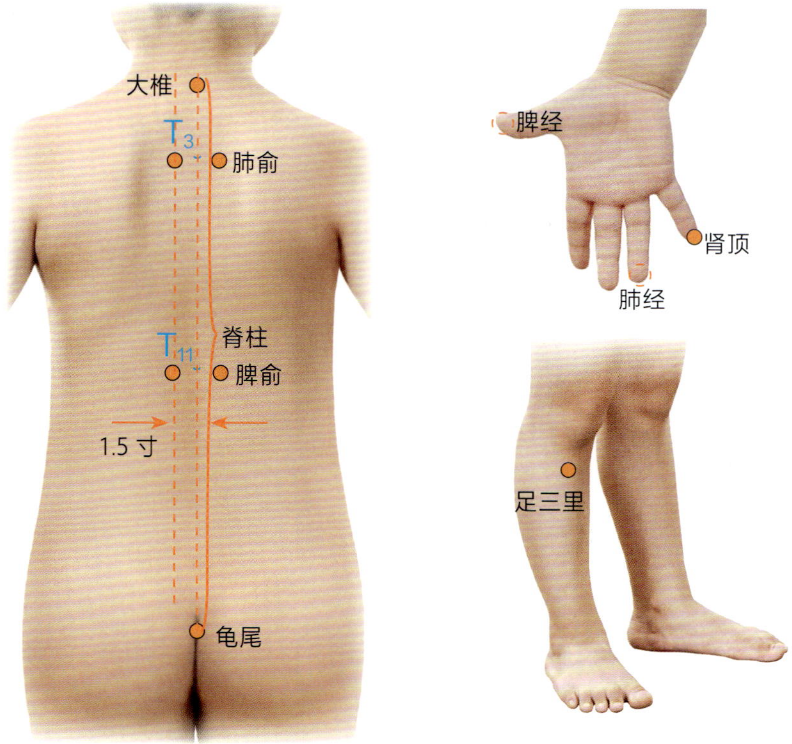

经典配穴

脾经：拇指末节指腹。
肺经：无名指掌面末节。
肾顶：小指顶端处。
足三里：膝盖外侧凹陷直下3寸，胫骨旁1寸处。
脊柱：大椎至尾骨端呈一直线。
脾俞：第11胸椎棘突下，旁开1.5寸处。
肺俞：第3胸椎棘突下，旁开1.5寸处。

按摩操作

补脾经：从拇指指尖向指根方向直推，推300次。
清肺经：从无名指指尖向指根方向推，推300次。
揉肾顶：用拇指指端揉，揉100次。
按揉足三里：用拇指指端按揉，按揉30次。
捏脊：小儿俯卧，按摩者用双手拇指、食指自小儿腰骶部开始把皮肤捏起，自下而上捏提至大椎穴处，捏10遍。
按揉脾俞：用两手拇指指腹或一手的食指和中指指端按揉，按揉30次。
揉肺俞：用两手拇指或食指指腹揉，揉30次。

33 开胃健脾

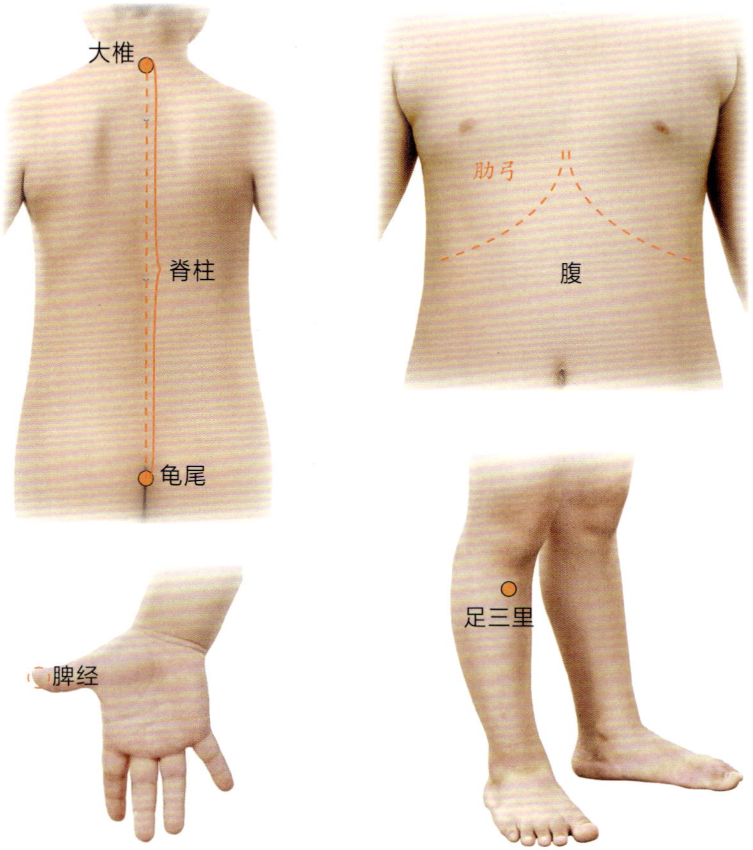

经典配穴

脾经：拇指末节指腹。
足三里：膝盖外侧凹陷直下3寸，胫骨旁1寸处。
腹：肋弓以下，肚脐以上。
脊柱：大椎至尾骨端呈一直线。

按摩操作

补脾经：从拇指指尖向指根方向直推，推200次。
按揉足三里：用拇指指端按揉，按揉100次。
摩腹：小儿仰卧，按摩者以全掌或食指、中指、无名指指腹摩上腹部，一般摩5分钟。
捏脊：小儿俯卧，按摩者用双手拇指、食指自小儿腰骶部开始把皮肤捏起，自下而上捏提至大椎穴处。一般捏3~5遍，以脊柱两侧皮肤微有潮红为有效。

32 Spontaneous Sweating and Night Sweat

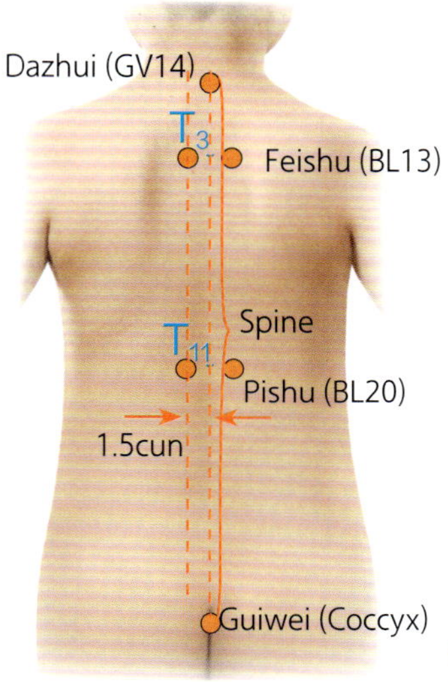

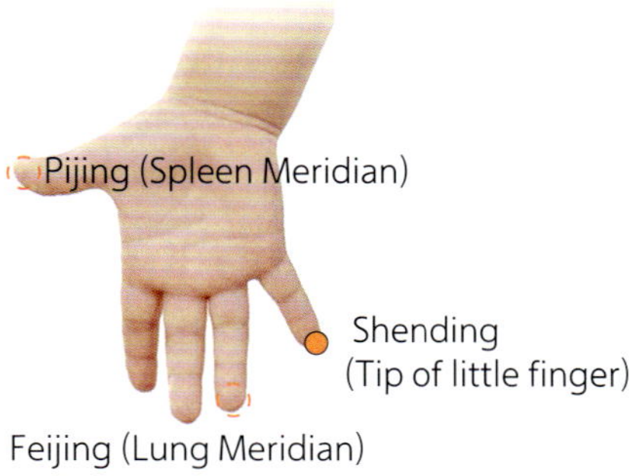

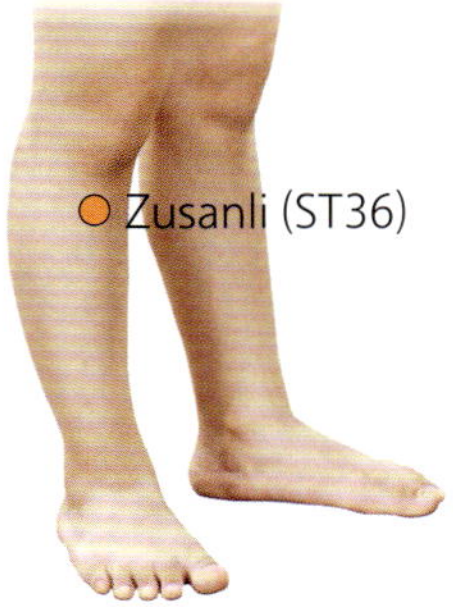

Classic Acupoints Matching

Pijing (Spleen Meridian): The finger pulp of the distal segment of thumb.
Feijing (Lung Meridian): The distal segment of the palm of ring finger.
Shending (Tip of little finger): At the tip of little finger.
Zusanli (ST36): 3 cun directly below the depression of the lateral side of the knee, 1 cun lateral to the tibia.
Spine: The straight line between Dazhui (GV14) to the end of coccygeal bone.
Pishu (BL20): 1.5 cun lateral to the spinous process of the 11th thoracic vertebra.
Feishu (BL13): 1.5 cun lateral to the spinous process of the 3rd thoracic vertebra.

Massage Manipulations

Tonify Pijing (Spleen Meridian): Push directly Pijing (Spleen Meridian) from the tip to the root of the thumb for 300 times.
Clear Feijing (Lung Meridian): Push from the tip to the root of ring finger for 300 times.
Knead Shending (Tip of little finger): Knead the point with the fingertip of the thumb for 100 times.
Press-knead Zusanli (ST36): Press-knead the point with the fingertip of the thumb for 30 times.
Pinch Spine: Let the child lie in prone position. Pinch the skin from bottom to top with the thumb and index finger of 2 hands starting from the lumbosacral region to Dazhui (GV14) for generally 10 times.
Press-knead Pishu (BL20): Press-knead the point with the finger pulp of the 2 thumbs or tips of index and middle fingers of 1 hand for 30 times.
Knead Feishu (BL13): Knead the point with the finger pulps of the thumbs or index fingers of the 2 hands for 30 times.

33 Stimulating Stomach and Invigorating Spleen

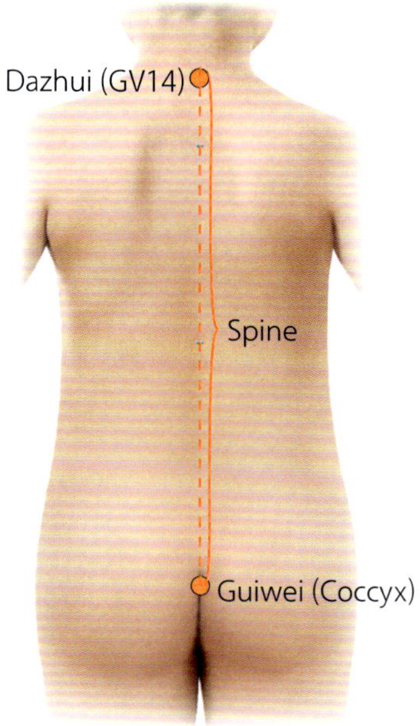

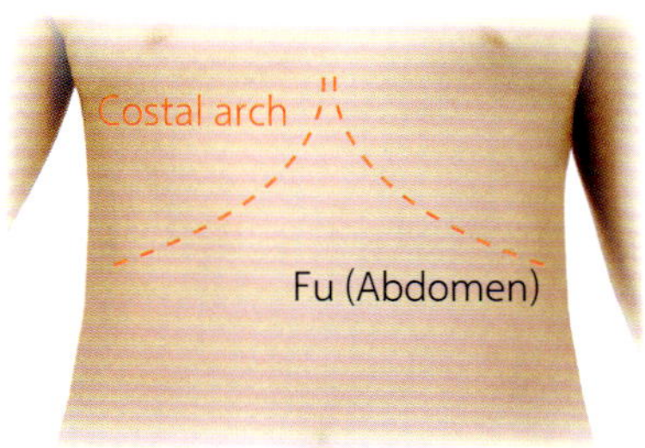

Classic Acupoints Matching

Pijing (Spleen Meridian): The finger pulp of the distal segment of thumb.
Zusanli (ST36): 3 cun directly below the depression of the lateral side of the knee, 1 cun lateral to the tibia.
Fu (Abdomen): Below the costal arch, above the umbilicus.
Spine: The straight line between Dazhui (GV14) to the end of coccygeal bone.

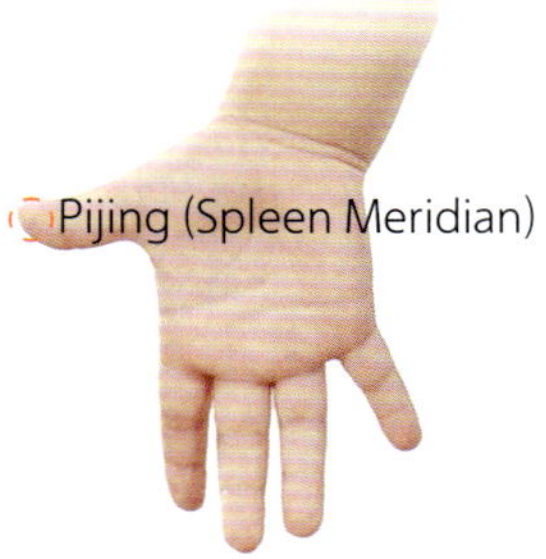

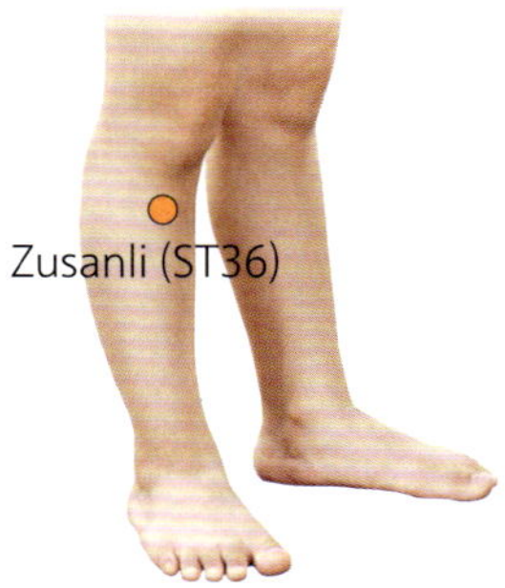

Massage Manipulations

Tonify Pijing (Spleen Meridian): Push directly Pijing (Spleen Meridian) from the tip to the root of the thumb for 200 times.
Press-knead Zusanli (ST36): Press-knead the point with the fingertip of the thumb for 100 times.
Rub Fu(Abdomen): Let the child lie in supine position. Rub the upper abdomen with the whole palm or the finger pulp of index, middle and ring fingers for generally 5 minutes.
Pinch Spine: Let the child lie in prone position. Pinch the skin from bottom to top with the thumb and index finger of 2 hands starting from the lumbosacral region to Dazhui (GV14) for generally 3 to 5 times until the skin in both sides of spine shows slightly flush as an effective manipulation.

34 宣通鼻窍

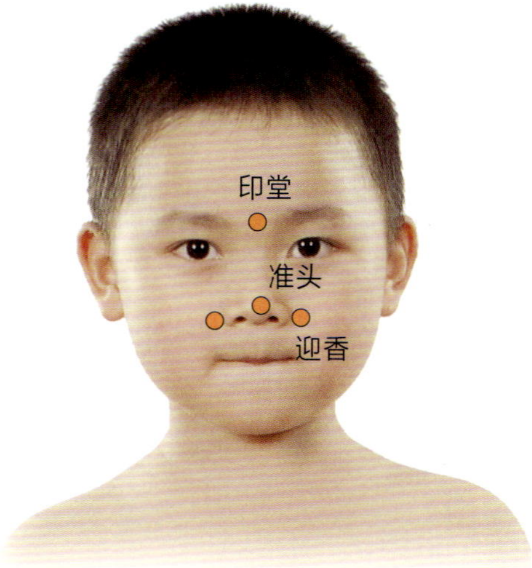

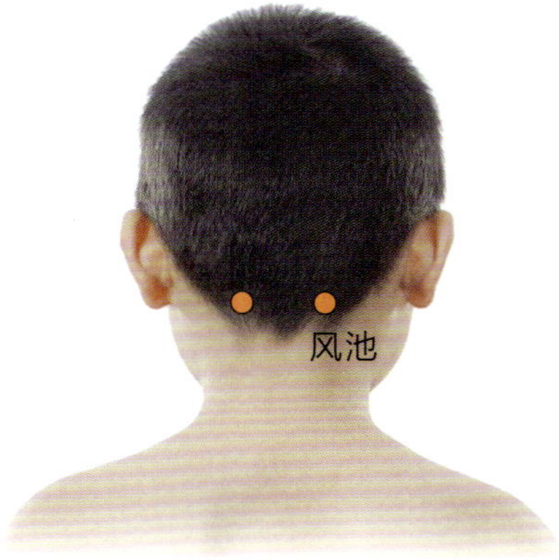

经典配穴

准头：在鼻尖中央。
风池：颈后枕骨下大筋外侧凹陷中。
迎香：鼻翼旁 0.5 寸，鼻唇沟中。
印堂：两眉内侧端连线的中点处。

按摩操作

掐准头：按摩者一手扶小儿头部以固定，另一手以拇指或食指指甲掐，掐 5 下。
揉准头：用中指指腹揉，揉 20 下。
揉风池：按摩者站在小儿身后，以一手扶小儿头顶，另一手的拇指和其余四指相对用力，揉 50 次。
拿风池：按摩者站在小儿身后，以一手扶小儿头顶，另一手的拇指和其余四指相对用力，一松一紧地拿捏本穴。
揉迎香：用食指、中指两指或两拇指指端按揉两侧穴位，揉 30 次。
揉印堂：用食指或拇指指端按揉两侧穴位，揉 30 次。
黄蜂入洞：按摩者用一手扶小儿头部，用另一手食指、中指两指指端在小儿两鼻孔下缘揉动。

35 清肺祛痰

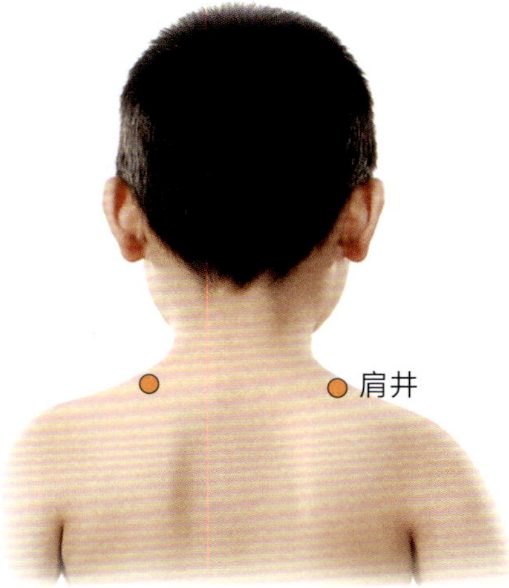

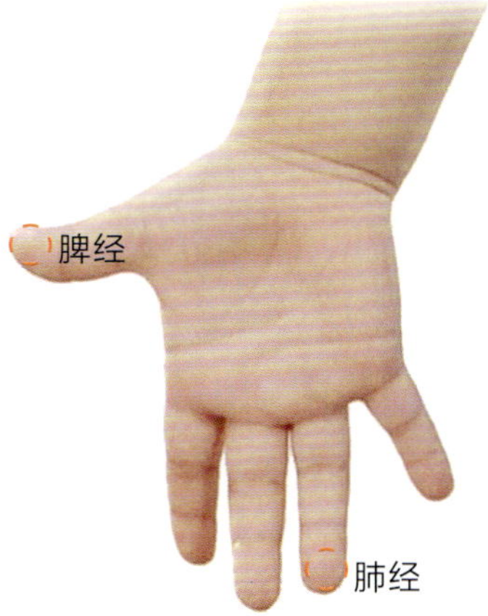

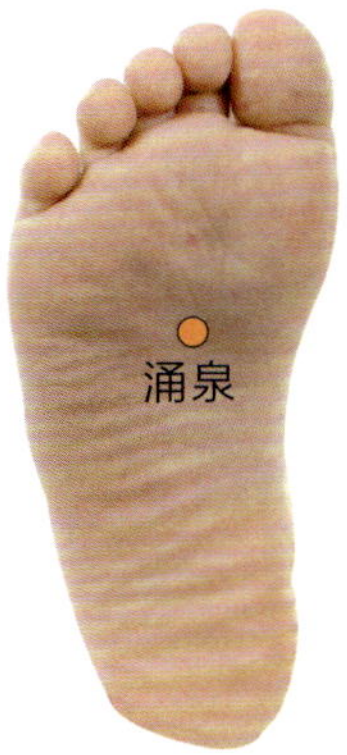

经典配穴

脾经：拇指末节指腹。
肺经：无名指掌面末节指腹。
涌泉：足掌心，屈指时呈凹陷处。
肩井：大椎与肩峰最高点连线的中点处。

按摩操作

补脾经：从拇指指尖向指根方向直推，推 100 次。
清肺经：从无名指末节指纹向指尖方向推，推 300 次。
揉涌泉：用拇指指腹按揉，以透热为度。
拿肩井：小儿取坐位，按摩者用拇指与食指、中指两指对称用力提拿本穴，拿 5 次。

34 Relieving Stuffy Nose

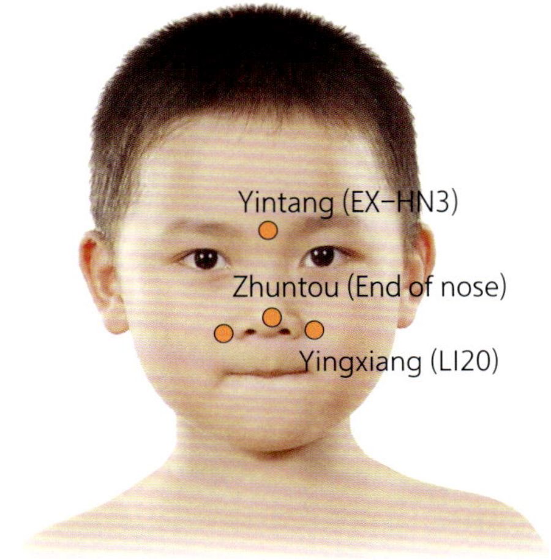

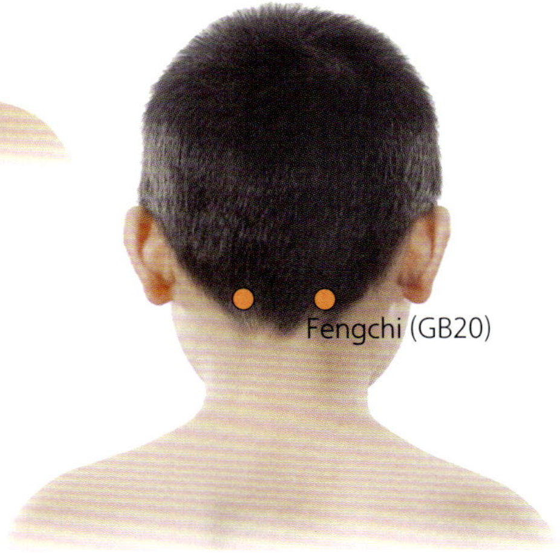

Classic Acupoints Matching

Zhuntou (End of nose): At the center of the nasal tip.
Fengchi (GB20): In the depression of the lateral side of the great tendon below the occipital bone behind the neck.
Yingxiang(LI20): 0.5 cun lateral to the nasal ala, in the nasolabial fold.
Yintang (EX-HN3): At the midpoint of the line between the medial side of the 2 eyebrows.

Massage Manipulations

Pinch Zhuntou (End of nose): Hold the head of the child for stability with 1 hand. Pinch the point with the nail of the thumb or index finger of the other hand for 5 times.
Knead Zhuntou (End of nose): Knead the point with the finger pulp of the middle finger for 20 times.
Knead Fengchi (GB20): Stand behind the child. Hold the vertex of the child with 1 hand. Exert proper strength with the thumb and other 4 fingers of the other hand to knead the point for 50 times.
Grasp Fengchi (GB20): Stand behind the child. Hold the vertex of the child with 1 hand. Exert proper strength with the thumb and other 4 fingers of the other hand to grasp and pinch the point.
Knead Yingxiang (LI20): Press-knead the point in both sides with the fingertips of the index and middle fingers or the 2 thumbs for 30 times.
Knead Yintang (EX-HN3): Press-knead the point in both sides with the fingertip of the index finger or the thumb for 30 times.
Manipulation of Huangfeng Rudong (Wasp entering the cavity): Hold the head of the child with one hand. Knead the inferior border of the 2 nares of the child with the fingertips of the index and middle fingers of the other hand.

35 Clearing Lung and Expelling Phlegm

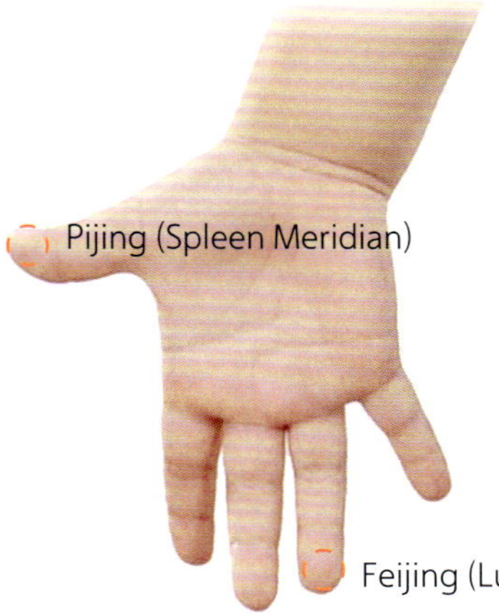

Classic Acupoints Matching

Pijing (Spleen Meridian): The finger pulp of the distal segment of the thumb.
Feijing (Lung Meridian): The finger pulp of the palm of the distal segment of ring finger.
Yongquan (KI1): In the depression of the sole when bend the toes.
Jianjing (GB21): The midpoint of the line between Dazhui (GV 14) to the peak of acromion.

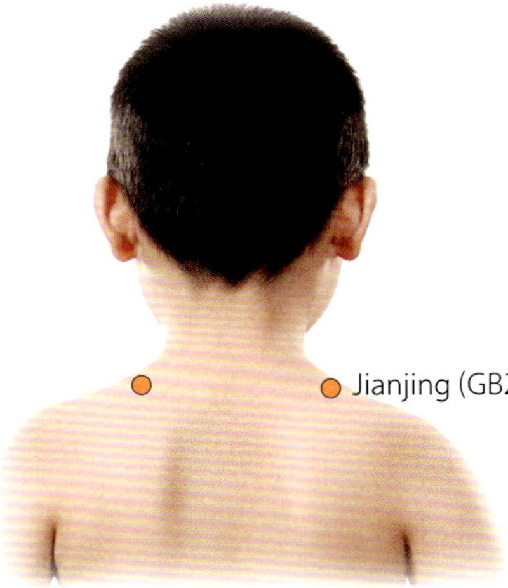

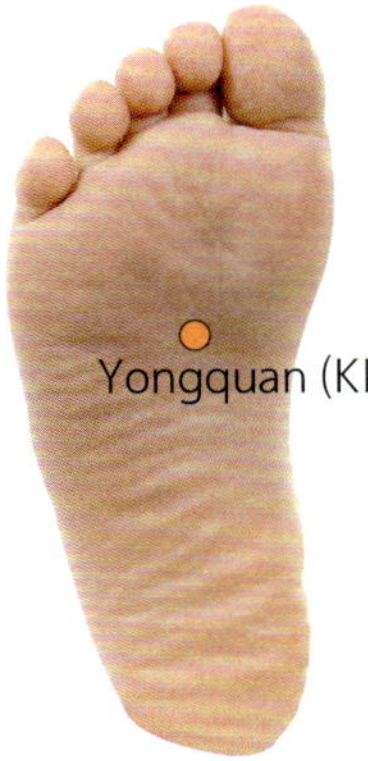

Massage Manipulations

Tonify Pijing (Spleen Meridian): Push directly Pijing (Spleen Meridian) from the tip to the root of the thumb for 100 times.
Clear Feijing (Lung Meridian): Push from the fingerprint of the distal segment of ring finger to the fingertip for 300 times.
Knead Yongquan (KI1): Press-knead the point with the finger pulp of the thumb until the skin feels warm.
Grasp Jianjing (GB21): Let the child take a sitting position. Exert strength symmetrically with the thumb, index and middle fingers to lift and grasp the point for 5 times.

36 通窍聪耳

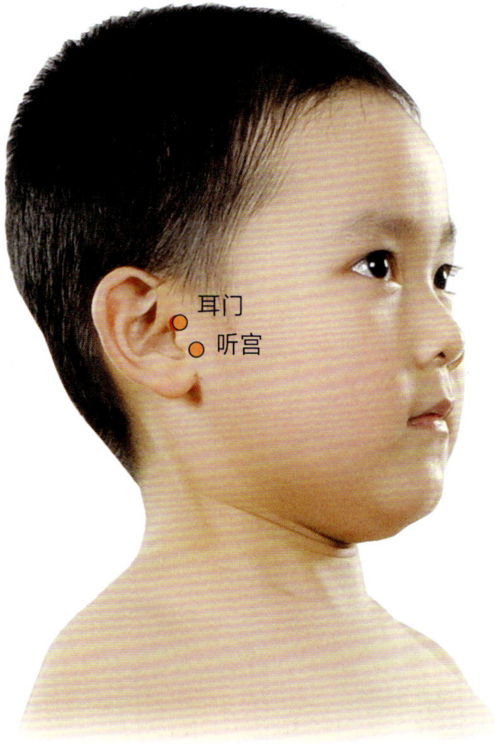

经典配穴

听宫：耳屏正中与下颌骨髁突之间的凹陷中。

耳门：耳屏上切迹前，下颌骨髁突后缘，张口凹陷处。

按摩操作

按压听宫：用食指指腹按压，按压30次。

揉耳门：用食指指腹揉，揉30次。

揉耳郭：用拇指和食指揉动耳郭，至耳郭发热。

拉耳垂：用拇指、食指捏住耳垂，向下拉动，拉30次。

摩擦双耳：用双手掌摩擦双耳，至耳朵发热。

37 清睛明目

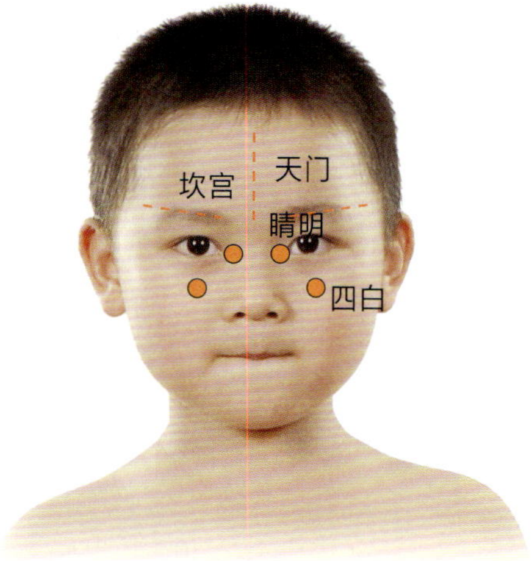

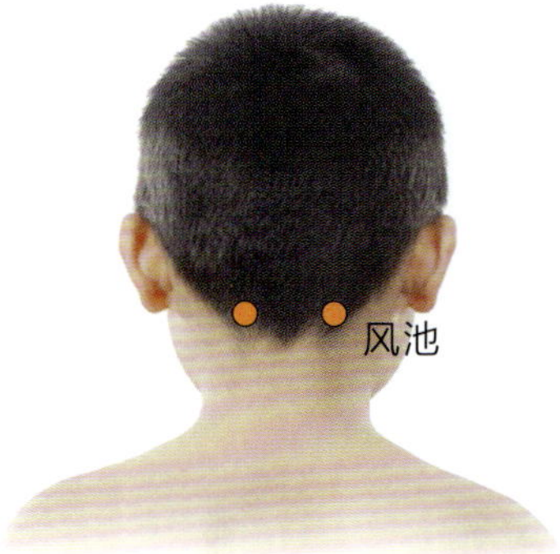

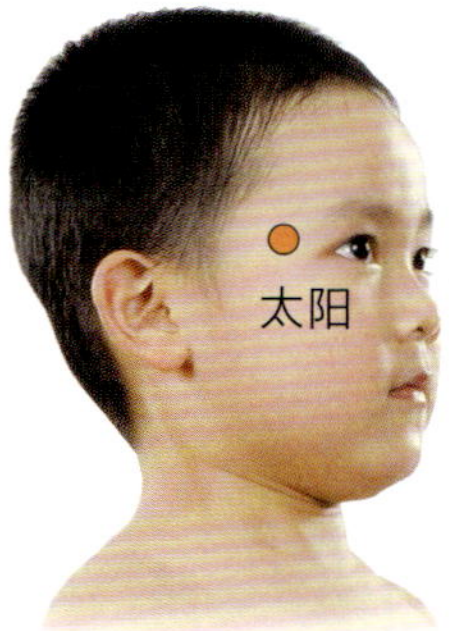

经典配穴

坎宫：从眉头起沿眉向眉梢呈一横线。

睛明：目内眦内上方框内侧壁凹陷中。

四白：瞳孔直下，眶下孔处。

太阳：眉梢与眼外角连线的中点。

风池：颈后枕骨下大筋外侧凹陷中。

天门：眉心至前发际呈一直线。

按摩操作

推坎宫：亦称分阴阳，两拇指自眉头向眉梢分推，推30次。

按睛明：用食指指腹按，按30次。

揉四白：用拇指或食指指腹揉，揉30次。

揉太阳：用拇指或食指指腹揉，两侧各揉30次。

按风池：用拇指或食指指腹按，按50次。

开天门：两拇指自下而上地交替直推，推50次。

36 Relieving Stuffy Orifices and Enhancing Hearing

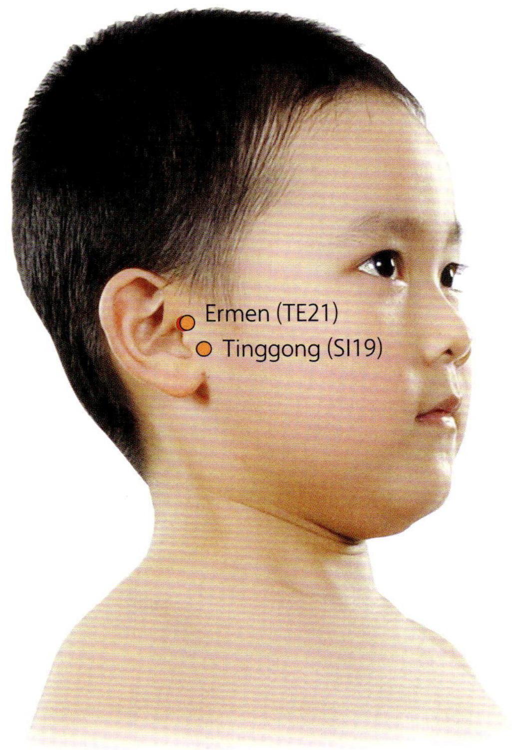

Classic Acupoints Matching

Tinggong (SI19): In the depression between the middle of tragus and the mandible condyle.
Ermen (TE21): Near the the supratragic notch, in the depression of the posterior border of the mandible condyle when open the mouth.

Massage Manipulations

Press Tinggong (SI19): Press the point with the finger pulp of the index finger for 30 times.
Knead Ermen (TE21): Knead it with the finger pulp of the index finger for 30 times.
Knead auricle: Knead the auricle with the thumb and index finger until some heat builds up.
Pull earlobe: Pinch the earlobe with the thumb and index finger. Then pull it downward for 30 times.
Rub the 2 ears: Rub the 2 ears with the 2 hands until the heat builds up.

37 Clearing Eyes and Improving Eyesight

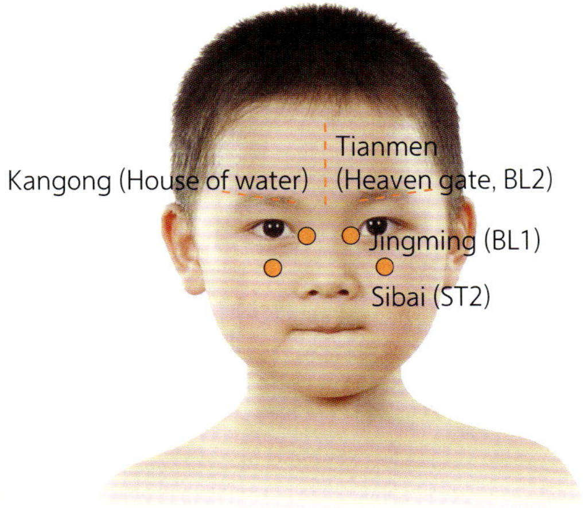

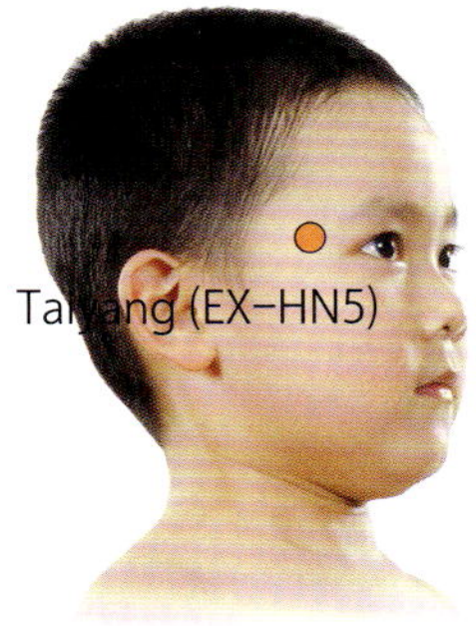

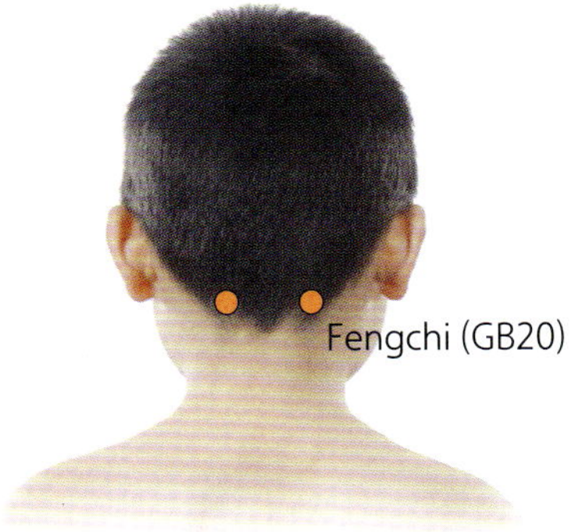

Classic Acupoints Matching

Kangong (House of water): The transverse line starting from the brow tip to the brow end along the brow.
Jingming (BL1): In the depression of the medial wall of the medial superior Inner canthus.
Sibai (ST2): Directly below the pupil, at the infraorbital foramen.
Taiyang (EX-HN5): The midpoint of the line between the brow tip to the outer canthus.
Fengchi (GB20): In the depression of the lateral side of the great tendon below the occipital bone behind the neck.
Tianmen (Heaven gate, BL2): The line between the midpoint of the 2 eyebrows and the anterior hairline.

Massage Manipulations

Push Kangong (House of water): Push from the brow tip to the brow end with the 2 thumbs for each side for 30 times, also called Yin and Yang seperation.
Press Jingming (BL1): Press the point with the finger pulp of index finger for 30 times.
Knead Sibai (ST2): Knead the point with the finger pulp of the thumb or index finger for 30 times.
Knead Taiyang (EX-HN5): Knead the point with the finger pulp of the thumb or index finger for respective 30 times in both sides of the head.
Press Fengchi (GB20): Knead the point with the finger pulp of the thumb or index finger for 50 times.
Open Tianmen (Heaven gate, BL2): Push directly and alternatively from bottom to top with the 2 thumbs for 50 times.

38 益智增聪

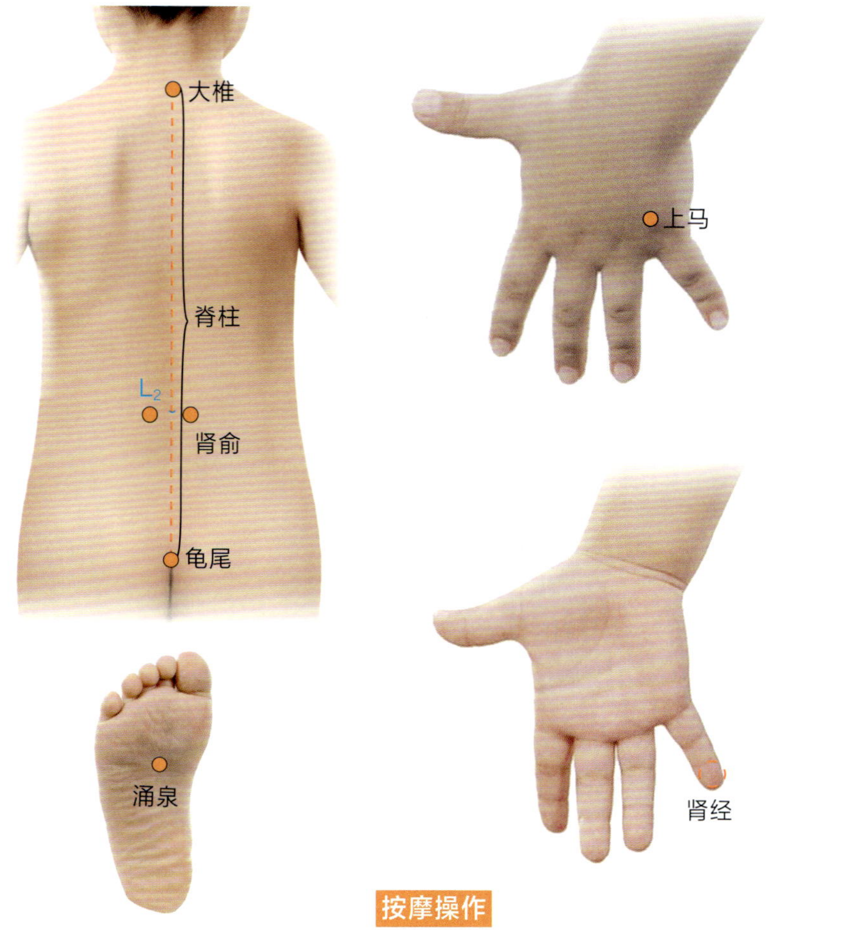

经典配穴

肾经：小指末节指腹。
上马：手背，无名指及小指之间，指掌关节后的凹陷中。
涌泉：足掌心，屈指时呈凹陷处。
脊柱：大椎至尾骨端呈一直线。
肾俞：第 2 腰椎下旁开 1.5 寸处。

按摩操作

补肾经：旋推或自指根直推至指尖，推 100 次。
揉上马：用手指指腹揉，揉 100 次。
揉涌泉：用拇指指腹按揉，以透热为度。
捏脊：小儿俯卧，按摩者用双手拇指、食指自小儿腰骶部开始把皮肤捏起，自下而上捏提至大椎穴处。捏 3~5 遍，以脊柱两侧皮肤微有潮红为有效。
揉肾俞：用两拇指端揉两侧穴位，揉 50 次。

39 壮骨增高

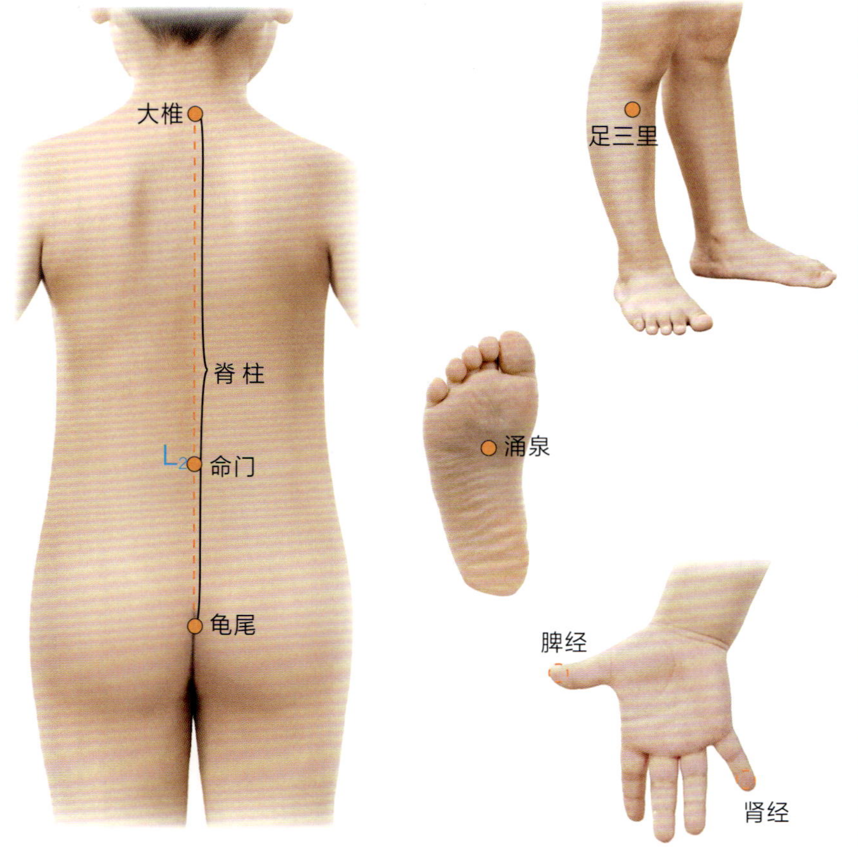

经典配穴

脾经：拇指末节指腹。
肾经：小指末节指腹。
足三里：膝盖外侧凹陷直下 3 寸，胫骨旁 1 寸处。
涌泉：足掌心，屈指时呈凹陷处。
脊柱：大椎至尾骨端呈一直线。
命门：第 2 腰椎棘突下。

按摩操作

补脾经：从拇指指尖向指根方向直推，推 100 次。
补肾经：旋推或自指根直推至指尖，推 100 次。
按揉足三里：用拇指指端按揉，按揉 100 次。
按揉涌泉：用拇指指腹按揉，以酸胀、透热为度。
捏脊：小儿俯卧，按摩者用双手拇指、食指自小儿腰骶部开始把皮肤捏起，自下而上捏提至大椎穴处。捏 3~5 遍，以脊柱两侧皮肤微有潮红为有效。
揉命门：用拇指或者食指指腹揉，揉 50 次。

38 Reinforcing Mental Development

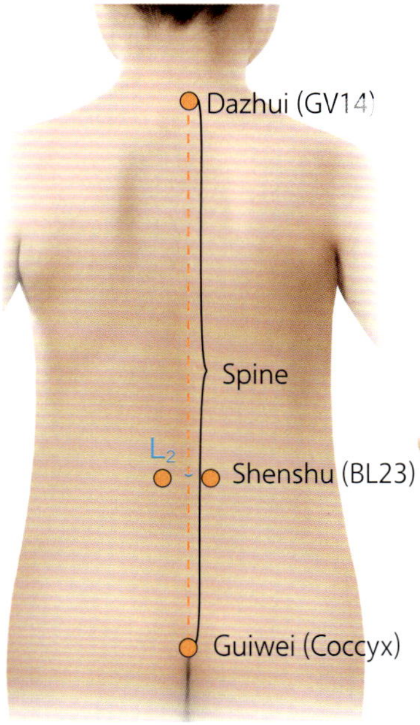

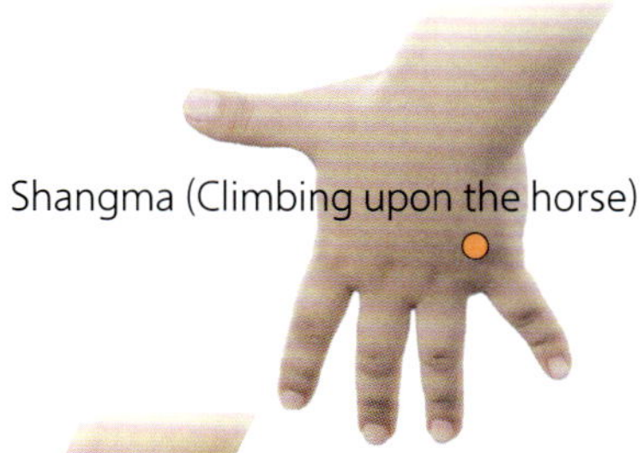

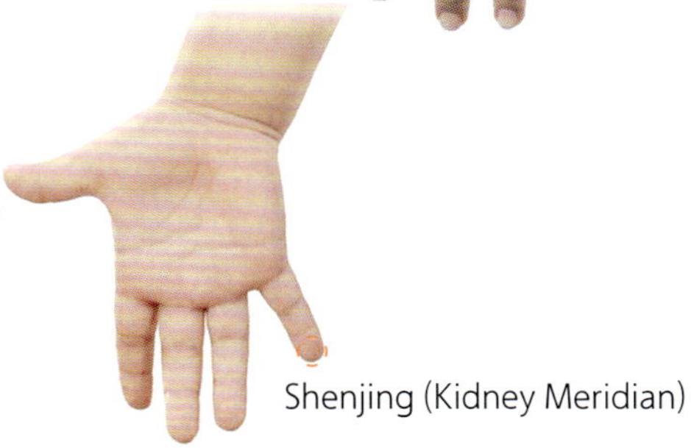

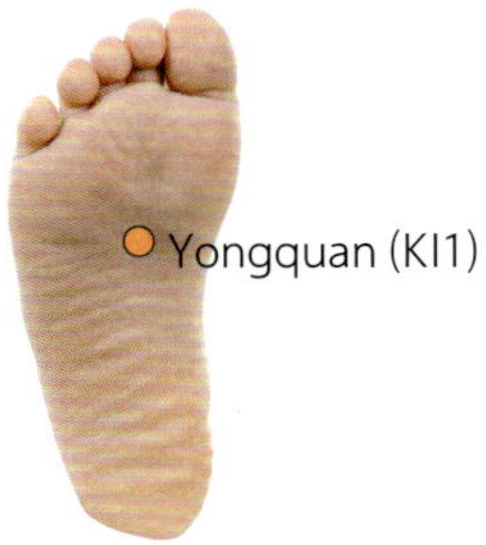

Classic Acupoints Matching

Shenjing (Kidney Meridian): The finger pulp of the distal segment of little finger.
Shangma (Climbing upon the horse): On the dorsum of hand, between the ring and little fingers, in the depression below the metacarpophalangeal joint.
Yongquan (KI1): In the depression of the sole when bend the toes.
Spine: The straight line between Dazhui (GV14) to the end of coccygeal bone.
Shenshu (BL23): 1.5 cun lateral to the depression below the spinous process of the 2nd lumbar vertebra.

Massage Manipulations

Tonify Shenjing (Kidney Meridian): Rotate-push or push directly from the root to the tip of the finger for 100 times.
Knead Shangma (Climbing upon the horse): Knead the point with the finger pulp for 100 times.
Knead Yongquan (KI1): Press-knead the point with the finger pulp of the thumb until the skin feels warm.
Pinch Spine: Let the child lie in prone position. Pinch the skin from bottom to top with the thumb and index finger of 2 hands starting from the lumbosacral region to Dazhui (GV 14) for generally 3 to 5 times until the skin in both sides of spine shows slightly flush as an effective manipulation.
Knead Shenshu (BL23): Knead the point in both sides with the fingertips of the 2 thumbs for 50 times.

39 Strengthening Bones and Increasing Height

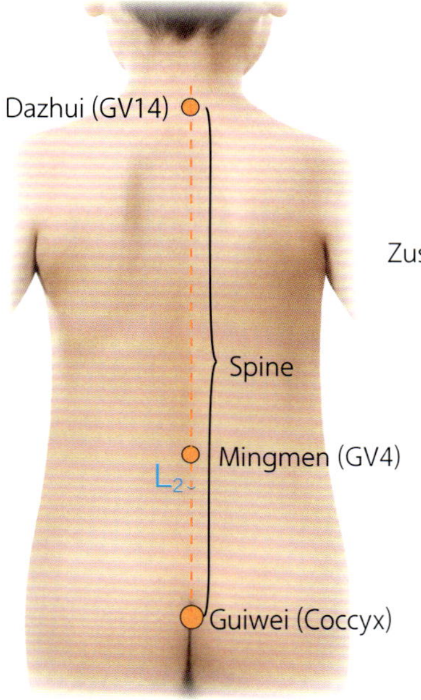

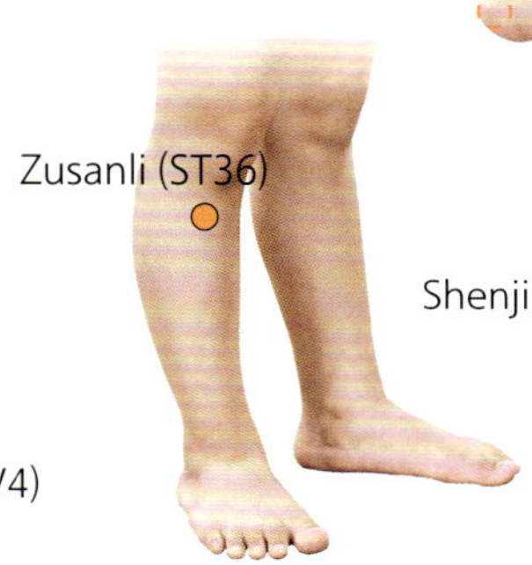

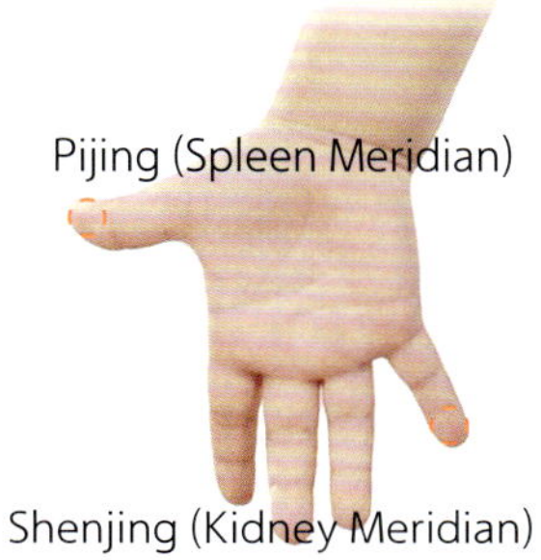

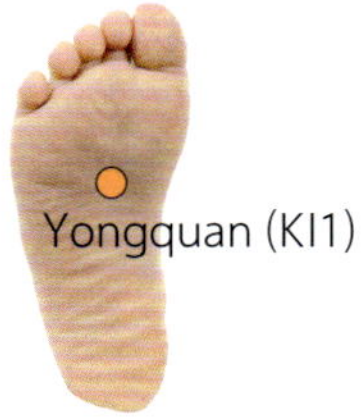

Classic Acupoints Matching

Pijing (Spleen Meridian): The finger pulp of the distal segment of thumb.
Shenjing (Kidney Meridian): The finger pulp of the distal segment of little finger.
Zusanli (ST36): 3 cun directly below the depression of the lateral side of the knee, 1 cun lateral to the tibia.
Yongquan (KI1): In the depression of the sole when bend the toes.
Spine: The straight line between Dazhui (GV14) to the end of coccygeal bone.
Mingmen (GV4): In the depression below the spinous process of the 2nd lumbar vertebra.

Massage Manipulations

Tonify Pijing (Spleen Meridian): Push directly Pijing (Spleen Meridian) from the tip to the root of the thumb for 100 times.
Tonify Shenjing (Kidney Meridian): Rotate-push or push directly from the root to the tip of the finger for 100 times.
Press-knead Zusanli (ST36): Press-knead the point with the fingertip of the thumb for 100 times.
Press-knead Yongquan (KI1): Press-knead the point with the finger pulp of the thumb until the skin feels soreness, distension and warm.
Pinch Spine: Let the child lie in prone position. Pinch the skin from bottom to top with the thumb and index finger of 2 hands starting from the lumbosacral region to Dazhui (GV 14) for generally 3 to 5 times until the skin in both sides of spine shows slightly flush as an effective manipulation.
Knead Mingmen (GV4): Knead the point with the finger pulp of the thumb or index finger for 50 times.

40 保健强身

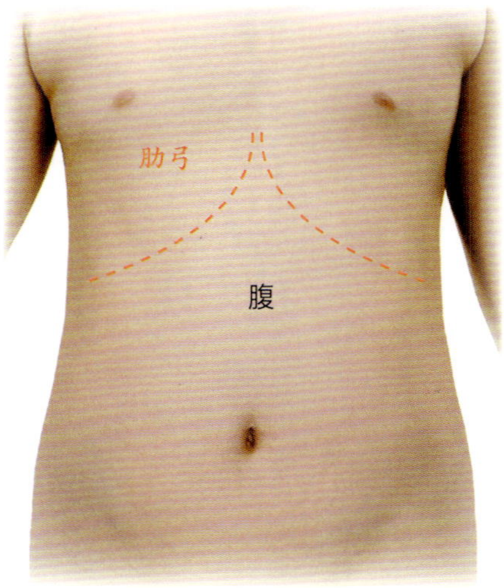

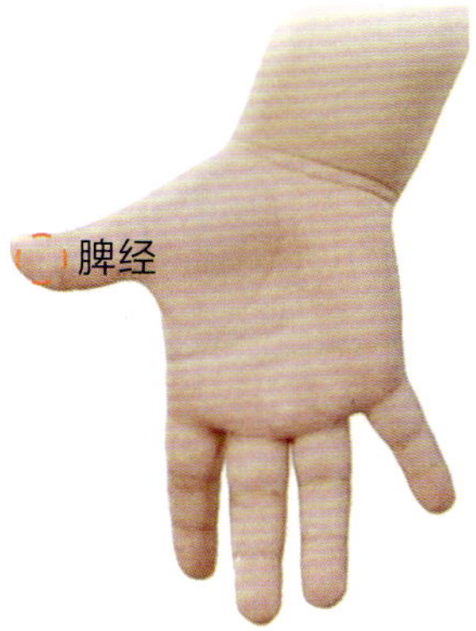

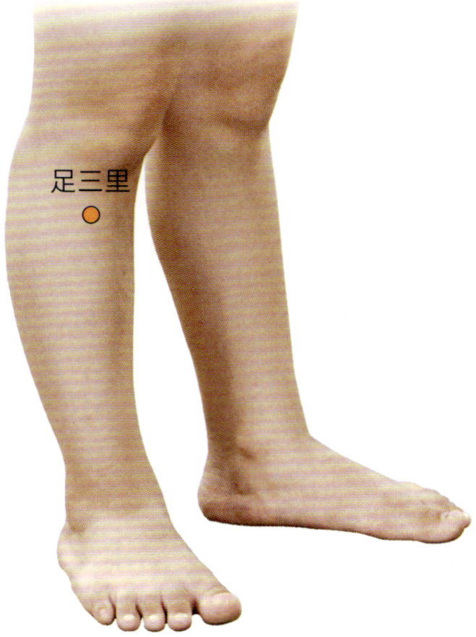

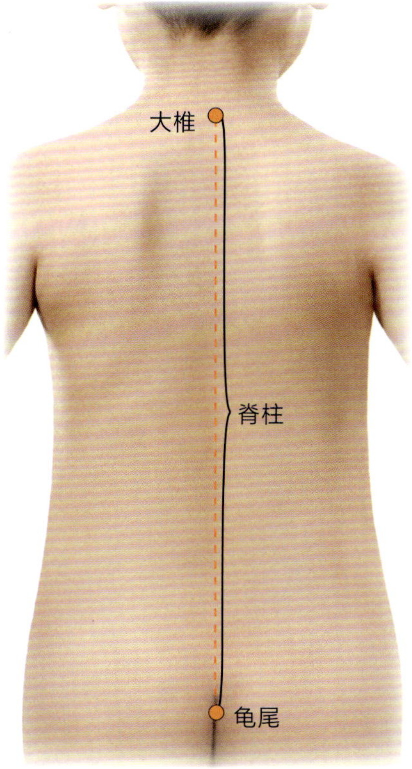

经典配穴

脾经：拇指末节指腹。
腹：肋弓以下，肚脐以上。
足三里：膝盖外侧凹陷直下 3 寸，胫骨旁 1 寸处。
脊柱：大椎至尾骨端呈一直线。

按摩操作

补脾经：从拇指指尖向指根方向直推，推 100 次。
摩腹：小儿仰卧，按摩者以全掌或食指、中指、无名指指腹摩上腹部，一般摩 5 分钟。
按揉足三里：用拇指指端按揉，按揉 200 次。
捏脊：小儿俯卧，按摩者用双手拇指、食指自小儿腰骶部开始把皮肤捏起，自下而上捏提至大椎穴处。捏 3~5 遍，以脊柱两侧皮肤微有潮红为有效。

40 Health Protection and Body Building

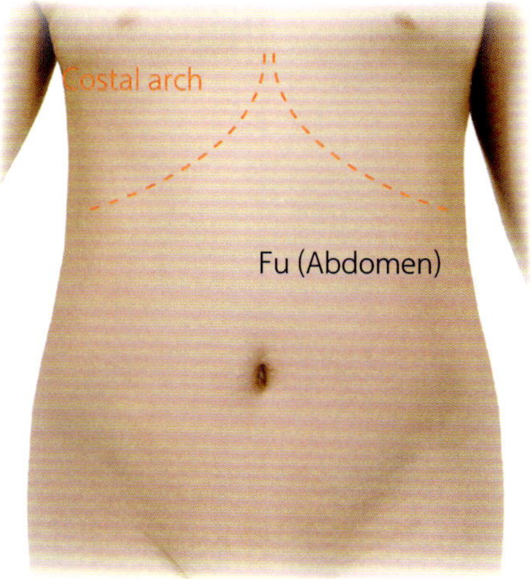

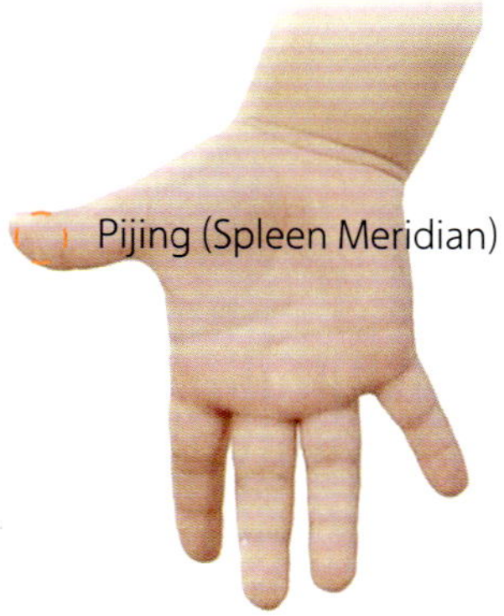

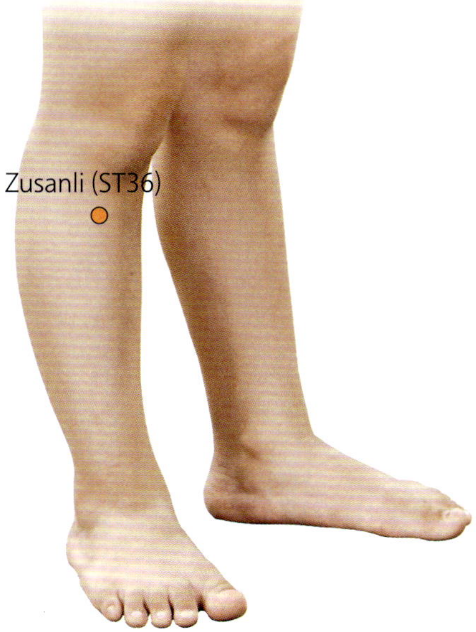

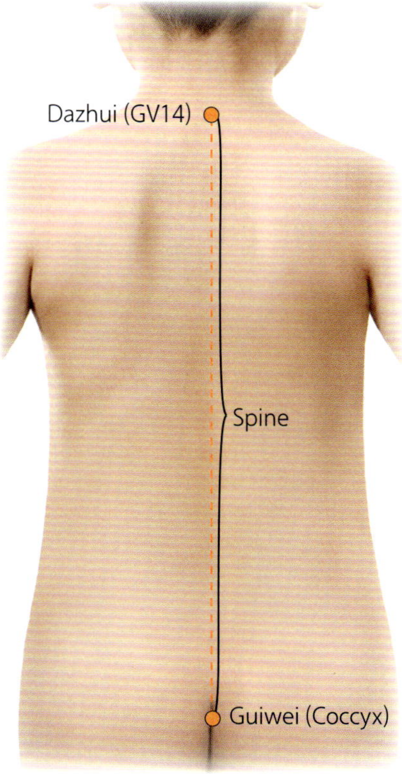

Classic Acupoints Matching

Pijing (Spleen Meridian): The finger pulp of the distal segment of thumb.
Fu (Abdomen): Below the costal arch, above the umbilicus.
Zusanli (ST36): 3 cun directly below the depression of the lateral side of the knee, 1 cun lateral to the tibia.
Spine: The straight line between Dazhui (GV14) to the end of coccygeal bone.

Massage Manipulations

Tonify Pijing (Spleen Meridian): Push directly Pijing (Spleen Meridian) from the tip to the root of the thumb for 100 times.
Rub Fu (Abdomen): Let the child lie in supine position. Rub the upper abdomen with the whole palm or the finger pulp of index, middle and ring fingers for generally 5 minutes.
Press-knead Zusanli (ST36): Press-knead the point with the fingertip of the thumb for 200 times.
Pinch Spine: Lie in prone position. Pinch the skin from bottom to top with the thumb and index finger of 2 hands starting from the lumbosacral region to Dazhui (GV14) for generally 3 to 5 times until the skin in both sides of spine shows slightly flush as an effective manipulation.

Three-Dimension

Colored Diagrams for

Meridians and Acupoints

(Chinese-English Edition)

三维经络穴位全彩图集

(中英对照版)

编　著　（按姓氏笔画排序）

老中医养生堂　刘嘉瑶
许博捷　杨丽雯
余骏腾　张金金
张晓雯　张淑巧
陈谷超　林　芳
段牡薇　贾荣曼
高玉伟　郭修兵
曹柏川　曹琳琰

Body Reflex Zones

人体反射区

编　著　（按姓氏笔画排序）

刘嘉瑶　杨丽雯
张晓雯　陈谷超
段牡薇　高玉伟
郭修兵

海峡出版发行集团 | 福建科学技术出版社
THE STRAITS PUBLISHING & DISTRIBUTING GROUP | FUJIAN SCIENCE & TECHNOLOGY PUBLISHING HOUSE

目录 CONTENTS

第一章　足部反射区及穴位 6
Chapter 1：Reflex Zones and Acupoints in Foot

第二章　手部反射区及穴位 56
Chapter 2：Reflex Zones and Acupoints in Hand

第三章　耳部反射区 122
Chapter 3：Reflex Zones in Ear

本书特色与使用说明

1. 收录人体五大反射区的定位、主治和按摩方法，大图大字，图文对照，兼具图书和挂图的优点。

2. 结合 AR 技术展示头、脊柱、手、足等身体四大部位的相关经脉循行和穴位取穴方法，形象直观。读者通过扫描并关注“健康乐读汇”微信公众号，按提示下载客户端，扫描识别码即可观看。

3. 收录 48 种常见病症的超速效对症按摩，简单实用疗效佳。

Features and Instructions

1.The book includes the location of 5 reflex zones in human body, indications and massage manipulations with bold images and characters, as well as text and diagram for better and clear understanding.

2.The relative meridian circulation and point-choosing on the head, spine, hand and foot are displayed vividly and straightforwardly in the book, combined with AR technology. Readers may scan the QR code in back cover and register on WeChat public account of ***Happy Reading on Health***. Download the client App under the instructions and you can read after scanning the identification code.

3.Super quick-acting symptomatic massage manipulations for 48 common syndromes are included. It is simple and practical with well curative effect.

第一章 足部反射区及穴位

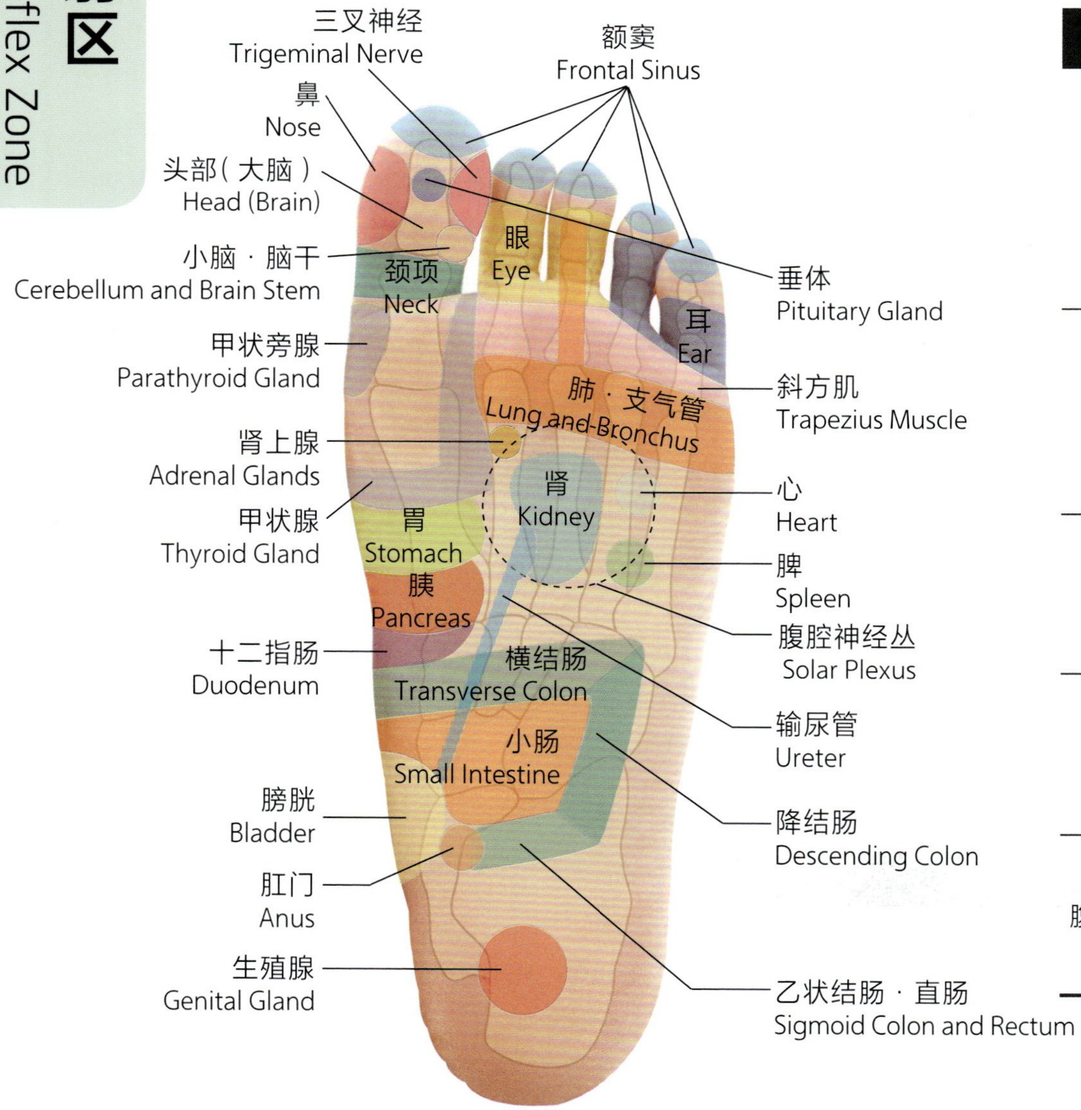

反射区	定 位	主 治
肾上腺	双足底脚掌中央第 1、2 跖趾关节所形成的“人”字形交叉点略偏外侧处	消炎、止痛、止喘、抗过敏、抗休克，适用于风湿性关节炎、甲状腺功能亢进或低下及其他内分泌疾患
肾	双足底脚掌中央第 2、3 跖骨与跖趾关节所形成的“人”字形交叉点后方凹陷处	泌尿系统疾患，以及水肿、风湿性关节炎、肾性高血压等疾病
输尿管	双足底，肾反射区与膀胱反射区之间，呈斜线状的一个弧形带状区域	尿路结石、前列腺炎、前列腺增生、排尿困难等泌尿系统病症
膀胱	双足底与足内侧交界处，足舟骨下方，拇展肌侧旁，足内踝前方	膀胱疾患及其他泌尿系统疾患
腹腔神经丛	双足底的中心，分布在肾反射区附近的、大致呈一圆形的区域	腹胀、腹泻、便秘、胃肠痉挛、反酸等

Chapter 1:
Reflex Zones and Acupoints in Foot

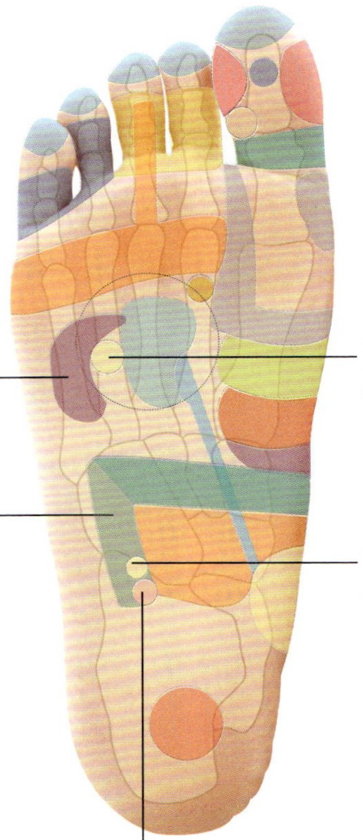

Reflex Zone	Location	Indications
Adrenal Glands	In the lateral part of the cross point of a herringbone pattern, formed by the 1st and 2nd metatarsophalangeal joints of the central soles	It is anti-inflammatory; pain-relieving; antasthmatic; anaphylactic; and antishocking. It indicated with rheumarthritis, hyperactivity or hypoactivity of thyroid and other endocrine disease
Kidney	In the rear sunken part of the cross point of a herringbone pattern, formed by the 2nd and 3rd metatarsal bones and the metatarsophalangeal joints of the central soles	Urinary diseases; edema; rheumatic arthritis; renal hypertension
Ureter	In the soles between the Kidney and Bladder reflex zone, the oblique arc-shaped band zone	Urinary diseases such as urolithiasis; prostatitis; prostatic hyperplasia and dysuria
Bladder	In the junction of the bottom and inside of feet, below the navicular bone, the side of abductor pollicis, and the front of the inside ankle	Vesical disease and other urinary diseases
Solar Plexus	In the central bottom part of feet, in the Kidney reflex zone, shaped like a circle	Abdominal distension; diarrhea; constipation; gastrointestinal spasm; acid regurgitation and so on

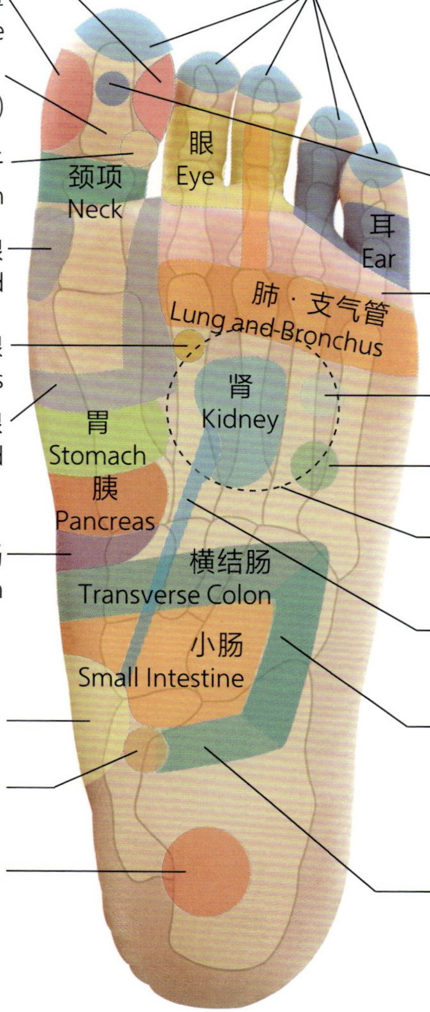

续表

反射区	定 位	主 治
额窦	双足底，10 个脚趾的趾端	头痛、头晕、失眠，以及鼻、眼、耳、口腔等部位的疾患
垂体	双足拇趾趾腹的中央	内分泌疾患、儿童发育不良、儿童智能低下、围绝经期综合征等，刺激该反射区还具有抗衰老作用
小脑 · 脑干	双足拇趾趾腹根部，近第 2 趾的一侧	小脑疾患、高血压、头痛、失眠、眩晕、肌肉紧张、肌腱关节疾病
三叉神经	双足拇趾趾腹中部，靠近第 2 趾的一侧	偏头痛、三叉神经痛、面瘫、面肌痉挛、腮腺炎及头面部其他疾患
鼻	双足拇趾内侧面，自拇趾趾腹内侧缘延伸到拇趾背面趾甲根部，呈“L”形的区域	鼻部各种疾患及上呼吸道感染
头部（大脑）	双足拇趾的整个趾腹	脑出血、脑梗死及其后遗症、脑震荡、头痛、头晕、失眠、神经衰弱、神志不清、大脑萎缩及帕金森病等

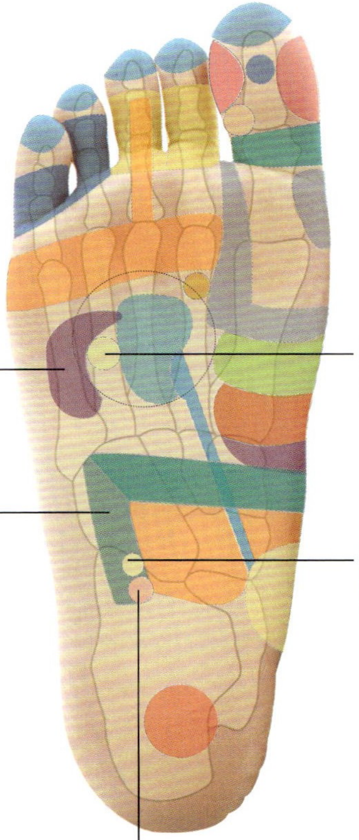

Continued

Reflex Zone	Location	Indications
Frontal Sinus	In the soles, the end of toes	Headache; dizziness; insomnia; and diseases in nose, eyes, ear and mouth
Pituitary Gland	In the central hallux pulp of feet	Endocrine diseases; dysplasia and mental retardation of children; perimenopausal syndrome. It stimulate the reflex zone and have anti–aging function
Cerebellum and Brain Stem	The root of hallux pulp of feet, in the side of the 2nd toe	Cerebellum disease; hypertension; headache; insomnia; dizziness; muscular tension; and tendon joints diseases
Trigeminal Nerve	In the central part of hallux pulp of feet, near the 2nd toe	Migraine headache; trigeminal neuralgia; facial paralysis; facial spasm; parotitis and other diseases in head and face
Nose	In the lateral part of hallux of feet, extended to the root of the back side of hallux, shaped like "L"	Nose diseases and infection of the upper respiratory tract
Head (Brain)	The whole toe pulp of feet	Cerebral hemorrhage; cerebral infarction and its sequels; concussion of brain; headache; dizziness; insomnia; neurosism; obnubilation; cerebral atrophy; parkinson disease, and so on

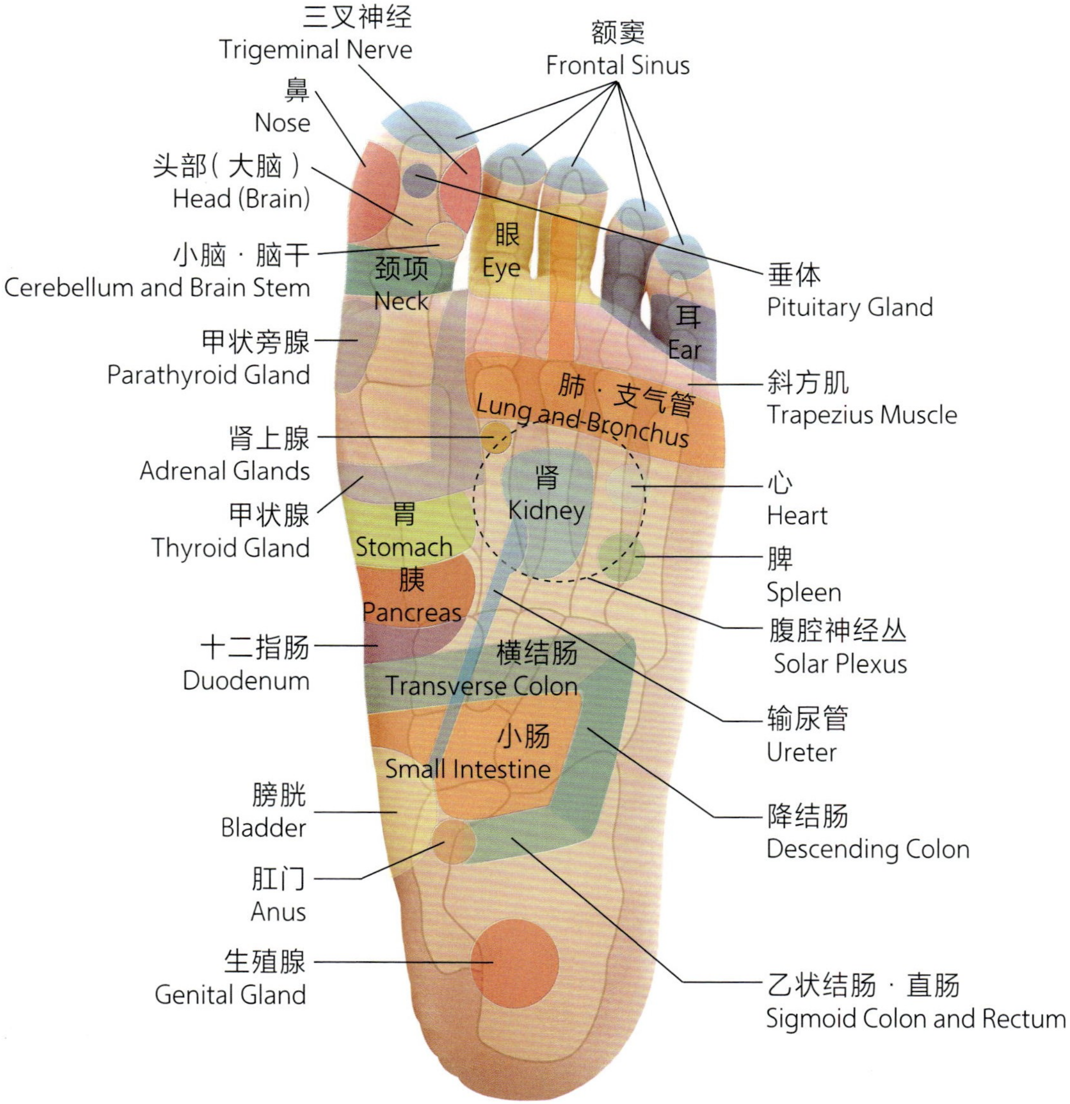

续表

反射区	定 位	主 治
颈项	双足底拇趾根部横纹处	颈椎病、落枕、颈部软组织损伤
眼	双足底，第 2、3 趾额窦反射区下方至中节趾骨底面之间的区域	眼部各种疾患（近视、远视、青光眼、白内障等）
耳	双足底，第 4、5 趾额窦反射区下方至中节趾骨底面之间的区域	耳部各种疾患（中耳炎、耳鸣、耳聋、重听等）
甲状旁腺	双足底内侧缘，第 1 跖趾关节前方凹陷处	缺钙症状（筋骨酸痛、手足麻痹或痉挛），指甲易断，中老年缺钙、骨质疏松，癫痫急性发作（用重手法强刺激）
甲状腺	双足底，第 1、2 趾间缝向后延伸，再转向内侧，呈弧形带状包围着第 1 跖骨小头	甲状腺功能亢进或低下、甲状腺炎、甲状腺肿大、肥胖症
斜方肌	双足底，第 2、3、4、5 趾后方约呈一拇指宽的横带状区域	颈项部及肩背部酸痛、落枕、上肢酸痛无力或麻痹等

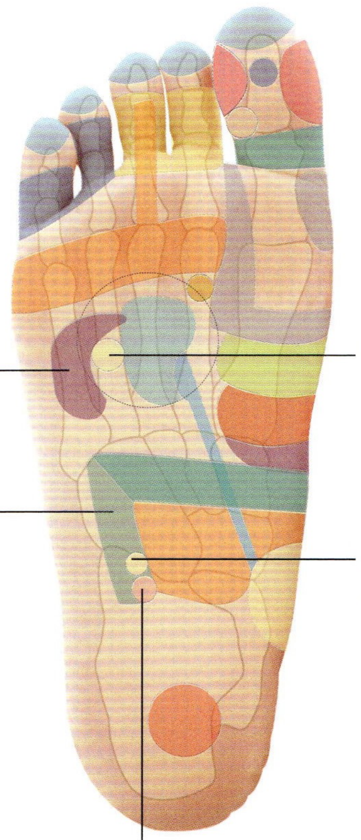

Continued

Reflex Zone	Location	Indications
Neck	The strip zone of the root of hallux in the soles	Cervical spondylopathy; stiff neck; and soft tissue injury of neck
Eye	The soles, the 2nd and 3rd toe of frontal sinus below the reflex zone, to the bottom of intermediate phalanges	Eye diseases (myopia, hyperopia, glaucoma, cataract and so on)
Ear	The soles, the 4th and 5th toe of frontal sinus below the reflex zone, to the bottom of intermediate phalanges	Ear diseases (tympanitis, tinnitus, deafness, hearing impairment and so on)
Parathyroid Gland	Inside of the soles, in the depression of the 1st metatarsophalangeal joint	Calcium deficiency (soreness of tendon and bone, paralysis and spasm of hand and foot); brittle nails; calcium deficiency of middle-aged people; osteoporosis; acute seizures (stimulating with strong measures)
Thyroid Gland	The soles, from the 1st and 2nd interphalangeal toe, backwards and turn to inside, surrounding the 1st metatarsal head shaped like a curved ribbon	Hyperactivity or hypoactivity of thyroid gland; thyreoitis; goiter; and obesity
Trapezius Muscle	The soles, a thumb's width of band zone in the back of the 2nd, 3rd, 4th, and 5th toe	Soreness in neck; shoulder and back; stiff neck; soreness; weakness or paralysis of upper limb and so on

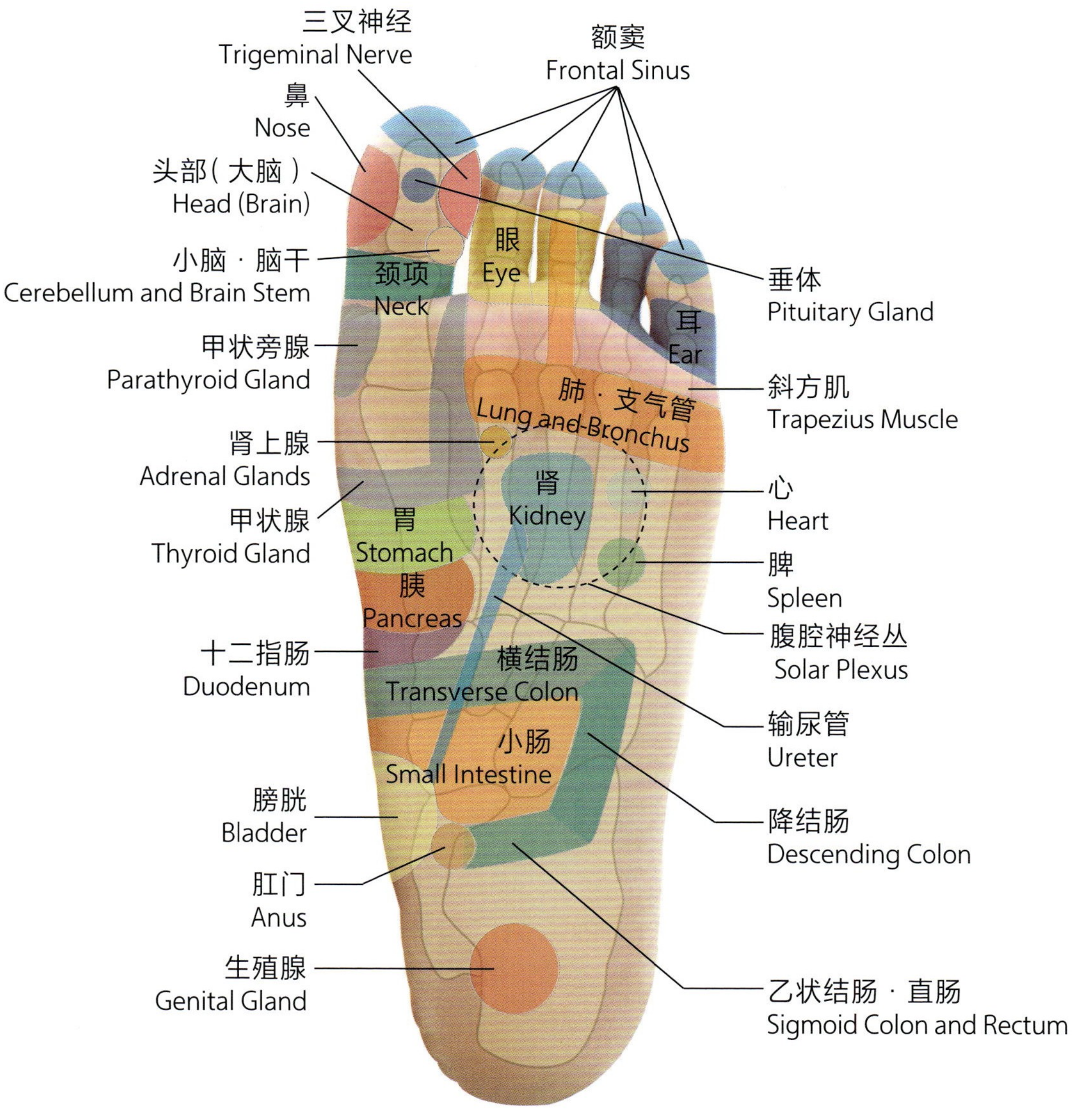

续表

反射区	定 位	主 治
肺 · 支气管	双足底，斜方肌反射区的后方约一拇指宽的横带状区域。自横带中部向第 3 趾延伸呈一竖条状区域是支气管敏感带	肺炎、支气管炎、哮喘、肺气肿等呼吸系统疾患
心	左足底，第 4、5 跖骨体之间，肺反射区下方（足跟方向）	循环系统疾患如心律不齐、心前区疼痛、心肌炎、冠心病、高脂血症、动脉硬化、高血压、低血压等
脾	左足底，第 4、5 跖骨体之间，心反射区向足跟方向约一横指处	贫血、皮肤病、食欲不振、消化不良、发热、各种炎症等，刺激该反射区还有增强免疫功能的功效
胃	双足底内侧第 1 跖骨头的后方，宽度约一横指的区域	消化系统疾患如恶心、呕吐、腹胀、胃痛、胃酸过多、消化不良、急慢性胃肠炎、胃溃疡、胃下垂等
胰	双足底内侧，第 1 跖骨体靠近跗跖关节处，胃反射区与十二指肠反射区之间，宽度约一横指的区域	糖尿病、消化不良、胰腺炎等

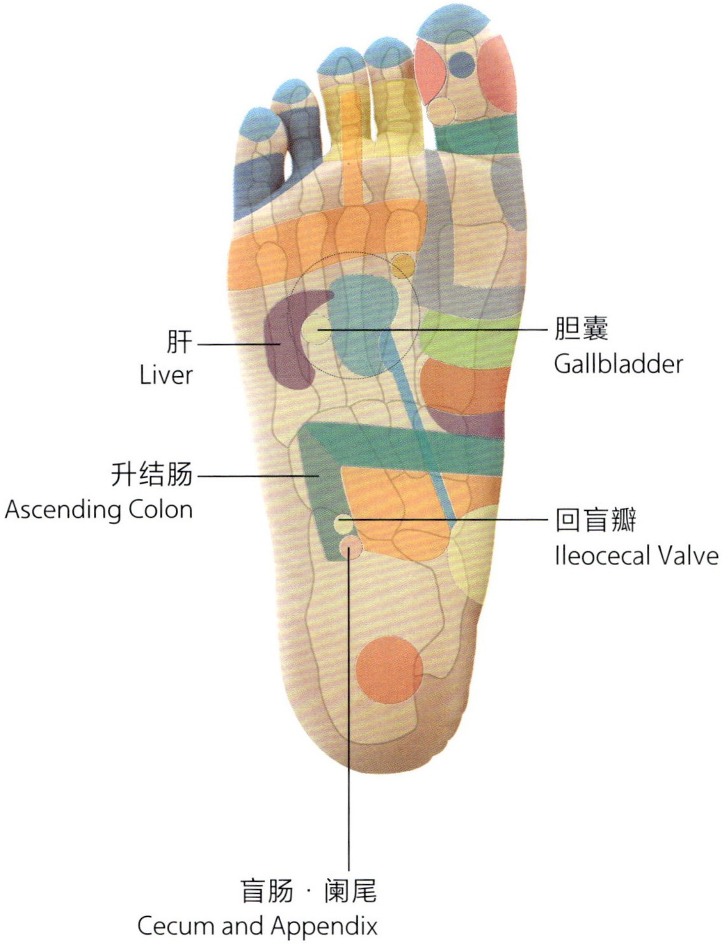

Continued

Reflex Zone	Location	Indications
Lung and Bronchus	The soles, a cross band zone behind the trapezius muscle of a thumb's width, in the middle of which is a sensitive zone of bronchus shaped a vertical strip zone extended to the 3rd toe	Pulmonary diseases such as pneumonia; bronchitis; asthma; pulmonary emphysema
Heart	The left soles, between the 4th and 5th metatarsals, below the reflex zone of Lung (toward the heel)	Diseases of circulatory system, such as arrhythmia, precardial pain, myocarditis, coronary heart disease, hyperlipidemia, arteriosclerosis, hypertension, hypotension and so on
Spleen	The left soles, between the 4th and 5th metatarsals, 1 thumb wide away from the Heart reflex zone on the side of the heel	Anemia; dermatosis; loss of appetite; indigestion; pyrexia; inflammations. Stimulating this reflex zone can enhance body immunity
Stomach	Inner sides of both soles, at the back of the 1st metatarsals, zone of approximately 1 finger's width	Diseases of digestive system such as nausea, vomiting, abdominal distension, stomachache, excessive gastric acid, indigestion, acute and chronic gastroenteritis, gastric ulcer, gastroptosis and so on
Pancreas	Inner sides of both soles, at the 1st metatarsals, close to the tarsometatarsal joints, between the Stomach reflex zone and the Duodenum reflex zone, about 1 finger' s width	Indications include diabetes mellitus; indigestion; pancreatitis and so on

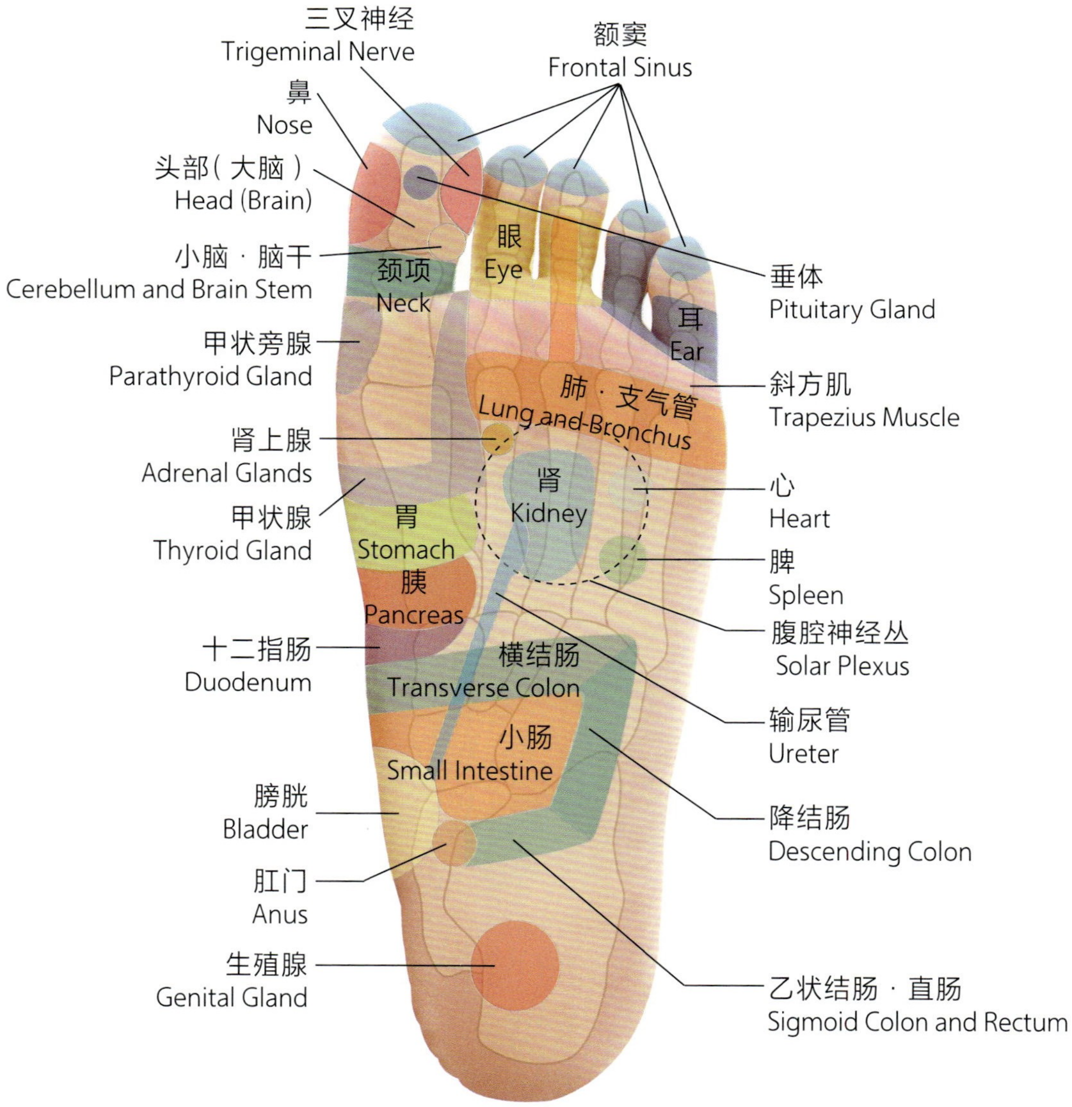

续表

反射区	定 位	主 治
十二指肠	双足底内侧，第 1 跗跖关节前，胰反射区的后方	腹胀、腹痛、消化不良、食欲不振、食物中毒等
小肠	双足底中部凹入区域，被升结肠、横结肠、降结肠、乙状结肠 · 直肠等反射区所包围	胃肠胀气、腹痛、腹泻、急慢性肠炎等
横结肠	双足底中部，横跨足掌呈一横带状的区域	腹痛、腹泻、肠炎、便秘等
降结肠	左足底，与足外侧平行的竖条状区，上接横结肠反射区，止于足跟骨外侧前缘	腹痛、腹泻、肠炎、腹胀、便秘等
乙状结肠 · 直肠	左足底，跟骨前缘一横带状区域	直肠息肉、腹泻、便秘、便血
肛门	左足底，足跟的前缘，乙状结肠 · 直肠反射区的末端	便秘、痔疮、瘘管、脱肛、肛裂、痔疮术后恢复

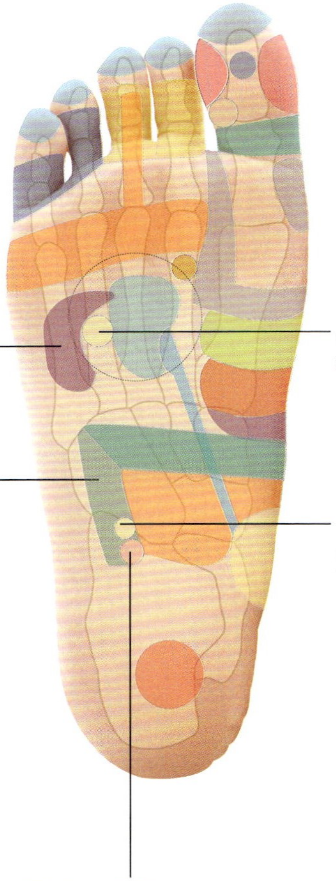

Continued

Reflex Zone	Location	Indications
Duodenum	Inner sides of both soles, in front of the 1st tarsometatarsal joint, at the back of the Pancreas reflex zone	Abdominal distension; abdominal pain; indigestion; loss of appetite and food poisoning
Small Intestine	The recessed zone in the middle of both soles, surrounded by the reflex zone of Ascending Colon, Transverse Colon, Descending Colon, Sigmoid Colon and the Rectum	Flatulence; abdominal pain; diarrhea; acute and chronic enteritis and so on
Transverse Colon	In the middle of both soles, the zone horizontally across the sole shaped like a belt	Abdominal pain; diarrhea; enteritis; constipation and so on
Descending Colon	In the left sole, the vertical strip zone parallel to the lateral foot, straightly below the Transverse Colon reflex zone and end at the lateral frontal edge of the heel	Abdominal pain; diarrhea; enteritis; constipation and so on
Sigmoid Colon and Rectum	In the left sole, the horizontal strip zone in the frontal edge of the heel	Rectal polyp; diarrhea; constipation and hematochezia
Anus	In the left sole, the frontal edge of the heel, at the end of the Sigmoid Colon and Rectum reflex zone	Constipation; hemorrhoids; fistula; rectocele; anal fissure; hemorrhoids; postoperative recovery

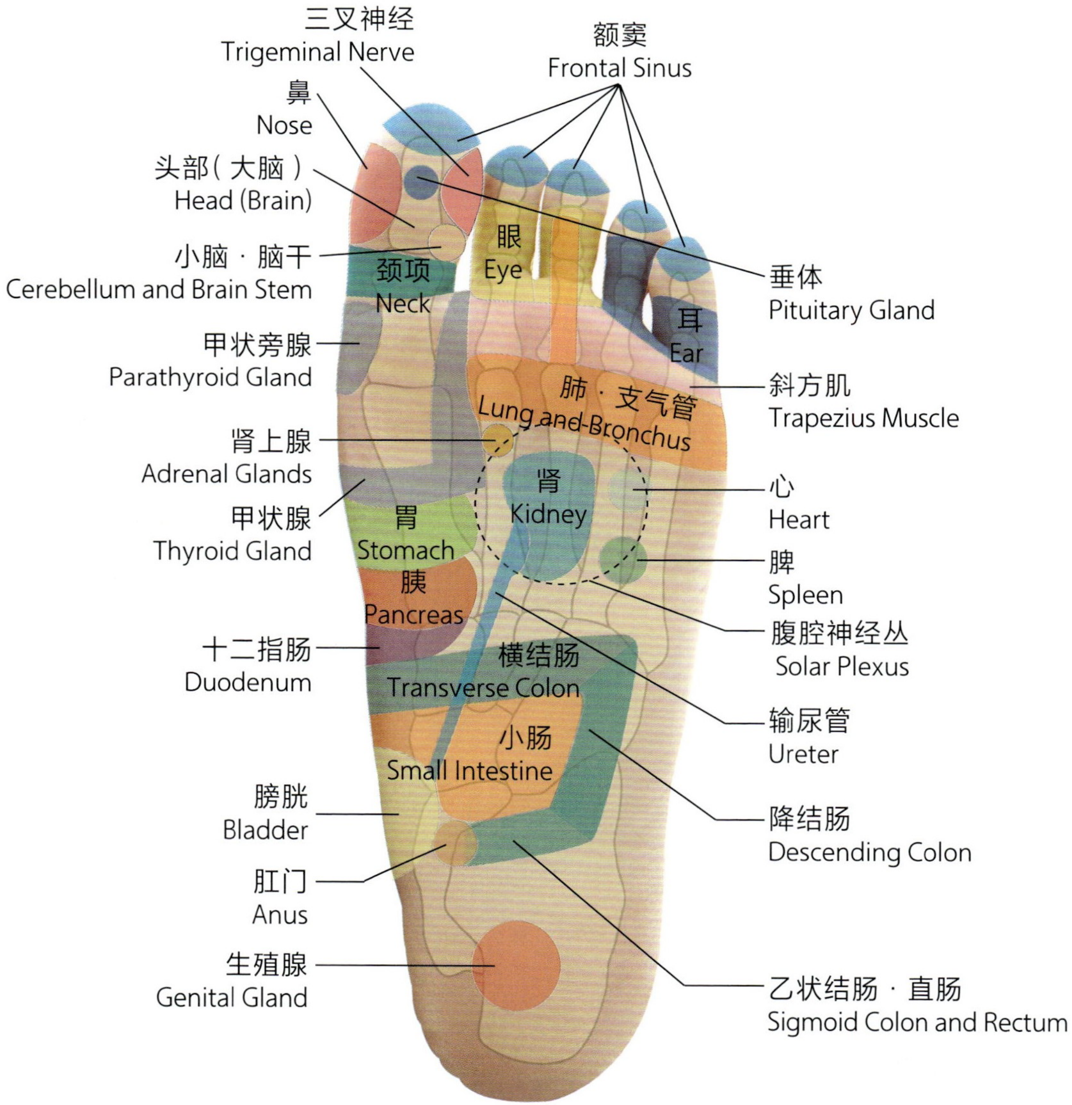

续表

反射区	定 位	主 治
生殖腺	双足底，足跟中央处	性功能低下、不孕、围绝经期综合征、月经不调、痛经、子宫肌瘤、不育、阳痿、早泄、睾丸炎
肝	右足底，第 4、5 跖骨体之间	肝炎、肝硬化、肝肿大、脂肪肝等
胆囊	右足底，第 4、5 跖骨体间近第 4 跖骨处，肝反射区的内下方	胆结石、胆囊炎、黄疸等
盲肠 · 阑尾	右足底，第 4、5 趾间垂直线上，跟骨前缘	腹胀、消化不良、阑尾炎、阑尾术后疼痛
回盲瓣	右足底，跟骨前缘的外侧，盲肠 · 阑尾反射区的上方（脚趾方向）	腹胀、腹痛、消化不良，可促进术后肠蠕动恢复
升结肠	右足底，自跟骨前缘沿骰骨外侧至第 5 跖骨底与足外侧平行的带状区	腹痛、腹泻、肠炎等

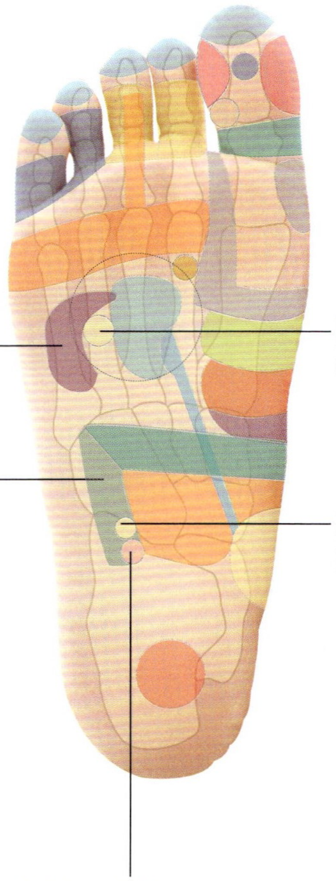

Continued

Reflex Zone	Location	Indications
Genital Gland	In both soles, in the middle of the heel	Sexual dysfunction; infertility; perimenopausal syndrome; abnormal menstruation; dysmenorrhea; myoma of uterus; sterility; impotence; premature ejaculation and testitis
Liver	In the right sole, between the 4th and the 5th metatarsals	Hepatitis; cirrhosis; hepatomegaly; fatty liver and so on
Gallbladder	In the right sole, between the 4th and the 5th metatarsals (closer to the 4th metatarsal), in the medial side below the Liver reflex zone	Gallstones; cholecystitis and jaundice
Cecum and Appendix	In the right sole, in the vertical line between the 4th and the 5th metatarsals, in the frontal edge of heel	Abdominal distension; indigestion; appendicitis and appendix postoperative pain
Ileocecal Valve	In the right sole, at the lateral frontal side, above the Cecum and Appendix reflex zone (on the side of toes)	Abdominal distension; abdominal pain; indigestion. And stimulating the reflex zone can promote the recovery of bowel movements after surgery.
Ascending Colon	In the right sole, the strip zone that is parallel to the lateral foot from the frontal edge of the heel to the bottom of the 5th metatarsal along the lateral side of the cuboid	Abdominal pain; diarrhea; enteritis and so on

超简单足底反射区按摩

Super-easy Massage in Sole Reflex Zone

肾上腺

用拇指指端或食指近侧指间关节施力按压 3~5 次

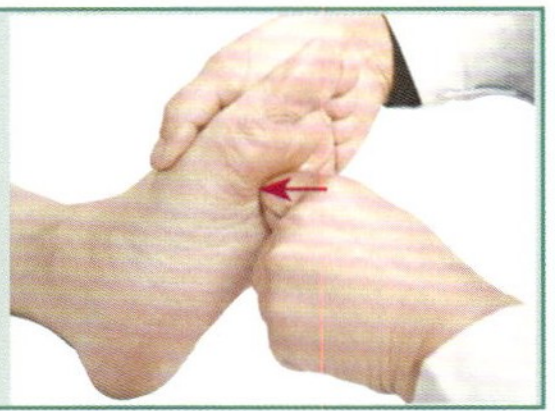

肾

用拇指指腹或食指近侧指间关节施力，先深按，不抬起，再沿着足心向足跟方向推按 3~5 次

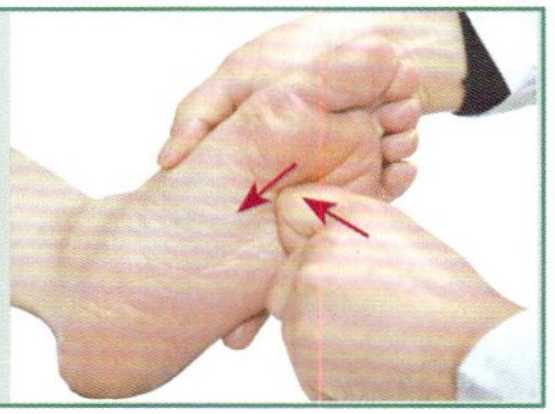

输尿管

用拇指指腹或食指近侧指间关节施力，先深按，不抬起，再从肾反射区向膀胱反射区方向慢慢推按 3~5 次

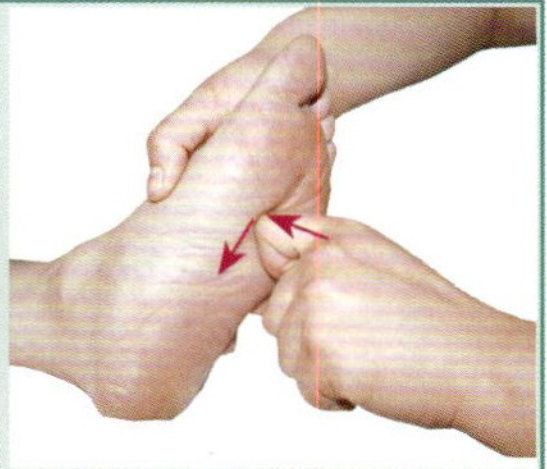

膀胱

用拇指指腹或食指近侧指间关节施力，定点向深部按压，并在定点周围揉按 3~5 次

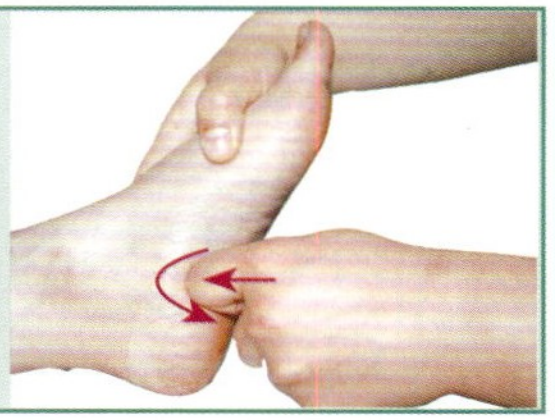

腹腔神经丛

用拇指指腹或食指近侧指间关节施力，沿反射区作半圆形推按 3~5 次

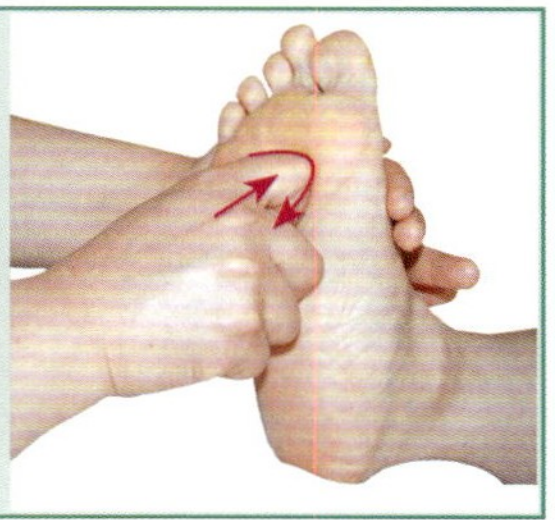

额窦

用拇指指端或拇指指间关节或食指近侧指间关节沿趾端做横向按压，亦可自趾端向趾根方向推按 3~5 次

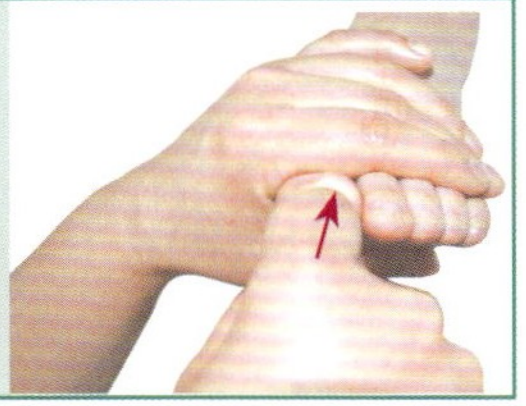

垂体

用拇指指端或食指近侧指间关节施力，定点向深部按压 3~5 次

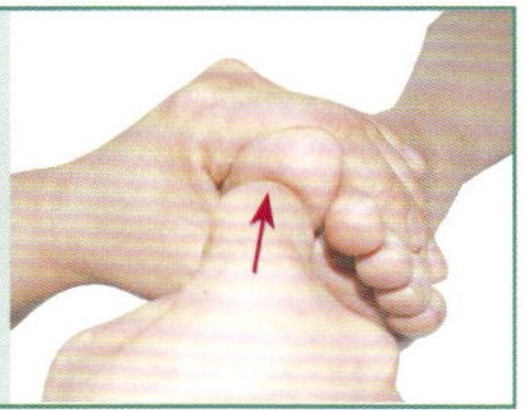

小脑·脑干

用拇指指端或食指近侧指间关节施力，定点向深部按压 3~5 次

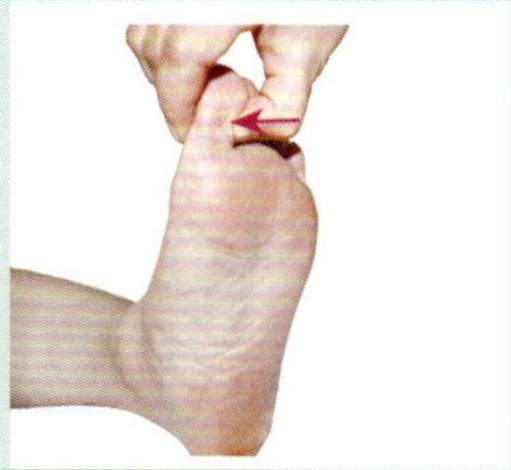

三叉神经

用拇指指端或食指近侧指间关节施力，自拇趾趾端向趾根方向推按 3~5 次

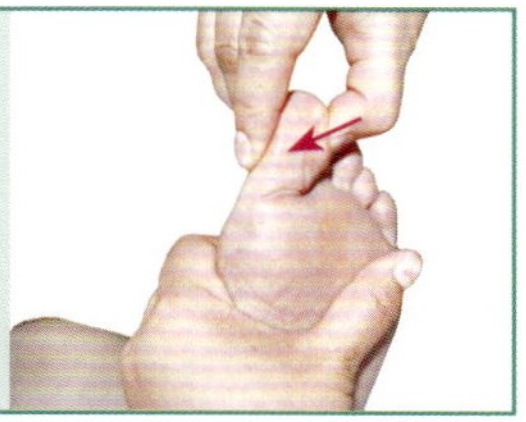

鼻

用拇指指端或食指近侧指间关节施力按压 3~5 次

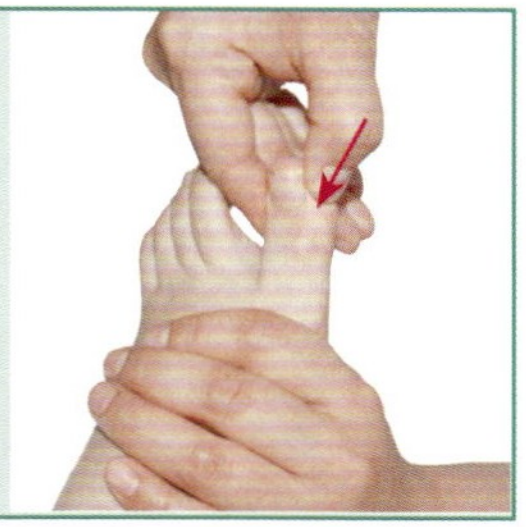

Adrenal Gland

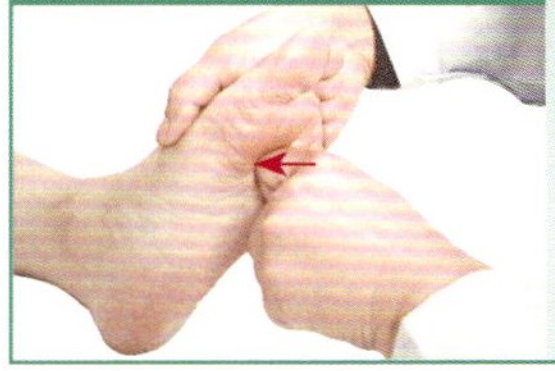

Press 3 to 5 times with the thumb tip or the proximal knuckle of the index finger

Kidney

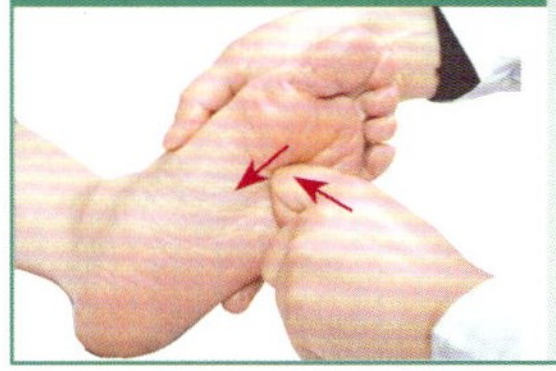

Deep press with the thumb pulp or the proximal knuckle of the index finger. Do not lift. Press towards the heel along the middle line

Ureter

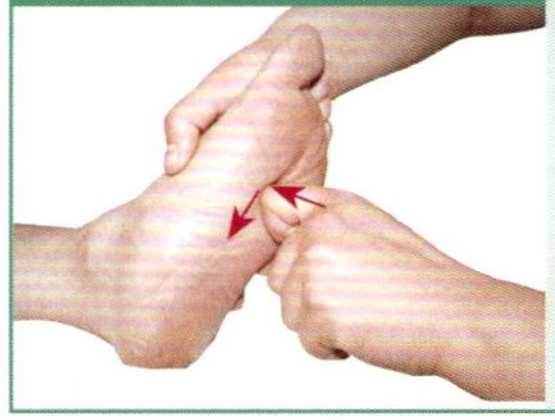

Deep press with the thumb pulp or the proximal knuckle of the index finger. Do not lift. Then slowly press and press 3 to 5 times from Kidney reflex zone to the Bladder reflex zone

Bladder

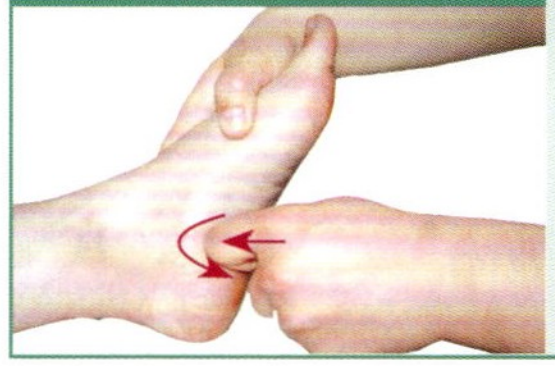

Deep press on 1 point with the thumb pulp or the proximal knuckle of the index finger. Then knead around the point 3 to 5 times

Celiac Plexus

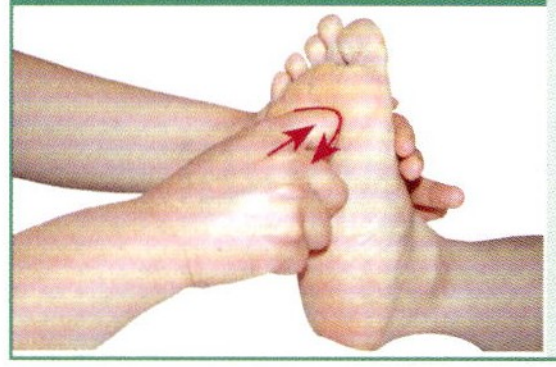

Press 3 to 5 times round the Celiac Plexus reflex zone for half circle with the thumb pulp or the proximal knuckle of the index finger

Frontal Sinus

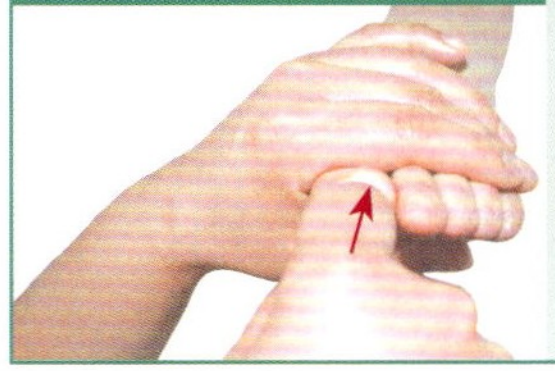

Press 3 to 5 times with the thumb tip or knuckle or the proximal knuckle of the index finger along the toe ends, or press from the toe end to the toe root

Pituitary Gland

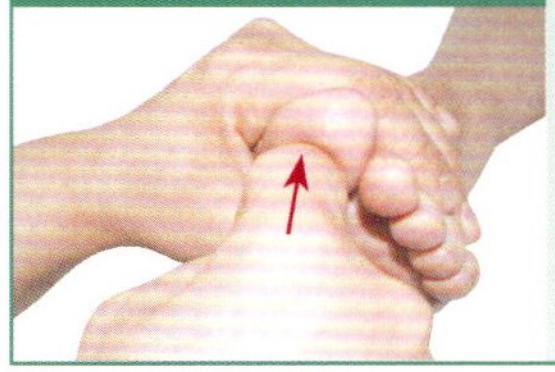

Press deep on the fixed point 3 to 5 times with the thumb tip or the proximal knuckle of the index finger

Cerebellum and Brainstem

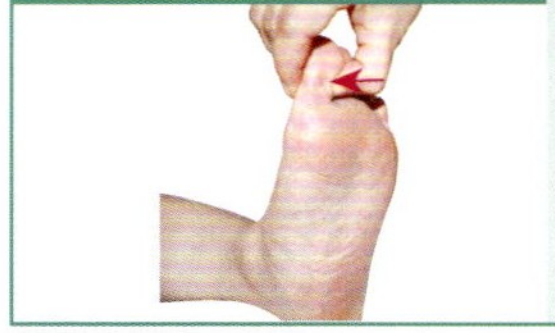

Press deep on the fixed point 3 to 5 times with the thumb tip or the proximal knuckle of the index finger

Nervi Trigeminus

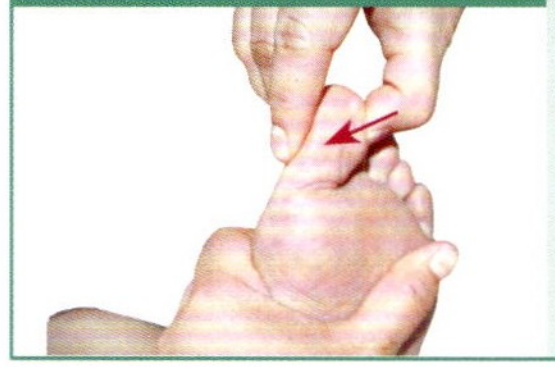

Press and press from the toe end to the toe root 3 to 5 times with the thumb tip or the proximal knuckle of the index finger

Nose

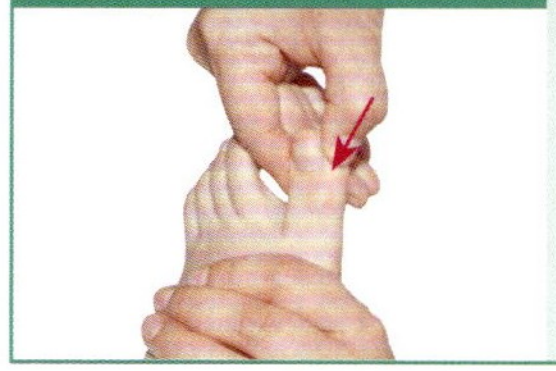

Press 3 to 5 times with the thumb tip or the proximal knuckle of the index finger

头部（大脑）

用拇指指端或食指近侧指间关节施力，由趾端向趾根方向按压 3~5 次

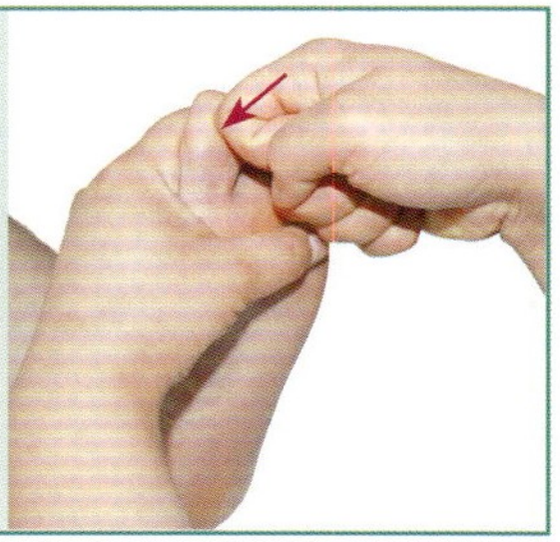

颈项

用拇指指端沿着拇趾根部推按 3~5 次

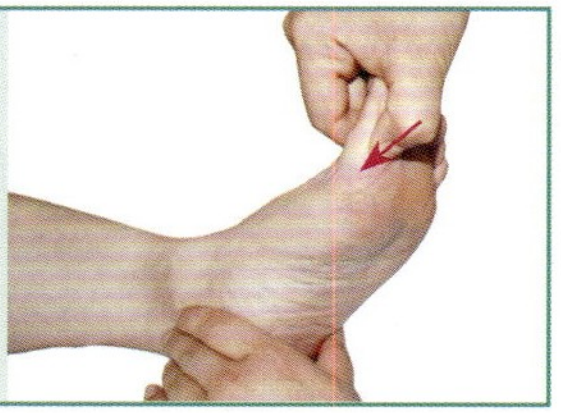

眼

用拇指指端由趾端向趾根方向推按；然后用拇指或食指的近侧指间关节施力，在第 2、3 趾底面根部的内侧和外侧分别深按 3~5 次

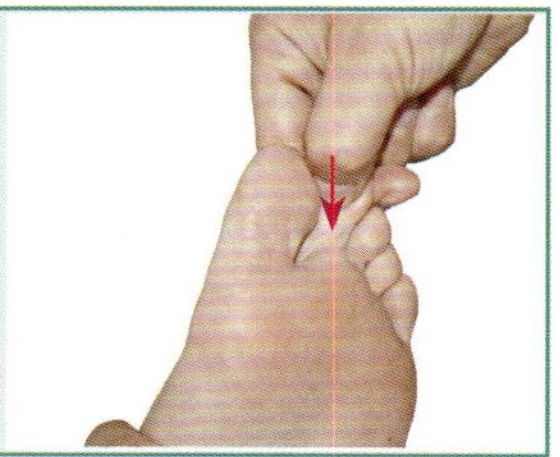

耳

用拇指指端由趾端向趾根方向推按；然后用拇指或食指近侧指间关节施力，在第 4、5 趾底面根部的内侧和外侧分别深按 3~5 次

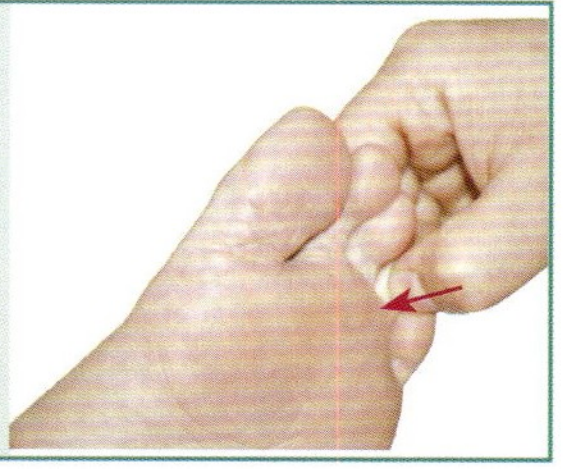

甲状旁腺

用拇指指端或食指近侧指间关节施力按压 3~5 次

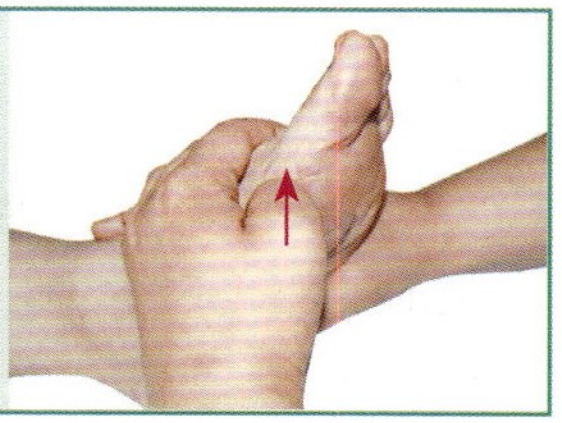

甲状腺

用拇指指端或拇指指间关节或食指近侧指间关节沿反射区按压 3~5 次

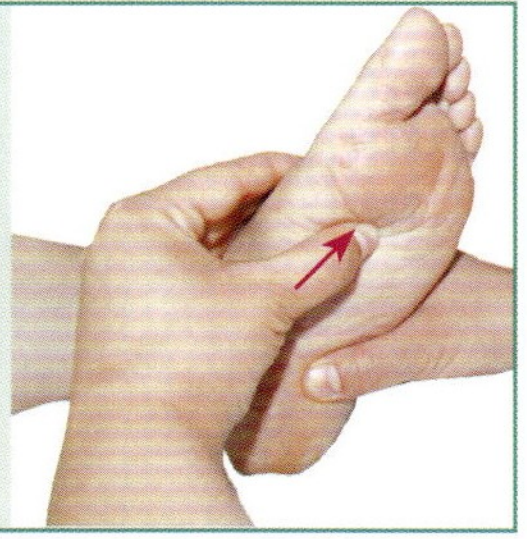

斜方肌

用拇指指端或拇指指间关节或食指近侧指间关节施力，沿反射区按压 3~5 次

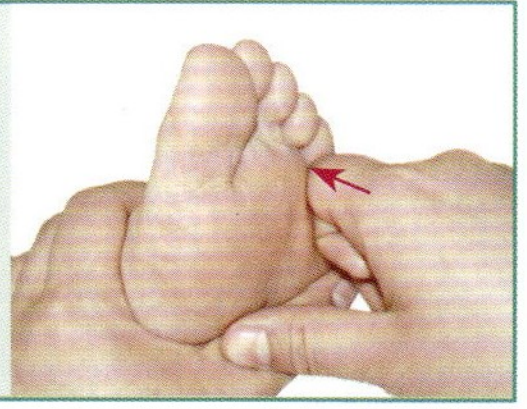

肺·支气管

用拇指指端或食指近侧指间关节施力，沿反射区纵向或横向按压 3~5 次

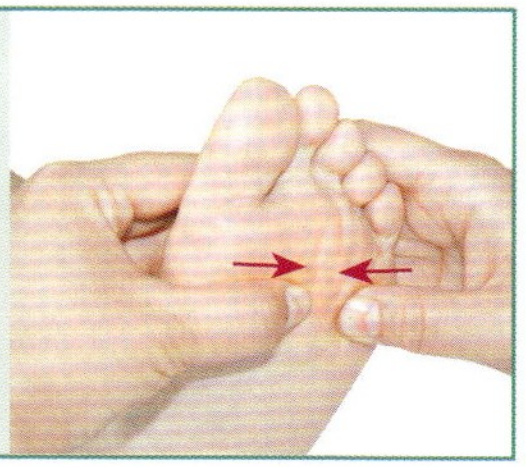

心

以拇指指腹或食指近侧指间关节施力，先轻后重，根据患者的承受程度逐渐加强力量

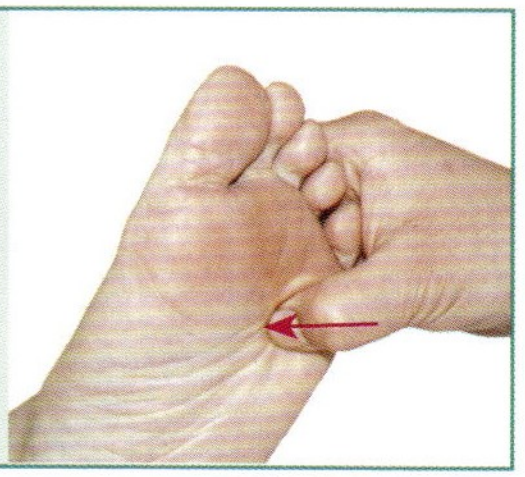

脾

以拇指指端或食指近侧指间关节施力，在反射区处定点按

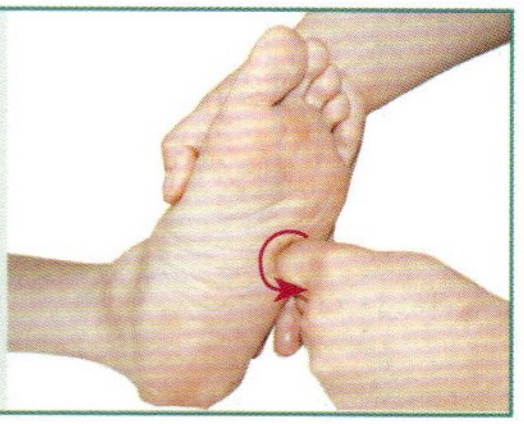

Head (Brain)

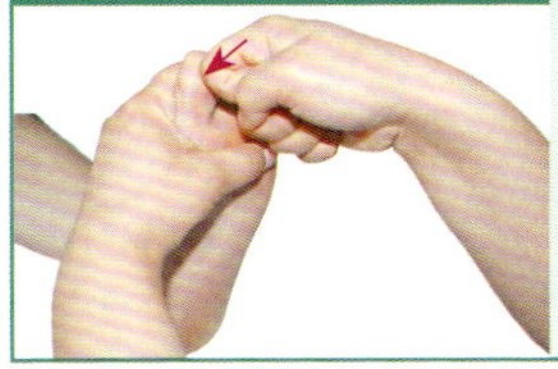

Press from the toe end to the toe root 3 to 5 times with the thumb tip or the proximal knuckle of the index finger

Neck

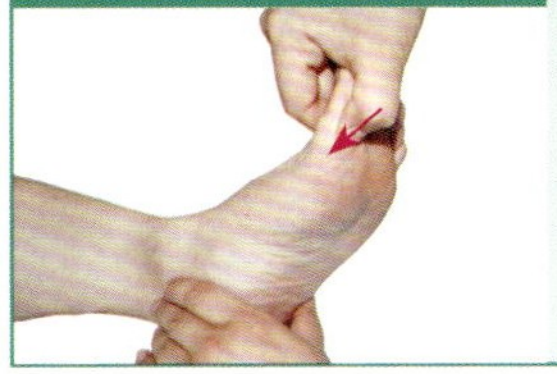

Press and press 3 to 5 times along the toe root with thumb tip

Eye

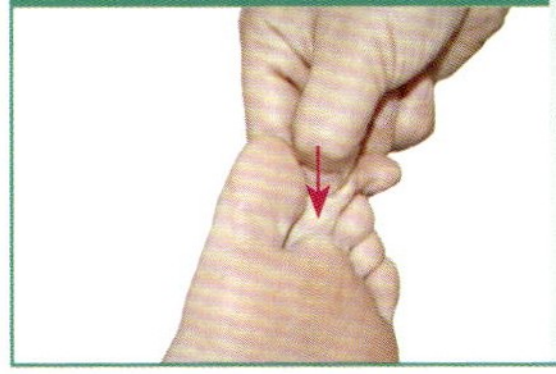

Press and press from the toe end to the toe root with the thumb tip; then press deep on the inner and outer sides of the bottom of the 2nd and the 3rd toes respectively for 3 to 5 times with the proximal knuckle of the thumb or index finger

Ear

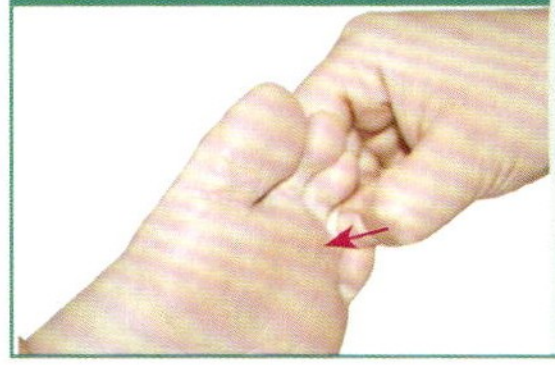

Press and press from the toe end to the toe root with the thumb tip; then press deep on the inner and outer sides of the bottom of the 4th and 5th toes respectively for 3 to 5 times with the proximal knuckle of the thumb or index finger

Parathyroid Gland

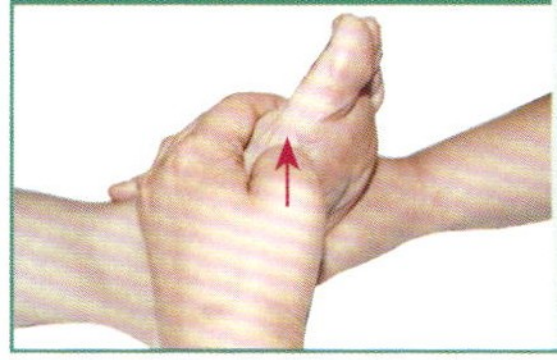

Press 3 to 5 times with the thumb tip or the proximal knuckle of the index finger

Thyroid Gland

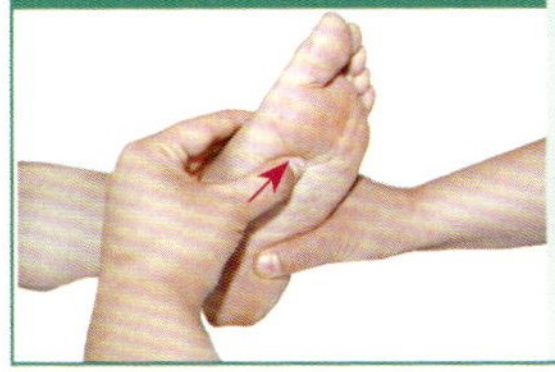

Press 3 to 5 times along the reflex zone with the thumb tip or knuckle or the proximal knuckle of the index finger

Trapezius

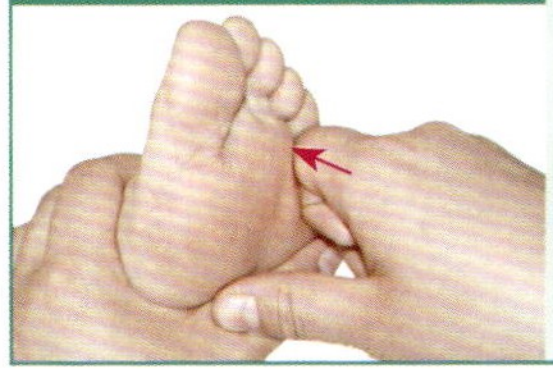

Press 3 to 5 times along the reflex zone with the thumb tip or knuckle or the proximal knuckle of the index finger

Lung and Bronchus

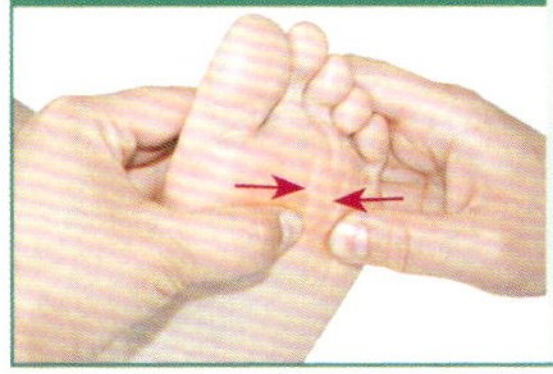

Press 3 to 5 times along the reflex zone vertically and horizontally with the thumb tip or the proximal knuckle of the index finger

Heart

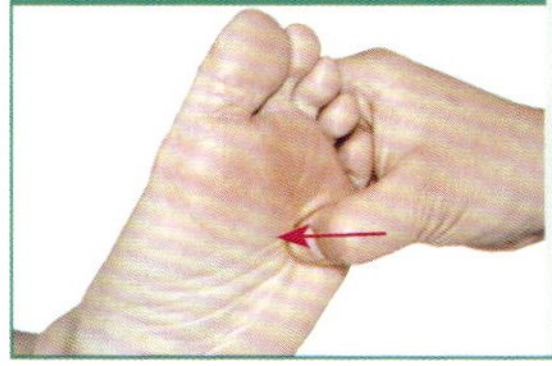

Press with the thumb pulp or the proximal knuckle of the index finger, gently at first and heavily later. The increase of force should be made according to the tolerance of the patient

Spleen

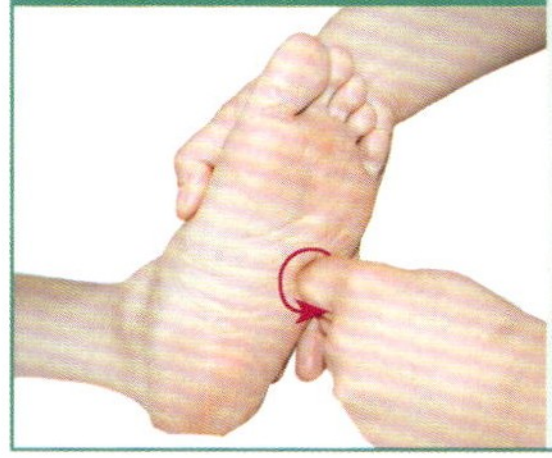

Press on the fixed point in the reflex zone with the thumb tip or the proximal knuckle of the index finger

胃

以拇指指腹或食指近侧指间关节施力按压 3~5 次

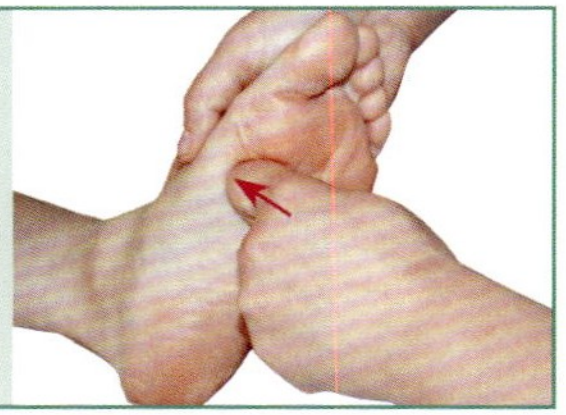

胰

以拇指指腹或食指近侧指间关节施力按压 3~5 次

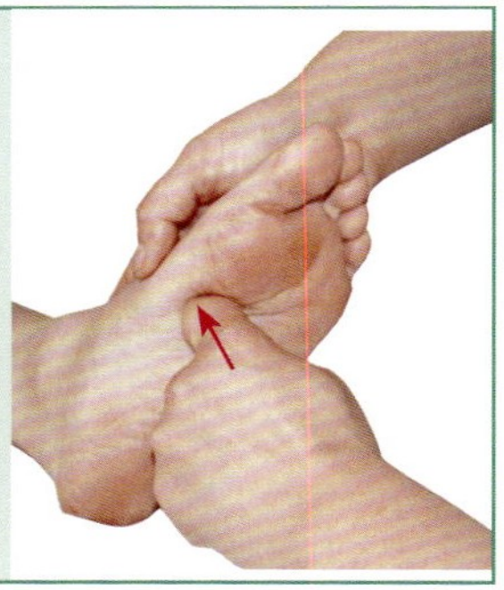

十二指肠

用拇指指腹或食指近侧指间关节施力按压 3~5 次。

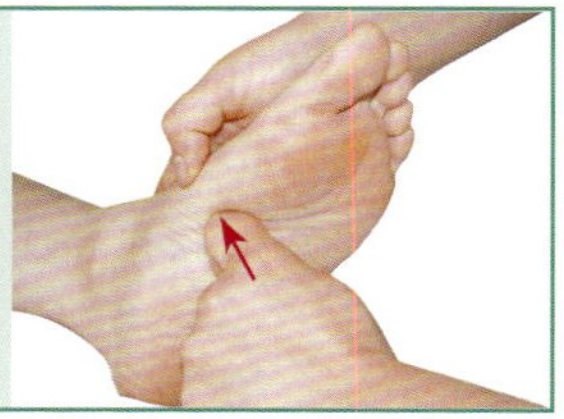

小肠

以拇指指腹，或食指、中指及无名指近侧指间关节自足心向足跟方向推按 3~5 次

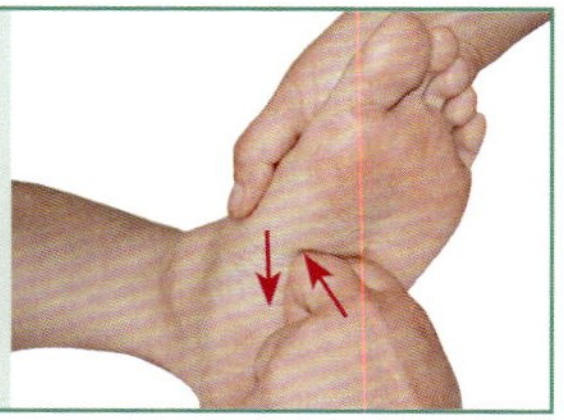

横结肠

以拇指指腹，或食指近侧指间关节沿反射区施力，左足自足内侧向外侧，右足自足外侧向内侧，分别推按 3~5 次

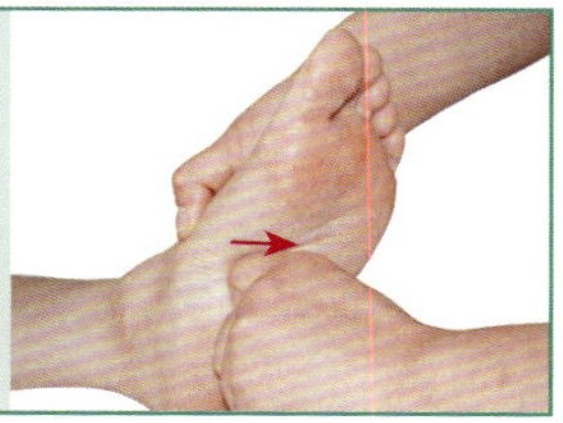

降结肠

以拇指指端或食指近侧指间关节向足跟方向按压 3~5 次

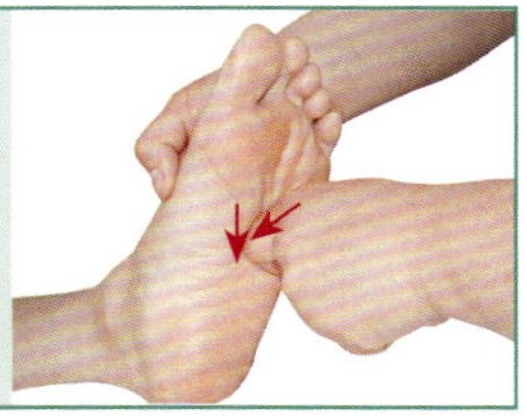

乙状结肠·直肠

以拇指指端或食指近侧指间关节自足外侧向足内侧按压 3~5 次

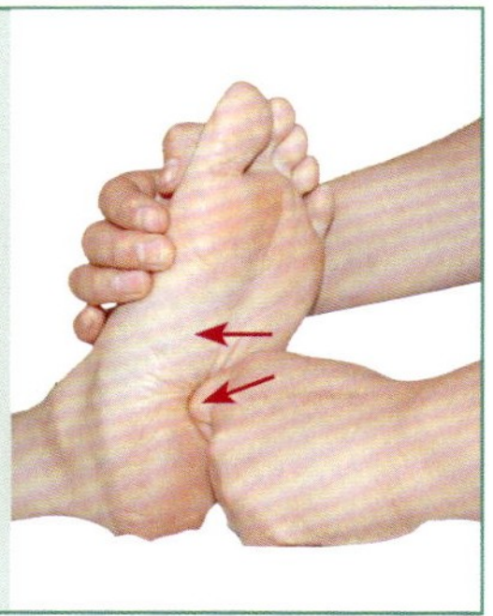

肛门

以拇指指端或食指近侧指间关节作定点揉按 3~5 次

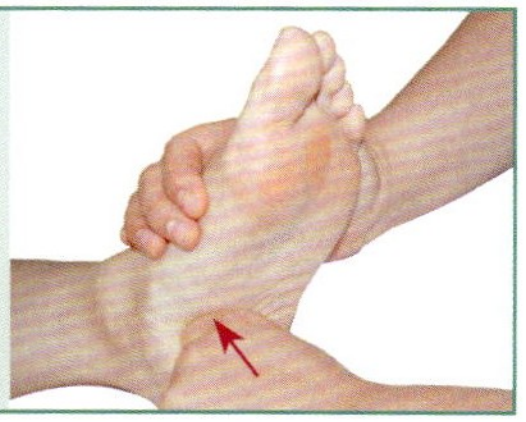

生殖腺

以拇指指端或食指近侧指间关节施力按揉 3~5 次

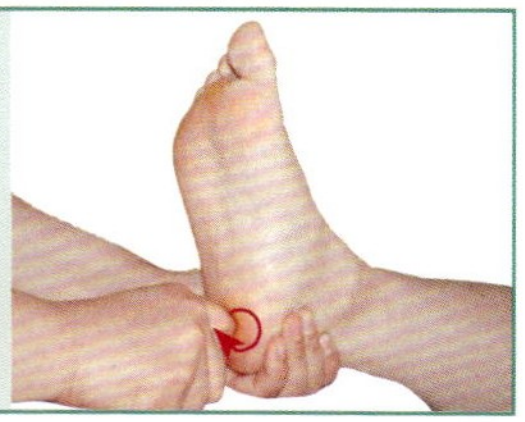

肝

以拇指指端或以食指近侧指间关节施力按压 3~5 次

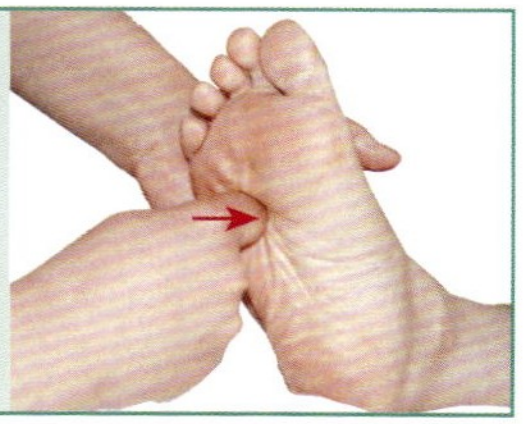

Stomach

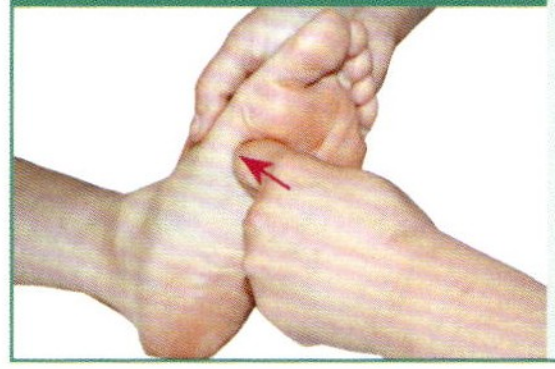

Press 3 to 5 times with the thumb pulp or the proximal knuckle of the index finger

Pancreas

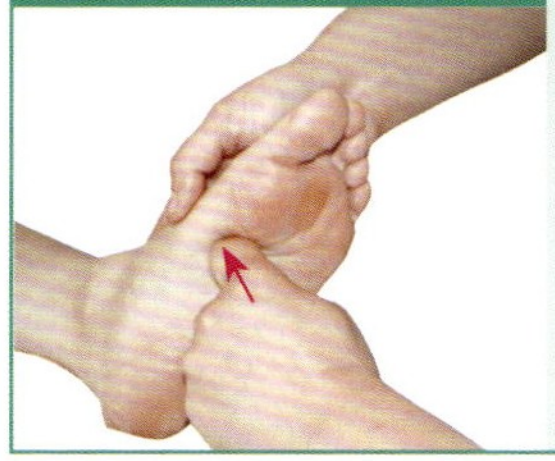

Press 3 to 5 times with the thumb pulp or the proximal knuckle of the index finger

Duodenum

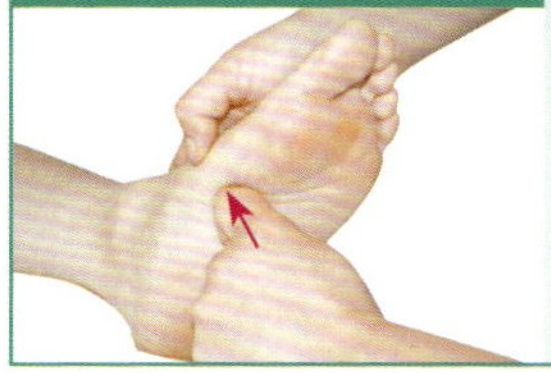

Press 3 to 5 times with the thumb pulp or the proximal knuckle of the index finger

Small Intestine

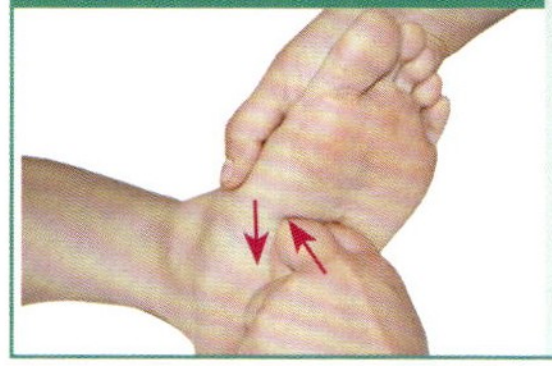

Press and press from the center of the sole to the heel 3 to 5 times with the thumb pulp or the proximal knuckle of the index finger or middle finger or ring finger

Transverse Colon

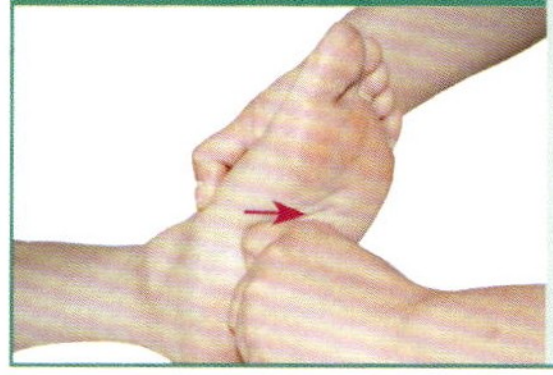

Press and press from left medial sole to lateral , and from right lateral sole to medial respectively 3 to 5 times with the thumb pulp or the proximal knuckle of the index finger

Descending Colon

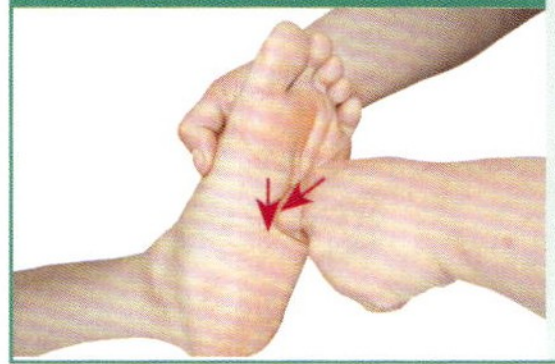

Press 3 to 5 times towards the heel with thumb tip or the proximal knuckle of the index finger

Sigmoid Colon and Rectum

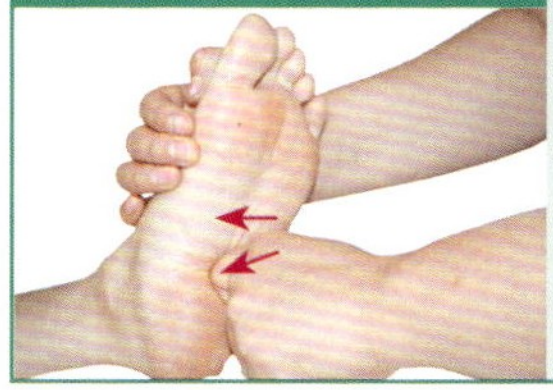

Press 3 to 5 times from lateral sole to medial sole with thumb tip or the proximal knuckle of the index finger

Anus

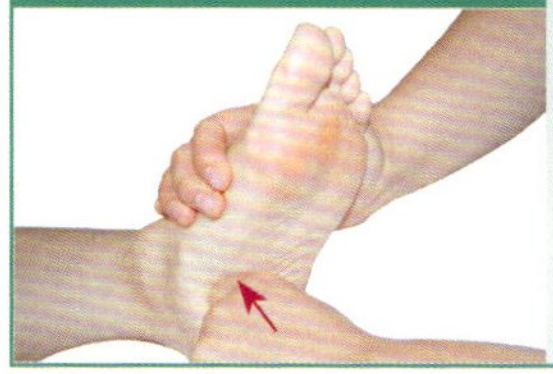

Press 3 to 5 times on fixed point with thumb tip or the proximal knuckle of the index finger

Genital Gland

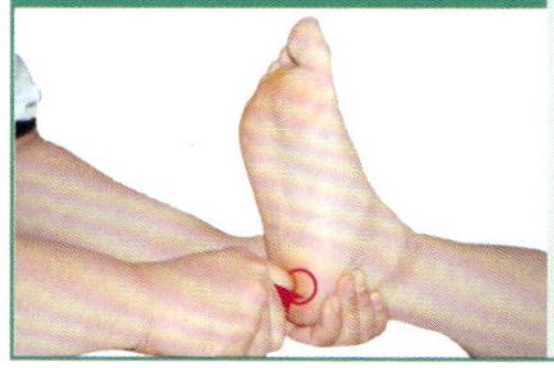

Press 3 to 5 times with thumb tip or the proximal knuckle of the index finger

Liver

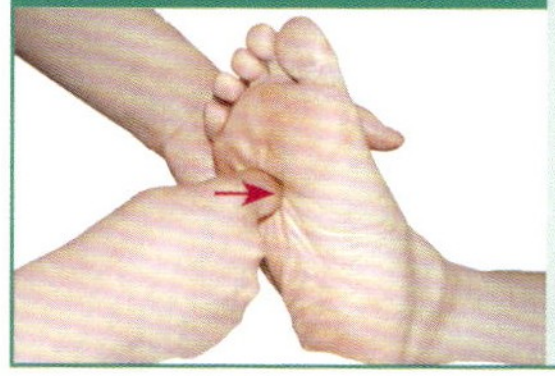

Press 3 to 5 times with thumb tip or the proximal knuckle of the index finger

胆囊

以拇指指端或食指近侧指间关节施力按压 3~5 次

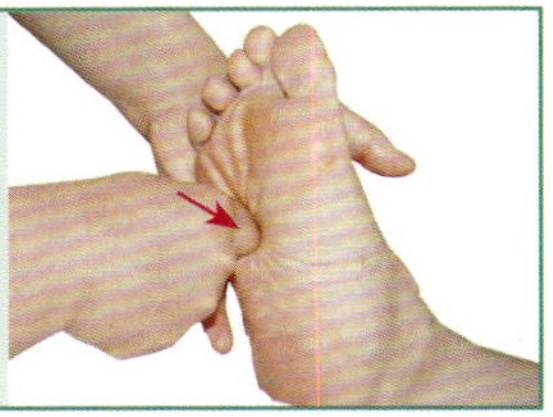

回盲瓣

以拇指指端或食指近侧指间关节施力按压 3~5 次

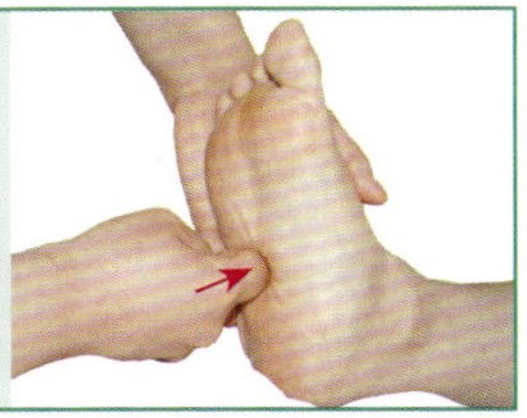

盲肠·阑尾

以拇指指端或食指近侧指间关节施力按压 3~5 次

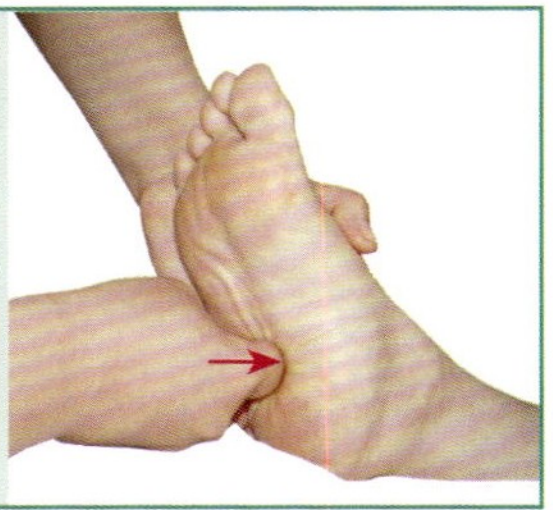

升结肠

以拇指指端或食指近侧指间关节施力，由足跟向足趾方向推按 3~5 次

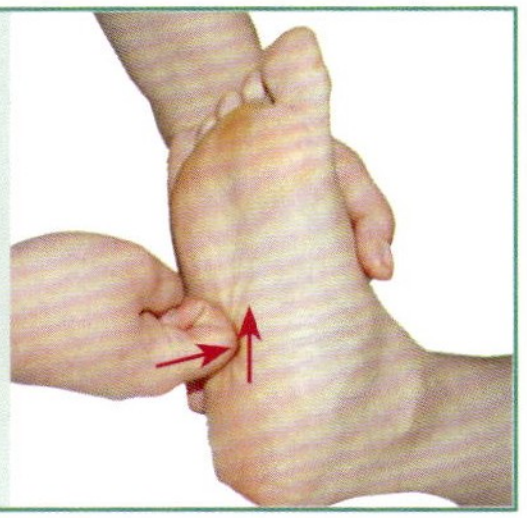

Gallbladder

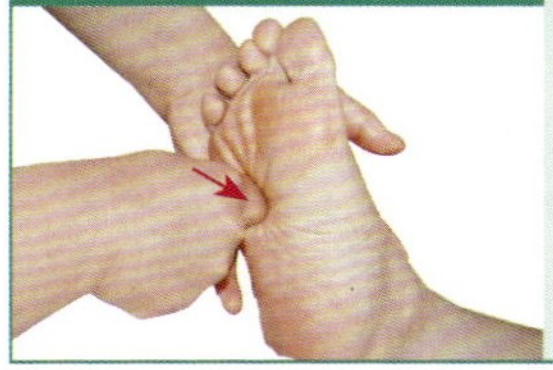

Press 3 to 5 times with thumb tip or the proximal knuckle of the index finger

Ileocecal Valve

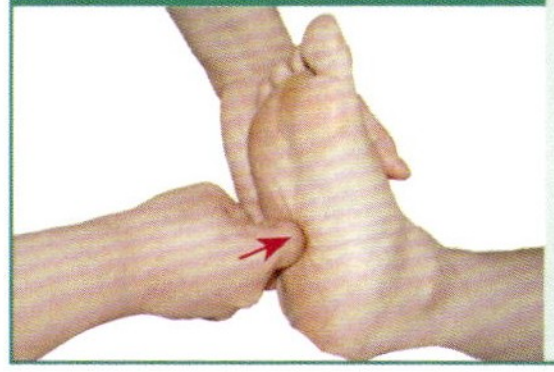

Press 3 to 5 times with thumb tip or the proximal knuckle of the index finger

Cecum and Appendix

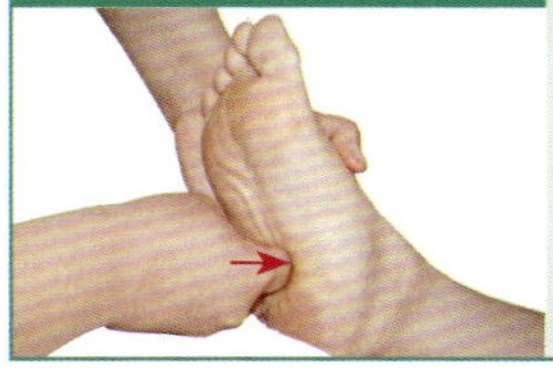

Press 3 to 5 times with thumb tip or the proximal knuckle of the index finger

Ascending Colon

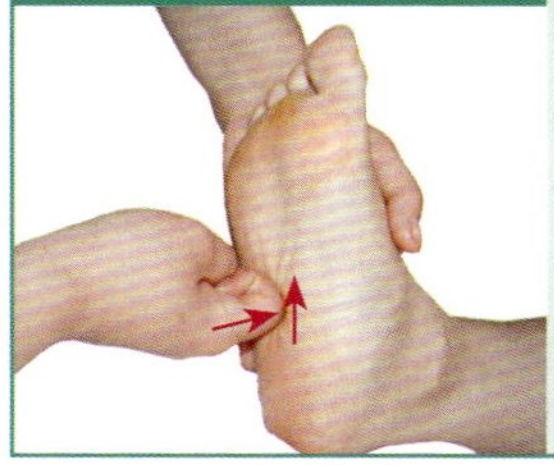

Press and press from the heel to the toes 3 to 5 times with thumb tip or the proximal knuckle of the index finger

足内侧反射区

Medial Foot Reflex Zone

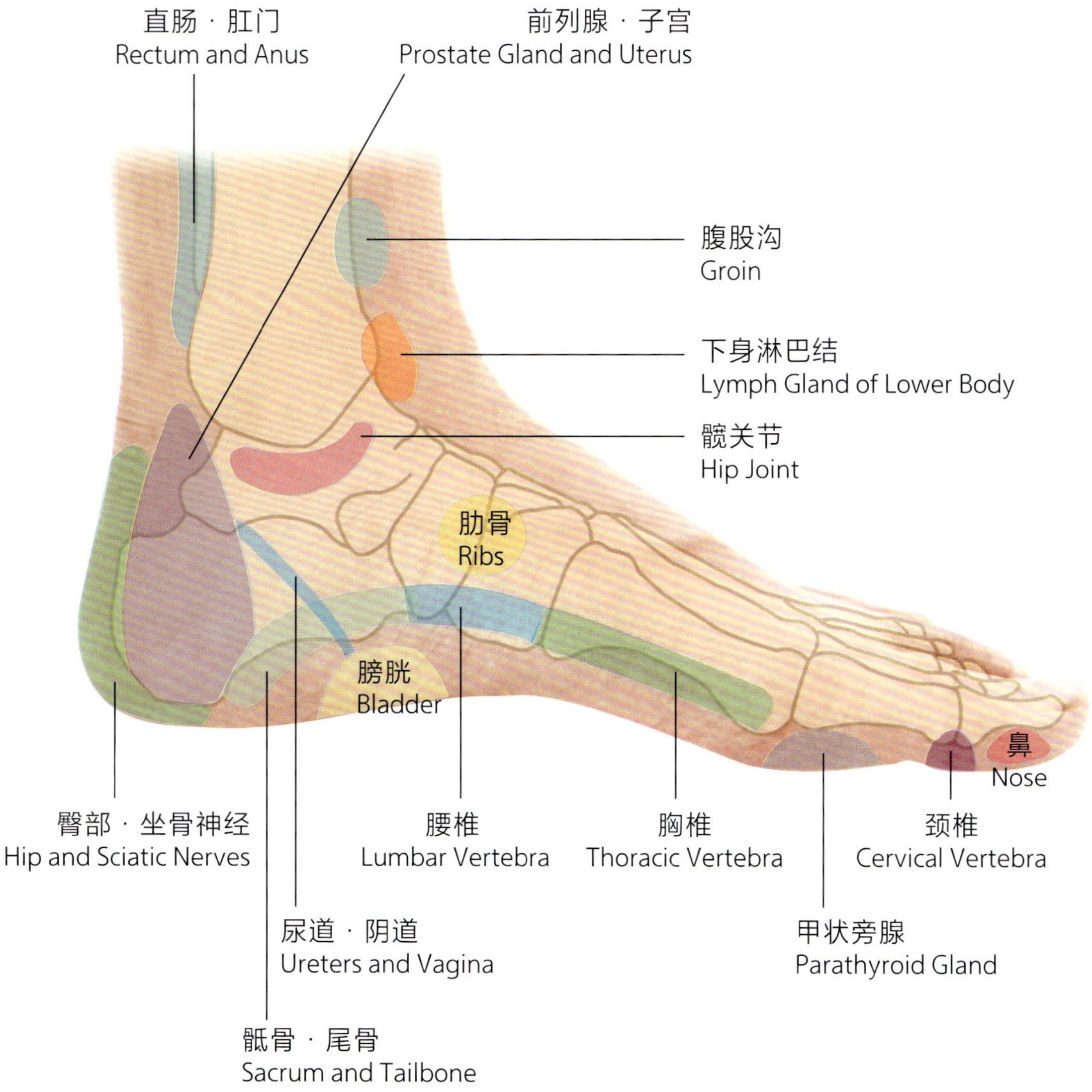

反射区	定位	主治
颈椎	双足拇趾根部横纹内侧尽头处	颈项酸痛、颈项僵硬、落枕及各种颈椎病变（包括骨质增生及因颈椎病引起的手麻、手痛等）
胸椎	双足弓内侧缘，从第1跖骨头到跖骨粗隆处	肩背酸痛、胸椎疾病、心脏病、肾病、肺部疾病

Reflex Zone	Location	Indications
Cervical Vertebra	At the end of the medial crease that is at the root of the great toes	Neck sore; pain and rigidity; stiff neck and all kinds of pathological changes of cervical vertebra (hyperstosis and hand numbness and pain caused by cervical spondylopathy)
Thoracic Vertebra	The zone on the medial edge of arch of feet, from the 1st metatarsal to metatarsal protrusion	Shoulder and back sore and pain; disease of thoracic vertebra; heart disease; nephropathy and pulmonary disease

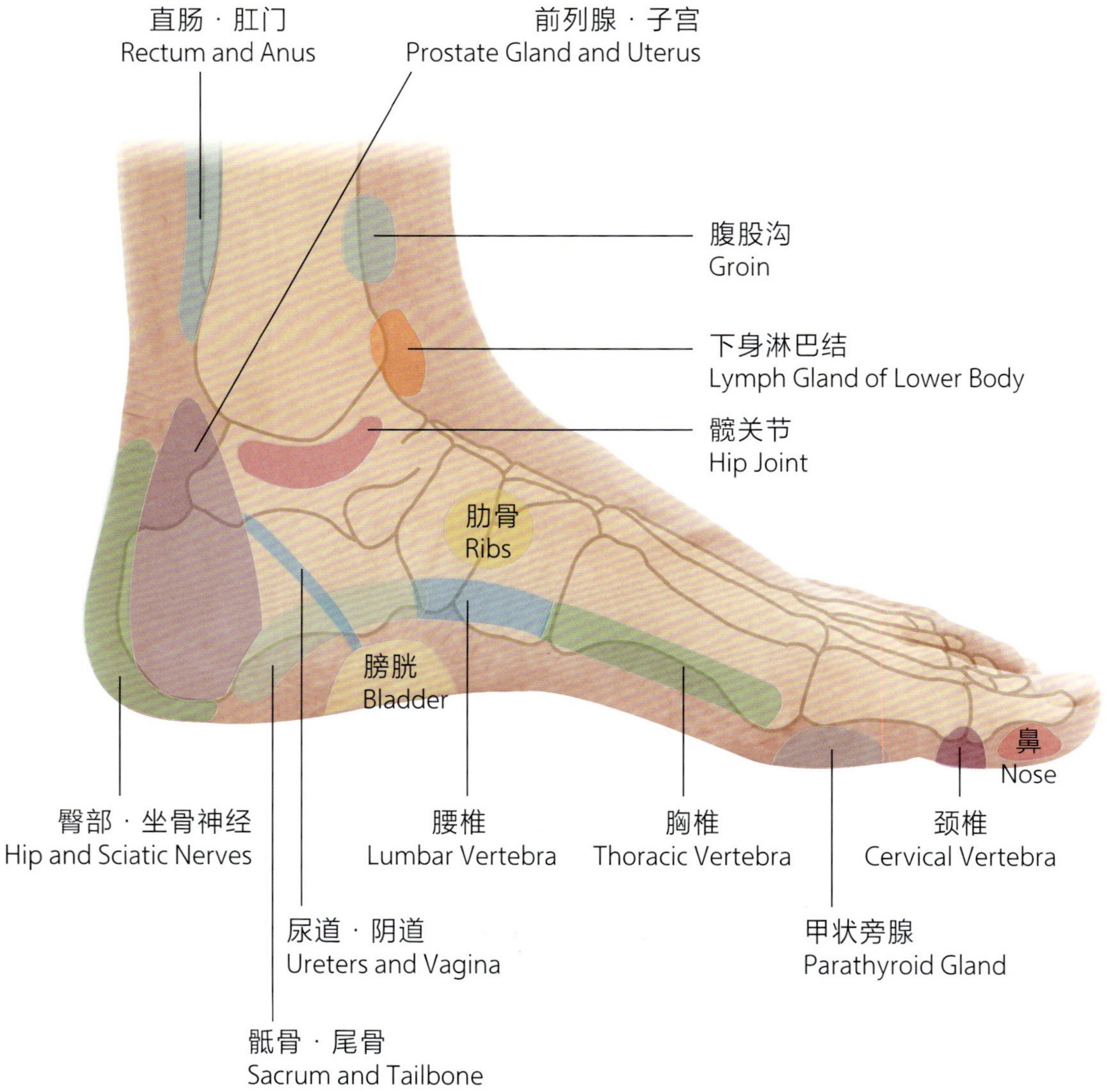

续表

反射区	定 位	主 治
腰椎	双足弓内侧缘，内侧楔骨至足舟骨的下方。上接胸椎反射区，下连骶骨 · 尾骨反射区	急性腰扭伤、腰背酸痛、腰椎间盘突出症、骨质增生及其他腰椎疾患
骶骨 · 尾骨	腰椎反射区的后方，双足弓内侧缘自舟骨后方起，经距骨下方至跟骨前缘	骶尾骨骨质增生、骶尾骨损伤、坐骨神经痛
臀部 · 坐骨神经	双足内侧足跟后缘上行至内踝下的带状区域	坐骨神经痛、脚麻
前列腺 · 子宫	双足跟内侧，内踝后下方的三角形区域	前列腺肥大、前列腺炎，子宫肌瘤、宫颈炎、子宫下垂、痛经、月经不调等

Continued

Reflex Zone	Location	Indications
Lumbar Vertebra	The zone on the medial edge of arch of feet, from entocuneiform to the bottom of navicular bone. It' s immediately below the Thoracic Vertebra reflex zone and above the Sacrum and Tailbone reflex zone	Acute lumbar sprain; lumbar and back sore and pain; protrusion of lumbar intervertebral disc; hyperostosis and other diseases of lumbar vertebra
Sacrum and Tailbone	The zone at the back of the Lumbar Vertebra reflex zone, beginning at the navicular bone, via the inferior side of the talus to the frontal edge of the heel along the medial edge of the arch of feet	Hyperostosis and injury of sacrum and tailbone; sciatica
Hip and Sciatic Nerves	The strip zone above the medial inferior edge of the heel and below the medial malleolus	Sciatica; numbness in feet
Prostate Gland and Uterus	The triangular zone inside the medial heel and on the posterior inferior side of the medial malleolus	Prostatomegaly; prostatitis; myoma of uterus; cervicitis; hysteroptosis; dysmenorrhea; abnormal menstruation; and so on

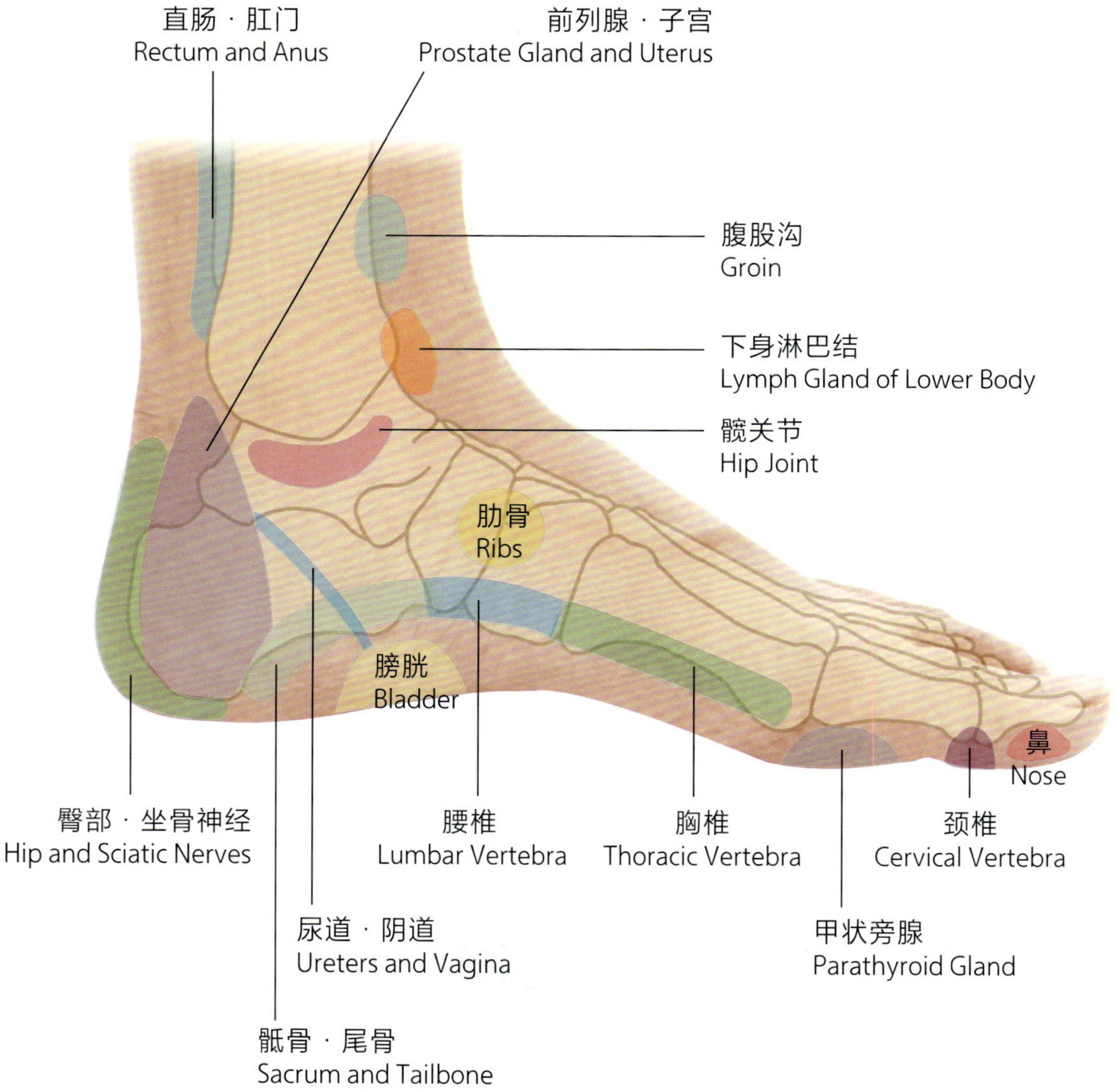

续表

反射区	定位	主治
尿道·阴道	双足跟内侧，自膀胱反射区斜向后上方延伸至足舟骨与距骨之间的带状区域	阴道炎、排尿困难、尿路感染等
髋关节	双足内踝的下缘呈弧形的带状区域	髋关节痛、坐骨神经痛、腰背痛
直肠·肛门	两小腿内侧，胫骨内侧后方，内踝后方向上延伸四横指的带状区域	痔疮、便秘、脱肛、直肠炎症、肛裂
腹股沟	双足胫骨内侧略前方，内踝尖上方两横指的凹陷处	腹股沟疝、阳痿、早泄、不孕、不育、月经不调、闭经

Continued

Reflex Zone	Location	Indications
Ureters and Vagina	The strip zone inside the medial heel and on the oblique superior side of the Bladder reflex zone until the zone between the navicular bone and the talus	Vaginitis; dysuresia; urinary tract infection and so on
Hip Joint	The strip zone below the medial malleolus of feet which is shaped like an arch	Hip joint pain; sciatica; lumbago and backache
Rectum and Anus	The strip zone that is on the medial side of the shanks and on the medial posterior side of the tibia and that is 4 fingers' width above the posterior side of the medial malleolus	Hemorrhoids; constipation; rectocele; rectitis and anal fissure
Groin	2 fingers wide recessed zone that is slightly on the anterior side of the medial tibia and above the tip of the medial malleolus	Inguinal hernia; impotence; premature ejaculation; infertility; sterility; abnormal menstruation and amenorrhea

超简单足内侧反射区按摩

Super-easy Massage in Medial Foot Reflex Zone

颈椎

以拇指指端按揉 3~5 次，或食指、中指弯曲成钳状夹住被按摩者的拇趾根部，以食指侧缘在反射区位置上施力按压 3~5 次

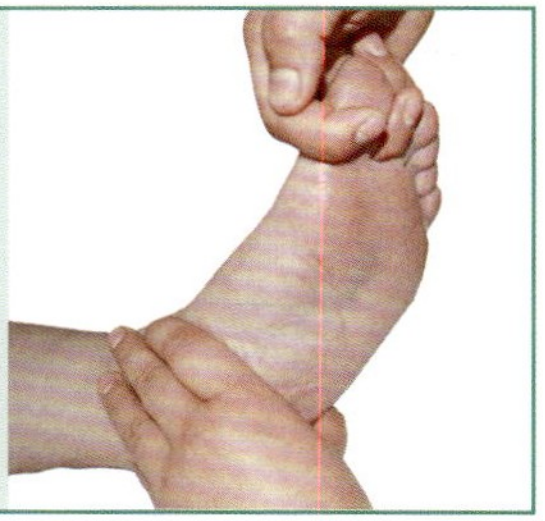

胸椎

以拇指指腹或拇指指端施力揉按 3~5 次

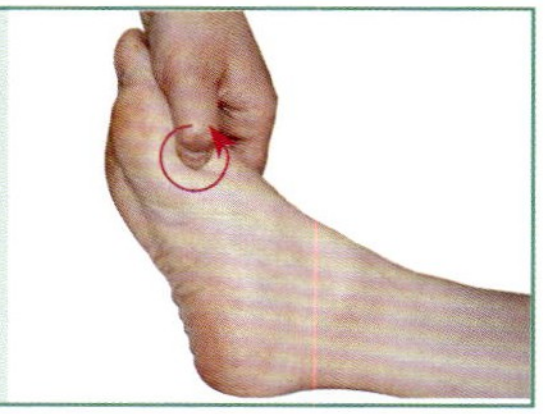

腰椎

以拇指指腹或食指指端施力按压 3~5 次

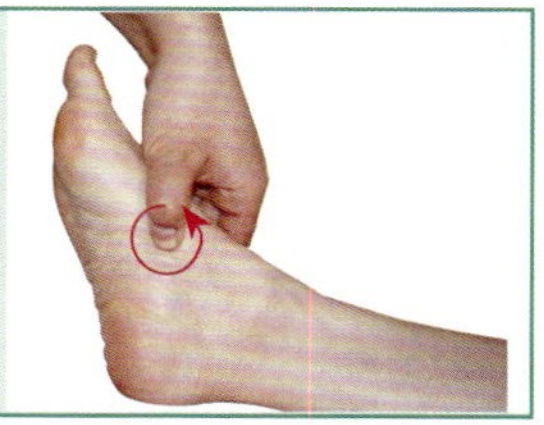

骶骨 · 尾骨

以拇指指腹或食指指端施力按压 3~5 次

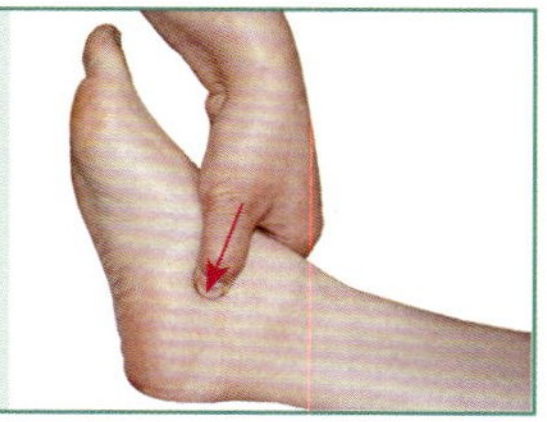

臀部 · 坐骨神经

以拇指固定在脚掌跟部，食指弯曲呈镰刀状，以食指侧缘施力，沿脚后跟自上而下刮压至足跟内侧缘，操作 3~5 次

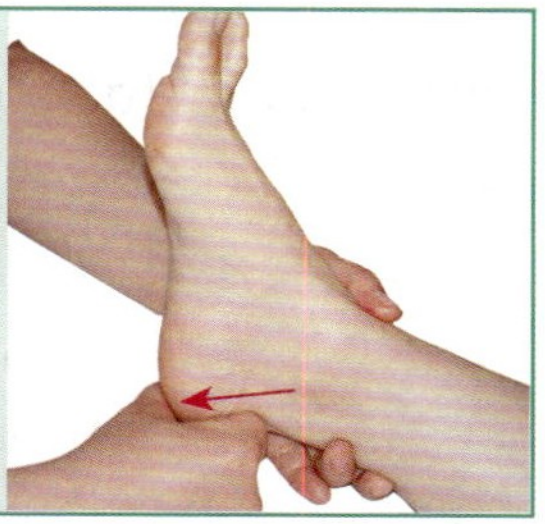

前列腺 · 子宫

以拇指指腹或食指侧缘施力按压 3~5 次

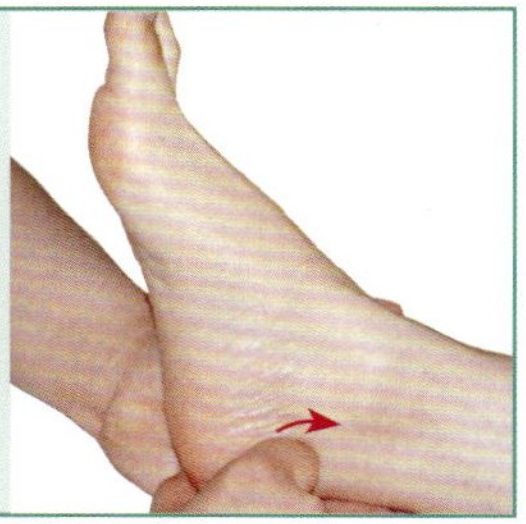

尿道 · 阴道

以拇指指腹或指端施力按压 3~5 次

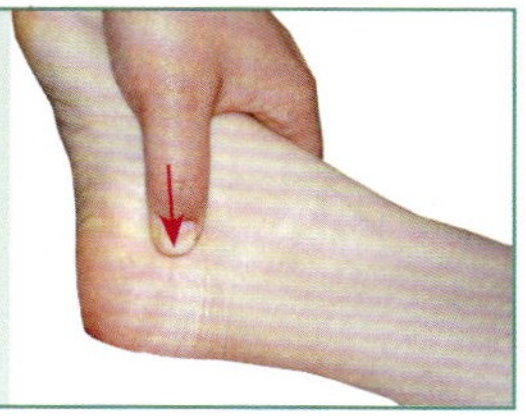

髋关节

以拇指指腹或指端施力，沿着内踝下缘推按 3~5 次

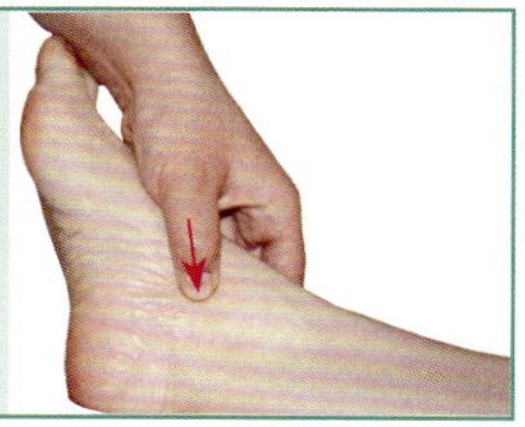

直肠 · 肛门

以拇指指腹或食指近侧指间关节施力按压 3~5 次

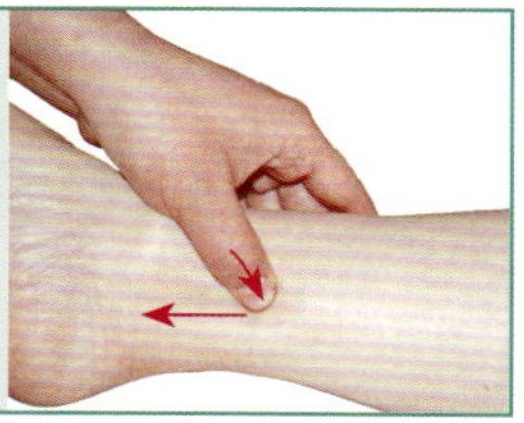

腹股沟

以拇指指腹或指端施力，定点揉按 3~5 次

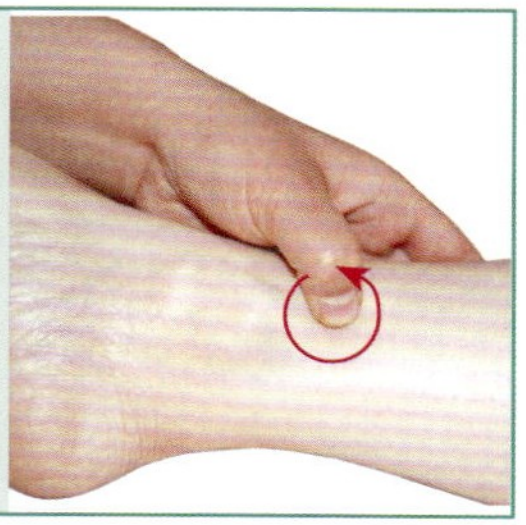

Cervical Vertebra

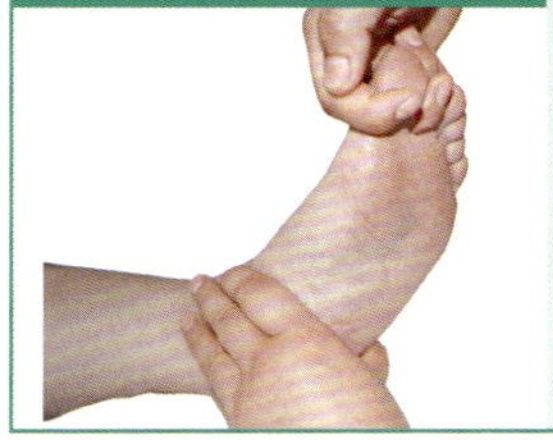

Using the thumb tip to press and knead for 3 to 5 times or using bending index finger and middle finger to pinch the bottom of participant's great toe, then pressing the reflex zone for 3 to 5 times by using index finger

Thoracic Vertebra

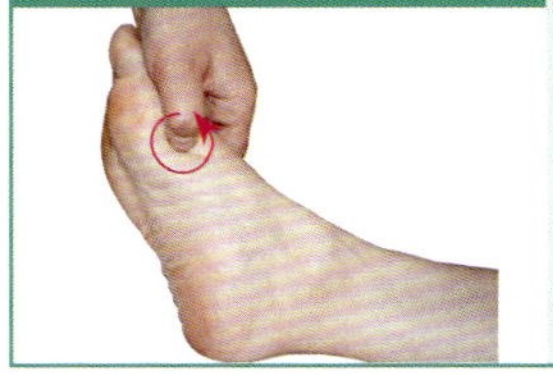

Using thumb pulp or the fingertip to knead and press for 3 to 5 times

Lumbar Vertebra

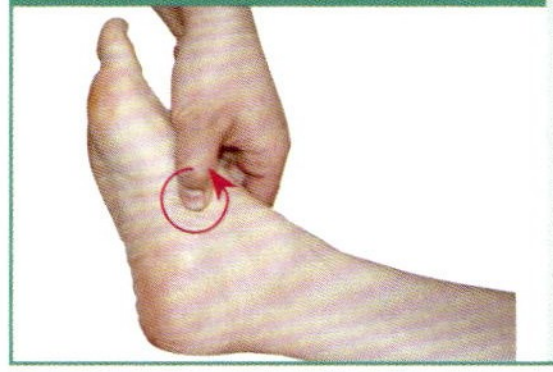

Using thumb pulp or index finger tip to press for 3 to 5 times

Sacrum and Coccyx

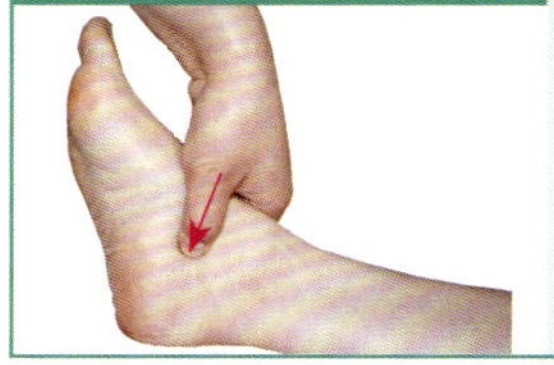

Using thumb pulp or index finger tip to press for 3 to 5 times

Buttock and Sciatic Nerves

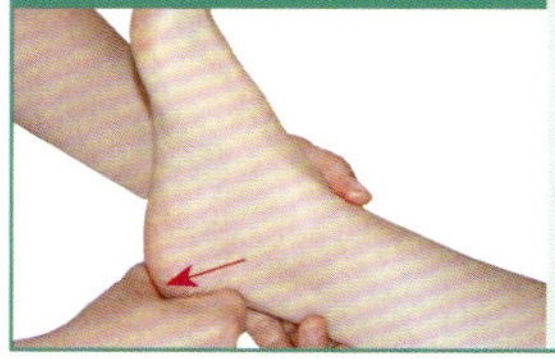

Making the thumb fixed on under the heel, using the bending index finger to scrap to the inside of heel for 3 to 5 times

Prostate Gland and Uterus

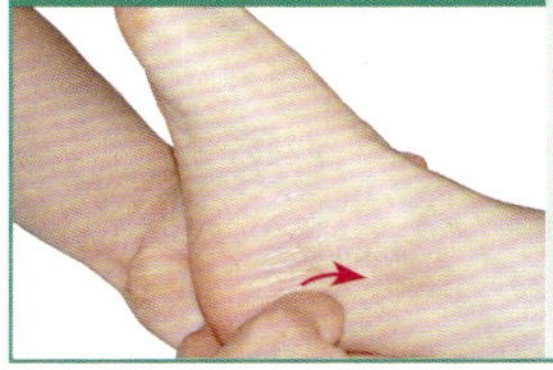

Pressing for 3 to 5 times by thumb pulp or medial side of index finger

Urethra and Vagina

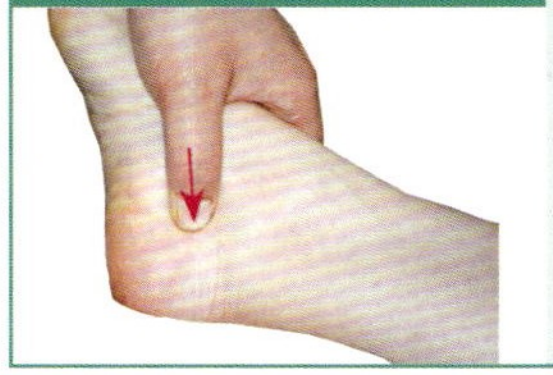

Using thumb pulp or fingertip to press for 3 to 5 times

Hip Joint

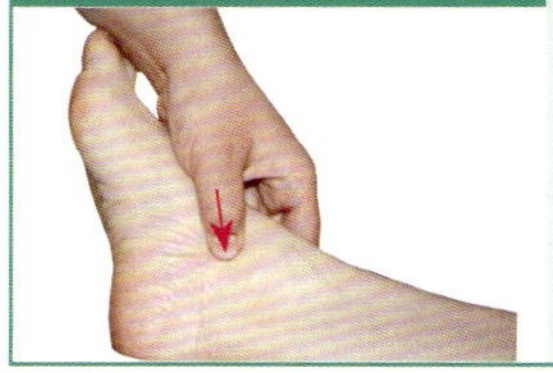

Pressing along the line under medial malleolus by thumb pulp or the fingertip for 3 to 5 times

Rectum and Anus

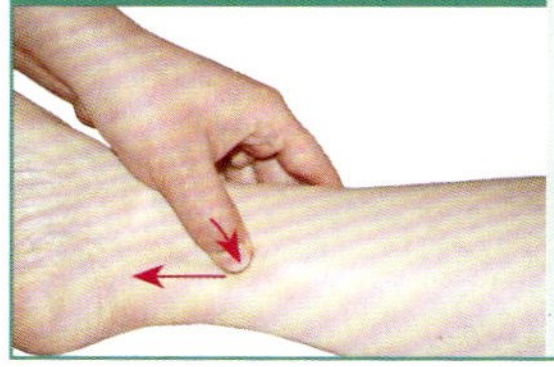

Pressing for 3 to 5 times by thumb pulp or index finger's metacarpophalangeal joint

Groin

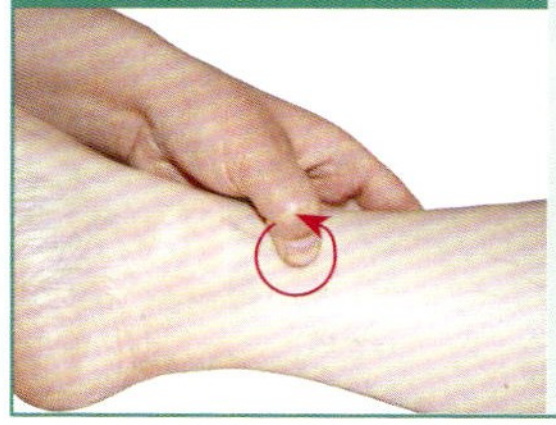

Using thumb pulp or fingertip to acupoint-knead and acupoint-press for 3 to 5 times

足外侧反射区
Lateral Foot Reflex Zone

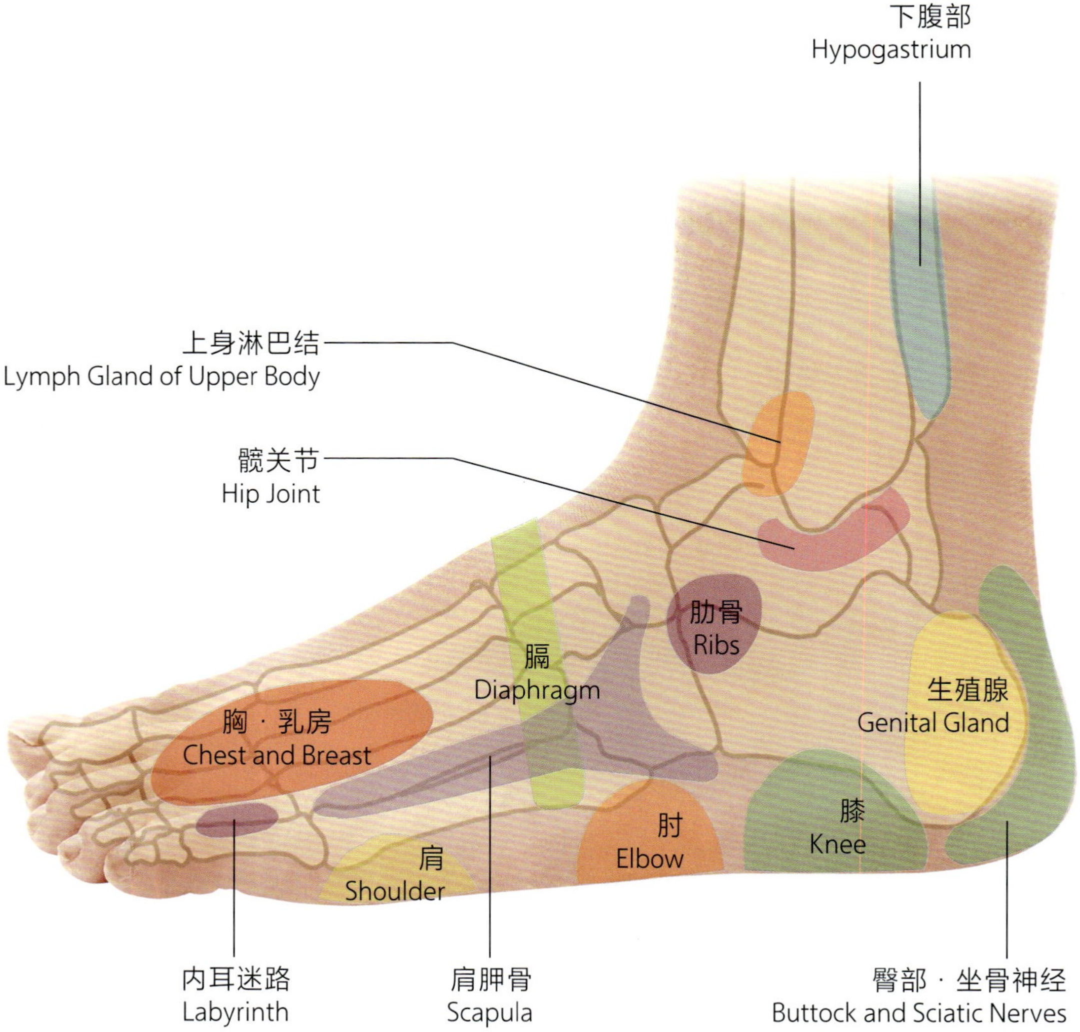

反射区	定 位	主 治
生殖腺	双足外踝后下方，跟腱前方的三角形区域	性功能低下、不孕、围绝经期综合征、月经不调、痛经、阳痿、早泄及其他生殖系统疾患
膝	双足外踝下方，骰骨与跟骨前缘形成的凹陷处	膝关节炎、膝关节痛等膝部及下肢疾患
肘	双足外侧第 5 跖骨粗隆前、后凹陷处	肘关节软组织损伤、肘关节酸痛、肘关节炎等肘部及上肢疾患
肩	双足第 5 跖趾关节后方凹陷处	肩周炎、肩酸痛、手臂无力、手麻等肩部及上肢疾患
肩胛骨	双足第 4、5 跖骨间延伸到骰骨处稍向两侧分开的带状区域	肩背酸痛、肩周炎、肩关节活动障碍等肩胛部疾患
髋关节	双足外踝的下缘呈弧形的区域	髋关节痛、坐骨神经痛、腰背痛等疾患
下腹部	双足腓骨外后方向上延伸四横指的带状区域	妇科疾患，如月经不调、痛经等
臀部 · 坐骨神经	双足外侧脚跟后缘上行至外踝下的带状区域	坐骨神经痛、脚麻

Reflex Zone	Location	Indications
Genital Gland	Triangle zone below and behind the lateral malleolus, and in the front of achilles tendon	Sexual dysfunction; infertility; perimenopausal syndrome; menstrual disorders; dysmenorrhea; impotence; premature ejaculation and other reproductive system disorders
Knee	Depression under the lateral malleolus, located to anterior border of cuboid bone and calcaneus	Knee osteoarthritis; knee pain; knee and lower limb disorders
Elbow	Depression located before and after lateral tuberosity of the 5th metatarsal bone	Elbow joint soft tissue injury; elbow joint aching pain; elbow arthritis and other elbow and upper limb disorders
Shoulder	Depression located after the 5th metatarsophalangeal joint	Periarthritis humeroscapularis; shoulder aching pain; weakness, numbness in the hand arm and other shoulder and upper limb disorders
Scapula	Band-shaped region which is tend to divide into 2 parts between the 4th and the 5th metatarsal bone and cuboid bone	The shoulder aching pain; periarthritis humeroscapularis; shoulder joint movement disorder and other scapular disorders
Hip Joint	Arc-shaped region under lateral malleolus	Hip joint pain; sciatica; low back pain and other disorders
Hypogastrium	Band-shaped region which is as wide as 4 fingers of a hand behind lateral surface of fibula	Gynecological diseases; such as menstrual disorders, dysmenorrhea and so on
Buttock and Sciatic Nerves	Band-shaped region between lateral heel and lateral malleolus	Sciatica; numbness in feet

超简单足外侧反射区按摩

Super-easy Massage in Lateral Foot Reflex Zone

生殖腺（足外侧）

以拇指指腹或食指侧缘施力按压 3~5 次

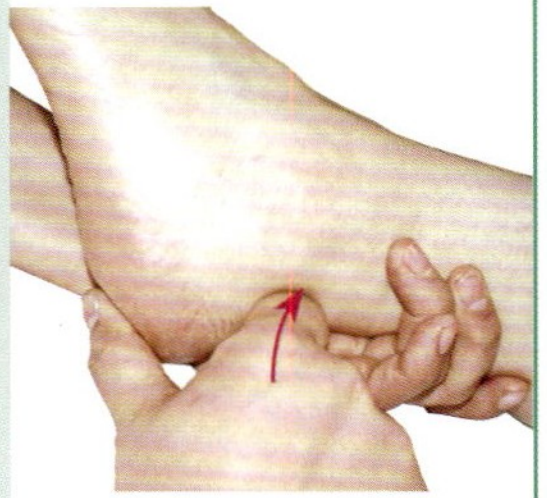

膝

以拇指指端或食指近侧指间关节，沿反射区半月形周边按压 3~5 次

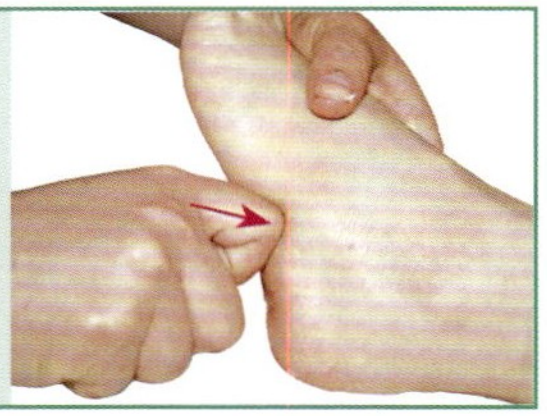

肘

以拇指指端，或食指、中指近侧指间关节施力按压 3~5 次

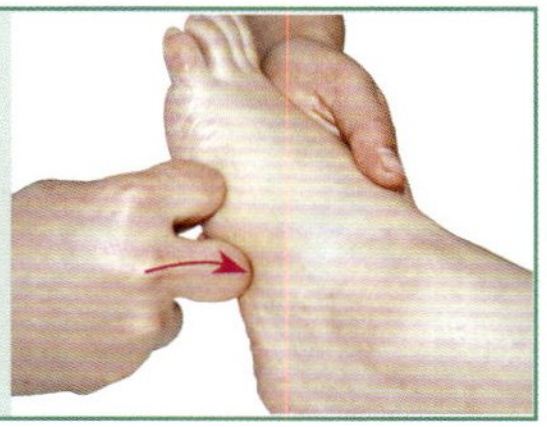

肩

以拇指指端或食指近侧指间关节施力按压 3~5 次

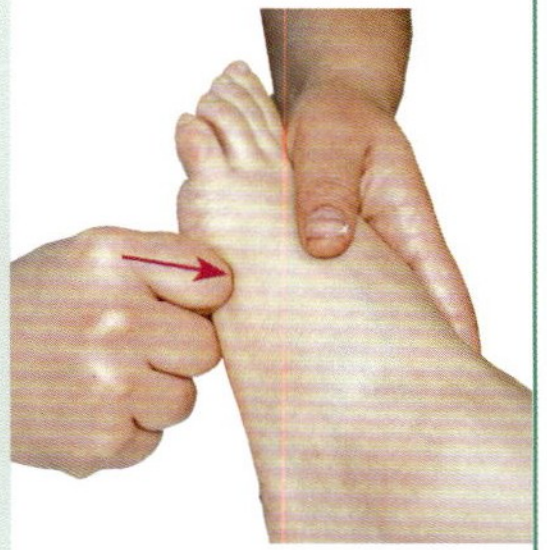

肩胛骨

以拇指指腹或指端施力推按 3~5 次

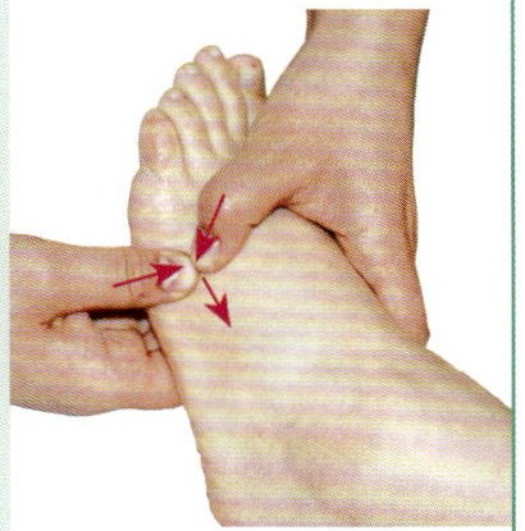

髋关节

以拇指指腹或指端施力，沿着外踝下缘推按 3~5 次

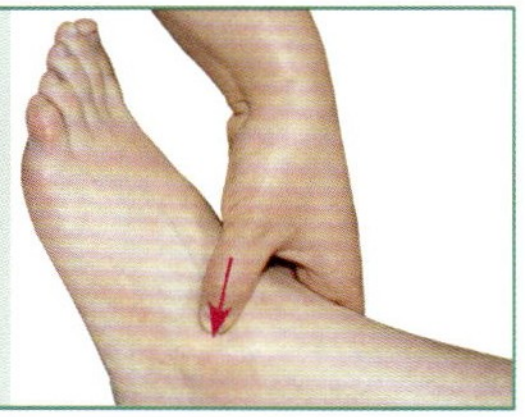

下腹部

以拇指指端，或食指、中指近侧指间关节施力按压 3~5 次

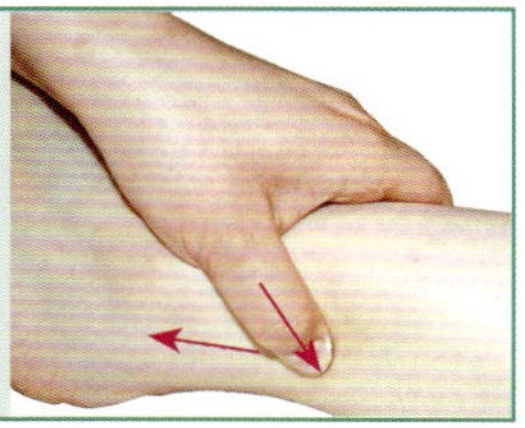

臀部·坐骨神经

以拇指固定在脚跟部，食指弯曲呈镰刀状，以食指侧缘施力，沿脚后跟自上而下刮压至足跟外侧缘，操作 3~5 次

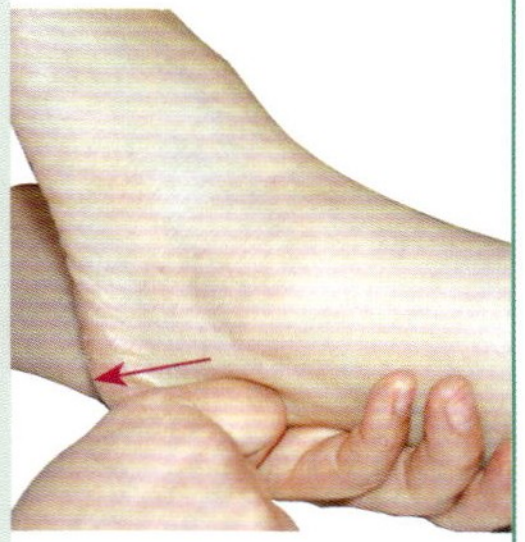

Genital Gland (Lateral border of foot)

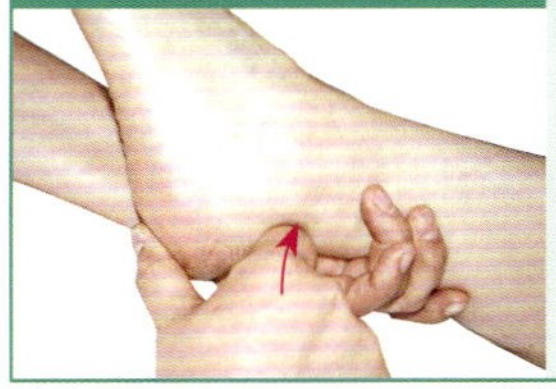

Pressing for 3 to 5 times by thumb pulp or medial side of index finger

Knee

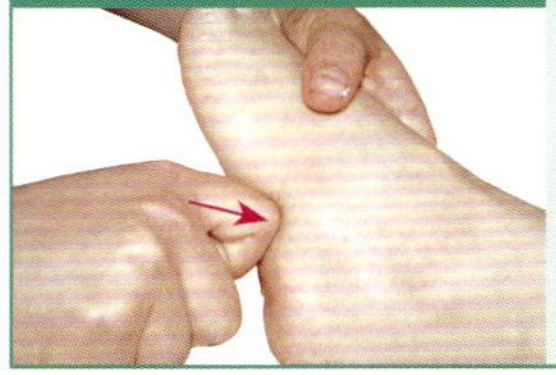

Pressing around the reflex zone which is like half-moon for 3 to 5 times by thumb tip or index finger' s metacarpophalangeal joint

Elbow

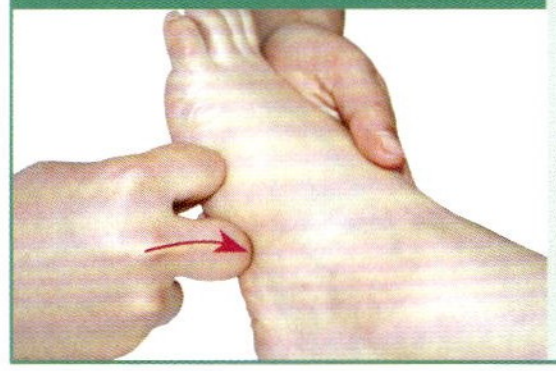

Pressing for 3 to 5 times by thumb tip or index finger' s and middle finger' s metacarpophalangeal joints

Shoulder

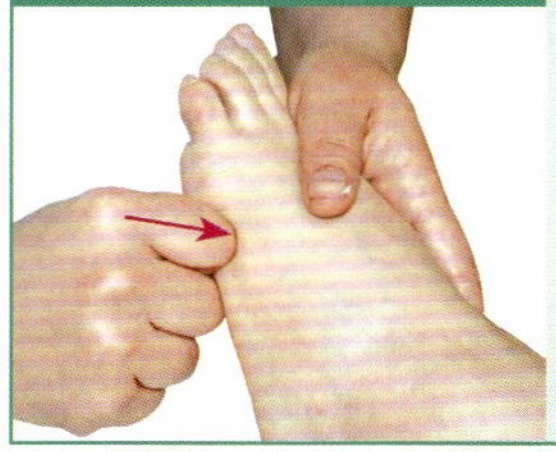

Pressing for 3 to 5 times by thumb fingertip or index finger' s metacarpophalangeal joint

Scapula

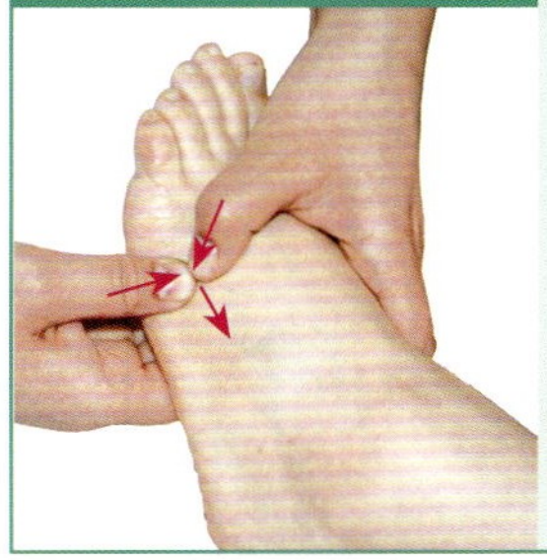

Using thumb pulp or fingertip to press for 3 to 5 times

Hip Joint

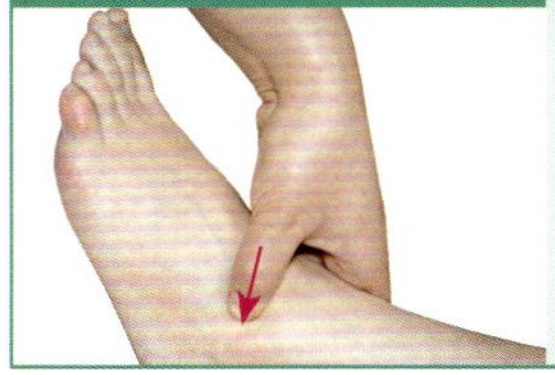

Using thumb pulp or fingertip to press and press the line under lateral malleolus for 3 to 5 times

Hypogastrium

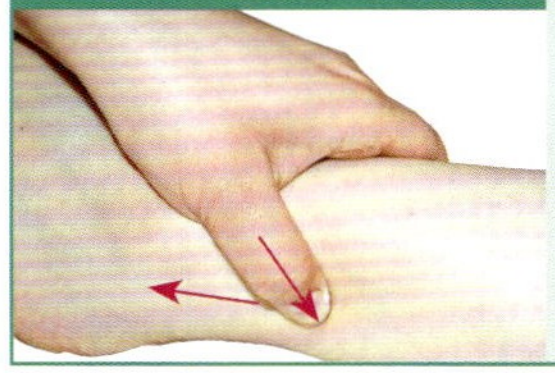

Pressing for 3 to 5 by thumb tip or index finger's and middle finger' s metacarpophalangeal joints

Buttock and Sciatic Nerves

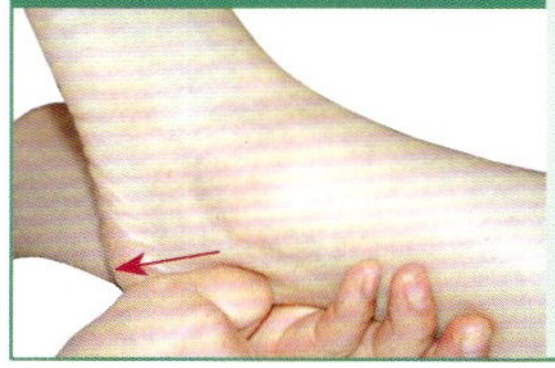

Making the thumb fixed on under the heel, using the bending index finger to scrap to the inside of heel for 3 to 5 times

足背反射区

Dorsal Foot Reflex Zone

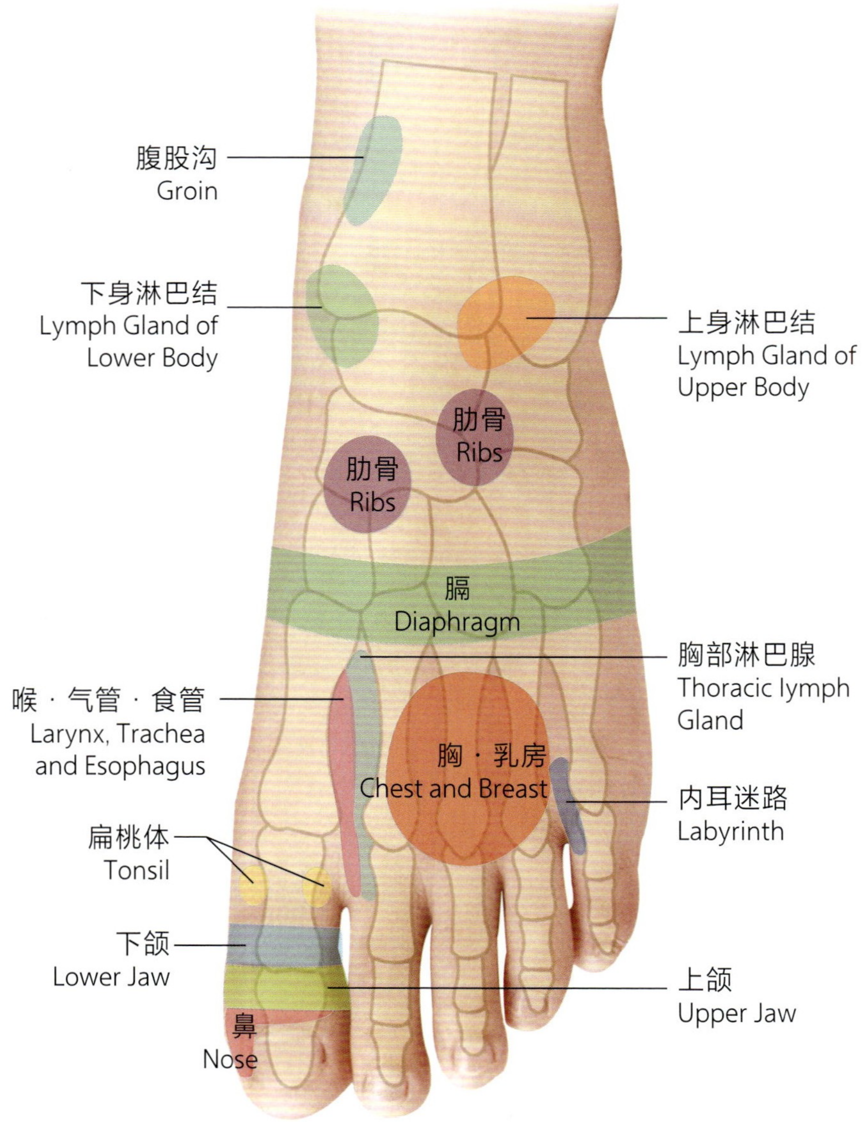

反射区	定 位	主 治
上颌	双足背拇趾趾间关节横纹前方的横带状区域	牙痛、牙周炎、牙龈炎、口腔溃疡、味觉障碍、打鼾等
下颌	双足背拇趾趾间关节横纹后方的横带状区域	牙痛、牙周炎、牙龈炎、口腔溃疡、味觉障碍、打鼾等
扁桃体	双足背拇趾的近节趾骨处，拇长伸肌腱的左右两侧	上呼吸道感染、扁桃体发炎、抵抗力下降
喉·气管·食管	双足背第 1、2 趾间缝至第 1、2 跖骨底，偏向内侧的带状区域	咽喉、气管及食管的各种炎症，各种原因引起的咳嗽、气喘、声音嘶哑等
胸部淋巴腺	双足背第 1、2 趾间缝至第 1、2 跖骨底，偏外侧的带状区域	上呼吸道感染及各种发热，炎症，免疫功能低下，胸部、子宫肿瘤等
内耳迷路	双足背第 4、5 趾间缝至第 4、5 跖趾关节间的凹陷处	眩晕、晕车、晕船、高血压、低血压、耳鸣等
胸·乳房	双足背第 2、3、4 趾蹼至第 2、3、4 跖骨底前所形成的圆形区域	乳腺炎、乳腺增生、乳腺肿瘤等
膈	双足背的中部，第 1~5 跖骨底与楔骨、骰骨之间，横跨足背的带状区域	膈肌痉挛、膈疝、腹胀、呕吐、哮喘
肋骨	内侧肋骨反射区在双足背内侧楔骨、中间楔骨与足舟骨间；外侧肋骨反射区在骰骨、足舟骨与距骨间	胸膜炎、肋骨的各种疾患，肩周炎
上身淋巴结	双足背，外踝的前下方，腓骨与距骨所形成的凹陷处	炎症、发热、肌瘤、囊肿，刺激该反射区还有增强免疫力、抗癌的功效
下身淋巴结	双足背，距骨与内踝形成的凹陷处	炎症、发热、肌瘤、囊肿，刺激该反射区还有增强免疫力、抗癌的功效

Reflex Zone	Location	Indications
Upper Jaw	The rectangular zone in the front of great toe joint	Toothache; periodontitis; gingivitis; oral ulcer; dysgeusia; snoring; and so on
Lower Jaw	The rectangular zone behind great toe joint	Toothache; periodontitis; gingivitis; oral ulcer; dysgeusia; snoring; and so on
Tonsil	The zone is beside the extensor pollicis longus muscle tendon and located on proximal phalanx of great toe	Upper respiratory tract infection; tonsil inflammation; decreased resistance
Larynx, Trachea and Esophagus	Lateral band-shaped zone between the 1st and the 2nd metatarsal bone	Various kinds of inflammation of the throat, trachea and esophagus; and cough; asthma; hoarseness; and so on
Thoracic Lymph Gland	Medial band-shaped zone between the 1st and the 2nd metatarsal bone	Upper respiratory tract infection and fever; inflammation; immune dysfunction; breast and uterus tumor; and so on
Labyrinth	The depression between the 4th and the 5th metatarsophalangeal joint	Dizziness; motion sickness; seasickness; hypertension; hypotension; tinnitus; and so on
Chest and Breast	Circular zone between which is made by the 2nd, 3rd and 4th toe bones beside the 2nd, 3rd and 4th metatarsal bones	Mastitis; hyperplasia of mammary; breast cancer; and so on
Diaphragm	In the middle of dorsum of foot, the band-shaped region which stretch across dorsum of foot between the base of metatarsal bone and cuneiform bone and cuboid bone	Diaphragmatic spasm; diaphragmatic hernia; abdominal distension; vomiting; asthma
Ribs	The Inner Rib reflex zone is between the medial cuneiform bone, intermediate cuneiform bone and navicular bone; Lateral Rib reflex zone is between the cuboid bone, navicular bone and talus	Pleurisy; various diseases of ribs; periarthritis humeroscapularis
Lymph Gland of Upper Body	Depression formed by fibula and talus under lateral malleolus	Inflammation; fever; fibroids; cyst. And stimulating the reflex zone can enhance immunity, have anti-cancer effect
Lymph Gland of Lower Body	Depression formed by talus and medial malleolus	Inflammation; fever; fibroids; cyst. And stimulating the reflex zone can enhance immunity, have anti-cancer effect

超简单足背反射区按摩

Super-easy Massage in Dorsal Foot Reflex Zone

上颌

以拇指指端或指间关节施力按压3~5次

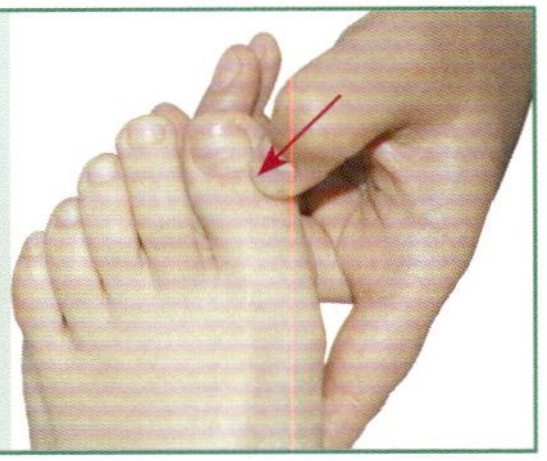

内耳迷路

以拇指指端或食指、中指指腹按压反射区3~5次

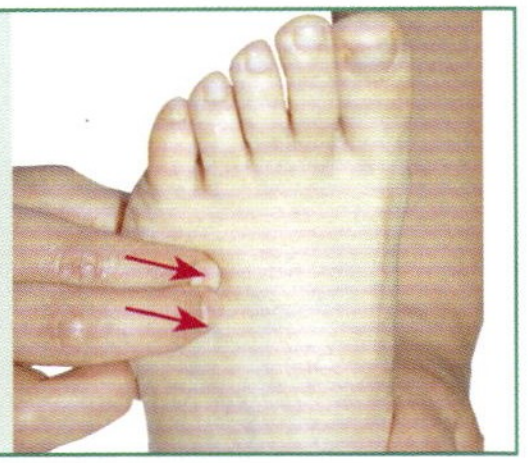

下颌

以拇指指端或食指近侧指间关节施力按压3~5次

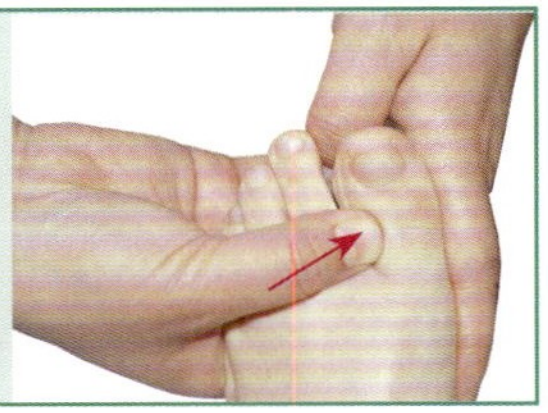

胸·乳房

以双手拇指指腹施力推按3~5次

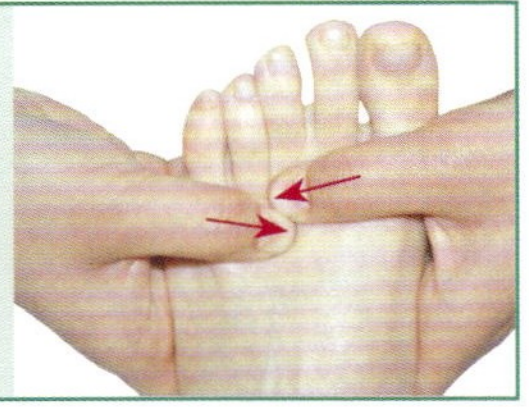

扁桃体

以拇指指端或食指近侧指间关节定点揉按3~5次

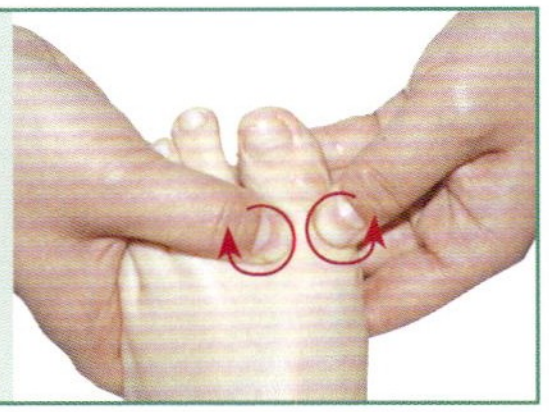

肋骨

以拇指指端或指腹施力，定点按3~5次

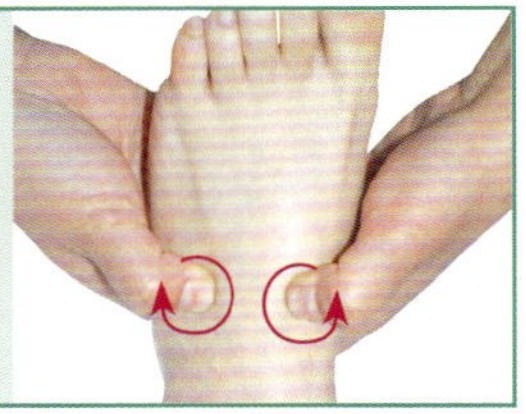

喉·气管·食管

食指、中指指腹按压反射区3~5次

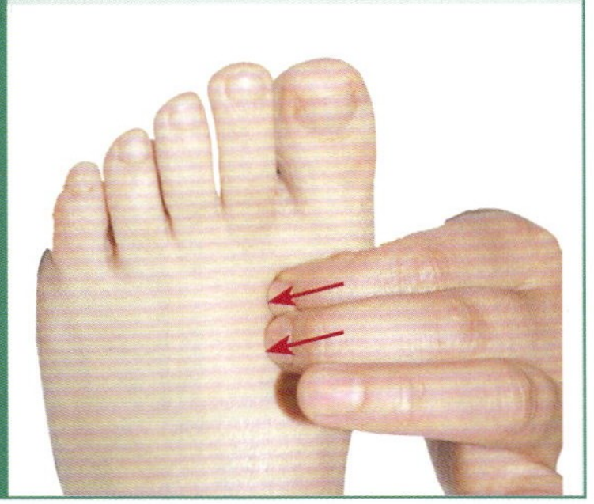

胸部淋巴腺

以拇指指端或食指、中指指腹按压反射区3~5次

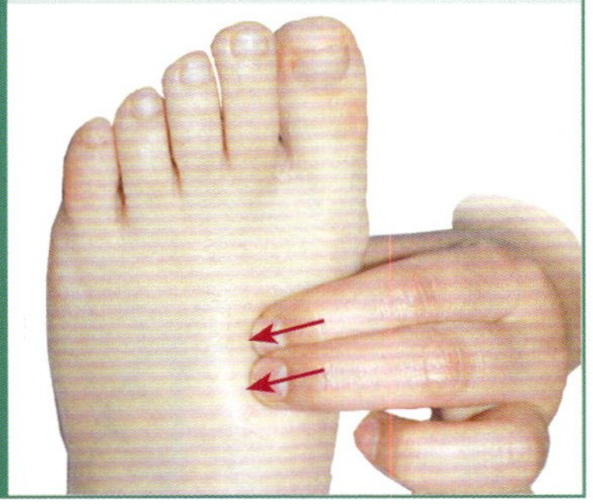

上身淋巴结

以拇指指端或以食指近侧指间关节施力，定点按3~5次

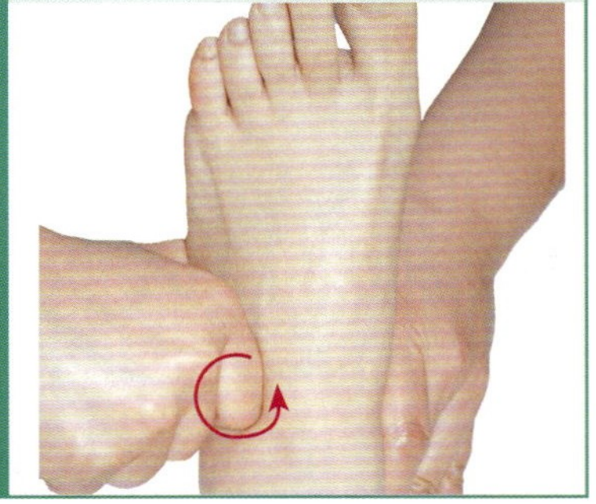

下身淋巴结

以拇指指端或以食指近侧指间关节施力，定点按3~5次

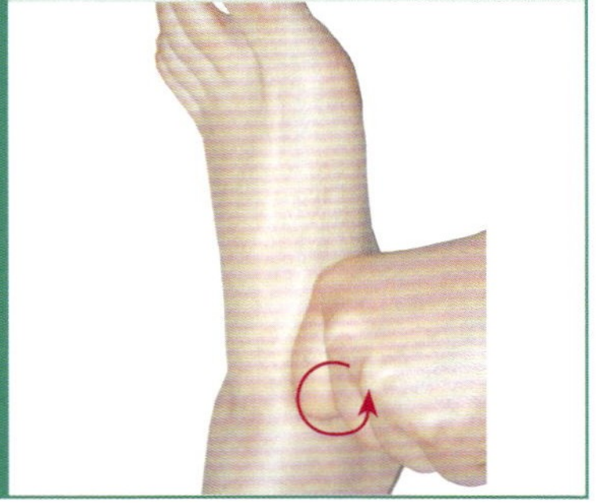

Upper Jaw

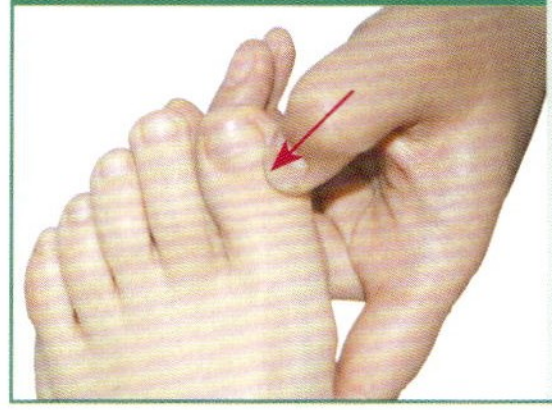

The power for massage comes from the thumb tip or the interphalangeal joint. Press 3 to 5 times

Lower Jaw

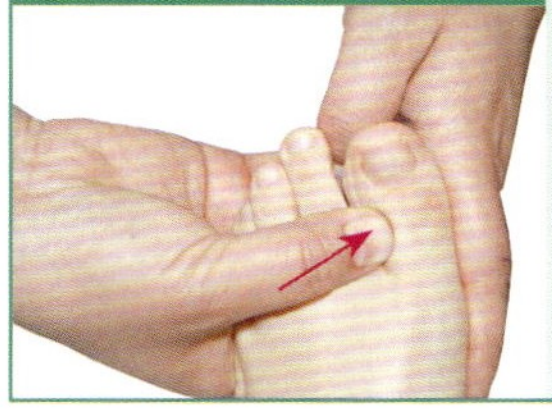

The power for massage comes from the thumb tip or the proximal interphalangeal joint of the index finger. Press 3 to 5 times

Tonsil

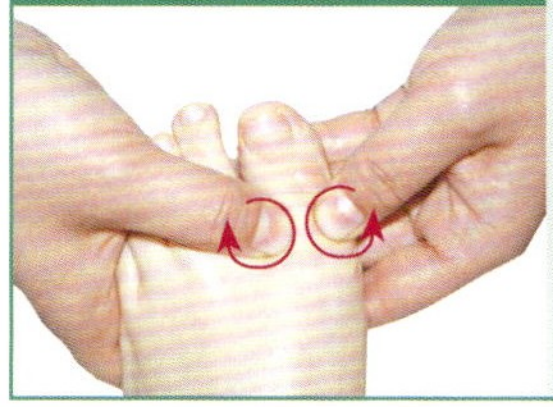

The power for massage comes from the thumb tip or the proximal interphalangeal joint of the index finger. Rub the fixed points for 3 to 5 times

Labyrinth

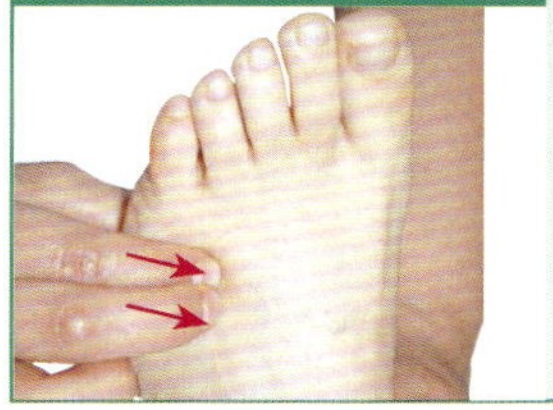

Press this reflex zone with the finger pulps of index finger and middle finger for 3 to 5 times

Chest and Breast

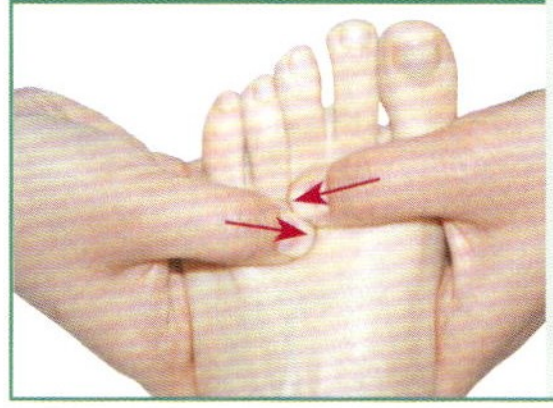

Press and press with the 2 thumb pulps for 3 to 5 times

Ribs

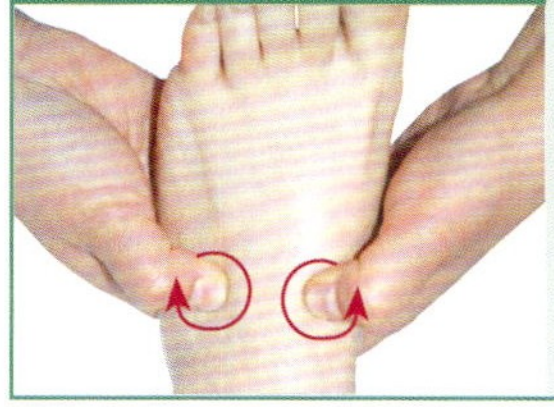

Press the fixed points with the thumb tip or the finger pulp for 3 to 5 times

Larynx, Trachea and Esophagus

Press the reflex zone with the finger pulps of index finger and middle finger for 3 to 5 times

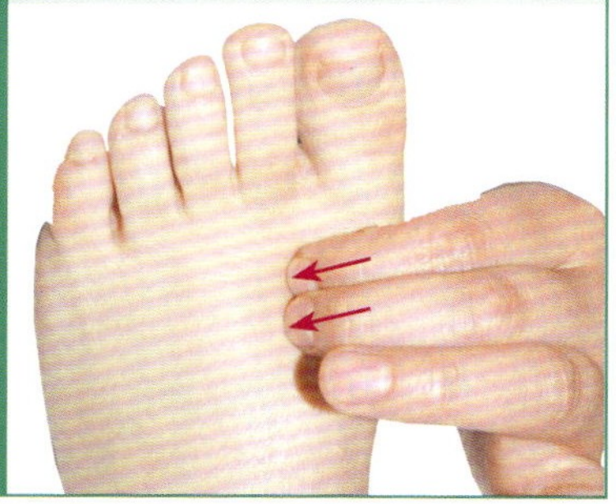

Thoracic Lymph Gland

Press this reflex zone with the thumb tip or the finger pulps of index finger and middle finger for 3 to 5 times

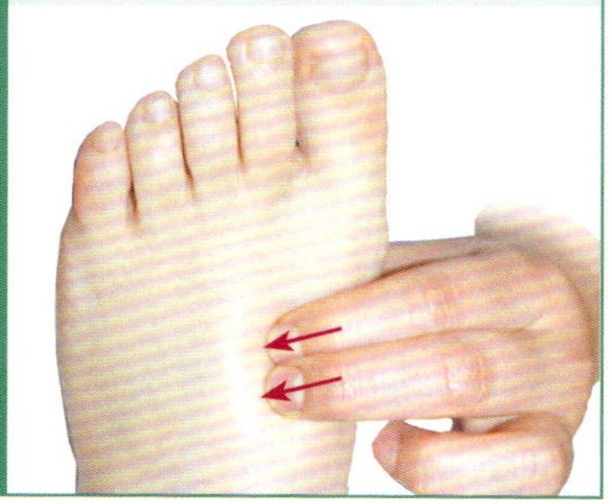

Lymph Gland of Upper Body

Press the fixed points with the thumb tip or the proximal interphalangeal joint of the index finger for 3 to 5 times

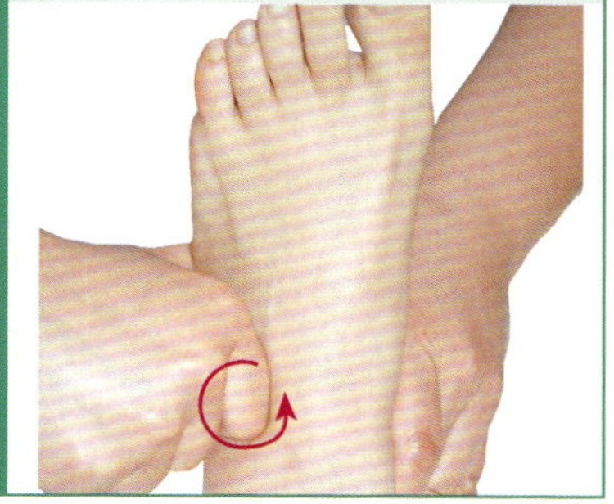

Lymph Gland of Lower Body

Press the fixed points with the thumb tip or the proximal interphalangeal joint of the index finger for 3 to 5 times

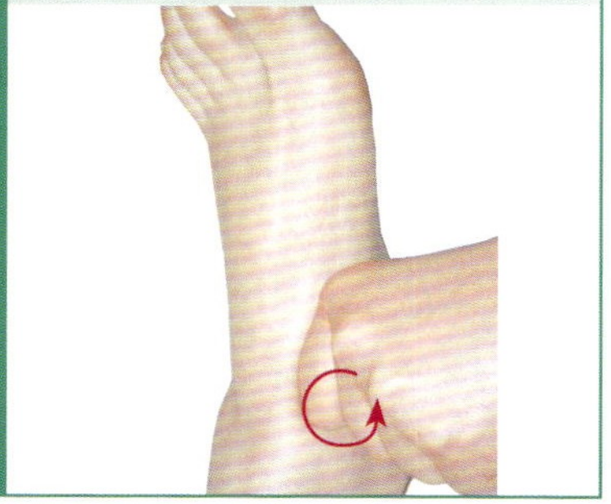

足部常用穴位
Common Foot Acupoints

足阳明胃经
Stomach Meridian of Foot-Yangming

足阳明胃经
Stomach Meridian of Foot-Yangming

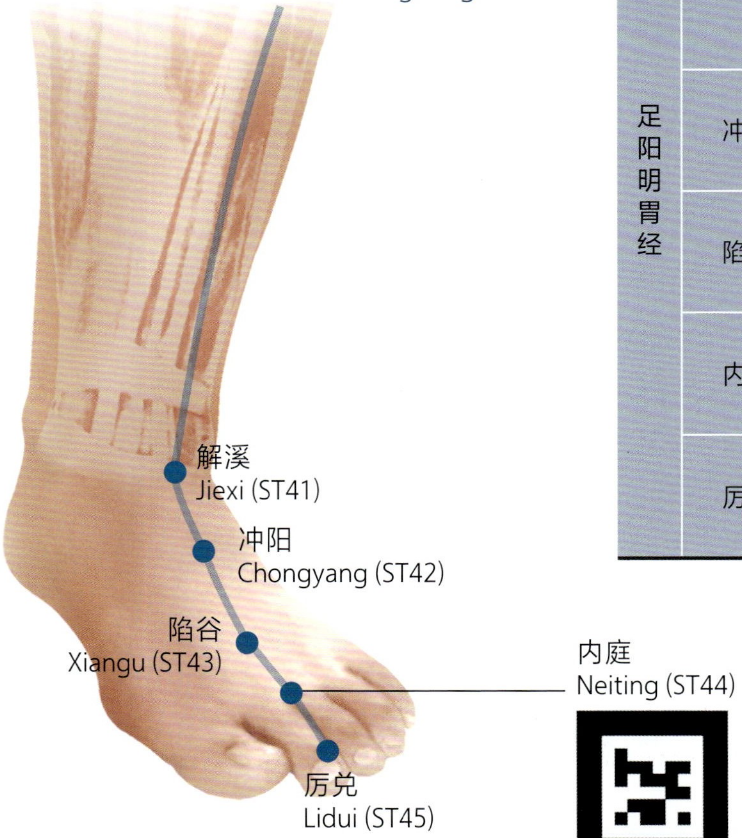

穴位		定位	主治
足阳明胃经	解溪	在踝部，踝关节前面中央凹陷中，当拇长伸肌腱与趾长伸肌腱之间 *取穴小窍门：令足趾上跷，显现足背部两肌腱，穴在两腱之间，相当于内、外踝尖连线的中点处	头痛、眩晕、癫狂、腹胀、便秘、下肢痿痹、足踝肿痛
	冲阳	在足背，第 2 跖骨基底部与中间楔状骨关节处，可触及足背动脉	胃痛、腹胀、面瘫、足背肿痛无力
	陷谷	在足背，当第 2、3 跖骨间，第 2 跖趾关节近端凹陷中	目赤肿痛、面部浮肿、足背肿痛
	内庭	在足背，第 2、3 趾间，趾蹼缘后方赤白肉际处	齿痛、咽喉肿痛、面瘫、热病、腹痛、腹胀、便秘、足背肿痛
	厉兑	在足趾，第 2 趾末节外侧，趾甲根角侧后方 0.1 寸（指寸）	齿痛、咽喉肿痛、面瘫、热病、癫狂、鼻出血、足背肿痛

Acupoints		Location	Indications
Stomach Meridian of Foot-Yangming	Jiexi (ST41)	The point is in the anterior articular depression of the ankle joint, between the tendons of extensor digitorum longus and hallucis longus Tip: Make your toes pointed up, and then you can see 2 tendons on the dorsum of foot. The point is between the 2 tendons, it also can be seen as the midpoint of the line from tip of the medial malleolus to tip of the lateral malleolus	Headache; dizziness; madness; abdominal distention; constipation; and flaccidity of the lower limbs; ankle pain
	Chongyang (ST42)	The point is on the dorsum of foot, at the 2nd metatarsal base and the middle cuneiform. You will feel the movement of the dorsalis pedis artery when massage this point	Stomachache; abdominal distention; facial paralysis; and swelling and weakness in dorsum of foot
	Xiangu (ST43)	The point is on the dorsum of foot, between the 2nd and the 3rd metatarsal bones, in the proximal depression of the 2nd metatarsophalangeal joint	Redness, swelling and pain of eyes; facial edema; and swelling pain in dorsum of foot
	Neiting (ST44)	The point is on the dorsum of foot, proximal to the web margin between the 2nd and the 3rd toes, at the junction of the red and white skin	Toothache; itchy and sore throat; facial paralysis; febrile disease; abdominal pain; abdominal distention; constipation; and swelling pain in dorsum of foot
	Lidui (ST45)	The point is on the lateral side of the 2nd toe, about 0.1 cun posterior to the corner of the nail	Toothache; itchy and sore throat; facial paralysis; febrile disease; madness; nosebleed; and swelling pain in dorsum of foot

足太阴脾经

Spleen Meridian of Foot-Taiyin

足太阴脾经

Spleen Meridian of Foot-Taiyin

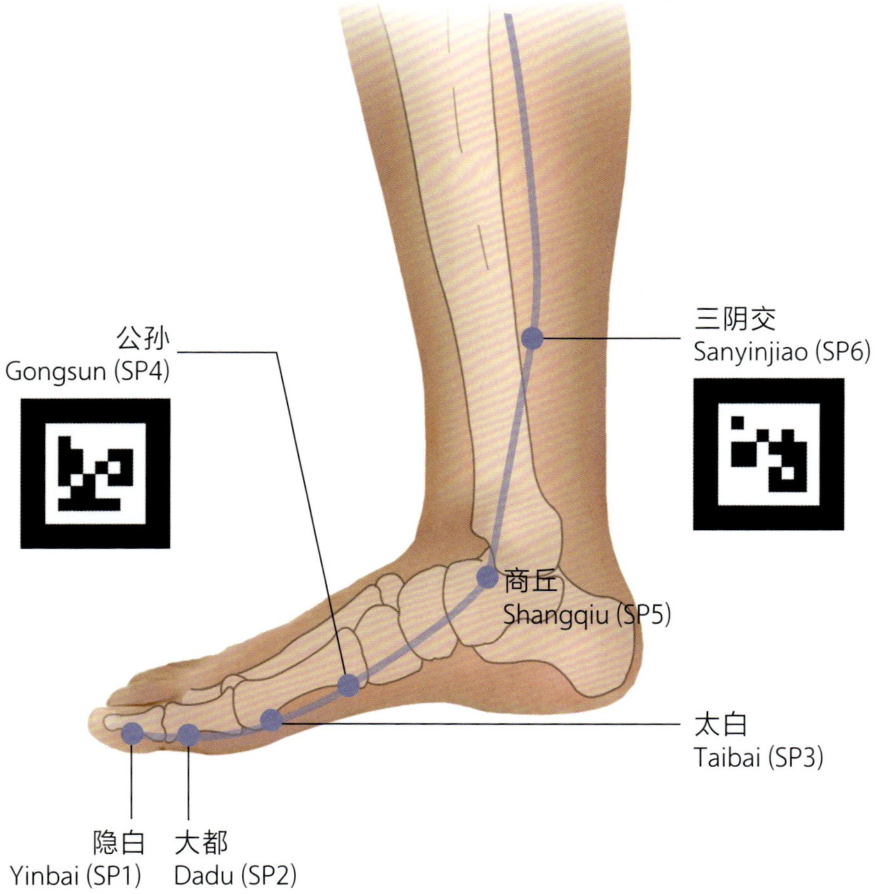

穴位		定位	主治
足太阴脾经	隐白	在足趾，拇趾末节内侧，趾甲根角侧后方 0.1 寸（指寸）	崩漏（突然阴道大量出血，或持续淋漓不断地出血）、月经过多、尿血、便血、腹胀、多梦
	大都	在足趾，第 1 跖趾关节远端赤白肉际凹陷中	腹胀、胃痛、泄泻、便秘、热病无汗
	太白	在跖区，第 1 跖趾关节近端赤白肉际凹陷中	胃痛、腹胀、腹痛、泄泻、便秘、纳呆（食欲不振）、脚趾关节痛
	公孙	在跖区，第 1 跖骨底的前下缘赤白肉际处 *取穴小窍门：沿太白向后推至一凹陷，即为本穴	胃痛、呕吐、腹胀、腹痛、泄泻、便秘、心痛、胸闷
	商丘	在踝区，内踝前下方，舟骨粗隆与内踝尖连线中点凹陷中 *取穴小窍门：内踝前缘垂线与内踝下缘横线的交点处	腹胀、泄泻、便秘、足踝肿痛、舌头强痛（僵硬疼痛）
	三阴交	在小腿内侧，内踝尖上 3 寸，胫骨内侧缘后际	月经不调、带下、难产、疝气、小便不利、遗尿、水肿、腹胀、泄泻、便秘、失眠、眩晕、下肢痿痹

Acupoints		Location	Indications
Spleen Meridian of Foot–Taiyin	Yinbai (SP1)	The point is on the medial side of the great toe, about 0.1 cun posterior to the corner of the nail	Metrorrhagia (suddenly massive uterine bleeding, or bleeding continuously); menorrhagia; hematuria; hemafecia; abdominal distention; and dreaminess
	Dadu (SP2)	The point is at toe, distal and inferior to the 1st metatarsophalangeal joint, in the depression of the junction of the red and white skin	Abdominal distention; stomachache; diarrhea; constipation; and febrile disease without sweating
	Taibai (SP3)	The point is proximal to the 1st metatarsophalangeal joint, in the depression of the junction of the red and white skin	Stomachache; abdominal distention; abdominal pain; diarrhea; constipation; anorexia (reduced appetite); and pain in the toe joint
	Gongsun (SP4)	The point is at metatarsal zone, in the depression distal and inferior to the base of the 1st metatarsal bone, at the junction of the red and white skin Tip: The point is in a depression behind Taibai (SP3)	Stomachache; vomiting; abdominal distention; abdominal pain; diarrhea; constipation; angina; chest tightness
	Shangqiu (SP5)	The point is in the depression distal and inferior to the medial malleolus, it also can be seen as the midpoint of the line from tuberositas ossis navicularis and the tip of the medial malleolus Tip: draw a perpendicular line at the front margin of the medial malleolus, and then find the distal margin line of the medial malleolus, the intersection of the 2 lines is Shangqiu (SP5)	Abdominal distention; diarrhea; constipation; swelling and pain in foot and ankle; and painful tongue (stiffening of the tongue)
	Sanyinjiao (SP6)	The point is on the inner side of shin, 3 cun above the tip of the medial malleolus, on the posterior border of the tibia	Irregular menstruation; leukorrheal diseases; difficult delivery; hernia; inhibited urinary; enuresis; edema; abdominal distention; diarrhea; constipation; insomnia; dizziness; and flaccidity of the lower limbs

足太阳膀胱经
Bladder Meridian of Foot-Taiyang

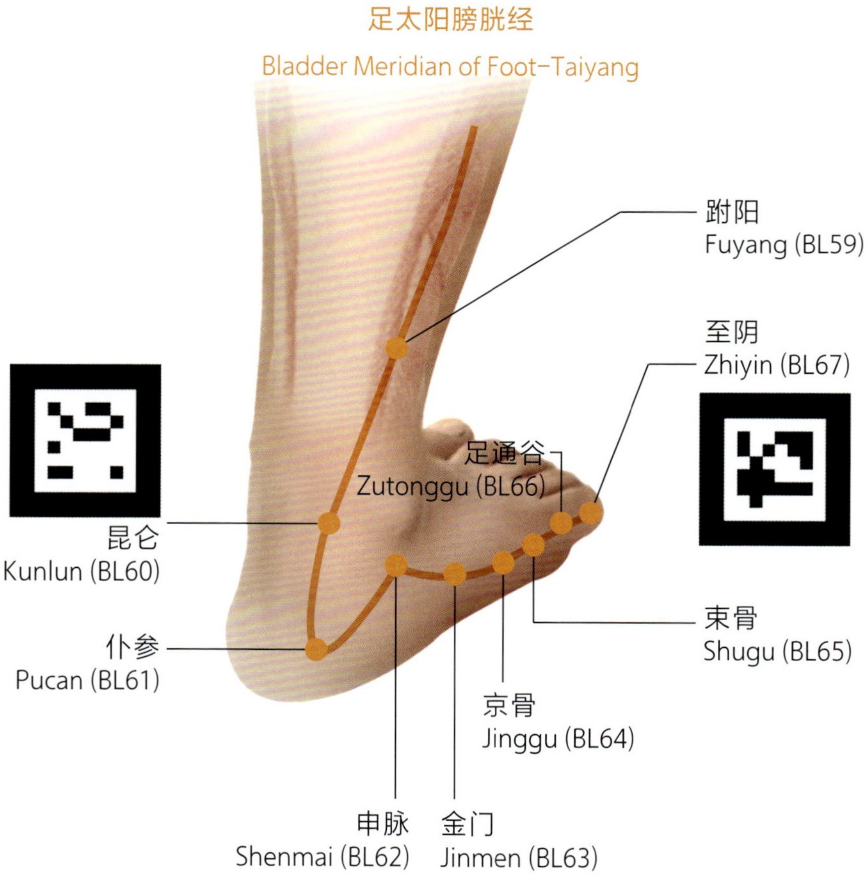

穴位		定位	主治
足太阳膀胱经	跗阳	在小腿后区，昆仑直上 3 寸，腓骨与跟腱之间	头痛、腰腿痛、下肢痿痹、外踝肿痛
	昆仑	在踝区，外踝尖与跟腱之间的凹陷中	头痛、项强、目眩、鼻塞、腰痛、足跟痛
	仆参	在跟区，昆仑直下，跟骨外侧，赤白肉际处	下肢痿痹、足跟痛、癫痫
	申脉	在踝区，外踝尖直下，外踝下缘与跟骨之间凹陷中	头痛、眩晕、失眠、目赤痛、眼睑下垂、腰腿痛、项强、足外翻
	金门	在足背，外踝前缘直下。第 5 跖骨粗隆后方，骰骨下缘凹陷中	腰痛、下肢痿痹、头痛、外踝肿痛
	京骨	在跖区，第 5 跖骨粗隆前下方，赤白肉际处 * 取穴小窍门：在足外侧缘，足跟与跖趾关节连线的中点处可触到明显隆起的骨，即第 5 跖骨粗隆	头痛、项强、目翳、癫痫、腰腿痛
	束骨	在跖区，第 5 跖趾关节的近端，赤白肉际处	头痛、项强、目眩、癫痫、腰腿痛
	足通谷	在跖区，第 5 跖趾关节的远端，赤白肉际处	头痛、项强、目眩、癫痫、腰腿痛
	至阴	在足趾，小趾末节外侧，趾甲根角侧后方 0.1 寸（指寸）	胎位不正、难产、头痛、目痛、鼻出血

Acupoints		Location	Indications
Bladder Meridian of Foot-Taiyang	Fuyang (BL59)	The point is on the posterior side of shin, between the fibula and the achilles tendon, 2 cun directly above Kunlun	Headache; pain in waist and lower extremities; flaccidity of the lower limbs; and swelling and pain on external malleolus
	Kunlun (BL60)	The point is in the depression between the apex of the external malleolus and the heel tendon	Headache; neck rigidity; dizziness; nasal congestion; low back pain; and heel pain
	Pucan (BL61)	The point is on the heel, below Kunlun (BL60). It is on the lateral calcaneus, at the junction of the red and white skin	Flaccidity of the lower limbs; heel pain; and epilepsy
	Shenmai (BL62)	The point is in the depression directly below the tip of the lateral malleolus, between the lower margin of lateral malleolus and calcaneus	Headache; dizziness; insomnia; painful redness of eyes; drooping eyelid; pain in waist and lower extremities; neck rigidity; and talipes valgus
	Jinmen (BL63)	The point is on the dorsum of foot, below the anterior lateral malleolus, behind the 5th metatarsal tuberosity, just in the depression of lower margin of cuboid	Lower back pain; weak wilting and pain in lower limbs; headache; and swelling and pain on external malleolus
	Jinggu (BL64)	The point is on distal and inferior to the 5th metatarsal tuberosity, at the junction of the red and white skin Tip: The point is on lateral margin of foot, You can obviously feel a raised bone (the 5th metatarsal tuberosity) at the midpoint of the line from heel and metatarsophalangeal joint	Headache; neck rigidity; eye screen; epilepsy; and pain in waist and lower extremities
	Shugu (BL65)	The point is proximal to the 5th metatarsophalangeal joint, at the junction of the red and white skin	Headache; neck rigidity; dizziness; epilepsy; and pain in waist and lower extremities
	Zutonggu (BL66)	The point is distal to the 5th metatarsophalangeal joint, at the junction of the red and white skin	Headache; neck rigidity; dizziness; epilepsy; and pain in waist and lower extremities
	Zhiyin (BL67)	The point is on the lateral aspect of the small toe, and 0.1 cun lateral and posterior to the corner of the toenail	Malposition of the fetus; difficult delivery; headache; eye pain; and nosebleed

足少阳胆经

Gallbladder Meridian of Foot-Shaoyang

足少阳胆经

Gallbladder Meridian of Foot-Shaoyang

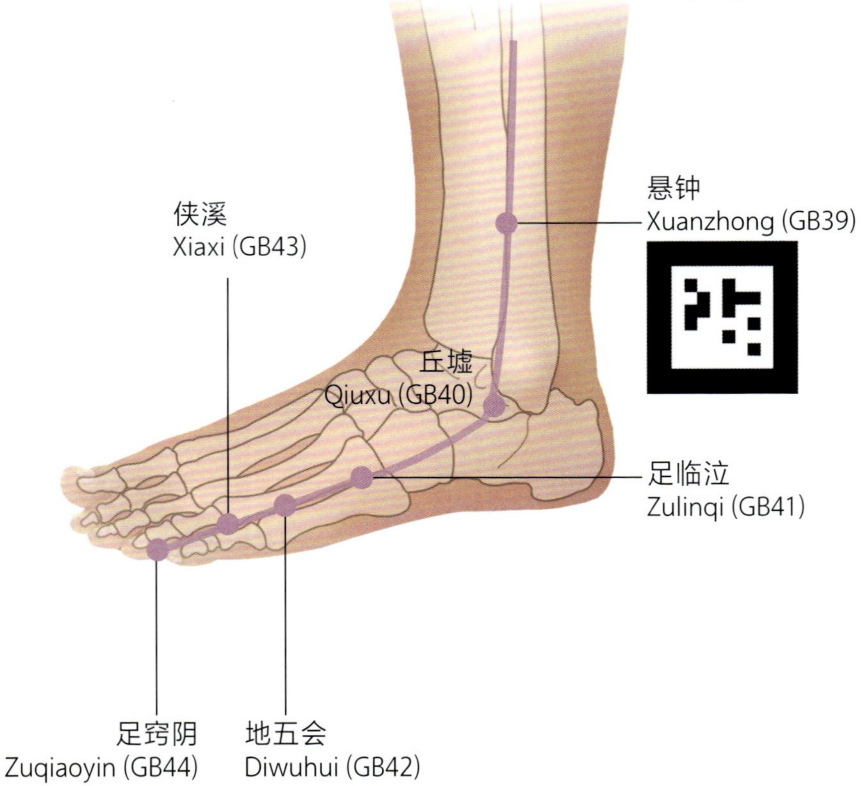

穴位		定位	主治
足少阳胆经	悬钟	在小腿外侧，外踝尖上 3 寸，腓骨前缘	下肢痿痹、胸胁胀痛、颈项强痛、偏头痛、膝髌肿痛
	丘墟	在踝区，外踝的前下方，趾长伸肌腱的外侧凹陷中 * 取穴小窍门：第 2~5 趾抗阻力伸展，可显现趾长伸肌腱	下肢痿痹、外踝肿痛、脚气、胸胁胀痛
	足临泣	在足背，第 4、5 跖骨底结合部的前方，第 5 趾长伸肌腱外侧凹陷中	足跗肿痛、胁肋疼痛、偏头痛、目赤肿痛
	地五会	在足背，第 4、5 跖骨间，第 4 跖趾关节近端凹陷中	足跗肿痛、胁肋疼痛、头痛、目赤、耳鸣、耳聋
	侠溪	在足背，第 4、5 趾间，趾蹼缘后方赤白肉际处	头痛、眩晕、目赤肿痛、耳鸣、耳聋、胸胁疼痛、乳痈（乳腺炎）
	足窍阴	在足趾，第 4 趾末节外侧，趾甲根角侧后方 0.1 寸（指寸）	足肿痛、胁痛、目赤肿痛、耳鸣、耳聋、头痛、失眠

Acupoints		Location	Indications
Gallbladder Meridian of Foot–Shaoyang	Xuanzhong (GB39)	The point is on the outside of shin, 3 cun above the tip of the lateral malleolus, anterior to the fibula	Flaccidity of the lower limbs; painful distension over hypochondrium; pain and rigidity of neck; migraine; and pain and swelling of knee cap
	Qiuxu (GB40)	The point is anterior and inferior to the external malleolus, in the depression on the lateral side of the tendon of extensor digitorum longus Tip: stretch the 2nd, 3nd, 4th, 5th toes forward, the tendon of extensor digitorum longus will be seen	Flaccidity of the lower limbs; pain on external malleolus; barbiers; and painful distension over hypochondrium
	Zulinqi (GB41)	The point is on the dorsum of foot, in front of the 4th and 5th metatarsal joints conction, in the depression of the lateral side of extensor digitorum longus	Pain in foot dorsum; rib pain; migraine; and redness, swelling and pain of eyes
	Diwuhui (GB42)	The point is on the dorsum of foot, between the 4th and 5th metatarsal bones, in the proximal depression of the 4th metatarsophalangeal joint	Pain in foot dorsum; rib pain; headache; red eyes; tinnitus; and deafness
	Xiaxi (GB43)	The point is on the dorsum of the foot, proximal to the web margin between the 4th and 5th toes, at the junction of the red and white skin	Headache; dizziness; redness,swelling and pain of eyes; tinnitus; deafness; rib pain; and mammary welling–abscesses (mammitis)
	Zuqiaoyin (GB44)	The point is on the distal and lateral side of 4th phalanx bone, about 0.1 cun posterior to the corner of the nail.	Foot swelling and pain; rib pain; redness, swelling and pain of eyes, tinnitus; deafness; headache; and insomnia

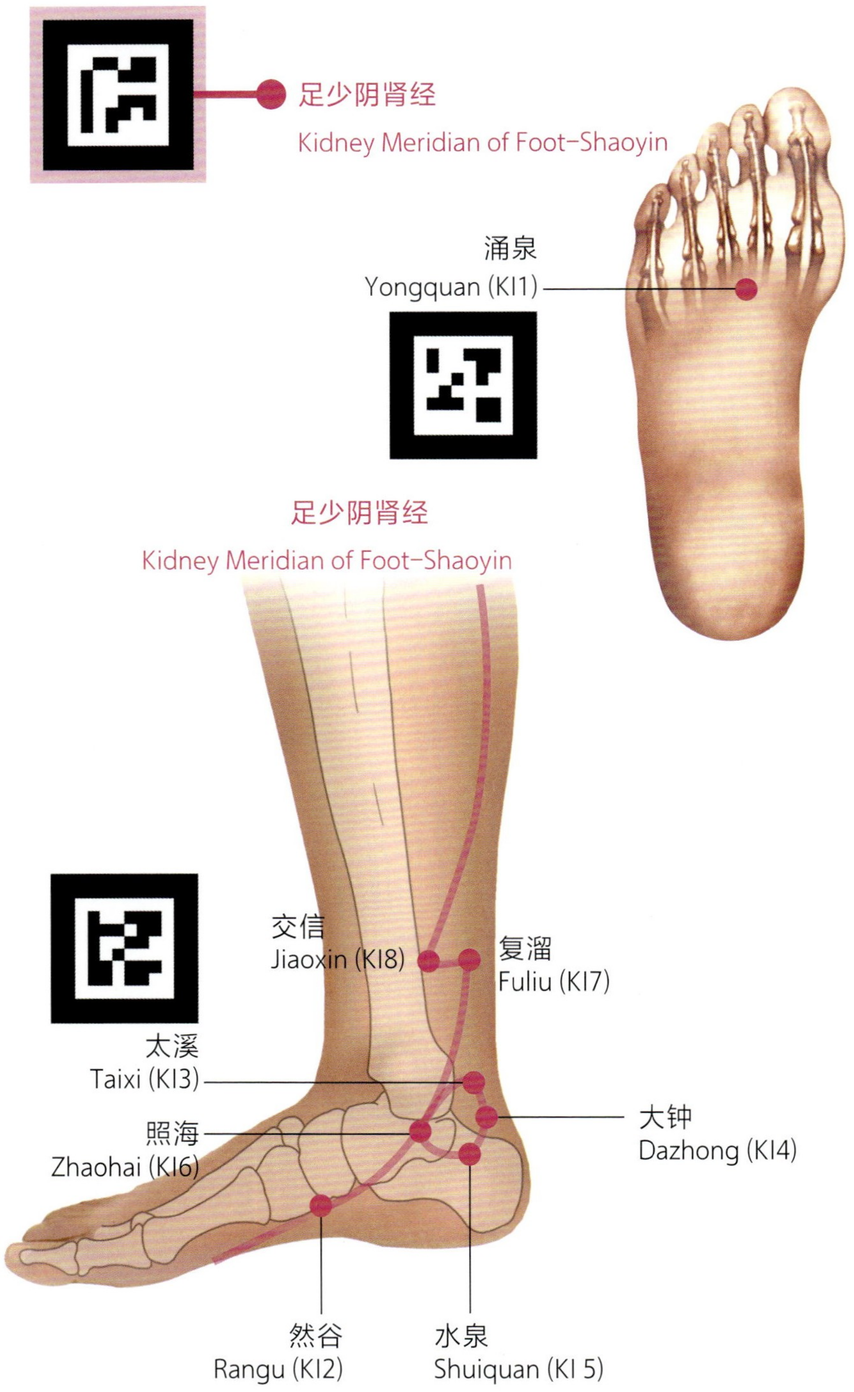

穴位		定位	主治
足少阴肾经	涌泉	在足底，屈足卷趾时足心最凹陷中 *取穴小窍门：卧位或伸腿坐位，卷足，约当足底第 2、3 趾蹼缘与足跟连线的前 1/3 与后 2/3 交点凹陷中	头顶痛、眩晕、昏厥、癫狂、失眠、便秘、小便不利、咽喉肿痛、失音、足心热
	然谷	在足内侧，足舟骨粗隆下方，赤白肉际处	月经不调、遗精、小便不利、泄泻、咽喉肿痛、咳血、牙关紧闭
	太溪	在踝区，内踝尖与跟腱之间的凹陷中	月经不调、遗精、阳痿、小便频数、消渴、泄泻、腰痛、头痛、耳鸣耳聋、咽喉肿痛、失眠、咳嗽、咳血
	大钟	在跟区，内踝后下方，跟骨上缘，跟腱附着部前缘凹陷中	癃闭、遗尿、便秘、咯血、气喘、嗜睡、足跟痛
	水泉	在跟区，太溪直下 1 寸，跟骨结节内侧凹陷中	月经不调、痛经、小便不利
	照海	在踝区，内踝尖下 1 寸，内踝下缘边际凹陷中 *取穴小窍门：由内踝尖向下推，至其下缘凹陷中	月经不调、痛经、带下、小便不利、咽喉痛、目赤肿痛、失眠
	复溜	在小腿内侧，内踝尖直上 2 寸，跟腱的前缘 *取穴小窍门：前平交信	水肿、腹胀、泄泻、盗汗、热病无汗或汗出不止
	交信	在小腿内侧，内踝尖上 2 寸，胫骨内侧缘后际凹陷中 *取穴小窍门：复溜前 0.5 寸	月经不调、崩漏、泄泻、便秘

Acupoints		Location	Indications
Kidney Meridian of Foot-Shaoyin	Yongquan (KI1)	The point is approximately at the most depression of the middle of the sole (excluding toe) Tip: lying or sitting with leg stretching and toes curled, in the depression of the anterior 1/3 and posterior 2/3 line from the web margin between the 2nd and 3rd toes to the heel	Vertex headache; dizziness; faint; madness; insomnia; constipation; inhibited urinary; sore swollen throat; loss of voice; and heat in the heart of the soles
	Rangu (KI2)	The point is on the inner side of foot, under the navicular tuberosity, at the junction of the red and white skin	irregular menstruation; seminal emission; inhibited urinary; diarrhea; sore swollen throat; hemoptysis; and folded jaw
	Taixi (KI3)	The point is in the depression between the prominence of the medial malleolus and heel tendon	irregular menstruation; seminal emission; frequent urination; diarrhea; lower back pain; headache; tinnitus; deafness; sore swollen throat; insomnia; cough; hemoptysis
	Dazhong (KI4)	The point is below and posterior to the medial malleolus, at the upper boundary of calcaneus, in the depression of front margin of calcaneal tendon attachment	Retention of urine; enuresis; constipation; hemoptysis; breathlessness; somnolence; and heel pain
	Shuiquan (KI5)	The point is on the heel, 1 cun below Taixi (KI3), in the depression of inner side of tuber calcanei	irregular menstruation; dysmenorrheal; inhibited urinary
	Zhaohai (KI6)	The point is 1 cun directly below the tip of the medial malleolus, in the depression of lower boundary of the medial malleolus Tip: find the tip of the medial malleolus, and then go down until touching the depression	Abnormal menstruation dysmenorrheal; leukorrheal diseases; inhibited urinary; sore throat; redness, swelling and pain of eyes; insomnia
	Fuliu (KI7)	The point is on the inner side of shin, 2 cun directly above the tip of the medial malleolus, at the front margin of calcaneal tendon Tip: Fuliu is at Jiaoxin (KI8) level	Edema; abdominal distention; diarrhea; night sweating; febrile disease without sweating or persistent sweating
	Jiaoxin (KI8)	The point is on the inner side of shin, 2 cun directly above the tip of the medial malleolus, in the depression of posterior border of the tibia Tip: the point is 0.5 cun posterior to Fuliu	irregular menstruation; metrorrhagia and metrostaxis; diarrhea; and constipation

足厥阴肝经

Liver Meridian of Foot-Jueyin

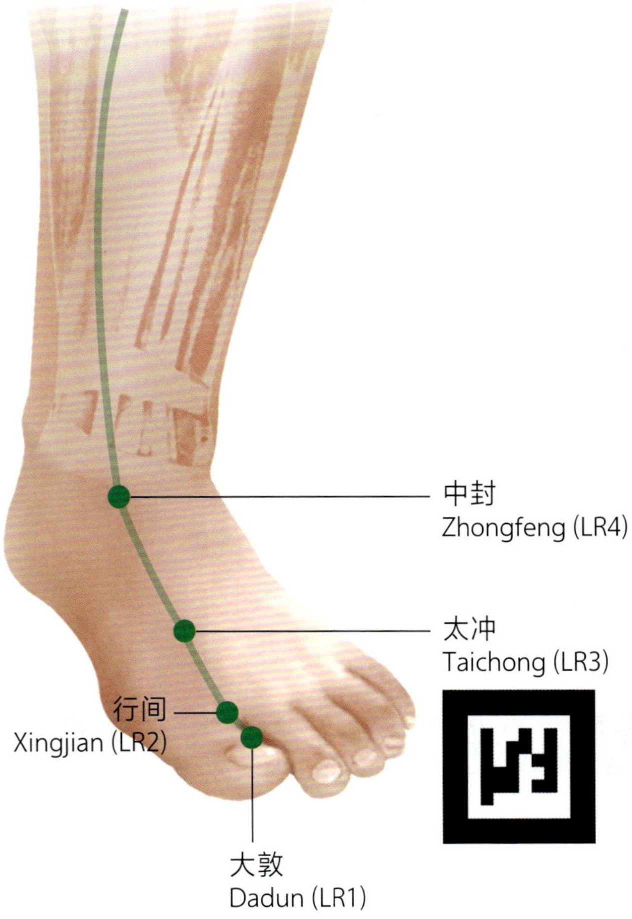

	穴位	定位	主治
足厥阴肝经	大敦	在足趾，大趾末节外侧，趾甲根角侧后方 0.1 寸	遗尿、癃闭、经闭、月经不调、疝气、癫痫
	行间	在足背，第 1、2 趾间，趾蹼缘后方赤白肉际处	头痛、目眩、目赤肿痛、月经不调、痛经、小便不利、中风、癫痫、胁肋疼痛、急躁易怒、黄疸
	太冲	在足背，第 1、2 跖骨间，跖骨底结合部前方凹陷中，或触及动脉搏动 * 取穴小窍门：从第 1、2 跖骨间向后推移至足背部的凹陷中取穴	头痛、目眩、目赤肿痛、耳鸣耳聋、呃逆、月经不调、崩漏、痛经、小便不利、中风、癫痫、胁肋疼痛、急躁易怒、黄疸、下肢痿痹、失眠
	中封	在踝区，内踝前，胫骨前肌肌腱的内侧凹陷中	腹痛、小便不利、疝气、下肢痿痹、足踝肿痛

Acupoints		Location	Indications
Liver Meridian of Foot-Jueyin	Dadun (LR1)	The point is on lateral side of the great toe, about 0.1 cun posterior to the corner of the nail	Enuresis; retention of urine; amenorrhea; irregular menstruation; mounting; epilepsy
	Xingjian (LR2)	The point is on the dorsum of foot, proximal to the web margin between the 1st and 2nd toes, at the junction of the red and white skin	Headache; dizziness; redness, swelling and pain of eyes; irregular menstruation; dysmenorrheal; inhibited urinary; wind stroke; epilepsy; rib pain; rashness; jaundice
	Taichong (LR3)	The point is on the dorsum of foot, between the 1st and the 2nd metatarsal bones, in the depression of the front of the metatarsal junction, you may feel the artery movement when massage this point Tip: find the point between the 1st and the 2nd metatarsal bones, and then go backward to a depression on dorsum pedis	Headache; dizziness; redness, swelling and pain of eyes; tinnitus; deafness; hiccough; irregular menstruation; metrorrhagia and metrostaxis; dysmenorrheal; inhibited urinary; wind stroke; epilepsy; rib pain; rashness; jaundice; flaccidity of the lower limbs; insomnia
	Zhongfeng (LR4)	The point is inferior to the medial malleolus, in the depression of tendon of tibialis anterior muscle	Abdominal pain; inhibited urinary; hernia; flaccidity of the lower limbs; ankle pain

超简单足部穴位按摩

Super-easy Massage of Foot Acupoints

解溪

用拇指按揉解溪穴 2 分钟，力度稍重。同法按揉对侧解溪穴。每日 2 次

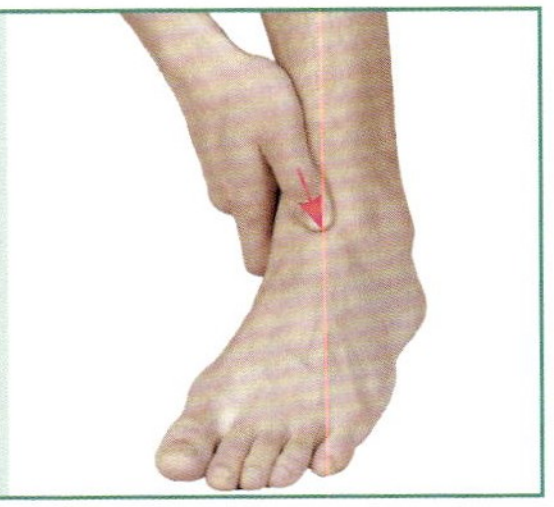

内庭

用拇指按揉内庭穴 2 分钟，力度稍重。同法按揉对侧内庭穴。每日 2 次

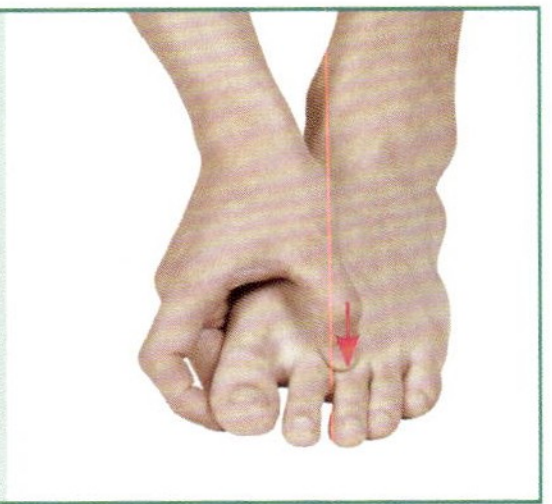

隐白

用拇指点按隐白穴 2 分钟，可停留片刻后放松，反复 5~6 下。同法按揉对侧隐白穴。每日 2 次

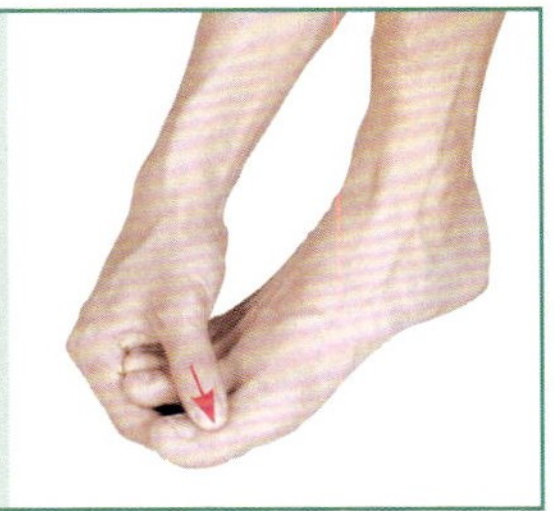

三阴交

用拇指用力按压三阴交穴，停留片刻后放松，反复 5~6 下。同法按压对侧三阴交穴。每日 2 次

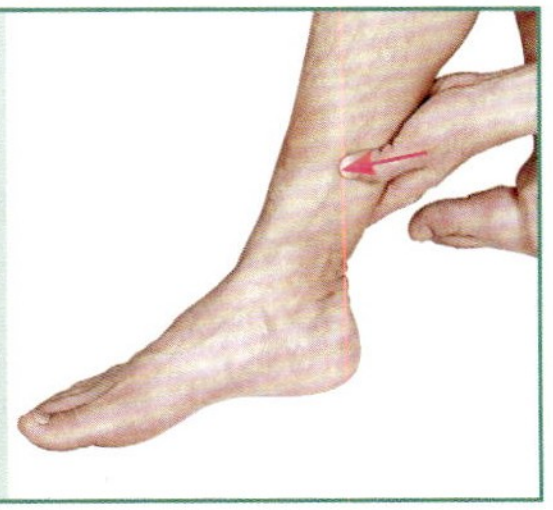

昆仑

用拇指和食指同时拿揉昆仑穴，力度稍重。同法拿揉对侧昆仑穴。每日 2 次

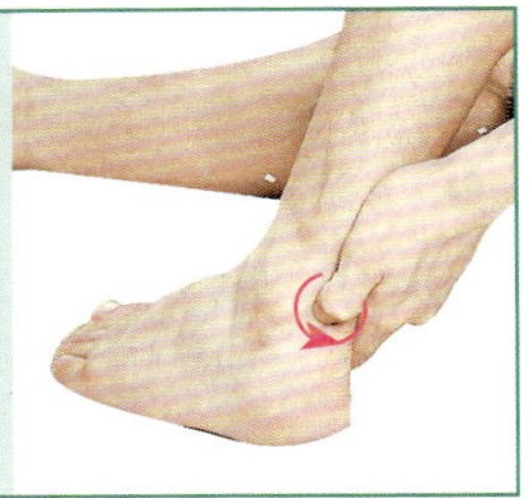

足通谷

用按摩棒点按足通谷穴，每分钟 30~50 下，力度适中，每次 2 分钟。同法点按对侧足通谷穴。每日 2 次

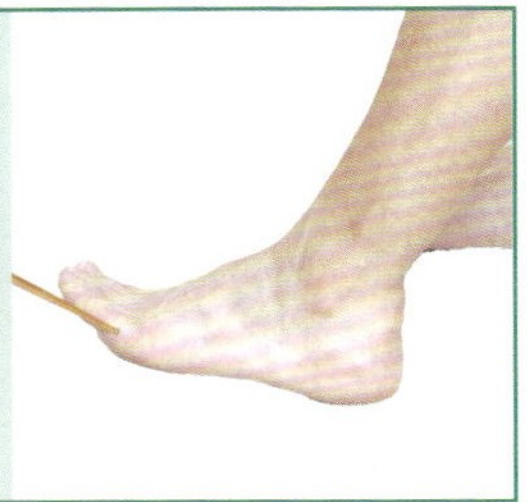

至阴

用拇指指尖掐揉至阴穴，力度可稍重，每分钟 30~50 下。同法按揉对侧至阴穴。每日 2 次

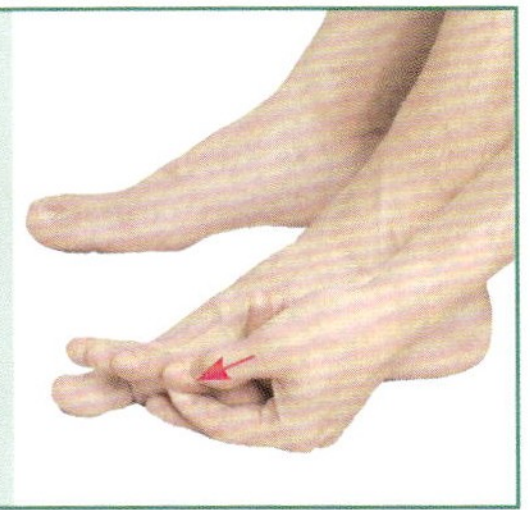

涌泉

用拇指按揉涌泉穴 2 分钟，力度稍重。同法按揉对侧涌泉穴。每日 2 次

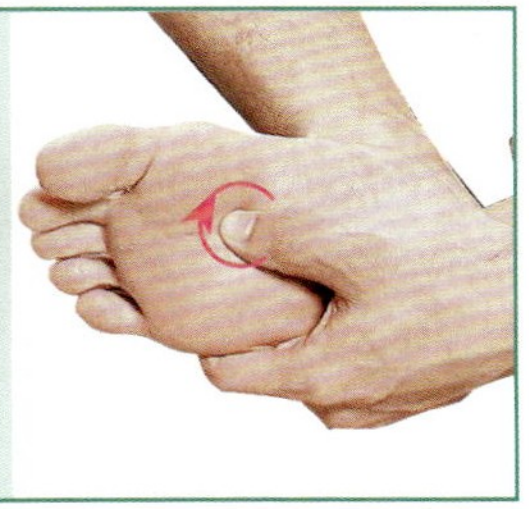

Jiexi (ST41)

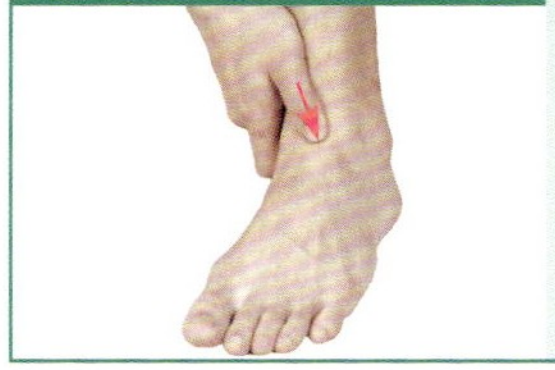

Pressing with thumb on Jiexi (ST41) point and rubbing for 2 minutes twice a day with slight stress. Massage opposite Jiexi (ST41) point by the same way

Neiting (ST44)

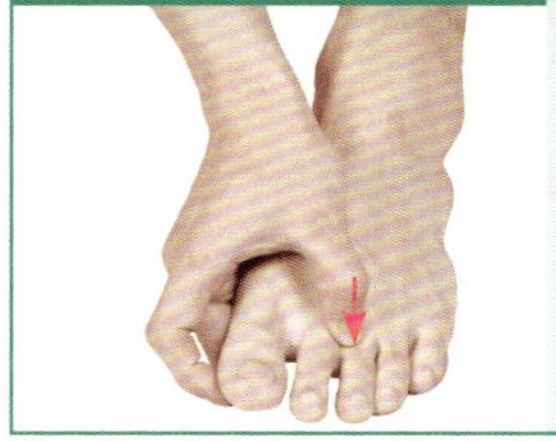

Pressing with thumb on Neiting (ST44) point and rubbing for 2 minutes twice a day with slight stress. Massage opposite Neiting (ST44) point by the same way

Yinbai (SP1)

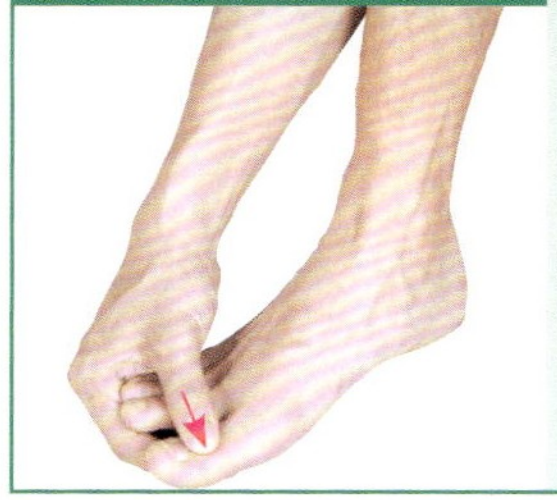

Pressing with thumb on Yinbai (SP1) point and rubbing for 2 minutes twice a day. You can hold the pressure on for several seconds at a time and then relax, and repeat this process for 5 to 6 times. Massage opposite Yinbai (SP1) point by the same way

Sanyinjiao (SP6)

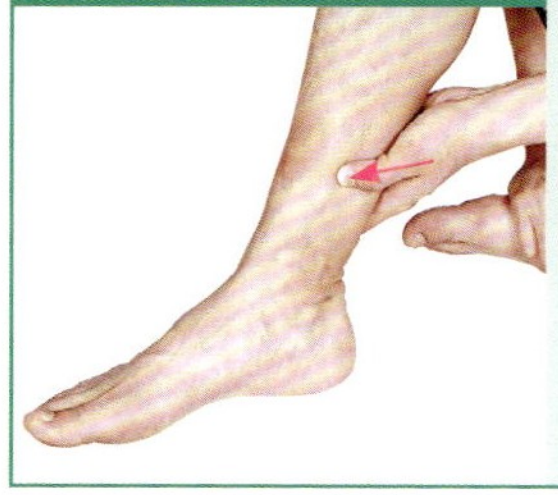

Pressing with thumb on Sanyinjiao (SP6) point and rubbing forcefully twice a day. You can hold the pressure on for several seconds at a time and then relax, and repeat this process for 5 to 6 times. Massage opposite Sanyinjiao (SP6) point by the same way

Kunlun (BL60)

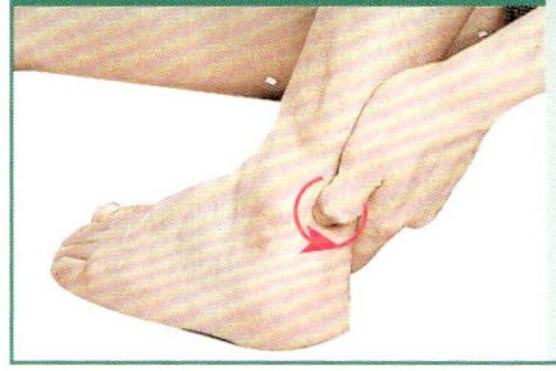

Pressing with thumb and index finger on Kunlun (BL60) point and rubbing with slight stress twice a day. Massage opposite Kunlun (BL60) point by the same way

Zutonggu (BL66)

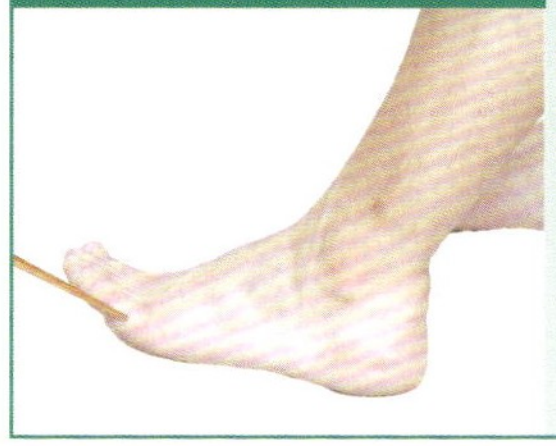

Pressing with massager on Zutonggu (BL66) point for 30 to 50 times per minute. Remember to press with moderate stress, twice a day. Massage opposite Zutonggu (BL66) point by the same way

Zhiyin (BL67)

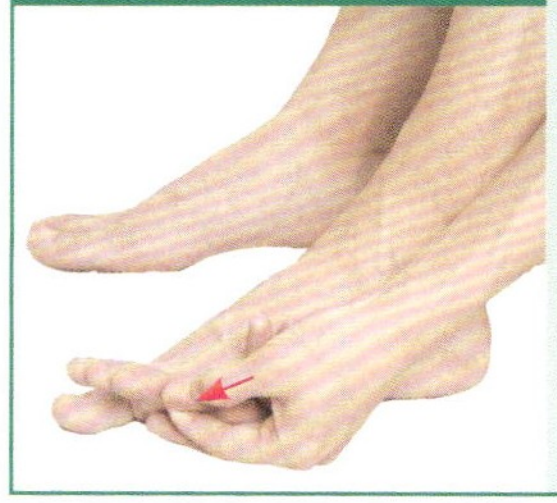

Pinch rubbing Zhiyin (BL67) point with tip of thumb, and you can rub with slight stress. Each minute rub 30 to 50 times, twice a day. Massage opposite Zhiyin (BL67) point by the same way

Yongquan (KI1)

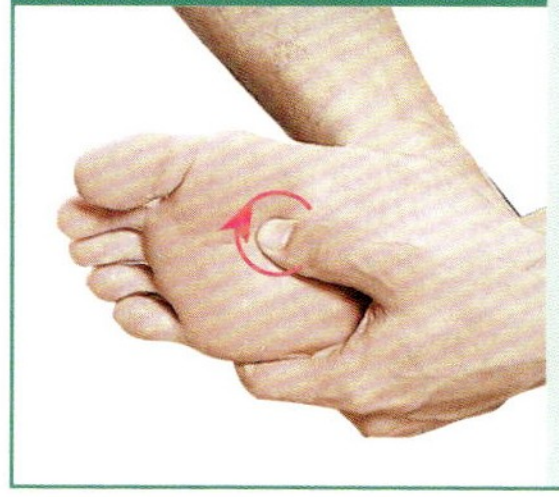

Pressing with thumb on Yongquan (KI1) point and rubbing with slight stress for 2 minutes twice a day. Massage opposite Yongquan (KI1) point by the same way

太溪

用拇指和食指同时拿揉太溪穴 2 分钟，力度稍重。同法按揉对侧太溪穴。每日 2 次

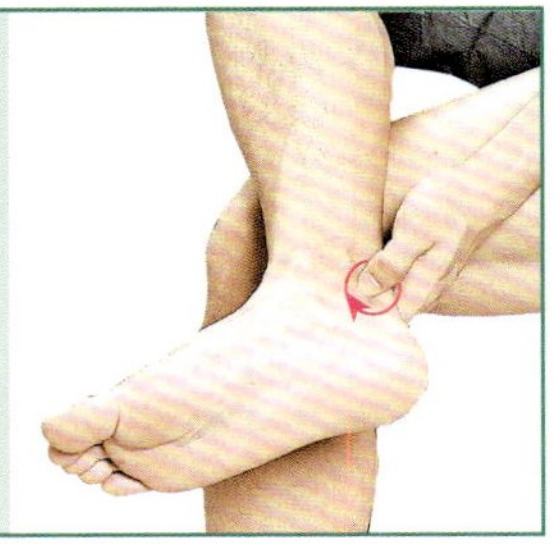

照海

用拇指按揉照海穴 2 分钟，力度稍重。同法按揉对侧照海穴。每日 2 次

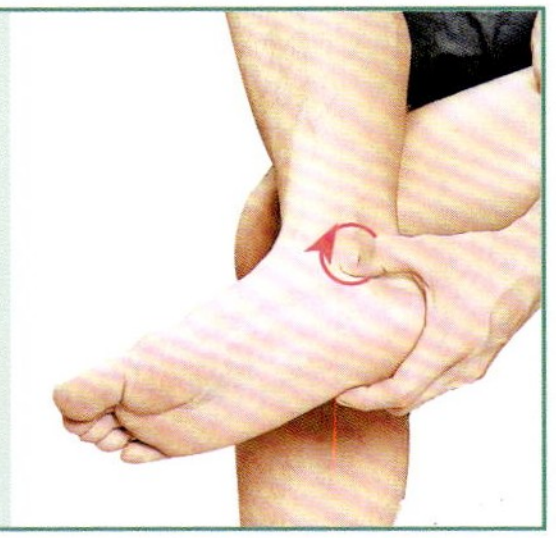

复溜

用拇指按揉复溜穴 2 分钟，力度稍重，同法按揉对侧复溜穴。每日 2 次

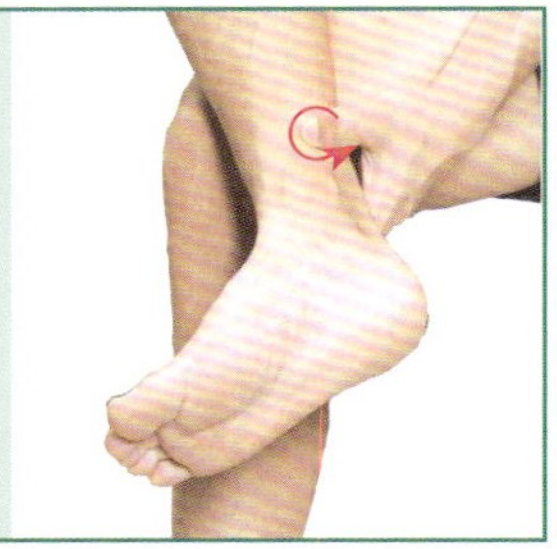

悬钟

用拇指点按悬钟穴 2 分钟，同法按揉对侧悬钟穴。每日 2 次

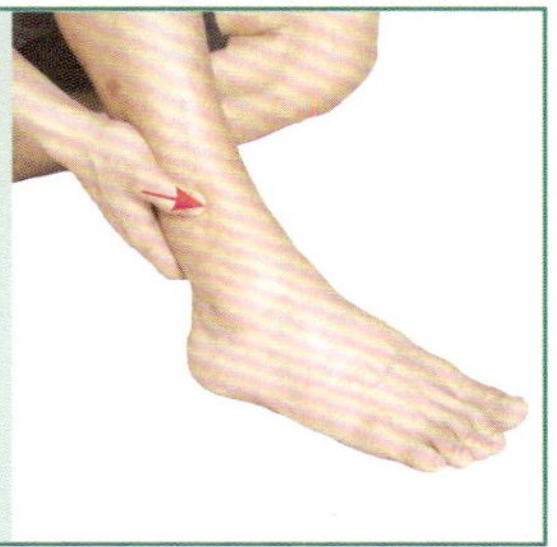

大敦

用拇指指端掐揉大敦穴，力度可稍重，每分钟 30~50 下。同法按揉对侧大敦穴。每日 2 次

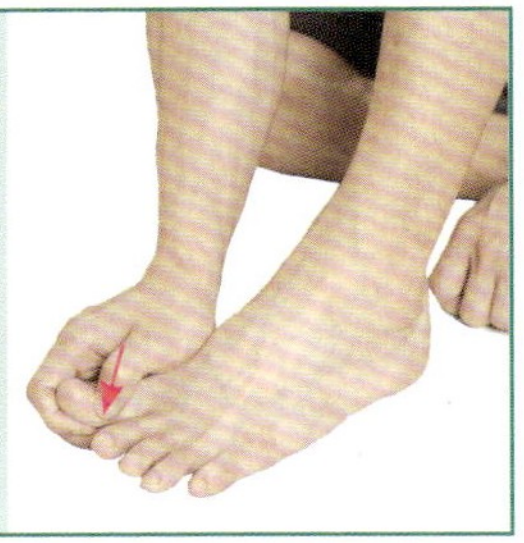

行间

用拇指指端掐揉行间穴，力度可稍重，每分钟 30~50 下。同法按揉对侧行间穴。每日 2 次

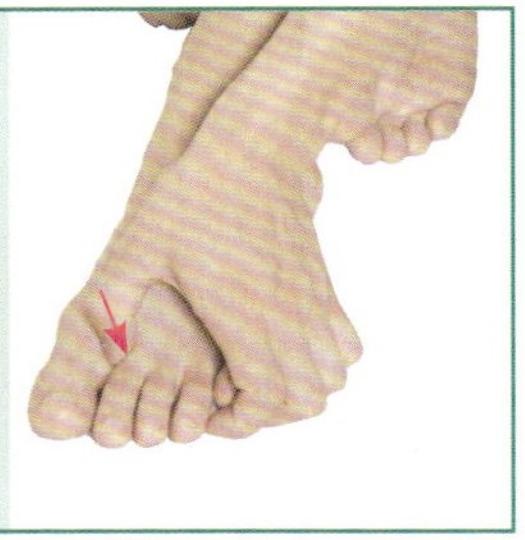

太冲

用拇指掐按太冲穴，停留片刻后放松，反复 5~6 下。同法掐按对侧太冲穴。每日 2 次

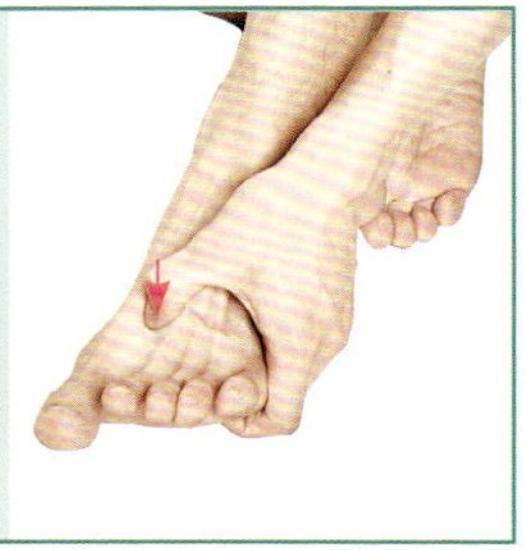

八风

用拇指指端掐揉八风穴，力度可稍重，每分钟 30~50 下。同法按揉对侧八风穴。每日 2 次

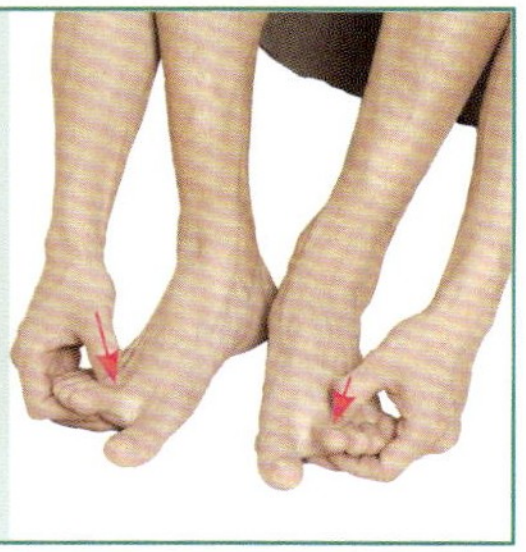

Taixi (KI3)

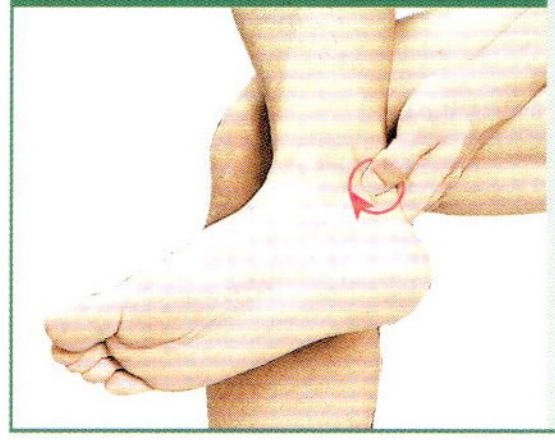

Pressing with thumb and index finger on Taixi (KI3) point and rubbing with slight stress for 2 minutes, twice a day. Massage opposite Taixi (KI3) point by the same way

Dadun (LR1)

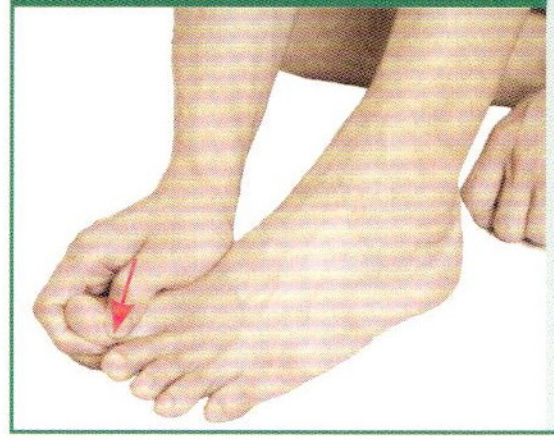

Pinch rubbing Dadun (LR1) point with thumb tip, and you can rub with slight stress. Each minute rub 30 to 50 times, twice a day. Massage opposite Dadun (LR1) point by the same way

Zhaohai (KI6)

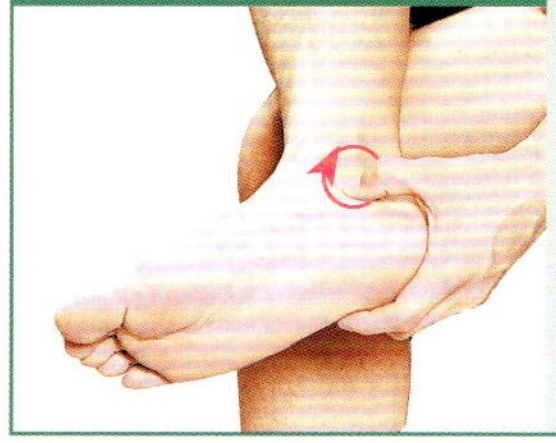

Pressing with thumb on Zhaohai (KI6) point and rubbing for 2 minutes twice a day with slight stress. Massage opposite Zhaohai (KI6) point by the same way

Xingjian (LR2)

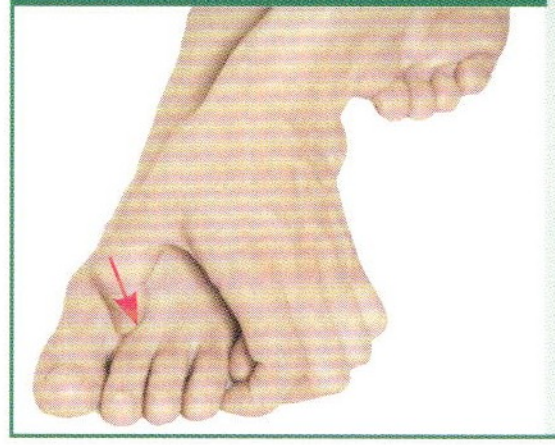

Pinch rubbing Xingjian (LR2) point with tip of thumb, and you can rub with slight stress. Each minute rub 30 to 50 times, twice a day. Massage opposite Xingjian (LR2) point by the same way

Fuliu (KI7)

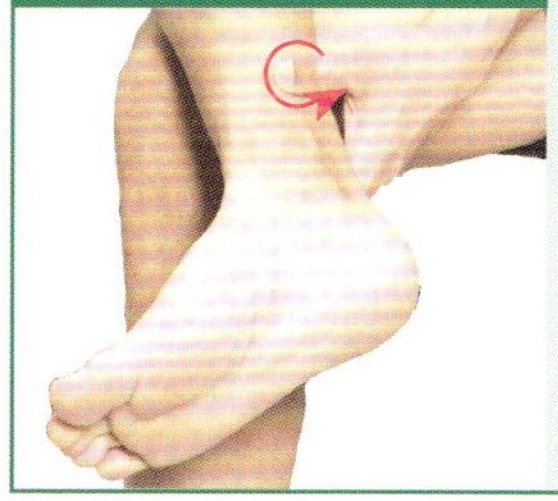

Pressing with thumb on Fuliu (KI7) point and rubbing for 2 minutes twice a day with slight stress. Massage opposite Fuliu (KI7) point by the same way

Taichong (LR3)

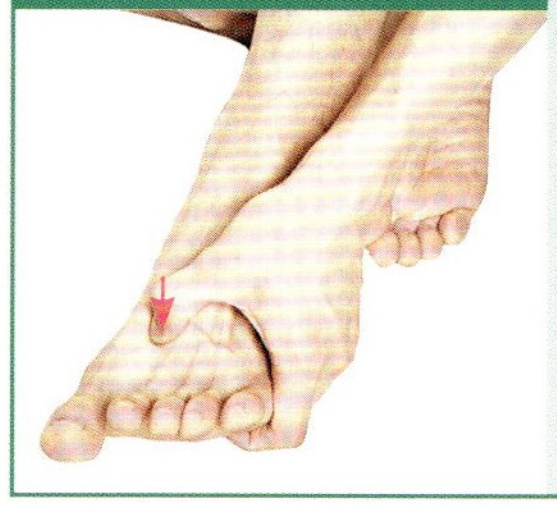

Pinch rubbing Taichong (LR3) point forcefully with thumb twice a day. You can hold the pressure on for several seconds at a time and then relax, and repeat this process for 5 to 6 times. Massage opposite Taichong (LR3) point by the same way

Xuanzhong (GB39)

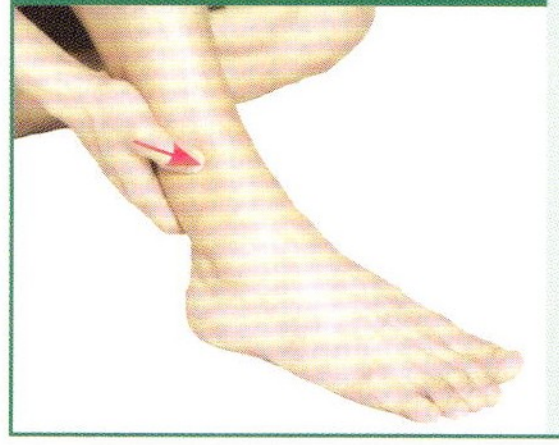

Pressing with thumb on Xuanzhong (GB39) point and rubbing for 2 minutes twice a day with slight stress Massage opposite Xuanzhong (GB39) point by the same way

Bafeng (EX-LE10)

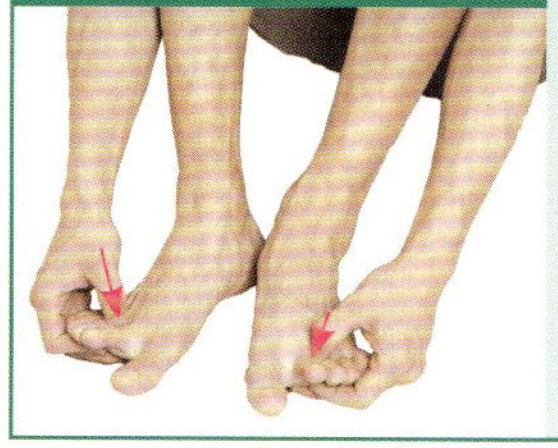

Pinch rubbing Bafeng (EX–LE10) point with tip of thumb, and you can rub with slight stress. Each minute rub 30 to 50 times, twice a day. Massage opposite Bafeng (EX–LE10) point by the same way

手掌面反射区 Palm Reflex Zone

第二章　手部反射区及穴位

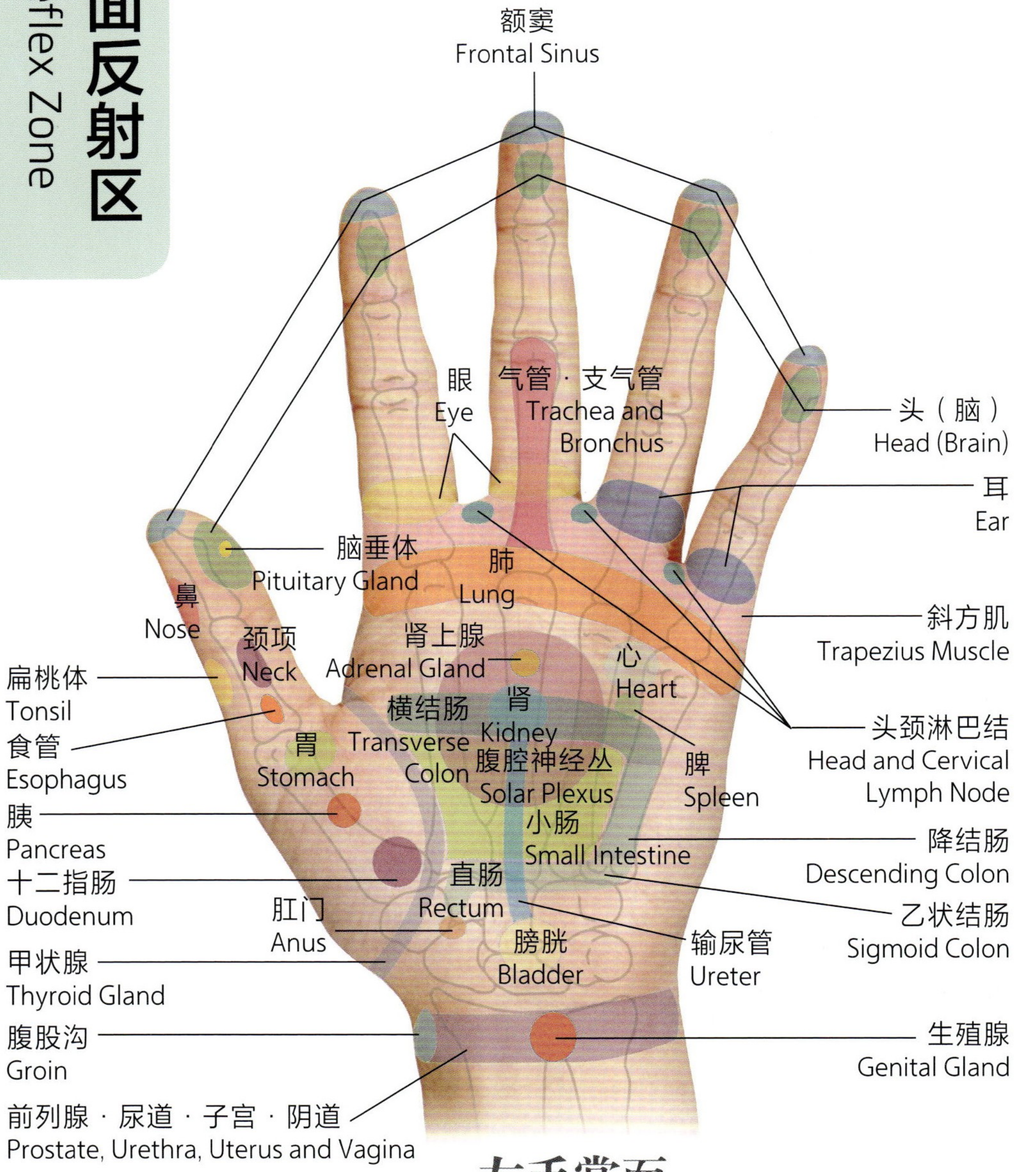

左手掌面
The left palm

反射区	定 位	主 治
头（脑）	双手掌面，10 个手指末节螺纹面	中风后遗症、脑震荡后遗症、高血压、头痛、头晕、神经衰弱
额窦	双手掌面，10 个手指尖	鼻窦炎、脑震荡后遗症、中风后遗症、头痛、头晕、神经衰弱
脑垂体	双手拇指指腹中心	内分泌功能失调、小儿发育不良、围绝经期综合征
眼	双手掌面和手背面第 2、3 指指根部	结膜炎、角膜炎、近视、远视、青光眼、白内障、眼出血
耳	双手掌面和手背面第 4、5 指指根部	中耳炎、耳鸣、耳聋、眩晕
鼻	双手拇指第 2 节（远节）指骨桡侧的中部，赤白肉际处	过敏性鼻炎、鼻出血、上呼吸道感染
扁桃体	双手拇指近节指骨桡侧的赤白肉际处，鼻反射区的近侧	扁桃体炎、上呼吸道感染、发热

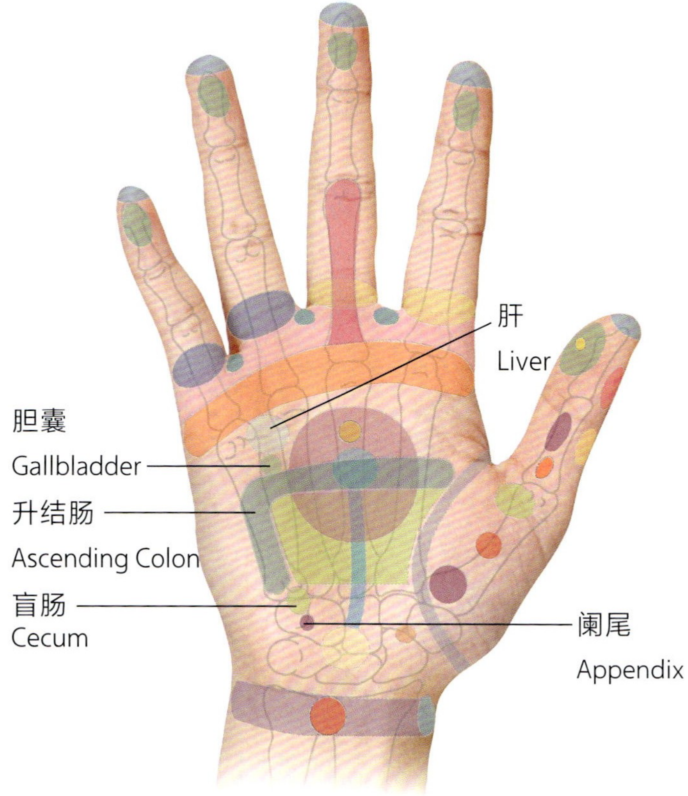

右手掌面
The right palm

Reflex Zone	Location	Indications
Head (Brain)	The reflex zone of Head (Brain) is on the 10 distal fingers of 2 palms	Sequelae of wind stroke; concussion sequelae; hypertension; headache; dizziness; and neurasthenia
Frontal Sinus	The reflex zone of Frontal Sinus is on the 10 finger tips of 2 palms	Sinusitis; concussion sequelae; sequelae of wind stroke; headache; dizziness; and neurasthenia
Pituitary Gland	The reflex zone of Pituitary Gland is on the center of 2 thumb pulps	Endocrine dysfunction; child dysplasia; and perimenopausal syndrome
Eye	The reflex zone of Eye is on the end of the 2nd and 3rd fingers of 2 palms and hand back	Conjunctivitis; keratitis; myopia; hyperopia; glaucoma; cataract; and vitreous hemorrhage
Ear	The reflex zone of Ear is on the end of the 4th and the 5th fingers of both sides of hands	Otitis media; tinnitus; deafness; and dizziness
Nose	The reflex zone of Nose is on the radial middle part of 2 distal thumbs, at the junction of the red and white skin	Allergic rhinitis; nosebleed; and upper respiratory infection
Tonsil	The reflex zone of Tonsil is on the radial part of proximal thumbs, at the junction of the red and white skin. It is proximal to the Nose reflex zone	Tonsillitis; upper respiratory infection; and fever

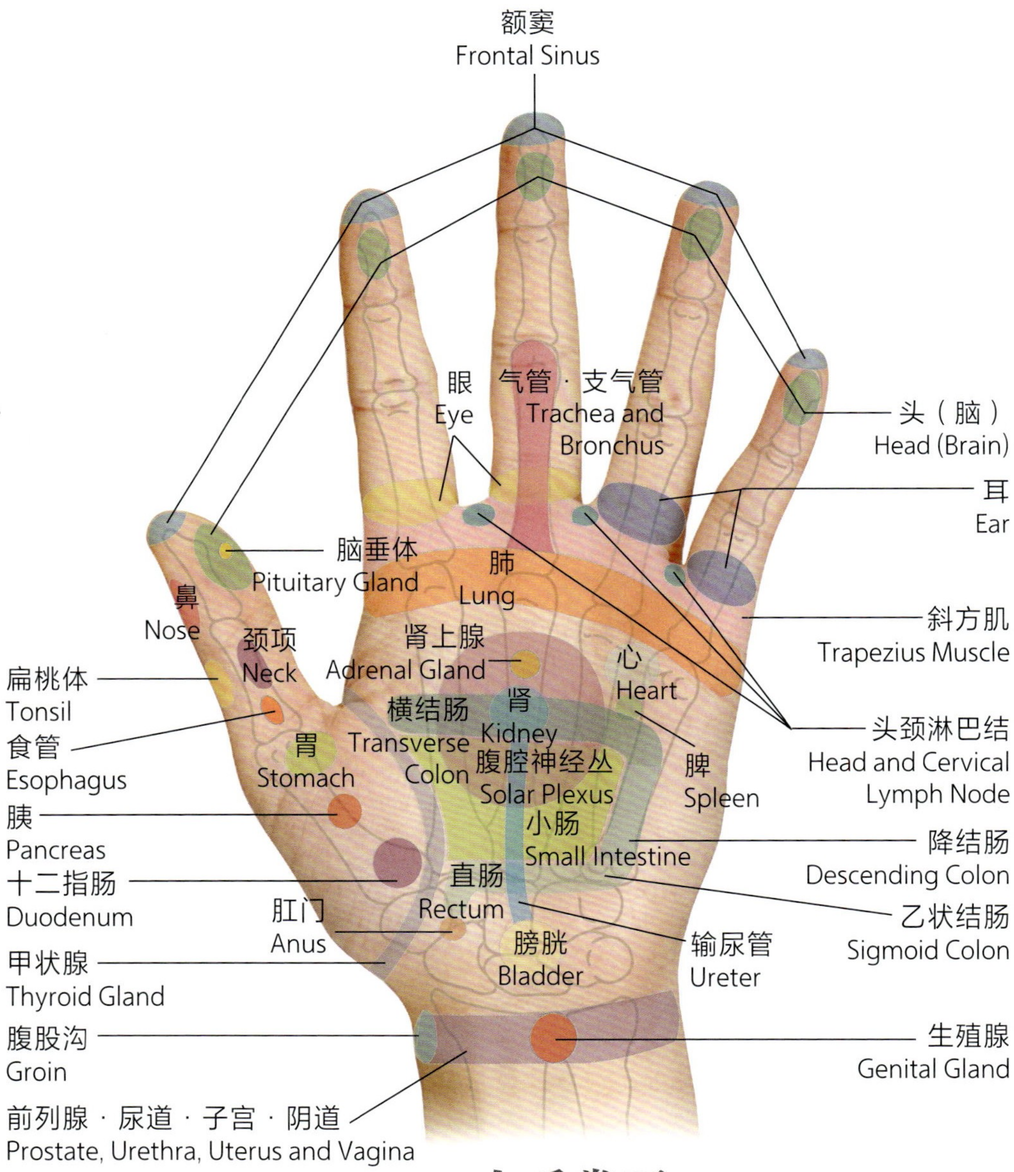

左手掌面
The left palm

续表

反射区	定位	主治
颈项	双手拇指掌面近节指骨中央	落枕、颈椎病、颈部酸痛、颈部僵硬、颈部软组织损伤
头颈淋巴结	在手掌面和手背面，第 2~5 指指根部间的凹陷处	眼、耳、舌、口腔、牙齿的疾患，甲状腺肿大，免疫力低下
斜方肌	双手掌面眼、耳反射区近侧，呈一弧形带状区域	落枕、颈部疼痛、背部酸痛、上肢疼痛、手指麻木无力
心	左手掌面第 4、5 掌骨之间，掌骨的远端，近掌骨头处	心绞痛、心肌梗死恢复期、心力衰竭恢复期、心律不齐、心功能不全等循环系统疾病
脾	左手掌面第 4、5 掌骨远端之间，心反射区的近侧	贫血、高血压、肌肉酸痛、消化不良、食欲不振
肺	双手掌面，横跨第 2、3、4、5 掌骨，为靠近掌指关节的带状区域	肺炎、支气管炎、肺气肿、肺结核

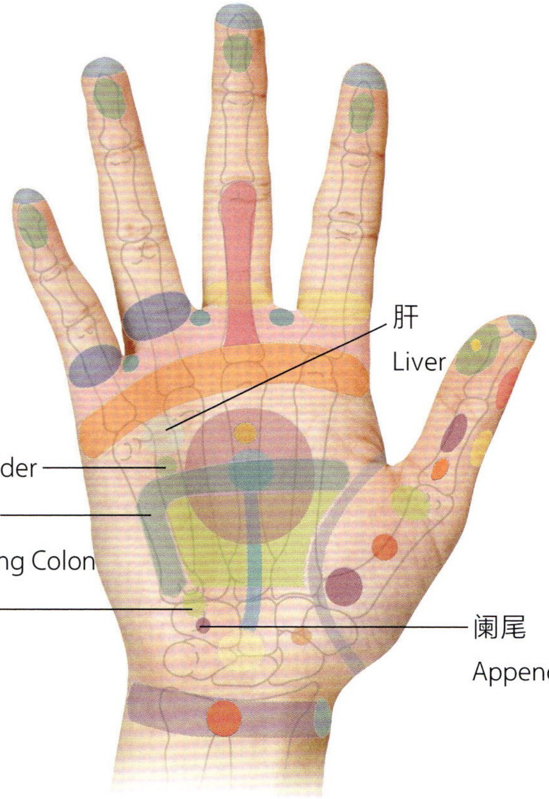

右手掌面
The right palm

Continued

Reflex Zone	Location	Indications
Neck	The reflex zone of Neck is on the center of the proximal thumbs of 2 palms	Stiff neck; cervical spondylopathy; soreness of neck; rigidity of the neck; soft tissue injury of the neck
Head and Cervical Lymph Node	The reflex zone of Cervical Lymph Node is in the depressions of the 2nd to the 5th finger roots of both sides of hands	Diseases of eyes, ears, tongue, mouth and teeth; thyroid enlargement; and hypoimmunity
Trapezius Muscle	The reflex zone of Trapezius Muscle is proximal to the Eye reflex zone and the Ear reflex zone. The zone is shown as an arc curve bounding	Stiff neck; pain in neck; soreness of back; pain in upper limbs; numbness and weakness of the extremities
Heart	The reflex zone of Heart is between the 4th and the 5th metacarpal bones, on the distal metacarpal bones, proximal to the head of metacarpal bones	Angina pectoris; recovery stage of myocardial infarction; recovery stage of heart failure; arrhythmia; cardiac insufficiency; and other circulation system disease
Spleen	Between the distal 4th and 5th metacarpal bones of the left palm, proximal to the Heart reflex zone	Anemia; hypertension; muscle pain; indigestion; loss of appetite
Lung	A zonal region which arches across the 2nd, 3rd, 4th, and 5th metacarpal bones of both palms, proximal to metacarpophalangeal joints	Pneumonia; bronchitis; emphysema; tuberculosis

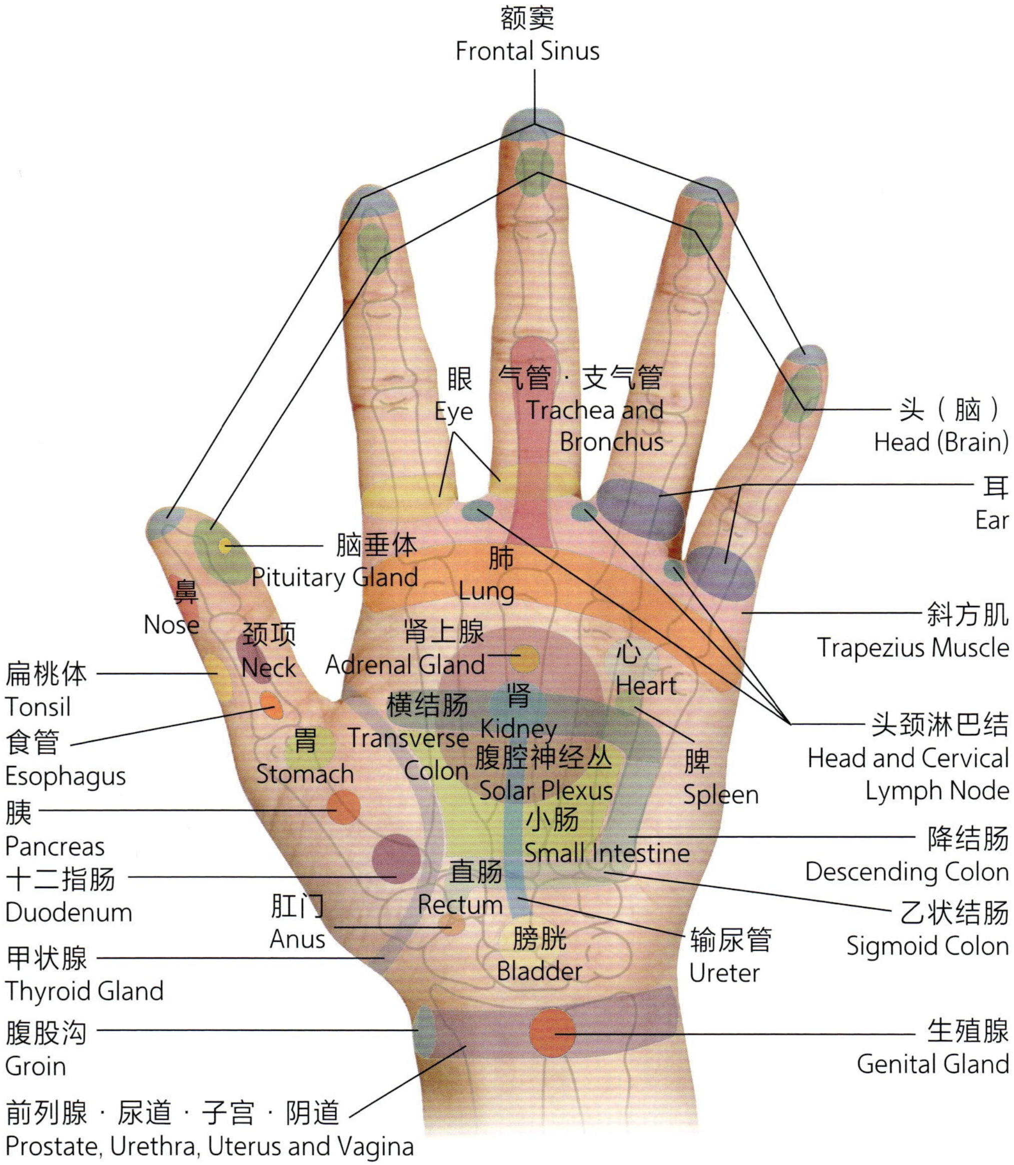

左手掌面
The left palm

续表

反射区	定位	主治
气管 · 支气管	双手掌面中指近节指骨，该反射区的近心端与肺反射区相连	肺炎、支气管炎
肝	右手掌面第 4、5 掌骨之间，掌骨的远端，近掌骨头处	肝区不适、肝炎、肝硬化、腹胀、腹痛、消化不良、高脂血症等
胆囊	右手掌面第 4、5 掌骨之间，肝反射区的近侧	胆囊炎、胆石症、厌食症、胃肠功能紊乱
甲状腺	双手掌面第 1 掌骨近心端至第 1、2 掌骨之间，再转向虎口边缘所形成的弧形带状区域	甲状腺功能亢进症、甲状腺功能低下症、单纯性甲状腺肿
腹腔神经丛	双手掌面第 2、3、4 掌骨之间的圆形区域	胃肠功能紊乱、腹胀、腹泻、胸闷、烦躁、神经衰弱
肾	双手掌面第 3 掌骨中部	急慢性肾炎、肾结石、肾功能不全、尿路结石、高血压、慢性支气管炎、前列腺炎、前列腺增生

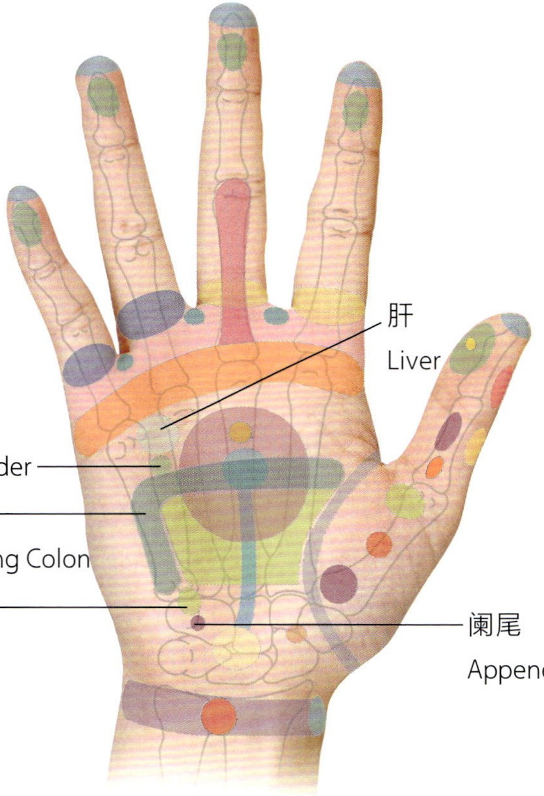

右手掌面
The right palm

Continued

Reflex Zone	Location	Indications
Trachea and Bronchus	On the proximal phalange of the middle finger of both palms, and the proximal part of this reflex zone is close to the Lung reflex zone	Pneumonia and bronchitis
Liver	Between the 4th and 5th metacarpal bones of the right palm, distal to the metacarpal bones, proximal to head of metacarpal bone	Liver discomfort; hepatitis; liver cirrhosis; abdominal distension; abdominal pain; dyspepsia; hyperlipidemia and so on
Gallbladder	Between the 4th and 5th metacarpal bones of the right palm, proximal to the Liver reflex zone	Cholecystitis; cholelithiasis; anorexia; gastrointestinal dysfunction
Thyroid Gland	A zonal region which is from the proximal 1st metacarpal bone to the junction of 1st and 2nd metacarpal bones, and then turns to the part of the hand between the thumb and the index finger	Hyperthyroidism; hypothyroidism; simple goiter
Solar Plexus	A round zone which is formed by the 2nd, 3rd, and 4th metacarpal bones	Gastrointestinal dysfunction; abdominal distension; diarrhea; chest tightness; irritability; neurasthenia
Kidney	On the middle of the 3rd metacarpal bones of both palms	Acute and chronic nephritis; kidney stones; renal insufficiency; urinary calculi; hypertension; chronic bronchitis; prostatitis; benign prostatic hyperplasia

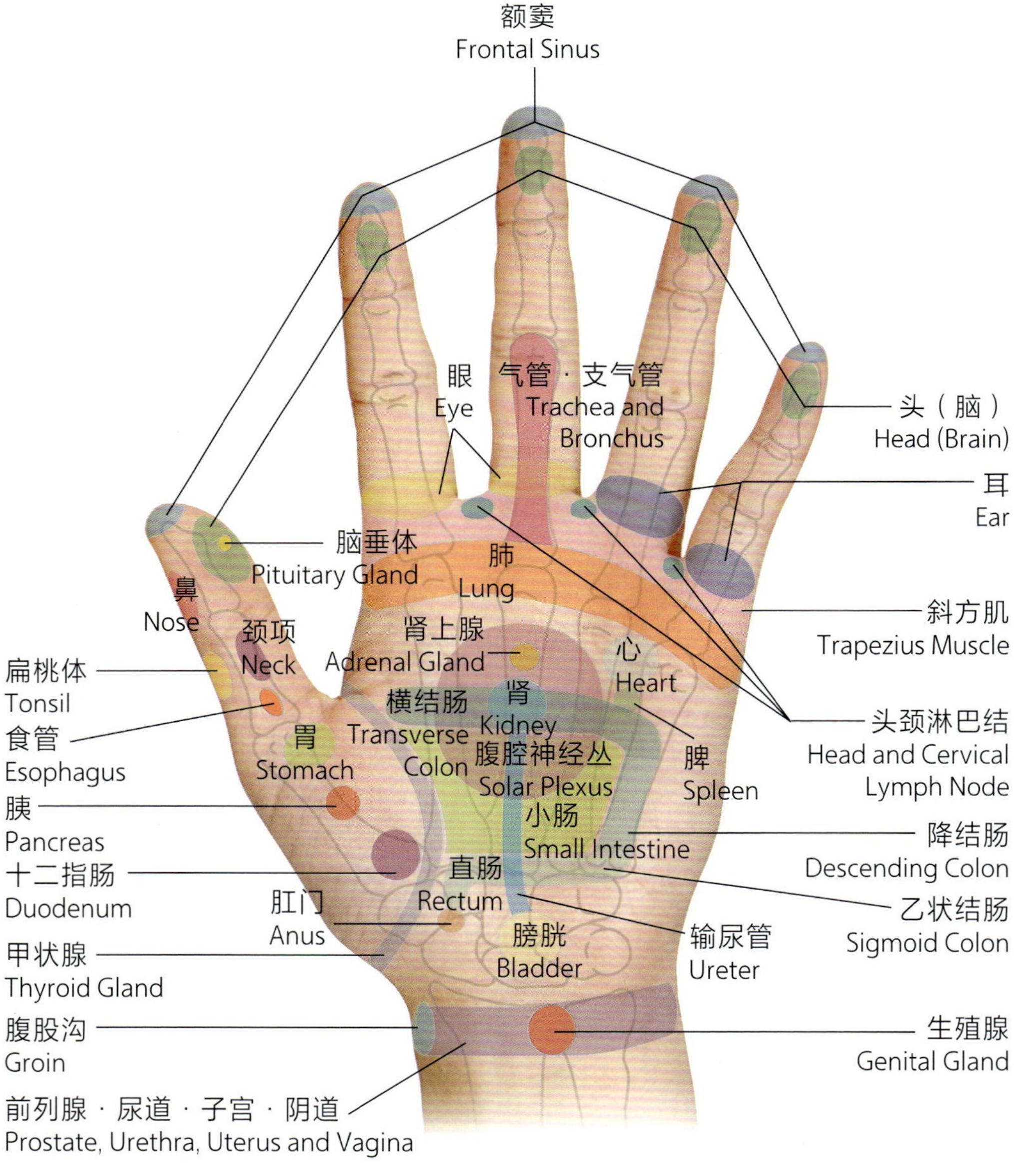

左手掌面
The left palm

续表

反射区	定位	主治
肾上腺	双手掌面第3掌骨中上段，肾反射区的远侧	肾上腺皮质功能不全、过敏性哮喘、心律不齐、风湿性关节炎
膀胱	双手掌面大、小鱼际交接处的凹陷中	输尿管结石、泌尿系统感染（症状特征为尿频、尿急、尿痛、尿液异常和腰痛）
输尿管	双手掌面中部肾反射区与膀胱反射区之间的条形带状区域	输尿管结石、泌尿系统感染、肾积水、高血压
生殖腺	双手掌侧腕横纹中点处，相当于大陵穴处	性功能低下、月经不调、围绝经期综合征
前列腺·尿道·子宫·阴道	双手掌侧腕横纹处生殖腺反射区两侧的带状区域	前列腺炎、泌尿系统感染、子宫肌瘤、宫颈炎、阴道炎、白带异常、尿道炎
腹股沟	双手掌侧腕横纹的桡侧端	生殖系统疾病，在男性包括排尿异常、脓尿、性功能障碍、不育症、前列腺增生等，在女性常见的有阴道炎、宫颈炎、子宫内膜炎

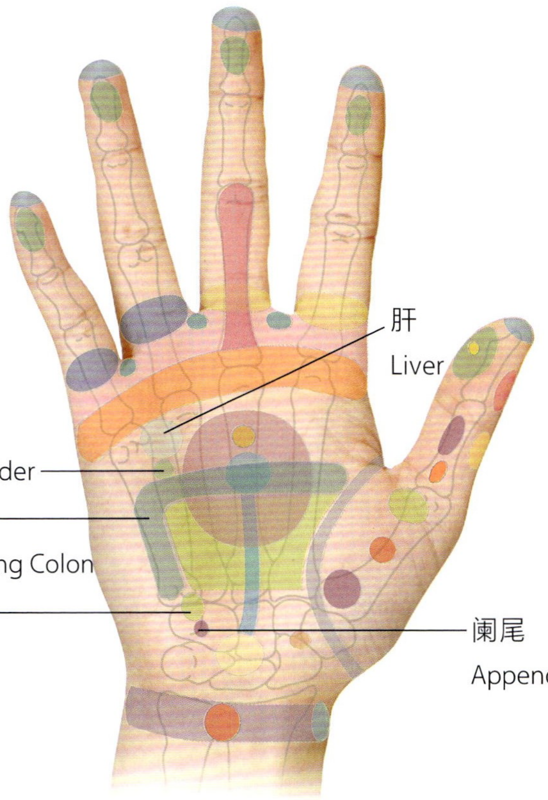

右手掌面
The right palm

Continued

Reflex Zone	Location	Indications
Adrenal Gland	On the mid-upper 3rd metacarpal bone of both palms, distal to the Kidney reflex zone	Adrenal insufficiency; arrhythmia; allergic asthma; rheumatoid arthritis
Bladder	In the depression of the junction of thenar eminence and antithenar	Ureteral calculi; urinary tract infection (symptoms: frequent micturition, urgency and dysuria, urine abnormalities and low back pain)
Ureter	A zonal region which from the middle the Kidney reflex zone to the Bladder reflex zone of both palms	Ureteral calculi; urinary system infection; hydronephrosis; hypertension
Genital Gland	On the midpoint of wrist creases of both palms, also can be seen as Daling (PC7)	Low sexual function; irregular menstruation; perimenopausal syndrome
Prostate, Urethra, Uterus and Vagina	A zonal region which on both sides of the Genital Gland reflex zone	Prostatitis; urinary system infection; uterine fibroids; cervicitis; vaginitis; abnormal leucorrhea; urethritis
Groin	Radial side of wrist crease on palmaris on both hands	Male reproductive system diseases include voiding dysfunction, pyuria, sexual dysfunction, infertility, hyperplasia of prostate; and common female reproductive system diseases, like vaginitis, cervicitis, endometritis

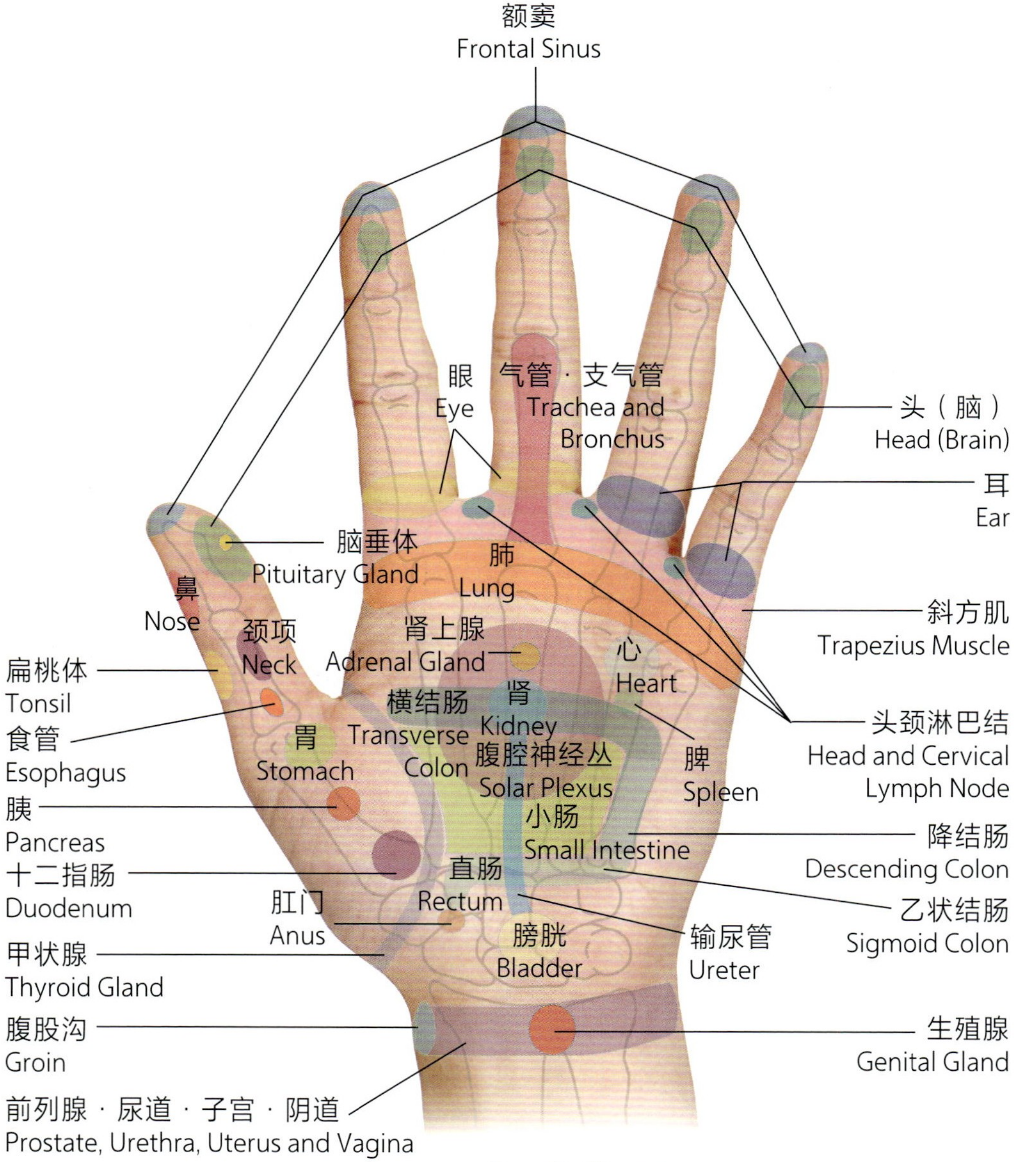

左手掌面
The left palm

续表

反射区	定 位	主 治
食管	双手掌面拇指近节指骨近端，颈项反射区的近侧	食管肿瘤、食管炎
胃	双手掌面第 1 掌骨体远端	胃痛、消化不良、呕吐、腹胀、胃酸分泌过多
十二指肠	双手掌面第 1 掌骨体近心端	消化不良、十二指肠溃疡、食欲不振
胰	双手掌面胃反射区与十二指肠反射区之间，约当第 1 掌骨体中部	胰腺炎、消化不良
小肠	双手掌面中部凹陷中，各结肠反射区所包围的区域	肠炎、腹痛、胃肠功能紊乱、消化不良、失眠、贫血
盲肠	右手掌面第 4、5 掌骨底与钩骨结合部的尺侧	腹泻、腹胀、便秘、阑尾炎、术后腹胀
阑尾	右手掌面盲肠反射区的近侧	阑尾炎及其术后康复

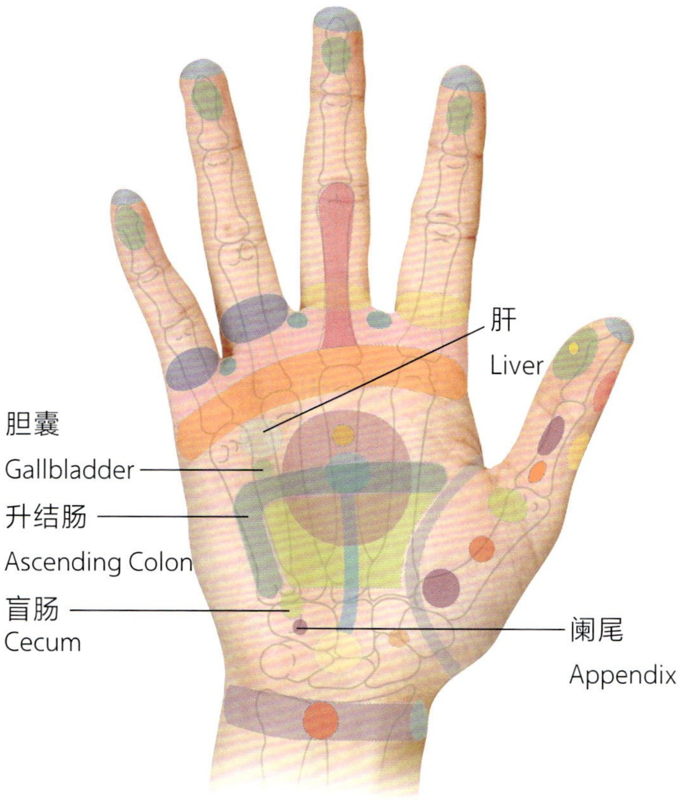

右手掌面
The right palm

Continued

Reflex Zone	Location	Indications
Esophagus	Close beside proximal phalanx of thumb and close to Neck reflex zone on both hands	Esophageal neoplasms; esophagitis
Stomach	Distal side of the 1st metacarpal bone on both hands	Stomach pain; indigestion; vomiting; abdominal distension; excessive gastric acid secretion
Duodenum	Proximal part of the 1st metacarpal bone on both hands	Indigestion; duodenal ulcer; loss of appetite
Pancreas	Between the Stomach reflex zone and Duodenum reflex zone at almost the middle of the 1st metacarpal bone on both hands	Pancreatitis; indigestion
Small Intestine	In the central depression of the palm, the zone which is circled by all colon reflex zones on both hands	Enteritis; abdominal pain; gastrointestinal dysfunction; indigestion; insomnia; anemia
Cecum	The ulnar side of the zone formed by the 4th, the 5th base of metacarpal bones and hamate on right palm	Diarrhea; abdominal distension; constipation; appendicitis; postoperative abdominal distension
Appendix	Proximal of Cecum reflex zone on right palm	Appendicitis and postoperative rehabilitation

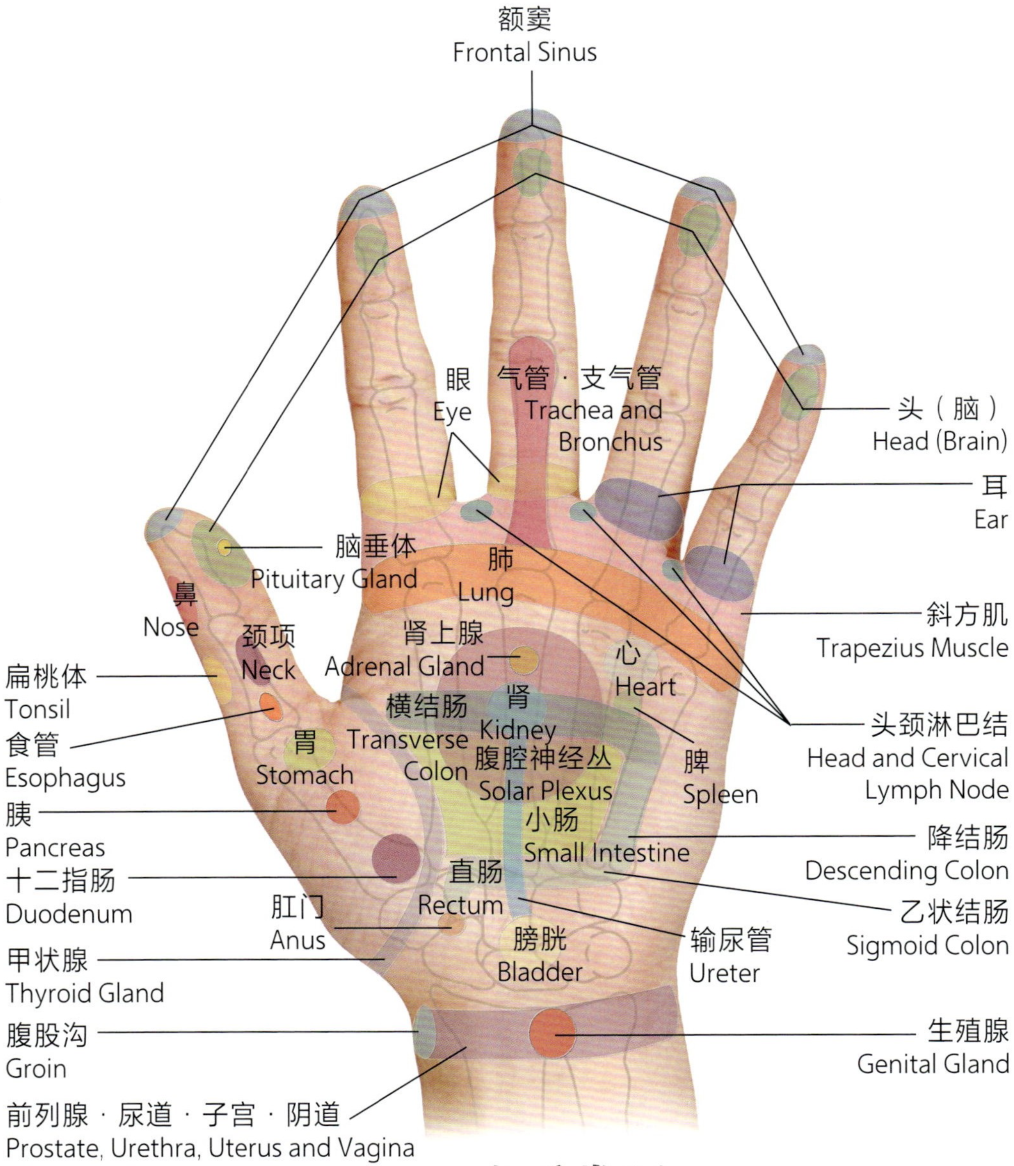

左手掌面
The left palm

续表

反射区	定 位	主 治
升结肠	右手掌面，第 5 掌骨近心端至中部的尺侧缘	腹胀、腹痛、便秘、消化不良、结肠炎
降结肠	左手掌面第 5 掌骨中部至近心端的尺侧缘	腹胀、腹痛、便秘、消化不良、结肠炎、痔疮
横结肠	双手掌面的带状区域。在左手掌为虎口与降结肠反射区之间的带状区域，在右手掌为虎口与升结肠反射区之间的带状区域	腹胀、腹痛、便秘、消化不良、结肠炎
乙状结肠	左手掌面，为腕掌关节处的带状区域，起始于第 5 掌骨与钩骨相交接处	便秘、结肠炎、直肠炎
肛门	左手掌面乙状结肠反射区的末端	肛周炎、痔疮、肛裂、便秘
直肠	左手掌面，连接乙状结肠反射区与肛门反射区的带状区域	痔疮、肛裂、便血、便秘、脱肛

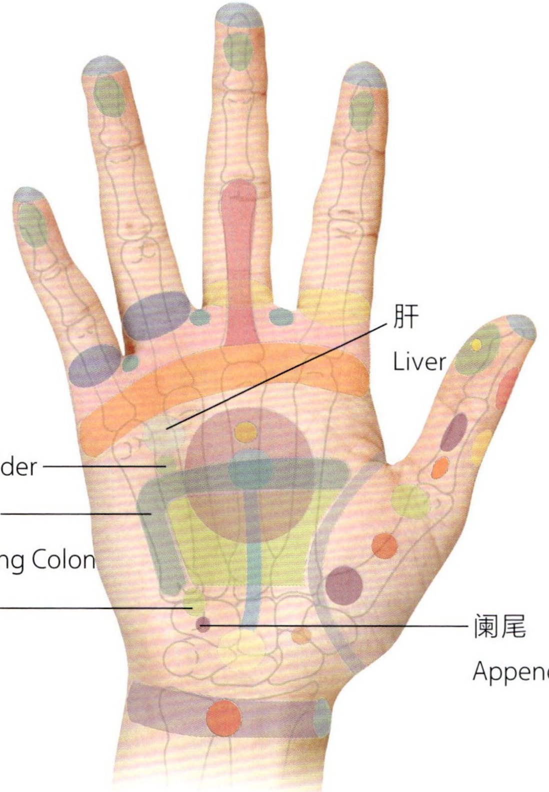

右手掌面
The right palm

Continued

Reflex Zone	Location	Indications
Ascending Colon	Ulnar side of the zone between proximal and the middle part of the 5th metacarpal bone on the right palm	Abdominal distension; abdominal pain; constipation; dyspepsia; colitis
Descending Colon	Ulnar side of the zone between proximal and the middle part of the 5th metacarpal bone on the left palm	Abdominal distension; abdominal pain; constipation; dyspepsia; colitis; hemorrhoids
Transverse Colon	A zonal region of both palms, which is formed from the part of the hand between the thumb and the index finger to the Descending Colon reflex zone (left palm)/ the Ascending Colon reflex zone (right palm)	Abdominal distension; abdominal pain; constipation; dyspepsia; colitis
Sigmoid Colon	A zonal region on volar carpal joint, which is from the junction of the 5th metacarpal bone and hamate	Constipation; colitis; proctitis
Anus	On the end part of the Sigmoid Colon reflex zone. This reflex zone is on the left palm	Anusitis; hemorrhoids; anal fissure; constipation
Rectum	On the left palm, and it is a zonal region which connects the Sigmoid Colon reflex zone to the Anus reflex zone	Hemorrhoids; anal fissure; hematochezia; constipation; rectal prolapse

超简单手掌面反射区按摩

Super-easy Massage in Palm Reflex Zone

头（脑）

从指尖向指根方向推 10~15 次

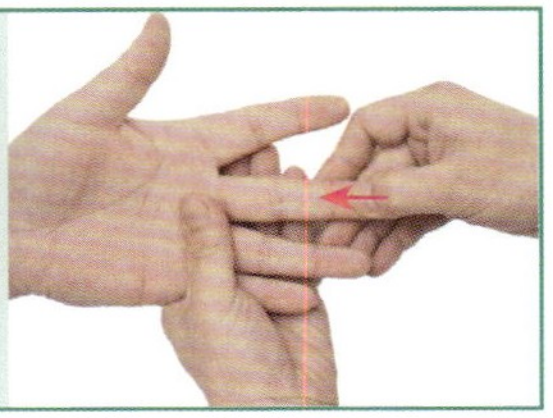

心

向手指方向推 10~20 次

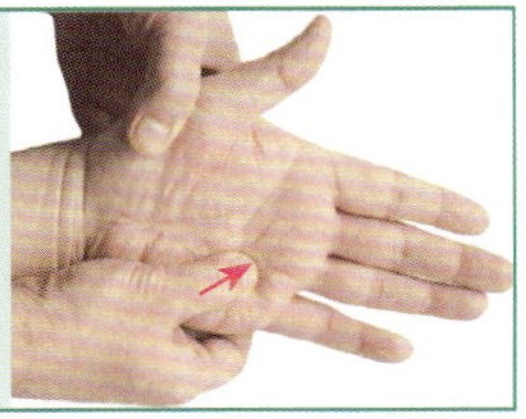

脑垂体

掐 5~10 次

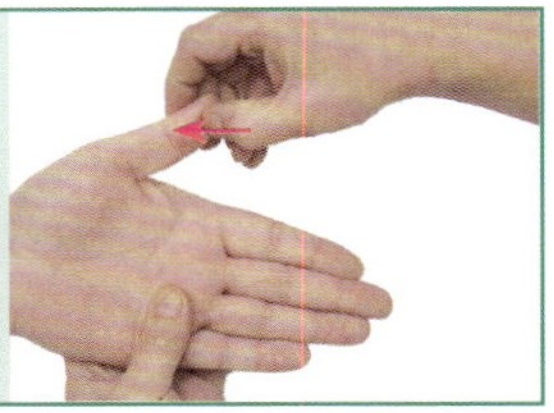

肺

横推 10~15 次

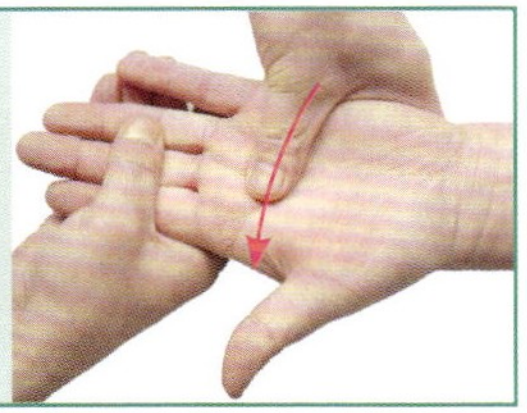

耳

横推 20 次

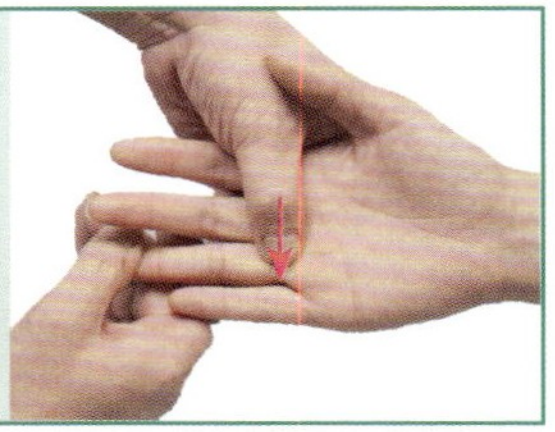

肝

点按 10 次

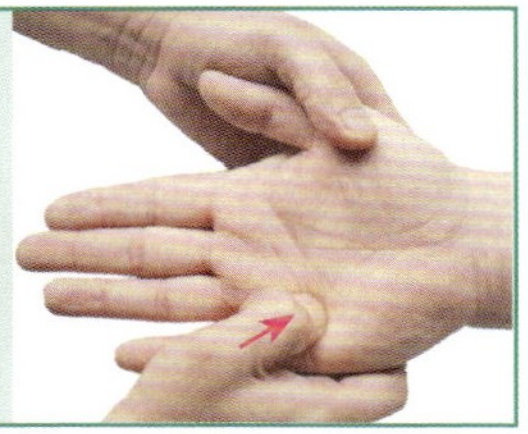

扁桃体

向指尖方向推 10~20 次

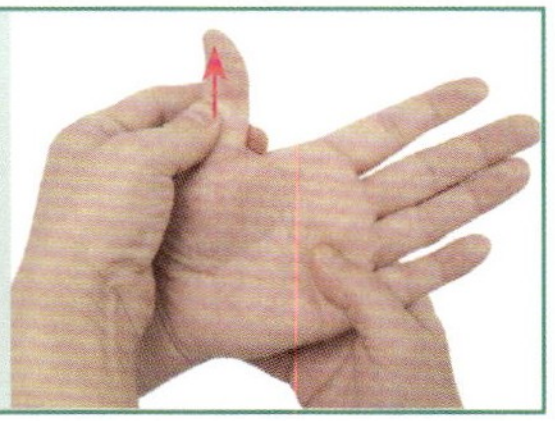

甲状腺

按揉 20~25 次

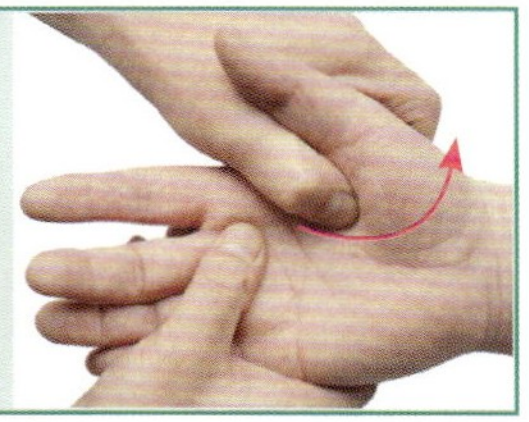

头颈淋巴结

点掐 5~10 次

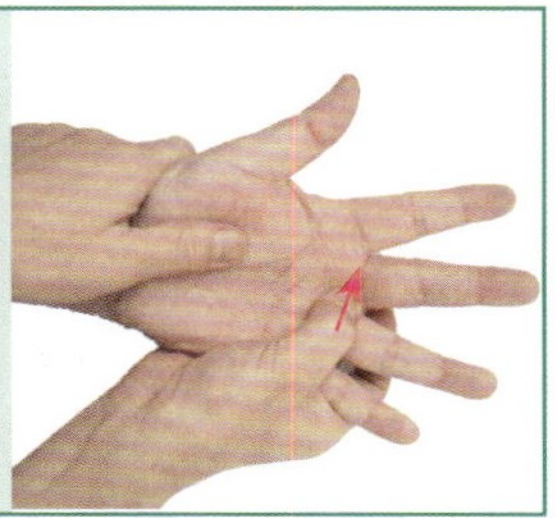

肾

点按 10~15 次

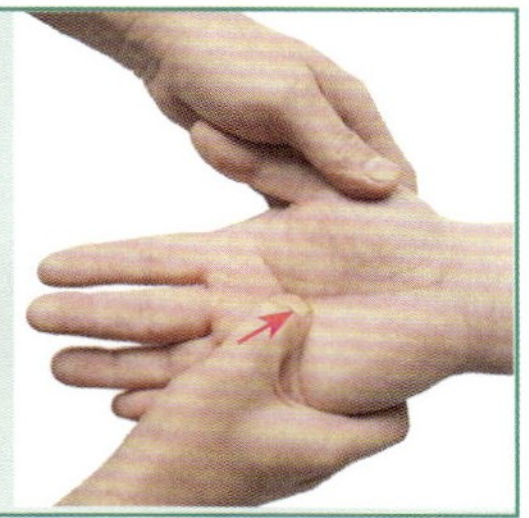

Head(Brain)

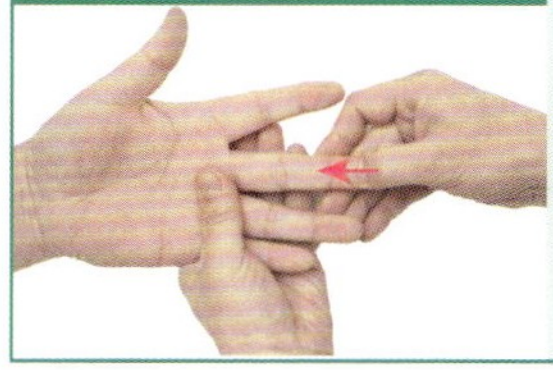

Pressing the finger from the tip to the bottom for 10 to 15 times

Pituitary Gland

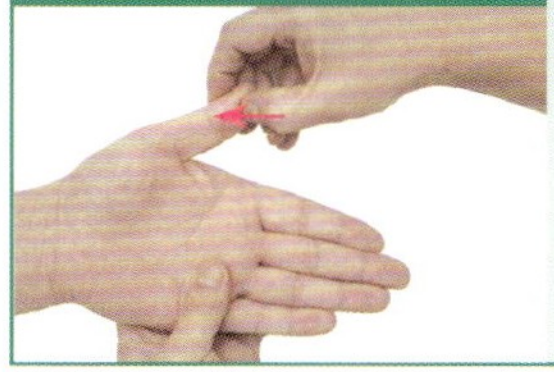

Pinching for 5 to 10 times

Ear

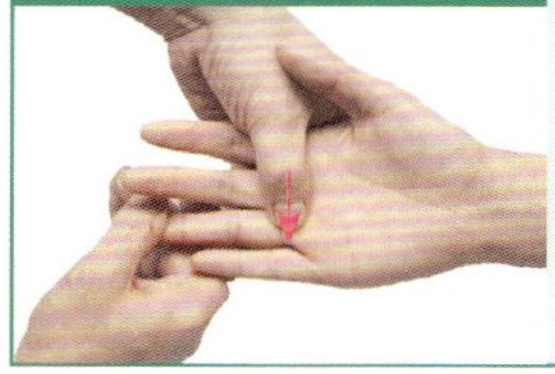

Pressing for 20 times

Tonsil

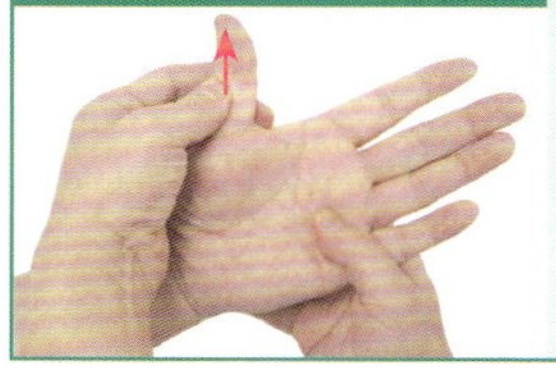

Pressing to the fingertip for 10 to 20 times

Head and Cervical Lymph Node

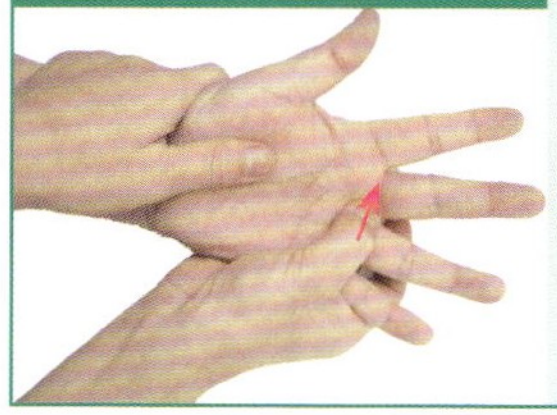

Acupoint-pinching for 5 to 10 times

Heart

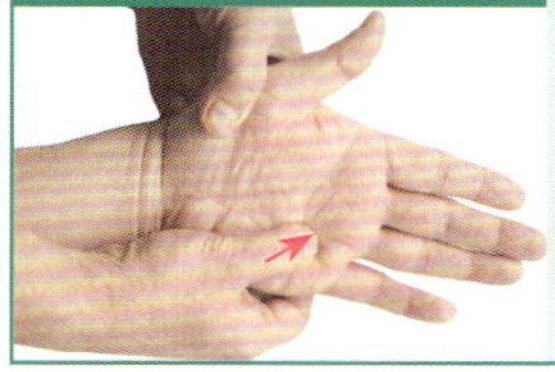

Pressing to the finger for 10 to 20 times

Lung

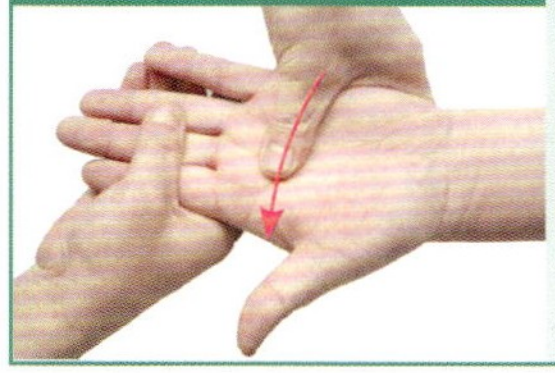

Pushing in horizontal direction 10 to 15 times

Liver

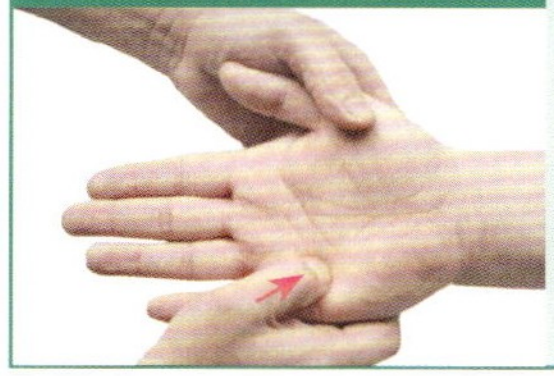

Acupoint-pressing for 10 times

Thyroid Gland

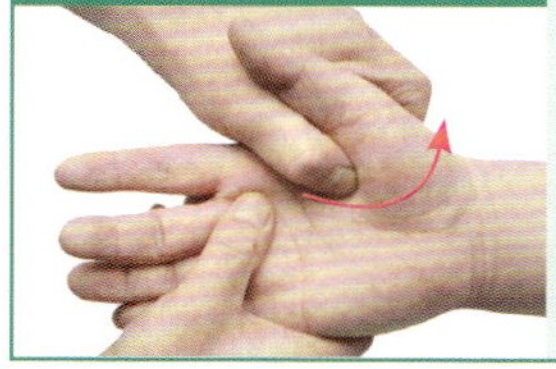

Pressing and kneading for 20 to 25 times

Kidney

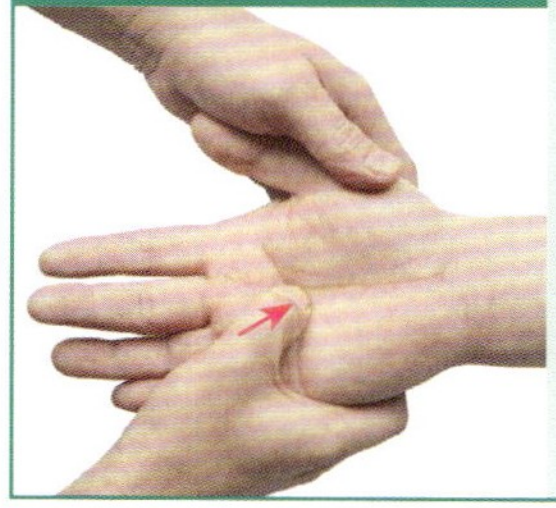

Acupoint-pressing for 10 to 15 times

额窦

用拇指指端点按 8~10 次

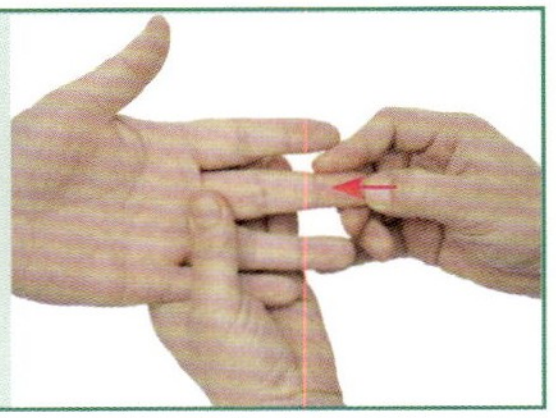

眼

横推 20 次

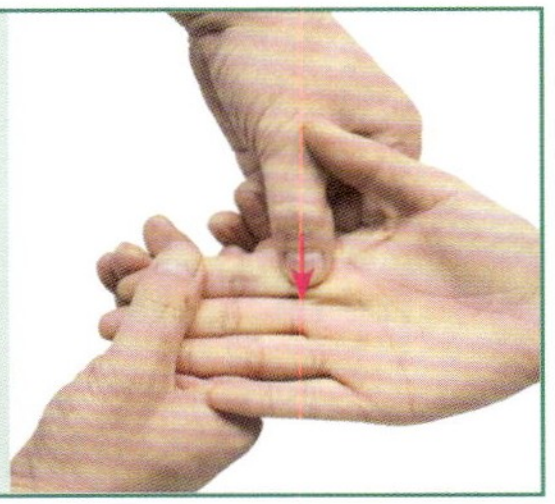

鼻

点按 15~20 次

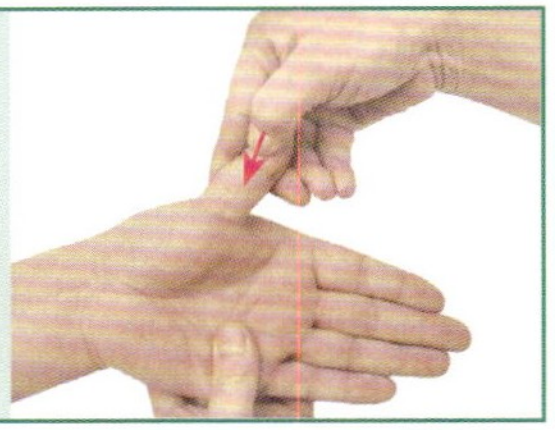

颈项

向指根方向推 10~15 次

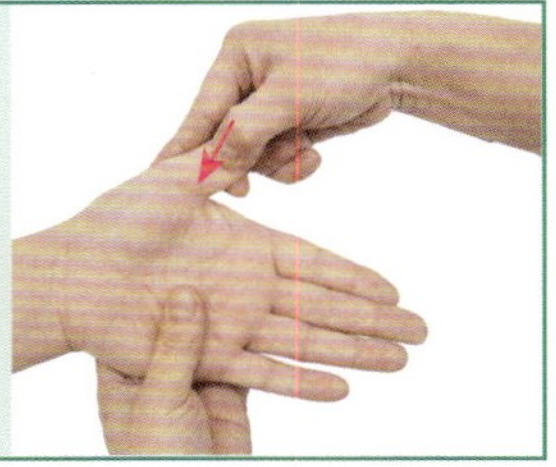

斜方肌

从尺侧向桡侧推 10~15 次

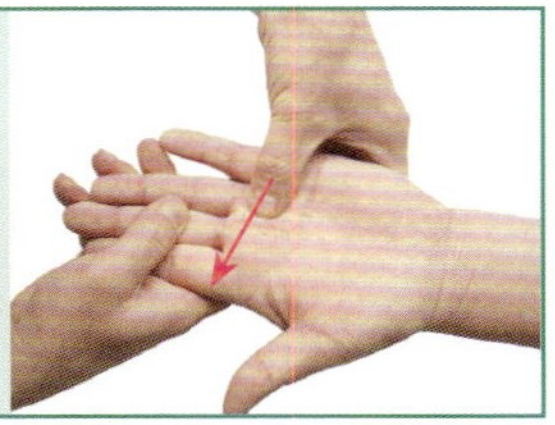

脾

点按 20~25 次

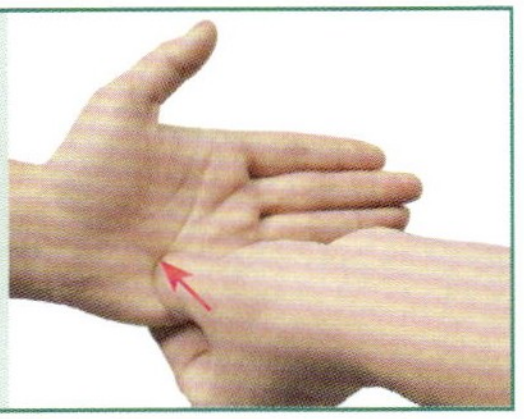

气管·支气管

向腕侧推 10~15 次

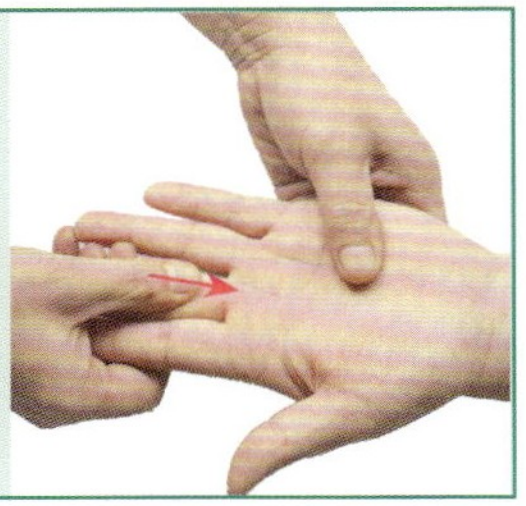

胆囊

点按 10~15 次

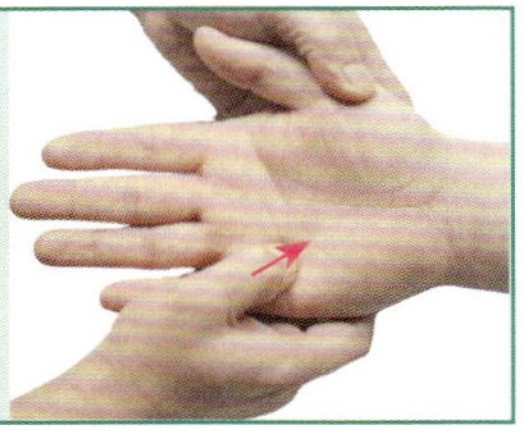

腹腔神经丛

围绕肾反射区两侧向手腕方向推 10~15 次

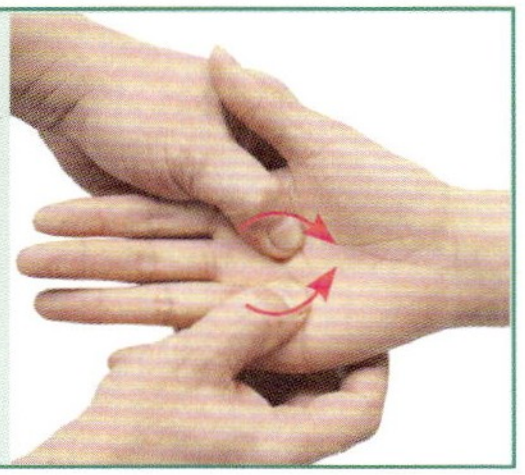

肾上腺

点按 10~15 次

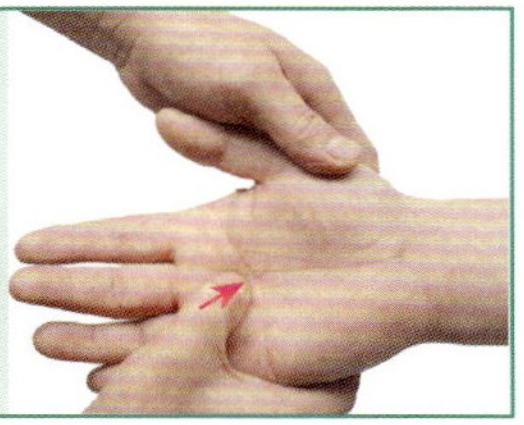

Frontal Sinus

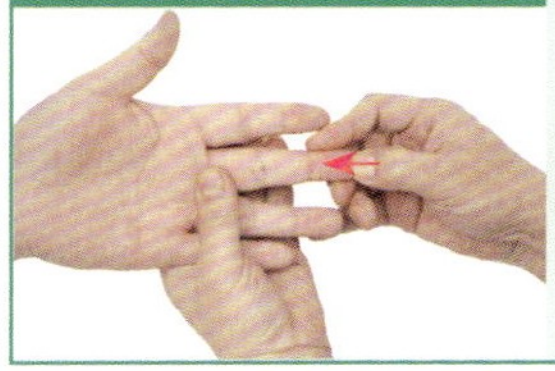

Using thumb fingertips to press for 8 to 10 times

Eye

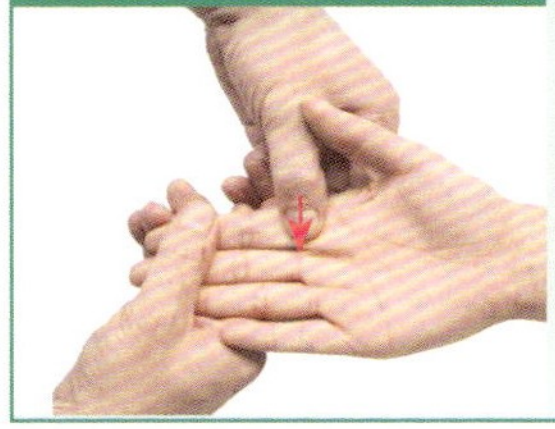

Pushing in horizontal direction for 20 times

Nose

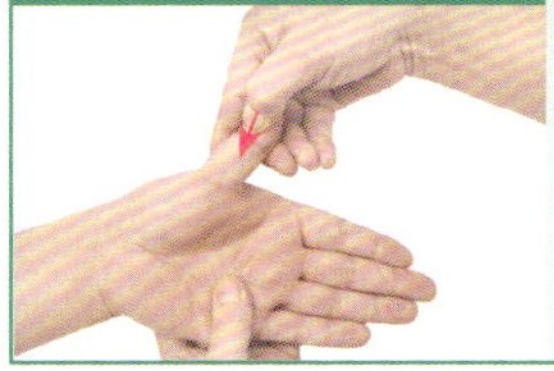

Acupoint-pressing for 10 to 15 times

Neck

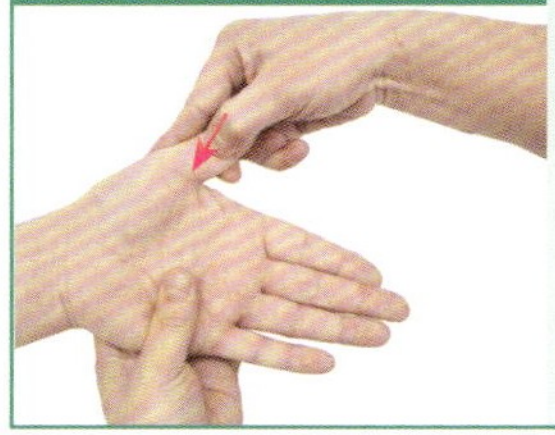

Pressing to the bottom of finger for 10 to 15 times

Trapezius

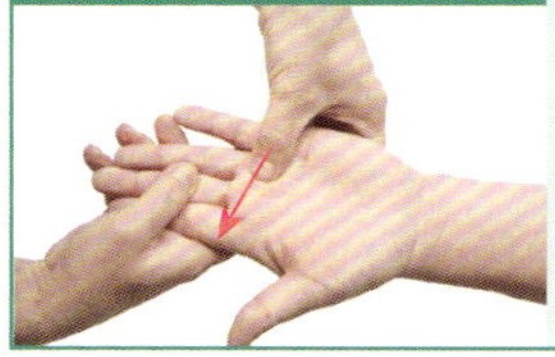

Pressing from the side of ulna to radius for 10 to 15 times

Spleen

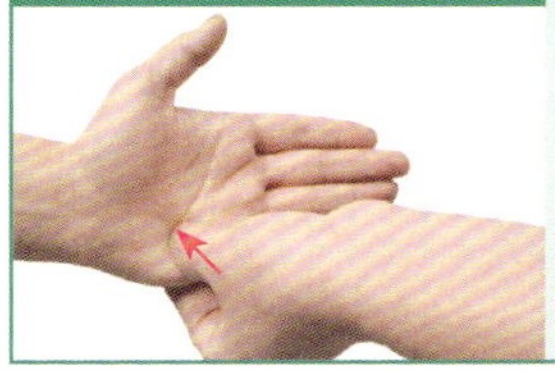

Acupoint-pressing for 20 to 25 times

Trachea and Bronchus

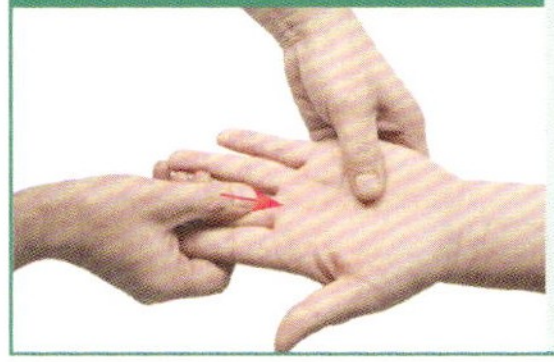

Pressing to the wrist for 10 to 15 times

Gallbladder

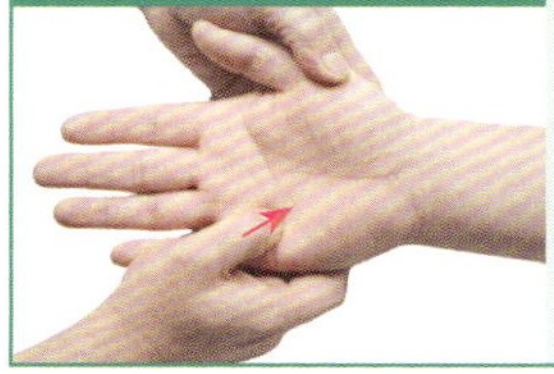

Acupoint-pressing for 10 to 15 times

Celiac Nervous Plexus

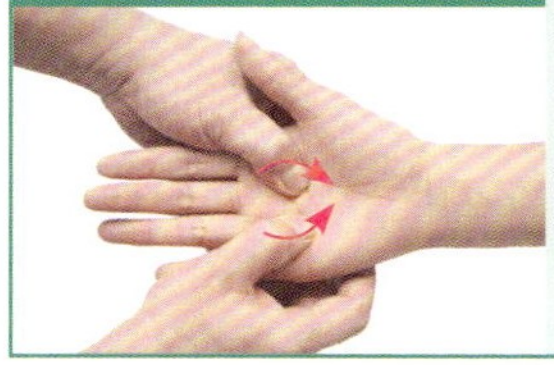

Pressing from the Zone circling the Kidney reflex zone to wrist for 10 to 15 times

Adrenal Gland

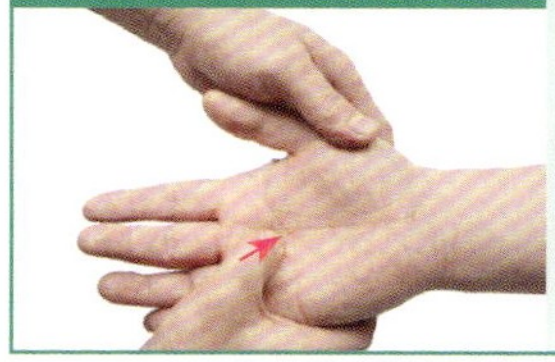

Acupoint-pressing for 10 to 15 times

膀胱

点按 10~15 次

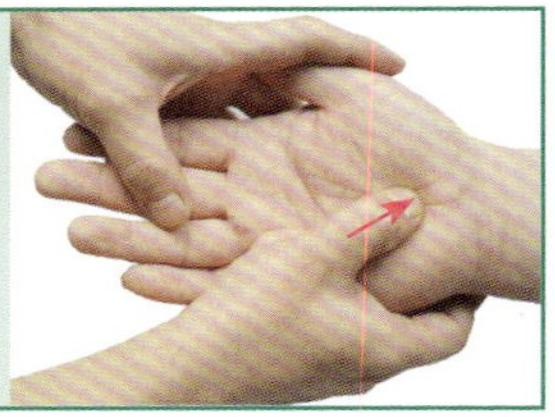

生殖腺

按揉 20~25 次

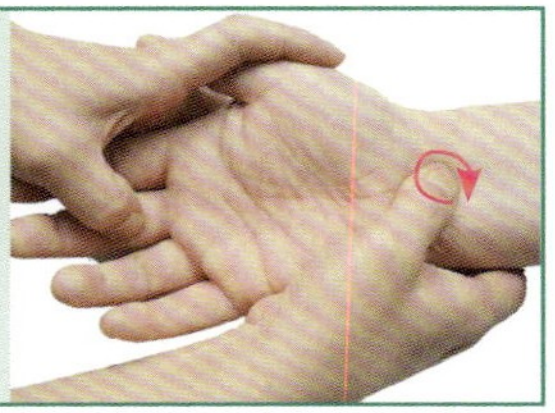

腹股沟

按揉 20~25 次

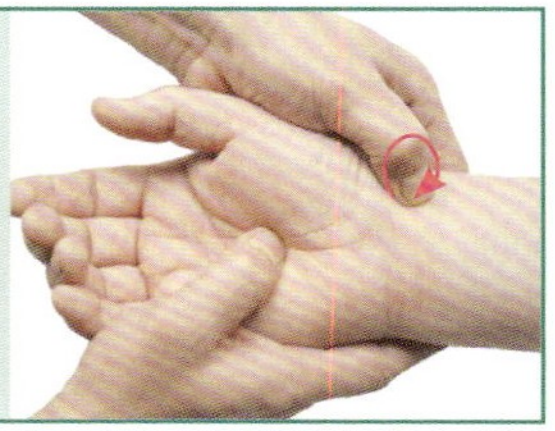

胃

向手腕方向推 10~15 次

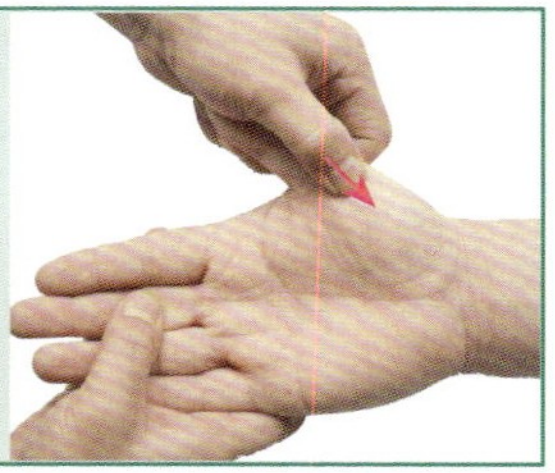

胰

向手腕方向推 10~15 次

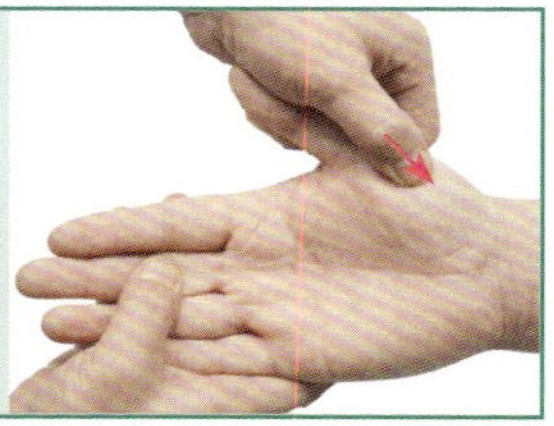

小肠

向手腕方向推 20~25 次

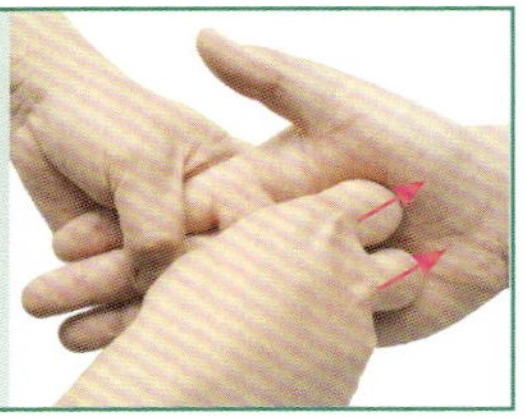

阑尾

点按 10 次

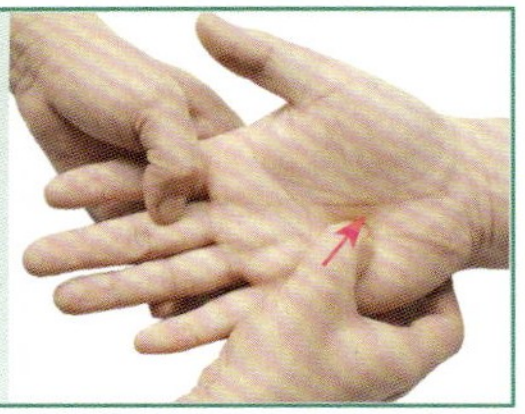

降结肠

向手腕方向推按 20~25 次

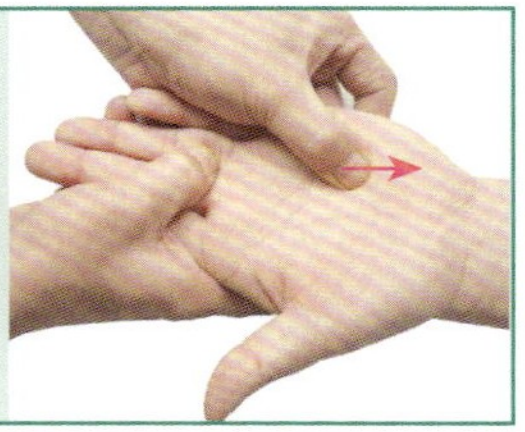

乙状结肠

由尺侧向桡侧推 20~25 次

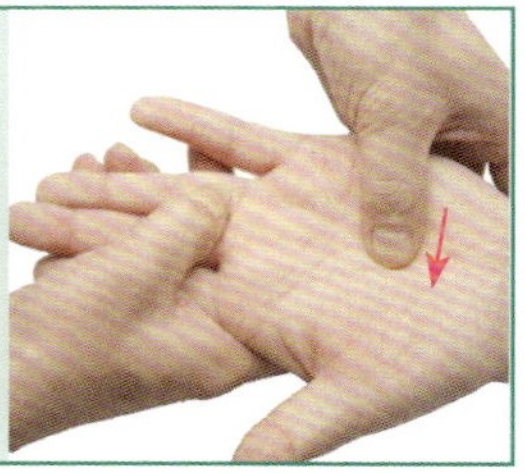

直肠

向手腕方向推 20 次

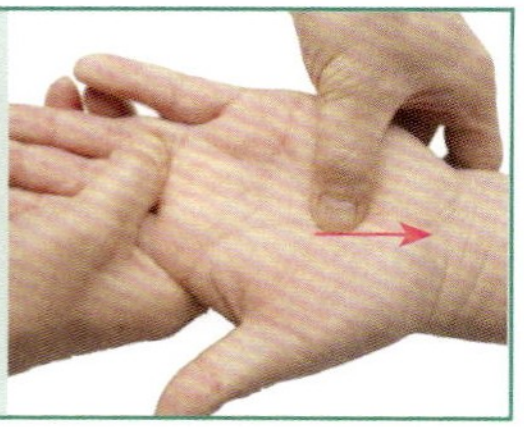

Bladder

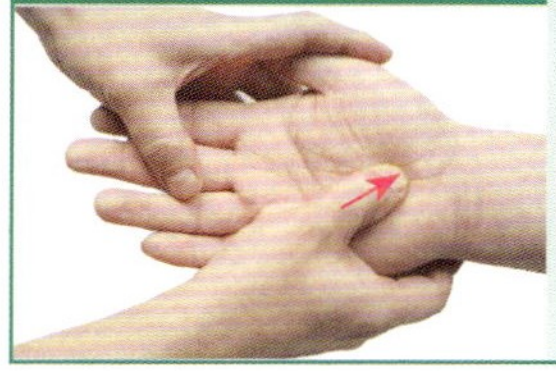

Acupoint-pressing for 10 to 15 times

Genital Gland

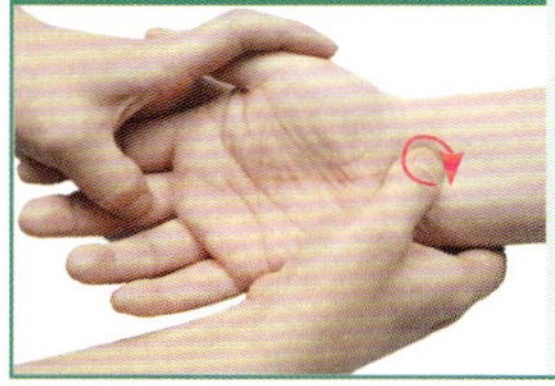

Pressing and kneading for 20 to 25 times

Groin

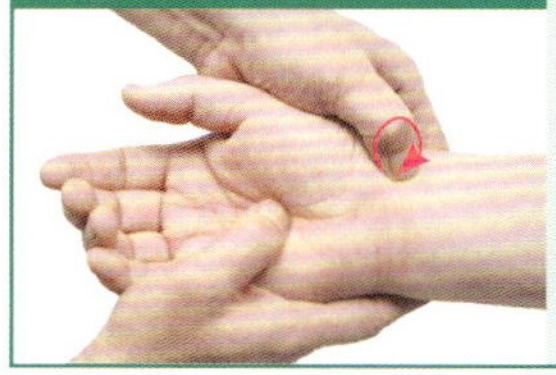

Pressing and kneading for 20 to 25 times

Stomach

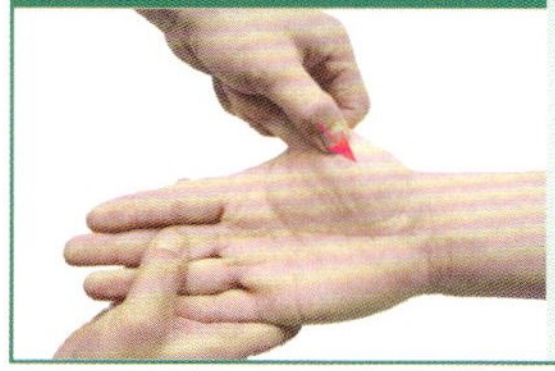

Pressing to wrist for 10 to 15 times

Pancreas

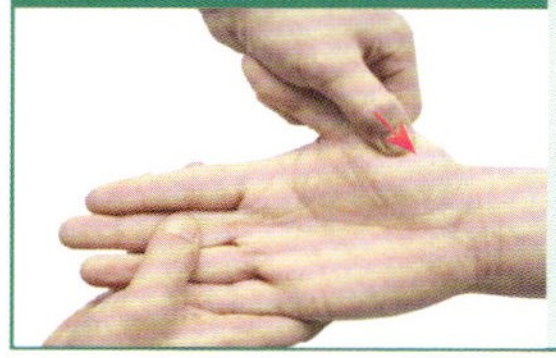

Pressing to wrist for 10 to 15 times

Small Intestine

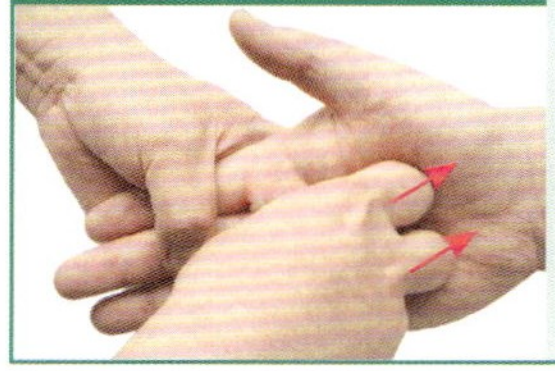

Pressing to wrist for 20 to 25 times

Appendix

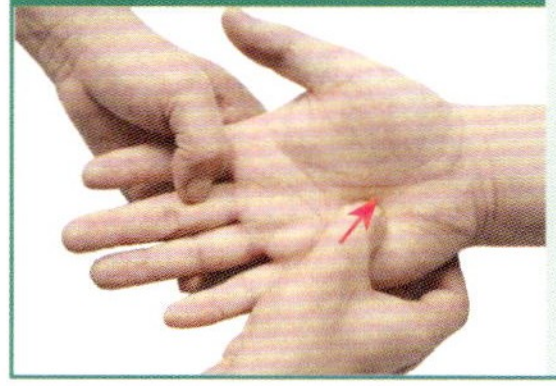

Acupoint-pressing for 10 times

Descending Colon

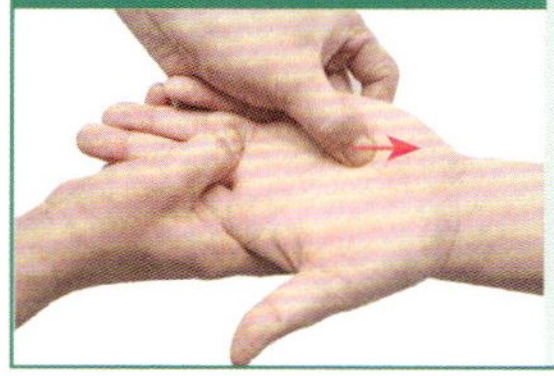

Pressing and pressing to wrist for 20 to 25 times

Sigmoid Colon

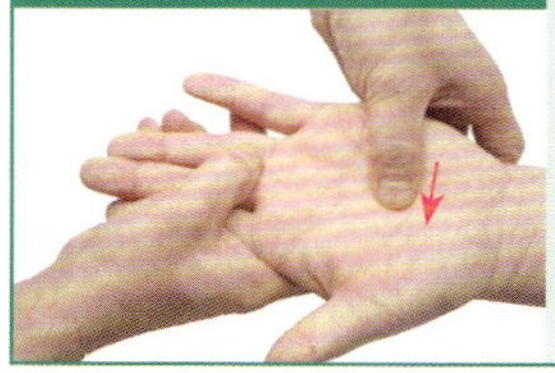

Pressing from the side of ulna to radius for 10 to 15 times

Rectum

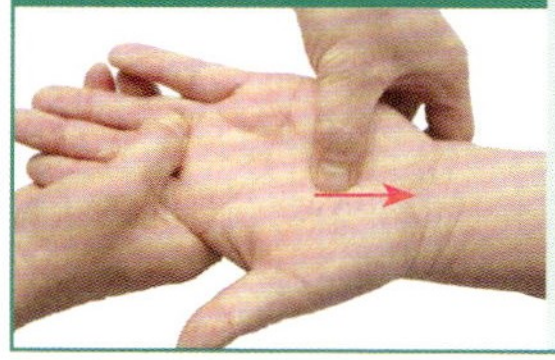

Pressing to wrist for 20 times

输尿管

用单指向手腕方向推 10~15 次

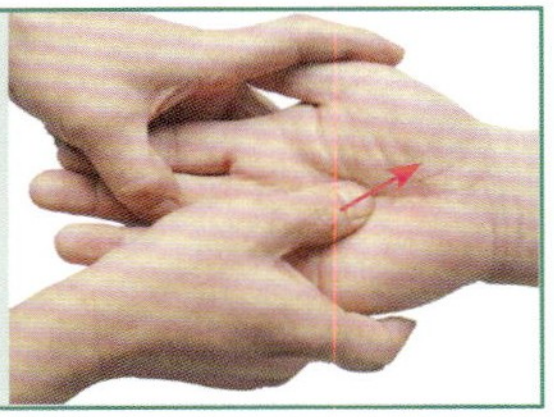

前列腺·尿道·子宫·阴道

由中间向两侧分推或由尺侧向桡侧推 20~30 次

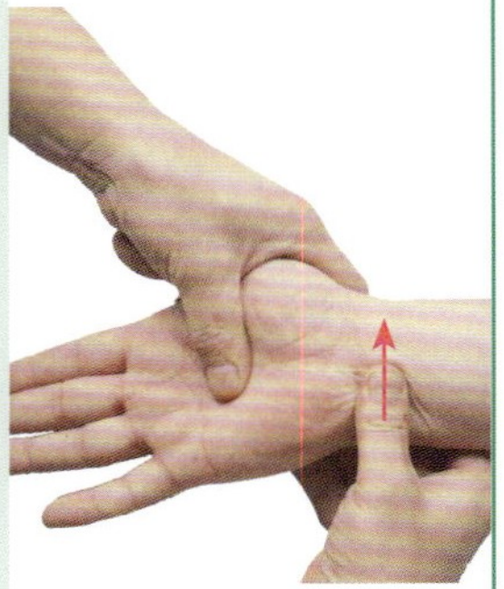

食管

向指根方向推 10~15 次

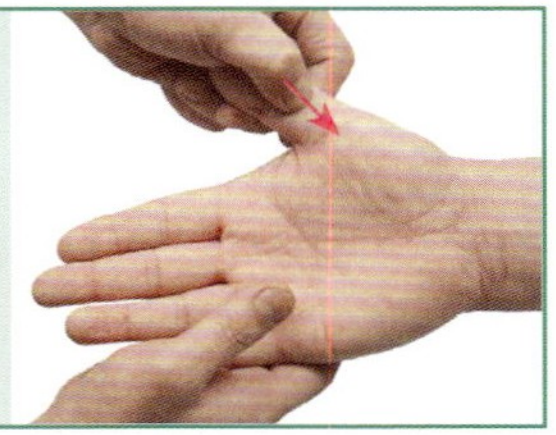

十二指肠

向手腕方向推 10~15 次

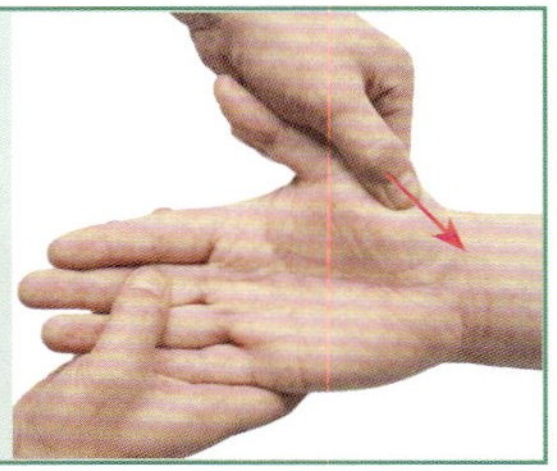

小肠

向手腕方向推 20~25 次

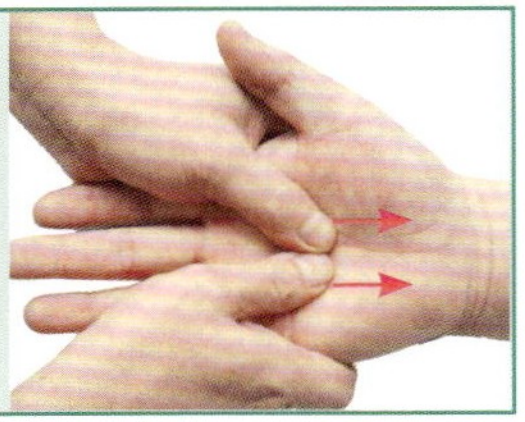

盲肠

掐 10~15 次

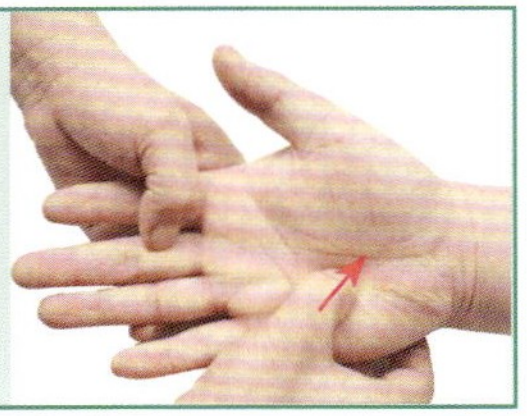

升结肠

向指尖方向推 20~25 次

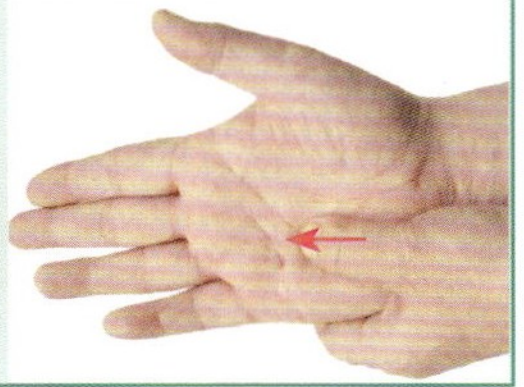

横结肠

由尺侧向桡侧推 20~25 次

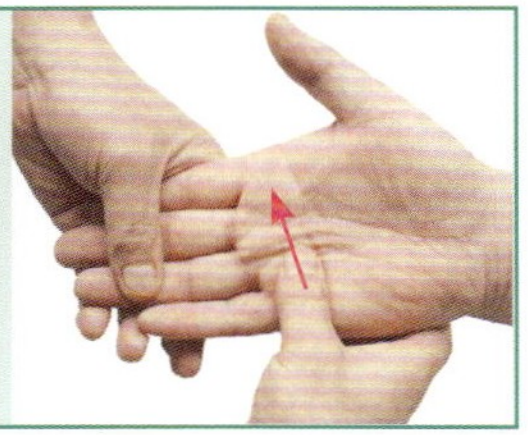

肛门

点按 10~15 次

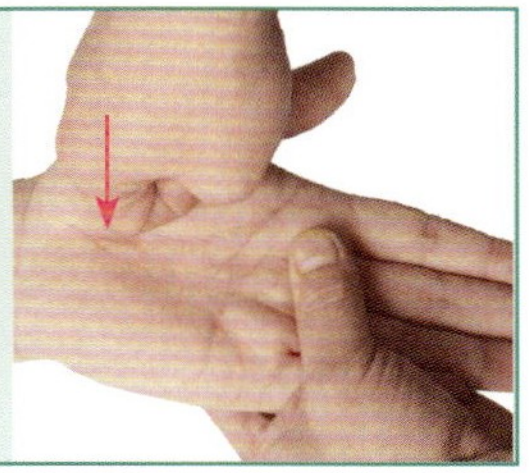

Ureter

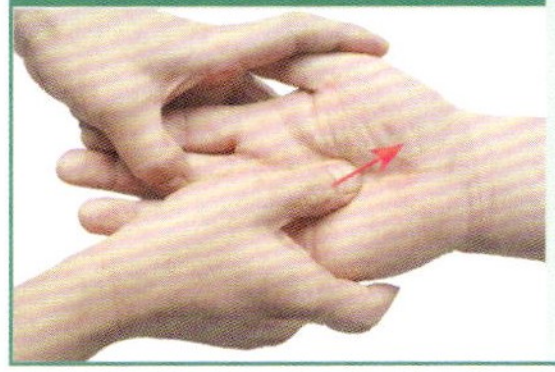

Pressing with 1 finger towards wrist for 10 to 15 times

Prostate, Urethra, Uterus and Vagina

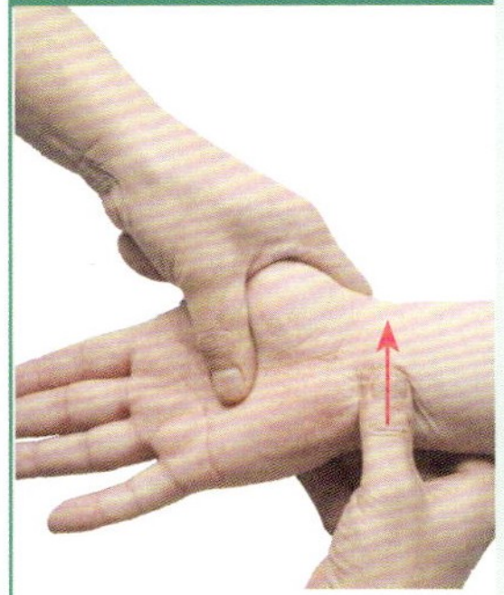

Pressing from middle to both sides or from ulnar side to radial side for 20 to 30 times

Esophagus

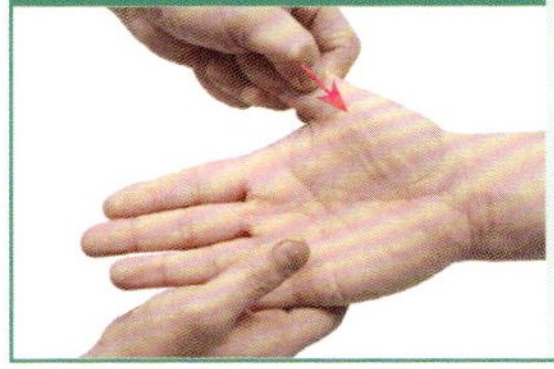

Pressing towards the roots for 10 to 15 times

Duodenum

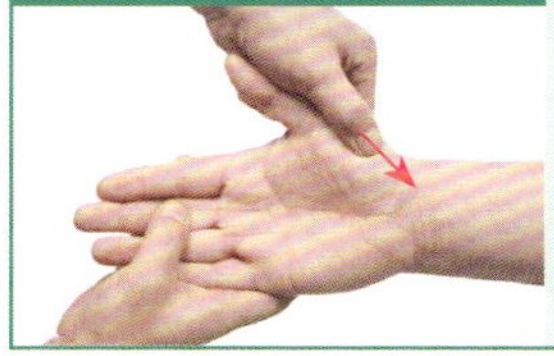

Pressing towards wrist for 10 to 15 times

Small Intestine

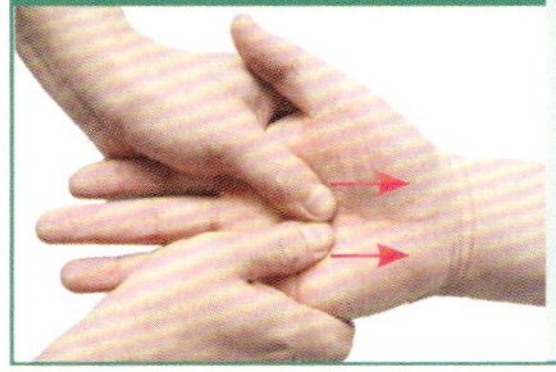

Pressing towards wrist for 20 to 25 times

Cecum

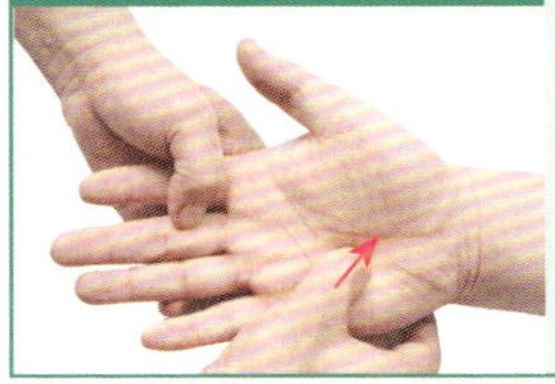

Fingernail pressing for 10 to 15 times

Ascending Colon

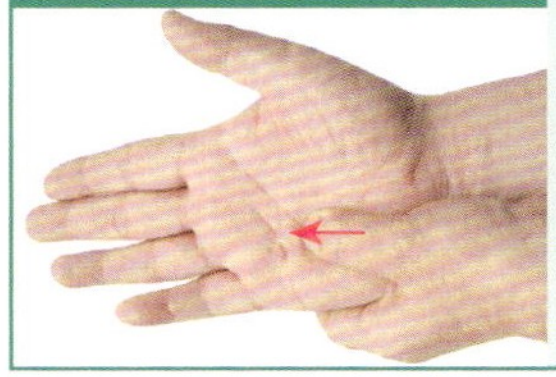

Pressing towards fingertips for 20 to 25 times

Transverse Colon

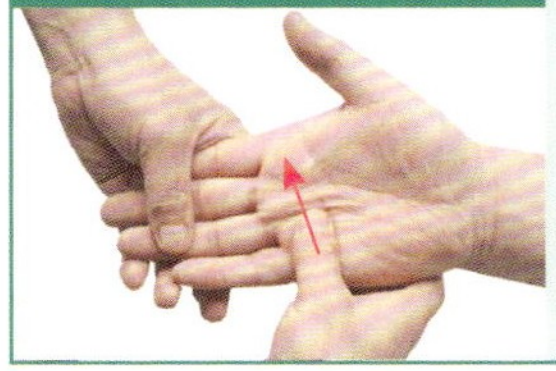

Pressing from ulnar side to radial side for 20 to 25 times

Anus

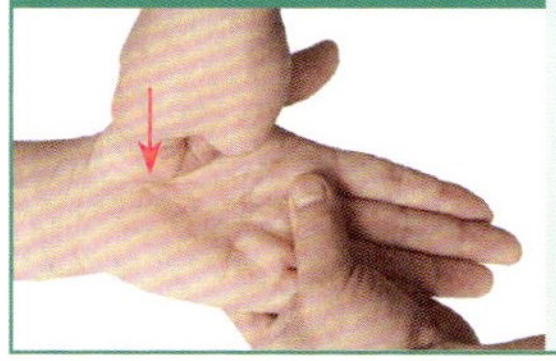

Point-pressing for 10 to 15 times

手背面反射区

Reflex Zone of the Back of the Hand

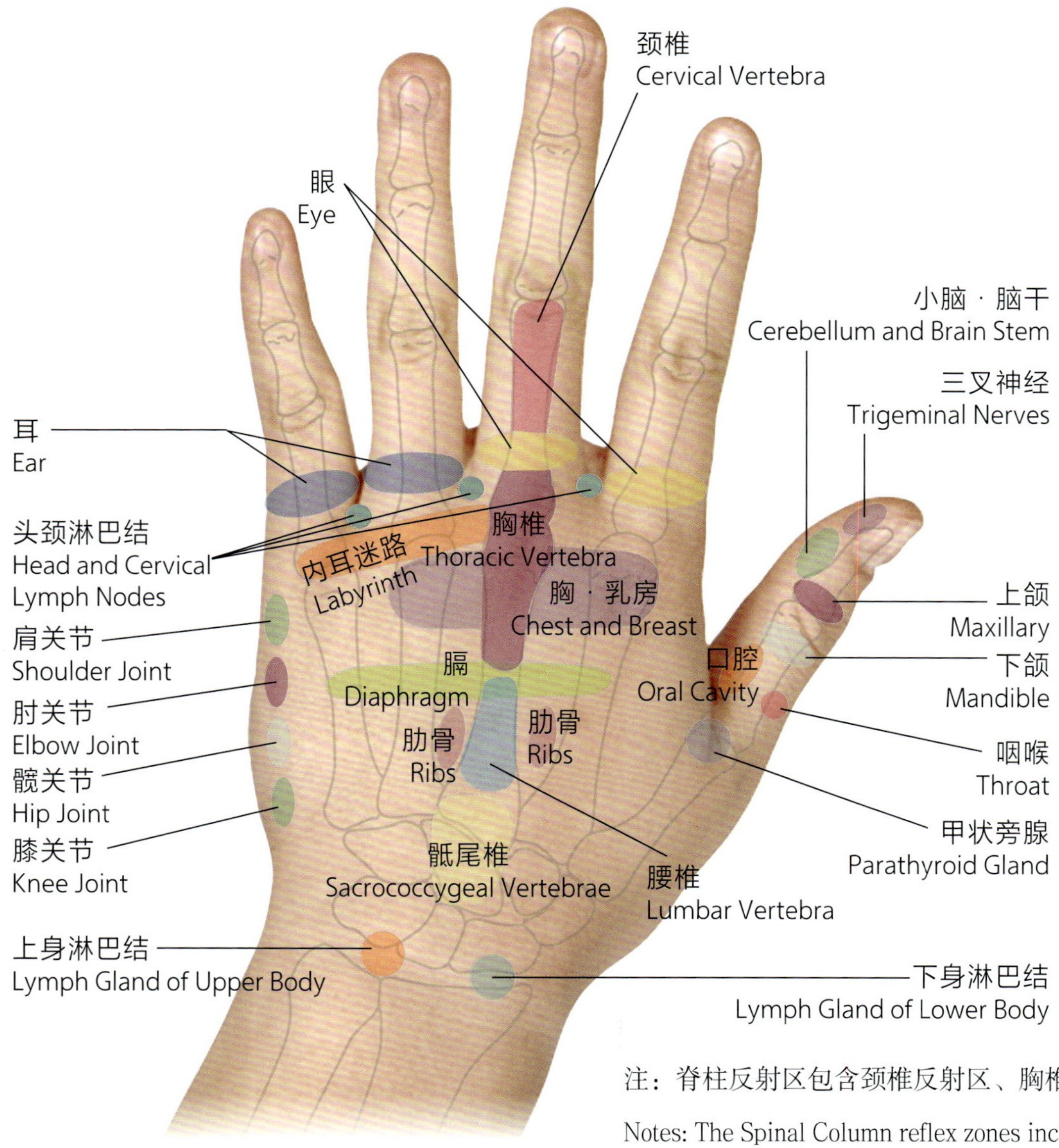

反射区	定位	主治
小脑 · 脑干	手掌面，拇指指腹尺侧	头痛、眩晕、失眠、记忆力减退、帕金森病
三叉神经	拇指末节指腹远端尺侧缘	偏头痛、牙痛、面瘫、三叉神经痛
上颌 · 下颌	双手拇指背侧，拇指指间关节横纹上下的带状区域，远侧为上颌，近侧为下颌	牙痛、颞颌关节炎、牙周炎
眼	双手掌面和手背面第 2、3 指指根部	结膜炎、角膜炎、近视、远视、青光眼、白内障、眼出血
耳	双手掌面和手背面第 4、5 指指根部	中耳炎、耳鸣、耳聋、眩晕
咽喉	双手拇指近节指骨背侧中央	气管炎、咽喉炎、咳嗽、声音嘶哑
口腔	双手拇指背侧，拇指近侧指间关节的尺侧缘	口腔溃疡、味觉异常、口唇疱疹
甲状旁腺	双手背面第 1 掌指关节背侧的凹陷处	甲状旁腺功能低下引起的缺钙症状如筋骨酸软、手足麻痹或痉挛等，白内障，癫痫

注：脊柱反射区包含颈椎反射区、胸椎反射区、腰椎反射区和骶尾椎反射区。

Notes: The Spinal Column reflex zones include reflex zones of Cervical Vertebra, Thoracic Vertebra, Lumbar Vertebra and Sacrococcygeal Vertebrae.

Reflex Zone	Location	Indications
Cerebellum and Brain Stem	Palm aspect, the ulnar side of thumb pulp	Headache; dizziness; insomnia; memory loss; Parkinson's disease
Trigeminal Nerves	Ulnar margin of distal thumb pulp	Migraine headache; toothache; facial paralysis; trigeminal neuralgia
Maxillary and Mandible	The dorsal sides of both thumbs, belt zone around the transverse crease on interphalangeal joint of the thumb, and the distal side as maxillary, the proximal side as mandible	Toothache; temporomandibular arthritis; periodontitis
Eye	On the palm and hand back, the root of the 2nd and the 3rd finger	Conjunctivitis; keratitis; myopia; hyperopia; glaucoma; cataract; vitreous hemorrhage
Ear	On the palm and hand back, the root of the 3rd and the 4th finger	Otitis media; tinnitus; deafness; vertigo
Throat	On the thumb, the center of the phalange back which near the joint	Tracheitis; pharyngolaryngitis; cough; hoarseness
Oral Cavity	The dorsal aspect of thumb, the ulnar side of proximal interphalangeal joint of the thumb	Oral ulcer; abnormal taste; herpes labialis
Parathyroid Gland	Hand back, the depression on dorsal side of the joint of the 1st metacarpal	Calcium deficiency symptoms caused by hypoparathyroidism such as aching sinews and bones; numbness or spasm of limbs; cataract; epilepsy

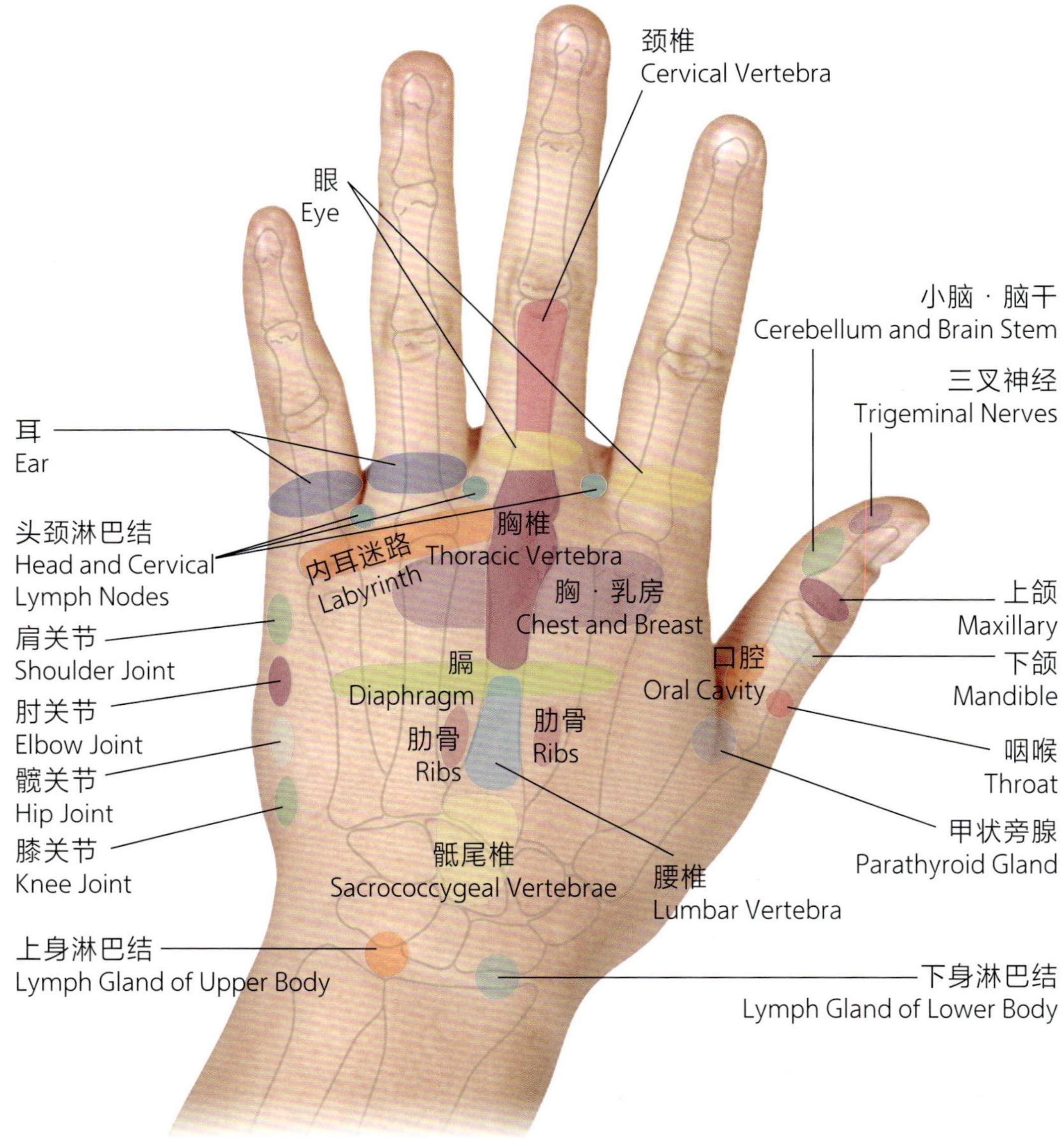

续表

反射区	定 位	主 治
头颈淋巴结	在手掌面和手背面，第2~5指指根部间的凹陷处	眼、耳、舌、口腔、牙齿等部位的疾病，淋巴结肿大，甲状腺肿大，免疫力低下
上身淋巴结	双手背面尺侧，月骨、三角骨与尺骨间的凹陷处	各种炎症、发热、免疫力低下
下身淋巴结	双手背面桡侧，舟骨与桡骨间的凹陷处	各种炎症、发热、免疫力低下
内耳迷路	双手背侧，横跨第3、4、5掌指关节的带状区域，第3、4、5指指根结合部	头晕、晕车晕船、耳鸣、高血压、低血压、平衡功能障碍
胸 · 乳房	手背面第2、3、4掌骨的中上部	乳腺炎、乳腺增生、乳腺癌、食管炎
膈	双手背面第2、3、4、5掌骨中部的带状区域	打嗝、腹痛、恶心、呕吐
脊柱	双手背侧中指第3指骨至腕部（含颈椎、胸椎、腰椎、骶尾椎）	颈椎病、落枕、背部不适、腰痛、腰肌劳损、腰椎间盘突出症
颈椎	双手背面，中指第1指骨远端2/3	颈椎病、落枕

Continued

Reflex Zone	Location	Indications
Head and Cervical Lymph Nodes	On the palm and hand back, the depression on the root of the 2nd to the 5th finger	Diseases of eyes, ears, tongue, mouth, teeth and other parts; lymph node enlargement; goiter; low immunity
Lymph Gland of Upper Body	Ulnar side of hand back, the depression among semilunare, ossa ulnare and ulna	Various inflammation; fever; low immunity
Lymph Gland of Lower Body	Radial side of hand back, the depression between radius and scaphoid	Various inflammation; fever; low immunity
Labyrinth	Dorsal side of hands, through the belt zone of the 3rd, 4th, 5th metacarpal joint, the joint part on the root of the 3rd, 4th, 5th finger	Dizziness; motion sickness; tinnitus; hypertension; hypotension; balance dysfunction
Chest and Breast	Hand back, the upper part of the 2nd, 3rd, 4th metacarpal	Mastitis; breast hyperplasia; breast cancer; esophagitis
Diaphragm	Hand back, the belt zone in the middle of the 2nd, 3rd, 4th, 5th metacarpal	Hiccups; abdominal pain; nausea; vomiting
Spinal Column	The dorsal aspect of hands, from the phalange of the middle finger to the wrist part(including Cervical Vertebra, Thoracic Vertebra, Lumbar Vertebra and Sacrococcygeal Vertebrae)	Cervical spondylopathy; stiff neck; back pain; lower back pain; lumbar muscle strain; lumbar disc protrusion
Cervical Vertebra	Hand back, the 2/3 part of the 1st phalange distal side of middle finger	Cervical spondylopathy; stiff neck

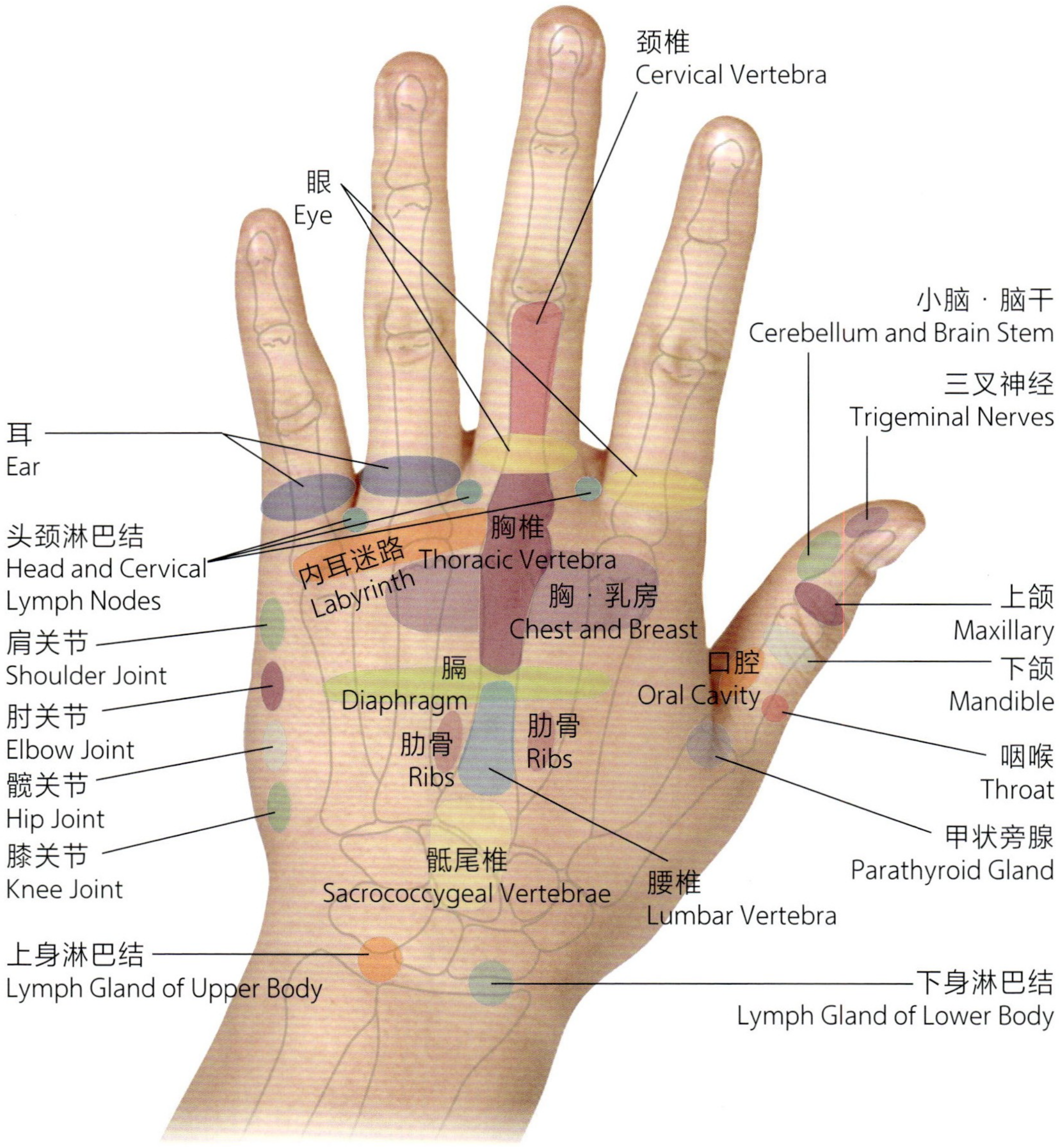

续表

反射区	定 位	主 治
胸椎	双手背面中指第 1 指骨近端 1/3 至第 3 掌骨中点	颈肩部软组织损伤、胸痛、胸闷
腰椎	双手背面胸椎反射区至骶尾椎反射区之间的部分	腰酸背痛、急性腰扭伤、慢性腰肌劳损、腰椎骨质增生、腰椎间盘突出症、坐骨神经痛
骶尾椎	双手背面脊柱反射区末端部分，腕掌关节结合处	坐骨神经痛、腰骶部劳损、便秘
肋骨	双手背面腰椎反射区两侧	肋骨骨折、肋软骨炎、胸痛、胸闷
肩关节	双手背面第 5 掌骨远端的尺侧缘，赤白肉际处	肩部疾病，包括肩周炎、肩部损伤、肩部肌肉痉挛
肘关节	双手背面第 5 掌骨尺侧远端 1/4 至 1/2 之间的区域	网球肘（肱骨外上髁炎）、肘部疼痛
髋关节	双手背面第 5 掌骨肘关节反射区与膝关节反射区之间的区域	髋关节痛、坐骨神经痛、腰背疼痛
膝关节	双手背面第 5 掌骨近端的尺侧缘	膝关节痛、膝关节炎

Continued

Reflex Zone	Location	Indications
Thoracic Vertebra	Hand back, from the 1/3 part of the 1st phalange distal side of the 3rd finger to the middle of the 3rd metacarpal	Soft tissue injury of neck and shoulder; chest pain; chest tightness
Lumbar Vertebra	Handback, between the Thoracic Vertebra reflex zone to the Sacrococcygeal Vertebrae reflect zone	Lumbar and back pain; acute lumbar sprain; chronic lumbar muscle strain; lumbar vertebra hyperplasia; lumbar disc protrusion; sciatica
Sacrococcygeal Vertebrae	Terminal part of the Spinal Column reflex zone, the joint part of carpal and metacarpal	Sciatica; lumbosacral strain; constipation
Ribs	Hand back, both sides of the Lumbar Vetebra reflex zone vertebra	Rib fracture; costal cartilage inflammation; chest pain; chest tightness
Shoulder Joint	Hand back, the ulnar margin of the 5th metacarpal distal side, border of the red and white skin	Shoulder diseases; including shoulder periarthritis, shoulder injury, shoulder muscle spasm
Elbow Joint	Hand back, between the 1/4 part and 1/2 part of ulnar side of the 5th metacarpal distal end	Tennis elbow (lateral epicondylitis of humerus); elbow pain
Hip Joint	Hand back, on the 5th metacarpal, between the reflex zone of Elbow Joint and Knee Joint	Hip pain; sciatica; lumbar pain
Knee Joint	Hand back, the ulnar margin of the 5th metacarpal proximal end	Knee pain; knee arthritis

超简单手背面反射区按摩

Super-easy Massage in Reflex Zone of the Back of the Hand

小脑·脑干

由指尖向指根方向推按 10~15 次

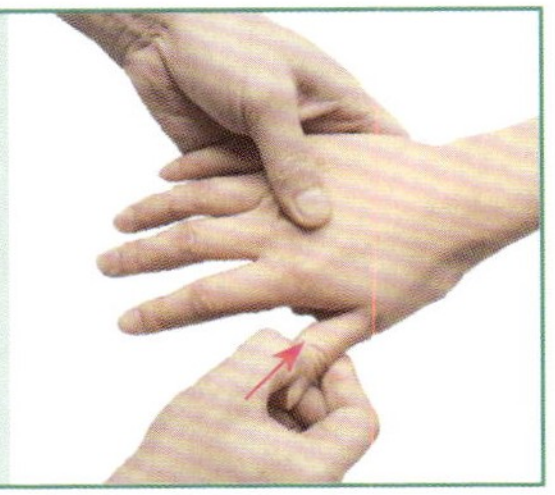

上颌

由尺侧向桡侧推 10~15 次

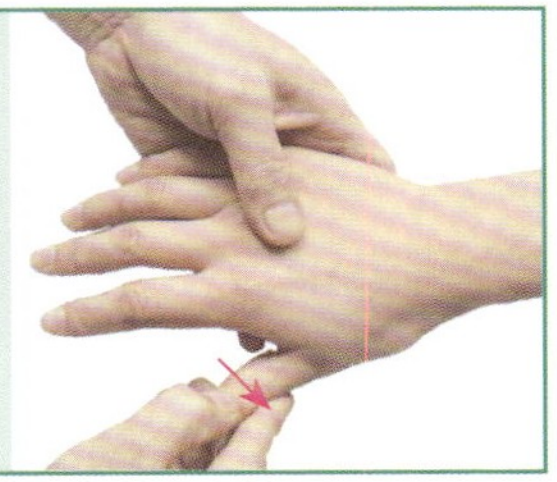

眼

横推 20 次

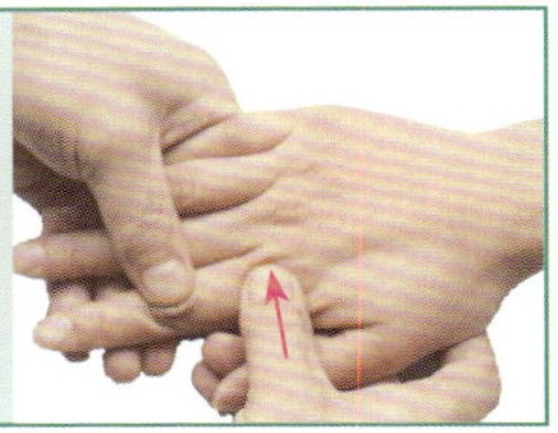

咽喉

点按 15~20 次

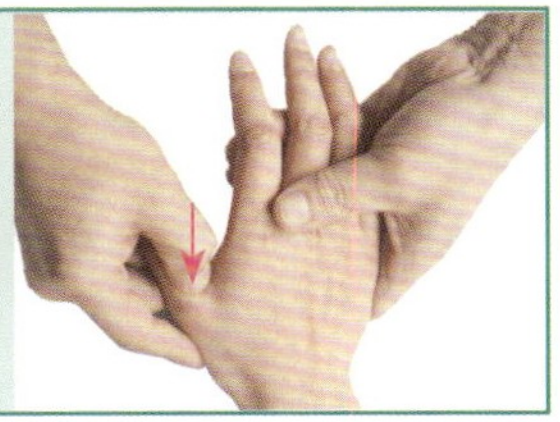

耳

横推 20 次

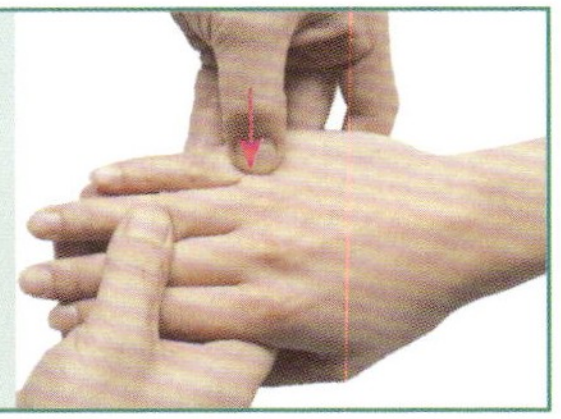

甲状旁腺

点按 20~25 次

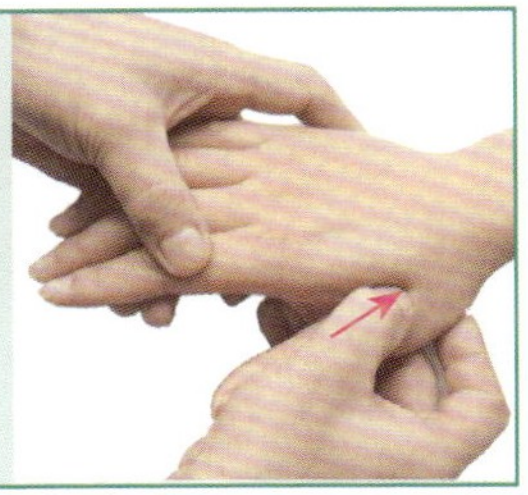

上身淋巴结

掐按或拨 15~20 次

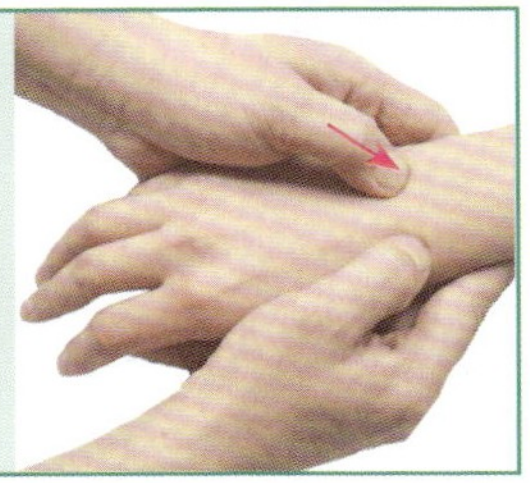

三叉神经

向虎口方向推按 10~15 次

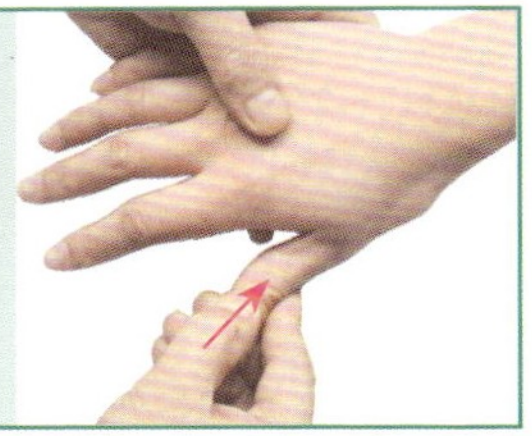

下颌

由尺侧向桡侧推 10~15 次

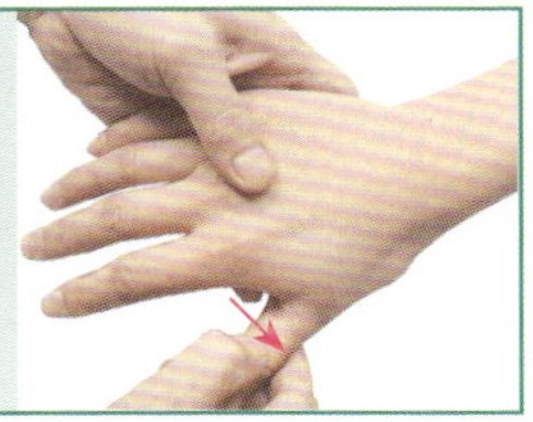

口腔

点按 15~20 次

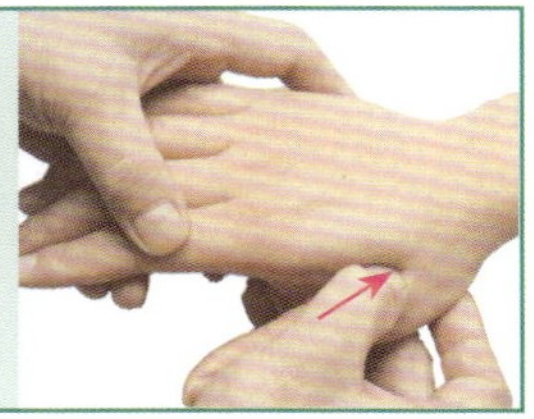

Cerebellum and Brain Stem

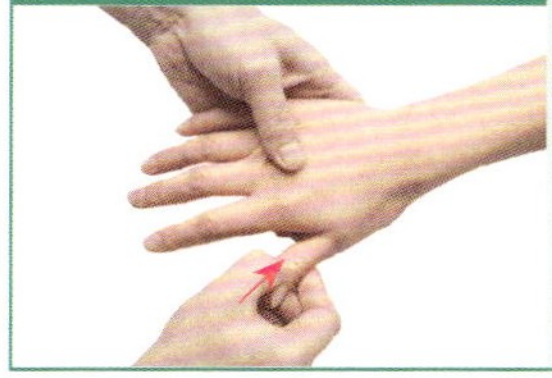

Pressing from fingertip to root for 10 to 15 times

Maxillary

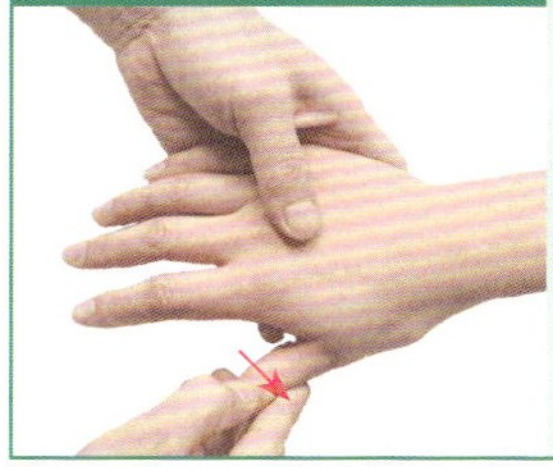

Pressing from ulnar side to radial side for 10 to 15 times

Eye

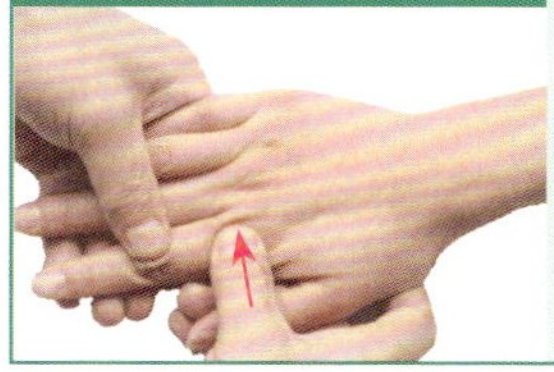

Pressing transversally for 20 times

Throat

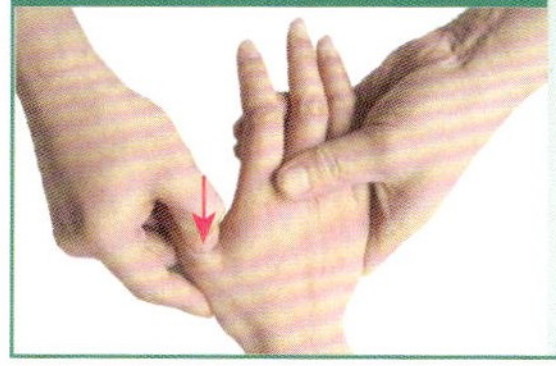

Point-pressing for 15 to 20 times

Ear

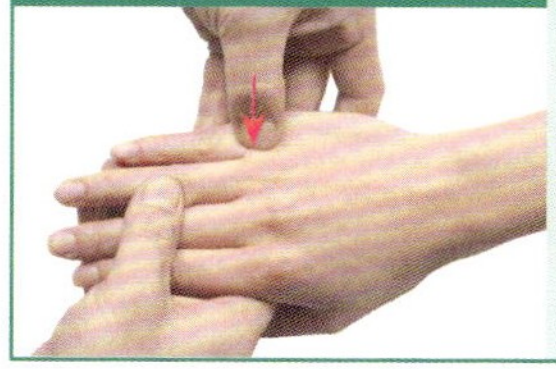

Pressing transversally for 20 times

Parathyroid Gland

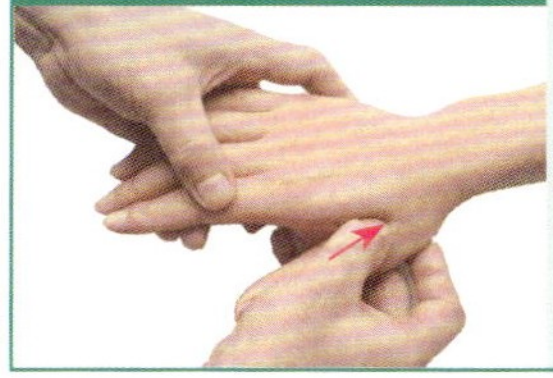

Point-pressing for 20 to 25 times

Lymph Gland of Upper Body

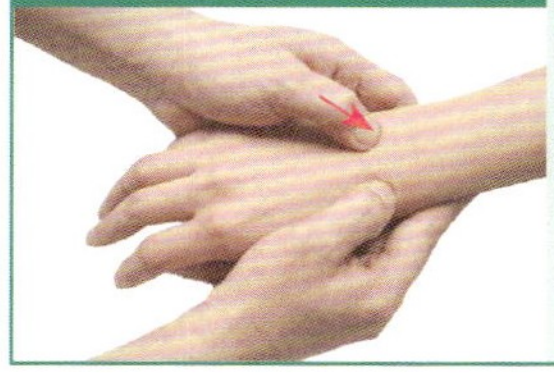

Fingernail pressing for 15 to 20 times

Trigeminal Nerves

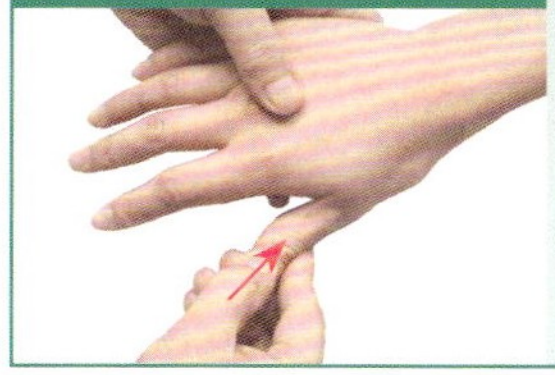

Pressing towards tiger' s mouth(region between the 1st and the 2nd metacarpal bones) for 10 to 15 times

Mandible

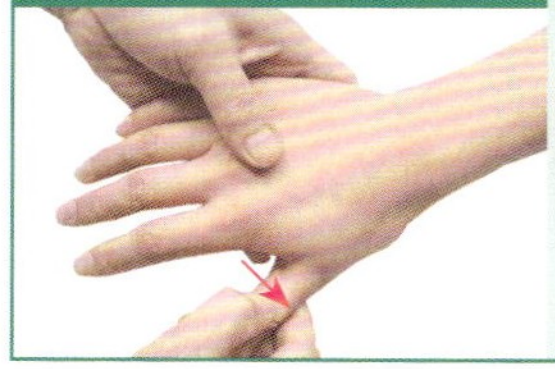

Pressing from ulnar side to radial side 10 to 15 times

Oral Cavity

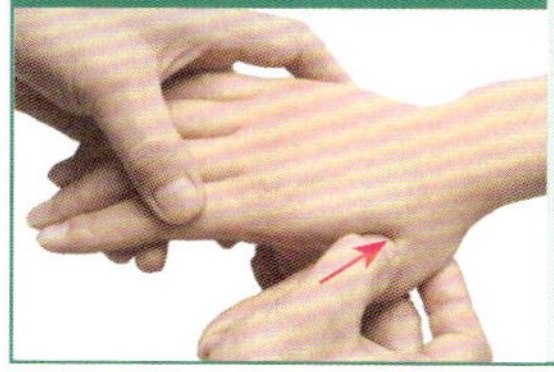

Point-pressing for 15 to 20 times

头颈淋巴结

点掐 5~10 次

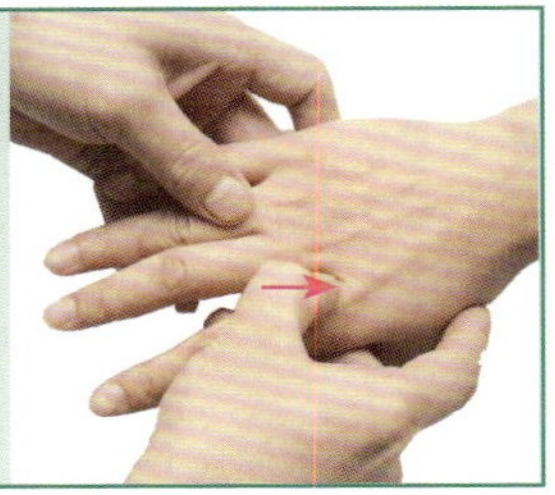

下身淋巴结

掐按或拨 15~20 次

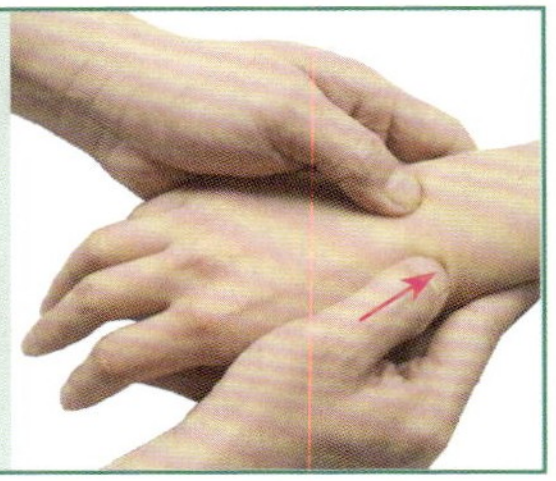

内耳迷路

横推 10~15 次

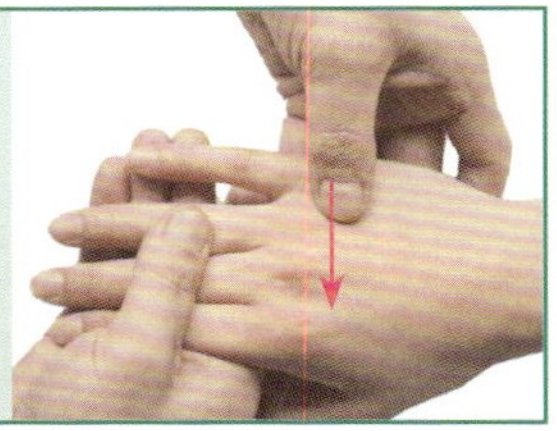

膈

双手拇指交叉推或以拇指推 20 次

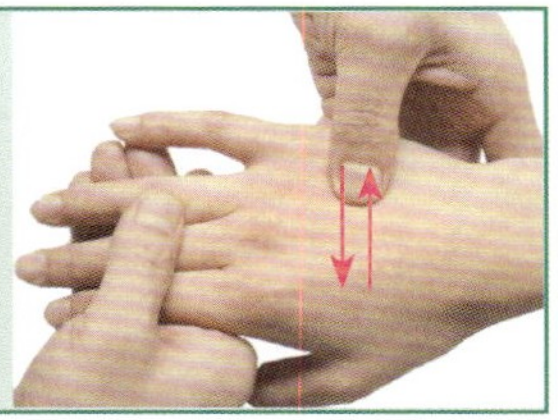

胸椎

向手腕方向推 20 次

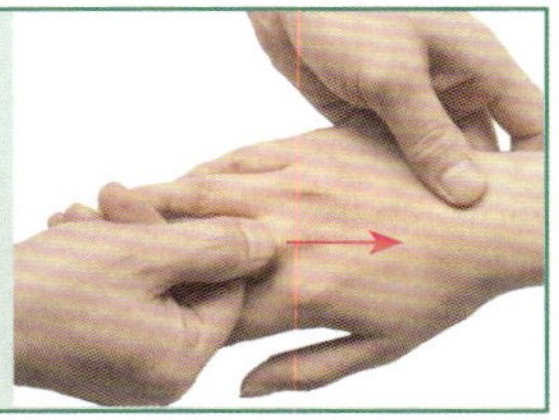

骶尾椎

向手腕方向推 20 次

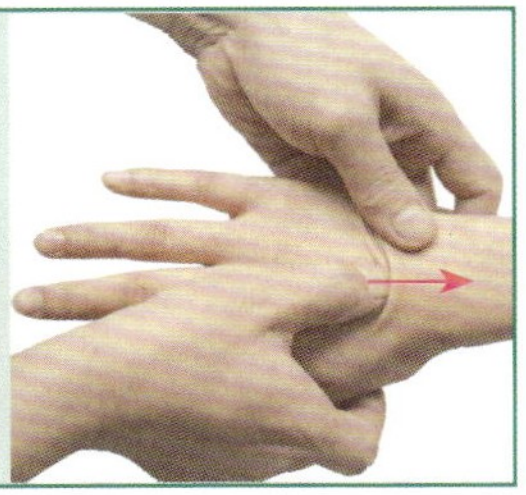

肩关节

按揉 20~25 次

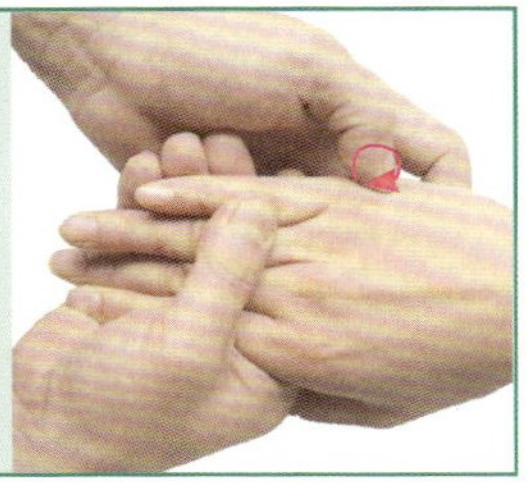

髋关节

按揉 10~15 次

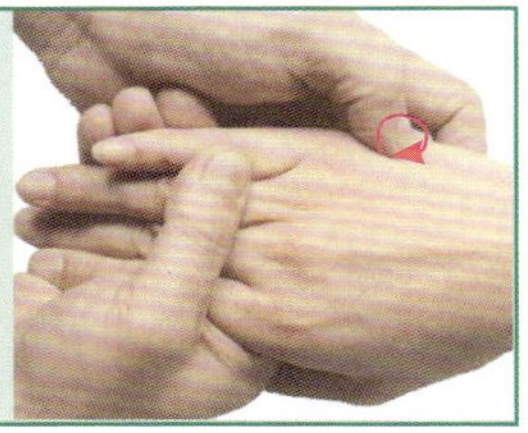

胸·乳房

从尺侧向桡侧推 15~20 次

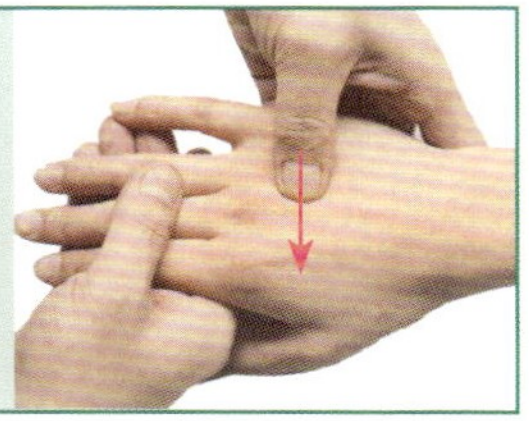

颈椎

向手腕方向推 20~25 次

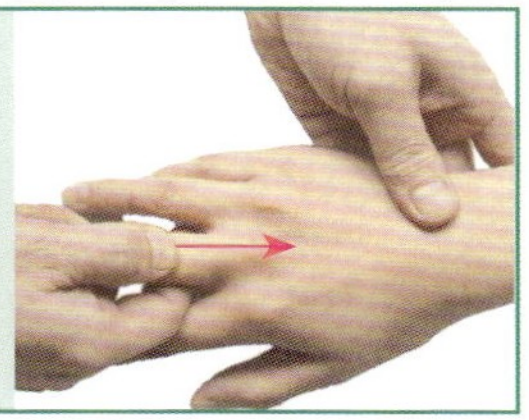

Cervical Lymph Nodes

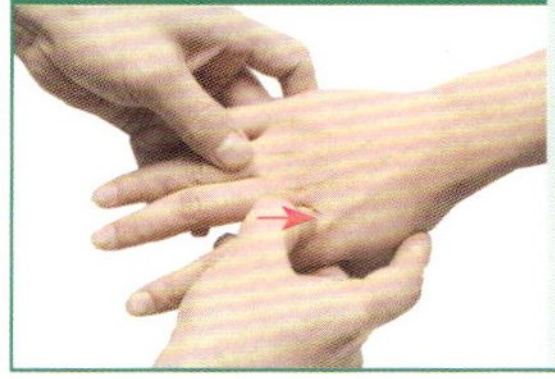

Fingernail pressing for 5 to 10 times

Lymph Gland of Lower Body

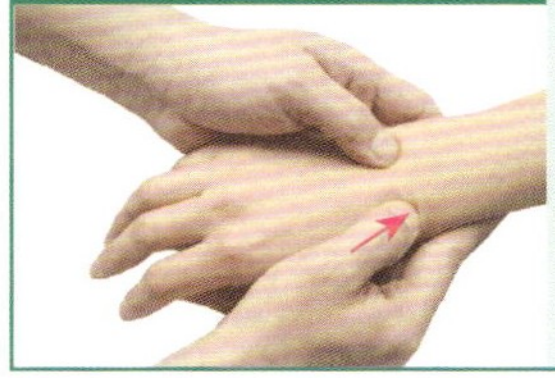

Fingernail pressing for 15 to 20 times

Labyrinth

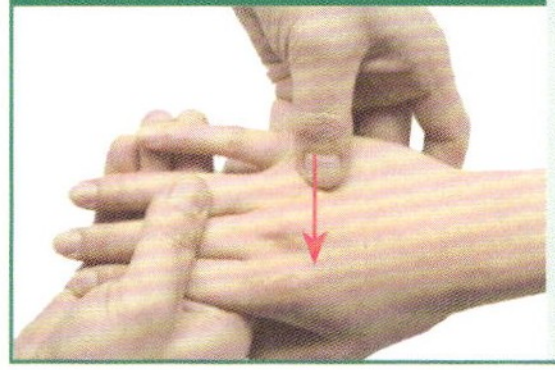

Pressing transversally for 10 to 15 times

Diaphragm

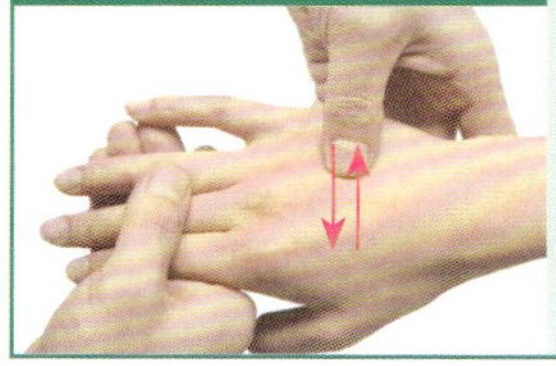

Thumbs cross pressing or single thumb pressing for 20 times

Thoracic Vertebra

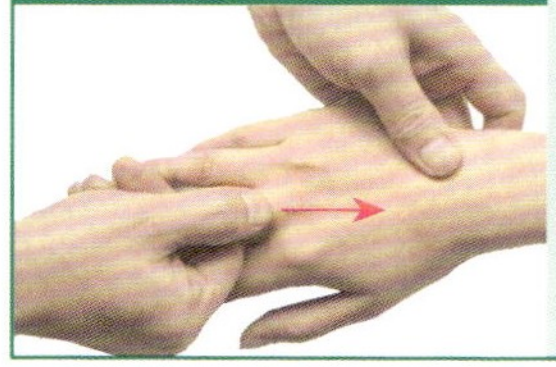

Pressing towards twist for 20 times

Sacrococcygeal Vertebrae

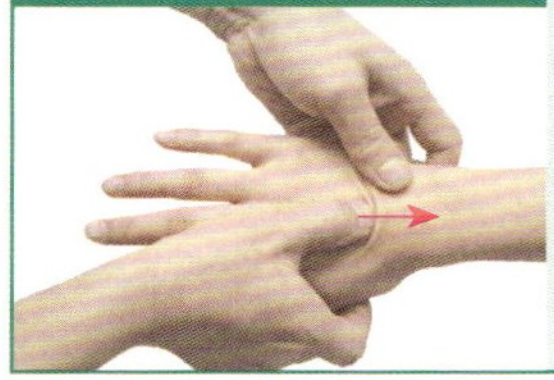

Pressing towards twist for 20 times

Shoulder Joint

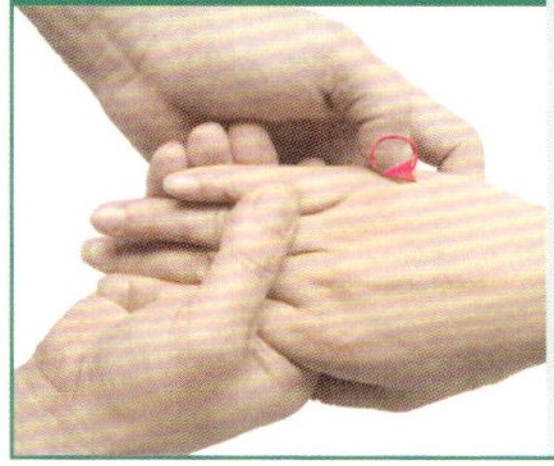

Pressing and kneading for 20 to 25 times

Hip Joint

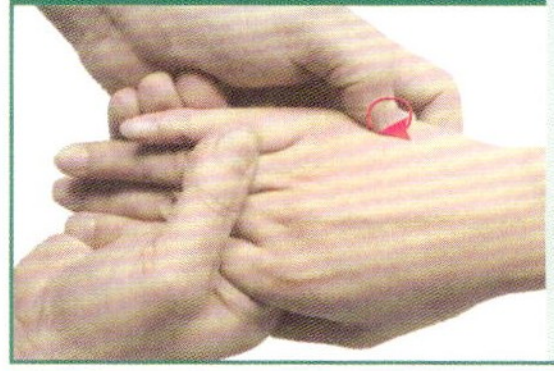

Pressing and kneading for 10 to 15 times

Chest and Breast

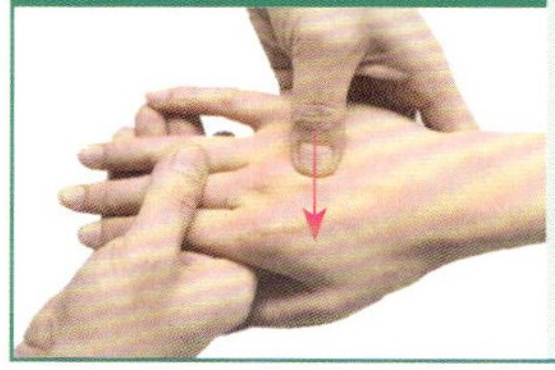

Pressing from ulnar side to radial side for 15 to 20 times

Cervical Vertebra

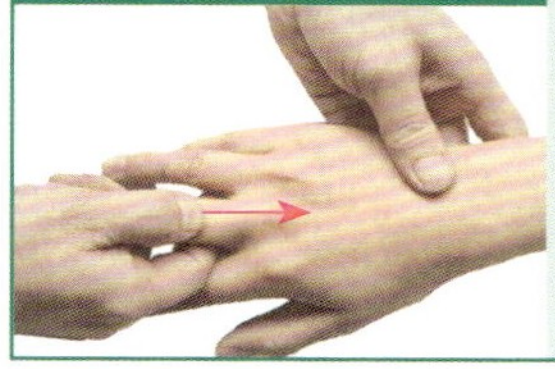

Pressing towards twist for 20 to 25 times

腰椎

向手腕方向推 20 次

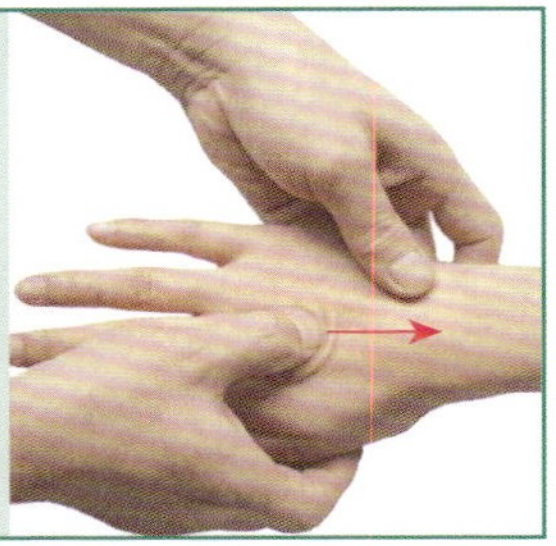

肋骨

点或揉拨 20~25 次

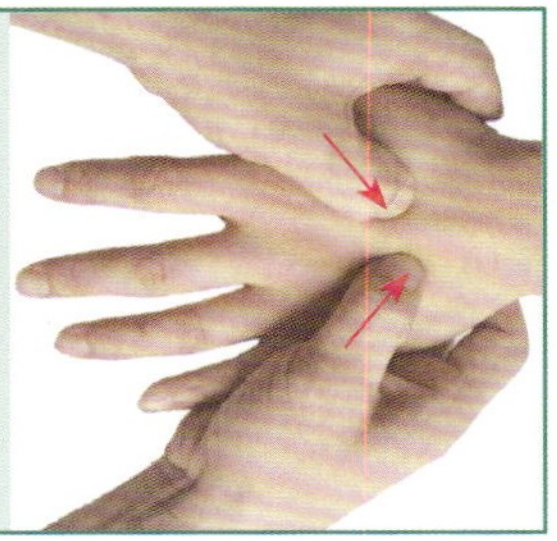

肘关节

按揉 10~15 次

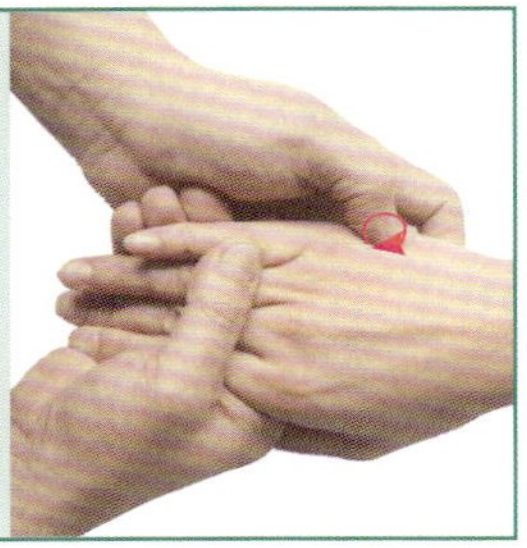

膝关节

按揉 10~15 次

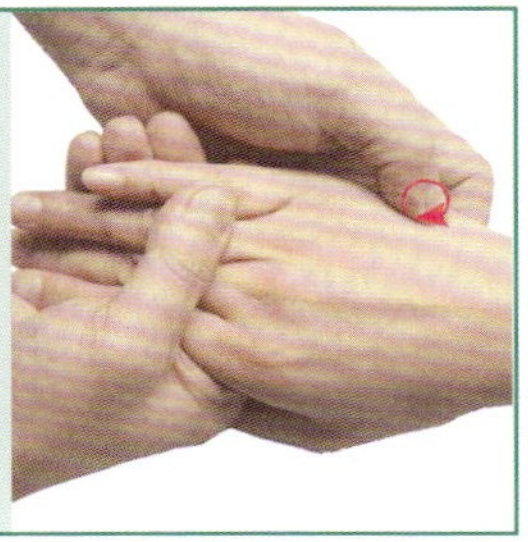

Lumbar Vertebra

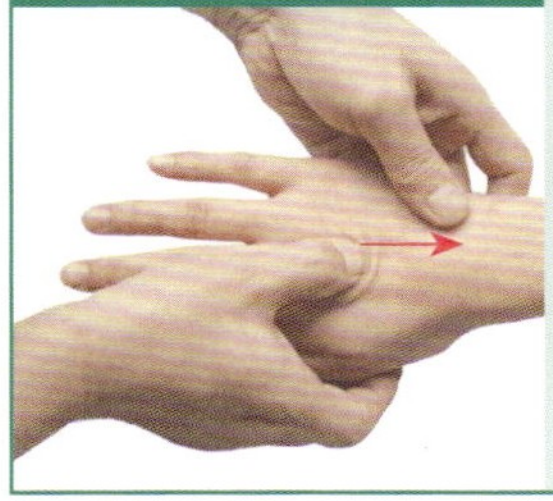

Pressing towards twist for 20 times

Ribs

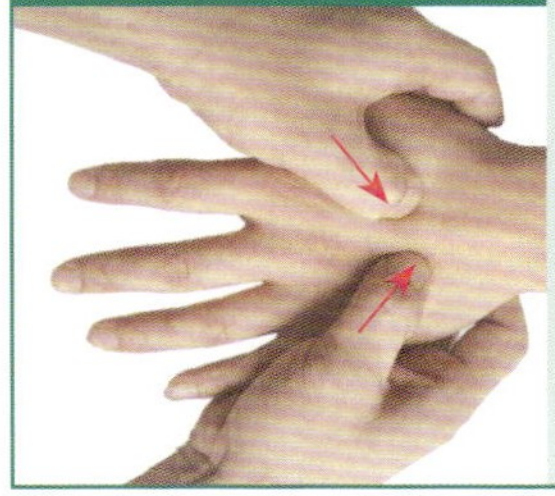

Point-pressing or kneading for 20 to 25 times

Elbow Joint

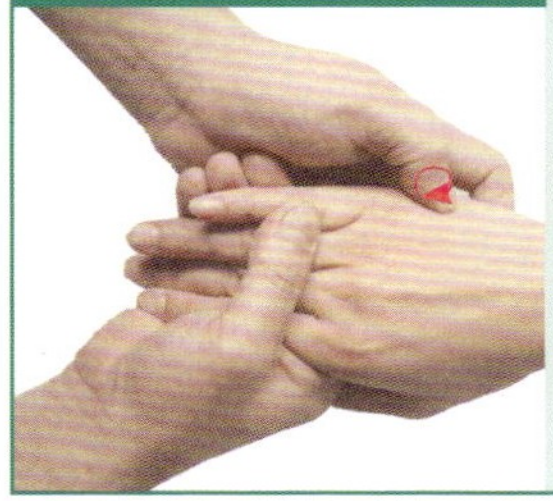

Pressing and kneading for 10 to 15 times

Knee Joint

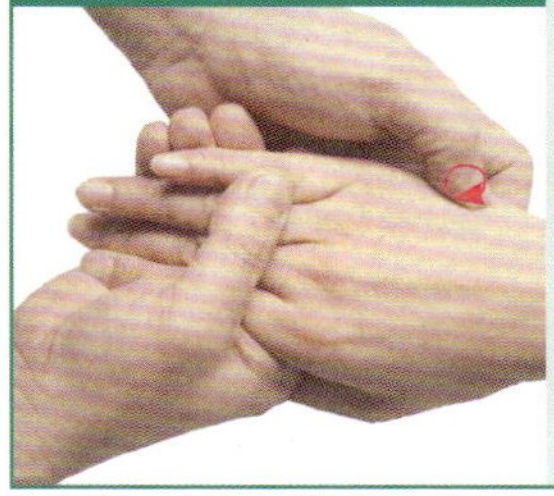

Pressing and kneading for 10 to 15 times

手掌面全息区

Holographic Palm Zone

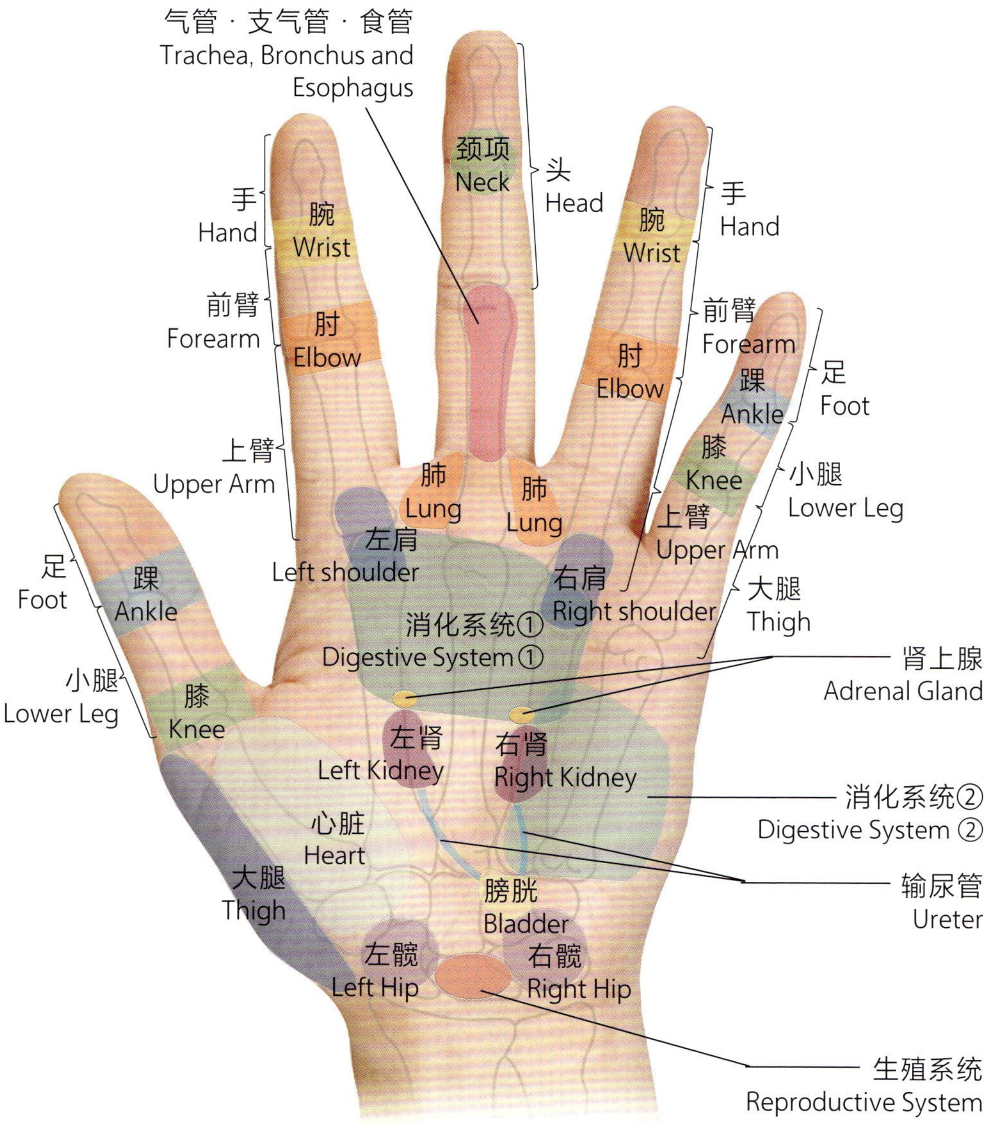

全身部位在手部的全息定位是诊病的基础，无论左手、右手均以靠大拇指侧为身体的左侧，靠小指侧为身体的右侧，以中指为身体的正中分界线。主要用于疾病的辅助诊断，提示相应部位可能存在的疾患。

全息区	定 位	反映疾病
头	双手掌面和背面，中指远节及中节指骨，包括脑、眼、耳、鼻、口腔等	相应的五官疾病
颈项	双手掌面中指远侧指间关节处	颈项部疾病
气管 · 支气管 · 食管	双手掌面中指近节指骨远端 2/3 处	气管、支气管及食管部位的疾病

The holographic location of body parts in hands is the basis for diagnosis. Whatever left hand or right hand, the thumb side is regarded as the left side of the body, the little finger as the right side of the body and the middle finger as the center of the body. The holographic zone is mainly used for diagnosing disease, suggesting that the potential existed disease in corresponding parts.

Holographic Zone	Location	Corresponding Diseases
Head	On the palm and back, the distal joint and middle joint of middle finger phalanges, including Brain, Eye, Ear, Nose, Oral Cavity and so on	Corresponding facial features diseases
Neck	On the palm, the distal side of interphalangeal joint of the middle finger	Neck diseases
Trachea and Bronchus and Esophagus	On the palm, the 2/3 part of proximal phalange distal side of middle finger	Diseases of the trachea; bronchus and esophagus

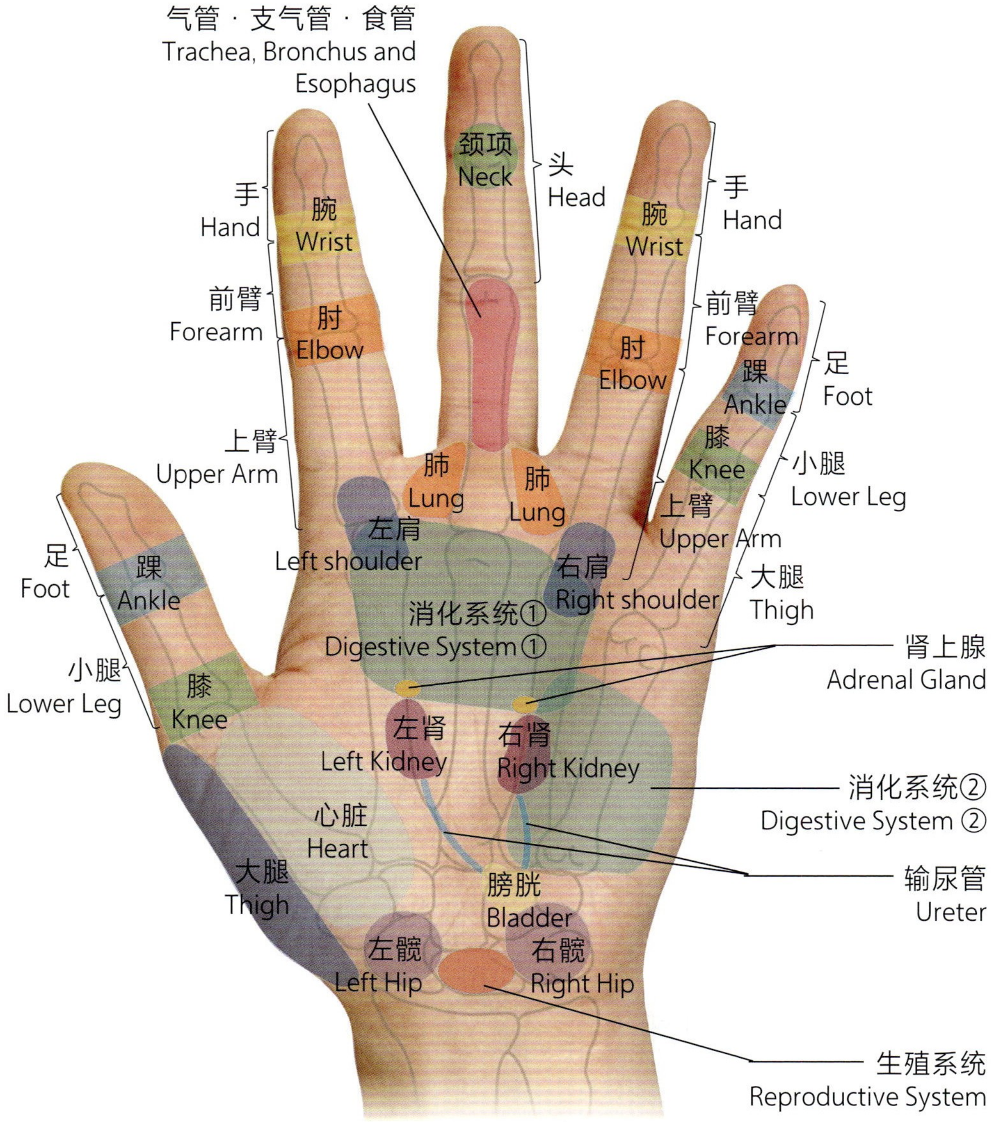

续表

全息区	定 位	反映疾病
肺	双手掌面中指近节指骨近端1/3 的两侧	肺部、气管、支气管部位的疾病
消化系统①	双手掌面第 2、3、4 掌骨的远端 1/2 处。包括胃、肝、胆、胰、脾及十二指肠区	相应各器官的疾病
消化系统②	双手掌面第 4、5 掌骨近端2/3 处。包括升结肠、横结肠、降结肠、乙状结肠、直肠、小肠、肛门区	相应各器官的疾病
肾	双手掌面，消化系统①区中部至掌根部横纹的竖直线的中部两侧，拇指侧为左肾区，小指侧为右肾区	肾及肾上腺等疾病
肾上腺	双手掌面肾区的远侧	肾及肾上腺疾病

Continued

Holographic Zone	Location	Corresponding Diseases
Lung	On the palm, the 1/3 part on both sides of proximal phalange distal side of middle finger	Diseases of the lungs; trachea; and bronchus
Digestive System ①	On the palm, the 1/2 part of the distal side of the 2nd, the 3rd, the 4th metacarpal, including Stomach, Liver, Gallbladder, Pancreas, Spleen and Duodenum	Diseases of corresponding organs
Digestive System ②	On the palm, the 2/3 part of the proximal side of the 4th, 5th metacarpal, including Ascending Colon, Transverse Colon, Descending Colon, Sigmoid Colon, Rectum, Small Intestine and Anus Region	Diseases of corresponding organs
Kidney	On the palm, the sides of the middle of vertical line between Digestive System ① middle part and transverse striation on the root of palm, and the thumb side as the Left Kidney, the little finger side as the Right Kidney	Diseases of kidney; adrenal and others
Adrenal Gland	On the palm, the distal side of the Kidney zone	Diseases of kidney and adrenal gland

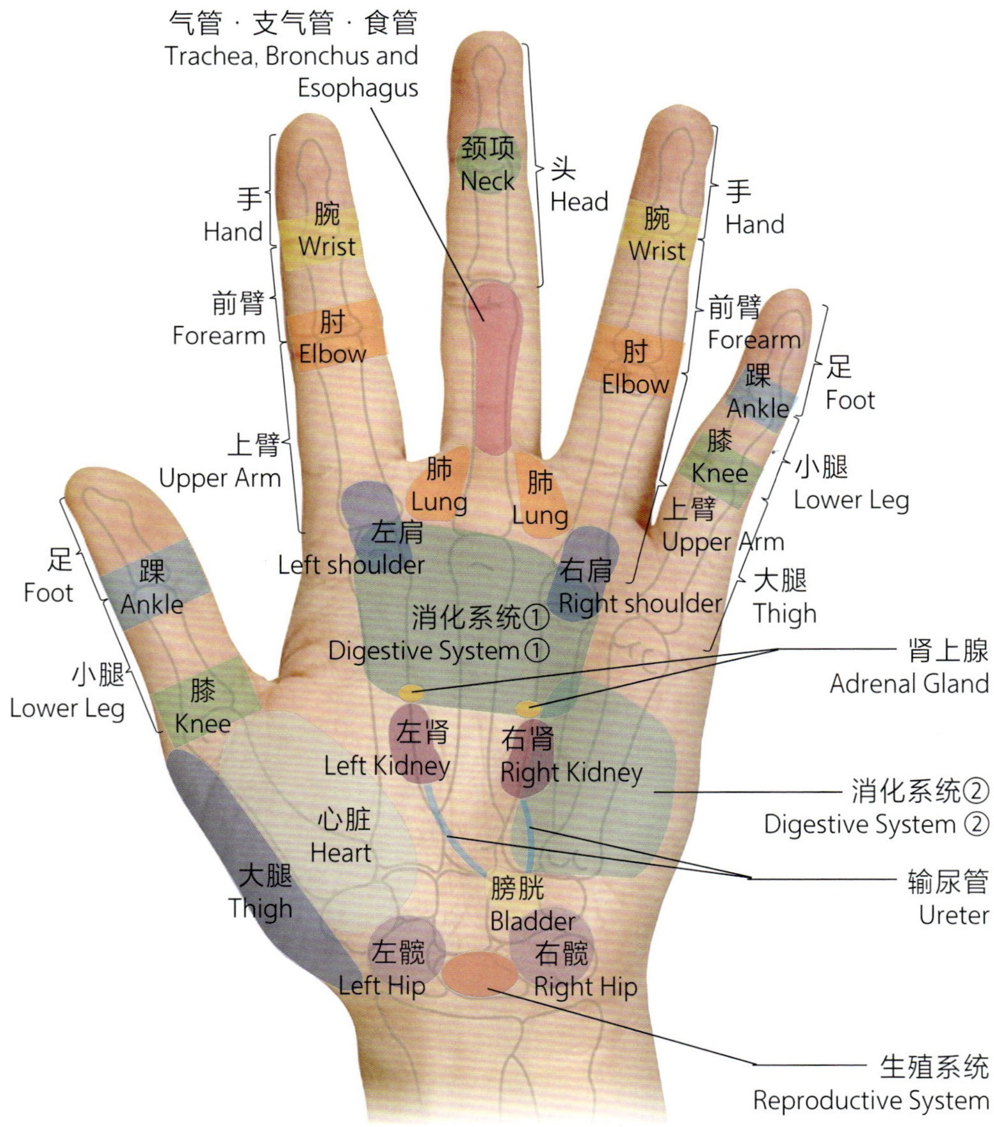

续表

全息区	定 位	反映疾病
膀胱	双手掌面中指掌骨与头状骨、钩骨之间	膀胱、尿道等泌尿系统疾病
输尿管	双手掌面肾区与膀胱区之间的带状区域	输尿管疾病
生殖系统	双手掌面，约当手掌的月骨区域	男性的前列腺疾病，女性的子宫、阴道、输卵管等妇科疾病
心脏	双手掌面的大鱼际处	心血管疾病
手	双手掌面和背面，食指、无名指的远节指骨	手部疾病
腕	双手掌面和背面，食指、无名指的远侧指间关节	手腕疾病
前臂	双手掌面和背面，食指、无名指的中节指骨	前臂疾病
肘	双手掌面和背面，食指、无名指的近侧指间关节	肘部疾病
上臂	双手掌面和背面，食指、无名指的近节指骨	上臂疾病
肩	双手掌面和背面，食指、无名指的掌指关节，食指掌指关节为左肩区，无名指掌指关节为右肩区	肩部疾病
足	双手掌面和背面，拇指、小指的远节指骨	足部疾病

Continued

Holographic Zone	Location	Corresponding Diseases
Bladder	On the palm, among the middle finger metacarpal, capitate and hamate	Bladder; urinary tract and other urinary system diseases
Ureter	On the palm, the belt zone between the Kidney reflex zone and Bladder reflex zone	Diseases of ureter
Reproductive System	On the palm, approximately equal to the lunate zone	Male prostate disease; women's uterus, vagina, fallopian tubes and other gynecological diseases
Heart	On the large fish's margin of the palm	Cardiovascular disease
Hand	On the palm and back, the distal phalange of the index finger and ring finger	Hand diseases
Wrist	On the palm and back, the distal interphalangeal joint of the index finger and ring finger	Wrist diseases
Forearm	On the palm and back, the middle phalange of the index finger and ring finger	Forearm diseases
Elbow	On the palm and back, the proximal interphalangeal joint of the index finger and ring finger	Elbow diseases
Upper Arm	On the palm and back, the proximal phalange of the index finger and ring finger	Upper arm diseases
Shoulder	On the palm and back, metacarpal joint of the index finger and ring finger, the index finger as the left shoulder and the ring finger as the right shoulder	Shoulder diseases
Foot	On the palm and back, the distal phalange of the thumb and little finger	Foot diseases

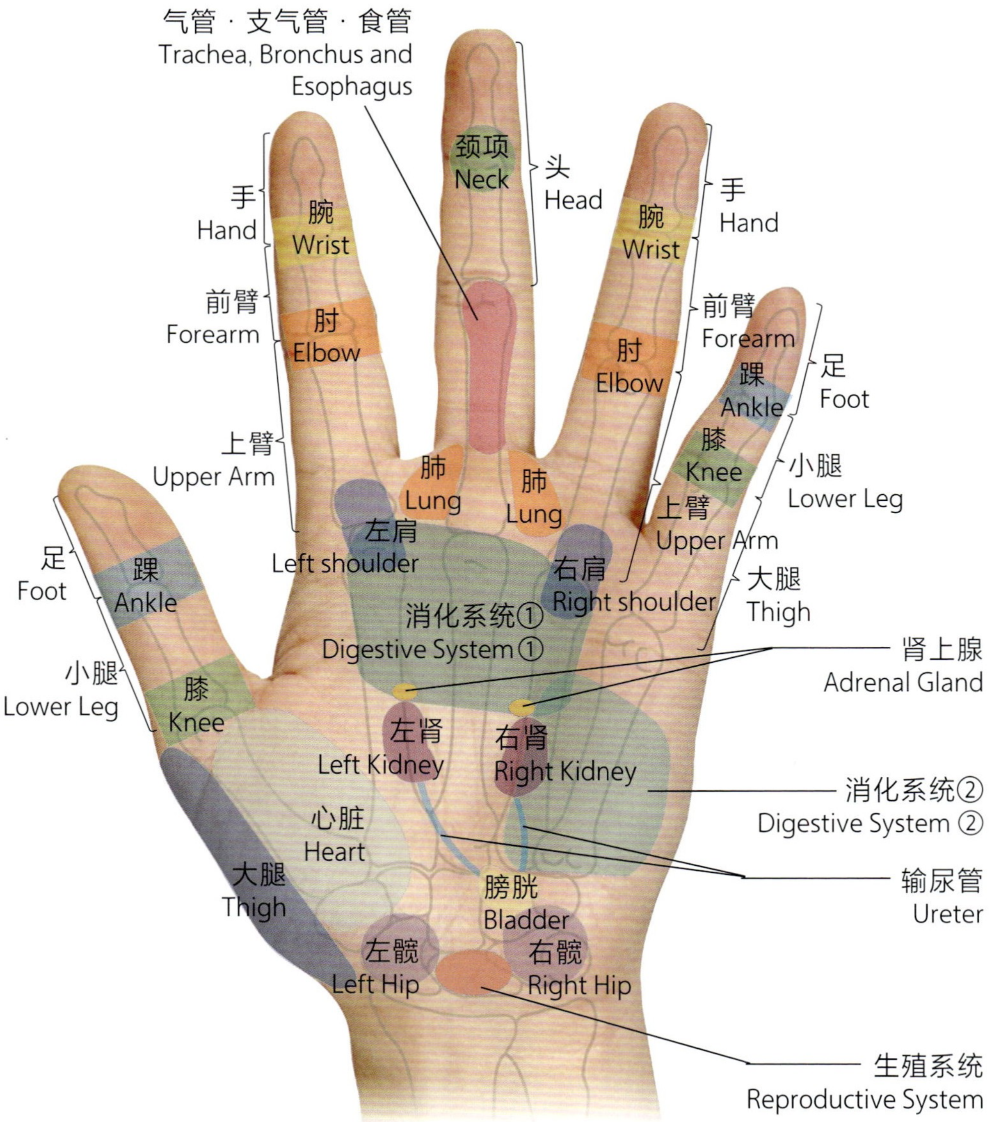

续表

全息区	定 位	反映疾病
踝	双手掌面和背面，拇指的指间关节和小指远侧指间关节	踝部疾病
小腿	双手掌面和背面，拇指近节指骨和小指中节指骨	小腿疾病
膝	双手掌面和背面，拇指掌指关节和小指的近侧指间关节	膝关节疾病
大腿	双手掌面和背面，拇指大鱼际桡侧缘，小指近节指骨及其近侧区域的尺侧缘	大腿疾病
髋	双手掌面大鱼际、小鱼际与腕横纹之间的区域，以及手背面与掌面相对应的区域，拇指侧为左髋区，小指侧为右髋区	髋部疾病

Continued

Holographic Zone	Location	Corresponding Diseases
Ankle	On the palm and back, the interphalangeal joint of the thumb and the distal interphalangeal joint of the little finger	Ankle diseases
Lower Leg	On the palm and back, the proximal phalange of thumb and the middle phalange of little finger	Leg diseases
Knee	On the palm and back, the metacarpal joint if thumb and proximal phalange joint of little finger	Knee joint diseases
Thigh	On the palm and back, the radial margin of the thumb's large fish's margin, the proximal phalange of little finger and ulnar margin of proximal region	Thigh diseases
Hip	The zone among large fish's margin, small fish's margin and wrist transverse crease on palms, and the corresponding region on the back. The thumb side as Left Hip and little finger side as Right Hip	Hip diseases

手背面全息区

Holographic Zone of the Back of the Hand

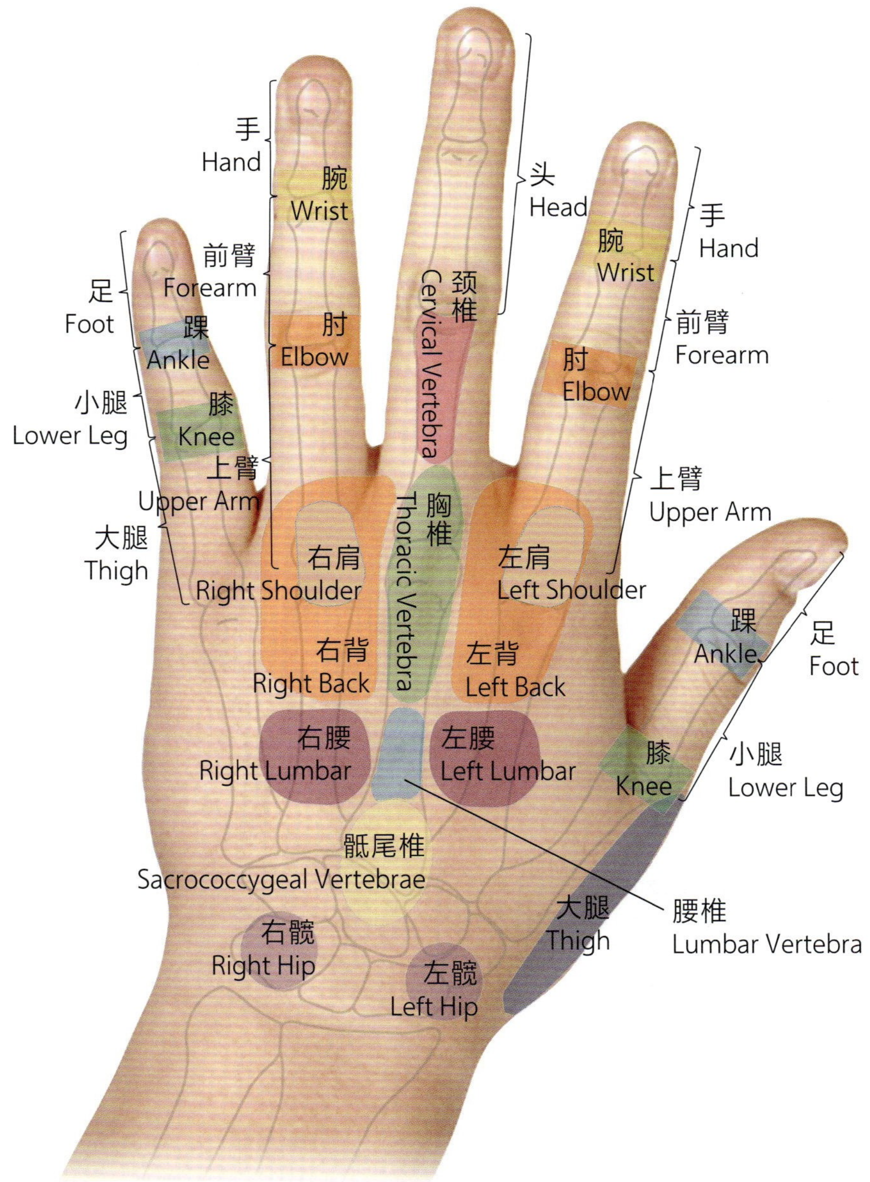

全身部位在手部的全息定位是诊病的基础，无论左手、右手均以靠大拇指侧为身体的左侧，靠小指侧为身体的右侧，以中指为身体的正中分界线。主要用于疾病的辅助诊断，提示相应部位可能存在的疾患。

全息穴	定 位	反映疾病
头	双手掌面和背面，中指远节及中节指骨。包括脑、眼、耳、鼻、口腔等区	相应的五官疾病
手	双手掌面和背面，食指、无名指的远节指骨	手部疾病
腕	双手掌面和背面，食指、无名指的远侧指间关节	手腕疾病
前臂	双手掌面和背面，食指、无名指的中节指骨	前臂疾病
肘	双手掌面和背面，食指、无名指的近侧指间关节	肘部疾病
上臂	双手掌面和背面，食指、无名指的近节指骨	上臂疾病
肩	双手掌面和背面，食指、无名指的掌指关节，食指掌指关节为左肩区，无名指掌指关节为右肩区	肩部疾病
足	双手掌面和背面，拇指、小指的远节指骨	足部疾病
踝	双手掌面和背面，拇指的指间关节和小指远侧指间关节	踝部疾病
小腿	双手掌面和背面，拇指近节指骨和小指中节指骨	小腿疾病

The holographic location of body parts in hands is the basis for diagnosis. Whatever left hand or right hand, the thumb side is regarded as the left side of the body, the little finger as the right side of the body and the middle finger as the center of the body. The holographic zone is mainly used for diagnosing disease, suggesting that the potential existed diseases in corresponding parts.

Holographic Zone	Location	Corresponding Diseases
Head	On the palm and back, the distal joint and middle joint of middle finger phalanges, including Brain, Eye, Ear, Nose, Oral Cavity and so on	Corresponding facial diseases
Hand	On the palm and back, the distal phalange of the index finger and ring finger	Hand diseases
Wrist	On the palm and back, the distal interphalangeal joint of the index finger and ring finger	Wrist diseases
Forearm	On the palm and back, the middle phalange of the index finger and ring finger	Forearm diseases
Elbow	On the palm and back, the proximal interphalangeal joint of the index finger and ring finger	Elbow diseases
Upper Arm	On the palm and back, the proximal phalange of the index finger and ring finger	Upper arm diseases
Shoulder	On the palm and back, metacarpal joint of the index finger and ring finger, the index finger as the Left Shoulder and the ring finger as the Right Shoulder	Shoulder diseases
Foot	On the palm and back, the distal phalange of the thumb and little finger	Foot diseases
Ankle	On the palm and back, the interphalangeal joint of the thumb and the distal interphalangeal joint of the little finger	Ankle diseases
Lower Leg	On the palm and back, the proximal phalange of thumb and the middle phalange of little finger	Lower leg diseases

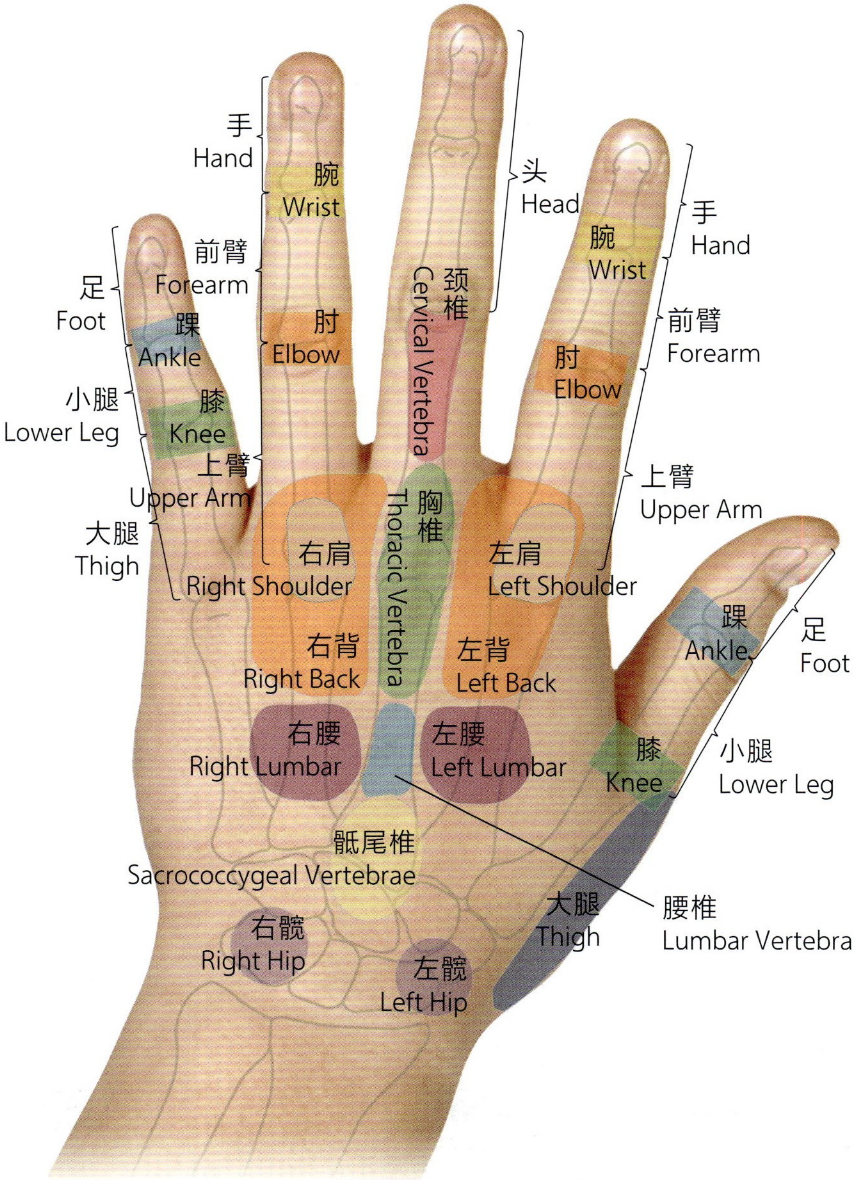

续表

全息穴	定 位	反映疾病
膝	双手掌面和背面，拇指掌指关节和小指的近侧指间关节	膝关节疾病
大腿	双手掌面和背面，拇指大鱼际桡侧缘，小指近节指骨及其近侧区域的尺侧缘	大腿疾病
髋	双手掌面大鱼际、小鱼际与腕横纹之间的区域，以及手背与掌面相对应的区域，拇指侧为左髋区，小指侧为右髋区	髋部疾病
颈椎	双手背面中指近节指骨远端 2/3 处	颈椎疾病
胸椎	双手背面中指近节指骨近端 1/3 至第 3 掌骨的远端 1/2 的区域	胸椎疾病
腰椎	双手背面，第 3 掌骨胸椎全息区与骶尾椎全息区之间	腰、腰肌及腰骶椎的疾病
骶尾椎	双手背面，第 3 掌骨近心端与腕骨关节之间的区域	骶尾椎疾病
背	胸椎全息区两侧的区域，拇指侧为左背区，小指侧为右背区	背部疾病
腰	腰椎全息区的两侧，拇指侧为左腰区，小指侧为右腰区	腰部疾病

Continued

Holographic Zone	Location	Corresponding Diseases
Knee	On the palm and back, the metacarpal joint if thumb and proximal phalange joint of little finger	Knee diseases
Thigh	On the palm and back, the radial margin of the thumb's large fish's margin, the proximal phalange of little finger and ulnar margin of proximal region	Thigh diseases
Hip	The zone among large fish's margin, small fish's margin and wrist transverse crease on palms, and the corresponding region on the back. The thumb side as Left Hip and little finger side as Right Hip	Hip diseases
Cervical Vertebra	The back of hand, the 2/3 part of distal side of the middle proximal phalange	Cervical diseases
Thoracic Vertebra	The back of hand, the zone form the 1/3 part of the proximal side of the middle proximal phalange to the 1/2 part of the distal side the 3rd metacarpal	Thoracic diseases
Lumbar Vertebra	The back of hand, between the Thoracic Vertebra holographic zone and Sacrococcygeal Vertebrae holographic zone of the 3rd metacarpal	Disease of lumbar; psoas muscle and lumbosacral vertebra
Sacrococcygeal Vertebrae	The back of hand, between the proximal side of the 3rd metacarpal and carpal joint	Sacrococcygeal diseases
Back	Both sides of the Thoracic Vertebra holographic zone, the thumb side as the Left Back, and little finger side as the Right Back	Back diseases
Lumbar	Both sides of the Lumbar Vertebra holographic zone, the thumb side as the Left Lumbar, and little finger side as the Right Lumbar	Lumbar diseases

手部全息穴
Holographic Acupoints of the Hand

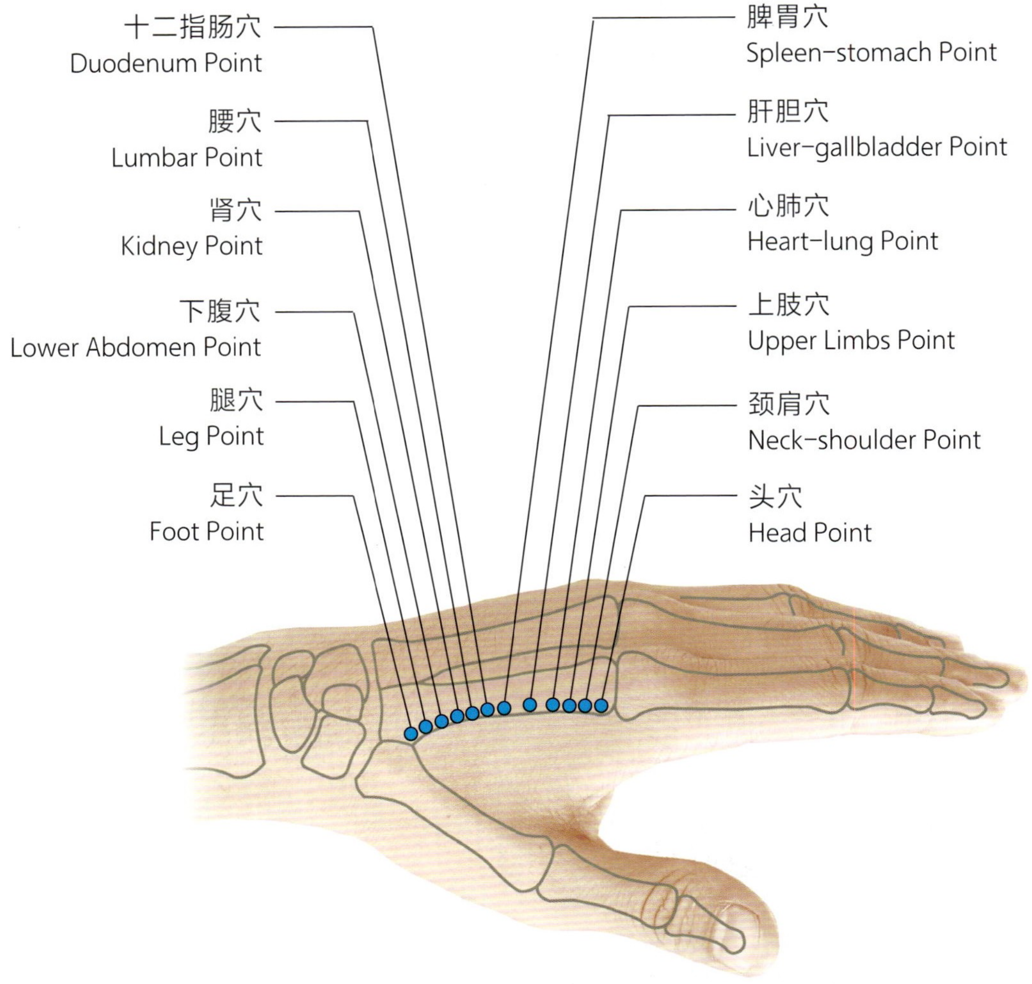

第 2 掌骨全息穴

Holographic acupoints of the 2nd metacarpal

第 2 掌骨全息穴为第 2 掌骨体桡侧从远心端的头穴到近心端的足穴依次排列的 12 穴。可以拇指端或指甲掐按全息穴来辅助治疗相应脏器的疾病。

全息穴	定 位	主 治
头穴	食指掌指关节桡侧后的凹陷处（第 2 掌骨头桡侧）	头痛、牙痛、三叉神经痛、急性结膜炎及头面、眼、耳、鼻、口、牙、脑等部位疾病
颈肩穴	第 2 掌骨体远端桡侧，头穴与上肢穴之间，将头穴与心肺穴间三等分，远端分点即是	颈肩、甲状腺、咽喉、气管上段、食管上段等部位疾病
上肢穴	第 2 掌骨体远端桡侧，颈穴与心肺穴之间，将头穴与心肺穴间三等分，近端分点即是	肩、上肢、肘、腕、手及食管中段的疾病
心肺穴	第 2 掌骨体远端桡侧，头穴与脾胃穴连线中点	心、肺、胸、乳房、气管下段、食管下段及背部疾病
肝胆穴	第 2 掌骨体中段桡侧，脾胃穴与心肺穴连线中点	肝胆疾病
脾胃穴	第 2 掌骨体中段桡侧，头穴与足穴连线中点	脾、胃及胰脏疾病

The 2nd metacarpal holographic points are the sequence of 12 points on the radial side of the 2nd metacarpal from the distal end of the Head point to the proximal end of the Foot point. You can press holographic points with thumb or fingernail to help the adjuvant treatment of the corresponding organs disease.

Holographic Points	Location	Indications
Head Point	The depression of the radial side after the index finger metacarpophalangeal joint(radial side of the head of the 2nd metacarpal)	Headache; toothache; trigeminal neuralgia; acute conjunctivitis and diseases of head, eyes, ears, nose, mouth, teeth, brain and other parts
Neck-shoulder Point	The radial side of the distal end of the 2nd metacarpal, between Head point and Upper Limbs point, trisecting the zone between Head point and Heart-lung point, that is the distal point	Diseases of neck-shoudler, thyroid, throat, upper trachea, upper esophagus and other parts
Upper Limbs Point	The radial side of the distal end of the 2nd metacarpal, between Neck point and Heart-lung point, trisecting the zone between Head point and Heart-lung point, that is the proximal point	Diseases of the shoulder, upper limbs, elbow, wrist, hand and middle esophagus
Heart-lung Point	The radial side of the distal end of the 2nd metacarpal, the midpoint of the Head point and Spleen-stomach point	Diseases of heart, lung, chest, breast; lower respiratory tract; lower esophagus and back
Liver-gallbladder Point	The radial side of the middle part of the 2nd metacarpal, the midpoint of Spleen-stomach point and Heart-lung point	Liver-gallbladder diseases
Spleen-stomach Point	The radial side of the middle part of the 2nd metacarpal, the midpoint of Head point and Foot point	Spleen, stomach and pancreas diseases

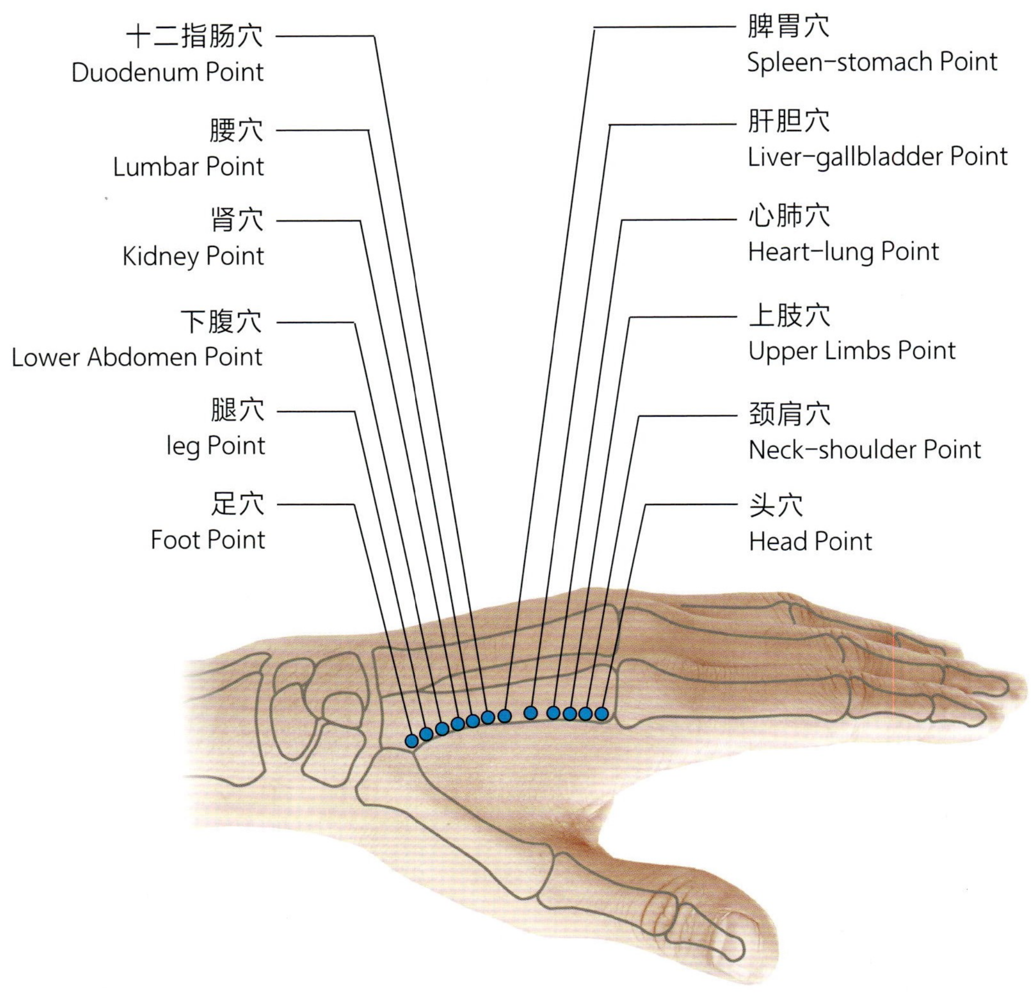

第 2 掌骨全息穴

Holographic acupoints of the 2nd metacarpal

续表

全息穴	定 位	主 治
十二指肠穴	第 2 掌骨体中段桡侧，脾胃穴与腰穴之间，将脾胃穴与肾穴间三等分，远端分点即是	十二指肠及结肠右曲部疾病
腰穴	第 2 掌骨体近端桡侧，十二指肠穴与肾穴之间，将脾胃穴与肾穴间三等分，近端分点即是	腰扭伤、腰腿痛、大肠与小肠疾病
肾穴	第 2 掌骨体近端桡侧，脾胃穴与足穴连线中点	肾、输尿管、大肠、小肠疾病
下腹穴	第 2 掌骨体近端桡侧，肾穴与腿穴之间，将肾穴与足穴间三等分，远端分点即是	下腹部、骶尾部、子宫、膀胱、结肠、直肠、阑尾、卵巢、阴道、睾丸、尿道、肛门等部位疾病
腿穴	第 2 掌骨体近端桡侧，下腹穴与足穴之间，将肾穴与足穴间三等分，近端分点即是	臀部、股部、膝关节等下肢疾病
足穴	第 2 掌骨底桡侧	足、踝部疾病

Continued

Holographic Points	Location	Indications
Duodenum Point	The radial side of the middle part of the 2nd metacarpal, between Spleen-stomach point and Lumbar point, trisecting the zone between Spleen-stomach point and Kidney point, that is the distal point	Duodenum diseases and colonic right flexure zone diseases
Lumbar Point	The radial side of the proximal end of the 2nd metacarpal, between Duodenum point and Kidney point, trisecting the zone between Spleen-stomach point and Kidney point, that is the proximal point	Lumbar sprain; lumbocrural pain; large intestine and small intestine diseases
Kidney Point	The radial side of the proximal end of the 2nd metacarpal, the midpoint of Spleen-stomach point and Foot point	Kidney, ureter, large intestine, small intestine diseases
Lower Abdomen Point	The radial side of the proximal end of the 2nd metacarpal, between Kidney point and Leg point, trisecting the zone between Kidney point and Foot point, that is the distal point	Diseases of lower abdomen, sacrococcygeal, uterus, bladder, colon, rectum, appendix, ovary, vagina, testis, urethra, anus and other parts
Leg Point	The radial side of the proximal end of the 2nd metacarpal, between Lower Abdomen point and Foot point, trisecting the zone between Kidney point and Foot point, that is the proximal point	Hip, thigh, knee and other lower limb diseases
Foot Point	The radial side of the end of the 2nd metacarpal	Foot and ankle diseases

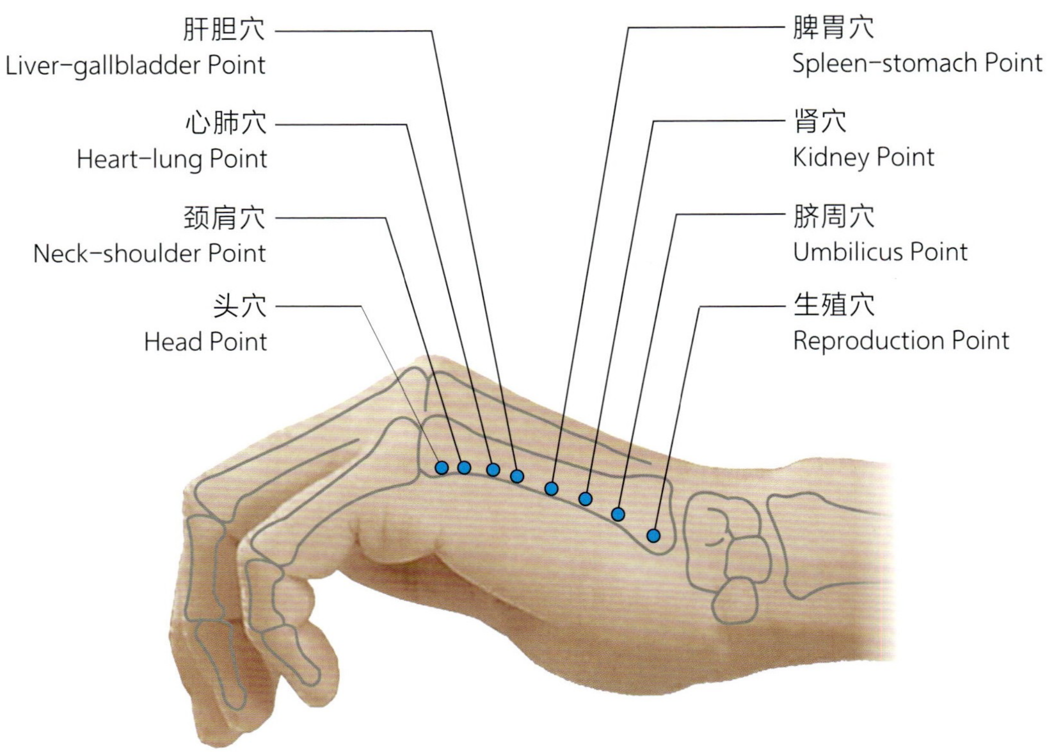

第 5 掌骨全息穴

Holographic acupoints of the 5th metacarpal

第 5 掌骨全息穴为第 5 掌骨尺侧从远心端的头穴到近心端的生殖穴依次排列的 8 穴。可以拇指端或指甲掐按全息穴来辅助治疗相应脏器的疾病。

全息穴	定 位	主 治
头穴	第 5 掌骨头尺侧	头面部及眼、耳、鼻、口腔等疾病
颈肩穴	第 5 掌骨体远端尺侧，头穴与心肺穴连线中点	肩周炎、肩部扭伤、落枕、颈椎病等
心肺穴	第 5 掌骨体远端尺侧，头穴与脾胃穴连线中点	心、肺、气管及胸背部疾病
肝胆穴	第 5 掌骨体中段尺侧，心肺穴与脾胃穴连线中点	肝胆疾病
脾胃穴	第 5 掌骨体中段尺侧，头穴与生殖穴连线中点	脾、胃、肌肉疾病
肾穴	第 5 掌骨体近端尺侧，脾胃穴与脐周穴之间，将脾胃穴与生殖穴间三等分，远端分点即是	遗尿等肾、膀胱及生殖系统疾病
脐周穴	第 5 掌骨体近端尺侧，肾穴与生殖穴之间，将脾胃穴与生殖穴间三等分，近端分点即是	结肠炎、小肠炎、腰扭伤
生殖穴	第 5 掌骨基底部尺侧	生殖系统疾病、肛周疾病、腰腿痛等

The 5th metacarpal holographic points are the sequence of 8 points on the ulnar side of the 5th metacarpal from the distal end of the Head point to the proximal end of the Reproductive point. You can press holographic points with thumb or fingernail to help the adjuvant treatment of the corresponding organs disease.

Holographic Points	Location	Indications
Head Point	The ulnar side of the head of the 5th metacarpal	Head and face, eyes, ears, nose, oral cavity and other diseases
Neck-shoulder Point	The ulnar side of the 5th metacarpal distal end, the midpoint between Head point and Heart-lung point	Periarthritis of shoulder; shoulder sprain; stiff neck; cervical spondylopathy; and so on
Heart-lung Point	The ulnar side of the 5th metacarpal distal end, the midpoint between Head point and Spleen-stomach point	Diseases of the heart, lung, trachea and chest and back
Liver-gallbladder Point	The ulnar side of the 5th metacarpal middle part, the midpoint between Heart-lung point and Spleen-stomach point	Hepatobiliary diseases
Spleen-stomach Point	The ulnar side of the 5th metacarpal middle part, the midpoint between Head point and Reproduction point	Spleen, stomach, muscle diseases
Kidney Point	The ulnar side of the 5th metacarpal proximal end, between Spleen-stomach point and Umbilicus point, trisecting the zone between Spleen-stomach point and Reproduction point, that is the distal point	Enuresis and diseases of kidney, bladder and reproductive system
Umbilicus Point	The ulnar side of the 5th metacarpal proximal end, between Kidney point and Reproductive point, trisecting the zone between Spleen-stomach point and Reproduction point, that is the proximal point	Colitis; enteritis; lumbar sprain
Reproduction Point	The ulnar side of the end of the 5th metacarpal	Reproductive system diseases; perianal disease; lumbus and leg pain; and so on

手部常用穴位

Common Hand Acupoints

手太阴肺经
Lung Meridian of Hand-Taiyin

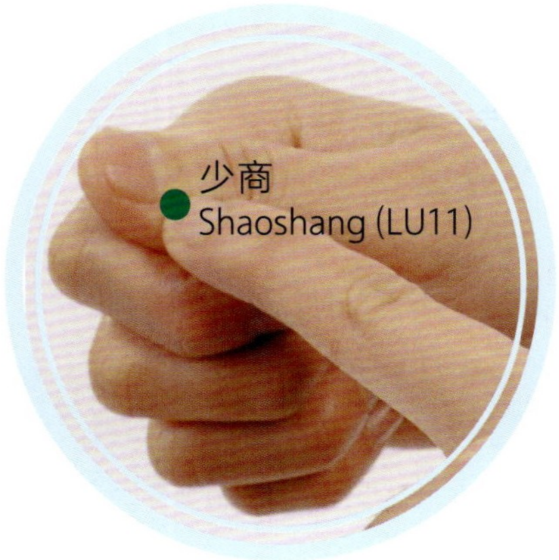

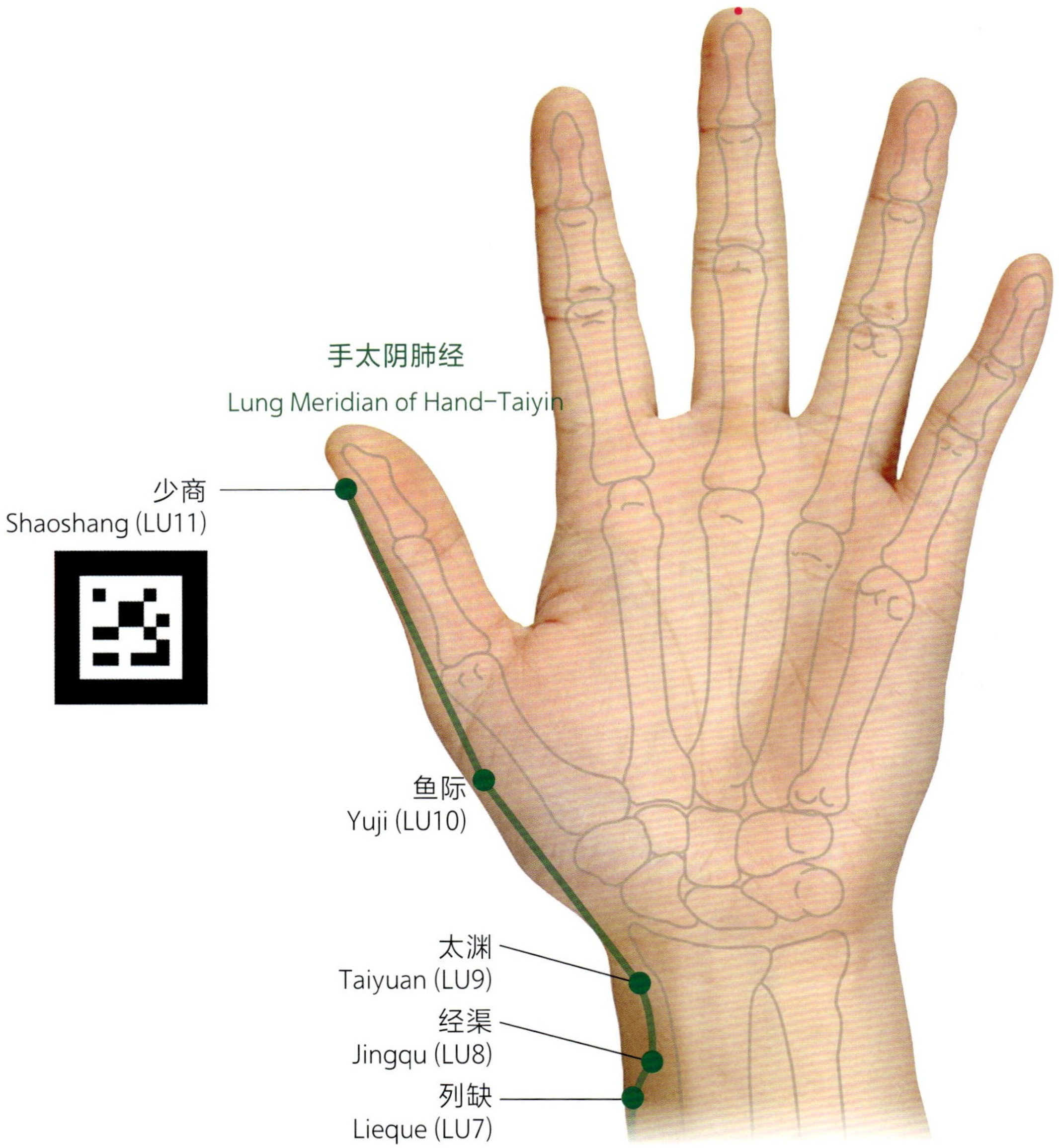

手掌面穴位

Acupoints in palm

穴位		定位	主治
手太阴肺经	少商	在手拇指末节桡侧，距指甲角 0.1 寸	咽喉肿痛、咳嗽、鼻出血、发热、昏迷
	鱼际	在手拇指本节（第 1 掌指关节）后凹陷处，第 1 掌骨中点桡侧，赤白肉际处	咳嗽、咯血、咽喉肿痛、声音嘶哑、发热
	太渊	在腕掌侧横纹桡侧，桡动脉搏动处	咳嗽、气喘、咳血、胸痛、咽喉肿痛、腕臂疼痛
	经渠	在前臂掌面桡侧，桡骨茎突与桡动脉之间凹陷处，腕横纹上 1 寸。桡骨茎突为桡骨下端的骨性隆起	咳嗽、气喘、胸痛、咽喉肿痛、腕关节疼痛
	列缺	在前臂桡侧缘，桡骨茎突上方，腕横纹上 1.5 寸，肱桡肌与拇长展肌腱之间。将两手虎口相交，一手食指压在另一手的桡骨茎突上，食指尖端到达的凹陷处，即为本穴	急性上呼吸道感染、头痛、颈项疼痛、咳嗽、气喘、咽喉肿痛、口眼歪斜、牙痛

Acupoints		Location	Indications
Lung Meridian of Hand-Taiyin	Shaoshang (LU11)	On the radial side of the thumb end and 0.1 cun lateral and posterior to the corner of the fingernail	Sore throat; cough; nasal bleeding; fever; coma
	Yuji (LU10)	The depression of the 1st thumb metacarpal, the midpoint of the radial side of the 1st metacarpal, the border of the red and white skin	Cough; hemoptysis; sore throat; hoarseness; fever
	Taiyuan (LU9)	On the radial side of carpal crease, where the radial pulse is throbbing	Cough; asthma; hemoptysis; chest pain; sore throat; wrist and arm pain
	Jingqu (LU8)	The radial side of the palm aspect of forearm, the depression between the styloid process of the radius and radial pulse, and 1 cun above the carpal crease. The styloid process of the radius is a bony eminence of lower radius	Cough; asthma; chest pain; sore throat; wrist pain
	Lieque (LU7)	Radial side of forearm, superior to the styloid process of the radius, and 1.5 cun above the carpal crease; or, between the brachioradialis muscle and abductor pollicis longus. When the index finger and the thumbs of both hands are crossed with the index finger of 1 hand placed on the styloid process of the radius of the other, the depression right under the tip of the index finger is the acupoint	Acute upper respiratory tract infection; headache; neck pain; cough; asthma; sore throat; facial palsy; toothache

手厥阴心包经
Pericardium Meridian of Hand-Jueyin

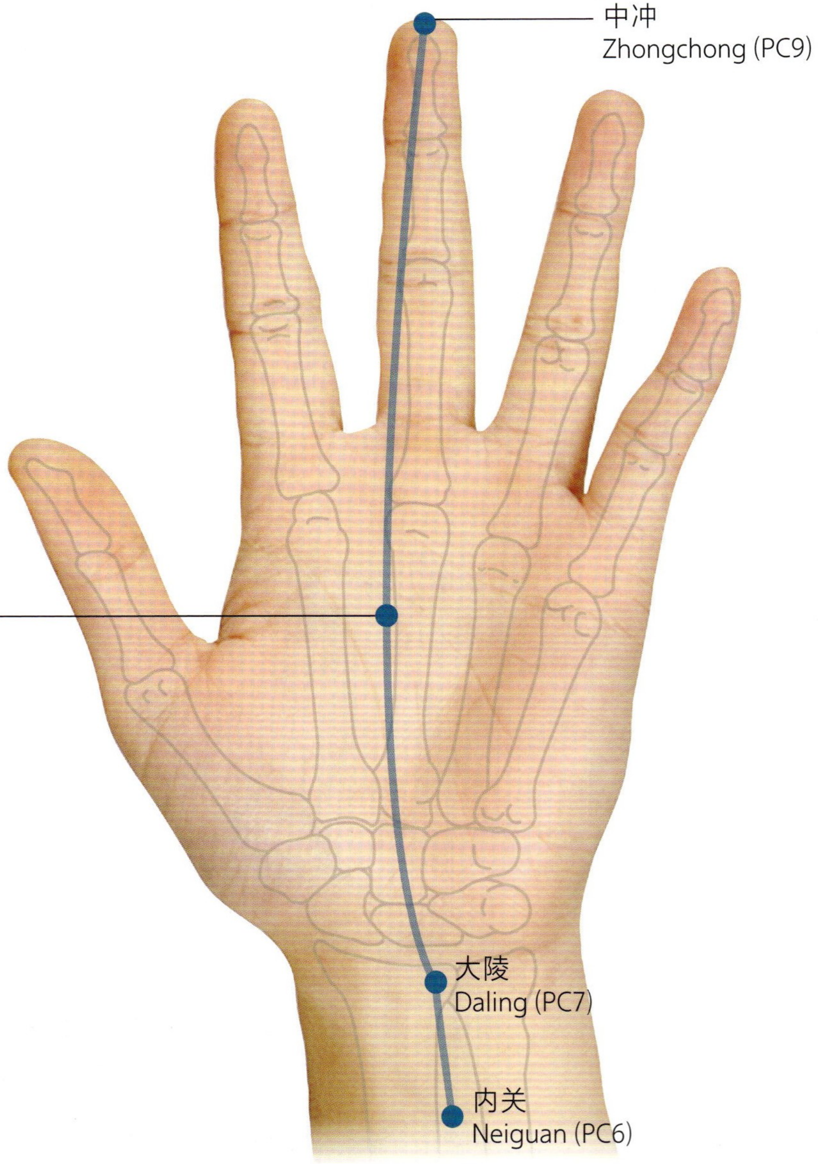

手掌面穴位
Acupoints in palm

穴位		定位	主治
手厥阴心包经	中冲	在手中指末节尖端中央	中风昏迷、中暑昏厥、心绞痛、烦躁
	劳宫	在手掌心，在第 2、3 掌骨之间偏于第 3 掌骨，握拳屈指时中指尖处	中风昏迷、中暑、心绞痛、口腔溃疡、口臭
	大陵	在腕掌横纹的中点处，掌长肌腱与桡侧腕屈肌腱之间。掌长肌腱和桡侧腕屈肌腱为手臂掌侧可触摸到的两条条索状筋，握拳屈腕时明显可见	心绞痛、心悸、胃痛、呕吐、胸胁痛、腕关节疼痛
	内关	在前臂掌侧，腕横纹上 2 寸即三横指（食指、中指、无名指），掌长肌腱与桡侧腕屈肌腱（手臂内侧可触摸到的两条条索状筋，握拳用力屈腕时可见）之间	心绞痛，心悸，胸痛，胃痛，呕吐，打嗝，失眠，眩晕，中风后遗症，哮喘，偏头痛，发热，产后血晕（产后突然头晕眼花，不能坐起，甚至不省人事），肘、臂疼痛

Acupoints		Location	Indications
Pericardium Meridian of Hand-Jueyin	Zhongchong (PC9)	On the midpoint of the middle fingertip	Wind stroke coma; heatstroke syncope; angina; irritability
	Laogong (PC8)	On the center of palm, between the 2nd and the 3rd metacarpal and near the 3rd one, at the tip of the middle finger when make a fist and the finger is flexed	Wind stroke coma; heatstroke; angina; oral ulcer; halitosis
	Daling (PC7)	On the midpoint of the metacarpal and carpal crease, between the tendons of palmaris longus and the flexor tendon of the ulnar wrist. The 2 tendons in the palm side of arm can be touched 2 strips of cord like ribs, hard fist and wrist flexion is visible	Angina; palpitation; stomachache; vomiting; chest and rib pain; wrist pain
	Neiguan (PC6)	The palm aspect of the forearm, 2 cun, 3 horizontal fingers (index finger, middle finger, ring finger) above the carpal crease. Between the tendons of palmaris longus and the flexor tendon of the ulnar wrist(the medial arm can touch the 2 strips of cord like ribs, hard fist and wrist flexion is visible)	Angina; palpitation; chest pain; stomachache; vomiting; hiccups; insomnia; dizziness; sequelae of wind stroke; asthma; migraine; fever; postpartum fainting (postpartum sudden dizziness, unable to sit up, and even become unconscious); elbow and arm pain

手少阴心经
Heart Meridian of Hand-Shaoyin

经外奇穴
Extra Point

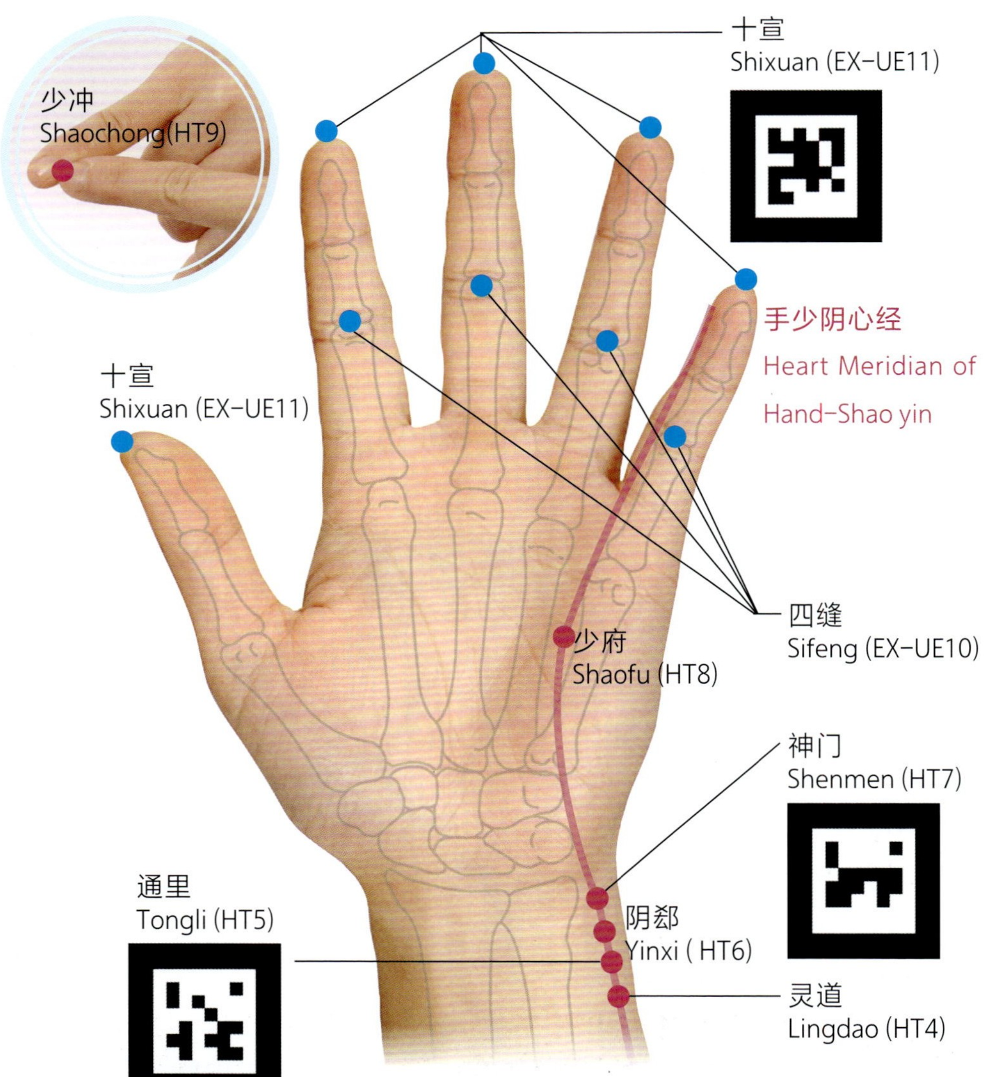

手掌面穴位
Acupoints in palm

穴位		定位	主治
手少阴心经	少冲	在小指末节桡侧，距指甲角 0.1 寸	心悸、胸闷、胸胁痛、发热、昏迷
	少府	在手掌面，第 4、5 掌骨之间，握拳时小指尖处	心悸、胸痛、小便不利、遗尿、阴部瘙痒
	神门	在腕部，腕掌侧横纹尺侧端，尺侧腕屈肌腱（手前臂手小指侧可触摸到的大筋）的桡侧凹陷处	胸闷、心悸、健忘、失眠、胸胁痛
	阴郄	在前臂掌侧，尺侧腕屈肌腱的桡侧缘，腕横纹上 0.5 寸	心绞痛、惊悸、吐血、声音嘶哑
	通里	在前臂掌侧，尺侧腕屈肌腱的桡侧缘，腕横纹上 1 寸	心悸，声音嘶哑，腕、臂疼痛
	灵道	在前臂掌侧，尺侧腕屈肌腱的桡侧缘，腕横纹上 1.5 寸	胸闷、声音嘶哑
经外奇穴	十宣	两手十指尖端，距指甲约 0.1 寸，左右手各 5 穴	中风（卒中）、中暑、各种原因所致的休克、小儿惊厥、扁桃体炎、咽喉肿痛、指端麻木
	四缝	手掌面，第 2 指至第 5 指的近侧指间关节横纹中点，左右手各 4 穴	小儿消化不良、腹胀、腹泻、丹毒、小儿百日咳、小儿遗尿

Acupoints		Location	Indications
Heart Meridian of Hand-Shaoyin	Shaochong(HT9)	On the radial aspect of the little finger, and 0.1 cun lateral to the corner of the fingernail	Palpitation; thoracic oppression; chest and rib pain; fever; coma
	Shaofu (HT8)	On the palm, between the 4th, the 5th metacarpal, the point on the little fingertip when making a fist	Palpitations; chest pain; dysuria; enuresis; genital itching
	Shenmen (HT7)	The wrist, on the palmar ulnar end of the transverse crease of the wrist, and on the radial aspect of the depression of flexor tendon of the ulnar wrist (the touchable large tendon in the forearm of little finger side)	Thoracic oppression; palpitation; forgetfulness; insomnia; chest and rib pain
	Yinxi (HT6)	The palm aspect of the forearm, on the radial aspect of the flexor tendon of the ulnar wrist, and 0.5 cun above the carpal crease	Angina; palpitation; hematemesis; hoarseness
	Tongli (HT5)	The palm aspect of the forearm, on the radial aspect of the flexor tendon of the ulnar wrist, and 1 cun above the carpal crease.	Palpitation; hoarseness; wrist and arm pain
	Lingdao (HT4)	The palm aspect of the forearm, on the radial aspect of the flexor tendon of the ulnar wrist, and 1.5 cun above the carpal crease	Thoracic oppression; hoarness
Extra Points	Shixuan (EX-UE11)	On the tips of the 10 fingers, 0.1 cun among fingernail, 5 points on each side	Wind stroke; heatstroke; shock due to various causes; child fright reversal; tonsillitis; sore throat; finger numbness
	Sifeng (EX-UE10)	On the palm, the midpoint of the proximal interphalangeal joint transverse crease of the 2nd to the 5th finger	Children with indigestion; bloating; diarrhea; infantile erysipelas; whooping cough; infantile enuresis

手阳明大肠经
Large Intestine Meridian of Hand-Yang ming

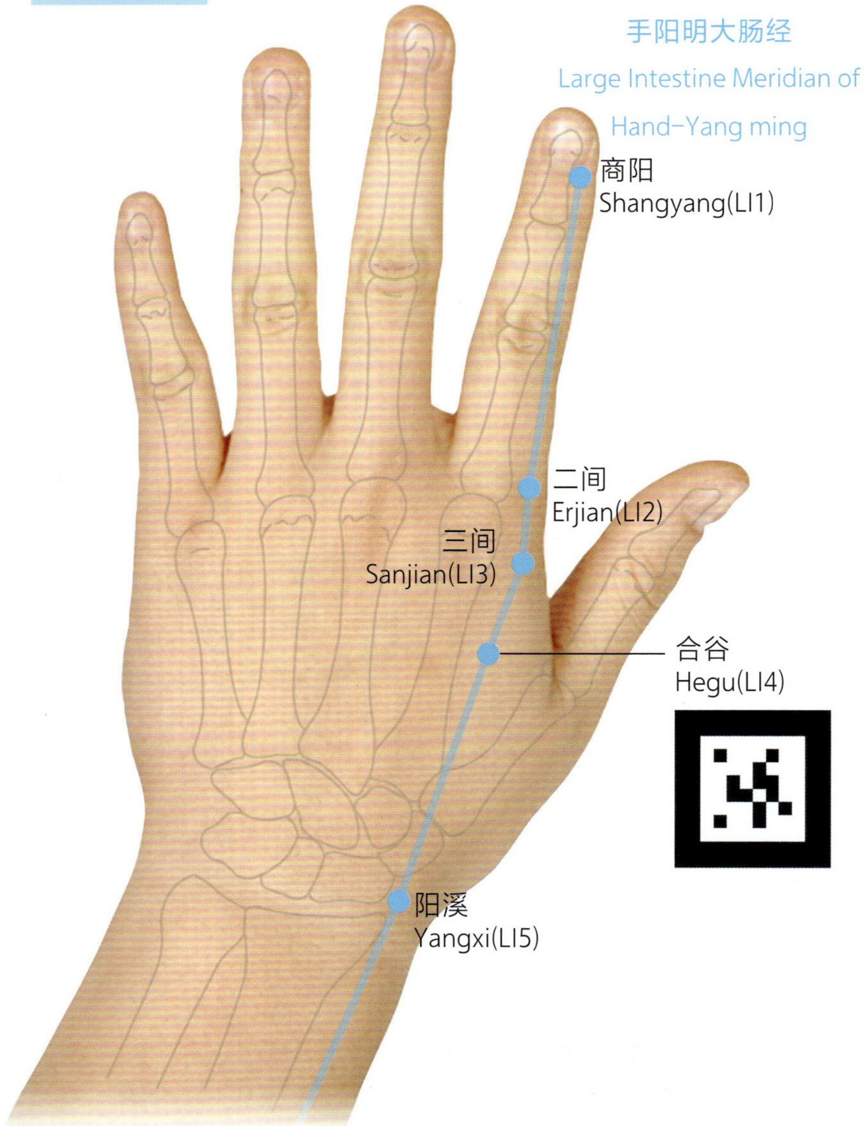

手背面穴位
Acupoints on the dorsum of the hand

穴位		定位	主治
手阳明大肠经	商阳	在手食指末节桡侧，距指甲角 0.1 寸	耳聋、牙痛、咽喉肿痛、手指麻木、发热、昏迷
	二间	微握拳，在第 2 掌指关节前桡侧凹陷中。微握拳，手食指掌指关节前缘桡侧皮肤皱褶顶点，触之有凹陷处即为本穴	目昏、鼻出血、牙痛、口歪、咽喉肿痛、发热
	三间	微握拳，在第 2 掌指关节后，桡侧凹陷处。微握拳，在手食指掌指关节后缘桡侧的掌背交界线（赤白肉际）处	咽喉肿痛、牙痛、腹胀、眼痛、腹泻
	合谷	在手背，第 1、2 掌骨间，第 2 掌骨桡侧的中点处。可以另一手的拇指指间横纹正对虎口指蹼缘上，屈指，拇指尖所指之处	头痛、目赤肿痛、鼻出血、牙痛、口眼歪斜、耳聋、流行性腮腺炎、咽喉肿痛、发热、多汗、腹痛、便秘、经闭
	阳溪	在腕背横纹桡侧，拇指掌骨的根部凹陷处。手拇指向上翘时，当拇短伸肌腱与拇长伸肌腱之间的凹陷中	头痛、目赤肿痛、耳聋、耳鸣、齿痛、咽喉肿痛、腕关节疼痛

Acupoints		Location	Indications
Large Intestine Meridian of Hand-Yangming	Shangyang(LI1)	On the radial side of the thumb end, and 0.1 cun lateral and posterior to the corner of the fingernail	Deafness; toothache; sore throat; finger numbness; fever; coma
	Erjian(LI2)	Slightly making a fist, in the depression of the radial side before the 2nd metacarpal; slightly making a fist, wrinkle vertex on the radial side of the front of index finger metacarpophalangeal joint, touching with depression is the point	Dizziness; epistaxis; toothache; mouth askew; sore throat; fever
	Sanjian(LI3)	Slightly making a fist, in the depression of the radial side after the 2nd metacarpal; slightly making a fist, on the margin of palm and back (border of the red and white skin) on the radial side of the trailing edge of index finger metacarpophalangeal joint	Sore throat; toothache; abdominal distension; sore eyes; diarrhea
	Hegu(LI4)	The dorsum of the hand, between the 1st and the 2nd metacarpal bone, and in the midpoint of the radial side of the metacarpal bone; or the transverse crease of interphalangeal joint of one thumb are placed on the stretched tiger's mouth between the thumb and index finger of the other hand, and the acupoint is where the tip of the thumb touches	Headache; redness,swelling and pain of eyes; epistaxis; toothache; deviated eyes and mouth; deafness; mumps; sore throat; fever; sweating; abdominal pain; constipation; amenorrhea
	Yangxi(LI5)	On the radial side of the dorsal transverse crease of the wrist, the depression part in the root of the thumb metacarpal, and in the depression between the tendons of the short extensor and long extensor of the thumb when the thumb is upward	Headache; redness,swelling and pain of eyes; deafness; tinnitus; toothache; sore throat; wrist pain

手少阳三焦经

Triple Energizer Meridian of Hand-Shaoyang

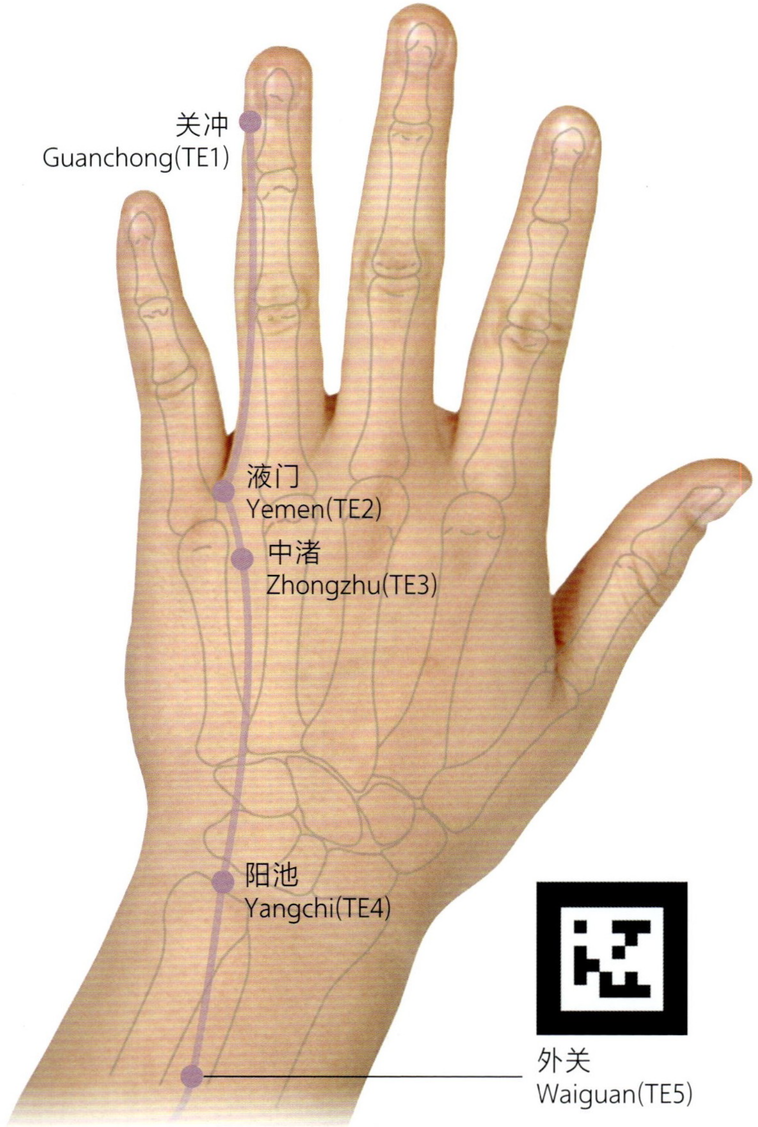

手背面穴位

Acupoints on the dorsum of the hand

手少阳三焦经

Triple Energizer Meridian of Hand-Shaoyang

穴位		定位	主治
手少阳三焦经	关冲	在手无名指末节尺侧，距指甲角 0.1 寸（指寸）	头痛、耳聋、耳鸣、发热、烦躁
	液门	在手背部，第 4 、5 指间，指蹼缘后方赤白肉际处	头痛、目赤、耳痛、耳鸣、耳聋、咽喉炎、手臂痛
	中渚	在手背部，无名指本节（掌指关节）的后方，第 4 、5 掌骨间凹陷处	头痛、头晕、耳聋、耳鸣、肩背及肘臂酸痛、手指不能屈伸、发热
	阳池	在腕背横纹中，指总伸肌腱的尺侧缘凹陷处。由第 4 掌骨向上推至腕关节横纹的凹陷处	腕关节疼痛、肩臂痛、耳聋、糖尿病、口干、咽喉炎
	外关	在前臂背侧，阳池与肘尖的连线上，腕背横纹上 2 寸即三横指（食指、中指、无名指），尺骨与桡骨之间	发热、头痛、颊痛、耳聋、耳鸣、目赤肿痛、肩背痛、肘臂屈伸不利、手指疼痛

Acupoints		Location	Indications
Triple Energizer Meridian of Hand-Shaoyang	Guanchong(TE1)	The ulnar side of the ring finger' s last phalange, 0.1 cun away from the nail angle	Headache; deafness; tinnitus; fever; irritability
	Yemen(TE2)	On the dorsum of the hand, between the 4th and 5th finger, on the border of the red and white skin after fingerweb edge	Headache; red eyes; earache; tinnitus; deafness; sore throat; arm pain
	Zhongzhu(TE3)	On the dorsum of the hand, posterior to the metacarpophalangeal joint, in the depression between the 4th and the 5th metacarpal bones	Headache; dizziness; deafness; tinnitus; pain in the shoulder and elbow; finger flexion and extension inability; fever
	Yangchi(TE4)	On transverse crease of wrist back, the depression of the ulnar side of the extensor tendon. The depression can be pressed from the 4th metacarpal to the carpal transverse crease	Wrist pain; shoulder pain; deafness; diabetes; dry mouth; sore throat
	Waiguan(TE5)	Dorsal side of forearm, on the line joining Yangchi(TE4) and the tip of elbow, 2 cun above the dorsal transverse crease, between the ulna and radius	Fever; headache; cheek pain; deafness; tinnitus; redness, swelling and pain of eyes; shoulder pain; elbow flexion and extension disadvantages; finger pain

手太阳小肠经
Small Intestine Meridian of hand-Taiyang

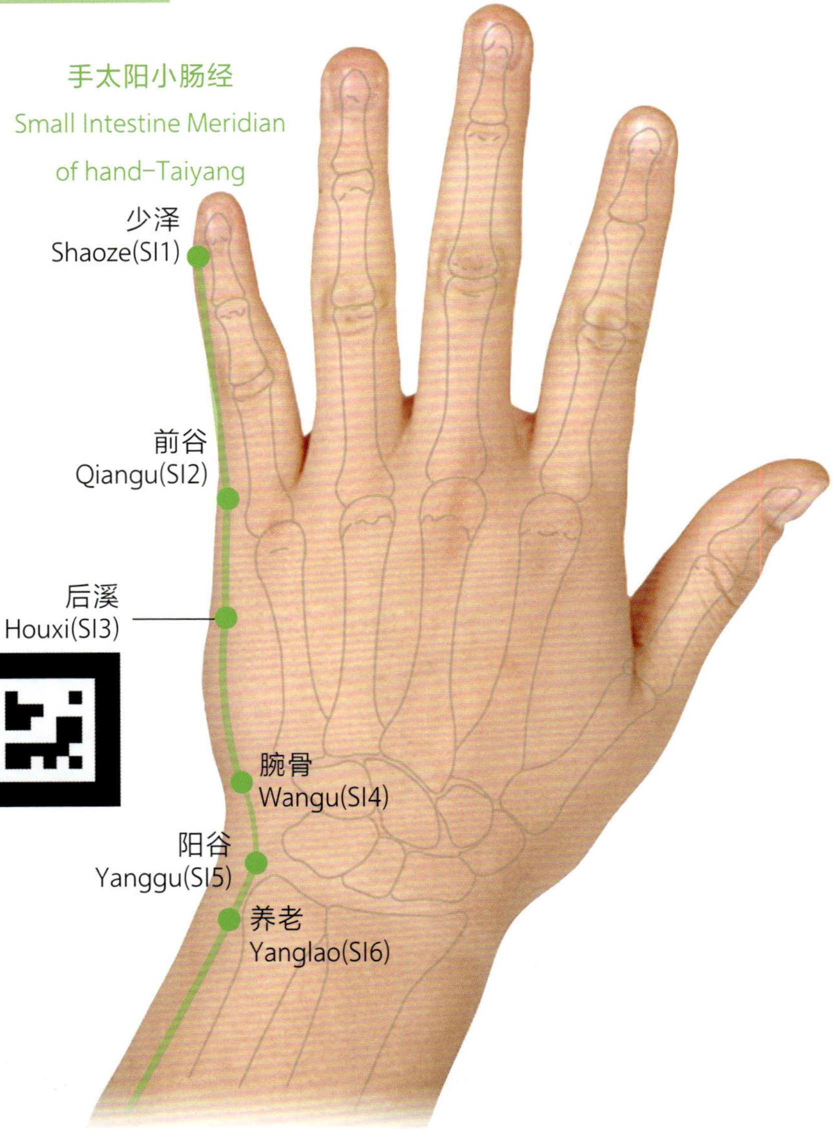

手背面穴位
Acupoints on the dorsum of the hand

穴位		定位	主治
手太阳小肠经	少泽	在小指末节尺侧，距指甲角 0.1 寸	头痛、咽喉肿痛、乳腺炎、乳汁少、昏迷、发热
	前谷	在手掌尺侧，微握拳，小指本节（第 5 指掌关节）前的掌指横纹头赤白肉际处	头痛、目痛、耳鸣、咽喉肿痛、乳汁少、发热
	后溪	在手掌尺侧，微握拳，小指本节（第 5 指掌关节）后的远侧掌横纹头赤白肉际，掌纹消失处	头痛、耳聋、咽喉肿痛、腰背痛、疟疾、手指及肘臂疼痛
	腕骨	在手掌尺侧，第 5 掌骨基底与钩骨之间的凹陷处，赤白肉际	头项疼痛、耳鸣、黄疸、发热、手指及腕关节疼痛
	阳谷	在手腕尺侧，尺骨茎突与三角骨之间的凹陷处	头痛、目眩、耳鸣、耳聋、发热、腕关节疼痛
	养老	在前臂背面尺侧，尺骨小头（手腕尺侧可摸到的一凸起高骨）近端桡侧凹陷中。掌心向下，用另一手指按在此高骨上，然后掌心转向胸部，手指滑入的骨缝中，即为本穴	视物不清、肩背及肘臂酸痛

Acupoints		Location	Indications
Small Intestine Meridian of Hand-Taiyang	Shaoze(SI1)	On the ulnar aspect of the little finger, and 0.1 cun lateral to the corner of the fingernail	Headache; sore throat; mastitis; breast milk deficiency; coma; fever
	Qiangu(SI2)	On the ulnar aspect of the palm, slightly making a fist, on the border of the red and white skin of the metacarpal crease in front of the 5th metacarpophalangeal joint, and at the border of the red and white skin	Headache; eye pain; tinnitus; sore throat; breast milk deficiency; fever
	Houxi(SI3)	On the ulnar aspect of the palm, slightly making a fist, on the border of the red and white skin of the distal side of metacarpal crease posterior to the 5th metacarpophalangeal joint, where the palmar crease disappear	Headache; deafness; sore throat; back pain; malaria; finger and arm pain
	Wangu(SI4)	On the ulnar aspect of the palm, the depression between the end of the 5th metacarpal and hamatum, border of the red and white skin	Head pain; tinnitus; jaundice; fever; finger and wrist pain
	Yanggu(SI5)	On the ulnar aspect of the palm, the depression between the styloid process of the ulna and pyramidal bone	Headache; dizziness; tinnitus; deafness; fever; pain in the wrist
	Yanglao(SI6)	On the ulnar side of the forearm dorsum, the depression on the radial side of the proximal end of capitulum ulnae (a raised high bone of the wrist ulnar side which can be touched). Palm down, with another finger in this high bone, and then palm to the chest, the finger slipped into the bone seam, that is the point	Blurred vision; shoulder and elbow pain

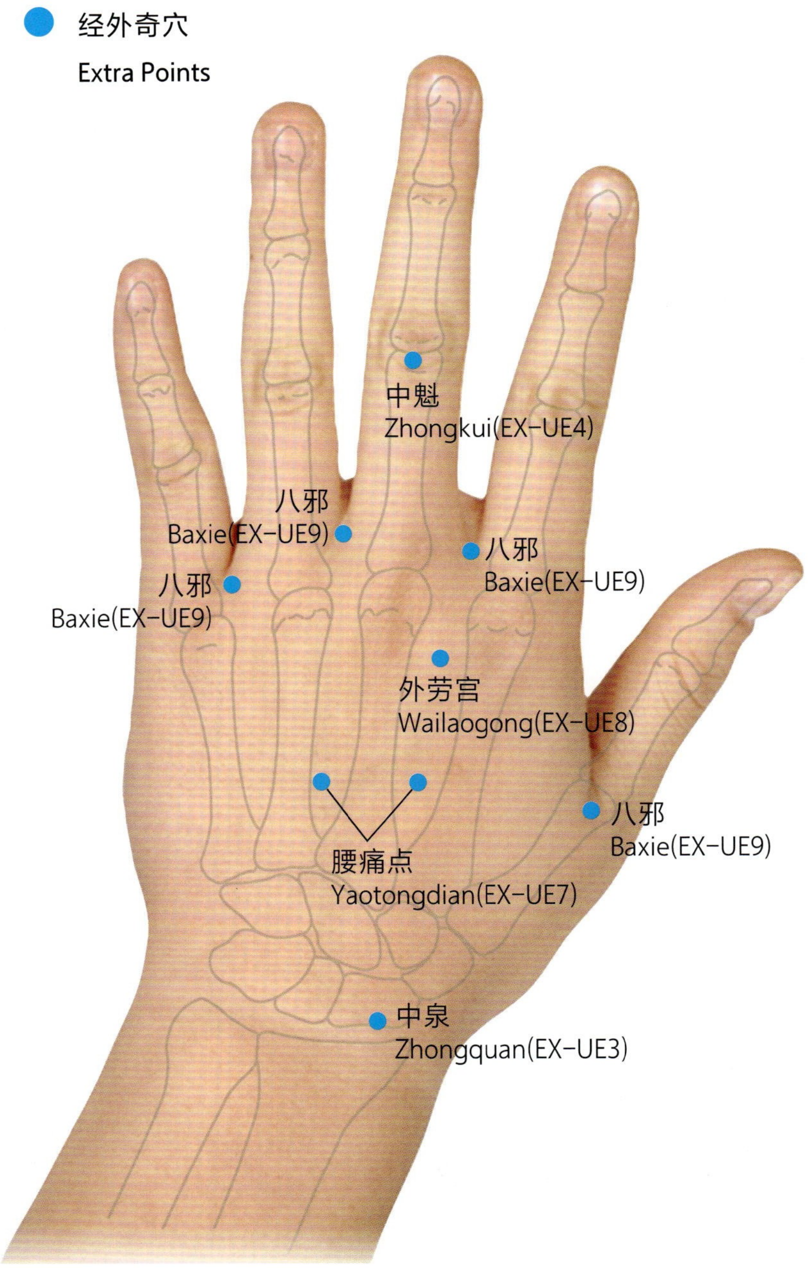

手背面穴位
Acupoints on the dorsum of the hand

穴位		定位	主治
经外奇穴	外劳宫	在手背第 2、3 掌骨间，从掌指关节向后 0.5 寸，即拇指半横指处	急慢性胃肠炎、掌指麻痹、五指不能屈伸、新生儿破伤风、手背红肿疼痛
	腰痛点	在手背，第 2、3 掌骨及第 3、4 掌骨之间，腕横纹与掌指关节中点处，左右各 2 穴	急性腰扭伤
	中泉	手腕背侧横纹中，指总伸肌腱桡侧的凹陷处	胃痛、吐血、胸闷、咳嗽、气喘、胃痉挛、腹胀、中风（卒中）、脑出血、腕关节炎、前臂诸肌痉挛或麻痹、癔病、疝气
	八邪	手指背侧，微握拳，第 1~5 指间，指蹼缘后方赤白肉际处，左右共 8 穴	烦躁、头痛、颈项痛、咽痛、齿痛、毒蛇咬伤、破伤风、手指麻木、手背红肿等手指关节疾病
	中魁	手中指背侧近侧指间关节的中点处	打嗝、呕吐、反胃、食欲不振、鼻出血、牙痛、白癜风

Acupoints		Location	Indications
Extra Points	Wailaogong(EX-UE8)	On the dorsum of the hand, between the 2nd and the 3rd metacarpal bones, 0.5 cun posterior to the metacarpophalangeal joint	Acute and chronic gastroenteritis; metacarpophalangeal paralysis; finger flexion and extension inability; neonatal tetanus; sore red swollen hands
	Yaotongdian(EX-UE7)	On the dorsum of the hand, between the 2nd and the 3rd and between the 3th and the 4th metacarpal bones, at the midpoint of the line joining the transverse crease of the wrist and the metacarpophalangeal joint, 2 acupoints each hand	Acute lumbar sprain
	Zhongquan(EX-UE3)	On the transverse crease of the wrist dorsum, the depression on the radial side of extensor tendon	Stomach pain; vomiting; chest pain; cough; asthma; stomach cramps; abdominal distension; wind stroke (Zu-zhong); cerebral hemorrhage; wrist arthritis; forearm muscles spasm or paralysis; hysteria; hernia
	Baxie(EX-UE9)	On the dorsum of the hand, slightly making a fist, among the 1st to the 5th finger, on the border of the red and white skin after fingerweb edge, 8 points in all	Irritability; headache; neck pain; sore throat; toothache; snake bites; tetanus; numbness of the finger; red swollen hands and other finger joints diseases
	Zhongkui(EX-UE4)	Midpoint of the dorsal middle finger's proximal interphalangeal joint	Hiccups; vomiting; nausea; loss of appetite; epistaxis; toothache; vitiligo

超简单手部穴位按摩

Super-easy Massage in Hand acupoints

少商

用拇指指尖掐揉该穴位，力度可稍重，每分钟 30~50 下。同法按揉对侧少商穴

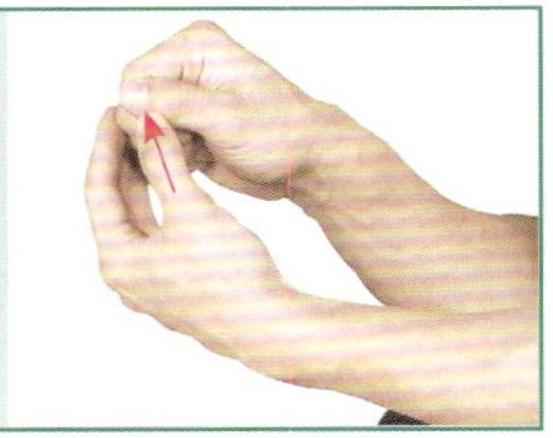

鱼际

用拇指按揉鱼际穴 2 分钟，力度稍重。同法按揉对侧鱼际穴。每日 2 次

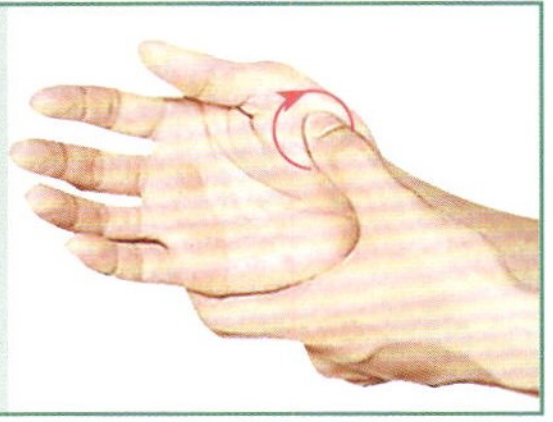

太渊

用拇指按压太渊穴，停留片刻后放松，反复 5~6 下，力度稍重。同法按压对侧太渊穴。每日 2 次

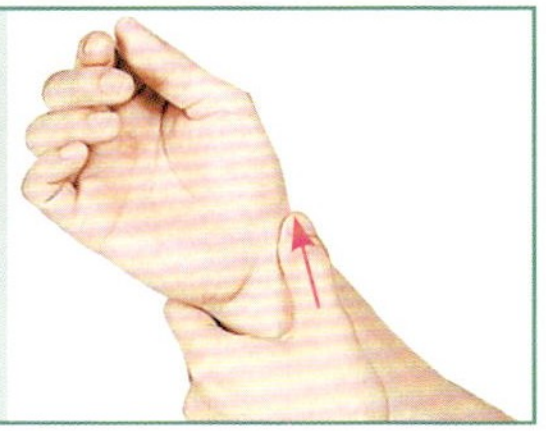

列缺

用拇指按揉列缺穴 2 分钟，力度稍重。同法按揉对侧列缺穴。每日 2 次

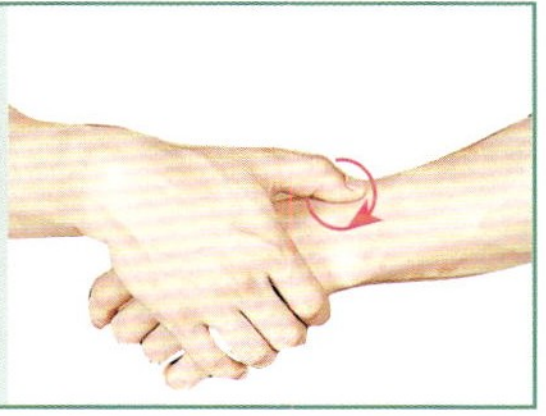

劳宫

用拇指按揉劳宫穴 2 分钟，力度稍重。同法按揉对侧劳宫穴。每日 2 次

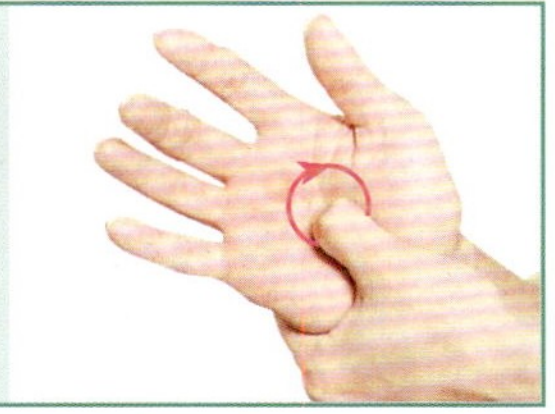

大陵

用拇指稍用力按压大陵穴，停留片刻后放松，反复 5~6 下。同法按压对侧大陵穴。每日 2 次

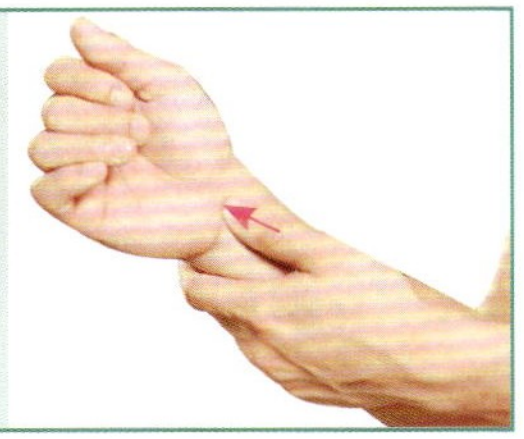

内关

用拇指稍用力按压内关穴，停留片刻后放松，反复 5~6 下。同法按压对侧内关穴。每日 2 次

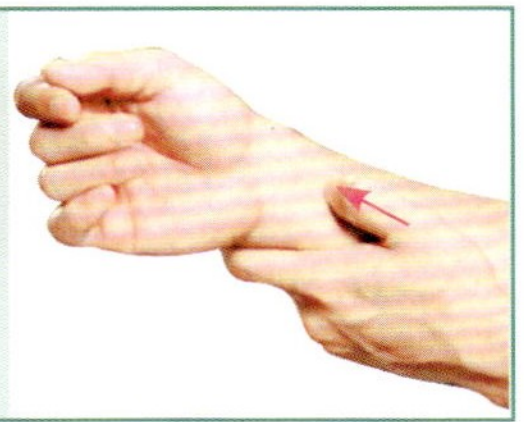

少府

用拇指稍用力按压少府穴，停留片刻后放松，反复 5~6 下。同法按压对侧少府穴。每日 2 次

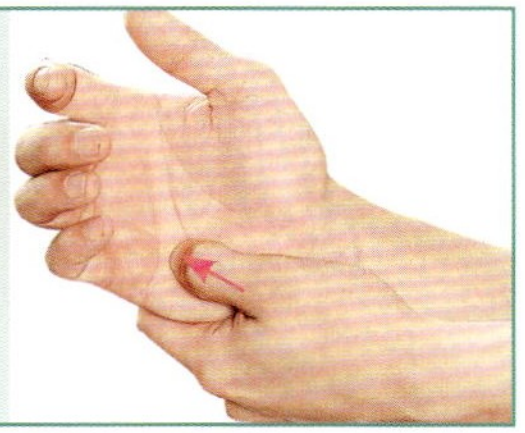

神门

用拇指稍用力按压神门穴，停留片刻后放松，反复 5~6 下。同法按压对侧神门穴。每日 2 次

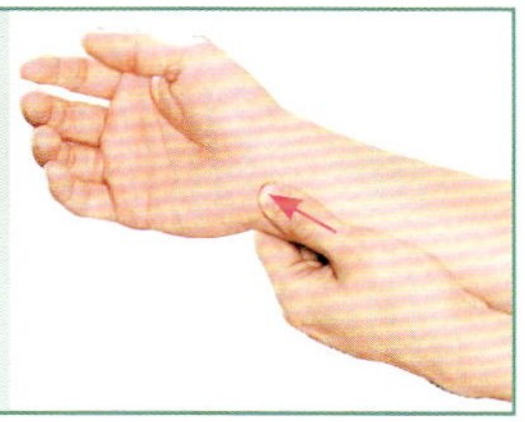

商阳

用拇指指尖掐揉该穴位，力度可稍重，每分钟 30~50 下。同法按揉对侧商阳穴

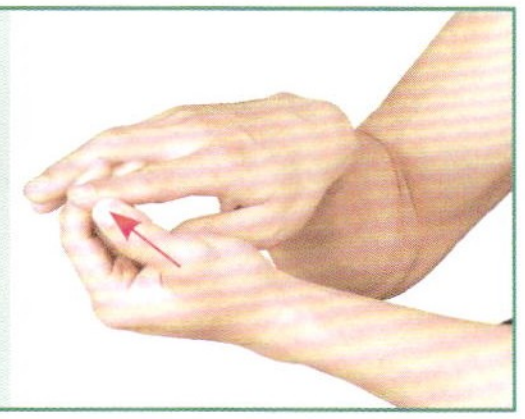

Shaoshang (LU11)

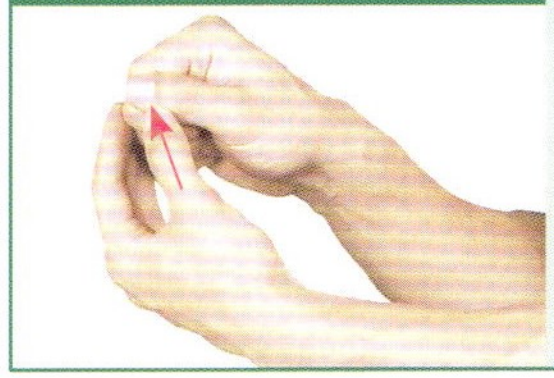

Pinching and rubbing with fingertip of the thumb for 30 to 50 times. Strength can be slightly heavier. The same method to knead the contralateral acupoints

Yuji (LU10)

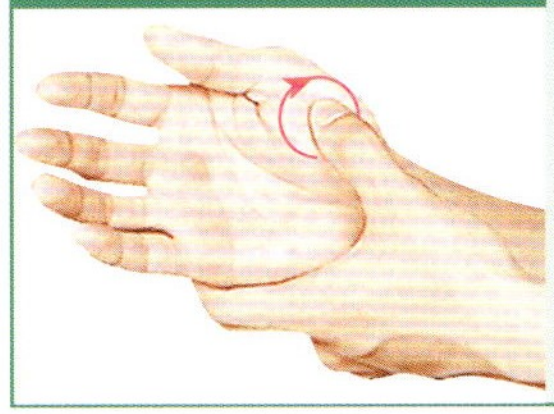

Kneading Yuji (LU10) with thumb for 2 minutes. Strength can be slightly heavier. The same method to knead the contralateral acupoints

Taiyuan (LU9)

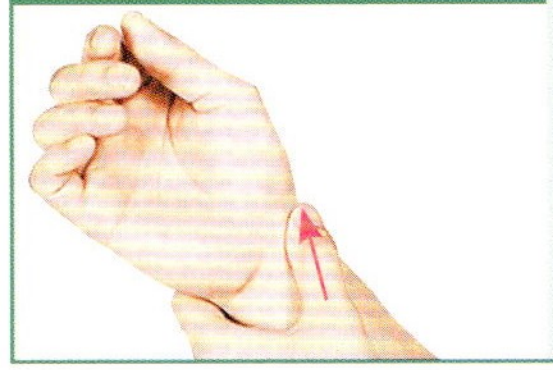

Pressing Taiyuan (LU9) with thumb, keep it for a while and relax. Repeat it for 5 to 6 times, strength can be slightly heavier. The same method to press the contralateral acupoint, 2 times each day

Lieque (LU7)

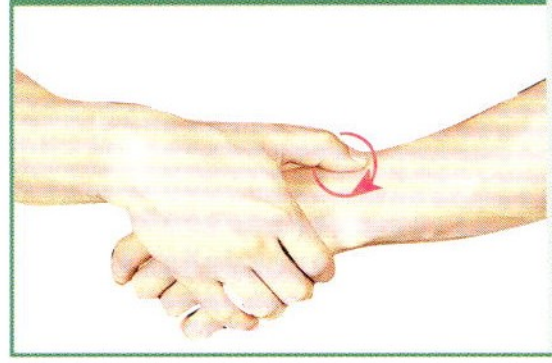

Kneading Lieque (LU7) with thumb for 2 minutes, strength can be slightly heavier. The same method to knead the contralateral acupoint, 2 times each day

Laogong (PC8)

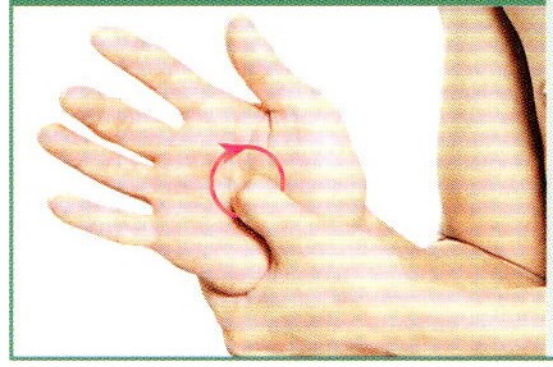

Kneading Laogong (PC8) with thumb for 2 minutes, strength can be slightly heavier. The same method to knead the contralateral acupoint, 2 times each day

Daling (PC7)

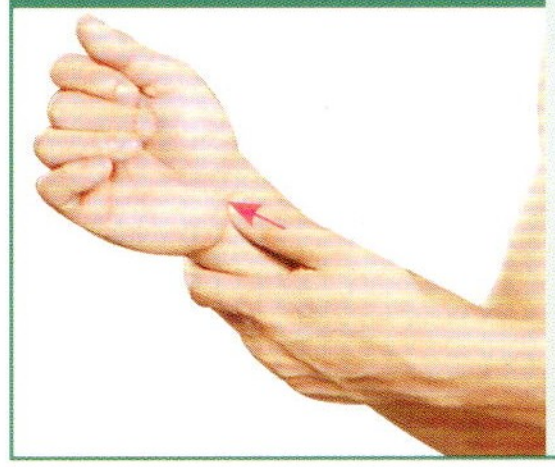

Pressing Daling (PC7) in heavier strength with thumb, keep it for a while and relax. Repeat it for 5 to 6 times. The same method to press the contralateral acupoint, 2 times each day

Neiguan (PC6)

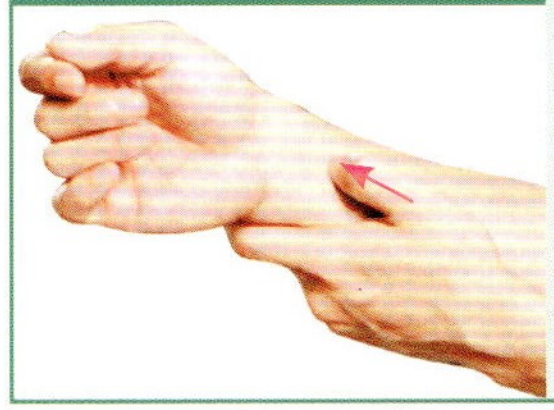

Pressing Neiguan (PC6) in heavier strength with thumb, keep it for a while and relax. Repeat it for 5 to 6 times. The same method to press the contralateral acupoint, 2 times each day

Shaofu (HT8)

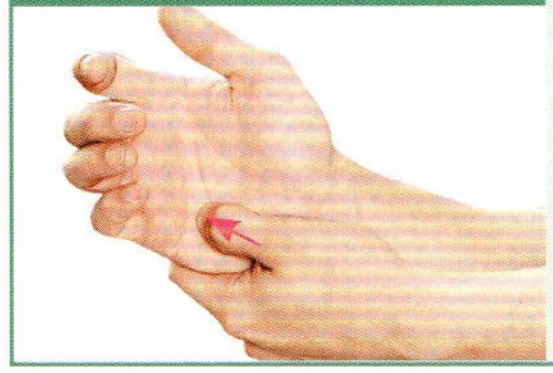

Pressing Shaofu (HT8) in heavier strength with thumb, keep it for a while and relax. Repeat it for 5 to 6 times. The same method to press the contralateral acupoint, 2 times each day

Shenmen (HT7)

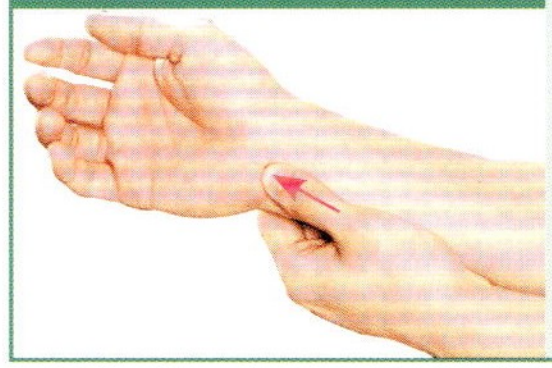

Pressing Shenmen (HT7) in heavier strength with thumb, keep it for a while and relax. Repeat it for 5 to 6 times. The same method to press the contralateral acupoint, 2 times each day

Shangyang(LI1)

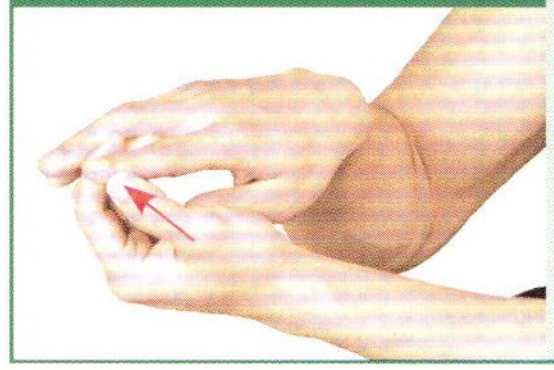

Pinching and rubbing with fingertip of the thumb, strength can be slightly heavier, 30 to 50 times each minute. The same method to knead the contralateral acupoint

合谷

用拇指用力按压合谷穴，停留片刻后放松，反复 5~6 下。同法按压对侧合谷穴。每日 2 次

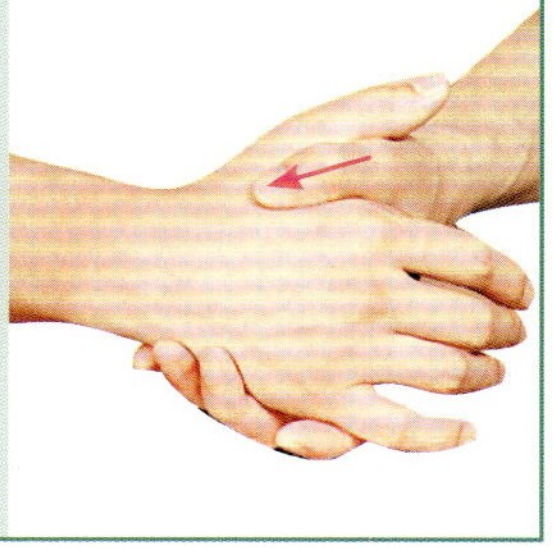

外关

用拇指稍用力按压外关穴，停留片刻后放松，反复 5~6 下。同法按压对侧外关穴。每日 2 次

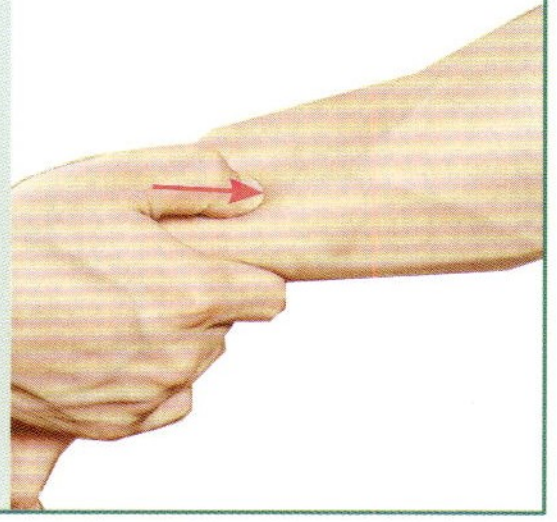

少泽

用拇指指尖掐揉少泽穴，力度可稍重，每分钟 30~50 下。同法按揉对侧少泽穴。每日 2 次

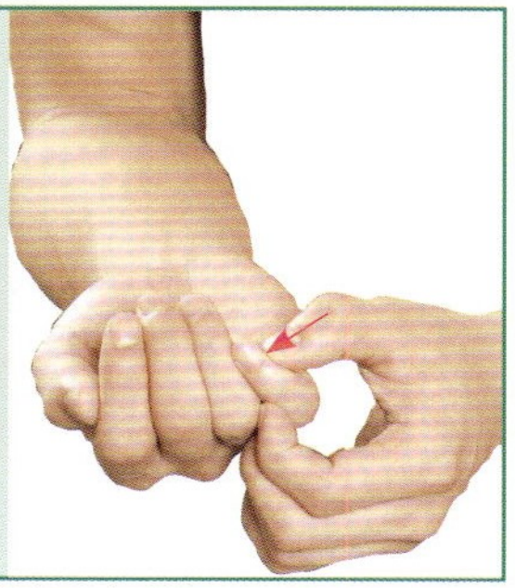

十宣

先用拇指指甲掐按十宣穴 30 下，掐后再按揉 30 下，力度稍重

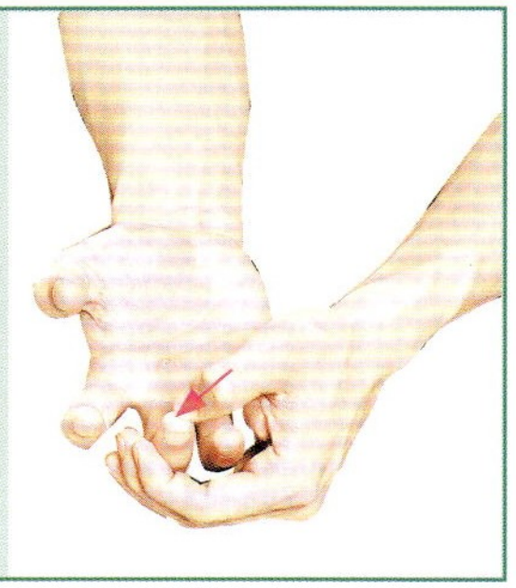

腰痛点

用拇指点揉腰痛点 2 分钟，力度适中。每日 2 次

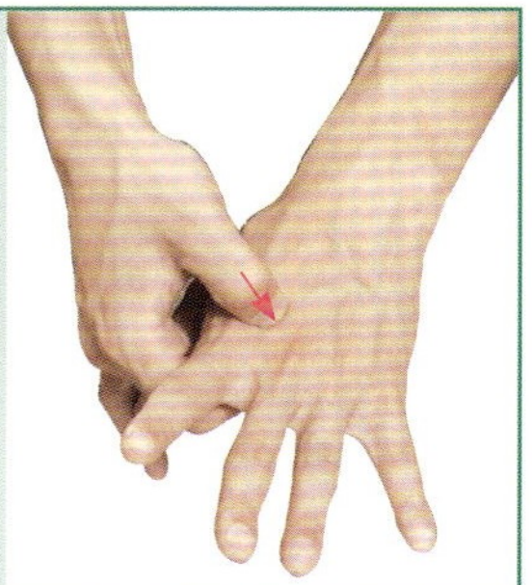

Hegu(LI4)

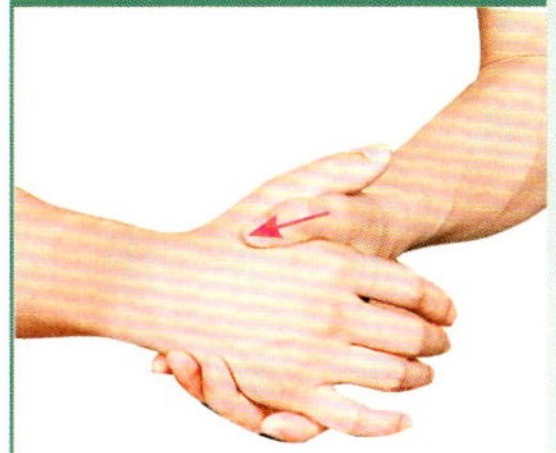

Pressing Hegu(LI4) in heavier strength with thumb, keep it for a while and relax. Repeat it for 5 to 6 times. The same method to press the contralateral acupoint, 2 times each day

Waiguan(TE5)

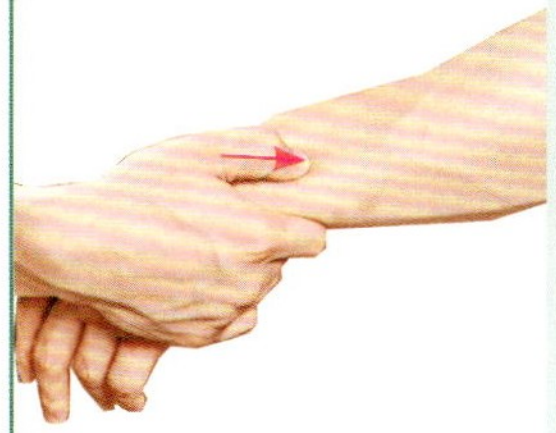

Pressing Waiguan(TE5) in heavier strength with thumb, keep it for a while and relax. Repeat it for 5 to 6 times. The same method to press the contralateral acupoint, 2 times each day

Shaoze(SI1)

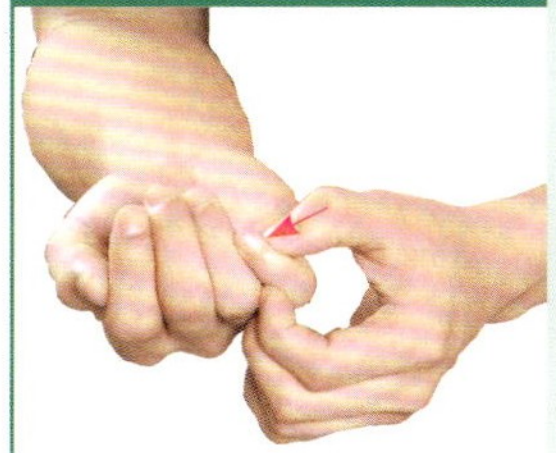

Pinching and rubbing Shaoze(SI1) with fingertip of the thumb, strength can be slightly heavier, 30 to 50 times each minute. The same method to knead the contralateral acupoint

Shixuan (EX-UE11)

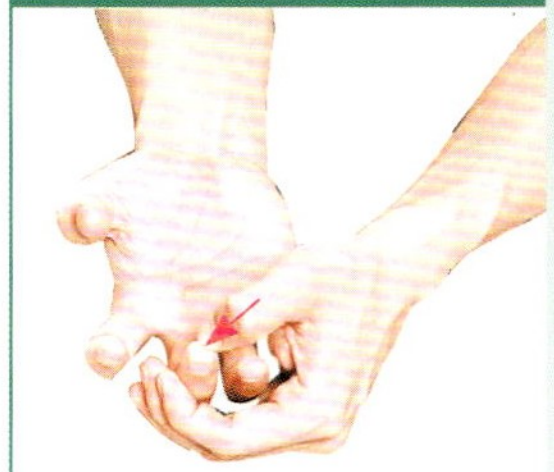

Fingernail pressing Shixuan (EX-UE11) with fingernail of the thumb for 30 times, and then kneading for 30 times. Strength can be slightly heavier

Yaotongdian (EX-UE7)

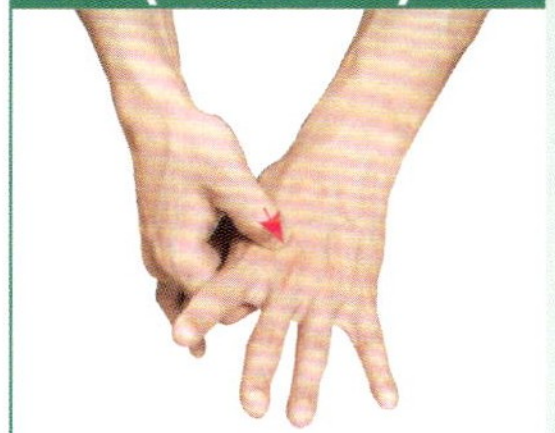

Point-pressing with thumb for 2 minutes with moderate strength, 2 times each day

第三章　耳部反射区

耳部各部位名称图解
Illustration of Ear Structure

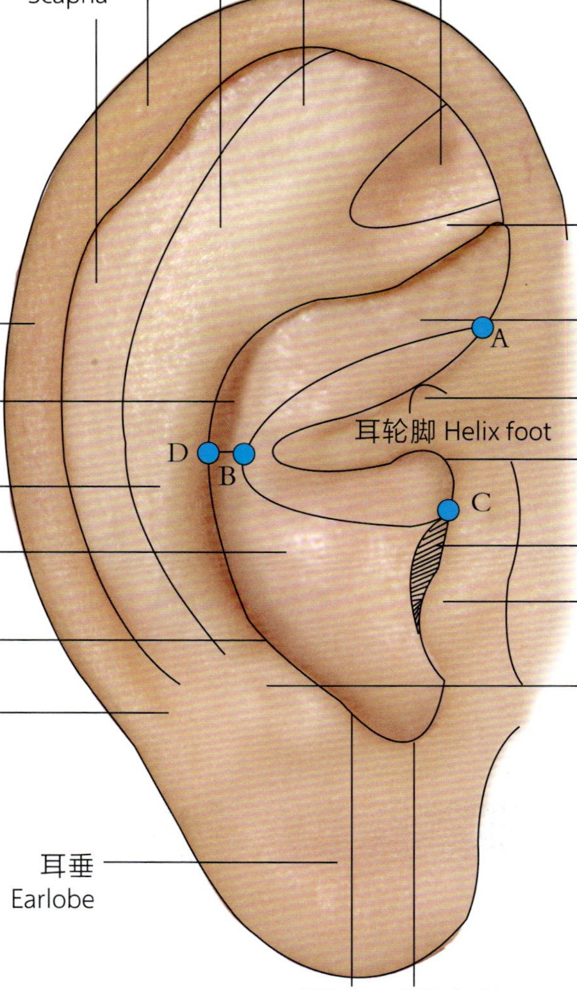

部位名称	定 位
耳垂	耳郭下部无软骨的部分
耳轮	耳郭外侧边缘的卷曲部分
耳轮脚	耳轮深入耳甲的部分
耳轮脚棘	耳轮脚和耳轮之间的隆起
耳轮结节	耳轮外上方的膨大部分
耳轮尾	耳轮向下移行于耳垂的部分
对耳轮	与耳轮相对呈“Y”字形的隆起部，由对耳轮体、对耳轮上脚和对耳轮下脚三部分组成
对耳轮体	对耳轮下部呈上下走向的主体部分
对耳轮上脚	对耳轮向上分支的部分
对耳轮下脚	对耳轮向前分支的部分
轮屏切迹	对耳轮与对耳屏之间的凹陷处
耳舟	耳轮与对耳轮之间的凹沟
三角窝	对耳轮上、下脚与相应耳轮之间的三角形凹窝
耳甲	部分耳轮和对耳轮、对耳屏、耳屏及外耳门之间的凹窝。由耳甲艇、耳甲腔两部分组成
耳甲艇	耳轮脚以上的耳甲部
耳甲腔	耳轮脚以下的耳甲部

Name of each part	Location
Earlobe	The lower part of the auricle without cartilage
Helix	Crimped portion of the outside edge of the auricle
Helix foot	Deep part of helix into concha
Spine of the helix foot	The bulge between the foot of the helix and helix
Auricular tubercle	The swollen part above the outside of helix
Helix tail	Part of helix down to the earlobe
Antihelix	“Y” shaped bulge relative to the helix, combining with body of the antihelix, superior antihelix crus and inferior antihelix crus
Body of the antihelix	The main body part of antihelix lower part with up and down direction
Superior antihelix crus	The upward part of the branch of the antihelix
Inferior antihelix crus	The forward part of the branch of the antihelix
Tragus–Helix incisura	The depression between antihelix and antitragus
Scapha	The groove between helixs
Triangular fossa	The triangle concave formed by superior, inferior antihelix crus and corresponding helix
Concha	The concave formed by part of helix, antitragus, tragus and external auditory canal, combing with superior concha and auricular cavity
Superior concha	The concha part above the foot of helix
Auricular cavity	The concha part below the foot of helix

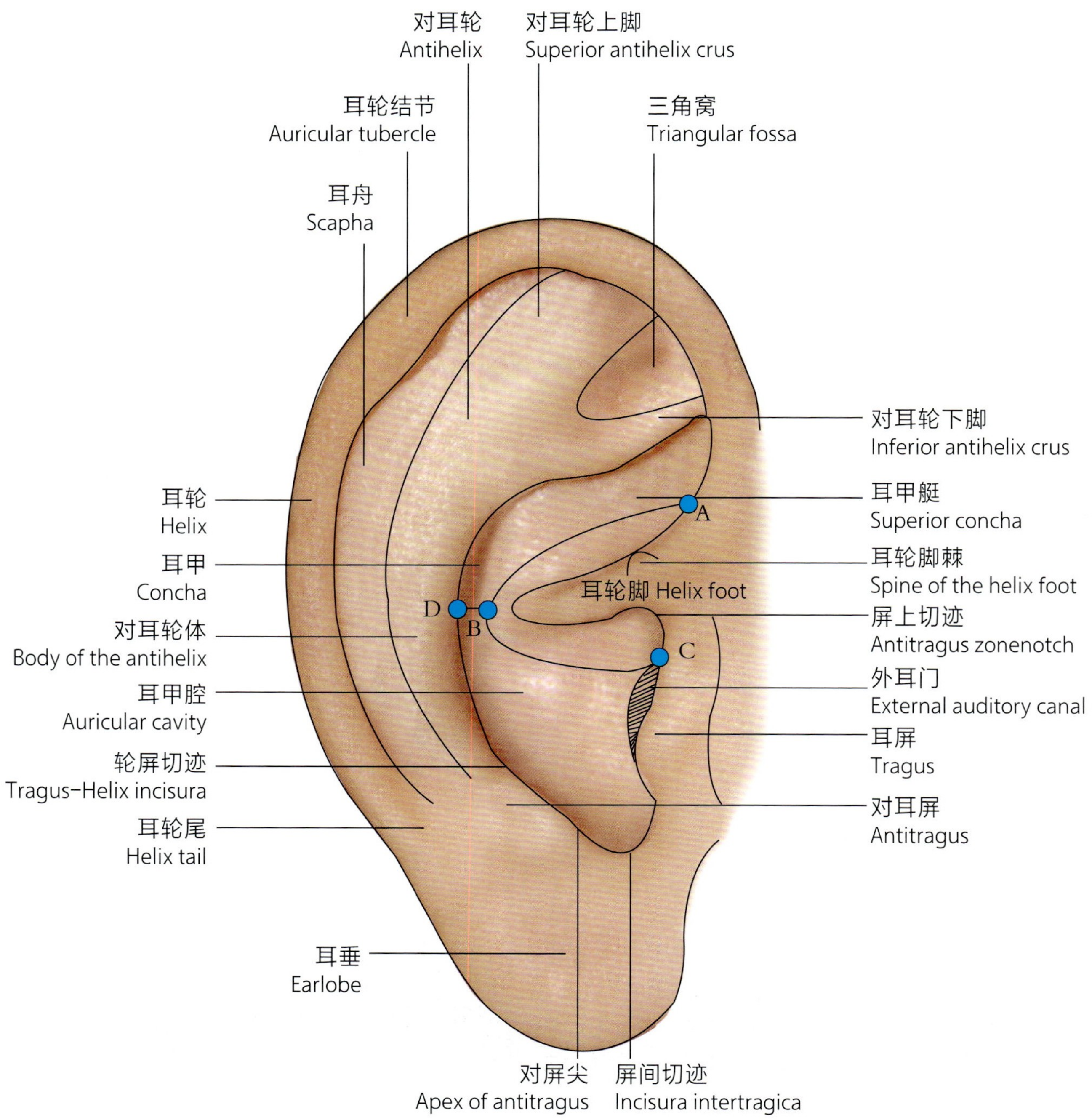
对耳轮
Antihelix
对耳轮上脚
Superior antihelix crus
耳轮结节
Auricular tubercle
三角窝
Triangular fossa
耳舟
Scapha
对耳轮下脚
Inferior antihelix crus
耳轮
Helix
耳甲艇
Superior concha
A
耳甲
Concha
耳轮脚棘
Spine of the helix foot
耳轮脚 Helix foot
D
B
屏上切迹
Antitragus zonenotch
对耳轮体
Body of the antihelix
C
外耳门
External auditory canal
耳甲腔
Auricular cavity
耳屏
Tragus
轮屏切迹
Tragus-Helix incisura
对耳屏
Antitragus
耳轮尾
Helix tail
耳垂
Earlobe
对屏尖
Apex of antitragus
屏间切迹
Incisura intertragica

续表

部位名称	定 位
耳屏	耳郭前方呈瓣状的隆起
屏上切迹	耳屏与耳轮之间的凹陷处
对耳屏	耳垂上方、与耳屏相对的瓣状隆起
对屏尖	对耳屏游离缘隆起的顶端
屏间切迹	耳屏和对耳屏之间的凹陷处
外耳门	耳甲腔前方的孔窍

Continued

Name of each part	Location
Tragus	The petal shaped bulge in front of auricle
Antitragus zonenotch	The depression between tragus and helix
Antitragus	The petal shaped bulge above earlobe, the opposite of tragus
Apex of antitragus	The top of antitragus free margin bulge
Incisura intertragica	The depression between the tragus and antitragus
External auditory canal	A canal in front of auricular cavity

耳部反射区
Ear Reflex Zone

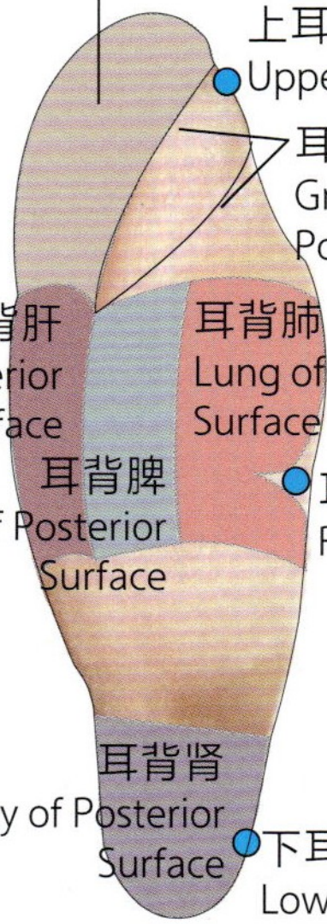

耳背面反射区
Reflex Zones of the Dorsum of the Ear

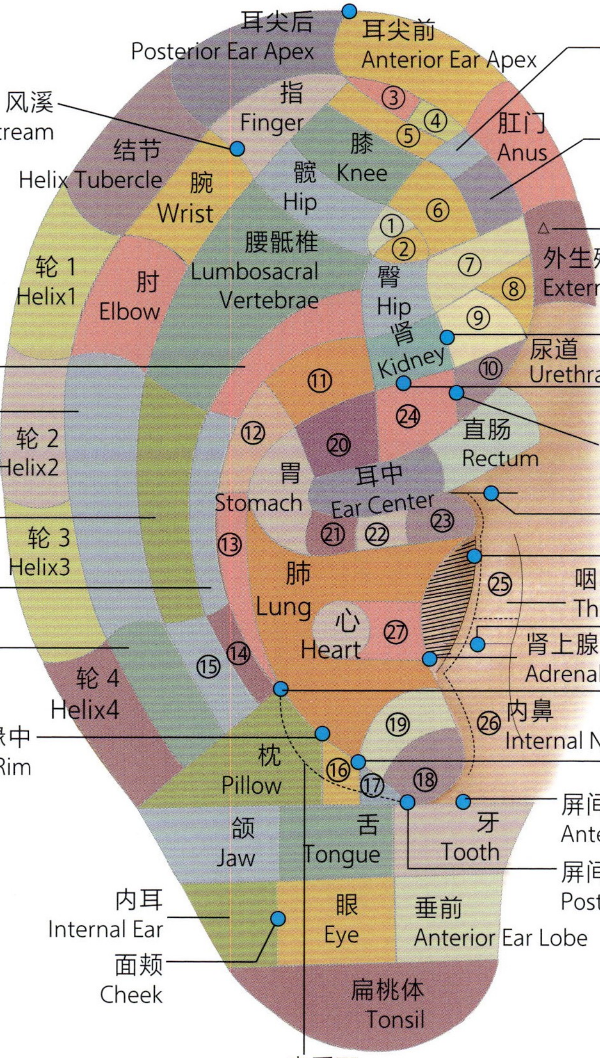

耳正面反射区
Reflex Zones of the Front of the Ear

①神门 Shenmen
②盆腔 Pelvic Cavity
③趾 Toe
④跟 Heel
⑤踝 Ankle
⑥角窝中 Middle Triangular Fossa
⑦坐骨神经 Sciatic Nerves
⑧艇角 Angle of Superior Concha
⑨膀胱 Bladder
⑩大肠 Large Intestine
⑪胰胆 Pancreaticobiliary
⑫肝 Liver
⑬脾 Spleen
⑭颈 Neck
⑮颈椎 Cervical Vertebra
⑯颞 Temporal
⑰额 Forehead
⑱内分泌 Endocrine
⑲三焦 Triple Energizer
⑳十二指肠 Duodenum
㉑贲门 Cardia
㉒食道 Esophagus
㉓口 Mouth
㉔小肠 Small Intestine
㉕上屏 Upper Tragus
㉖下屏 Lower Tragus
㉗气管 Trachea

反射区	定 位	主 治
耳中	在耳轮脚处	呃逆、荨麻疹、皮肤瘙痒、小儿遗尿、咯血、出血性疾病
直肠	在耳轮脚棘前上方的耳轮处	便秘、腹泻、脱肛、痔疮
尿道	在直肠上方的耳轮处	尿频、尿急、尿痛、尿潴留
外生殖器	在对耳轮下脚前方的耳轮处	睾丸炎、附睾炎、外阴瘙痒
肛门	在三角窝前方的耳轮处	痔疮、肛裂
耳尖前	在耳郭向前对折上部尖端的前部	发热、高血压
耳尖	在耳郭向前对折的上部尖端处	发热、高血压、急性结膜炎、睑腺炎、牙痛、失眠
耳尖后	在耳郭向前对折上部尖端的后部	发热、高血压
结节	在耳轮结节处	头晕、头痛、高血压

Reflex Zone	Location	Indications
Ear Center	On the foot of the helix	Hiccup; urticaria; pruritus; child enuresis; hemoptysis; hemorrhagic disease
Rectum	On the helix up front spine of the helix foot	Constipation; diarrhea; rectal prolapse and hemorrhoids
Urethra	On the helix above rectum zone	Frequent urination; urgency; dysuria; urinary retention
External Genitalia	On the helix above inferior antihelix crus	Orchitis; epididymitis; vulva pruritus
Anus	On the helix above Triangular fossa	Hemorrhoids; anal fissure
Anterior Ear Apex	In front of the tip of the upper auricular forward fold	Fever; hypertension
Ear Apex	On the tip of the upper auricular forward fold	Fever; hypertension; acute conjunctivitis; stye; toothache; insomnia
Posterior Ear Apex	In the posterior part of the upper auricular forward fold	Fever; hypertension
Helix Tubercle	On the auricular tubercle	Dizziness; headache; hypertension

续表

反射区	定 位	主 治
轮 1	在耳轮结节下方的耳轮处	发热、扁桃体炎、上呼吸道感染
轮 2	在轮 1 区下方的耳轮处	发热、扁桃体炎、上呼吸道感染
轮 3	在轮 2 区下方的耳轮处	发热、扁桃体炎、上呼吸道感染
轮 4	在轮 3 区下方的耳轮处	发热、扁桃体炎、上呼吸道感染
指	在耳舟上方处	甲沟炎、手指麻木和疼痛
腕	在指区的下方处	腕部疼痛
风溪	在耳轮结节前方，指区与腕区之间	荨麻疹、皮肤瘙痒、过敏性鼻炎
肘	在腕区的下方处	肱骨外上髁炎、肘部疼痛
肩	在肘区的下方处	肩关节周围炎、肩部疼痛
锁骨	在肩区的下方处	肩关节周围炎
跟	在对耳轮上脚前上部	足跟痛
趾	在耳尖下方的对耳轮上脚后上部	甲沟炎、趾部疼痛
踝	在趾、跟区下方处	踝关节扭伤
膝	在对耳轮上脚的中 1/3 处	膝关节疼痛、坐骨神经痛
髋	在对耳轮上脚的下 1/3 处	髋关节疼痛、坐骨神经痛、腰骶部疼痛
坐骨神经	在对耳轮下脚的前 2/3 处	坐骨神经痛、下肢瘫痪
交感	在对耳轮下脚前端与耳轮内缘交界处	胃肠痉挛、心绞痛、胆绞痛、输尿管结石、自主神经功能紊乱
臀	在对耳轮下脚的后 1/3 处	坐骨神经痛、臀筋膜炎
腹	在对耳轮体前部上 2/5 处	腹痛、腹胀、腹泻、急性腰扭伤、痛经、产后宫缩痛
腰骶椎	在腹区后方	腰骶部疼痛

Continued

Reflex Zone	Location	Indications
Helix1	On the helix below the auricular tubercle	Fever; tonsillitis; upper respiratory tract infection
Helix2	On the helix below Helix1	Fever; tonsillitis; upper respiratory tract infection
Helix3	On the helix below Helix2	Fever; tonsillitis; upper respiratory tract infection
Helix4	On the helix below Helix3	Fever; tonsillitis; upper respiratory tract infection
Finger	Above scapha	Paronychia; finger numbness and pain
Wrist	Below finger zone	Wrist pain
Wind Stream	Above auricular tubercle, between the finger zone and wrist zone	Urticaria; pruritus; allergic rhinitis
Elbow	Below wrist zone	Lateral epicondylitis, elbow pain
Shoulder	Below elbow zone	Periarthritis of shoulder; shoulder pain
Clavicle	Below shoulder zone	Periarthritis of shoulder
Heel	Up front superior antihelix crus	Heel pain
Toe	Below ear tip and above superior antihelix crus	Paronychia; the pain
Ankle	Below toe zone and heel zone	Ankle sprain
Knee	Middle 1/3 part of superior antihelix crus	Knee pain; sciatica
Hip	Lower 1/3 part of superior antihelix crus	Hip pain; sciatica; lumbosacral pain
Sciatic Nerves	Upper 2/3 part of inferior antihelix crus	Sciatica; lower limb paralysis
Sympathetic	The border of the front end of antihelix and inner edge of helix	Gastrointestinal spasm; angina; biliary colic; ureteral calculi; autonomic dysfunction
Hip	Lower 1/3 part of inferior antihelix crus	Sciatica; gluteal fasciitis
Abdomen	Upper 2/5 part of frontal body of the antihelix	Abdominal pain; abdominal distension; diarrhea; acute lumbar sprain; dysmenorrhea; uterine contraction pain
Lumbosacral Vertebrae	Behind the abdomen zone	Lumbosacral pain

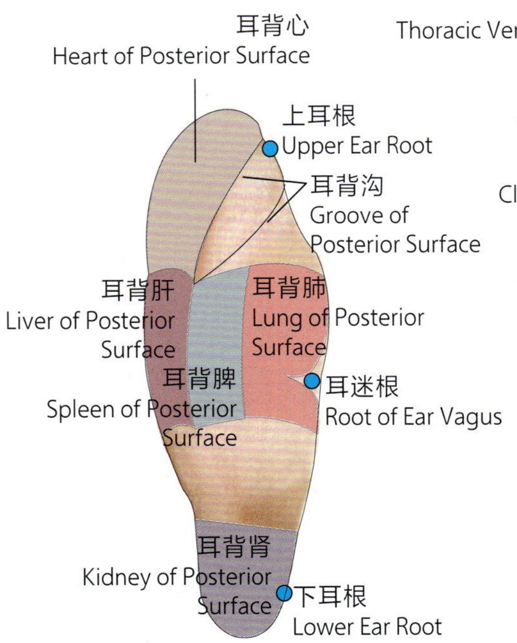

耳背面反射区

Reflex Zones of the Dorsum of the Ear

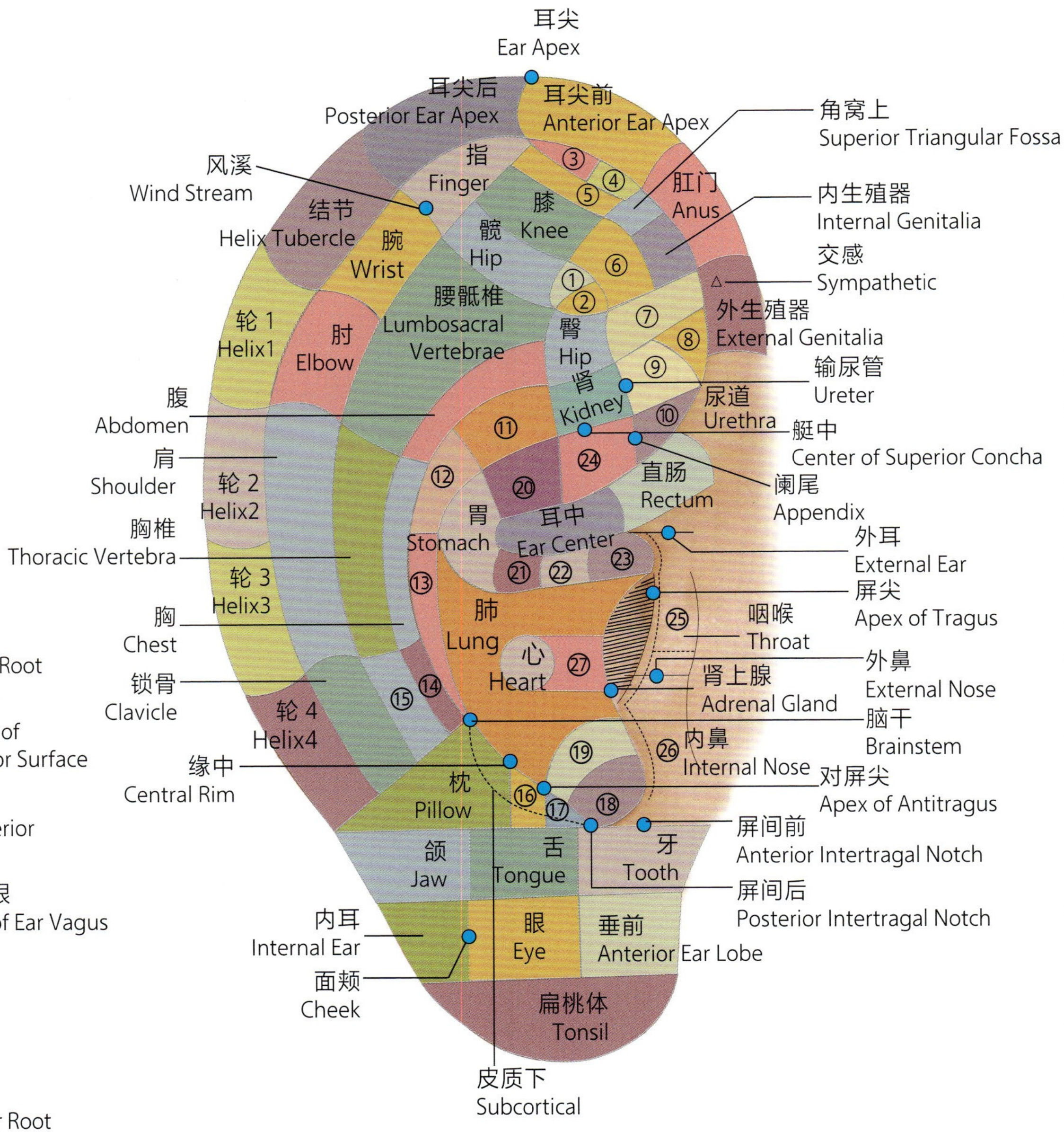

耳正面反射区

Reflex Zones of the Front of the Ear

①神门 Shenmen
②盆腔 Pelvic Cavity
③趾 Toe
④跟 Heel
⑤踝 Ankle
⑥角窝中 Middle Triangular Fossa
⑦坐骨神经 Sciatic Nerves
⑧艇角 Angle of Superior Concha
⑨膀胱 Bladder
⑩大肠 Large Intestine
⑪胰胆 Pancreaticobiliary
⑫肝 Liver
⑬脾 Spleen
⑭颈 Neck
⑮颈椎 Cervical Vertebra
⑯颞 Temporal
⑰额 Forehead
⑱内分泌 Endocrine
⑲三焦 Triple Energizer
⑳十二指肠 Duodenum
㉑贲门 Cardia
㉒食道 Esophagus
㉓口 Mouth
㉔小肠 Small Intestine
㉕上屏 Upper Tragus
㉖下屏 Lower Tragus
㉗气管 Trachea

续表

反射区	定 位	主 治
胸	在对耳轮体前部中 2/5 处	胸胁疼痛、肋间神经痛、胸闷、乳腺炎
胸椎	在胸区后方	胸痛、经前乳房胀痛、乳腺炎、产后泌乳不足
颈	在对耳轮体前部下 1/5 处	落枕、颈椎疼痛
颈椎	在颈区后方	落枕、颈椎病
角窝上	在三角窝前 1/3 的上部	高血压
内生殖器	在三角窝前 1/3 的下部	痛经、月经不调、白带过多、功能性子宫出血、阳痿、遗精、早泄
角窝中	在三角窝中 1/3 处	哮喘

Continued

Reflex Zone	Location	Indications
Chest	Middle 2/5 part of frontal body of the antihelix	Hypochondriac pain; intercostal nerve pain; chest tightness; mastitis
Thoracic Vertebra	Behind chest zone	Chest pain; premenstrual breast pain; mastitis; postpartum lactation deficiency
Neck	Lower 1/5 part of frontal body of the antihelix	Stiff neck; neck pain
Cervical Vertebra	Behind neck zone	Stiff neck; cervical spondylopathy
Superior Triangular Fossa	1/3 of the upper part in front of triangular fossa	Hypertension
Internal Genitalia	1/3 of the lower part in front of triangular fossa	Dysmenorrhea; irregular menstruation; leucorrhea excessive; dysfunctional uterine bleeding; impotence; spermatorrhea; premature ejaculation
Middle Triangular Fossa	1/3 of the middle of triangular fossa	Asthma

续表

反射区	定 位	主 治
神门	在三角窝后 1/3 的上部	失眠、多梦、戒断综合征、癫痫、高血压、神经衰弱
盆腔	在三角窝后 1/3 的下部	盆腔炎、附件炎
上屏	在耳屏外侧面上 1/2 处	咽炎、鼻炎
下屏	在耳屏外侧面下 1/2 处	鼻炎、鼻塞
外耳	在屏上切迹前方近耳轮部	外耳道炎、中耳炎、耳鸣
屏尖	在耳屏游离缘上部尖端	发热、牙痛、斜视
外鼻	在耳屏外侧面中部	鼻前庭炎、鼻炎
肾上腺	在耳屏游离缘下部尖端	低血压、风湿性关节炎、腮腺炎、链霉素中毒、眩晕、哮喘、休克
咽喉	在耳屏内侧面上 1/2 处	声音嘶哑、咽炎、扁桃体炎、失语、哮喘
内鼻	在耳屏内侧面下 1/2 处	鼻炎、上颌窦炎、鼻出血
屏间前	在屏间切迹前方耳屏最下部	咽炎、口腔炎
额	在对耳屏外侧面的前部	偏头痛、头晕
屏间后	在屏间切迹后方对耳屏前下部	额窦炎
颞	在对耳屏外侧面的中部	偏头痛、头晕
枕	在对耳屏外侧面的后部	头晕、头痛、癫痫、哮喘、神经衰弱
皮质下	在对耳屏内侧面	痛证、神经衰弱、假性近视、失眠
对屏尖	在对耳屏游离缘的尖端	哮喘、腮腺炎、睾丸炎、附睾炎、神经性皮炎
缘中	在对耳屏游离缘上，对屏尖与轮屏切迹之中点处	遗尿、内耳性眩晕、尿崩症、功能性子宫出血

Reflex Zone	Location	Indications
Shenmen(HT7)	1/3 of the upper part behind triangular fossa	Insomnia; dreaminess; withdrawal syndrome; epilepsy; hypertension; neurasthenia
Pelvic Cavity	1/3 of the lower part behind triangular fossa	Pelvic inflammation; annex inflammation
Upper Tragus	The upper 1/2 part outside of tragus	Pharyngitis; rhinitis
Lower Tragus	The lower 1/2 part outside of tragus	Rhinitis; nasal obstruction
External Ear	Above Antitragus zonenotch, near helix	Otitis externa; otitis media; tinnitus
Apex of Tragus	The top of upper part of antitragus free margin	Fever; toothache; strabismus
External Nose	The middle of the outside of tragus	Nasal vestibule inflammation; rhinitis
Adrenal Gland	The top of lower part of antitragus free margin	Hypotension; rheumatoid arthritis; mumps; streptomycin poisoning; dizziness; asthma; shock
Throat	The upper 1/2 part inside of tragus	Hoarseness; pharyngitis; tonsillitis; aphasia; asthma
Internal Nose	The lower 1/2 part inside of tragus	Rhinitis; sinusitis; nasal bleeding
Anterior Intertragal Notch	The lowest part of tragus in front of incisura intertragica	Pharyngitis; stomatitis
Forehead	The forepart of the outside of antitragus	Migraine; headache
Posterior Intertragal Notch	The lower part behind incisura intertragica, above antitragus	Frontal sinusitis
Temporal	The middle of the outside of antitragus	Migraine; headache
Pillow	The back of the outside of antitragus	Dizziness; headache; epilepsy; asthma; neurasthenia
Subcortical	The inside of antitragus	Pain syndrome; neurasthenia; pseudo myopia; insomnia
Apex of antitragus	The top of antitragus free margin	Asthma; mumps; orchitis; epididymitis; neurodermatitis
Central Rim	On the free margin of antitragus, the midpoint of the apex of antitragus and tragus-helix incisura	Enuresis; internal ear vertigo; diabetes insipidus; functional uterine bleeding

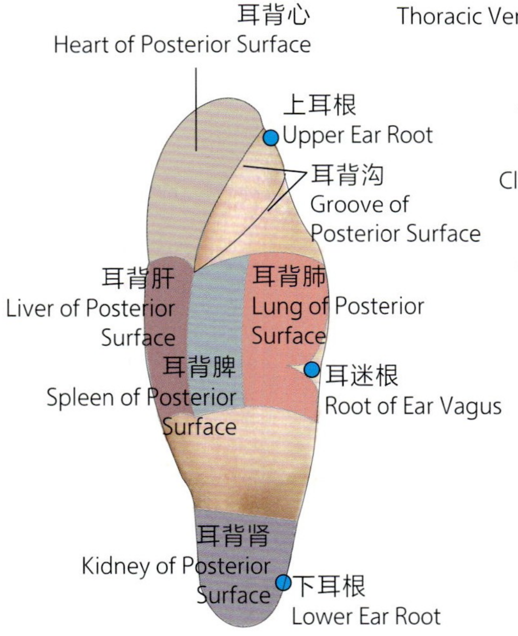

耳背面反射区

Reflex Zones of the Dorsum of the Ear

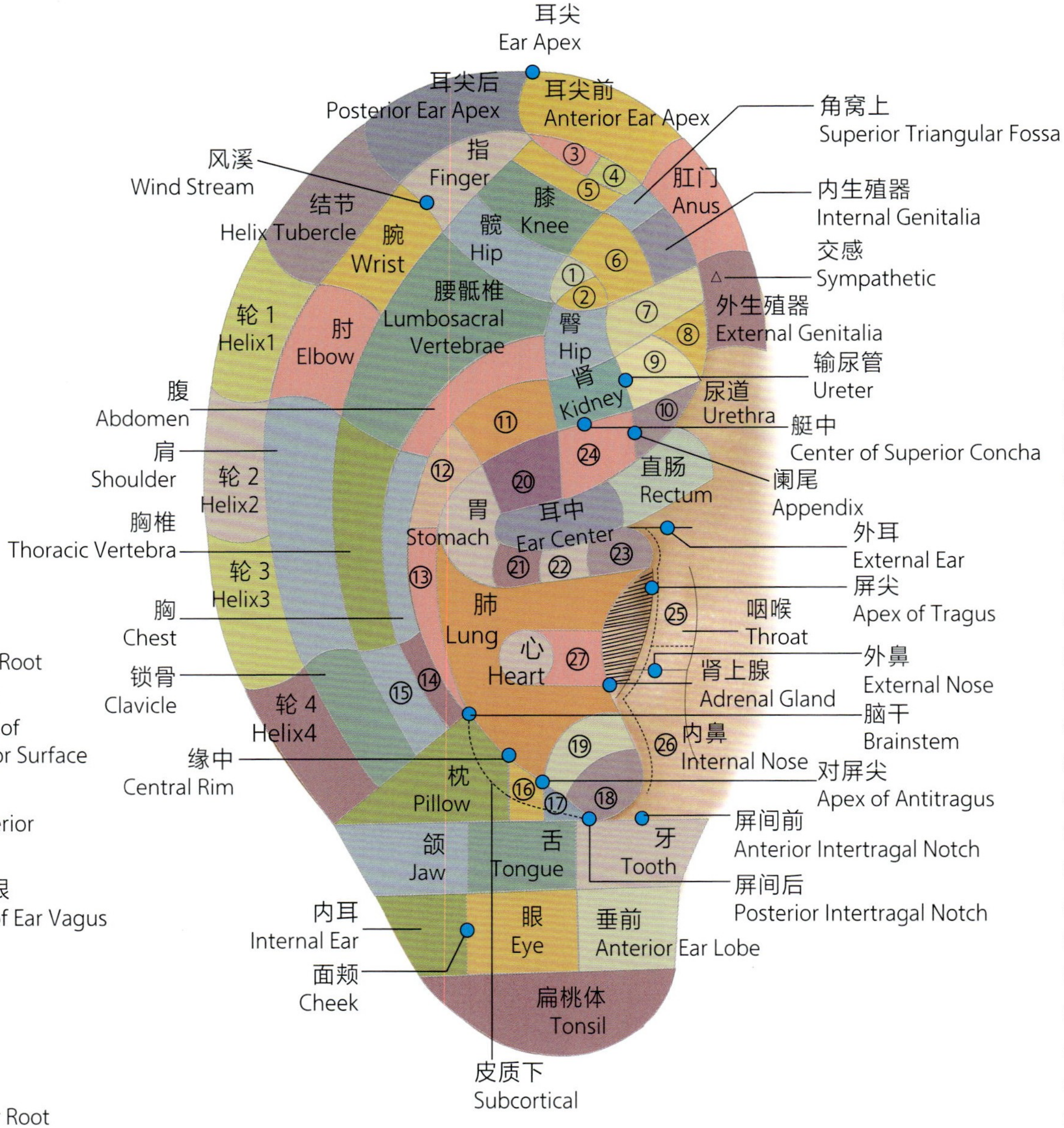

耳正面反射区

Reflex Zones of the Front of the Ear

①神门 Shenmen
②盆腔 Pelvic Cavity
③趾 Toe
④跟 Heel
⑤踝 Ankle
⑥角窝中 Middle Triangular Fossa
⑦坐骨神经 Sciatic Nerves
⑧艇角 Angle of Superior Concha
⑨膀胱 Bladder
⑩大肠 Large Intestine
⑪胰胆 Pancreaticobiliary
⑫肝 Liver
⑬脾 Spleen
⑭颈 Neck
⑮颈椎 Cervical Vertebra
⑯颞 Temporal
⑰额 Forehead
⑱内分泌 Endocrine
⑲三焦 Triple Energizer
⑳十二指肠 Duodenum
㉑贲门 Cardia
㉒食道 Esophagus
㉓口 Mouth
㉔小肠 Small Intestine
㉕上屏 Upper Tragus
㉖下屏 Lower Tragus
㉗气管 Trachea

续表

反射区	定 位	主 治
脑干	在轮屏切迹处	眩晕、后头痛、假性近视
口	在耳轮脚下方前 1/3 处	面瘫、口腔炎、胆囊炎、胆石症、戒断综合征、牙周炎、舌炎
食道	在耳轮脚下方中 1/3 处	食管炎、食管痉挛
贲门	在耳轮脚下方后 1/3 处	贲门痉挛、神经性呕吐
胃	在耳轮脚消失处	胃痉挛、胃炎、胃溃疡、消化不良、恶心呕吐、前额痛、牙痛、失眠
十二指肠	在耳轮脚及部分耳轮与 AB 线之间的后 1/3 处	十二指肠溃疡、胆囊炎、胆石症、幽门痉挛、腹胀、腹泻、腹痛
小肠	在耳轮脚及部分耳轮与 AB 线之间的中 1/3 处	消化不良、腹痛、腹胀、心动过速

Continued

Reflex Zone	Location	Indications
Brainstem	On the tragus–helix incisura	Vertigo; back pain; pseudo myopia
Mouth	The front 1/3 part behind the foot of the helix	Facial paralysis; stomatitis; cholecystitis; cholelithiasis; withdrawal syndrome; periodontitis; glossitis
Esophagus	The middle 1/3 part behind the foot of the helix	Esophagitis; esophageal spasm
Cardia	The behind 1/3 part behind the foot of the helix	Cardiac spasm; nervous vomiting
Stomach	Where the foot of the helix disappear	Stomach cramps; gastritis; gastric ulcer; indigestion; nausea and vomiting; forehead pain; toothache; insomnia
Duodenum	The behind 1/3 part of the zone among the foot of the helix, part of helix and AB line	Duodenal ulcer; cholecystitis; cholelithiasis; pyloric spasm; abdominal distension; diarrhea; abdominal pain
Small Intestine	The middle 1/3 part of the zone among the foot of the helix, part of helix and AB line	Dyspepsia; abdominal pain; abdominal distension; tachycardia

续表

反射区	定 位	主 治
大肠	在耳轮脚及部分耳轮与 AB 线之间的前 1/3 处	腹泻、便秘、咳嗽、牙痛、痤疮
阑尾	在小肠区与大肠区之间	单纯性阑尾炎、腹泻
艇角	在对耳轮下脚下方前部	前列腺炎、尿道炎
膀胱	在对耳轮下脚下方中部	膀胱炎、遗尿、尿潴留、腰痛、坐骨神经痛、后头痛
肾	在对耳轮下脚下方后部	腰痛、耳鸣、神经衰弱、肾盂肾炎、遗尿、遗精、阳痿、早泄、哮喘、月经不调
输尿管	在肾区与膀胱区之间	输尿管结石绞痛
胰胆	在耳甲艇的后上部	胆囊炎、胆石症、胆道蛔虫症、偏头痛、带状疱疹、中耳炎、耳鸣、急性胰腺炎
肝	在耳甲艇的后下部	胁痛、眩晕、经前期紧张、月经不调、围绝经期综合征、高血压、近视、单纯性青光眼
艇中	在小肠区与肾区之间	腹痛、腹胀、胆道蛔虫症
脾	在 BD 线下方，耳甲腔的后上部	腹胀、腹泻、便秘、食欲不振、功能性子宫出血、白带过多、内耳性眩晕
心	在耳甲腔正中凹陷处	心动过速、心律不齐、心绞痛、无脉症、神经衰弱、癔症、口舌生疮
气管	在心区与外耳门之间	哮喘、支气管炎
肺	在心区、气管区周围处	咳嗽、胸闷、声音嘶哑、皮肤瘙痒、荨麻疹、便秘、戒断综合征
三焦	在外耳门后下，肺区与内分泌区之间	便秘、腹胀、上肢外侧疼痛

Continued

Reflex Zone	Location	Indications
Large Intestine	The frontal 1/3 part of the zone among the foot of the helix, part of helix and AB line	Diarrhea; constipation; cough; toothache; acne
Appendix	Between small intestine zone and large intestine zone	Simple appendicitis; diarrhea
Angle of Superior Concha	The frontal part behind inferior antihelix crus	Prostatitis; urethritis
Bladder	The middle part behind inferior antihelix crus	Cystitis; urinary incontinence; urinary retention; lower back pain; sciatica; headache
Kidney	The back part behind inferior antihelix crus	Lower back pain; tinnitus; neurasthenia; pyelonephritis; spermatorrhea; enuresis; impotence; premature ejaculation; asthma; irregular menstruation
Ureter	Between Kidney zone and Bladder zone	Ureteral colic
Pancreaticobiliary	The behind upper part of superior concha	Cholecystitis; cholelithiasis; biliary ascariasis; migraine; herpes zoster; tinnitus; otitis media; acute pancreatitis
Liver	The behind lower part of superior concha	Rib pain; dizziness; premenstrual tension; irregular menstruation; perimenopausal syndrome; hypertension; myopia; simple glaucoma
Center of Superior Concha	Between Small Intestine zone and Kidney zone	Abdominal pain; abdominal distension; biliary ascariasis
Spleen	Below BD line, the behind upper part of auricular cavity	Abdominal distension; diarrhea; constipation; loss of appetite; dysfunctional uterine bleeding; excessive leucorrhea; internal ear vertigo
Heart	The depression in the center of auricular cavity	Tachycardia; arrhythmia; angina; pulseless disease; neurasthenia; hysteria; mouth sores
Trachea	Between heart zone and external auditory canal	Asthma; bronchitis
Lung	Around heart zone and trachea zone	Cough; chest tightness; hoarseness; pruritus; urticaria; constipation; withdrawal syndrome
Triple Energizer	The behind lower part of external auditory canal, between Lung zone and Endocrine zone	Constipation; abdominal distension; upper limb pain

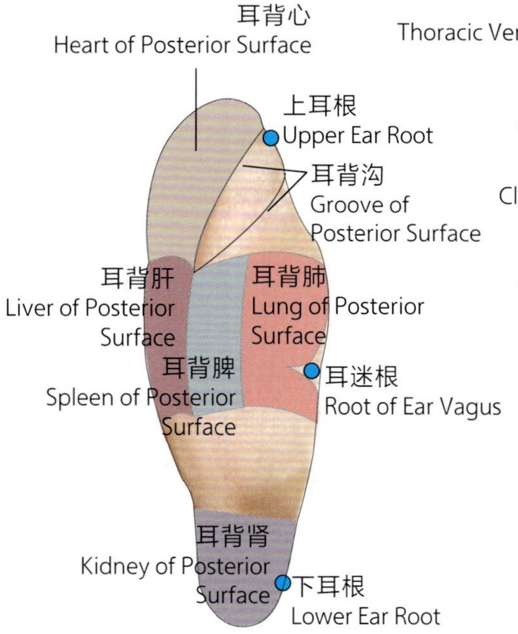

耳背面反射区

Reflex Zones of the Dorsum of the Ear

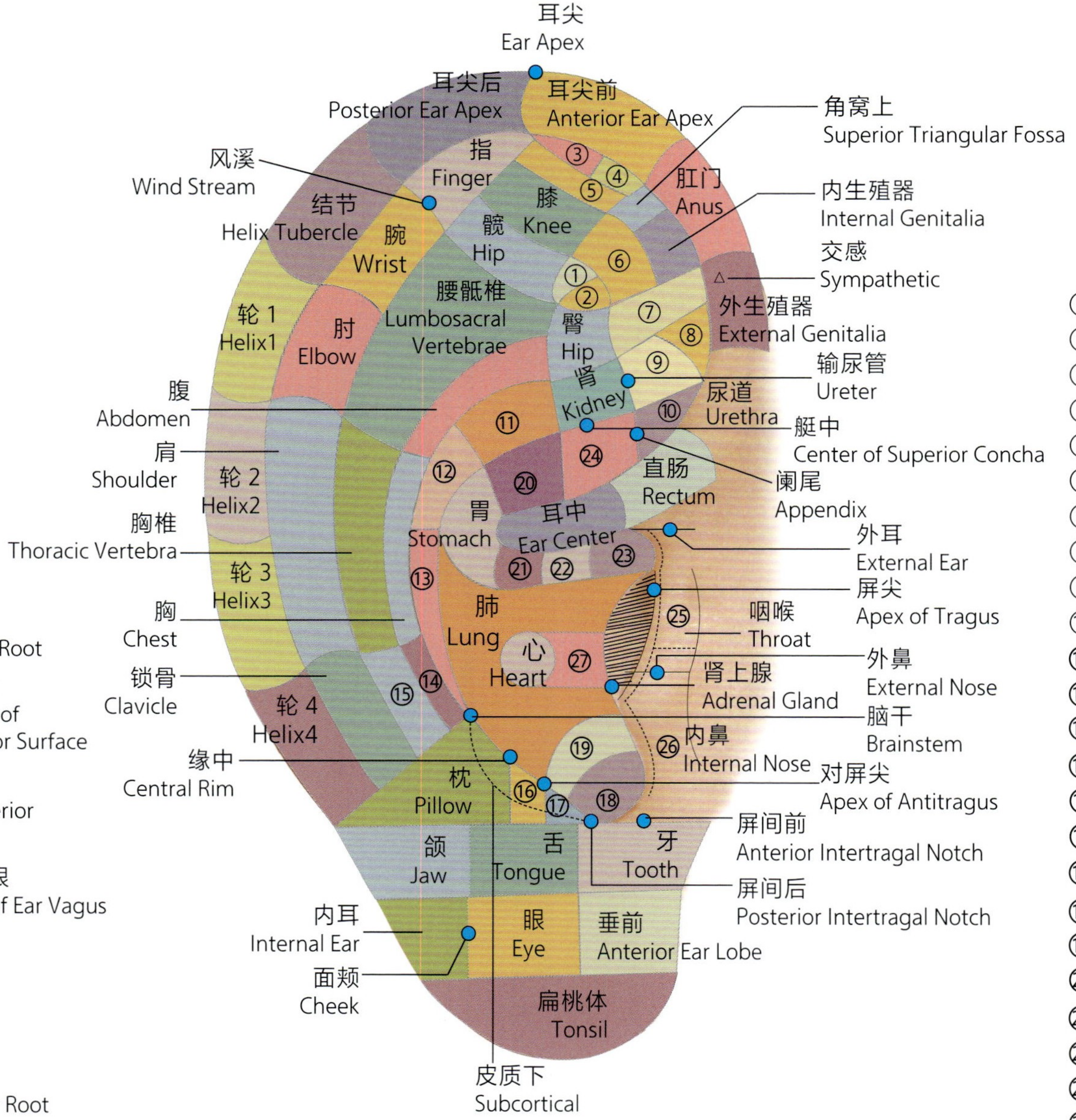

耳正面反射区

Reflex Zones of the Front of the Ear

①神门 Shenmen
②盆腔 Pelvic Cavity
③趾 Toe
④跟 Heel
⑤踝 Ankle
⑥角窝中 Middle Triangular Fossa
⑦坐骨神经 Sciatic Nerves
⑧艇角 Angle of Superior Concha
⑨膀胱 Bladder
⑩大肠 Large Intestine
⑪胰胆 Pancreaticobiliary
⑫肝 Liver
⑬脾 Spleen
⑭颈 Neck
⑮颈椎 Cervical Vertebra
⑯颞 Temporal
⑰额 Forehead
⑱内分泌 Endocrine
⑲三焦 Triple Energizer
⑳十二指肠 Duodenum
㉑贲门 Cardia
㉒食道 Esophagus
㉓口 Mouth
㉔小肠 Small Intestine
㉕上屏 Upper Tragus
㉖下屏 Lower Tragus
㉗气管 Trachea

续表

反射区	定 位	主 治
内分泌	在屏间切迹内，耳甲腔的底部	痛经、月经不调、围绝经期综合征、甲状腺功能减退或亢进
牙	在耳垂正面前上部	牙痛、牙周炎、低血压
舌	在耳垂正面中上部	舌炎、口腔炎
颌	在耳垂正面后上部	牙痛、颞下颌关节炎
垂前	在耳垂正面前中部	神经衰弱、牙痛
眼	在耳垂正面中央部	急性结膜炎、电光性眼炎、睑腺炎、近视
内耳	在耳垂正面后中部	内耳性眩晕、耳鸣、听力减退、中耳炎
面颊	在耳垂正面眼区与内耳区之间	面瘫、三叉神经痛、痤疮、扁平疣、面肌痉挛、腮腺炎
扁桃体	在耳垂正面下部	扁桃体炎、咽炎

Continued

Reflex Zone	Location	Indications
Endocrine	In incisura intertragica, the bottom of auricular cavity	Dysmenorrhea; irregular menstruation; perimenopausal syndrome; hypothyroidism or hyperthyroidism
Tooth	The frontal upper part in front of earlobe	Toothache; periodontitis; hypotension
Tongue	The middle upper part in front of earlobe	Glossitis; stomatitis
Jaw	The behind upper part in front of earlobe	Toothache; temporomandibular arthritis
Anterior Ear Lobe	The frontal middle part in front of earlobe	Neurasthenia; toothache
Eye	The center part in front of earlobe	Acute conjunctivitis; ophthalmia; hordeolum; myopia
Internal Ear	The behind middle part in front of earlobe	Internal ear vertigo; tinnitus; hearing loss; otitis media
Cheek	Between Eye zone and Internal Ear zone in front of earlobe	Facial paralysis; trigeminal neuralgia; acne; warts; hemifacial spasm; mumps
Tonsil	The lower part in front of earlobe	Tonsillitis; pharyngitis

续表

反射区	定位	主治
耳背心	在耳背上部	心悸、失眠、多梦
耳背肺	在耳背中内部	哮喘、皮肤瘙痒
耳背脾	在耳背中央部	胃痛、消化不良、食欲不振
耳背肝	在耳背中外部	胆囊炎、胆石症、胁痛
耳背肾	在耳背下部	头痛、头晕、神经衰弱
耳背沟	在对耳轮沟和对耳轮上、下脚沟处	高血压、皮肤瘙痒
上耳根	在耳郭与头部相连的最上处	鼻出血
耳迷根	在耳轮脚沟的耳根处	胆囊炎、胆石症、胆道蛔虫症、腹痛、腹泻、鼻塞、心动过速
下耳根	在耳郭与头部相连的最下处	低血压、下肢瘫痪、小儿麻痹后遗症

Continued

Reflex Zone	Location	Indications
Heart of Posterior Surface	The upper part of posterior surface	Palpitation; insomnia and dreaminess
Lung of Posterior Surface	The center inner part of posterior surface	Asthma; pruritus
Spleen of Posterior Surface	The center part of posterior surface	Stomach pain; indigestion; loss of appetite
Liver of Posterior Surface	The center outer part of posterior surface	Cholecystitis; cholelithiasis; rib pain
Kidney of Posterior Surface	The lower part of posterior surface	Headache; dizziness; neurasthenia
Groove of Posterior Surface	In the groove of antihelix and the groove of superior, inferior antihelix crus	Hypertension; pruritus
Upper Ear Root	The top between auricle and head zone	Epistaxis
Root of Ear Vagus	The root of ear in the groove of the foot of the helix	Cholecystitis; cholelithiasis; biliary ascariasis; abdominal pain; diarrhea; nasal congestion; tachycardia
Lower Ear Root	The bottom between auricle and head zone	Low blood pressure; lower limb paralysis; post–Polio Syndrome

超简单耳部反射区按摩

Super-easy Massage In Ear Reflex Zone

耳部反射区密密麻麻地分布在小小的耳朵上，全身的器官组织在耳部都有反射区投影，所以每天给耳朵做按摩，相当于给全身按摩了一遍。耳部反射区按摩的方法多以手或按摩棒对反射区进行按、点、掐、推等手法操作。

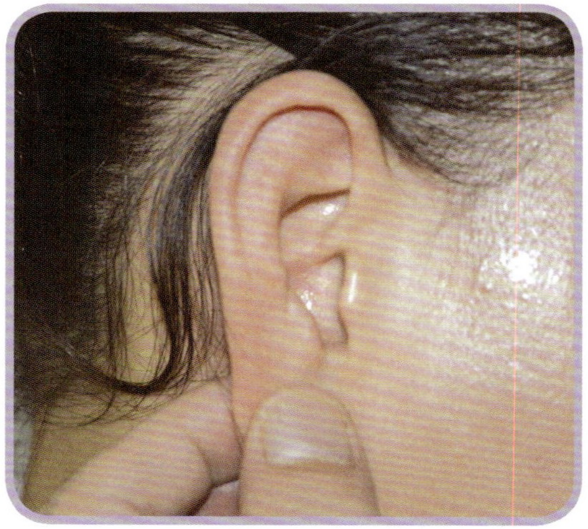

按法

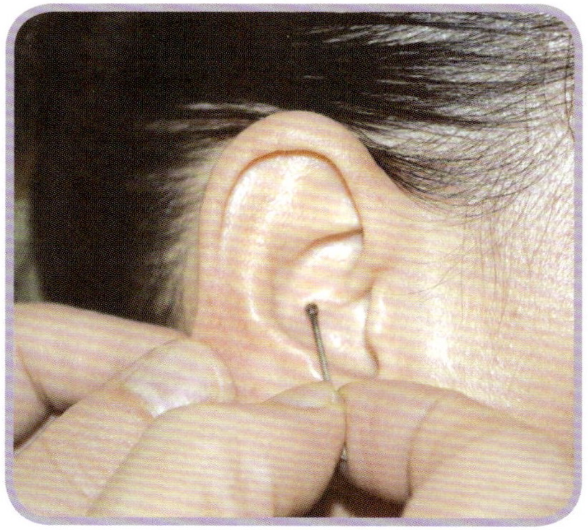

点法

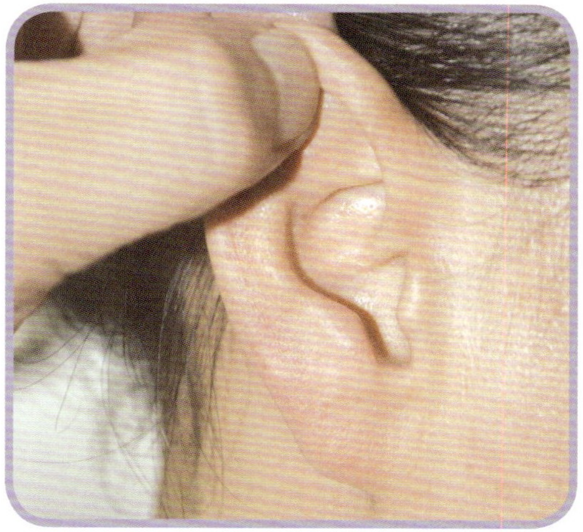

掐法

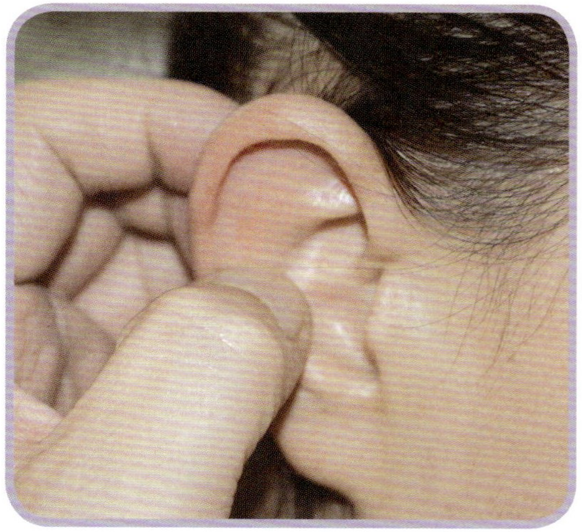

推法

The Ear reflex zone is densely distributed in the small ears, and systemic organ tissues have reflections in the ear, so massaging the ear every day is equivalent to massage the whole body. The ways of massaging Ear reflex zone include pressing, point-pressing, fingernail pressing and other operations with hand or massage stick.

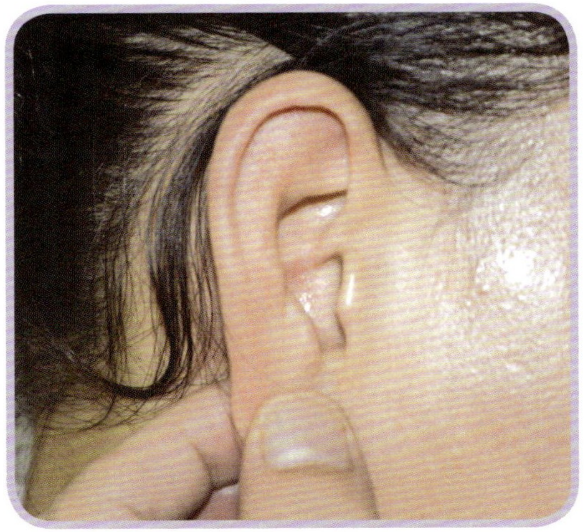

Pressing

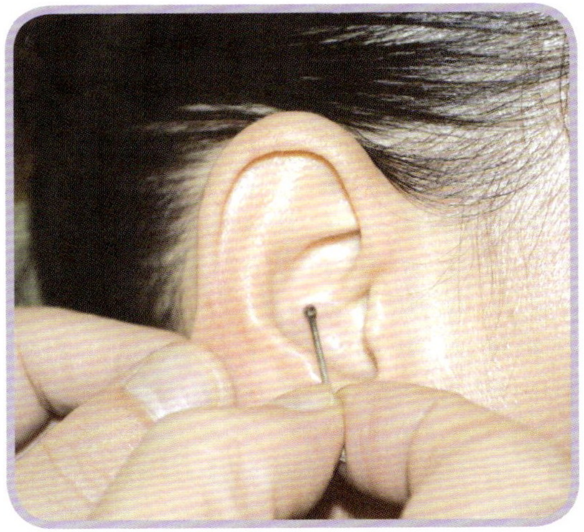

Point-pressing

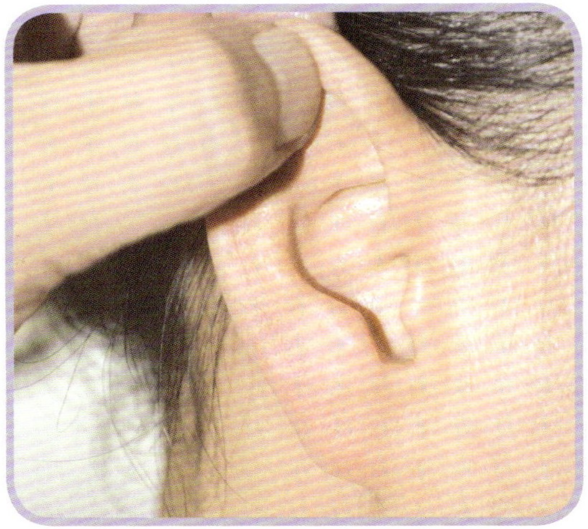

Fingernail pressing

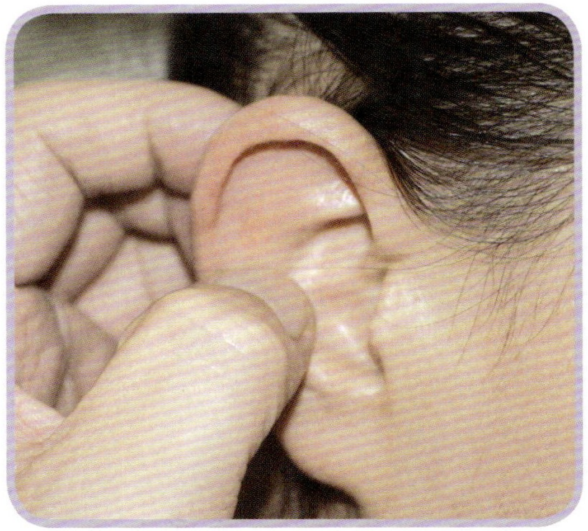

Pressing

面部反射区
Facial Reflex Zone

第四章 头面部反射区及穴位

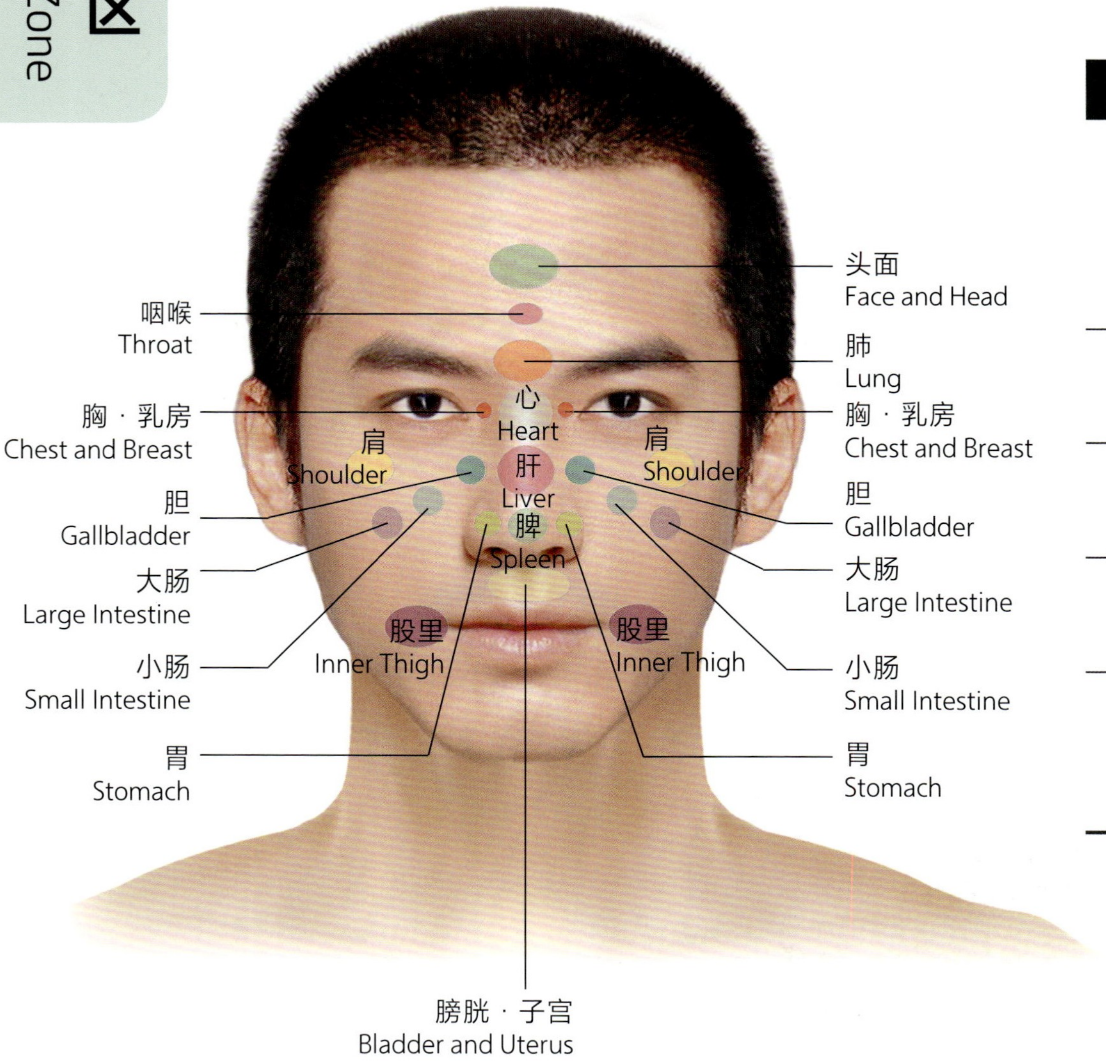

反射区	定 位	主 治
头面	额正中点	头面部感觉异常、面肌痉挛、偏头痛、颞颌关节炎、眩晕、周围性面瘫、听力减退、齿龈肿痛等
肺	两眉内端连线中点	感冒、咳嗽、哮喘、鼻炎等呼吸道疾患
咽喉	头面反射区与肺反射区连线中点	咽喉肿痛、咳嗽等
心	鼻梁最低处，两目内眦连线中点	心绞痛、心律不齐、失眠、胸闷等
肝	心反射区之下，两颧之间，鼻骨与鼻软骨交界处	胁痛、胆囊炎、腹胀等

Chapter 4: Reflex Zones and Acupoints in Head and Face

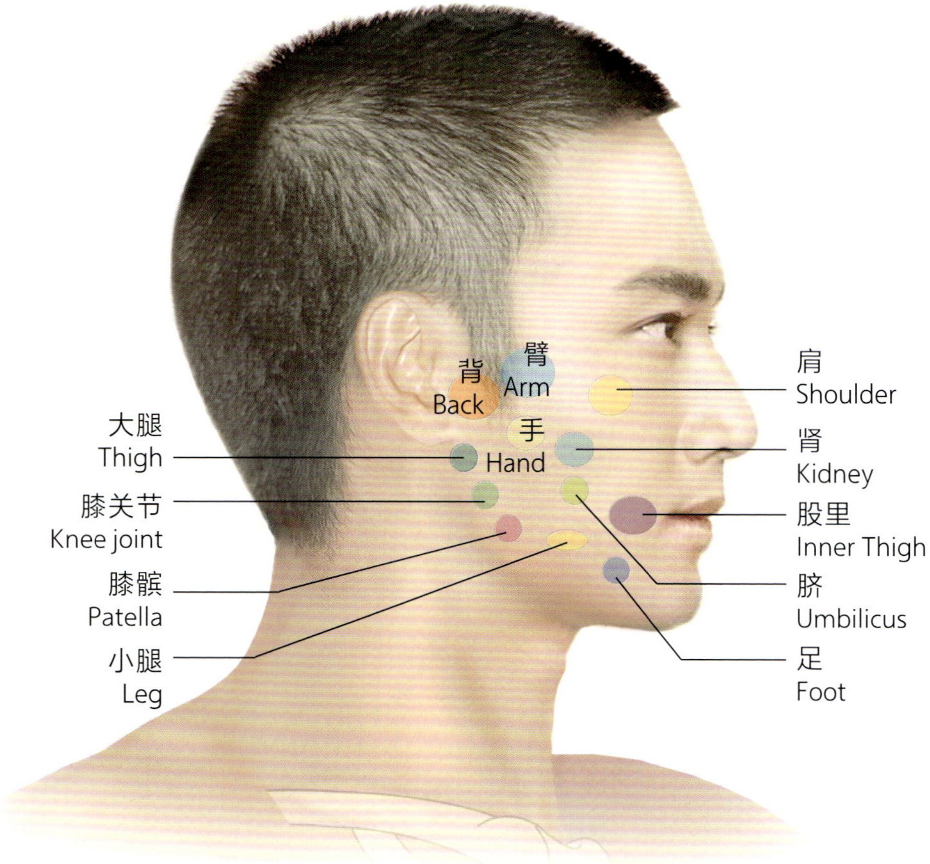

Reflex Zone	Location	Indications
Face and Head	It locates at the central point of the temple	Abnormal feeling of the head and the face; facial spasm; migraine; temporomandibular arthritis; dizziness; peripheral facial paralysis; poor hearing
Lung	It locates at the mid-point of the medial line between of 2 eyebrows	Cold; cough; asthma; rhinitis and other respiratory diseases; gingivitis
Throat	It locates at the mid-point of the medial line between the reflex zone of the Head and the Face and the refection zone of the Lung	Swelling and pain of throat; cough
Heart	It locates at the lowest portion of the nasal bridge, the mid-point of the inner canthus of each eye	Angina pectoris; arrhythmia; insomnia; oppression in the chest
Liver	It locates at the junction of nasal bone and the nasal cartilage between both malar bones below the reflex zone of the Heart	Rib pain; cholecystitis; abdominal distension

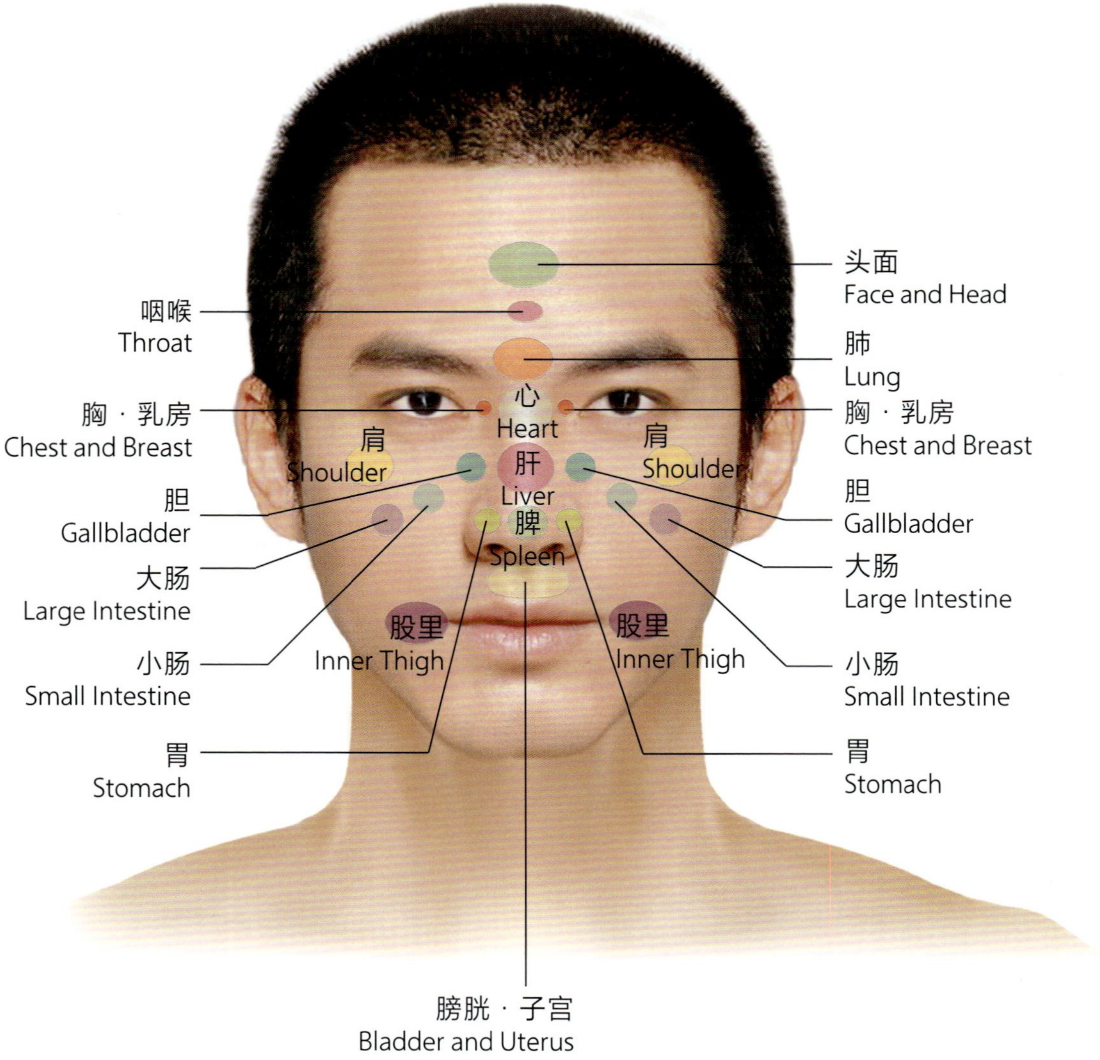

续表

反射区	定 位	主 治
脾	鼻尖处	食欲不振、消化不良、腹泻等
膀胱 · 子宫	人中沟中点	痛经、月经不调、尿频、多尿等
胸 · 乳房	心反射区与目内眦连线之中点	乳汁缺少、乳腺增生、胸闷等
胆	肝反射区两旁，内眼角直下	胆结石、黄疸、胁痛、胆囊炎、恶心、呕吐等
胃	脾反射区两旁，当鼻翼中央处	胃痛、呃逆、呕吐等
小肠	胆反射区、胃反射区连线中点外方，瞳孔直下	消化不良、腹泻等
肩	目外眦直下方，胆反射区外方	肩臂疼痛、上肢麻木等

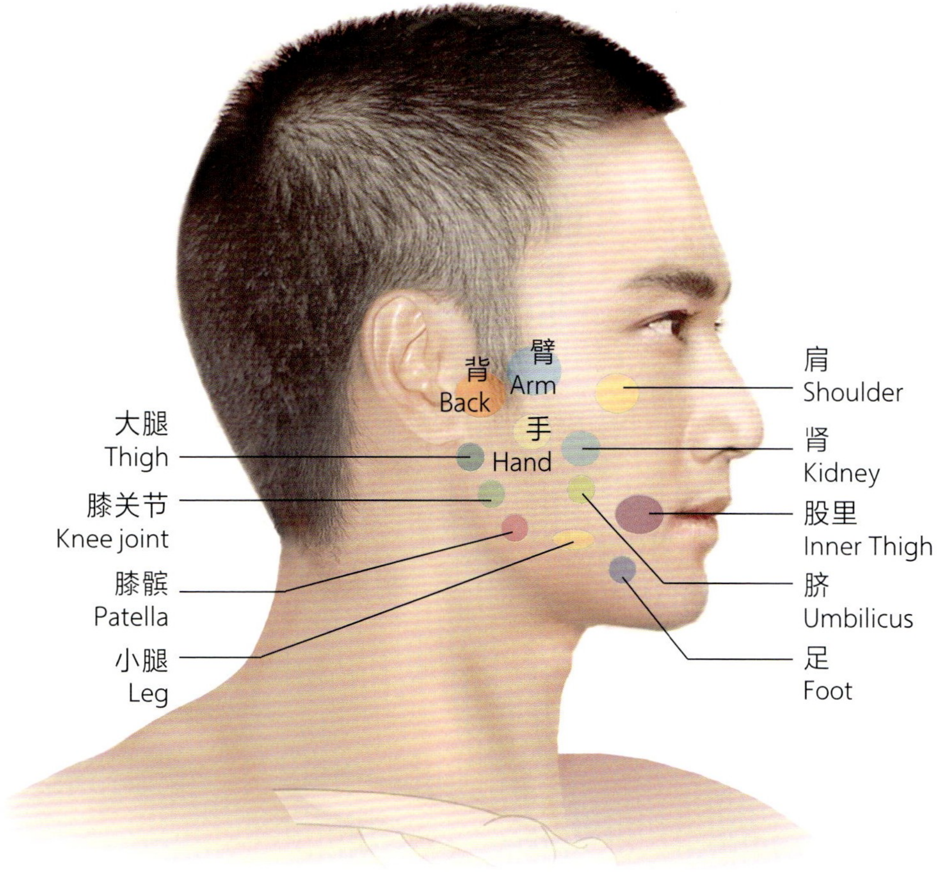

Continued

Reflex Zone	Location	Indications
Spleen	It locates at the tip of the nose	Bad appetite; dyspepsia; diarrhea
Bladder and Uterus	It locates at the mid-point of the groove of the philtrum	Dysmenorrhea; irregular menstruation; frequent urine; copious urine
Chest and Breast	It locates at the mid-point of the reflex zone of the Heart and the of the inner canthus of each eye	Lack of milk; hyperplasia of mammary glands; oppression in the chest
Gallbladder	It locates below straightly the medial angle of eyelid at the bilateral sides of the reflex zone of the Liver	Cholelithes; jaundice; rib pain; cholecystitis; nausea; vomiting
Stomach	It locates the center of the nose wing at the bilateral sides of the reflex zone of the Liver	Stomachache; hiccup; vomiting
Small Intestine	It locates at the lateral portion of the mid-point of the line between the reflex zone of the Gallbladder and the reflex zone of the Stomach	Dyspepsia; diarrhea
Shoulder	It locates straightly below the outer canthus at the lateral portion of the reflex zone of the Gallbladder	Pain in the shoulder and the arm; numbness of the upper limbs

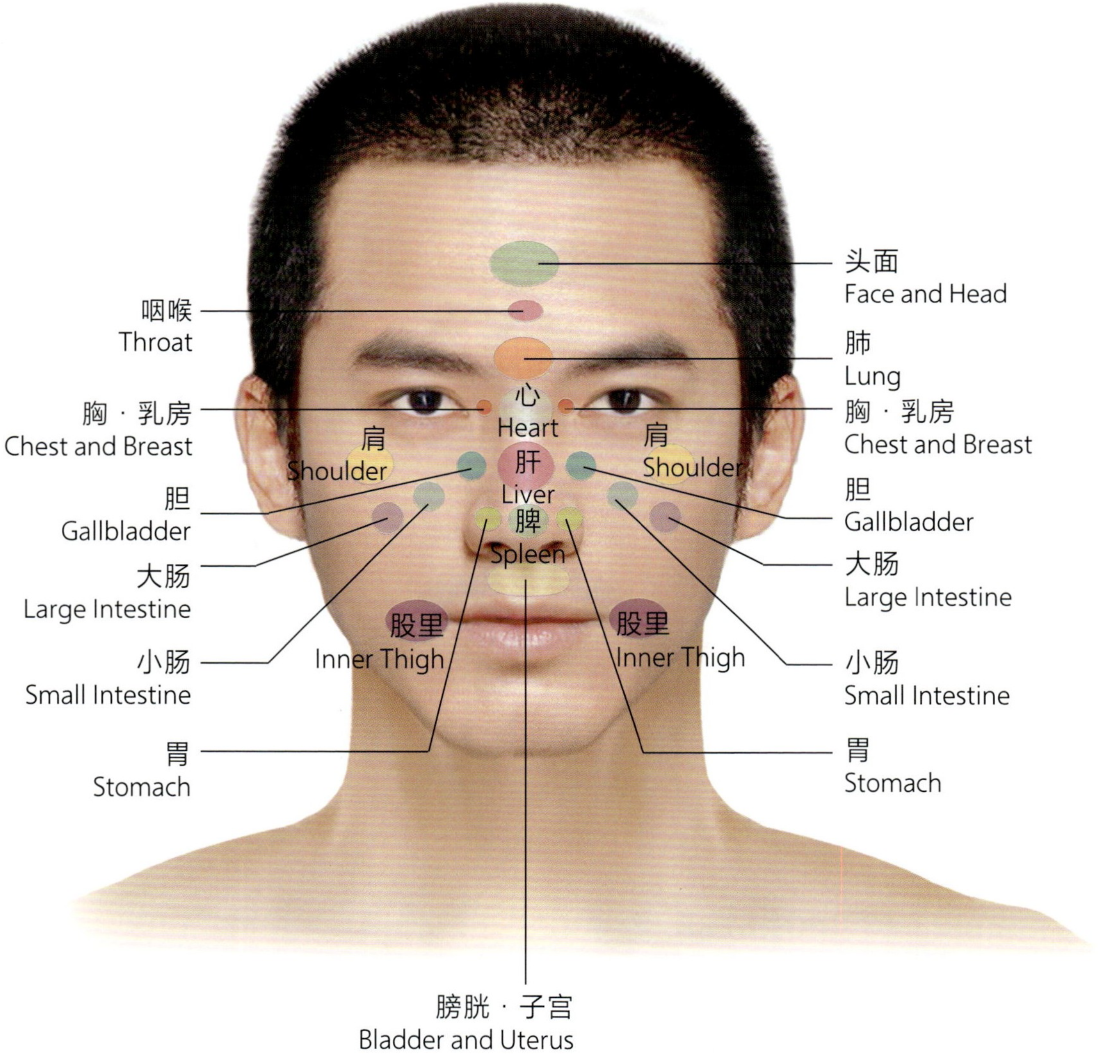

续表

反射区	定 位	主 治
大肠	目外眦直下方，颧骨下缘	结肠炎、便秘、腹痛、腹泻、痔疮、痢疾等
股里	口角旁开 0.5 寸，近地仓穴	股内侧痛
肾	大肠反射区外方颊部，约当鼻翼水平线与太阳穴直下垂线相交处	尿少、尿痛、尿频等
脐	肾反射区下 0.3 寸	腹痛、腹泻等
背	颊部中央外后方 1 寸处	颈背部软组织损伤、腰酸背痛等
臂	肩反射区外，下关穴直上	肩臂肿痛、麻木、无力等

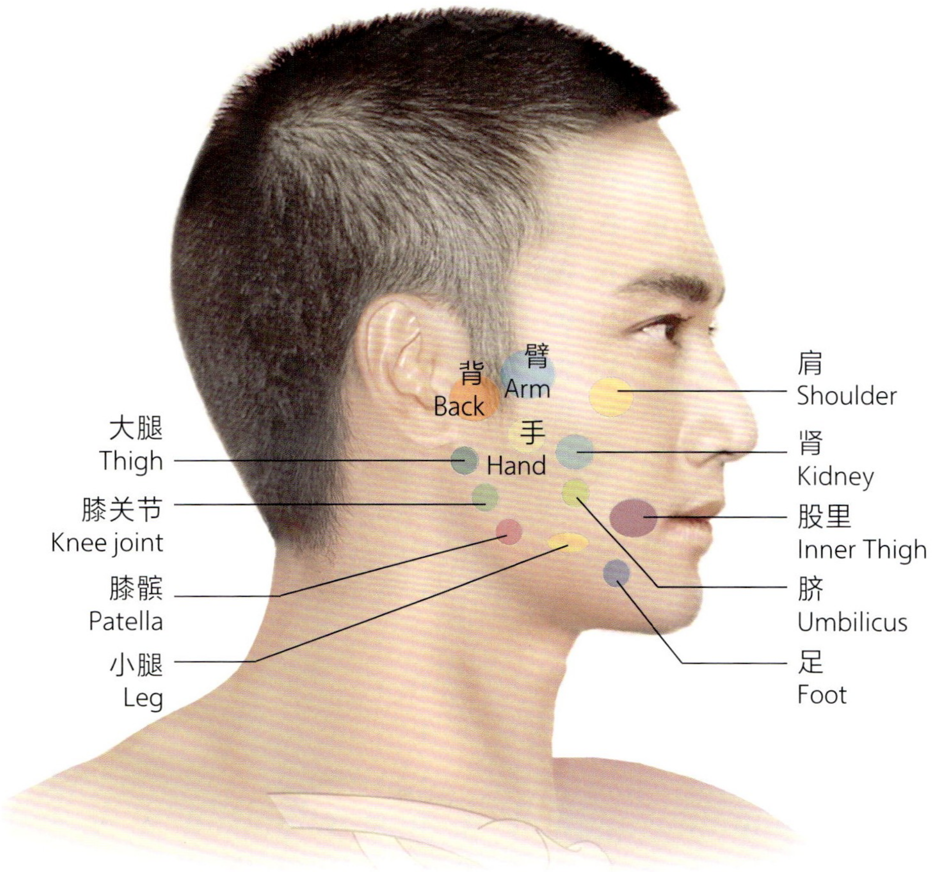

Continued

Reflex Zone	Location	Indications
Large Intestine	It locates straightly below the outer canthus at the border of the malar bone	Colitis; constipation; abdominal pain; diarrhea; hemorrhoids; dysentery and so on
Inner Thigh	0.5 cun next to the corner of the mouth, being close to the Dicang point	Pain in the internal hip
Kidney	The cheek of the lateral portion of the reflex zone of the Large Intestine, it locate about the junction of the waterline of the nose wing and the straight down line of the Taiyang point	Oliguria; painful urination; frequent urine
Navel	It locates 0.3 cun below the reflex zone of the Kidney	Abdominal pain; diarrhea and so on
Back	It locates at the portion 1 cun posterior to the lateral side of the central of the cheek	Soft tissue injury in the neck and back; soreness and pain in waist and back
Arm	It locates at the straight upside portion of the Xiaguan point at the inferior portion of the reflex zone of the Shoulder	Painful and swollen shoulder and arm; numbness; weakness

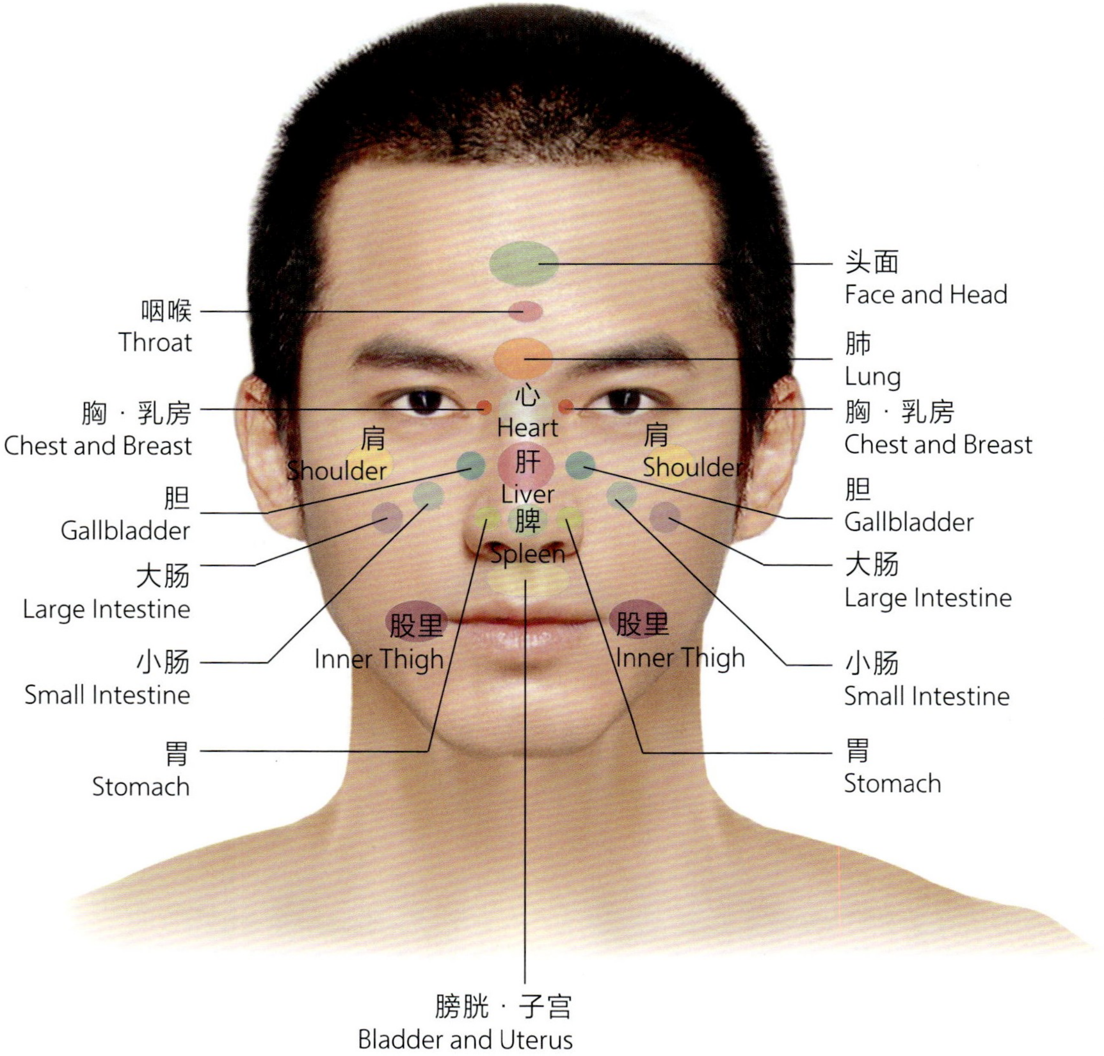

续表

反射区	定位	主治
手	臂反射区内下方，颧骨弓下缘处	手肿痛
大腿	耳垂与下颌角连线中上 1/3 处	大腿肌肉拉伤
膝关节	耳垂与下颌角连线中下 1/3 处	膝关节肿痛等
膝髌	下颌角上方凹陷处	膝关节损伤
小腿	下颌角前方	小腿疼痛、抽搐、肌肉酸痛
足	目外眦直下，下颌骨上缘	足部肿痛、足跟痛、足弓损伤等

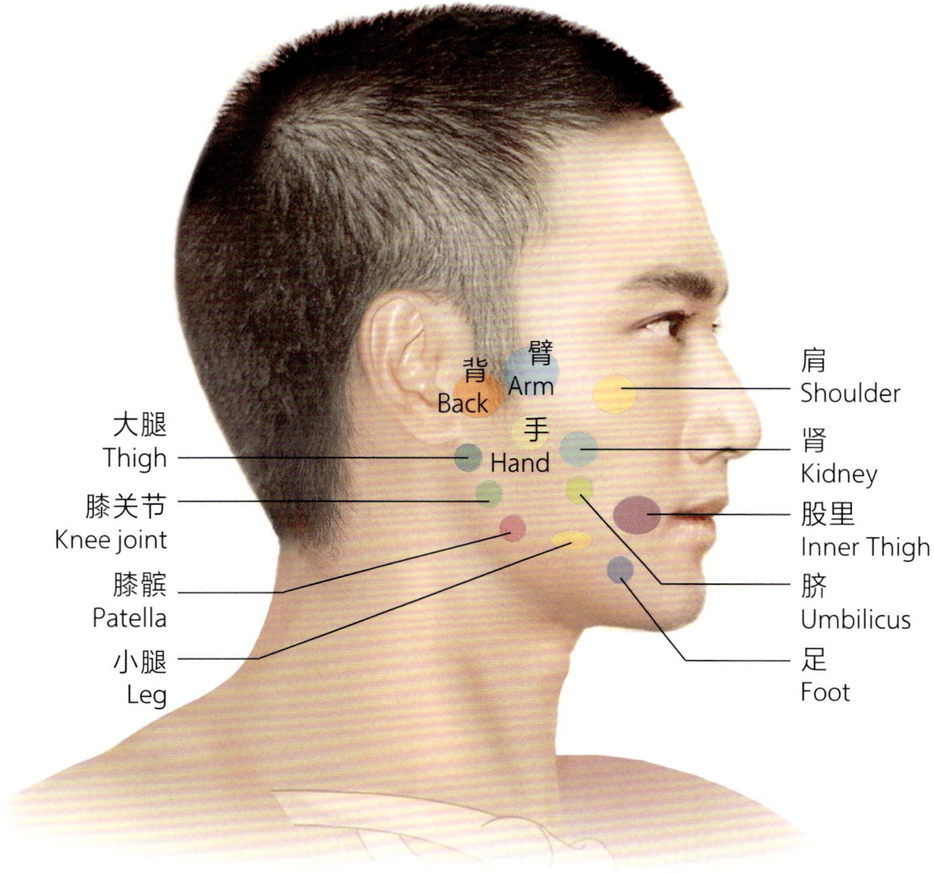

Continued

Reflex Zone	Location	Indications
Hand	It locates at the inferior border of the arch of the malar bone at the inferior portion inside the reflex zone of the Arm	Painful and swollen hands
Thigh	It locates at the superior 1/3 portion in the middle of the line between the earlobe and the lower mandible	Muscle sprain of thigh
Knee Joint	It locates at the inferior 1/3 portion in the middle of the line between the earlobe and the lower mandible	Painful and swollen knee joint and so on
Patella	It locates at the depression above the lower mandible	Injury of the knee joint
Leg	It locates anterior to the corner of the lower mandible	Pain in leg; convulsions; soreness in the muscles
Foot	It locates straightly below the outer canthus at the superior border of the lower jaw	painful and swollen foot; pain in heel; injury of the foot arch and so on

头面部常用穴位
Common Acupoints in Head and Face

手阳明大肠经
Large Intestine Meridian of Hand-Yangming

足太阳膀胱经
Bladder Meridian of Foot-Taiyang

足阳明胃经
Stomach Meridian of Foot-Yangming

任脉
Conception Vessel Meridian

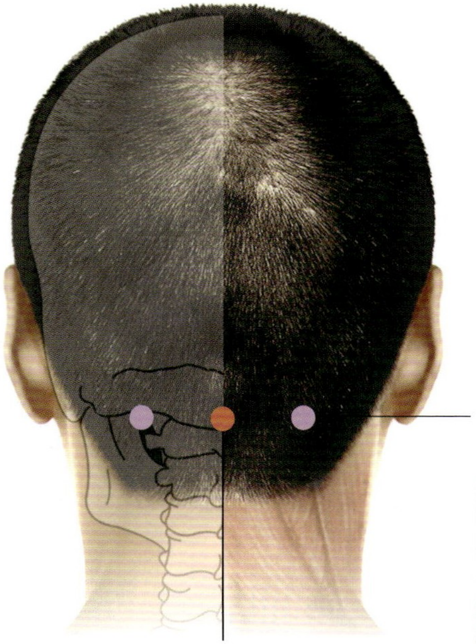

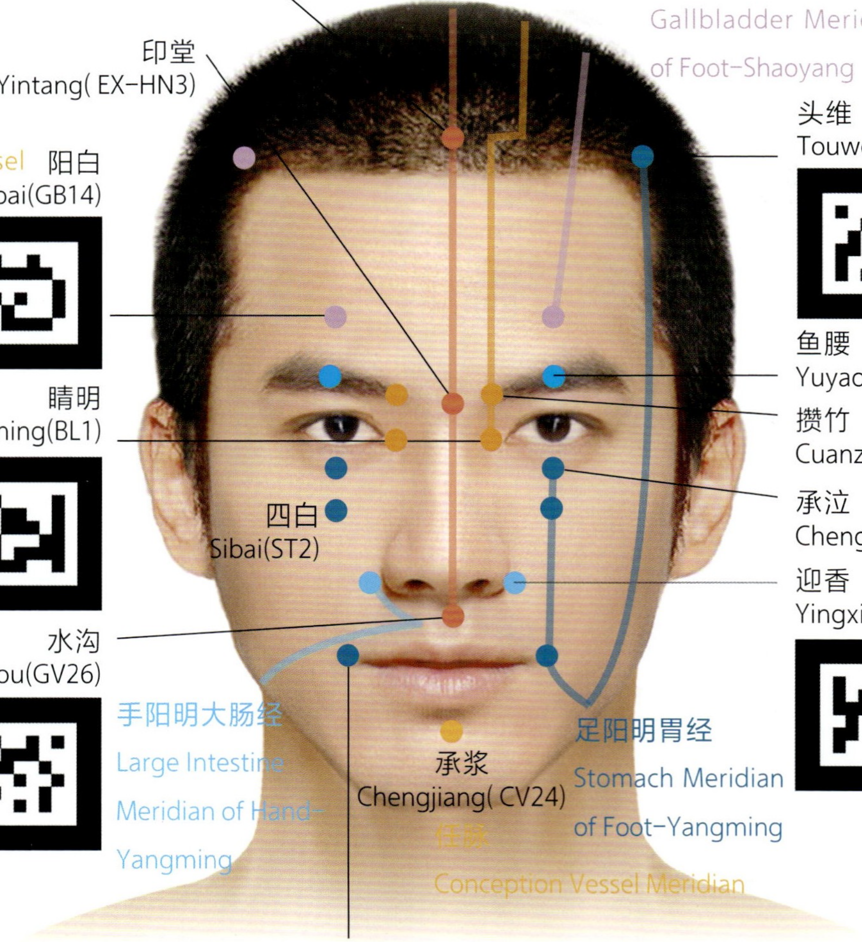

足少阳胆经
Gallbladder Meridian of Foot-Shaoyang

督脉
Governor Vessel Meridian

手太阳小肠经
Small Intestine Meridian of Hand-Taiyang

手少阳三焦经
Triple Energizer Meridian of Hand-Shaoyang

经外奇穴
Extra Points

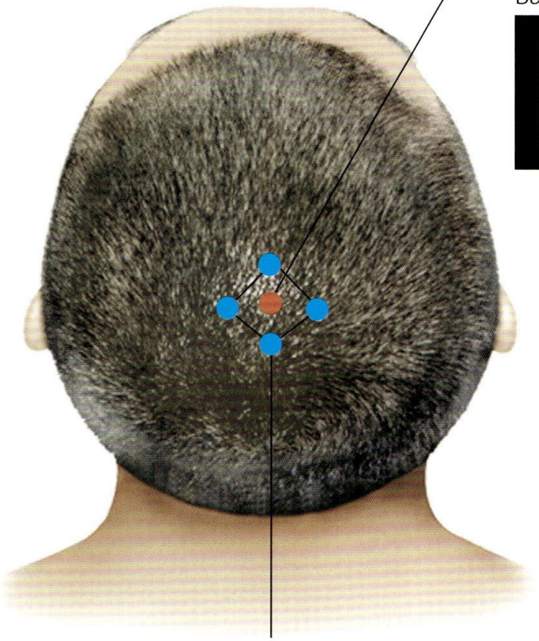

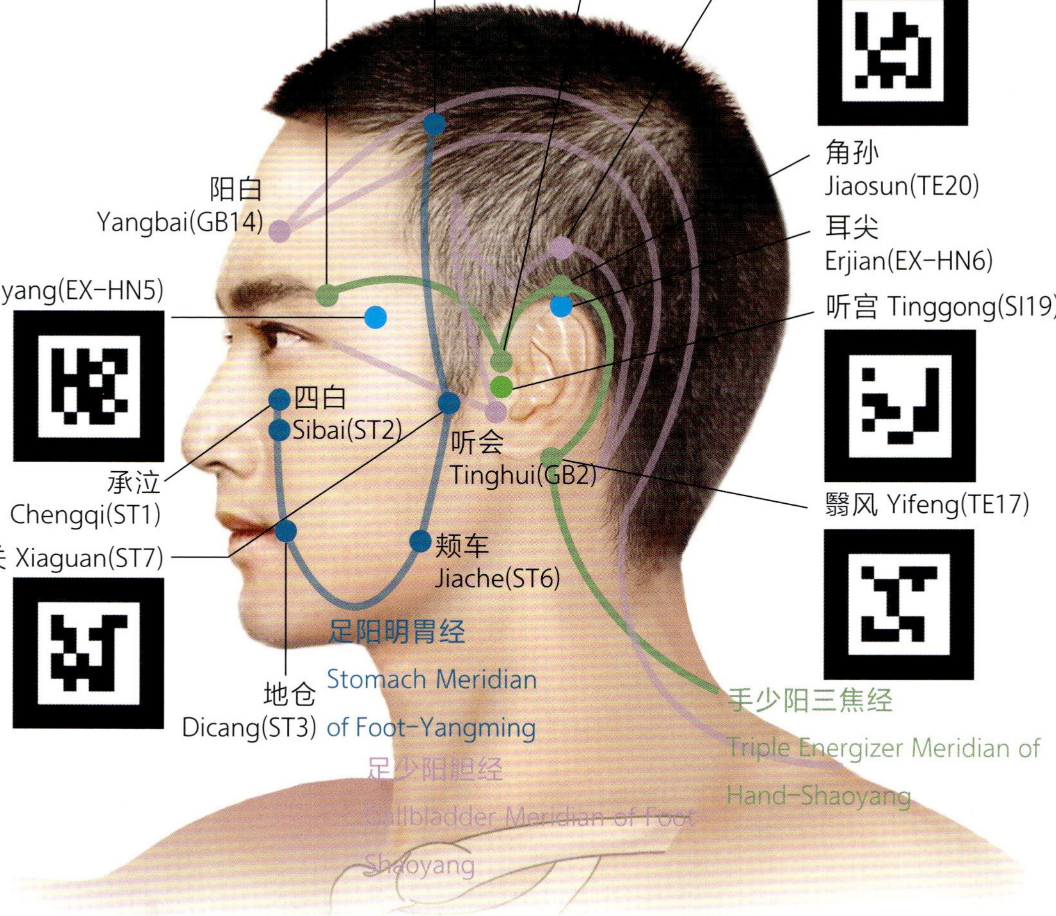

穴位		定位	主治
手阳明大肠经	迎香	在面部，鼻翼外缘中点旁，鼻唇沟中	鼻炎、口㖞、胆道蛔虫症
足阳明胃经	承泣	在面部，眼球与眶下缘之间，瞳孔直下	目赤肿痛、流泪、近视、眼睑抽动、面瘫、面肌痉挛
	四白	在面部，眶下孔处	目赤肿痛、眼睑瞤动、近视、面瘫、胆道蛔虫症、头痛、眩晕
	地仓	在面部，口角旁开 0.4 寸（指寸）	面瘫、面肌痉挛、眼睑瞤动
	颊车	在面部，下颌角前上方约一横指（中指） *取穴小窍门：沿下颌角角平分线上一横指，闭口咬紧牙时咬肌隆起，放松时按之有凹陷处	面瘫、颊肿、齿痛、口噤不语、颞下颌关节炎
	下关	在面部，颧弓下缘中央与下颌切迹之间凹陷中 *取穴小窍门：闭口，上关直下，颧弓下缘凹陷中	耳鸣、耳聋、齿痛、面瘫、颞下颌关节炎
	头维	在头部，额角发际直上 0.5 寸，头正中线旁开 4.5 寸	头痛、眩晕、目痛、眼睑瞤动、老年痴呆
手太阳小肠经	听宫	在面部，耳屏正中与下颌骨髁突之间的凹陷中	耳鸣耳聋、癫狂

Acupoints		Location	Indications
Large Intestine Meridian of Hand-Yangming	Yingxiang (LI 20)	On the face, lateral to the midpoint of the ala nasi exterior margin and in the nasolabial groove	Rhinitis; wry mouth; biliary ascariasis
Stomach Meridian of foot-Yangming	Chengqi(ST1)	On the face, between the eyeball and the infraorbital ridge, directly below the pupil	Redness,swelling and pain of eyes; tears; myopia; eyelid twitches; facial paralysis; facial spasm
	Sibai(ST2)	On the face, in the depression of the infraorbital foramen	Redness,swelling and pain of eyes; twisting of the eyelids; myopia; facial paralysis; biliary ascariasis; headache; vertigo
	Dicang(ST3)	On the face, 0.4 cun lateral to the corner of the mouth	Facial paralysis; facial spasm; twisting of the eyelids
	Jiache(ST6)	On the face, one finger-breadth anterosuperior to the mandibular angle *Tips: one finger above the bisector of mandibular angle, the masseter muscles bulged when close and bite tightly, and could touch the depression when relax	Facial paralysis; swollen cheek; toothache; folded jaw preventing speech; temporomandibular arthritis
	Xiaguan(ST7)	On the face, below the zygomatic arch and in the depression anterior to mandibular condyloid process *Tips: close your mouth, directly below Shangguan(GB3), the depression below the zygomatic arch	Tinnitus; hearing loss; toothache; facial paralysis; temporomandibular arthritis
	Touwei(ST8)	On the head, 0.5 cun directly above the frontal hairline, 4.5 cun lateral to head midline	Headache; dizziness; eye pain; headache; dizziness; eye pain; dementia; Alzheimer' s disease
Small Intestine Meridian of Hand-Taiyang	Tinggong(SI19)	On the face, the depression between the center of tragus and the condyloid process of the mandible	Tinnitus and deafness; mania

续表

穴位		定位	主治
足太阳膀胱经	睛明	在面部，目内眦内上方眶内侧壁凹陷中 *取穴小窍门：闭目，在目内眦内上方 0.1 寸的凹陷中	近视、目赤肿痛、目视不明、夜盲、目翳、急性腰痛
	攒竹	在面部，眉头凹陷中，额切迹处 *取穴小窍门：沿睛明直上至眉头边缘可触及一凹陷即为本穴	头痛、面瘫、腰痛、目视不明、眼睑瞤动、眼睑下垂、眉棱骨痛
手少阳三焦经	翳风	在颈部，耳垂后方，乳突下端前方凹陷中	耳鸣、耳聋、口㖞、牙关紧闭、齿痛、呃逆、颊肿
	角孙	在头部，耳尖正对发际处	目翳、齿痛、偏头痛、项强
	耳门	在耳区，耳屏上切迹与下颌骨髁突之间的凹陷中 *取穴小窍门：微张口，耳屏上切迹前的凹陷中	耳鸣、耳聋、齿痛
	丝竹空	在面部，眉梢凹陷中	目赤肿痛、眼睑瞤动、目眩、头痛、癫狂
足少阳胆经	听会	在面部，耳屏间切迹与下颌骨髁突之间的凹陷中 *取穴小窍门：张口，耳屏间切迹前方的凹陷中	耳鸣、耳聋、颞颌关节炎
	率谷	在头部，耳尖直上入发际 1.5 寸 *取穴小窍门：咀嚼时，以手按之有肌肉鼓动	头痛、眩晕、耳鸣、耳聋
	阳白	在头部，眉上 1 寸，瞳孔直上	头痛、眩晕、视物模糊、目痛、眼睑下垂、面瘫、眼睑瞤动
	风池	在颈后区，枕骨之下，胸锁乳突肌上端与斜方肌上端之间的凹陷中	头痛、眩晕、失眠、癫痫、中风、感冒、颈项强痛

Acupoints		Location	Indications
Bladder Meridian of Foot-Taiyang	Jingming(BL1)	On the face, the depression on medial orbital wall above the inner canthus *Tips: close eyes, the depression, 0.1 cun above the inner canthus	Myopia; redness, swelling and pain of eyes; visual unknown; night blindness; conjunctivitis; acute lumbago
	Cuanzhu(BL2)	On the face, the medial end of the eyebrow, the frontal notch *Tips: upright Jingming(BL1) to brow edge can touch a depression, that is the point	Headache; facial paralysis; lower back pain; dim vision; twisting of the eyelids; eyelid ptosis; eyebrow bone pain
Triple Energizer Meridian of Hand-Shaoyang	Yifeng(TE 17)	On the neck, posterior to the ear lobe, the depression on mastoid process inferior side	Tinnitus; deafness; wry mouth; trismus; toothache; hiccup; swollen the cheek
	Jiaosun(TE20)	On the head, directly above the ear apex within the hairline	Conjunctivitis; toothache; migraine; rigidity of the neck
	Ermen(TE21)	On the ear, the depression between the incisura supertragica and the condyloid process of the mandible *Tips: open mouth, the depression anterior to the incisura supertragica	Tinnitus; deafness; toothache
	Sizhukong(TE23)	On the face, in the depression at the lateral end of the eyebrow	redness, swelling and pain of eyes; twisting of the eyelids; dizziness; headache; madness
Gallbladder Meridian of Foot-Shaoyang	Tinghui(GB2)	On the face, the depression between incisura intertragica and condyloid process of the mandible *Tips: open mouth , the depression anterior to incisura intertragica	Tinnitus; deafness; temporomandibular joint arthritis
	Shuaigu(GB8)	On the head, 1.5 cun directly above the hairline *Tips: when chewing, pressing the point can touch muscle agitation	Headache; dizziness; tinnitus; deafness
	Yangbai(GB14)	On the head, 1 cun above the midpoint of the eyebrow, directly above the pupil	Headache; dizziness; blurred vision; eye pain; ptosis; facial paralysis; twisting of the eyelids
	Fengchi(GB20)	In the posterior cervical region, below the occipital, the depression between the upper ends of the sternocleidomastoid and upper ends of trapezius muscles	Headache; dizziness; insomnia; epilepsy; wind stroke; cold; painful stiff neck and nape

续表

穴位		定位	主治
督脉	风府	在颈后区，枕外隆凸直下，两侧斜方肌之间凹陷中 *取穴小窍门：正坐，头稍仰，使项部斜方肌松弛，从项后发际正中上推至枕骨而止即是本穴	头痛、眩晕、项强、中风不语、半身不遂、癫狂、目痛、咽喉肿痛
	百会	在头部，前发际正中直上 5 寸 *取穴小窍门：折耳，两耳尖向上连线的中点	头痛、眩晕、中风不语、癫狂、失眠、健忘、脱肛、久泻、胃下垂
	神庭	在头部，前发际正中直上 0.5 寸 *取穴小窍门：发际不明者，眉心直上 3.5 寸处取穴	头痛、眩晕、失眠、癫痫、鼻炎、目痛
	水沟	在面部，人中沟的上 1/3 与中 1/3 交点处	昏迷、晕厥、中风、癫狂、抽搐、面瘫、齿痛、鼻塞、牙关紧闭、急性腰扭伤、消渴、黄疸、全身水肿
	印堂	在头部，两眉毛内侧端中间的凹陷中	头痛、眩晕、失眠、小儿惊风、鼻塞、鼻炎、眉棱骨痛、目痛
任脉	承浆	在面部，颏唇沟的正中凹陷处	面瘫、齿龈肿痛、暴喑（突然失音）、消渴、癫痫
经外奇穴	四神聪	在头部，百会前后左右各旁开 1 寸，共 4 穴 *取穴小窍门：后神聪在前后发际正中连线的中点处	头痛、眩晕、失眠、健忘、癫痫
	鱼腰	在头部，瞳孔直上，眉毛中	目赤肿痛、目翳、眼睑下垂、眼睑瞤动、眉棱骨痛
	太阳	在头部，眉梢与目外眦之间，向后约一横指的凹陷中	头痛、目疾、齿痛、面痛、面瘫
	耳尖	在耳区，在外耳轮的最高点 *取穴小窍门：折耳向前时，耳郭上方的尖端处	目赤肿痛、目翳、睑腺炎、咽喉肿痛

Acupoints		Location	Indications
Governor Vessel Meridian	Fengfu(GV16)	In the posterior cervical region, directly below the external occipital protuberance, the depression between both sides trapezius muscles *Tips: sit straight, head slightly upward, relax trapezius muscle, after the median to stop is the point, pressing from median hairline behind the neck till occipital bone is the point	Headache; dizziness; rigidity of the neck; aneos; hemiplegia; mania; eye pain; sore throat
	Baihui(GV20)	On the head, 5 cun directly above the midpoint of the anterior hairline *Tips: fold the ears, the midpoint of the line of 2 tips of ears	Headache; dizziness; aneos; mania; insomnia; amnesia; prolapse of the rectum; enduring diarrhea; gastroptosia
	Shenting(GV24)	On the head, 0.5 cun directly above the midpoint of the anterior hairline *Tips: the unclear hairline, 3.5 cun directly above the eyebrows middle	Headache; dizziness; insomnia; epilepsy; rhinitis; eye pain
	Shuigou(GV26)	On the face, at the junction of the upper 1/3 and middle 1/3 of the philtrum	Syncope; wind stroke; coma; convulsions; paralysis; madness; toothache; nasal congestion; trismus; acute lumbar sprain; diabetes; jaundice; dropsy
	Yintang(EX-HN3)	On the head, the depression between the middle of 2 eyebrows medial ends	Headache; dizziness; insomnia; child fright wind; rhinitis; stuffy nose; brow bone pain; pain in the eyes
Conception Vessel Meridian	Chengjiang (CV24)	On the face, the depression of the center of the mentolabial groove	Facial paralysis; gingival swelling; sudden loss of voice; diabetes; epilepsy
Extra Points	Sishencong (EX-HN1)	On the parietal region, 1 cun anterior, posterior and lateral to Baihui,4 acupoints totally *Tips: on the midpoint of the connection line of the anterior and posterior middle hairline	Headache; dizziness; insomnia; amnesia; epilepsy
	Yuyao(EX-HN4)	On the head, directly above the pupil, in the center of the eyebrow	Redness, swelling and pain of eyes; conjunctivitis; drooping eyelids; twisting of the eyelids; eyebrow bone pain
	Taiyang(EX-HN5)	On the head, between the brow and the outer canthus, the depression after 1 finger	Headache; eye disease; toothache; facial pain; facial paralysis
	Erjian(EX-HN6)	On the ear region, the vertex of external helix *Tip: at the tip of the auricle when the ear folded forward	Redness, swelling and pain of eyes; conjunctivitis; stye; sore throat

超简单头面部穴位按摩

Super-easy Massage of Acupoints in Head and Face

迎香

用两手食指按揉两侧迎香穴 2 分钟，力度稍轻。每日 2 次

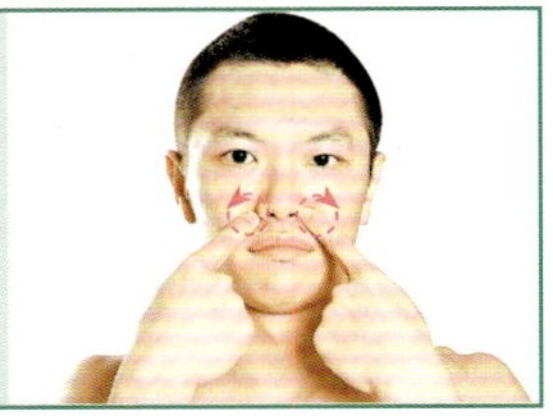

承泣

用两手食指按揉两侧承泣穴 2 分钟，力度稍轻。每日 2 次

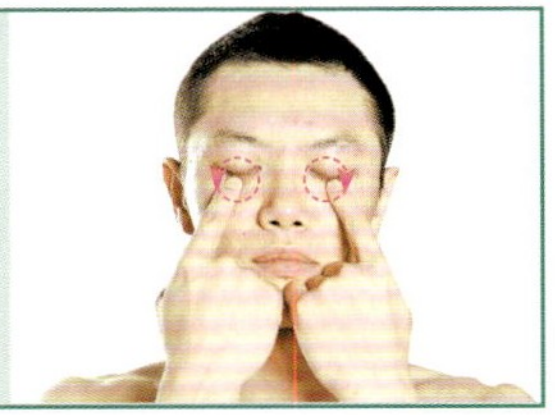

四白

用双手食指按压两侧四白穴，停留片刻后放松，反复 5~6 下，力度稍轻。每日 2 次

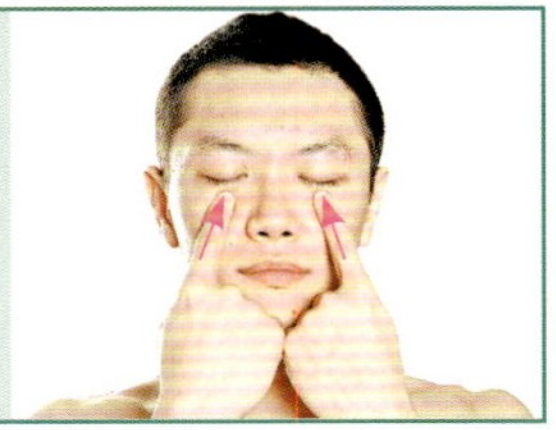

地仓

用食指稍用力按压地仓穴，停留片刻后放松，反复 5~6 下。同法按压对侧地仓穴。每日 2 次

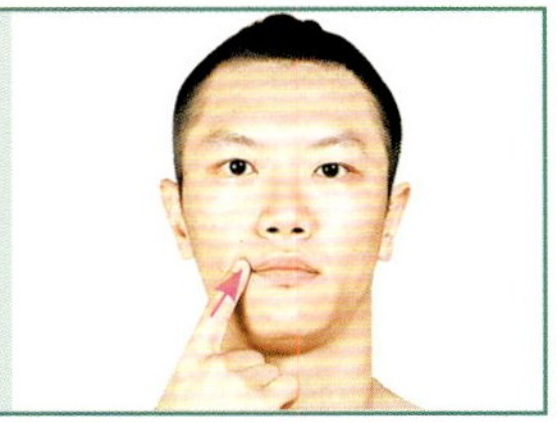

颊车

用双手食指稍用力按压两侧颊车穴，停留片刻后放松，反复 5~6 下。每日 2 次

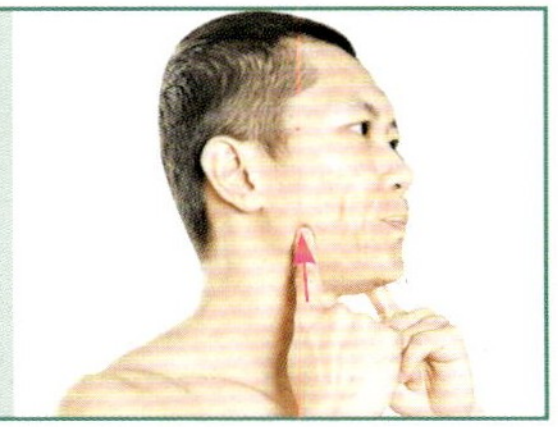

下关

用拇指稍用力按压下关穴，停留片刻后放松，反复 5~6 下。同法按压对侧下关穴。每日 2 次

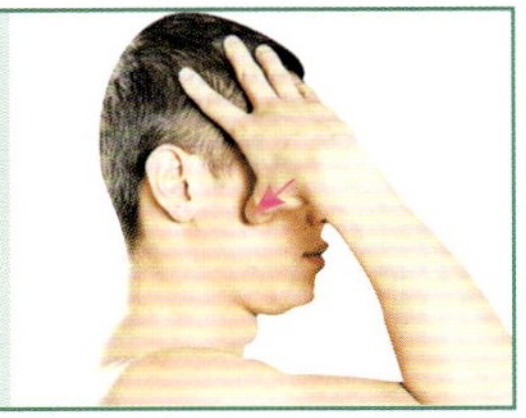

头维

用食指按揉头维穴 2 分钟，力度稍重。同法按揉对侧头维穴。每日 2 次

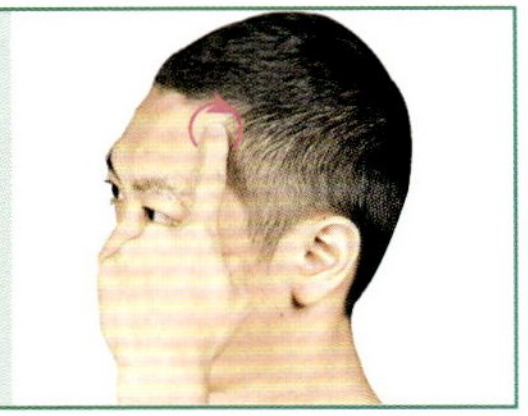

听宫

用食指稍用力按压听宫穴，停留片刻后放松，反复 5~6 下。同法按揉对侧听宫穴。每日 2 次

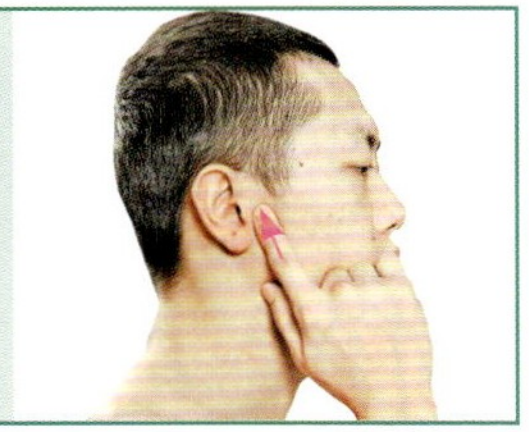

睛明

用双手拇指按揉两侧睛明穴 2 分钟，力度稍轻。每日 2 次

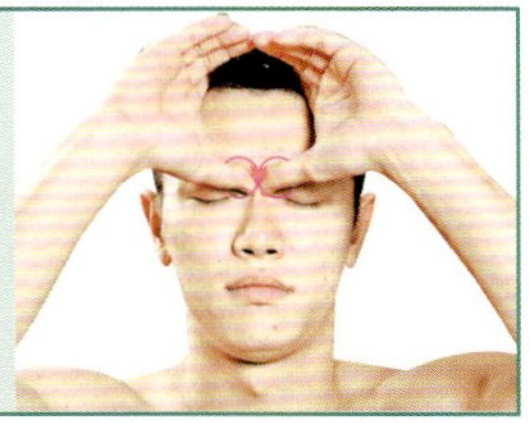

攒竹

将两手拇指按揉两侧攒竹穴 2 分钟，力度稍轻。每日 2 次

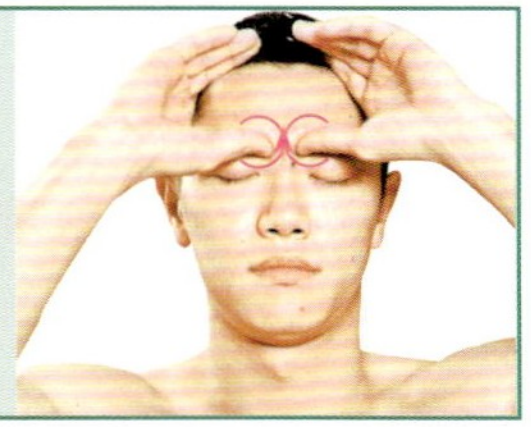

Yingxiang(LI20)

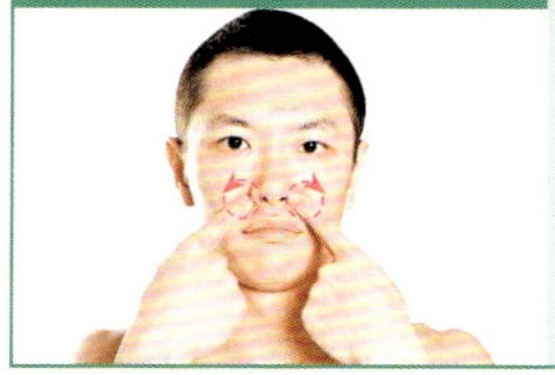

Kneading both sides Yingxiang(LI20) slightly with index fingers for 2 minutes, 2 times each day

Chengqi(ST1)

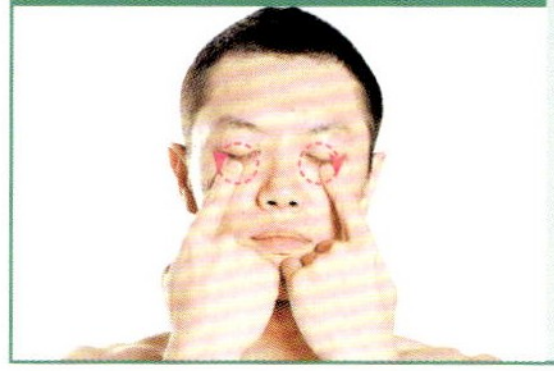

Kneading both sides Chengqi(ST1) slightly with index fingers for 2 minutes, 2 times each day

Sibai(ST2)

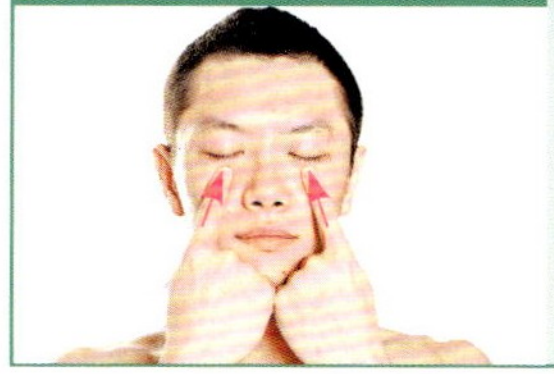

Pressing both sides Sibai(ST2) slightly with index fingers, keep for a while and relax, and repeat 5 to 6 times, 2 times each day

Dicang(ST3)

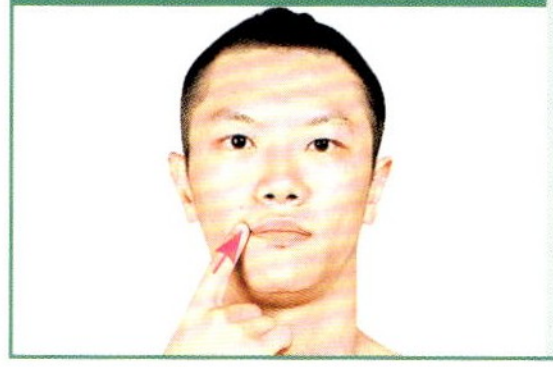

Pressing Dicang(ST3) a little heavily with index fingers, keep for a while and relax, and repeat 5 to 6 times. Apply the same way to press the other side, 2 times each day

Jiache(ST6)

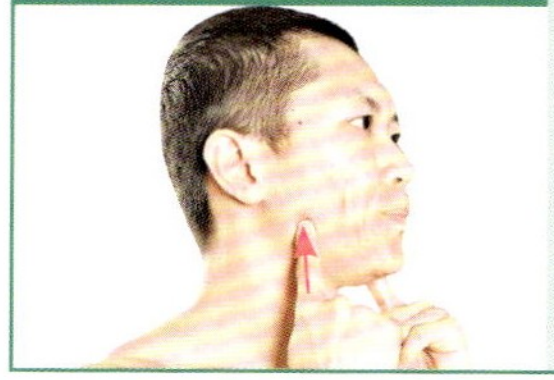

Pressing both sides Jiache(ST6) a little heavily with index fingers, keep for a while and relax, and repeat 5 to 6 times. Apply the same way to press the other side, 2 times each day

Xiaguan(ST7)

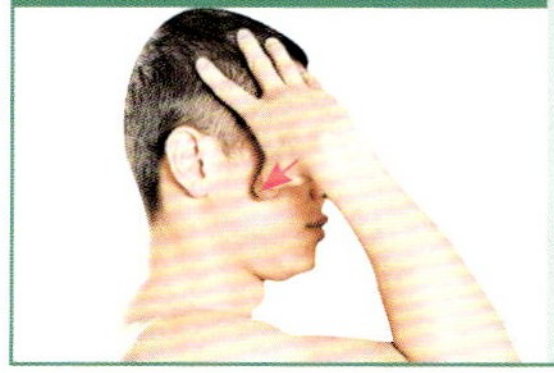

Pressing Xiaguan(ST7) a little heavily with thumbs, keep for a while and relax, and repeat 5 to 6 times. Apply the same way to press the other side, 2 times each day

Touwei(ST8)

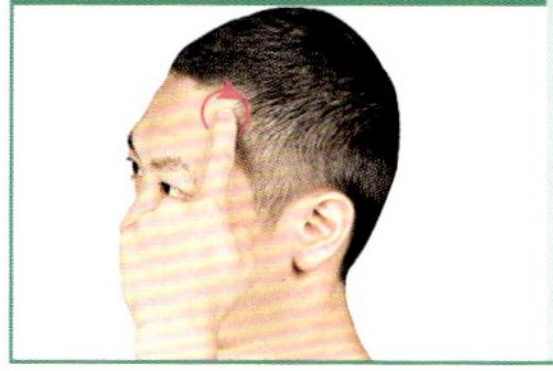

Kneading Touwei(ST8) a little heavily with index fingers for 2 minutes. Apply the same way to press the other side, 2 times each day

Tinggong(SI19)

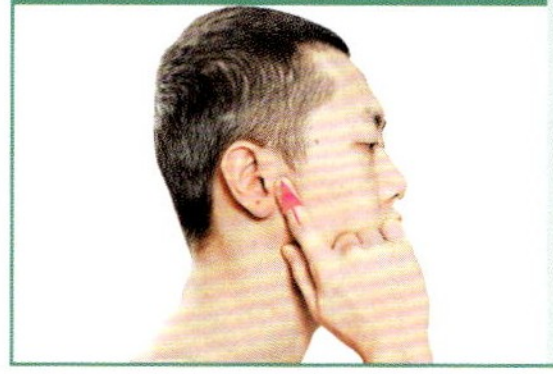

Pressing Tinggong(SI19) a little heavily with index fingers, keep for a while and relax, and repeat 5 to 6 times. Apply the same way to press the other side, 2 times each day

Jingming(BL1)

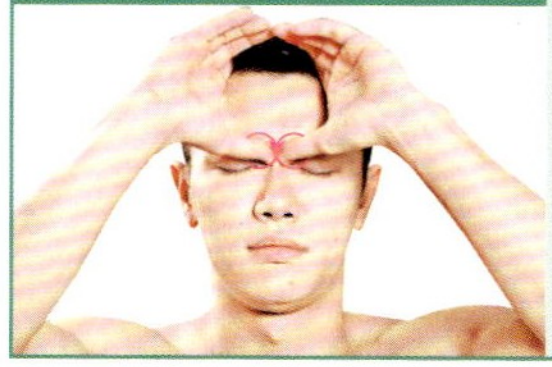

Kneading both sides Jingming(BL1) with thumbs slightly for 2 minutes, 2 times each day

Cuanzhu(BL2)

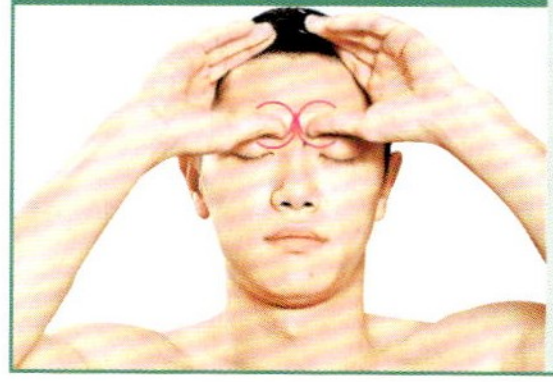

Kneading both sides Cuanzhu(BL2) with thumbs slightly for 2 minutes, 2 times each day

翳风

食、中二指并拢稍用力按压翳风穴，停留片刻后放松，反复 5~6 下。同法按压对侧翳风穴。每日 2 次

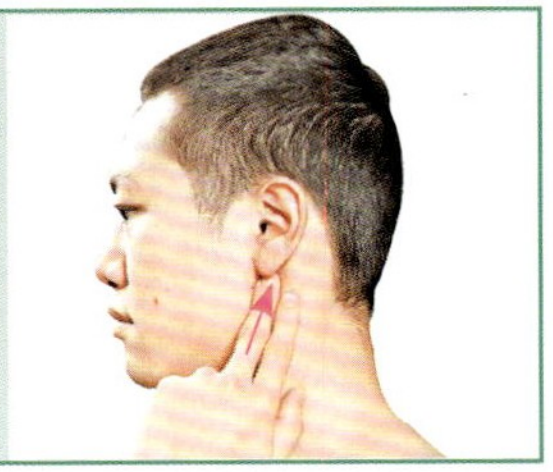

耳门

用食指按揉耳门穴 2 分钟，力度适中。同法按揉对侧耳门穴。每日 2 次

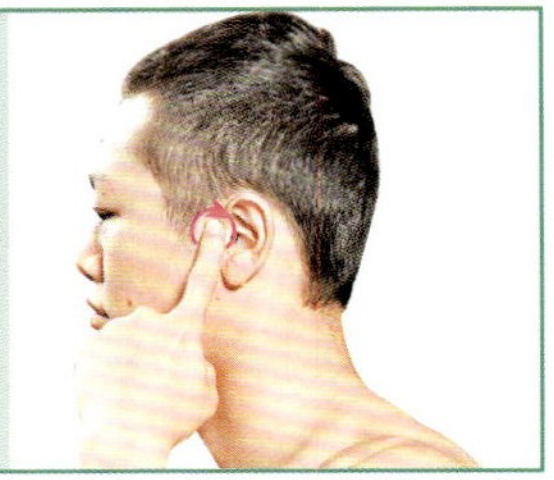

听会

用食指稍用力按压听会穴，停留片刻后放松，反复 5~6 下。同法按压对侧听会穴。每日 2 次

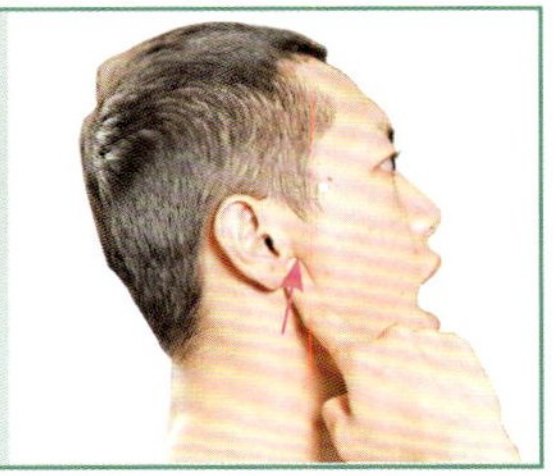

风池

两手拇指勾揉两侧风池穴 2 分钟，力度稍重。每日 2 次

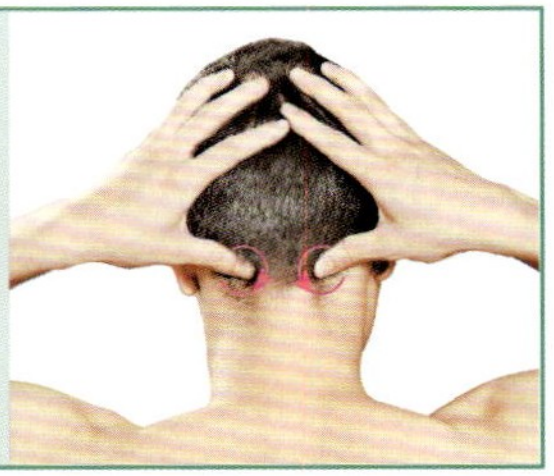

百会

两手食指重叠稍用力按压百会穴，停留片刻后放松，反复 5~6 下。每日 2 次

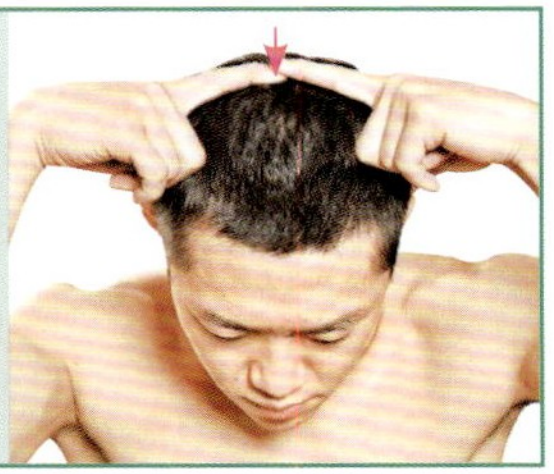

神庭

用拇指指端掐按神庭穴，力度可稍重，每分钟 30~50 下。每日 2 次

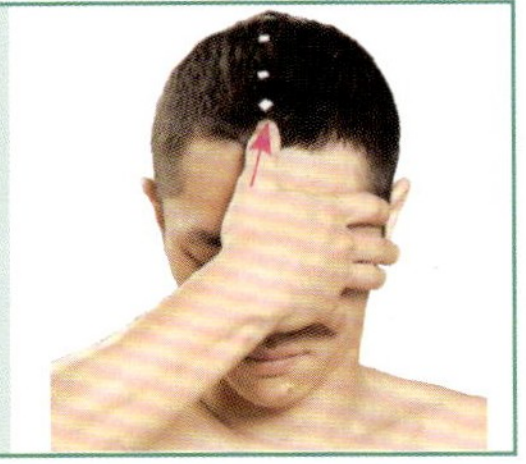

水沟

先用拇指指甲掐按水沟穴 30 下，掐后再揉按 30 下，力度稍重。每日 2 次

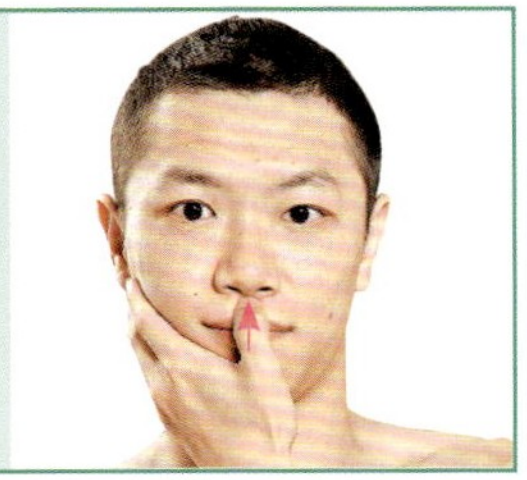

印堂

用拇指掐揉印堂穴 2 分钟，力度适中。每日 2 次

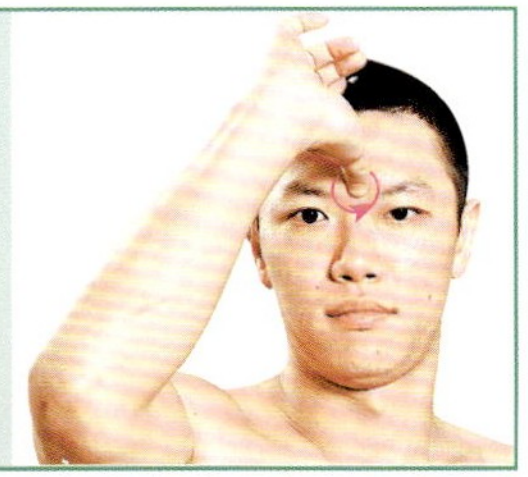

承浆

先用拇指掐按承浆穴 30 下，掐后再按揉 30 下，力度稍重，至有酸胀感。每日 2 次

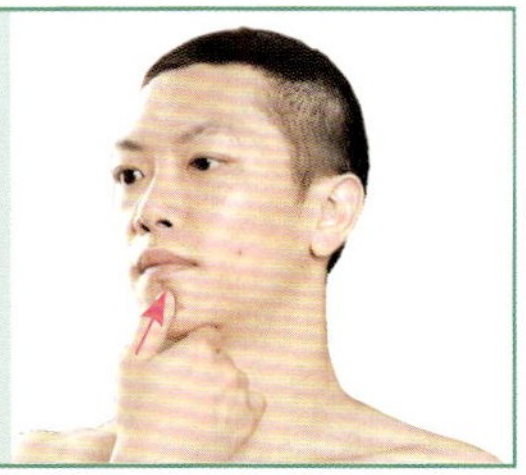

太阳

用两手拇指按揉两侧太阳穴 2 分钟，力度稍重。每日 2 次

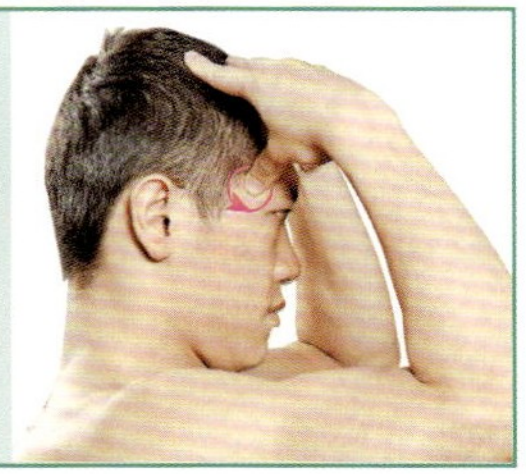

Yifeng(TE17)

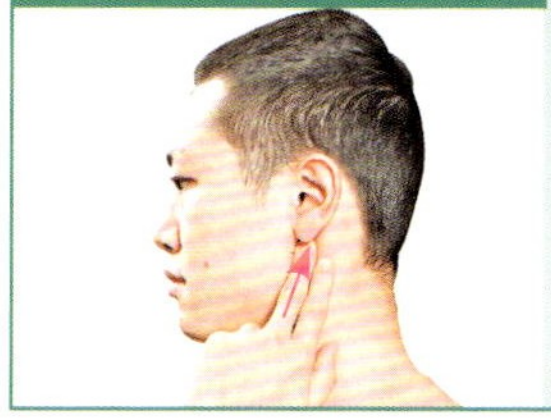

Pressing both sides Yifeng(TE17) a little heavily with index finger and middle finger, keep for a while and relax, and repeat 5 to 6 times. Apply the same way to press the other side, 2 times each day

Ermen(TE21)

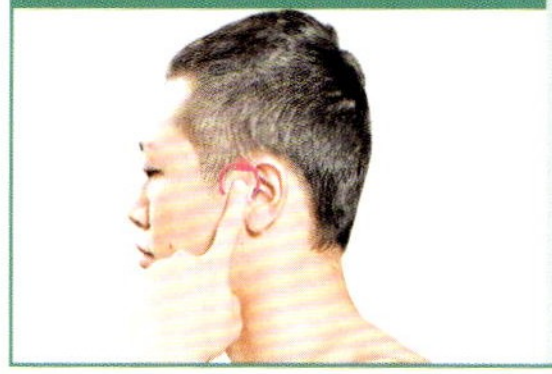

Kneading Ermen(TE21) with index finger for 2 minutes with moderate strength. Apply the same way to press the other side, 2 times each day

Tinghui(GB2)

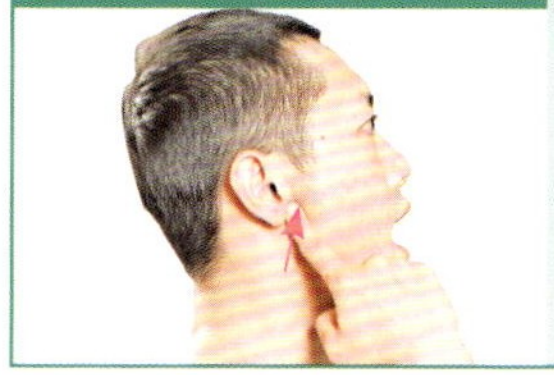

Pressing Tinghui(GB2) a little heavily with index finger, keep for a while and relax, and repeat 5 to 6 times. Apply the same way to press the other side, 2 times each day

Fengchi(GB20)

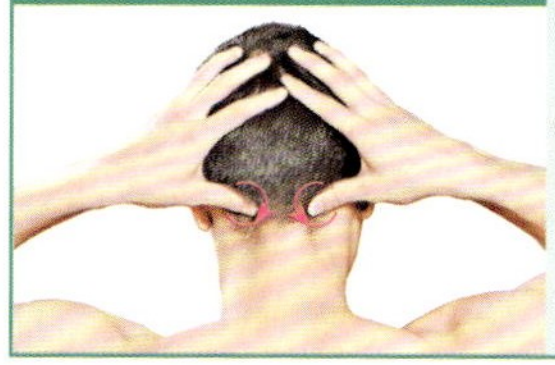

Kneading both sides Fengchi(GB20) a little heavily with thumbs for 2 minutes, 2 times each day

Baihui(GV20)

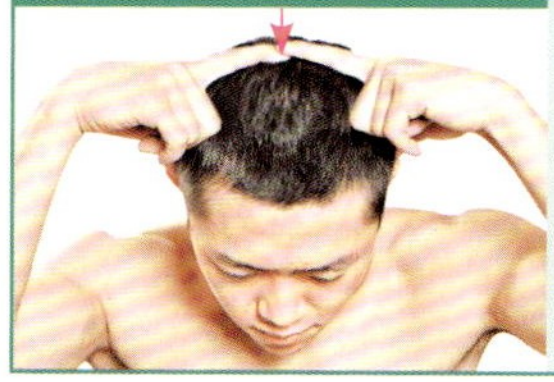

Pressing Baihui(GV20) a little heavily with overlap index fingers, keep for a while and relax, and repeat 5 to 6 times, 2 times each day

Shenting(GV24)

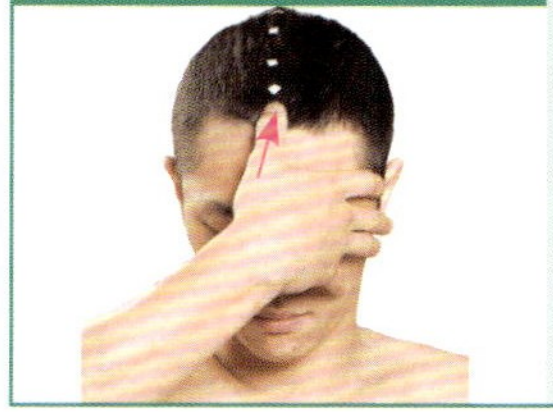

Fingernail pressing Shenting(GV24) a little heavily with thumb, 30 to 50 times one minute, 2 times a day

Shuigou(GV26)

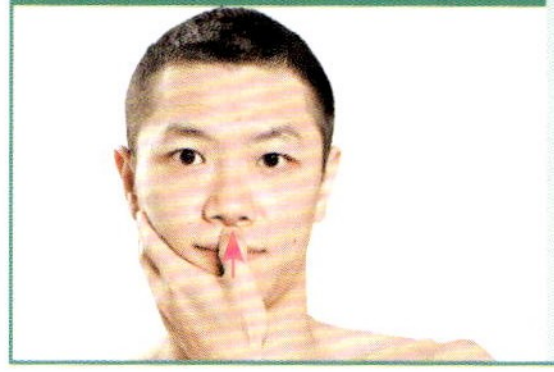

Fingernail pressing Shuigou(GV26) with thumb for 30 times, and then kneading a little heavily for 30 times, 2 times a day

Yintang(EX-HN3)

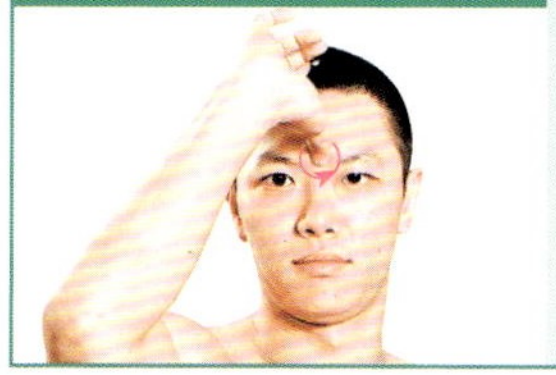

Pinch rubbing Yintang(EX-HN3) with thumb for 2 minutes with moderate strength, 2 times a day

Chengjiang(CV24)

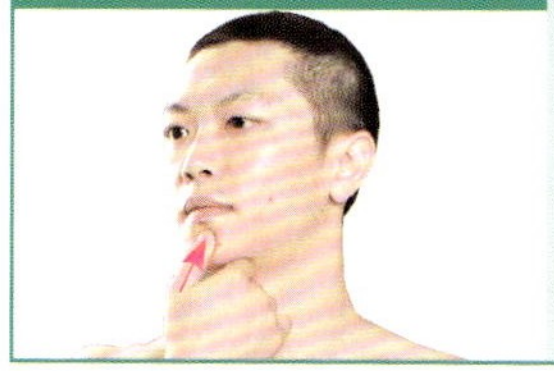

Fingernail pressing Chengjiang(CV24) with thumb for 30 times, and then kneading a little heavily 30 times till feeling acid and swell, 2 times a day

Taiyang(EX-HN5)

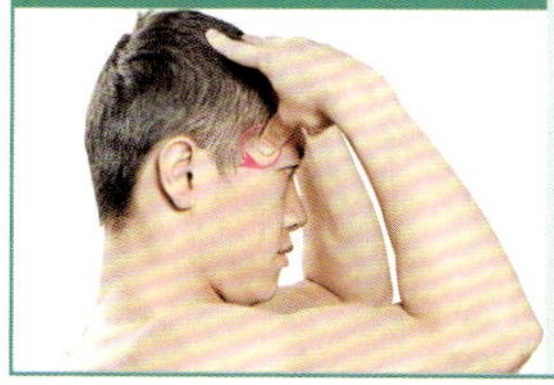

Kneading both sides Taiyang(EX-HN5) a little heavily with thumbs, 2 times a day

第五章　脊柱反射区及穴位

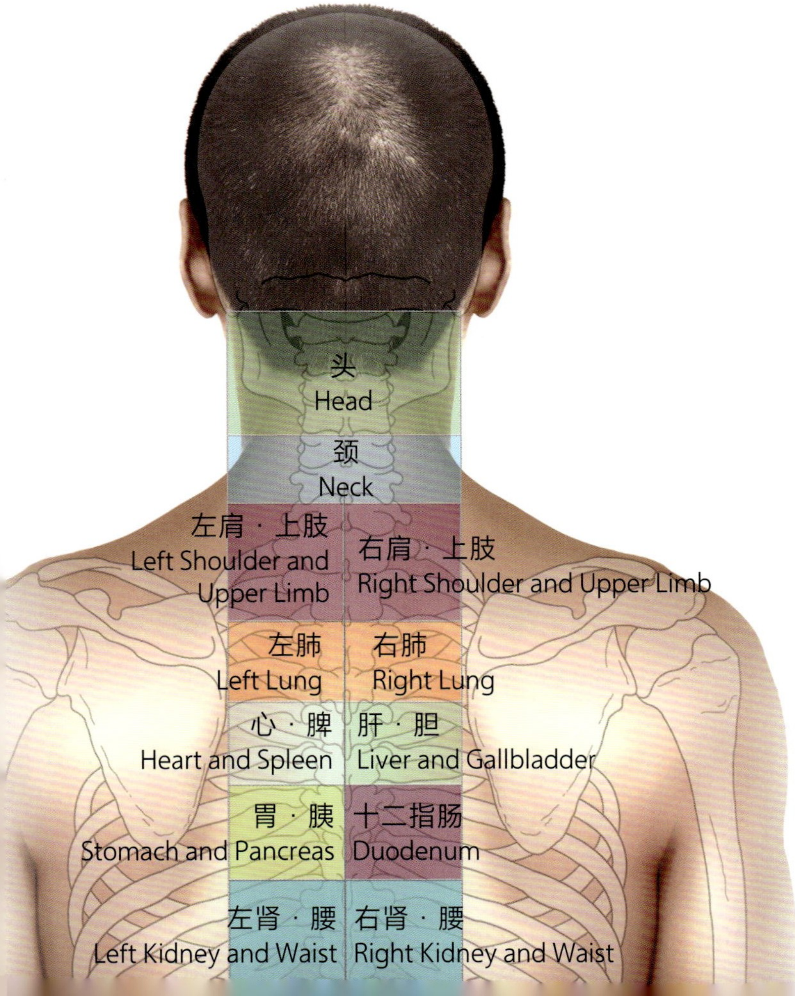

反射区	定位	主治
头	颈部第 1~4 颈椎区域	脑震荡、头痛、头晕、失眠、神经衰弱、神志不清、脑萎缩等
颈	颈部第 5~6 颈椎区域	颈椎病、落枕、颈部软组织损伤等颈部疾患
肩 · 上肢	在过肩胛内侧的垂线内，第 7 颈椎至第 2 胸椎区域。以后正中线为界，分为左、右肩 · 上肢反射区	肩周炎、肩酸痛、手臂无力、手麻等肩部及上肢疾患
肺	在过肩胛内侧的垂线内，第 3~4 胸椎区域。以后正中线为界，分为左、右肺反射区	肺部及支气管疾患如肺炎、支气管炎、哮喘、肺气肿等
心 · 脾	在过肩胛内侧的垂线内，第 5~6 胸椎左侧区域	心律不齐、心肌炎、冠心病、高血压、低血压等

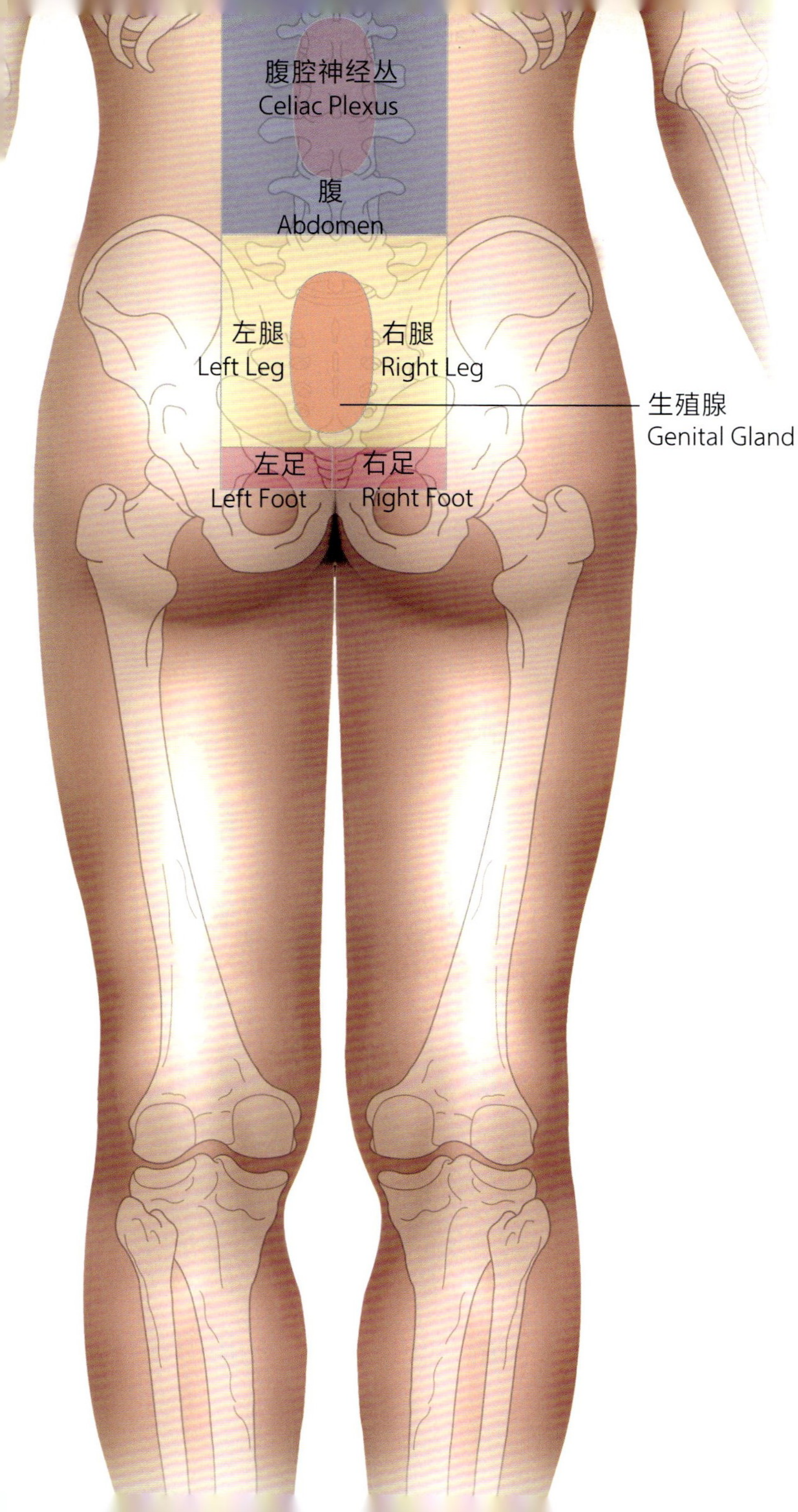

Chapter 5: Reflex Zones and Acupoints in Spine

Reflex Zone	Location	Indications
Head	The 1st to the 4th cervical region of cervix	Concussion; headache; dizziness; insomnia; neurasthenia; unconsciousness; brain atrophy and so on
Neck	The 5th to the 6th cervical region of cervix	Cervical spondylopathy; stiff neck; neck soft tissue injury and other neck disease
Shoulder and Limb	In a vertical inner side of the scapula, from the 7th cervical vertebra to the 2nd thoracic vertebra region. The midline is as boundary, dividing into left, right shoulder and upper limb	Periarthritis of shoulder; shoulder pain; arm weakness; numbness; and other shoulder and upper limb disorders
Lung	In a vertical inner side of the scapula, from the 3rd thoracic vertebra region to the 4th thoracic vertebra region. The midline is as boundary, dividing into Left, Right Lung reflex zones	Pulmonary and bronchial diseases such as pneumonia, bronchitis, asthma, emphysema and so on
Heart and Spleen	In a vertical inner side of the scapula, the left side of the 5th to the 6th thoracic vertebra region	Arrhythmia; myocarditis; coronary heart disease; hypertension; hypotension and so on.

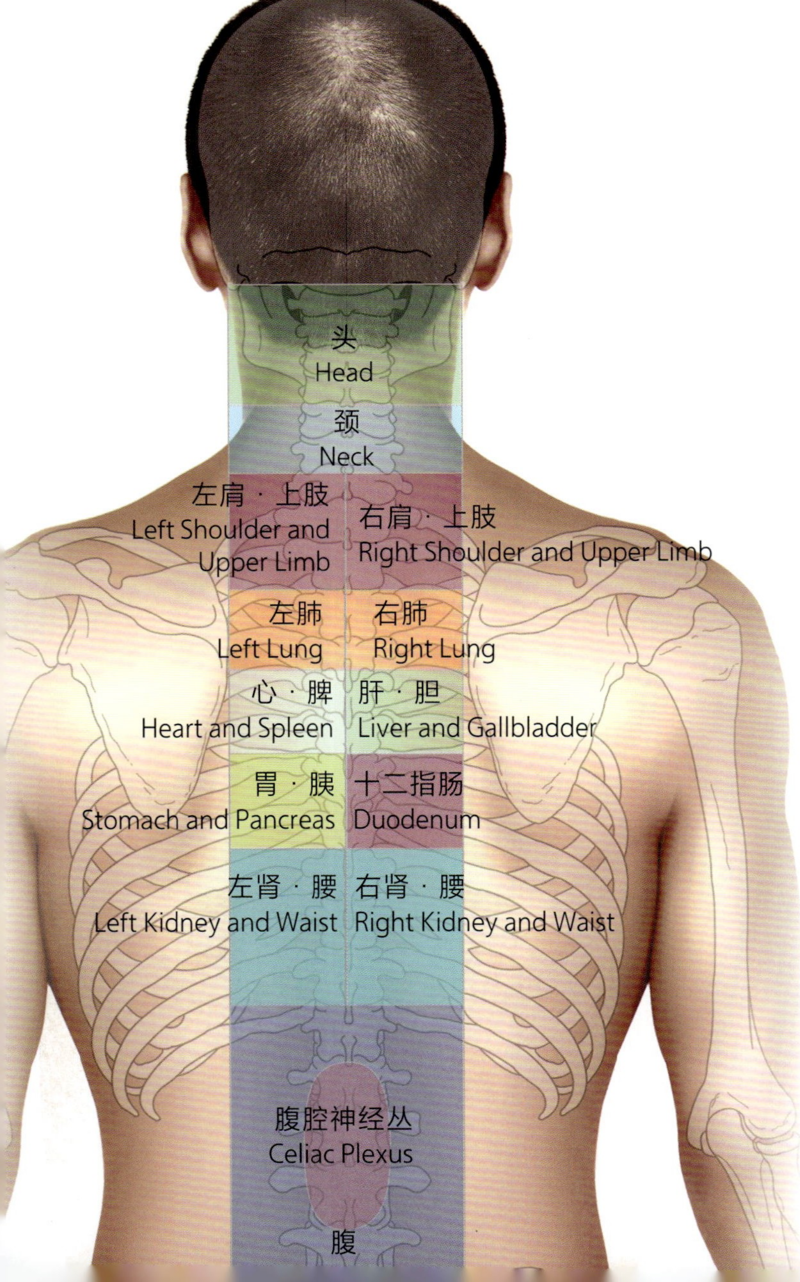

续表

反射区	定 位	主 治
肝 · 胆	在过肩胛内侧的垂线内，第 5~6 胸椎右侧区域	肝炎、肝肿大、脂肪肝、胆结石、胆囊炎、黄疸等
胃 · 胰	在过肩胛内侧的垂线内，第 7~8 胸椎左侧区域	恶心、呕吐、腹胀、胃痛、胃酸过多、糖尿病、消化不良、急慢性胃肠炎等
十二指肠	在过肩胛内侧的垂线内，第 7~8 胸椎右侧区域	腹胀、腹痛、消化不良 、食欲不振、食物中毒、胃及十二指肠溃疡等
肾 · 腰	在过肩胛内侧的垂线内，第 9~11 胸椎区域。以后正中线为界，分为左、右肾 · 腰反射区	水肿、腰痛、肾性高血压等
腹腔神经丛	第 1~3 腰椎的竖条状区域	刺激腹腔神经丛，可调节腹腔脏器功能，对腹胀、腹泻、胃肠痉挛、反酸、打嗝等有疗效

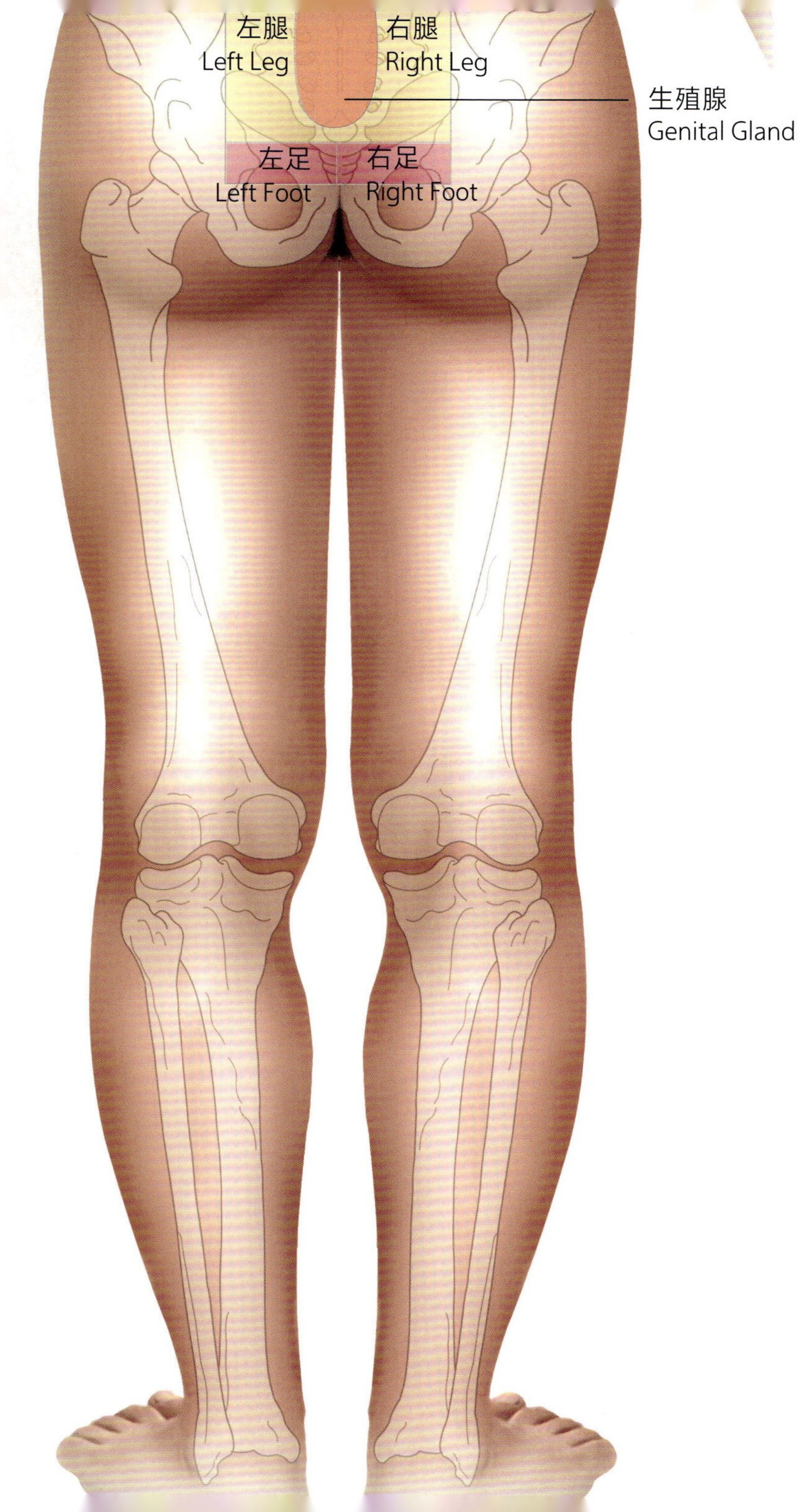

Continued

Reflex Zone	Location	Indications
Liver and Gallbladder	In a vertical inner side of the scapula, the right side of the 5th to the 6th thoracic vertebra region	Hepatomegaly, hepatitis, fatty liver, gallstones, cholecystitis, jaundice and so on
Stomach and Pancreas	In a vertical inner side of the scapula, the left side of the 7th to the 8th thoracic vertebra region	Nausea, vomiting, abdominal distention, stomach pain, heartburn, indigestion, diabetes, acute or chronic gastroenteritis and so on
Duodenum	In a vertical inner side of the scapula, the right side of the 7th to the 8th thoracic vertebra region	Abdominal distension, abdominal pain, indigestion, loss of appetite, food poisoning, gastric and duodenal ulcer and so on
Kidney and Waist	In a vertical inner side of the scapula, the 9th to the 11th thoracic vertebra region. The midline is as boundary, dividing into Left Kidney and Waist reflex zone, Right Kidney and Waist reflex zone	Edema; low back pain; renal hypertension
Celiac Plexus	The vertical strip zone of the 1st to the 3rd lumbar vertebra	Stimulating the coeliac plexus can regulate viscera function; working on abdominal distension; diarrhea; stomach cramps; acid regurgitation; belching and so on

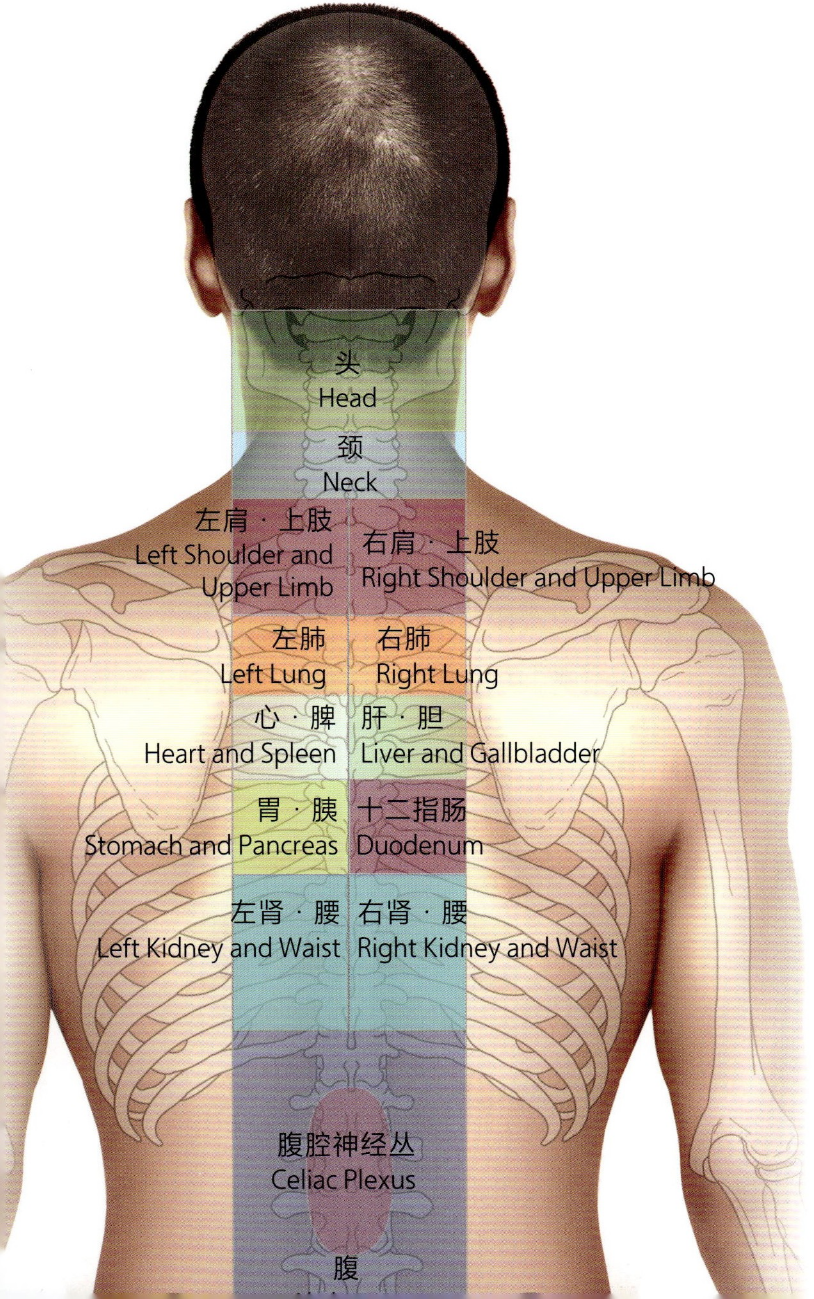

续表

反射区	定位	主治
腹	在过肩胛内侧的垂线内，第 12 胸椎至第 4 腰椎、腹腔神经丛以外的区域	妇科疾患如月经不调、痛经等
生殖腺	第 1~5 骶椎的竖条状区域	性功能低下、不孕症、围绝经期综合征、月经不调、痛经
腿	在过肩胛内侧的垂线内，第 5 腰椎至骶骨、生殖腺反射区以外的区域，以后正中线为界分为左、右腿反射区	坐骨神经痛、下肢麻木等
足	在过肩胛内侧的垂线内，尾骨区域	足部肿痛、足跟痛、足弓损伤等

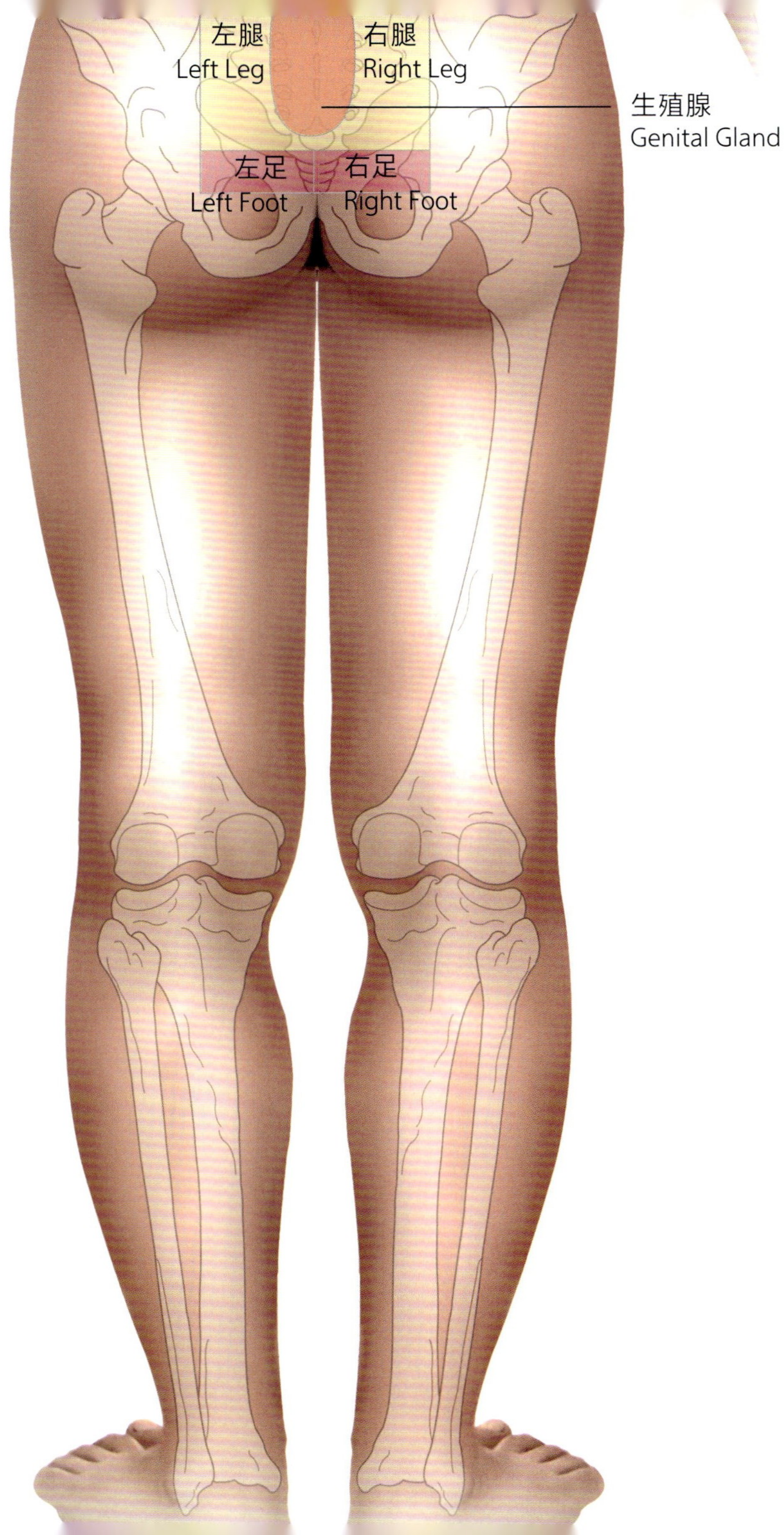

Continued

Reflex Zone	Location	Indications
Abdomen	In a vertical inner side of the scapula, from the 12th thoracic vertebra region to the 4th lumbar vertebra, except for Celiac plexus zone	Gynecological diseases such as irregular menstruation, dysmenorrhea, and so on
Genital Gland	The vertical strip zone of the 1st to the 5th sacral vertebra	Sexual dysfunction; infertility; perimenopausal syndrome; irregular menstruation; dysmenorrhea
Leg	In a vertical inner side of the scapula, from the 5th lumbar vertebra to sacral vertebra, except for Gonad reflex zone. The midline is as boundary, dividing into Left, Right Leg reflex zones	Sciatica, lower limb numbness and so on
Foot	In a vertical inner side of the scapula, the tailbone zone	Foot pain; heel pain; instep injury and so on

超简单脊柱反射区按摩

Super-easy Massage in Spine Reflex Zone

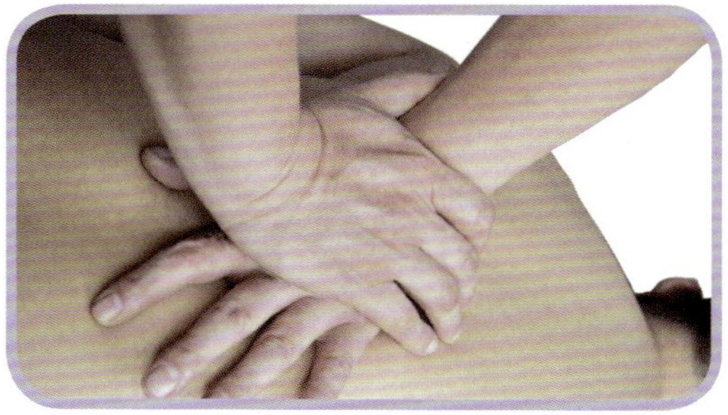

按法 · 叠掌按法

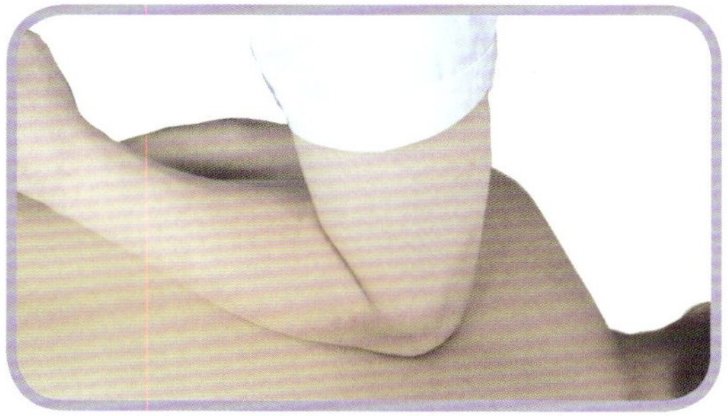

拨法 · 肘拨法

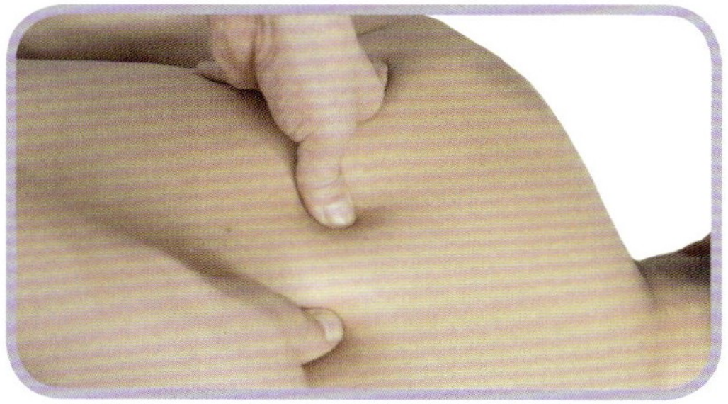

点法 2

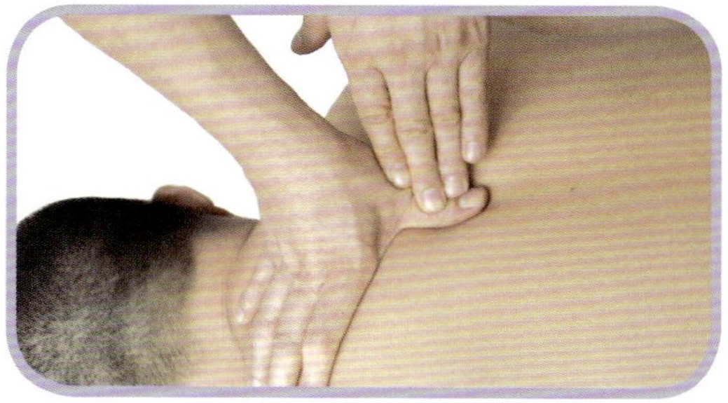

拨法 · 叠加指拨法

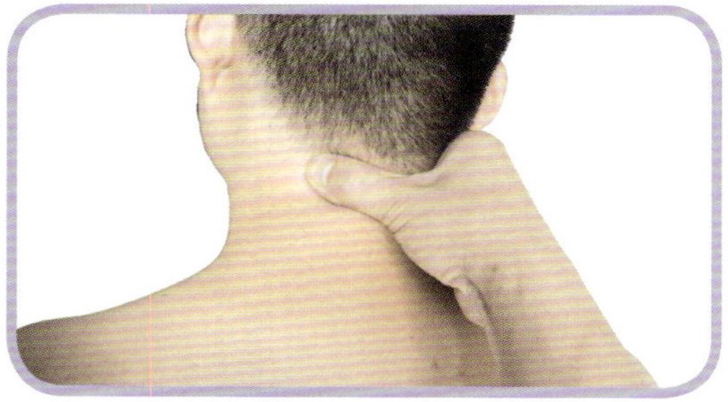

拨法 · 弹拨法

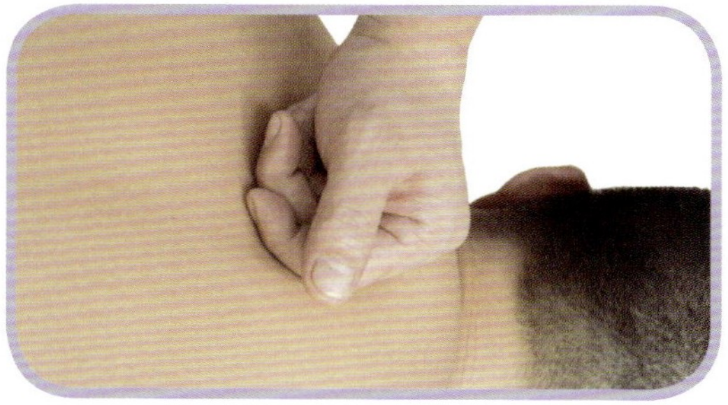

揿法

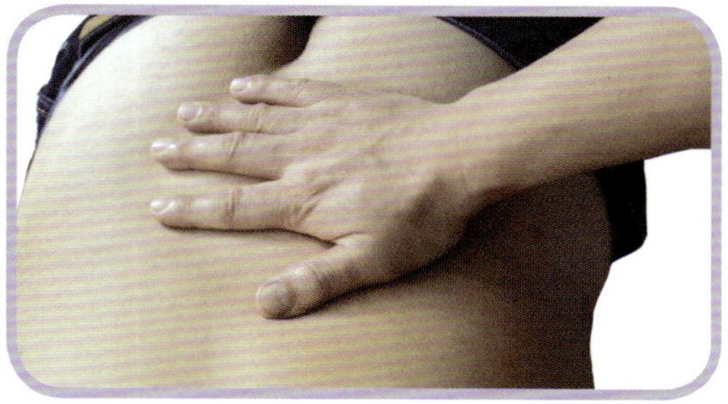

擦法

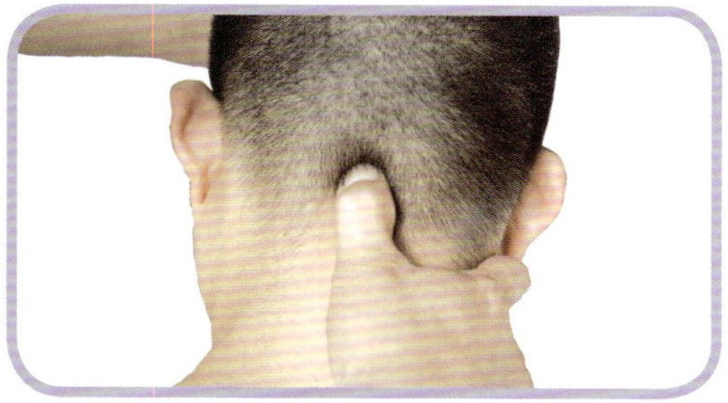

点法 1

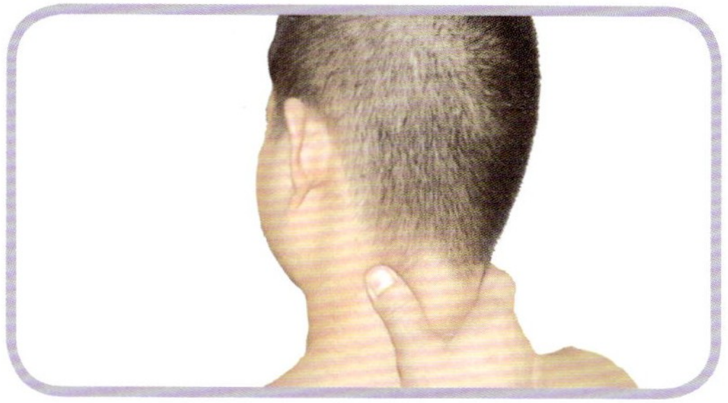

拿法

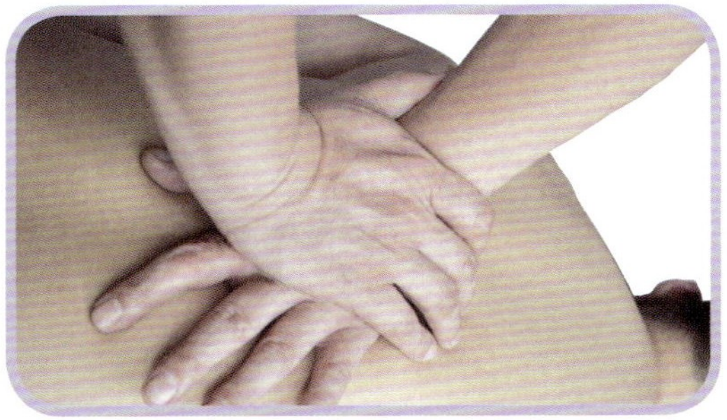
Pressing Manipulation: pressing manipulation with folded hands

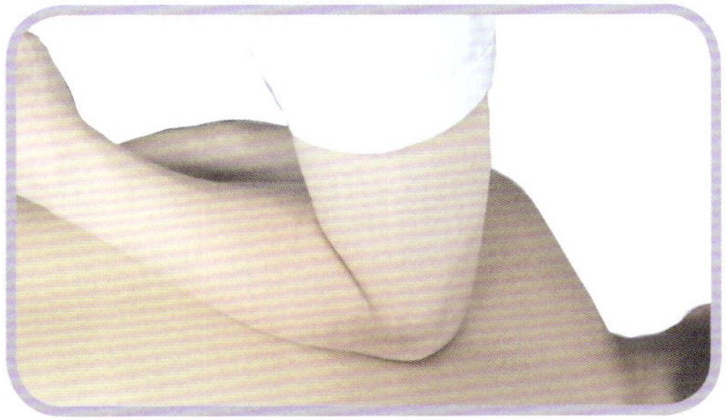
Drawing Manipulation: drawing manipulation with elbows

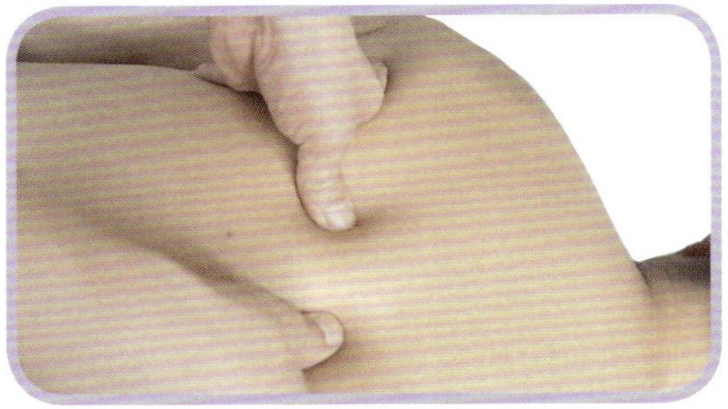
Pressing Manipulation 2

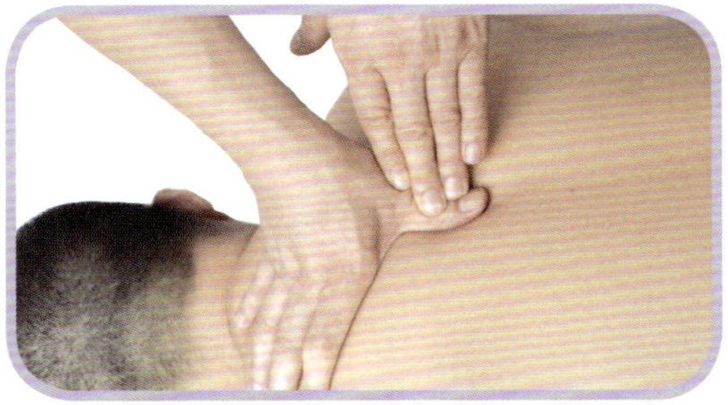
Drawing Manipulation: drawing manipulation with folded fingers

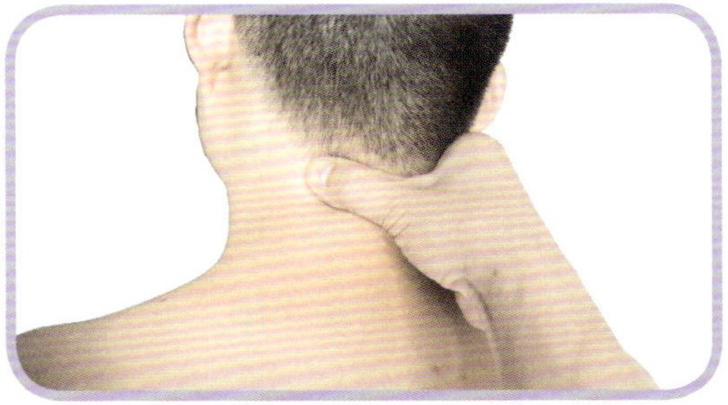
Drawing Manipulation: drawing manipulation with flicking

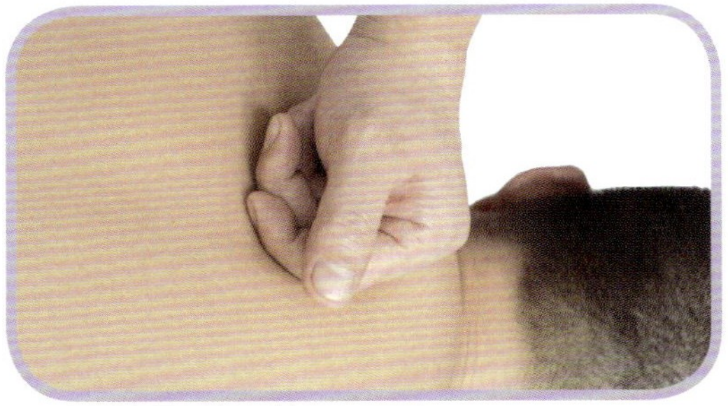
Rolling Manipulation

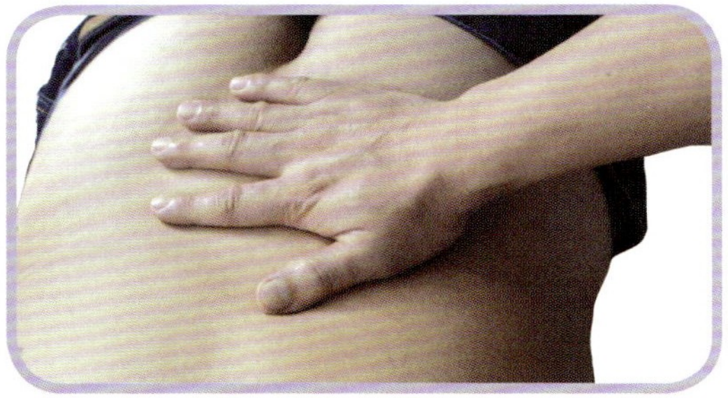
Scrubbing Manipulation

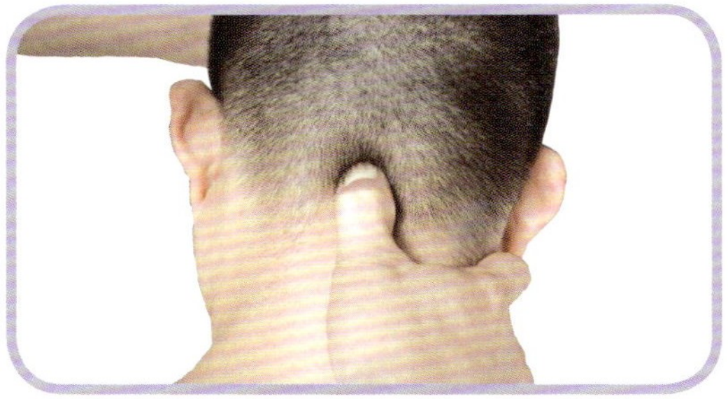
Pressing Manipulation 1

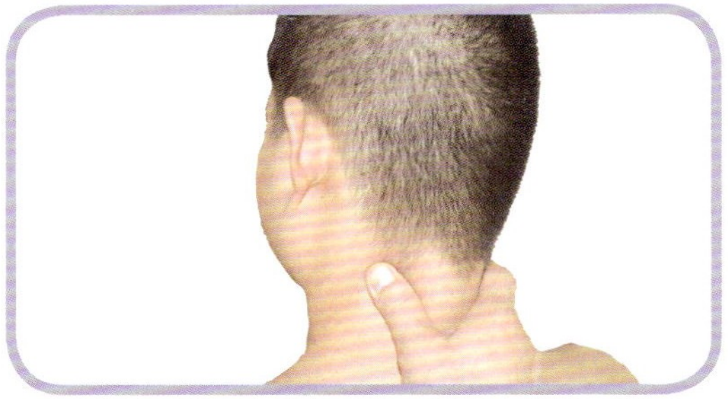
Grasping Manipulation

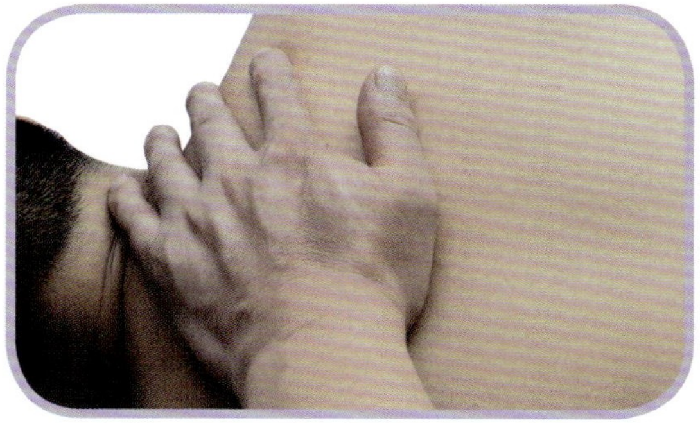

揉法 · 掌揉法

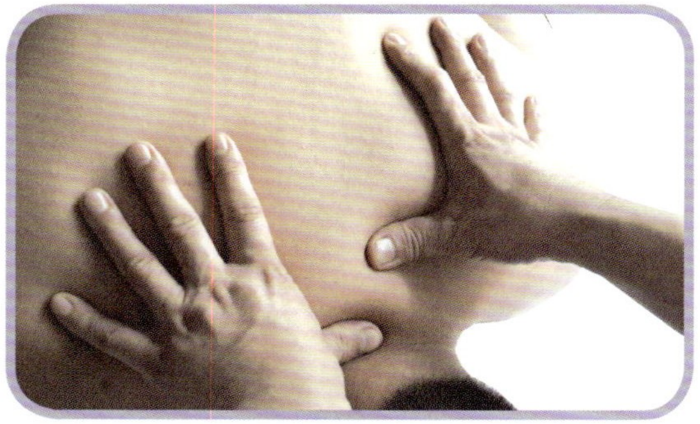

揉法 · 八卦揉法

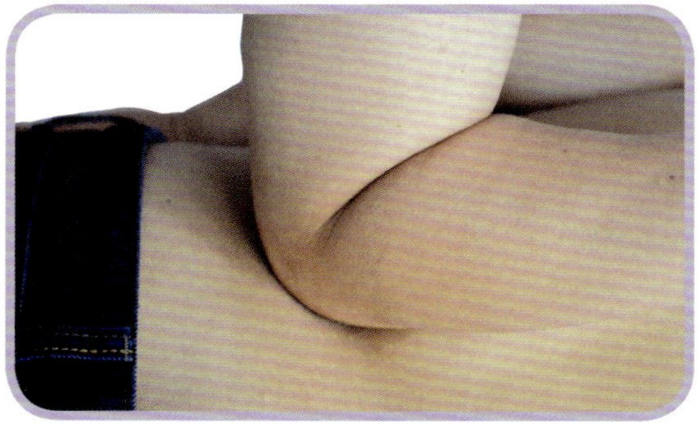

肘压法

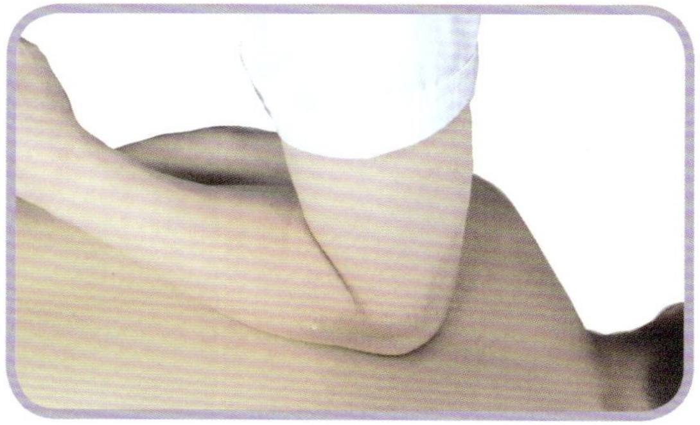

揉法 · 肘揉法

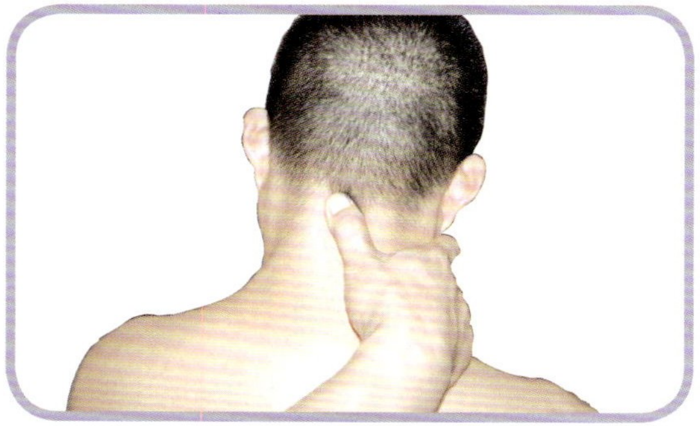

揉法 · 指揉法

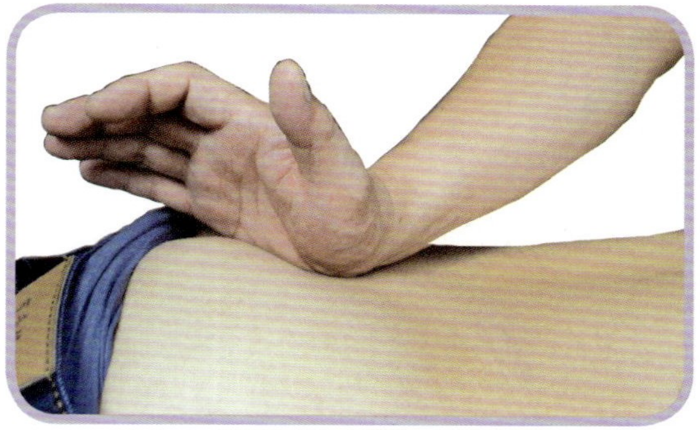

推法 · 小鱼际推法

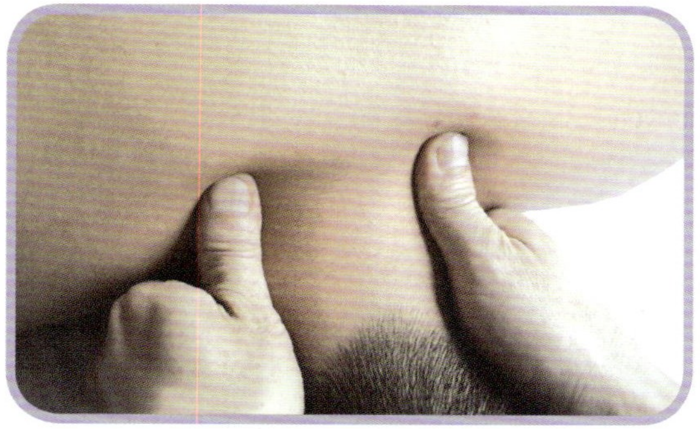

推法 · 分推法

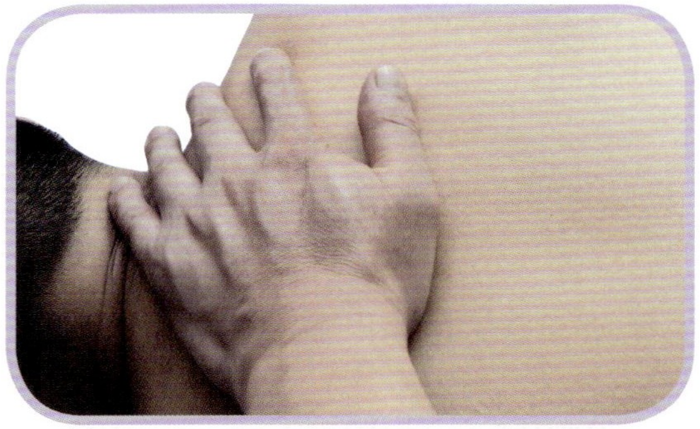

Kneading Manipulation: kneading manipulation with palm

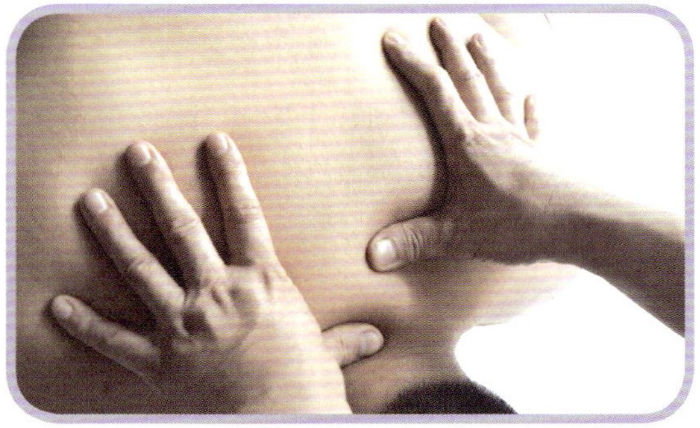

Kneading Manipulation: eight-diagram kneading manipulation

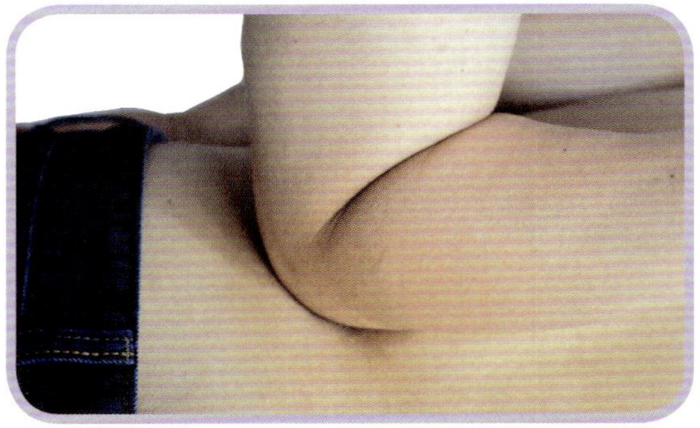

Pushing Manipulation with Elbow

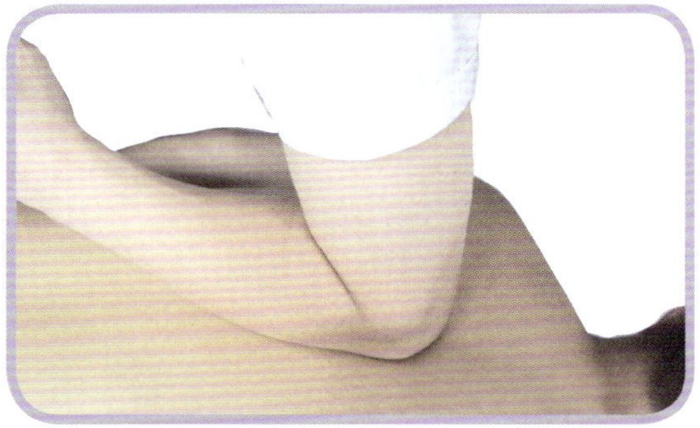

Kneading Manipulation: kneading manipulation with elbow

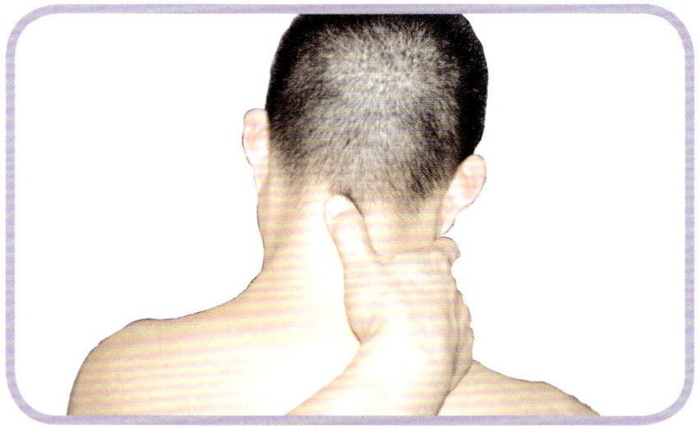

Kneading Manipulation: kneading manipulation with finger

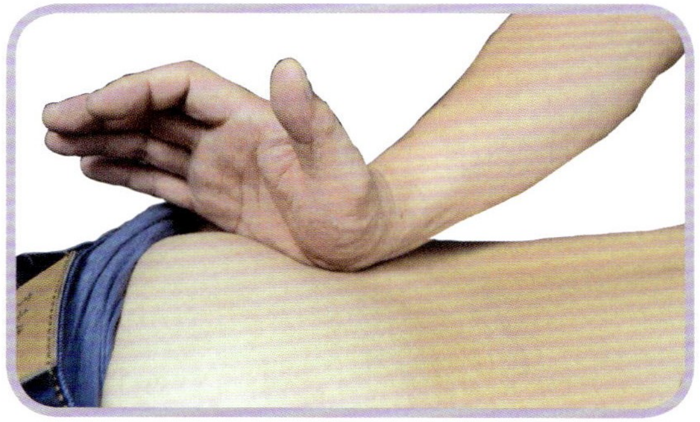

Pushing Manipulation: pushing manipulation with hypothenar

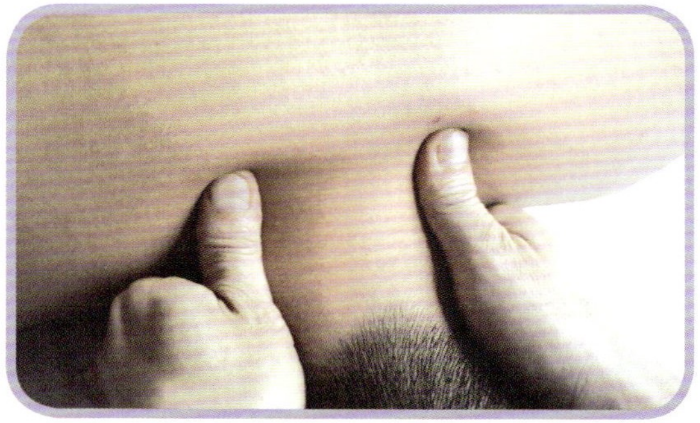

Pushing Manipulation: parting manipulation

脊背部常用穴位
Common Acupoints in the Back

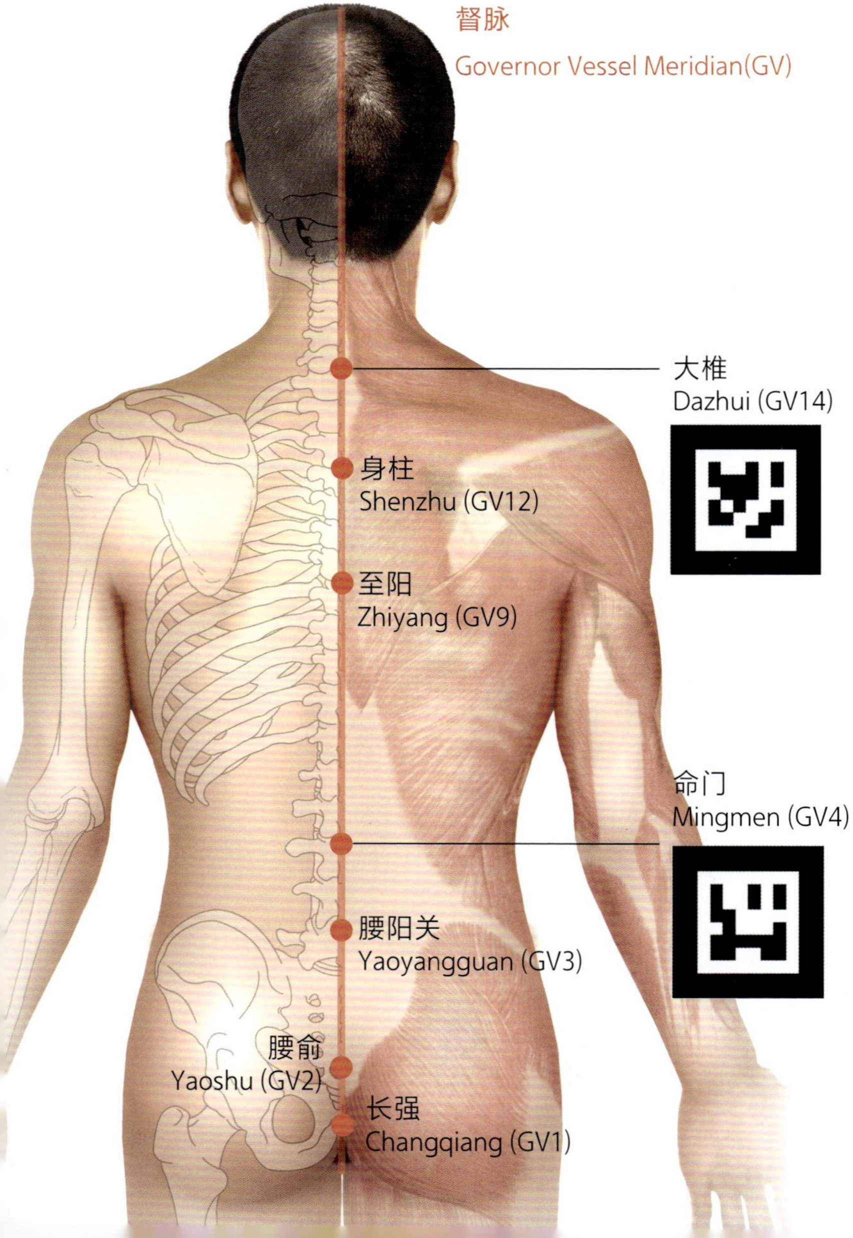

督脉
Governor Vessel Meridian

穴位		定位	主治
督脉	长强	在会阴部，尾骨下方，尾骨端与肛门连线的中点处	脱肛、泄泻、便秘、癫狂、腰骶痛、小儿痴呆
	至阳	在脊柱区，第 7 胸椎棘突下凹陷中，后正中线上	黄疸、胸胁胀痛、身热、咳嗽、气喘、脊背强痛
	身柱	在脊柱区，第 3 胸椎棘突下凹陷中，后正中线上	咳嗽、气喘、身热、癫痫、脊背强痛
	大椎	在脊柱区，第 7 颈椎棘突下凹陷中，后正中线上	热病、骨蒸盗汗、咳嗽、气喘、癫痫、小儿惊风、感冒、胃寒、风疹、头项强痛、体虚怕冷
	腰俞	在骶区，正对骶管裂孔，后正中线上 *取穴小窍门：臀裂正上方的小凹陷即骶管裂孔	腰脊疼痛、下肢痿痹、月经不调、脱肛、便秘、癫痫
	腰阳关	在脊柱区，第 4 腰椎棘突下凹陷中，后正中线上	腰脊疼痛、下肢痿痹、月经不调、带下、遗精、阳痿
	命门	在脊柱区，第 2 腰椎棘突下凹陷中，后正中线上	腰痛、下肢痿痹、遗精、阳痿、月经不调、带下、遗尿、尿频、泄泻

Acupoint		Location	Indications
Governor Vessel Meridian	Changqiang (GV1)	In the perineum portion, behind the coccyx, at the middle of the line between the coccyx end and the anus	Prolapse of rectum; diarrhea; constipation; madness; lumbar and sacral pain; pediatric dementia
	Zhiyang (GV9)	In the spinal portion, in the hollow of the spinous process of the 7th thoracic vertebra, on the posterior middle line	Jaundice; distension and pain in the chest and hypochondrium; fever; cough; asthma; strong spinal and back pain
	Shenzhu (GV12)	In the spinal portion, in the hollow of the spinous process of the 3rd thoracic vertebra, on the posterior middle line	Cough; asthma; fever; epilepsy; strong spinal and back pain
	Dazhui (GV14)	In the spinal portion, in the hollow of the spinous process of the 7th cervical vertebra, on the posterior middle line	Fever; night sweat with steaming bone; cough; asthma; epilepsy; infantile convulsion; cold; rubella; strong pain of the head and neck; sensation of chill with deficiency
	Yaoshu (GV2)	In the sacral portion, directly facing the sacral hiatus, on the posterior middle line Tips: the tiny hollow right above the anal cleft is the sacral hiatus	Lumbar and spinal pain; flaccid and paralytic lower body; irregular menstruation; Prolapse of rectum; constipation; epilepsy
	Yaoyangguan (GV3)	In the spinal portion, in the hollow of the spinous process of the 4th lumbar vertebra, on the posterior middle line	Lumbar and spinal pain; flaccid and paralytic lower body; irregular menstruation; leukorrhea; seminal emission; impotence
	Mingmen (GV4)	In the spinal portion, in the hollow of the spinous process of the 2nd cervical vertebra, on the posterior middle line	Lower back pain; flaccid and paralytic lower body; seminal emission; impotence; irregular menstruation; leucorrhea; enuresis; frequent urination; diarrhea

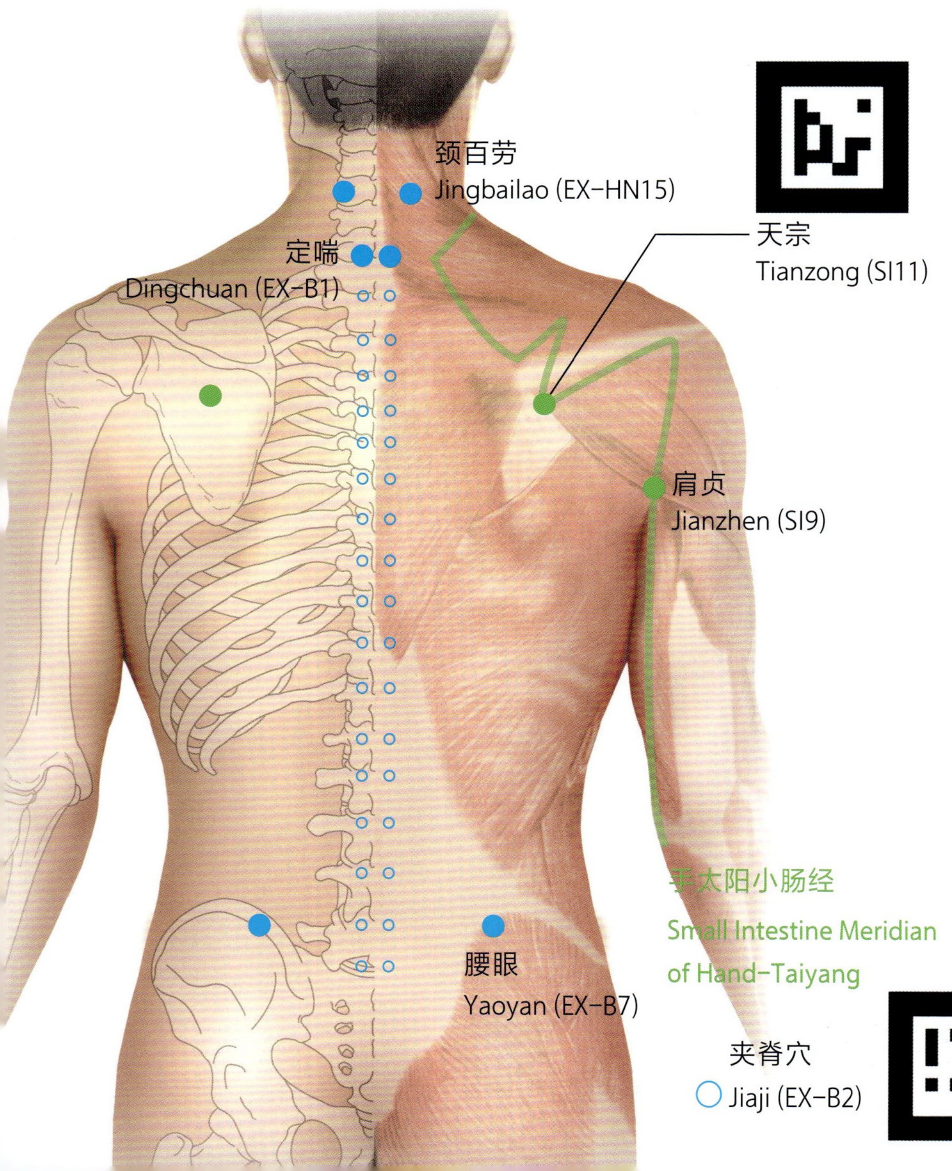

穴位		定位	主治
手太阳小肠经	肩贞	在肩胛区，肩关节后下方，腋后纹头直上 1 寸 * 取穴小窍门：腋后纹头直上 1 寸，三角肌后缘	肩背疼痛、手臂麻痛
	天宗	在肩胛区，肩胛冈中点与肩胛下角连线上 1/3 与下 2/3 交点凹陷中	肩胛疼痛、乳腺炎、气喘
经外奇穴	颈百劳	在颈部，第 7 颈椎棘突直上 2 寸，后正中线旁开 1 寸	颈项强痛、咳嗽、气喘、骨蒸潮热、盗汗
	定喘	在脊柱区，横平第 7 颈椎棘突下，后正中线旁开 0.5 寸 * 取穴小窍门：大椎旁开 0.5 寸	哮喘、咳嗽、落枕、肩背痛、上肢疼痛不举
	夹脊	在脊柱区，第 1 胸椎至第 5 腰椎棘突下两侧，后正中线旁开 0.5 寸，一侧 17 穴	胸 1~5 夹脊：心肺、胸部及上肢疾病；胸 6~12 夹脊：胃肠、脾、肝胆疾病；腰 1~5 夹脊：腰骶小腹部疾病及下肢疼痛
	腰眼	在腰区，横平第 4 腰椎棘突下，后正中线旁开约 3.5 寸凹陷中	腰痛、尿频、月经不调、带下

Acupoint		Location	Indications
Small Intestine Meridian of Hand-Taiyin	Jianzhen (SI9)	In the scapula portion, apposition behind and below shoulder joints, posterior armpit, 1cun straight up head. Tips: posterior armpit, 1 cun straight up head, back margin of deltoid	Shoulder and back pain; arm numbing pain
	Tianzong (SI11)	In the scapula portion, in the hollow situated at the crossover point of the upper 1/3 and the lower 2/3 of the line between the spine of scapula and the underhorn of the scapula	Scapula pain; mammitis; asthma
Extra Points	Jingbailao (EX-HN15)	In the neck portion, 2 cun straight up the spinous process of the 7th cervical vertebra, 1 cun beside the posterior middle line	heavy pain on neck; cough; asthma; steaming bone with tidal fever; night sweat
	Dingchuan （EX-B1）	In the spinal portion, behind the spinous process of the horizontal 7th cervical vertebra, 0.5 cun beside the posterior middle line Tips: 0.5 cun beside Dazhui (GV14)	Asthma; cough; stiff neck; shoulder and back pain; impotence and pain of upper body
	Jiaji (EX-B2)	In the spinal portion, both sides beside the spinous process from the 1st thoracic vertebra and the 5th lumbar vertebra, 0.5 cun beside the posterior middle line, 17 acupoints at one side	Chest 1 to 5 Jiaji (EX-B2): heart, lung, chest and diseases of upper body Chest 6 to 12 Jiaji (EX-B2): diseases of stomach and intestine, spleen, liver and gallbladder Waist 1 to 5: Jiaji (EX-B2): diseases of lumbosacral and lower abdomen portion, pain of lower body
	Yaoyan (EX-B7)	In the waist portion, behind the spinous process of the 4th horizontal lumbar vertebra, in the hollow 3.5 cun beside the posterior middle line	Lower back pain; frequent urine; irregular menstruation; leukorrhea

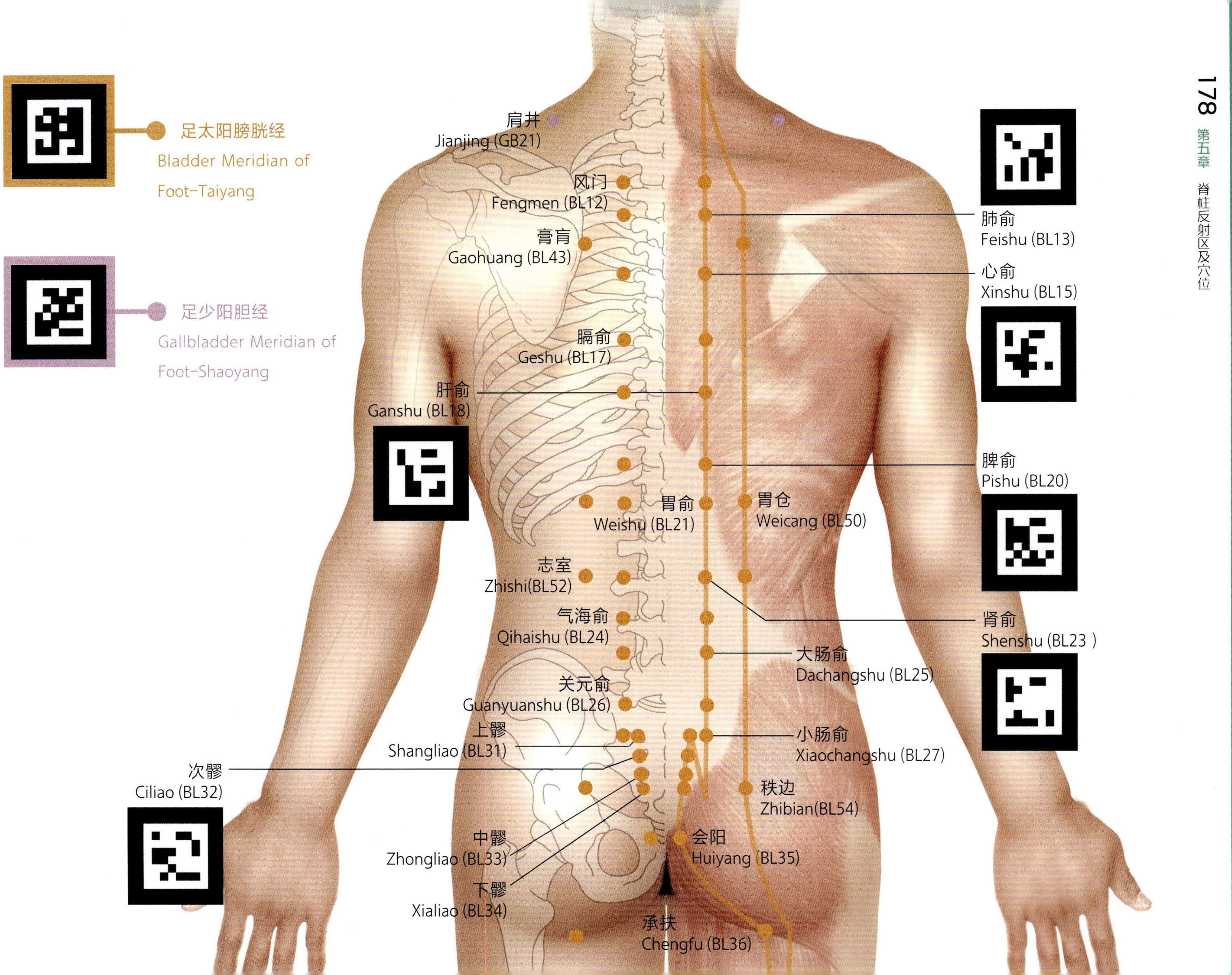
足太阳膀胱经
Bladder Meridian of Foot-Taiyang
足少阳胆经
Gallbladder Meridian of Foot-Shaoyang
肩井
Jianjing (GB21)
风门
Fengmen (BL12)
膏肓
Gaohuang (BL43)
膈俞
Geshu (BL17)
肝俞
Ganshu (BL18)
胃俞
Weishu (BL21)
志室
Zhishi(BL52)
气海俞
Qihaishu (BL24)
关元俞
Guanyuanshu (BL26)
上髎
Shangliao (BL31)
次髎
Ciliao (BL32)
中髎
Zhongliao (BL33)
下髎
Xialiao (BL34)
承扶
Chengfu (BL36)
会阳
Huiyang (BL35)
秩边
Zhibian(BL54)
小肠俞
Xiaochangshu (BL27)
大肠俞
Dachangshu (BL25)
肾俞
Shenshu (BL23)
胃仓
Weicang (BL50)
脾俞
Pishu (BL20)
心俞
Xinshu (BL15)
肺俞
Feishu (BL13)

穴位		定位	主治
足太阳膀胱经	风门	在脊柱区，第 2 胸椎棘突下，后正中线旁开 1.5 寸	咳嗽、发热、头痛、胸背痛
	肺俞	在脊柱区，第 3 胸椎棘突下，后正中线旁开 1.5 寸	咳嗽、气喘、鼻塞、盗汗、皮肤瘙痒、瘾疹
	心俞	在脊柱区，第 5 胸椎棘突下，后正中线旁开 1.5 寸	心痛、心悸、心烦、失眠、健忘、咳嗽、吐血
	膈俞	在脊柱区，第 7 胸椎棘突下，后正中线旁开 1.5 寸	胃脘痛、呕吐、饮食不下、呃逆、咳嗽、气喘、瘾疹
	肝俞	在脊柱区，第 9 胸椎棘突下，后正中线旁开 1.5 寸	黄疸、胁痛、目视不明、夜盲、吐血、眩晕、呃逆、癫狂
	脾俞	在脊柱区，第 11 胸椎棘突下，后正中线旁开 1.5 寸	腹胀、呕吐、泄泻、便血、消化不良、水肿、黄疸、背痛

Acupoints		Location	Indications
Bladder Meridian of Foot-Taiyang	Fengmen (BL12)	In the spinal portion, behind the spinous process of the 2nd thoracic vertebra, 1.5 cun beside the posterior middle line	Cough; fever; headache; chest and back pain
	Feishu (BL13)	In the spinal portion, behind the spinous process of the 3rd thoracic vertebra, 1.5 cun beside the posterior middle line	Cough; asthma; nasal congestion; night sweating; itching skin; urticaria
	Xinshu (BL15)	In the spinal portion, behind the spinous process of the 5th thoracic vertebra, 1.5 cun beside the posterior middle line	Heart pain; palpitation; vexation; insomnia; amnesia; cough; hematemesis
	Geshu (BL17)	In the spinal portion, behind the spinous process of the 7th thoracic vertebra, 1.5 cun beside the posterior middle line	Epigastric pain; Vomiting; poor diet; hiccup; cough; asthma; urticaria
	Ganshu (BL18)	In the spinal portion, behind the spinous process of the 9th thoracic vertebra, 1.5 cun beside the posterior middle line	Jaundice; rib pain; poor eyesight; nyctalopia; hematemesis; dizziness; hiccup; madness
	Pishu (BL20)	In the spinal portion, behind the spinous process of the 11th thoracic vertebra, 1.5 cun beside the posterior middle line	Abdominal distension; vomiting; diarrhea; blood stool; dyspepsia; edema; jaundice; back pain

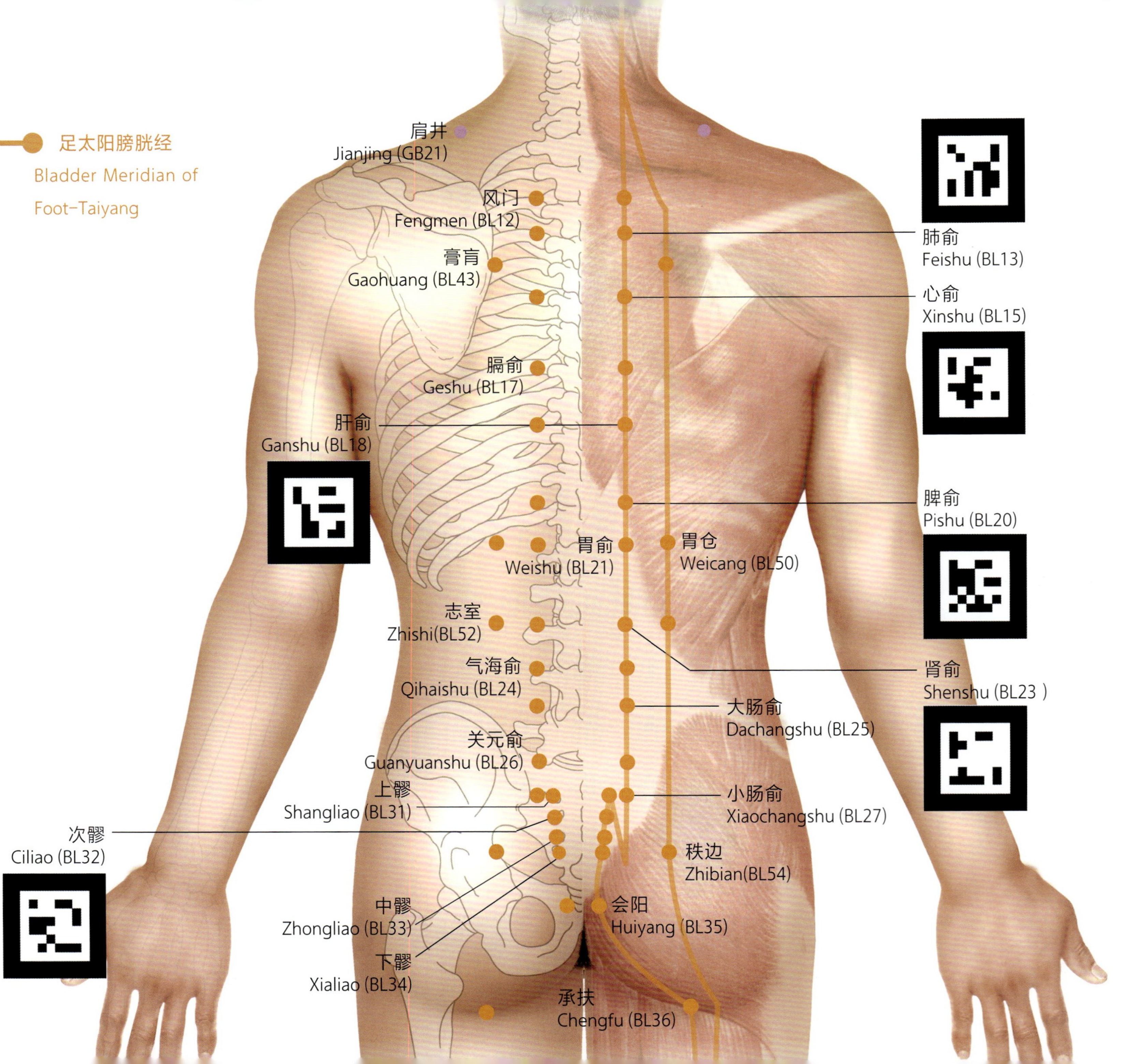
足太阳膀胱经
Bladder Meridian of Foot-Taiyang
肩井
Jianjing (GB21)
风门
Fengmen (BL12)
膏肓
Gaohuang (BL43)
膈俞
Geshu (BL17)
肝俞
Ganshu (BL18)
胃俞
Weishu (BL21)
志室
Zhishi(BL52)
气海俞
Qihaishu (BL24)
关元俞
Guanyuanshu (BL26)
上髎
Shangliao (BL31)
次髎
Ciliao (BL32)
中髎
Zhongliao (BL33)
下髎
Xialiao (BL34)
承扶
Chengfu (BL36)
会阳
Huiyang (BL35)
秩边
Zhibian(BL54)
小肠俞
Xiaochangshu (BL27)
大肠俞
Dachangshu (BL25)
肾俞
Shenshu (BL23)
胃仓
Weicang (BL50)
脾俞
Pishu (BL20)
心俞
Xinshu (BL15)
肺俞
Feishu (BL13)

续表

穴位		定位	主治
足太阳膀胱经	胃俞	在脊柱区，第 12 胸椎棘突下，后正中线旁开 1.5 寸	胃脘痛、腹胀、呕吐、胸胁痛
	肾俞	在脊柱区，第 2 腰椎棘突下，后正中线旁开 1.5 寸 * 取穴小窍门：先定第 12 胸椎棘突，下数第 2 个棘突即第 2 腰椎棘突	遗精、阳痿、月经不调、带下、遗尿、小便不利、水肿、耳鸣耳聋、气喘、腰痛
	气海俞	在脊柱区，第 3 腰椎棘突下，后正中线旁开 1.5 寸	腰痛、痛经、腹胀肠鸣、胃下垂
	大肠俞	在脊柱区，第 4 腰椎棘突下，后正中线旁开 1.5 寸	腰痛、腹胀、泄泻、便秘
	关元俞	在脊柱区，第 5 腰椎棘突下，后正中线旁开 1.5 寸	腹胀、泄泻、小便频数或不利、遗尿、腰痛

Continued

Acupoints		Location	Indications
Bladder Meridian of Foot-Taiyang	Weishu (BL21)	In the spinal portion, behind the spinous process of the 12th thoracic vertebra, 1.5 cun beside the posterior middle line	Epigastric pain; abodominal distension; vomiting; chest and rib pain
	Shenshu (BL23)	In the spinal portion, behind the spinous process of the 2nd lumbar vertebra, 1.5 cun beside the posterior middle line *Tip: first select the spinous process of the 12th lumbar vertebra, the 2nd spinous process counted downward is the 2nd spinous process of lumbar vertebra	Seminal emission; impotence; irregular menstruation; leukorrhea; enuresis; difficult urination; edema; tinnitus; deafness; asthma; lower back pain
	Qihaishu (BL24)	In the spinal portion, behind the spinous process of the 3rd lumbar vertebra, 1.5 cun beside the posterior middle line	Lower back pain; dysmenorrheal; abdominal distension with bowel sounds; gastroptosis
	Dachangshu (BL25)	In the spinal portion, behind the spinous process of the 4th lumbar vertebra, 1.5 cun beside the posterior middle line	Lower back pain; abdominal distension; diarrhea; costipation
	Guanyuanshu (BL26)	In the spinal portion, behind the spinous process of the 5th lumbar vertebra, 1.5 cun beside the posterior middle line	Abdominal distension; diarrhea; frequent or difficult urination; enuresis; lower back pain

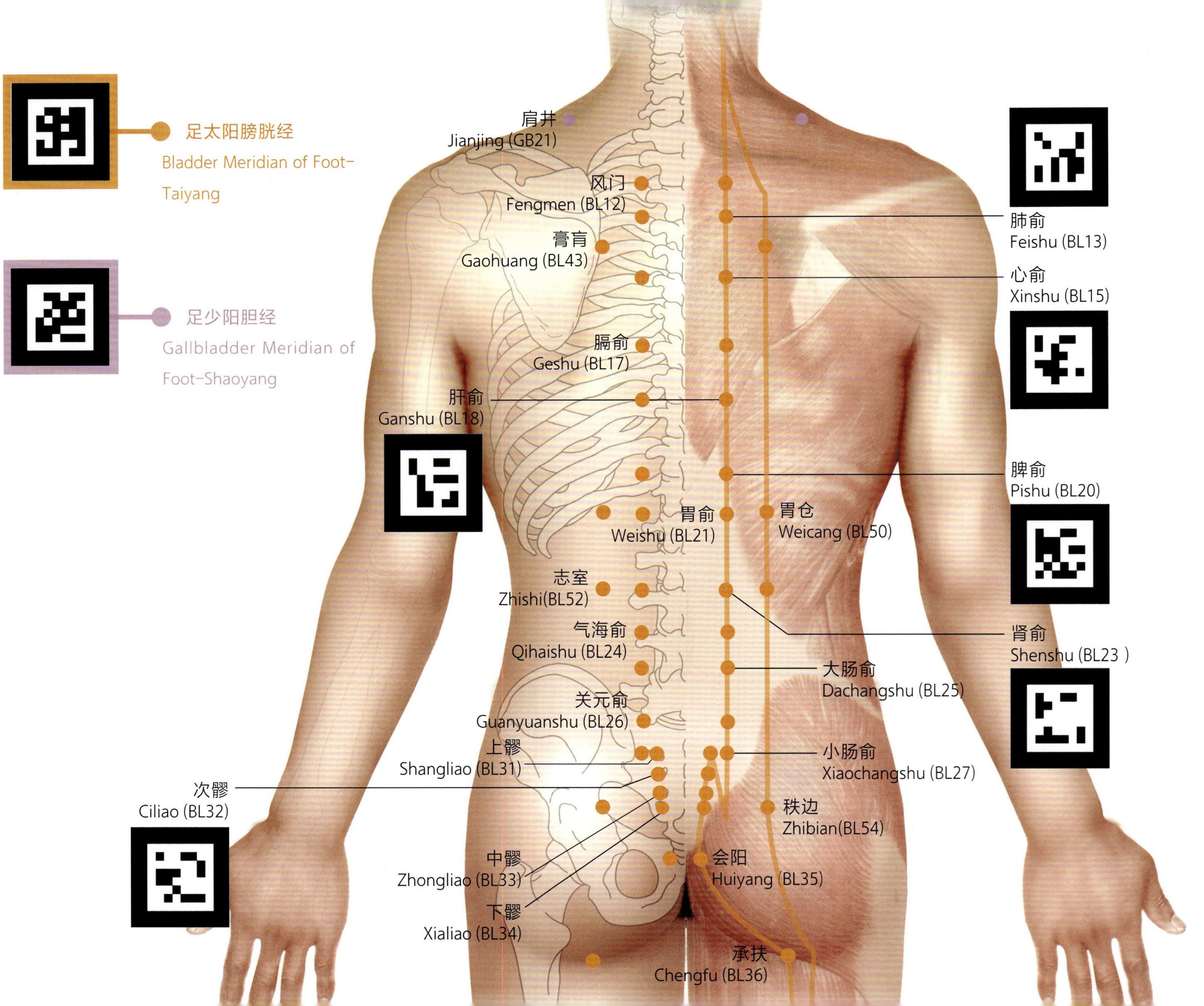
足太阳膀胱经
Bladder Meridian of Foot-Taiyang
足少阳胆经
Gallbladder Meridian of Foot-Shaoyang
肩井
Jianjing (GB21)
风门
Fengmen (BL12)
膏肓
Gaohuang (BL43)
膈俞
Geshu (BL17)
肝俞
Ganshu (BL18)
胃俞
Weishu (BL21)
志室
Zhishi(BL52)
气海俞
Qihaishu (BL24)
关元俞
Guanyuanshu (BL26)
上髎
Shangliao (BL31)
次髎
Ciliao (BL32)
中髎
Zhongliao (BL33)
下髎
Xialiao (BL34)
肺俞
Feishu (BL13)
心俞
Xinshu (BL15)
脾俞
Pishu (BL20)
胃仓
Weicang (BL50)
肾俞
Shenshu (BL23)
大肠俞
Dachangshu (BL25)
小肠俞
Xiaochangshu (BL27)
秩边
Zhibian(BL54)
会阳
Huiyang (BL35)
承扶
Chengfu (BL36)

续表

穴位		定位	主治
足太阳膀胱经	小肠俞	在骶区，横平第 1 骶后孔，骶正中嵴旁开 1.5 寸	遗精、遗尿、尿血、带下、腹痛、泄泻、腰痛
	上髎	在骶区，正对第 1 骶后孔处 * 取穴小窍门：次髎向上触摸到的凹陷即第 1 骶后孔	月经不调、带下、遗精、阳痿、大小便不利、腰脊痛
	次髎	在骶部，正对第 2 骶后孔中 * 取穴小窍门：髂后上棘与第 2 骶椎棘突连线的中点凹陷处，即第 2 骶后孔	月经不调、痛经、带下、遗精、阳痿、小便不利、腰脊痛、下肢痿痹

Continued

Acupoint		Location	Indications
Bladder Meridian of Foot-Taiyang	Xiaochangshu (BL27)	In the coccyx portion, the posterior hole of the 1st horizontal coccyx, 1.5 cun beside the ridge in the middle of the coccyx	Seminal emission; enuresis; hematuria; leucorrhea; abdominal pain; diarrhea, lower back pain
	Shangliao (BL31)	In the sacral portion, directly facing the 1sth posterior hole of the sacrum *Tips: the hollow above the Ciliao (BL32), the 1st posterior hole of the sacrum	Irregular menstruation; leukorrhea; seminal emission; impotence; fecal and urinary difficulty; lumbar and spinal pain
	Ciliao (BL32)	In the sacral portion, directly facing the 2nd posterior hole of the sacrum *Tips: the hollow in the middle of the line between posterior skeletons and the 2nd spinous process of the sacral vertebra, the 2nd sacral posterior hole	Irregular menstruation; dysmenorrheal; leukorrhea; seminal emission; impotence; difficult urination; lumbar and spinal pain; flaccid and paralytic lower body

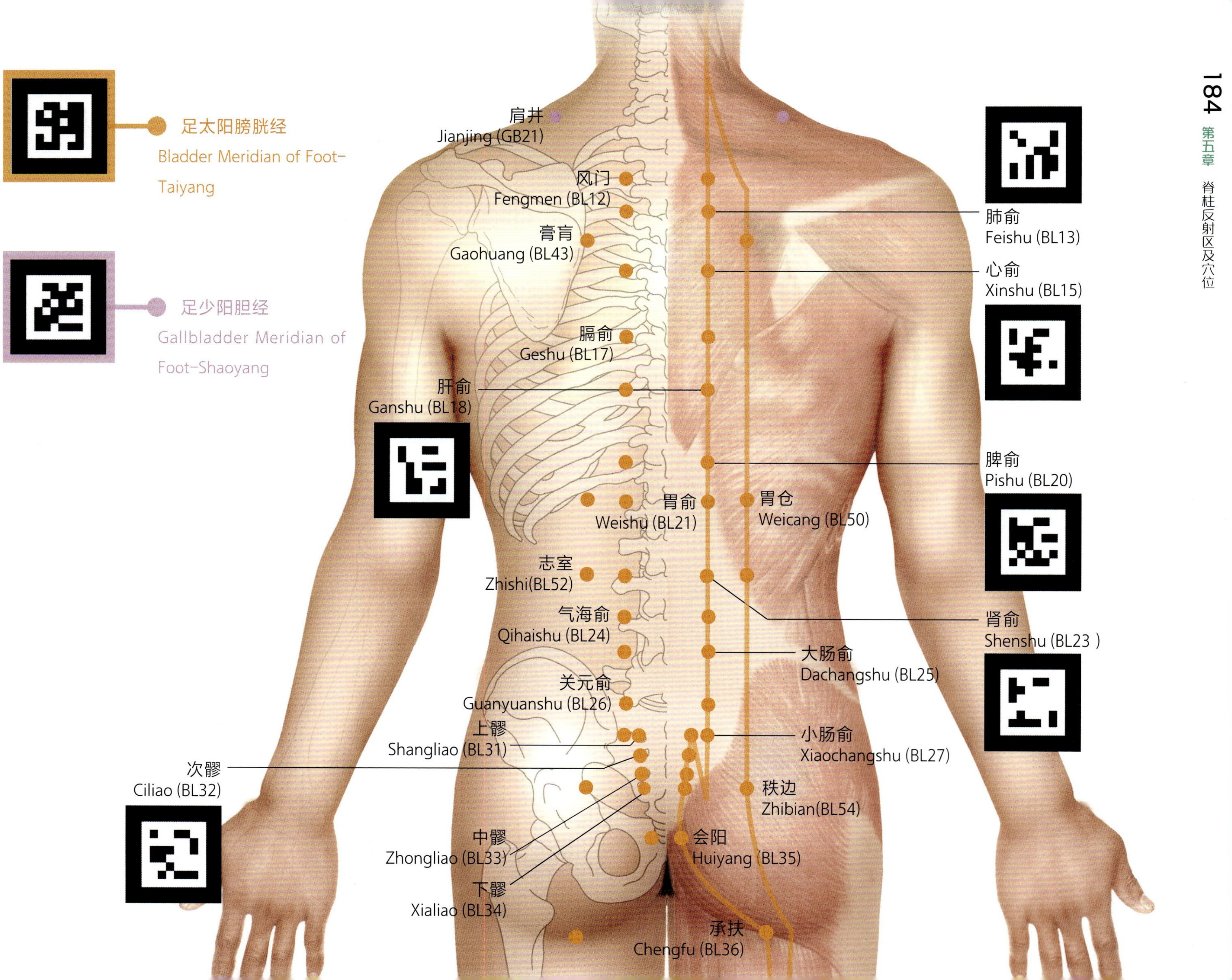
足太阳膀胱经
Bladder Meridian of Foot-Taiyang
足少阳胆经
Gallbladder Meridian of Foot-Shaoyang
肩井
Jianjing (GB21)
风门
Fengmen (BL12)
膏肓
Gaohuang (BL43)
膈俞
Geshu (BL17)
肝俞
Ganshu (BL18)
胃俞
Weishu (BL21)
志室
Zhishi(BL52)
气海俞
Qihaishu (BL24)
关元俞
Guanyuanshu (BL26)
上髎
Shangliao (BL31)
次髎
Ciliao (BL32)
中髎
Zhongliao (BL33)
下髎
Xialiao (BL34)
会阳
Huiyang (BL35)
承扶
Chengfu (BL36)
秩边
Zhibian(BL54)
胃仓
Weicang (BL50)
肺俞
Feishu (BL13)
心俞
Xinshu (BL15)
脾俞
Pishu (BL20)
肾俞
Shenshu (BL23)
大肠俞
Dachangshu (BL25)
小肠俞
Xiaochangshu (BL27)

续表

穴位		定位	主治
足太阳膀胱经	中髎	在骶部，正对第 3 骶后孔中 * 取穴小窍门：次髎向下触摸到的第 1 个凹陷，即第 3 骶后孔	月经不调、带下、小便不利、便秘、泄泻、腰痛
	下髎	在骶部，正对第 4 骶后孔中 * 取穴小窍门：次髎向下触摸到的第 2 个凹陷即第 4 骶后孔，横平骶管裂孔	小腹痛、腰骶痛、小便不利、带下、便秘
	会阳	在骶区，尾骨端旁开 0.5 寸 * 取穴小窍门：俯卧或跪伏位，按取尾骨下端旁软陷处取穴	泄泻、阳痿、带下
	承扶	在股后区，臀沟的中点	腰腿痛、下肢痿痹

Continued

Acupoint		Location	Indications
Bladder Meridian of Foot-Taiyang	Zhongliao (BL33)	In the sacral portion, directly facing the 3rd posterior hole of the sacrum *Tips: the 1st hollow behind the Ciliao (BL32), the 3rd posterior hole of the sacrum	Irregular menstruation; leukorrhea; difficult urination; constipation; diarrhea; lower back pain
	Xialiao (BL34)	In the sacral portion, directly facing the 4th posterior hole of the sacrum Tips: the 2nd hollow behind the Ciliao (BL32), the 4th posterior hole of the sacrum, the horizontal sacral hiatus	Lower abdominal pain; lumbar and sacral pain; difficult urination; leukorrhea; constipation
	Huiyang (BL35)	In the sacral portion, 0.5 cun beside the coccyx Tips: Lying prostrate or couched, select the acupoint at the soft hollow beside the bottom of the coccyx	Diarrhea; impotence; leukorrhea
	Chengfu (BL36)	At the posterior region of the thigh, in the middle of the gluteal fold	Lumbar and leg pain; flaccid and paralytic lower body

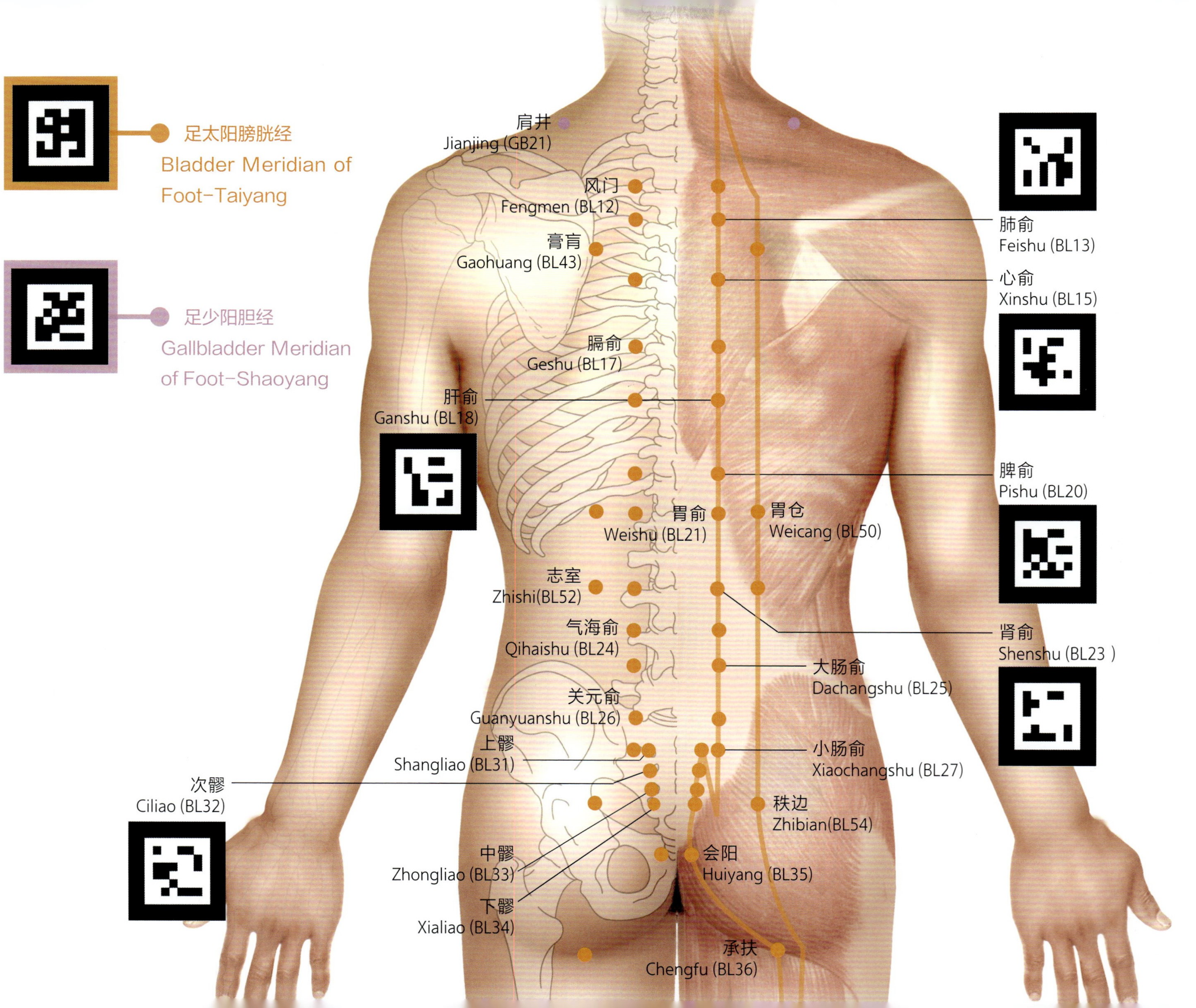
足太阳膀胱经
Bladder Meridian of Foot-Taiyang
足少阳胆经
Gallbladder Meridian of Foot-Shaoyang
肩井
Jianjing (GB21)
风门
Fengmen (BL12)
膏肓
Gaohuang (BL43)
膈俞
Geshu (BL17)
肝俞
Ganshu (BL18)
胃俞
Weishu (BL21)
胃仓
Weicang (BL50)
志室
Zhishi(BL52)
气海俞
Qihaishu (BL24)
关元俞
Guanyuanshu (BL26)
上髎
Shangliao (BL31)
次髎
Ciliao (BL32)
中髎
Zhongliao (BL33)
下髎
Xialiao (BL34)
会阳
Huiyang (BL35)
承扶
Chengfu (BL36)
秩边
Zhibian(BL54)
肺俞
Feishu (BL13)
心俞
Xinshu (BL15)
脾俞
Pishu (BL20)
肾俞
Shenshu (BL23)
大肠俞
Dachangshu (BL25)
小肠俞
Xiaochangshu (BL27)

续表

穴位		定位	主治
足太阳膀胱经	膏肓	在脊柱区，第 4 胸椎棘突下，后正中线旁开 3 寸	咳嗽、气喘、肺痨、健忘、遗精、虚劳（脏腑气血虚损所致的病症）
	胃仓	在脊柱区，第 12 胸椎棘突下，后正中线旁开 3 寸	胃脘痛、腹胀、水肿
	志室	在腰区，第 2 腰椎棘突下，后正中线旁开 3 寸	遗精、阳痿、遗尿、小便不利、水肿、月经不调、腰脊强痛
	秩边	在骶区，横平第 4 骶后孔，骶正中嵴旁开 3 寸	腰腿痛、下肢痿痹、便秘、小便不利、遗精、阳痿
足少阳胆经	肩井	在肩胛区，第 7 颈椎棘突与肩峰最外侧点连线的中点	颈项强痛、肩背疼痛、上肢不遂

Continued

Acupoint		Location	Indications
Bladder Meridian of Foot-Taiyang	Gaohuang (BL43)	In the spinal portion, behind the 4th spinous process of the thoracic vertebra, 3 cun beside the posterior middle line	Cough; asthma; pulmonary tuberculosis; amnesia; seminal emission; fatigue (the symptoms caused by the qi-blood deficiency of zang-fu organs)
	Weicang (BL50)	In the spinal portion, behind the 12th spinous process of the thoracic vertebra, 3 cun beside the posterior middle line	Epigastric pain; abdominal distension; edema
	Zhishi (BL52)	In the waist portion, behind the 2nd spinous process of the lumbar vertebra, 3 cun beside the posterior middle line	Seminal emission; impotence; enuresis; difficult urination; edema; irregular menstruation; lumbar and spinal pain
	Zhibian (BL54)	In the sacral portion, the 4th horizontal posterior sacral hole. 3 cun beside the middle ridge of the sacrum	Lumbar and leg pain; flaccid and paralytic lower body; difficult urination; seminal emission; impotence
Gallbladder Meridian of Foot-Shaoyang	Jianjing (GB21)	In the scapula portion, the middle of the line between the spinous process of the 7th cervical vertebra and the outermost point of the acromion	Stiffness and pain in neck; shoulder and back pain; hemiplegia

超简单脊柱穴位按摩

Super-easy Massage of Spine Acupoints

风门

用同侧中指端稍用力按压风门穴，停留片刻后放松，反复5~6下。同法按压对侧风门穴。每日2次

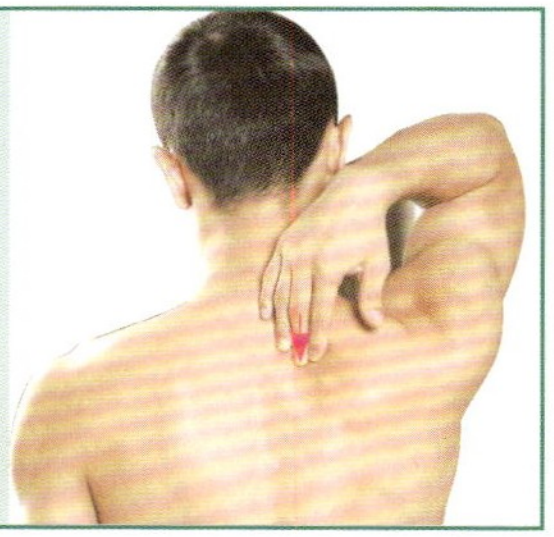

肺俞

将手抬起放于背后，用手指稍用力按压肺俞穴，停留片刻后放松，反复5~6下。同法按压对侧肺俞穴。每日2次

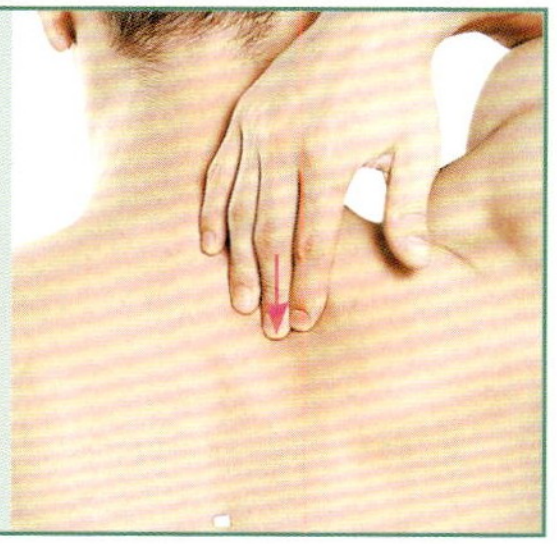

心俞

将手绕于背后，用拇指稍用力推按心俞穴，停留片刻后放松，反复5~6下。同法推按对侧心俞穴。每日2次

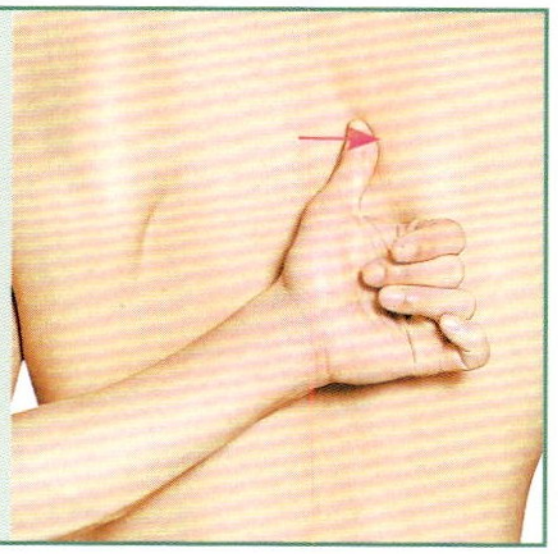

肝俞

一手握拳绕于背后，用掌指关节按揉肝俞穴2分钟，力度稍重。同法按揉对侧肝俞穴。每日2次

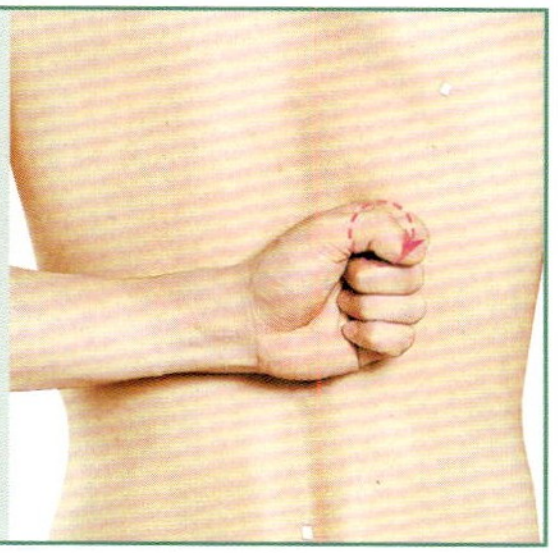

脾俞

双手握拳绕于背后，用掌指关节稍用力按压两侧脾俞穴，停留片刻后放松，反复5~6下。每日2次

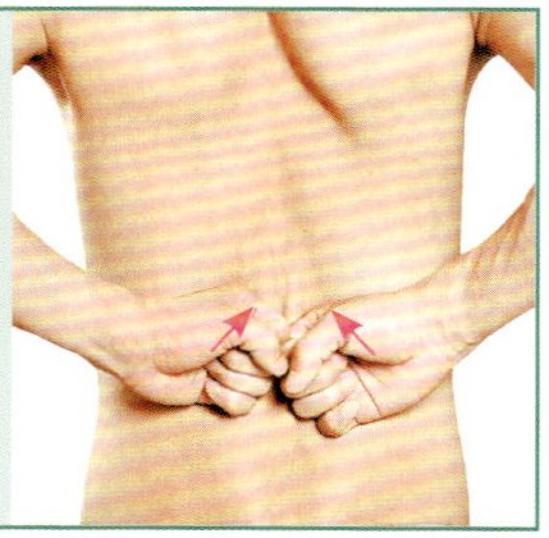

胃俞

两手握拳绕于背后，用掌指关节稍用力按压胃俞穴2分钟，停留片刻后放松，反复5~6下。同时按揉对侧胃俞穴每日2次

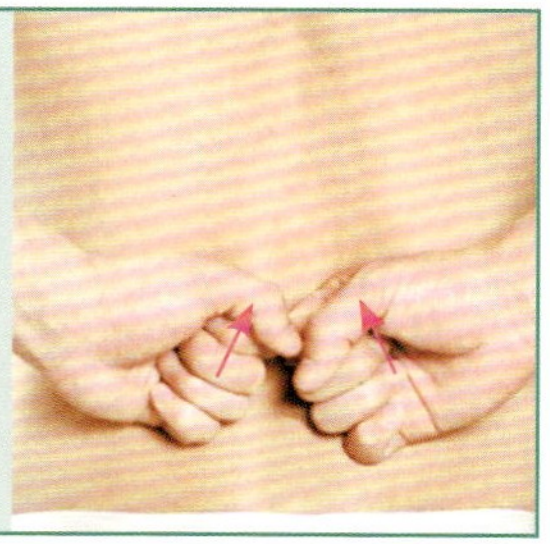

肾俞

双手握拳绕于背后，用掌指关节按揉两侧肾俞穴，力度稍重。每日2次

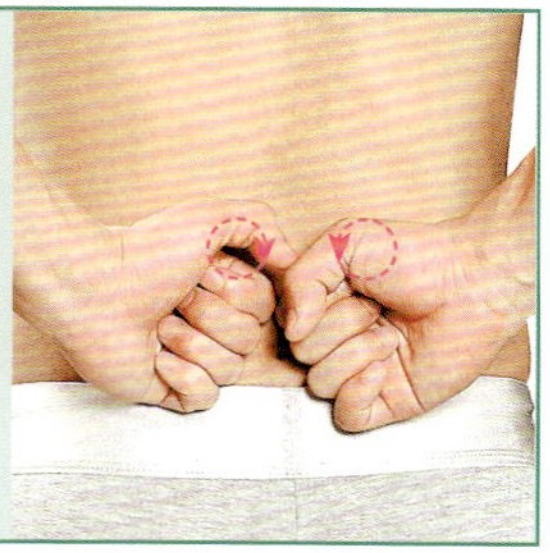

上髎

两手握拳绕于背后臀部，用掌指关节稍用力按揉两侧上髎穴2分钟。每日2次

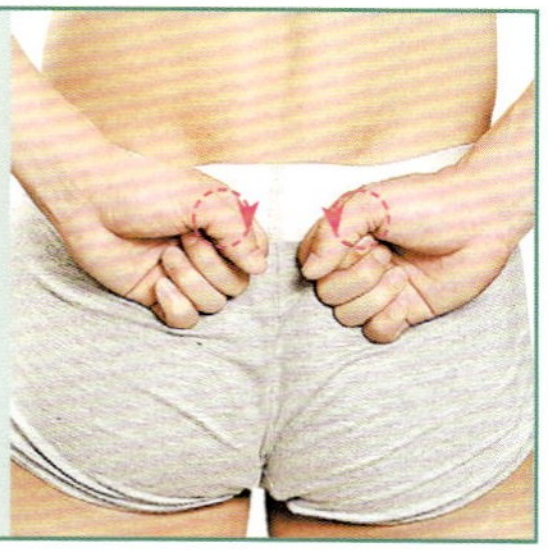

Fengmen (BL12)

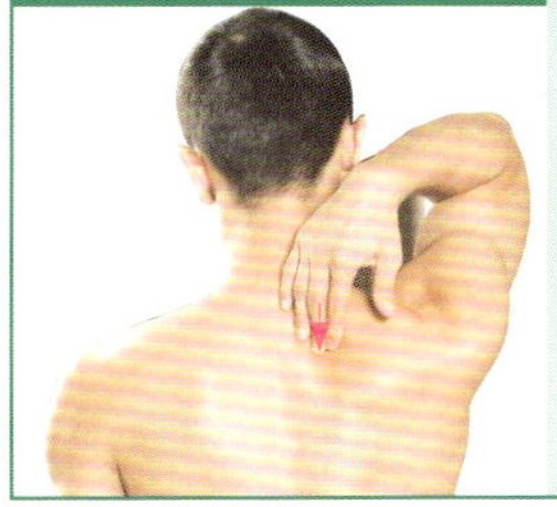

Press a little hard on the Fengmen (BL12) with the middle finger of the same side and relax after each short stay. Repeat 5 to 6 times and apply the same manipulation to the opposite Fengmen (BL12). The massage should be taken twice a day

Feishu (BL13)

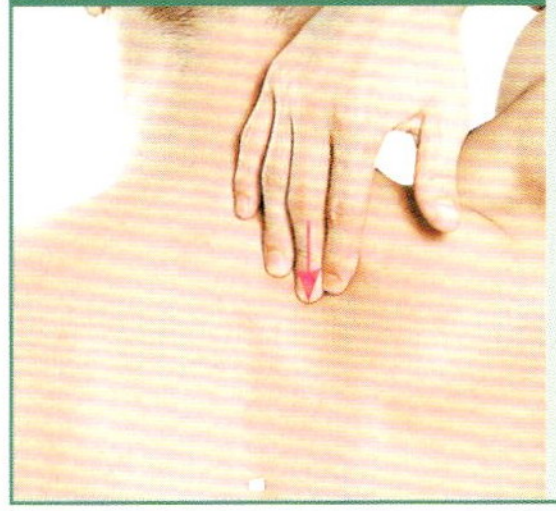

Raise your hand and place it at the back, and then use fingers to press hard on Feishu (BL13). Take a break after each short stay and the action should be repeated 5 to 6 times. Apply the same manipulation to the opposite Feishu (BL13) twice a day

Xinshu (BL15)

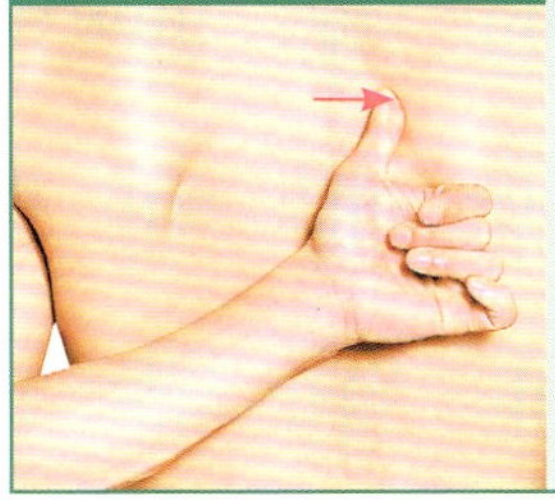

Wind your hand at the back and push the Xinshu (BL15) with a little pressure with thumbs repeatedly for 5 to 6 times and relax after each short stay. Apply the same manipulation to the opposite Xinshu (BL15) twice a day

Ganshu (BL18)

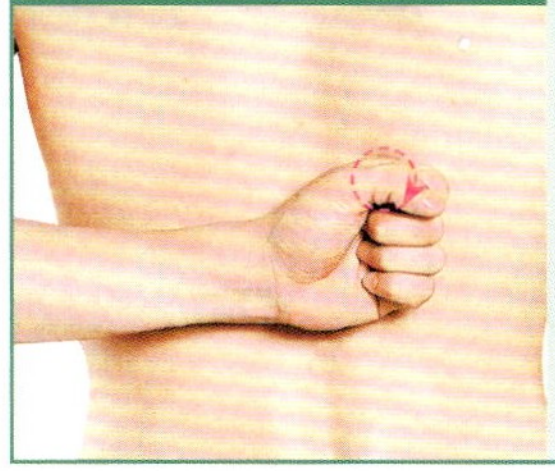

Twist your fist at the back and massage the Ganshu (BL18) with relatively heavy pressure using finger joints for 2 minutes. Apply the same manipulation to the opposite Ganshu (BL18) twice a day

Pishu (BL20)

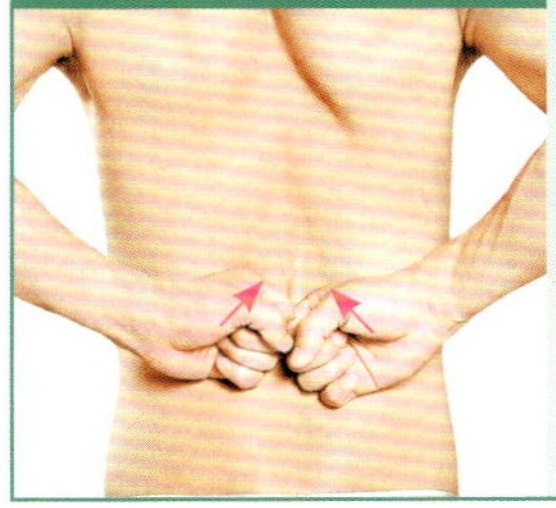

Place your 2 folded fists at the back and use finger joints to press hard on Pishu (BL20) on both sides repeatedly for 5 to 6 times. Relax after each short stay. The massage is supposed to be twice a day

Weishu (BL21)

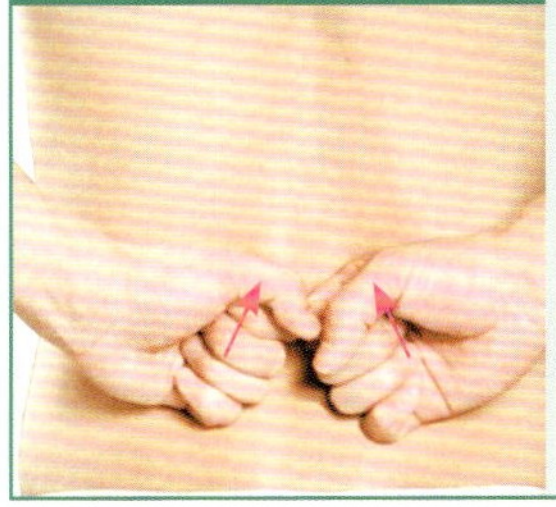

Place your 2 folded fists at the back and use finger joints to press hard on Weishu (BL21) on both sides for 2 minutes. Repeat it for 5 to 6 times and relax after each short stay. The massage is supposed to be twice a day

Shenshu (BL23)

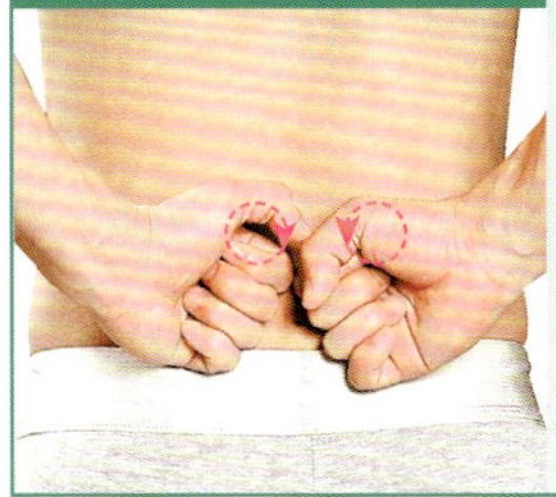

Place your 2 folded fists at the back and use finger joints to press hard on Shenshu (BL23) on both sides with relatively heavy pressure twice a day

Shangliao (BL31)

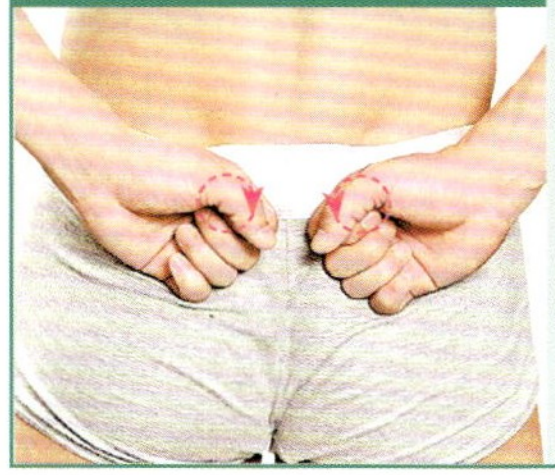

Fold your 2 fists and place them at the haunch portion, then use finger joints to press hard on 2 acupoints of Shangliao (BL31) on both sides for 2 minutes twice a day

承扶

用拇指按揉承扶穴 2 分钟，力度稍重。同法按揉对侧承扶穴。每日 2 次

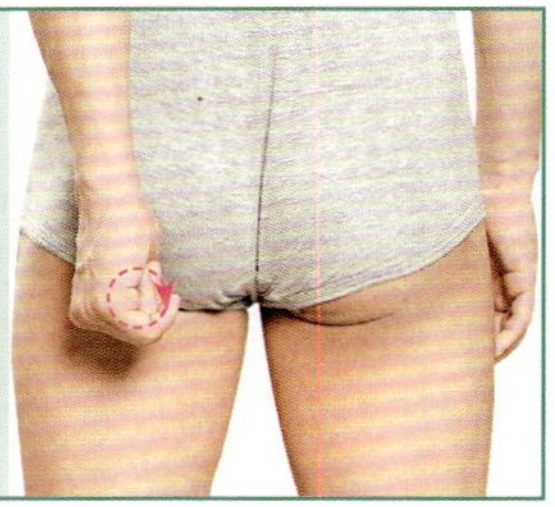

秩边

两手握拳绕于背后腰骶部，用掌指关节稍用力按揉两侧秩边穴 2 分钟。每日 2 次

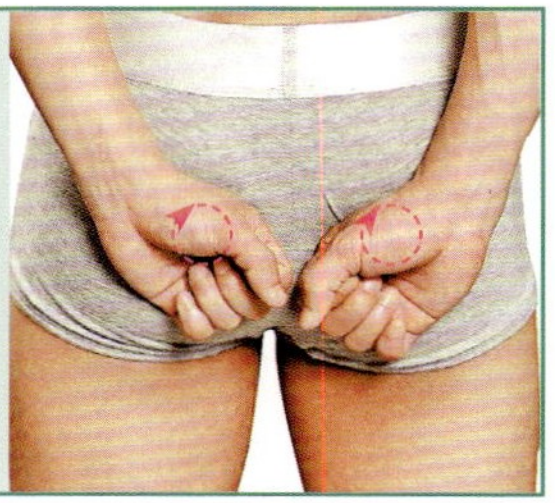

肩井

食、中二指并拢按揉肩井穴 2 分钟，力度稍重。同法按揉对侧肩井穴。每日 2 次

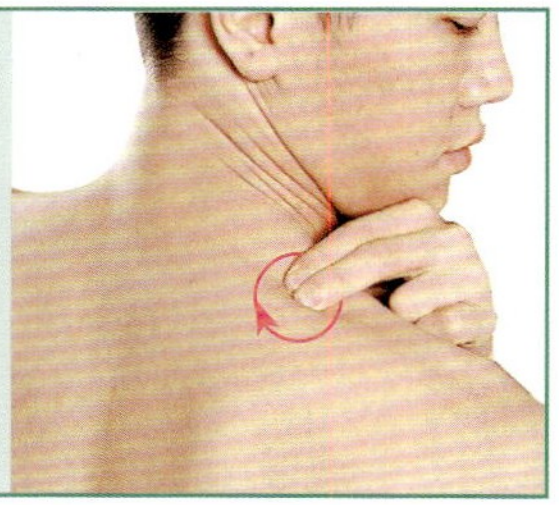

长强

手握拳绕于背后，用掌指关节按揉长强穴，力度稍重。每日 2 次

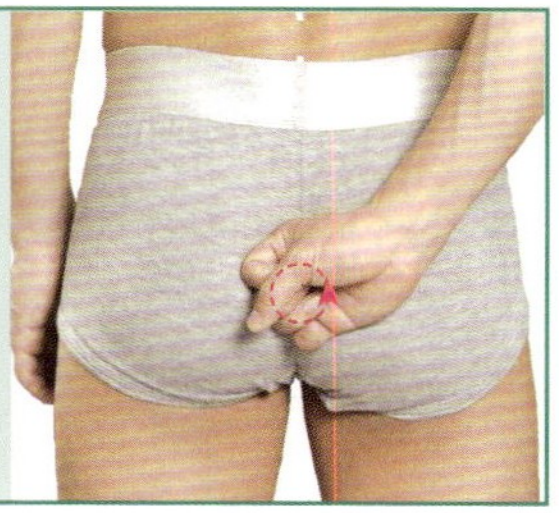

腰阳关

一手握拳绕于背后，用掌指关节稍用力按揉腰阳关穴 2 分钟。同法按揉对侧腰阳关穴。每日 2 次

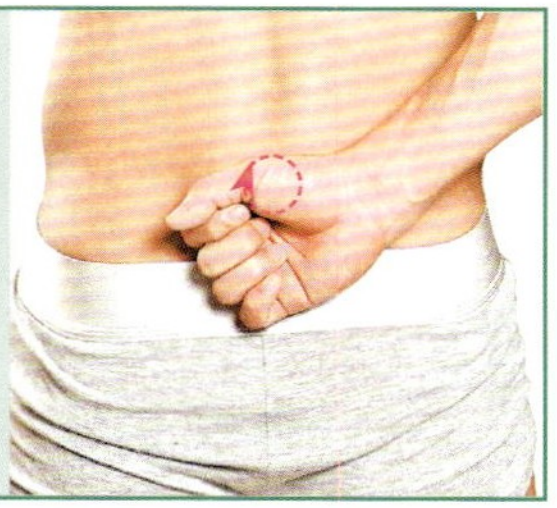

命门

一手握拳绕于背后，用掌指关节稍用力按揉命门穴 2 分钟。每日 2 次

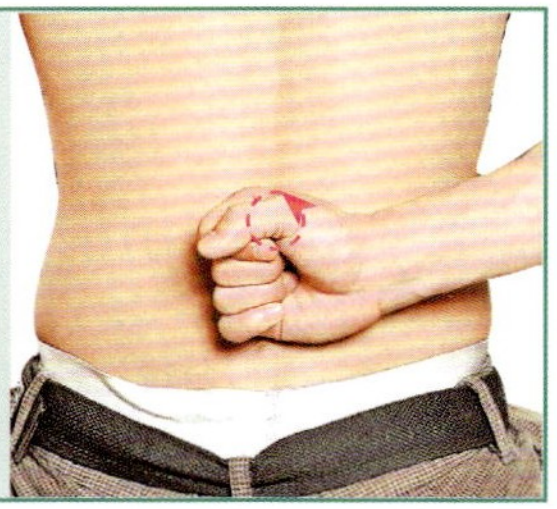

大椎

两手食指重叠用力按压大椎穴，停留片刻后放松，反复 5~6 下。每日 2 次

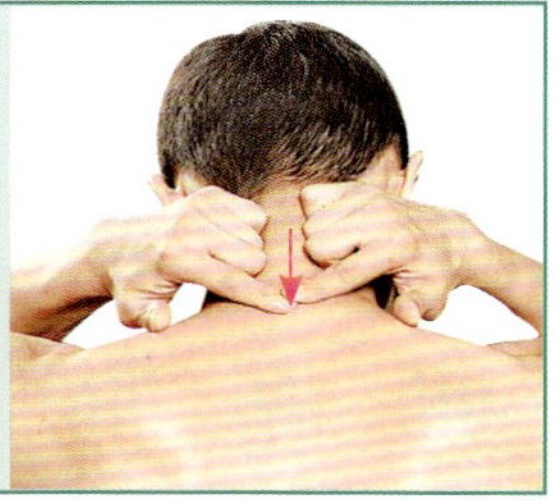

定喘

将手绕颈放于肩上，拇指稍用力按压定喘穴，停留片刻后放松，反复 5~6 下。同法按压对侧定喘穴。每日 2 次

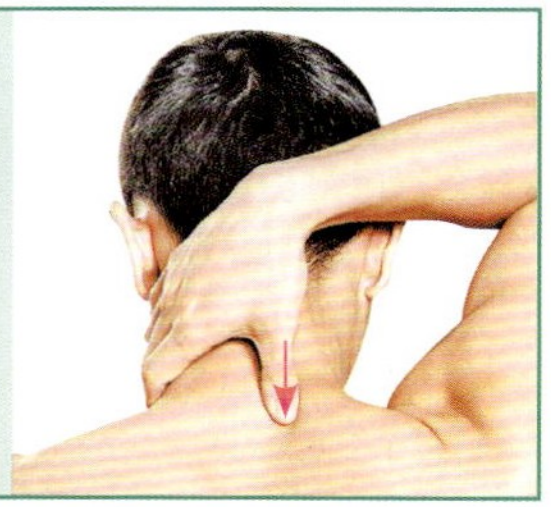

腰眼

用拇指稍用力按揉腰眼穴 2 分钟。同法按揉对侧腰眼穴。每日 2 次

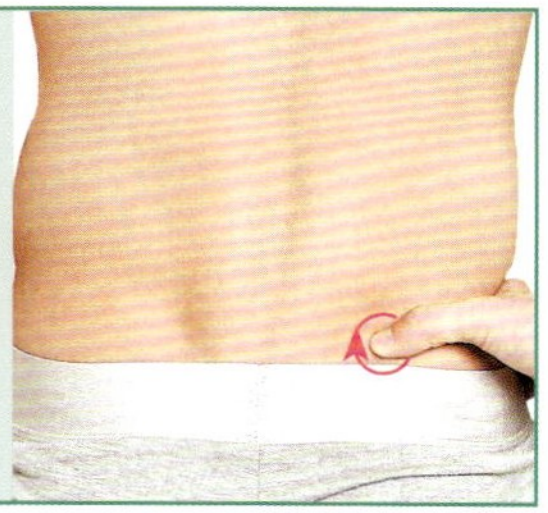

Chengfu (BL36)

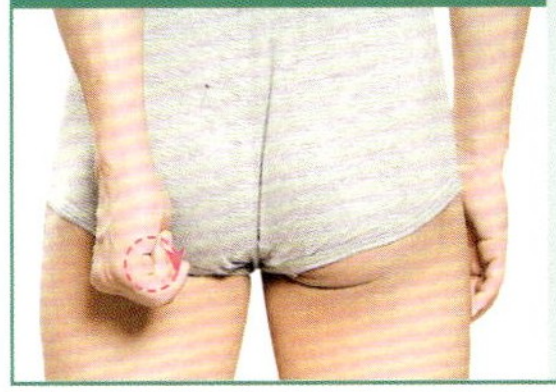

Use thumbs to massage the Chengfu (BL36) for 2 minutes with a little pressure twice a day. Apply the same manipulation to the opposite Chengfu (BL36)

Zhibian (BL54)

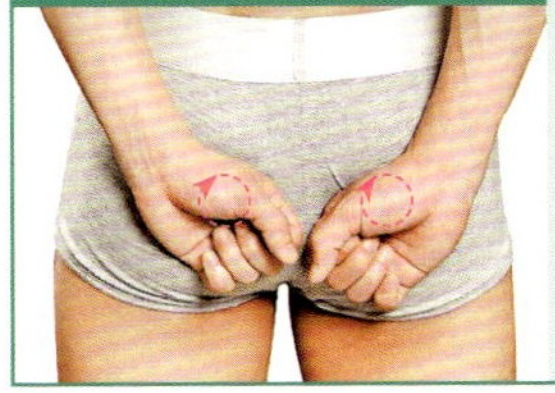

Fold your 2 fists at the lumbosacral portion, and use finger joints to press Zhibian (BL54) on both sides with a little pressure for 2 minutes twice a day

Jianjing (GB21)

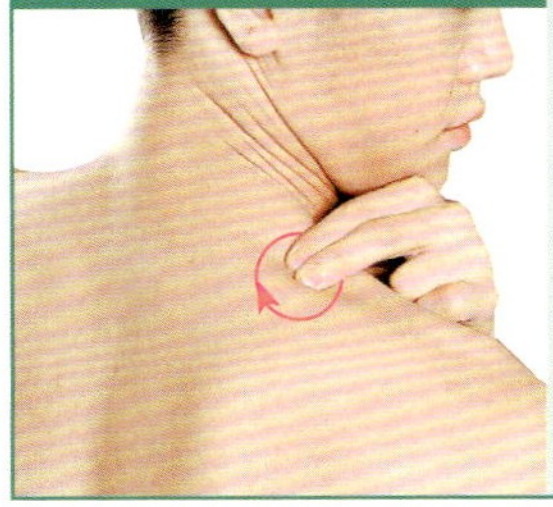

Fold your index finger and middle finger to massage the Jianjing (GB21) for 2 minutes with relatively heavy pressure twice a day and apply the same manipulation to the opposite one

Changqiang(GV1)

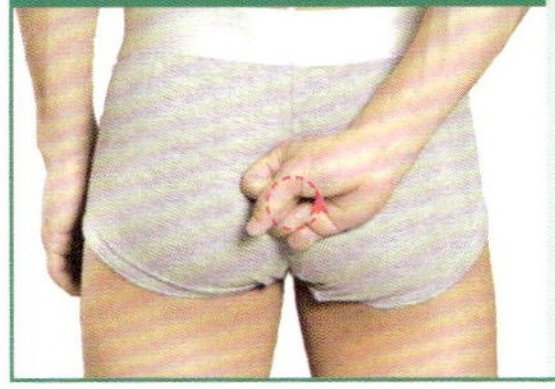

Fold your fists at the back and use finger joints to massage the Changqiang (GV1) with relatively heavy pressure twice a day

Yaoyangguan (GV3)

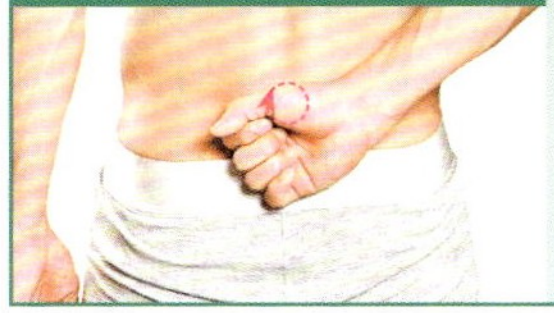

Fold a fist at the back and use finger joints to press hard on Yaoyangguan (GV3) for 2 minutes twice a day and apply the same manipulation on the opposite

Mingmen (GV4)

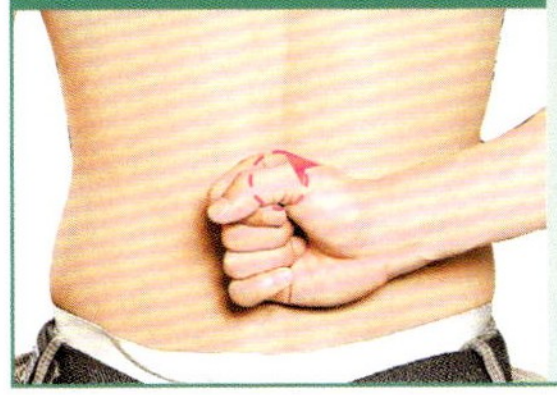

Fold a fist at the back and use finger joints to press hard on Mingmen (GV4) for 2 minutes twice a day

Dazhui (GV14)

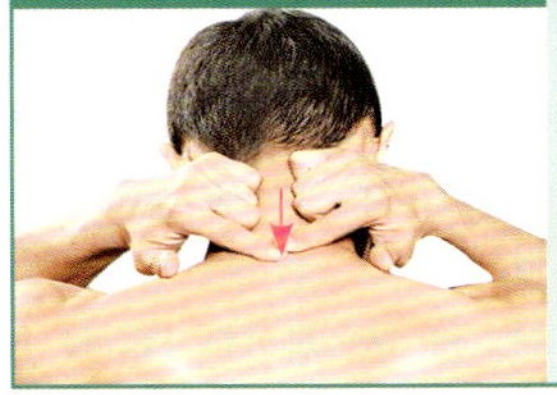

Fold 2 index fingers and press hard on Dazhui (GV14) and relax after each short stay repeatedly for 5 to 6 times twice a day

Dingchuan(EX-B1)

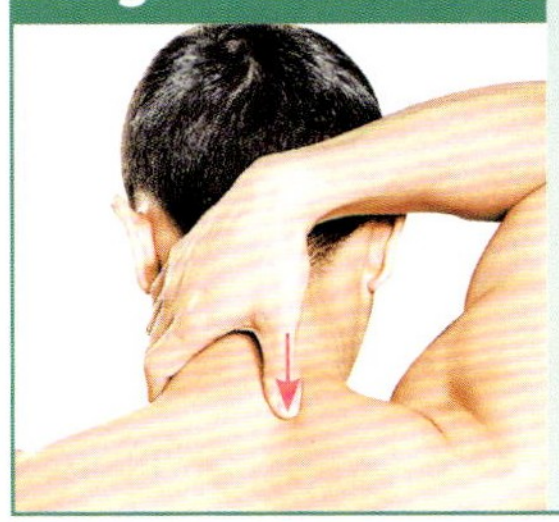

Place the hand on one side on the shoulder on the other side and use thumb to press hard on Dingchuan (EX-B1). Relax after each short stay and apply the same manipulation on the opposite Dingchuan (EX-B1). Repeat the massage for 5 to 6 times twice a day

Yaoyan (EX-B7)

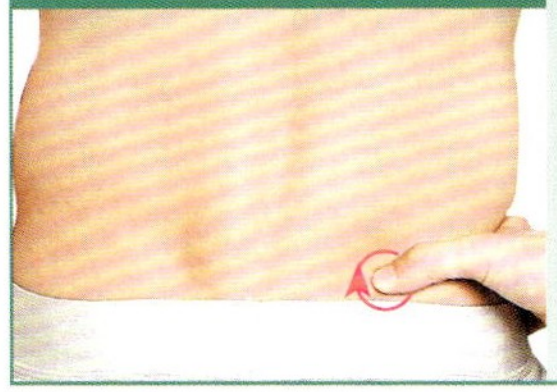

Use thumbs to press the Yaoyangguan (EX-B7) with relatively heavy pressure and apply the same manipulation on the opposite twice a day

第六章　超速效对症按摩

❶ 美颜祛痘

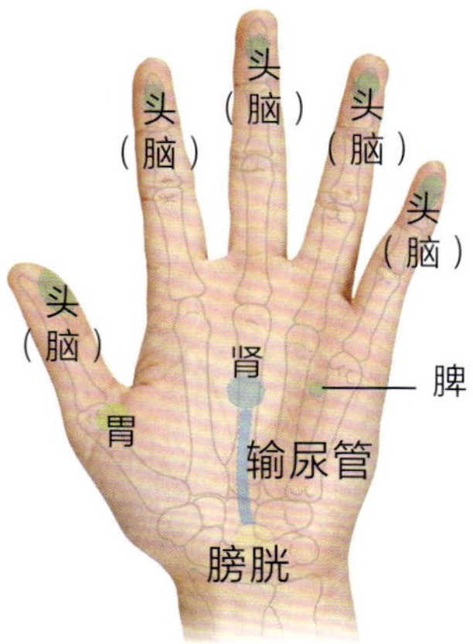

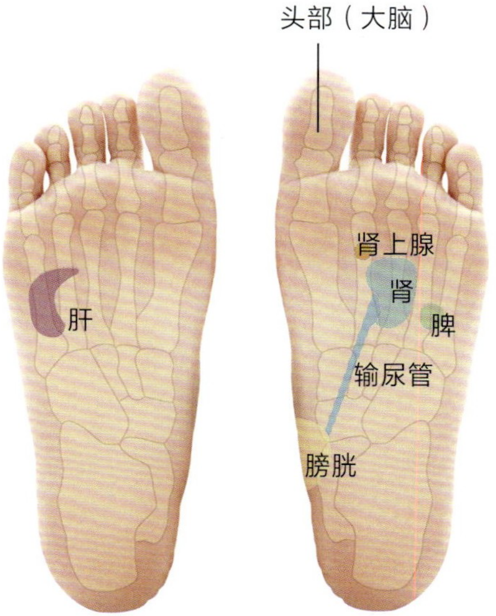

手部按摩

1. 点按脾、肾、胃反射区各 2~3 分钟，手法要由轻到重，再由重到轻，逐渐渗透。
2. 拇指指腹按揉输尿管、膀胱反射区各 2~3 分钟，每分钟 50~80 次。
3. 放松手部，拇指先轻轻按揉头（脑）反射区 2~3 分钟，再稍用力按此反射区，以局部有酸痛感为宜。

足部按摩

1. 泡脚至全脚放松后，按摩肾、输尿管、膀胱反射区各 2 分钟，以局部有热胀感为宜。
2. 用工具如铅笔点按头部（大脑）反射区 30~50 次，以局部有热胀感为宜。
3. 拇指从外向内推肝、脾反射区各 10~20 次，接着拇指由下至上推肾反射区 10~20 次。
4. 按摩肾上腺反射区 3~5 分钟，以局部有热胀感为宜。

❷ 美白祛皱

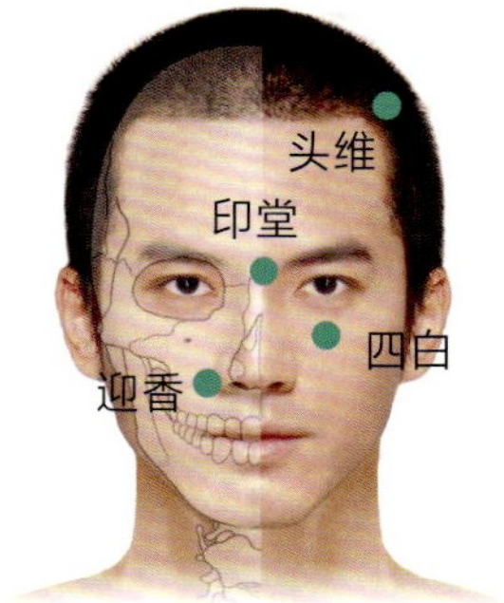

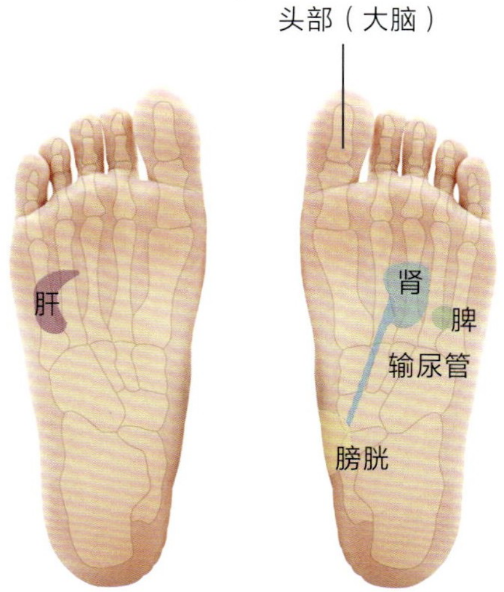

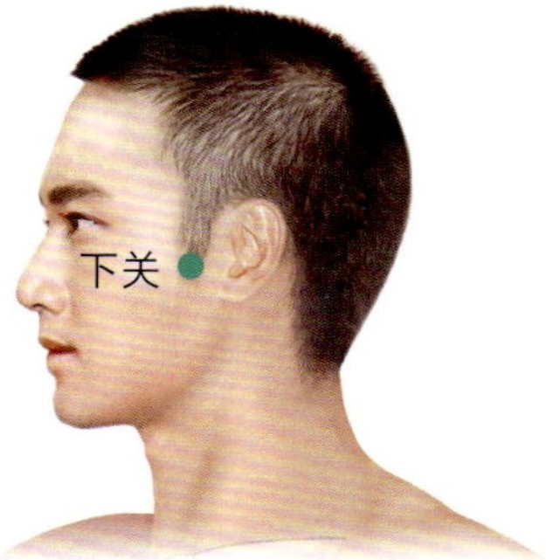

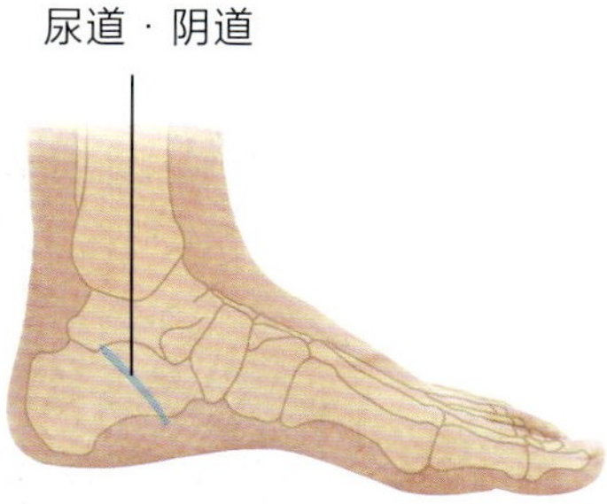

头面部按摩

1. 按揉头维、印堂穴各 30 次，手法宜轻。
2. 按揉迎香、四白、下关穴各 30 次，手法宜轻。
3. 双手合掌，用拇指及大鱼际从额头正中向两侧轻轻按摩，缓慢来回做 3 次。

足部按摩

1. 拇指指腹从趾尖向趾根方向推头部（大脑）反射区，以局部有热胀感为宜。
2. 泡脚至全脚放松后，按摩输尿管、膀胱、尿道·阴道反射区，以局部有酸胀感为宜。
3. 拇指推压肾、肝、脾反射区各 20~30 次，再次放松全足结束按摩，使按摩后身体的代谢废物及时排出体外。

1 Facial Beautification with Acne Treatment

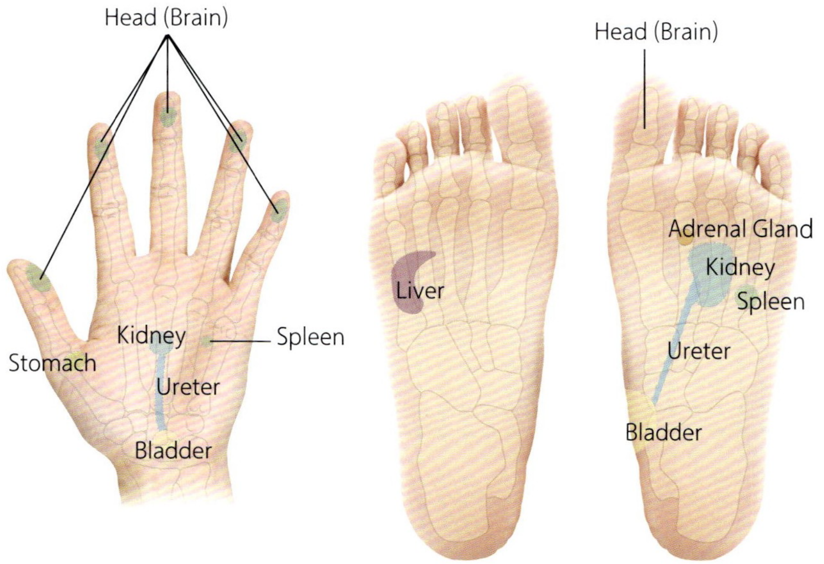

Hand Massage

1. Press the reflex zones of Spleen, Kidney and Stomach for 2 to 3 minutes and the manipulation should gradually penetrate from light to heavy and then heavy to light.
2. Massage the reflex zones of Ureter and Bladder with finger pulp each for 2 to 3 minutes, and there would be 50 to 80 times within every minute.
3. Relax your hands, and gently massage the reflex zones of Head (Brain) with thumbs. Then, put significant pressure on this region and it is preferred to have a local sense of aching pain.

Foot Massage

1. After taking a foot bath to have overall relaxation, massage the reflex zones of Kidney, Ureter and Bladder each for 2 minutes and a local sense of warmth and distension is preferable.
2. Press the reflex zone of Head (Brain) for 30 to 50 times with tolls such as pencils, and it is preferred to have a local sense of warmth and distension.
3. Massage the reflex zones of Liver and Spleen from the exterior to the interior with thumbs. Then, use the thumbs to massage the reflex zones of Kidney from the lower side to the upper side for 10 to 20 times.
4. Massage the reflex zone of Adrenal Gland for 3 to 5 minutes, and it is preferred to have a local sense of warmth and distension.

2 Whitening and Freckle Removal

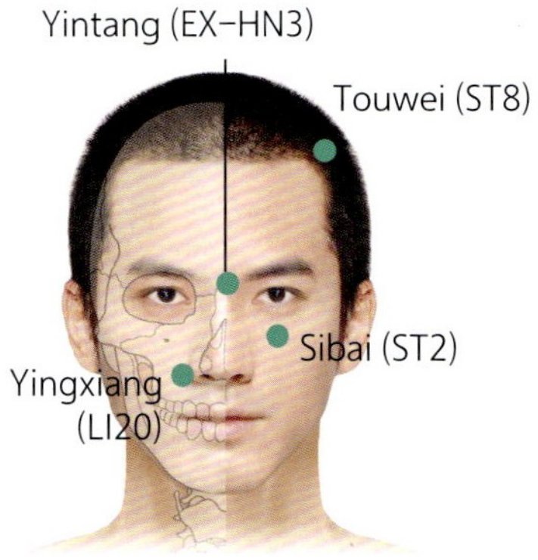

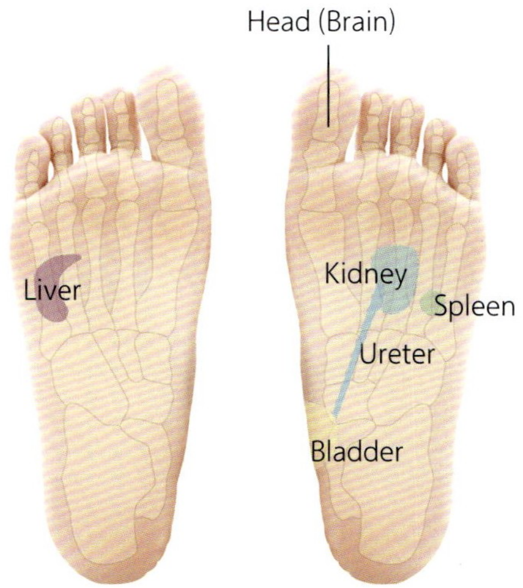

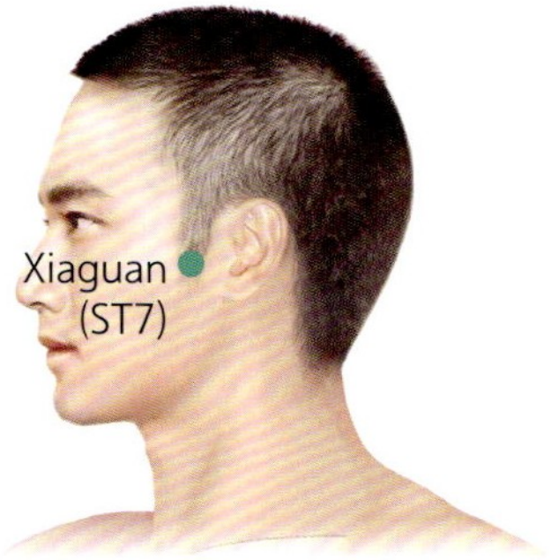

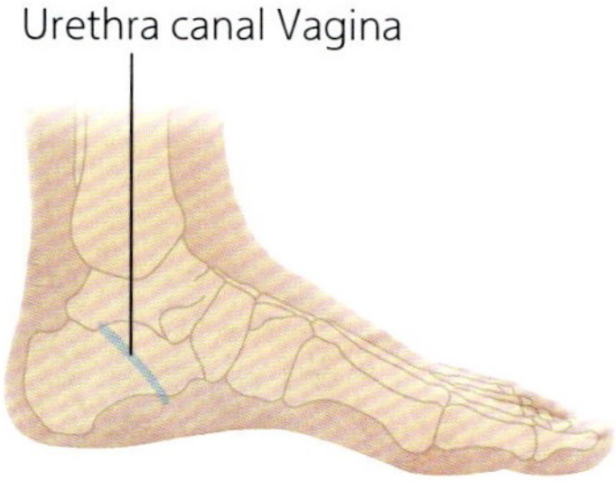

Head and Facial Massage

1. Massage the acupoints of Yintang (EX-HN3) and Touwei (ST8) gently for 30 times each.
2. Massage the acupoints of Yingxiang (LI20), Sibai (ST2) and Xiaguan (ST7) gently for 30 times each.
3. Use thumbs and the thenar to gently massage from the middle to both sides of the forehead with hands folded. The movements should be back and forth for 3 times.

Foot Massage

1. Massage the reflex zone of the Head (Brain) from the tip to root using finger pulp, and it is preferred that there appears a local sense of warmth and distension.
2. After taking a foot bath to have overall relaxation, massage the reflex zones of Ureter, Bladder, Urethra Canal and Vagina and it is preferred to have a local sense of soreness.
3. Using thumbs to press onto the reflex zones of Kidney, Liver and Spleen for 20 to 30 times each, and then end the massage with relaxing feet so that the metabolic waste could be eliminated out of the body in time.

3 乌发固脱

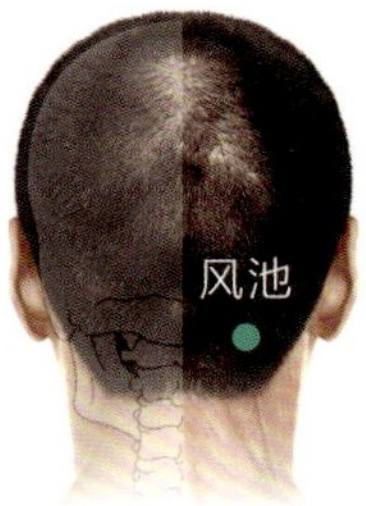

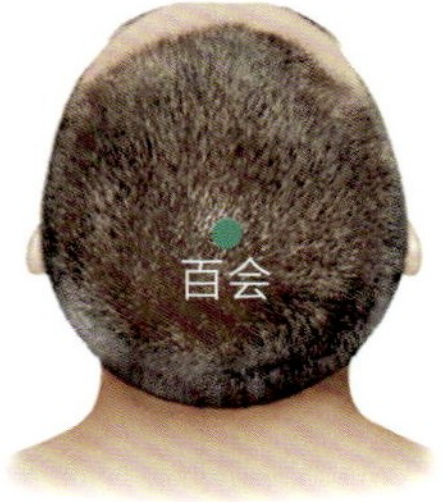

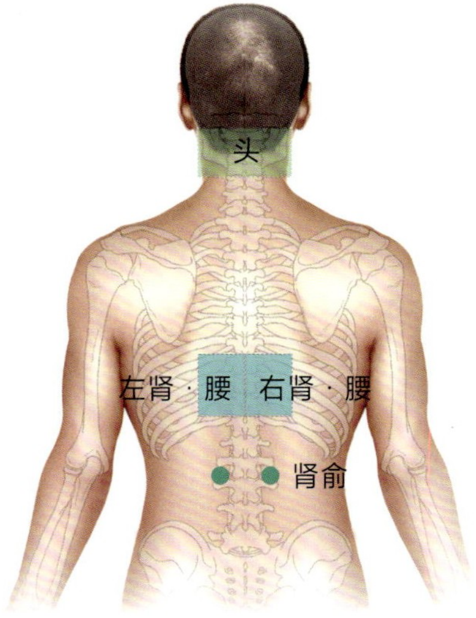

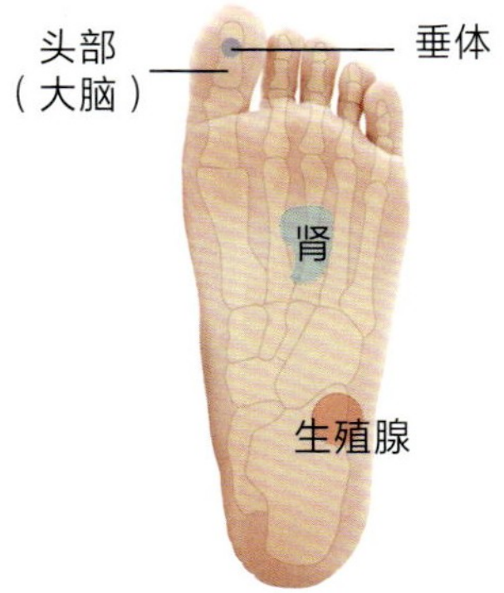

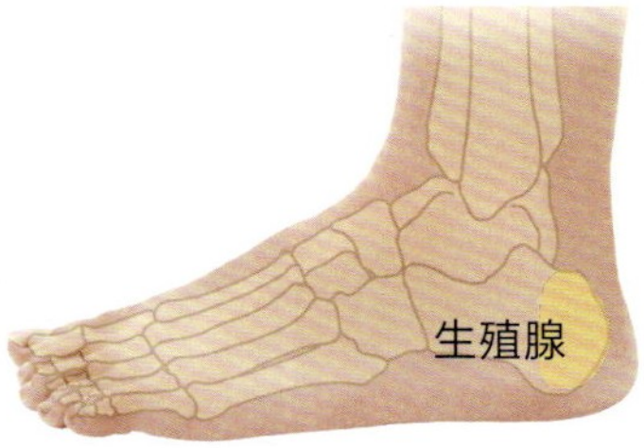

头面部按摩

1. 两手食指重叠稍用力按压百会穴 20 次，再顺时针按揉 20 次。
2. 两手食、中指并拢按揉两侧风池穴各 20 次，力度稍重，每次停留片刻后放松。

脊背按摩

1. 拇指点按肾俞穴 40~60 次。
2. 将两手对搓至发热后，搓擦腰背部 30~50 次。
3. 两手食指重叠稍用力按压肾·腰、头反射区各 5~6 次，每次停留片刻后放松。

足部按摩

1. 食指近侧指间关节依次刮压头部（大脑）反射区 3~5 次。
2. 按摩棒点按肾、垂体、生殖腺反射区各 3~5 分钟，以局部有酸胀感为宜。

4 缓解眼疲劳

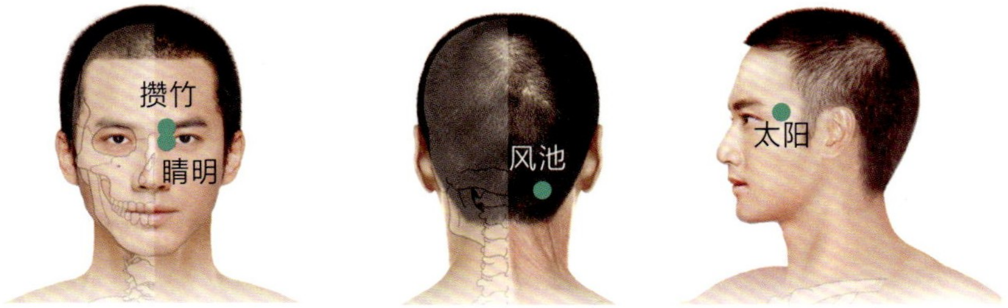

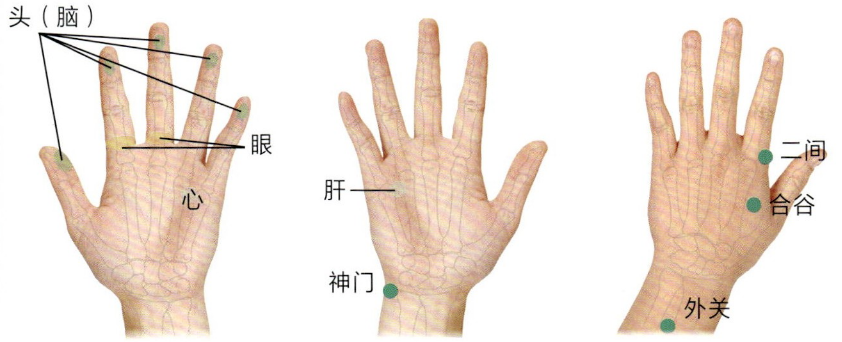

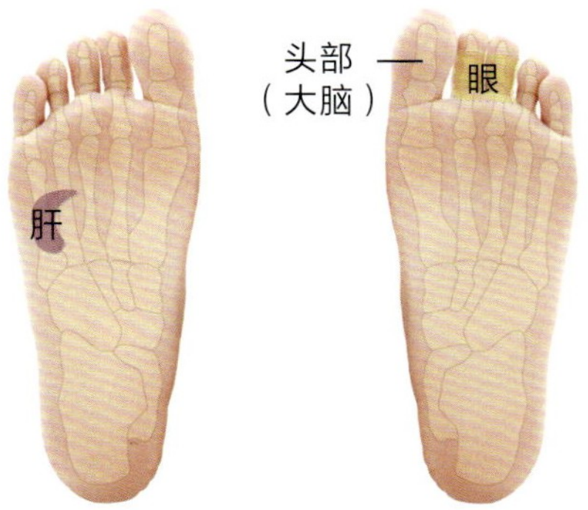

头面部按摩

1. 双手食指近侧指间关节分别按揉双侧睛明穴各 3~5 分钟。
2. 双手拇指指腹分别按揉双侧攒竹、太阳穴各 3~5 分钟。
3. 双手分别强压双侧风池穴 3~5 分钟。

手部按摩

1. 食指近侧指间关节按揉眼反射区 2~3 分钟，用力均匀，力度适中。
2. 放松手部，拇指轻轻按揉头（脑）、心、肝反射区，以局部有酸痛感为宜。
3. 点按合谷、外关、神门、二间穴，以被按摩者耐受为度。

足部按摩

1. 用工具如铅笔点按眼反射区 30~50 次。
2. 按摩头部（大脑）、肝反射区各 3~5 分钟。

3 Hair Blackening and Prevention for Hair Loss

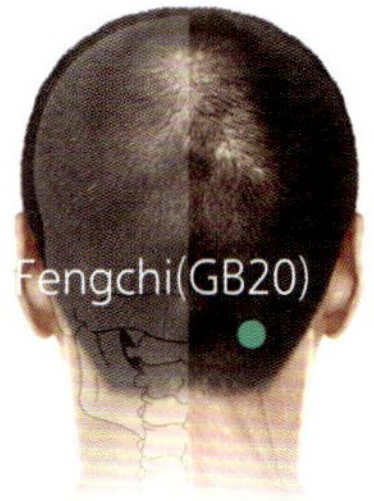

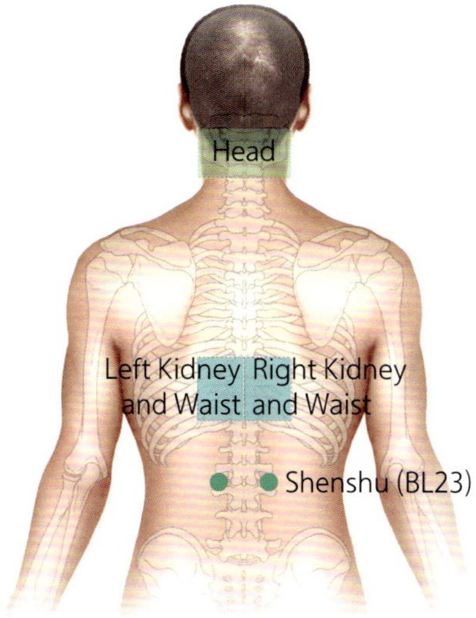

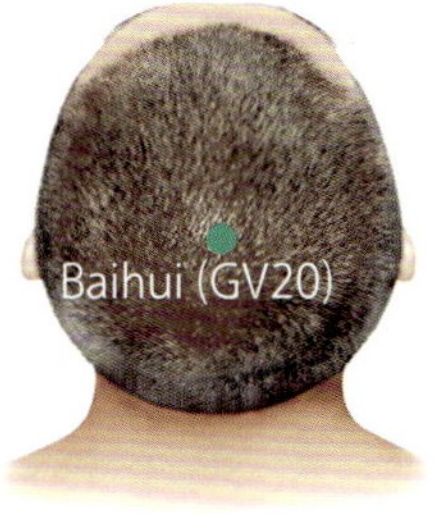

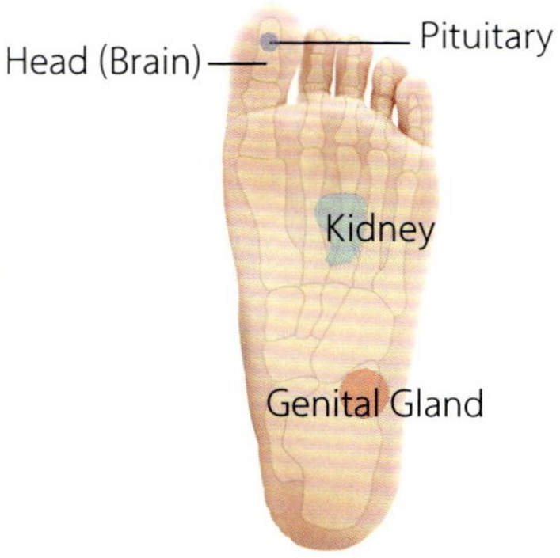

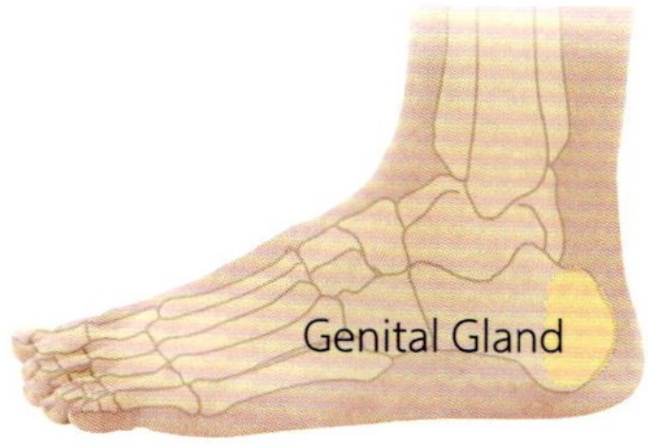

Head and Facial Massage

1. Use overlapped index finger to press Baihui(GV20) 20 times with a little bit pressure, and massage 20 times clockwise.
2. Massage Fengchi(GB20) on both sides each for 20 times with folded index fingers and middle fingers with a little bit pressure. There should be a relaxation after each massage.

Back Massage

1. Press Shenshu (BL23) for 40 to 60 times with thumbs.
2. After generating heat with folded hands, massage the waist and back 30 to 50 times.
3. Use overlapped index fingers to press hard on the reflex zones of Kidney, Waist and Head for 5 to 6 times. There should be a relaxation after each massage.

Foot Massage

1. Press and scratch the reflex zone of Head (Brain) for 3 to 5 times with interphalangeal joint at the proximal side of index fingers.
2. Press the reflex zones of Kidney, Pituitary and Genital Gland each for 3 to 5 minutes with massage stick. It is preferred to have a local soreness.

4 Visual Fatigue Alleviation

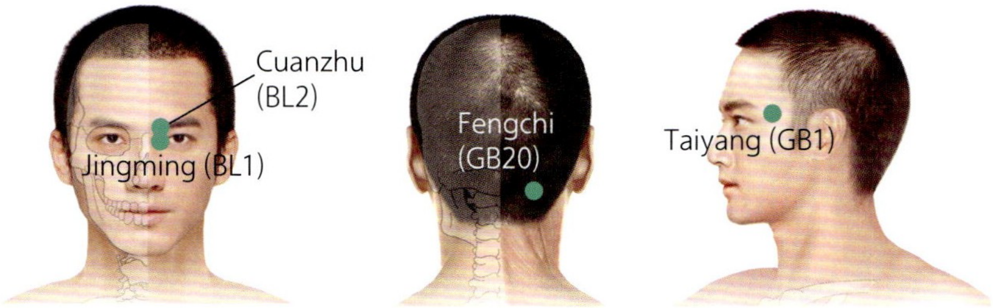

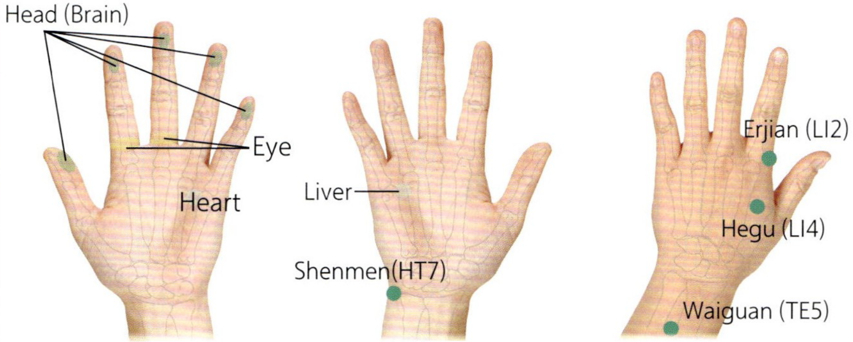

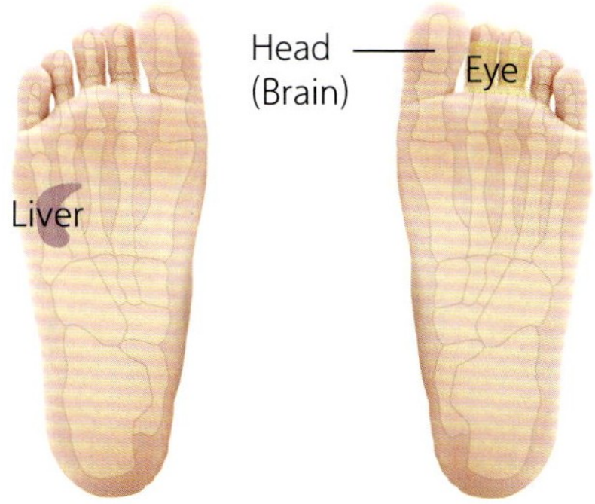

Head and Facial Massage

1. Massage Jingming (BL1) on both sides with interphalangeal joint at the proximal side of index fingers each for 3 to 5 minutes.
2. Massage Cuanzhu (BL2) and Taiyang (GB1) on both sides with thumbs for 3 to 5 minutes.
3. Press Fengchi (GB20) on both sides with great pressure for 3 to 5 minutes.

Hand Massage

1. Massage the reflex zone of Eye with interphalangeal joint at the proximal side of index fingers for 2 to 3 minutes with moderate pressure.
2. Relax your hands and gently massage the reflex zones of Head (Brain), Heart and Liver with thumbs. Local aching pain is preferable.
3. Press the acupoints of Hegu (LI4), Waiguan (TE5), Shenmen (HT7) and Erjian (LI2) taking the tolerance degree of the patient into consideration.

Foot Massage

1. Press Eye reflex zone with tools such as pencil for 30 to 50 times.
2. Massage the reflex zones of Head (Brain) and Liver each for 3 to 5 minutes.

5 缓解压力

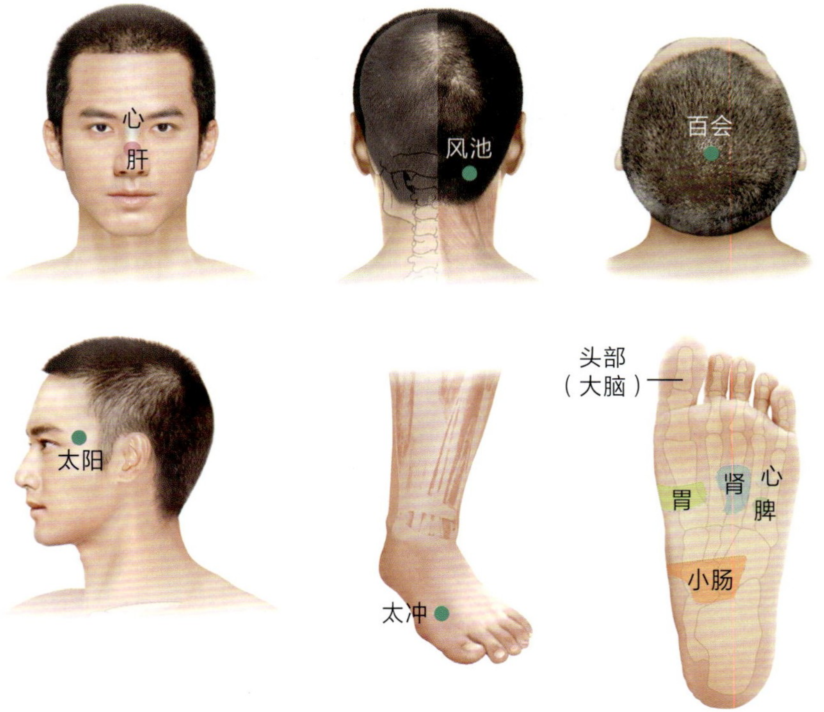

头面部按摩

1. 两手食指重叠稍用力按压心、肝反射区，反复 5~6 次，每次停留片刻后放松。
2. 两手食指指腹稍用力按压两侧太阳、百会穴各2分钟，力度稍重。同法按压对侧。
3. 两手食、中指并拢分别按揉两侧风池穴，力度稍重，每次停留片刻后放松。

足部按摩

1. 食指近侧指间关节刮压头部（大脑）、心、肾反射区 2~3 分钟。
2. 食指桡侧缘刮小肠、脾、胃反射区各 5 分钟。
3. 泡脚至全脚放松后，掐按太冲穴 5~6 次，以局部有酸胀感为宜。

6 益智健脑

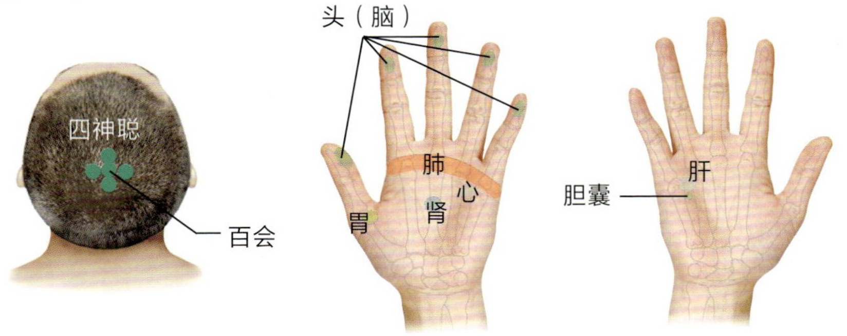

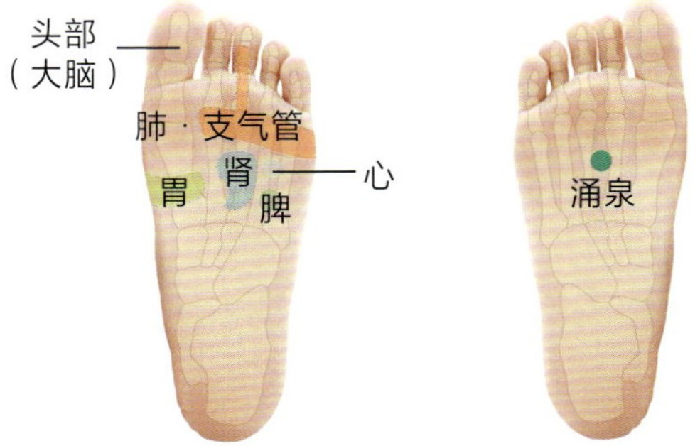

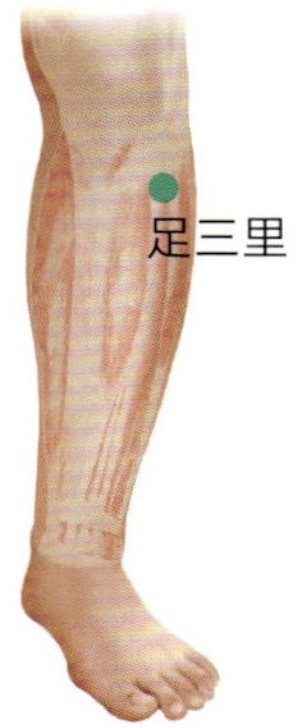

头面部按摩

1. 两手食指重叠稍用力按压百会穴，反复 5~6 次，每次停留片刻后放松。
2. 两手拇指指腹按压四神聪穴 1 分钟，力度稍重。

手部按摩

1. 左右手相互捻指，每指捻动 5 次。
2. 食指近侧指间关节点按头（脑）、心、肺反射区，力度适中，以局部有轻度胀痛为宜。
3. 点按胃、肝、胆囊、肾反射区，力度以被按摩者耐受为度。

足部按摩

1. 泡脚至全脚放松后，按摩头部（大脑）、心、肺 · 支气管反射区，以局部有酸胀感为宜。
2. 拇指或牙签束点按脾、胃反射区各 30~50 次，以局部有轻微胀痛为宜。
3. 拇指推压肾反射区 20~30 次，再次放松全足结束按摩，使按摩后身体的代谢废物及时排出体外。
4. 按揉涌泉、足三里穴各 2 分钟，力度稍重，反复 5~6 次，每次停留片刻后放松。

5 Pressure Relief

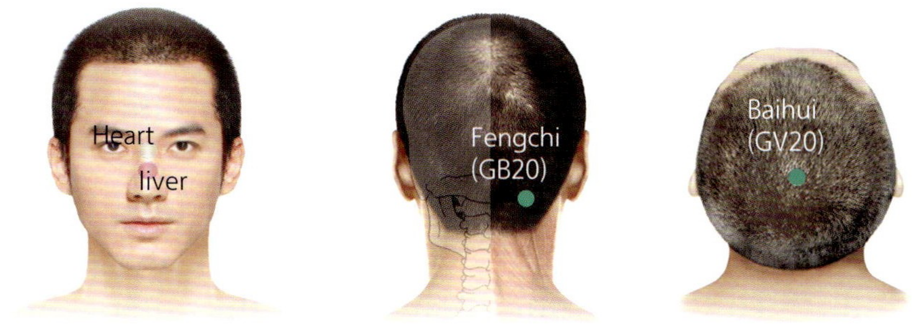

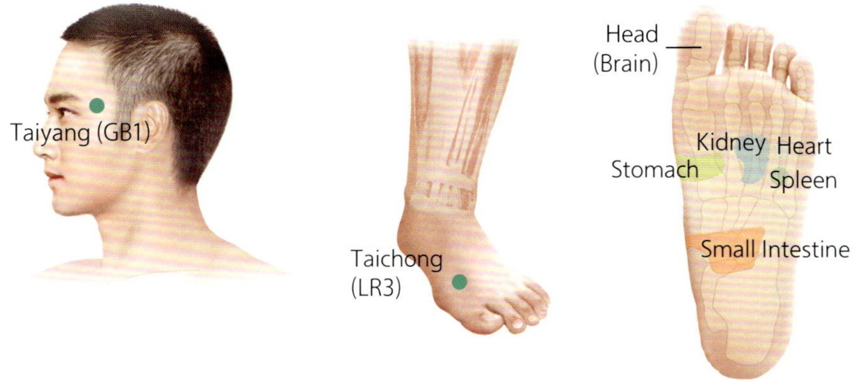

Head and Facial Massage

1. Press the reflex zones of Heart and Liver with a little bit pressure using both index fingers for 5 to 6 times. There is a relaxation after each manipulation.
2. Press Taiyang (GB1) and Baihui (GV20) with a little bit pressure using both index fingers for 2 minutes each. The same manipulation should be applied at the other side.
3. Use both folded index fingers and middle fingers to massage Fengchi (GB20) with a little bit pressure, and relax after each manipulation.

Foot Massage

1. Press and scratch the reflex zones of Head (Brain), Heart and Kidney with interphalangeal joint at the proximal side of index fingers for 2 to 3 minutes.
2. Scratch the reflex zones of Small Intestine, Spleen and Stomach each for 5 minutes with radical margins of index fingers each for 5 minutes.
3. After having overall relaxation with foot bath, nip Taichong (LR3) for 5 to 6 times.

6 Reinforcing Intelligence and Enhancing Brain

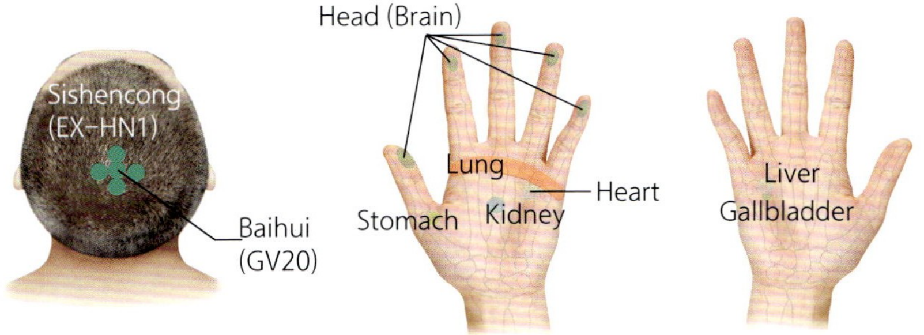

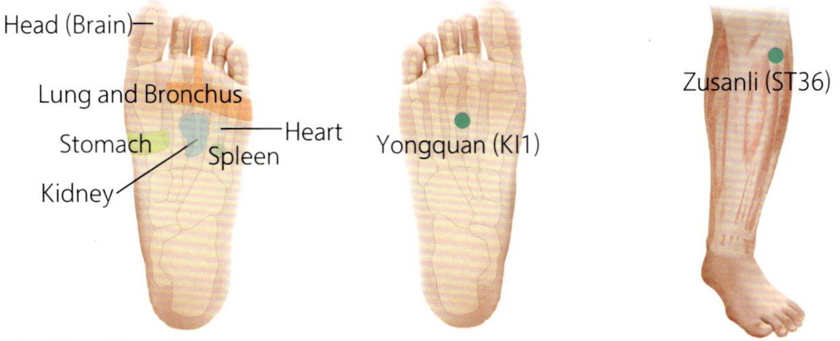

Head and Facial Massage

1. Use overlapped index fingers to press Baihui (GV20) with a little bit pressure for 5 to 6 minutes, and relax after every short stay.
2. Press hard on Sishenchong (EX-HN1) for 1 minute with both thumb pulps.

Hand Massage

1. Twist your fingers of both hands with 5 times at each finger.
2. Press the reflex zones of Head (Brain), Heart and Lung with moderate strength using interphalangeal joint at the proximal side of index fingers, and it is preferred to have a slight local distension.
3. Press the reflex zones of Stomach, Liver, Gallbladder and Kidney taking the patient' s tolerance degree into consideration.

Foot Massage

1. Massage the reflex zones of Head (Brain), Heart, Lung and Bronchus after overall relaxation due to a foot bath, and a local sense of soreness is preferred.
2. Press the reflex zones of Spleen and Stomach each for 30 to 50 times with thumbs or toothpicks, and it is preferred to have a slight local distension.
3. Press and massage the Kidney reflex zone for 20 to 30 times with thumbs, and take another foot relaxation to end the massage so that the metabolic waste could be eliminated as soon as possible after the massage.
4. Massage Yongquan (KI1) and Zusanli (ST36) each for 2 minutes with a little pressure for 5 to 6 minutes, and relax after each short manipulation.

7 增强免疫力

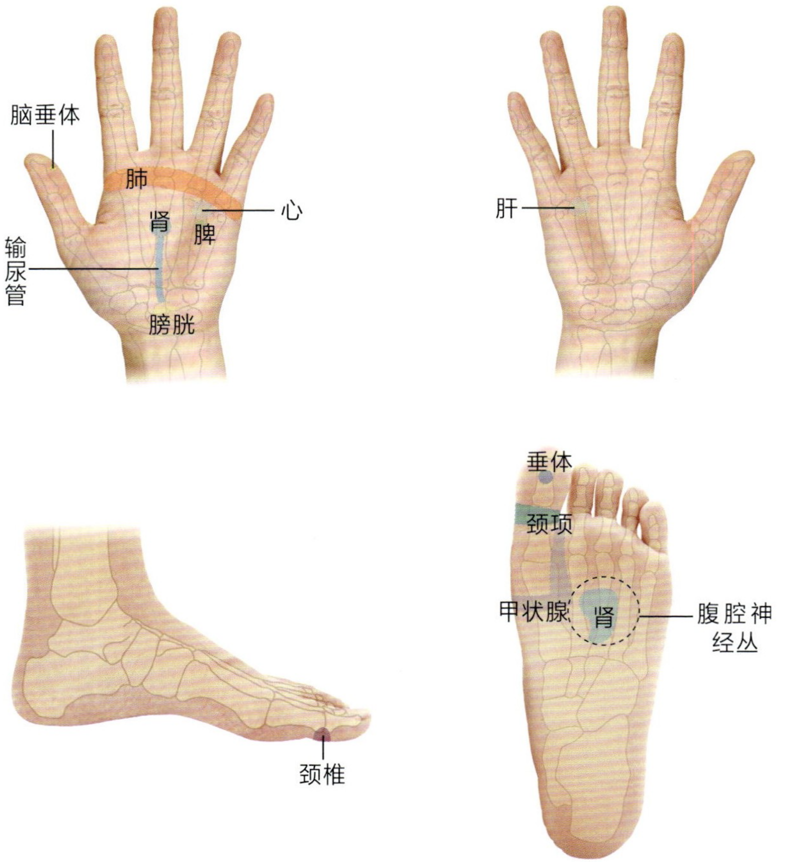

手部按摩

1. 推按肾、膀胱、输尿管反射区各20~30次，以局部有轻度胀痛为宜。
2. 拇指指腹按揉心、肝、肺、脑垂体、脾反射区各20~30次，力度以被按摩者能耐受为度。

足部按摩

1. 食指近侧指间关节推压甲状腺、腹腔神经丛反射区各10次，以局部有酸胀感为宜。
2. 拇指指腹按揉垂体、肾反射区各20次。
3. 食指、中指近侧指间关节推压颈椎、颈项反射区各10分钟，每分钟20~40次。

8 感冒

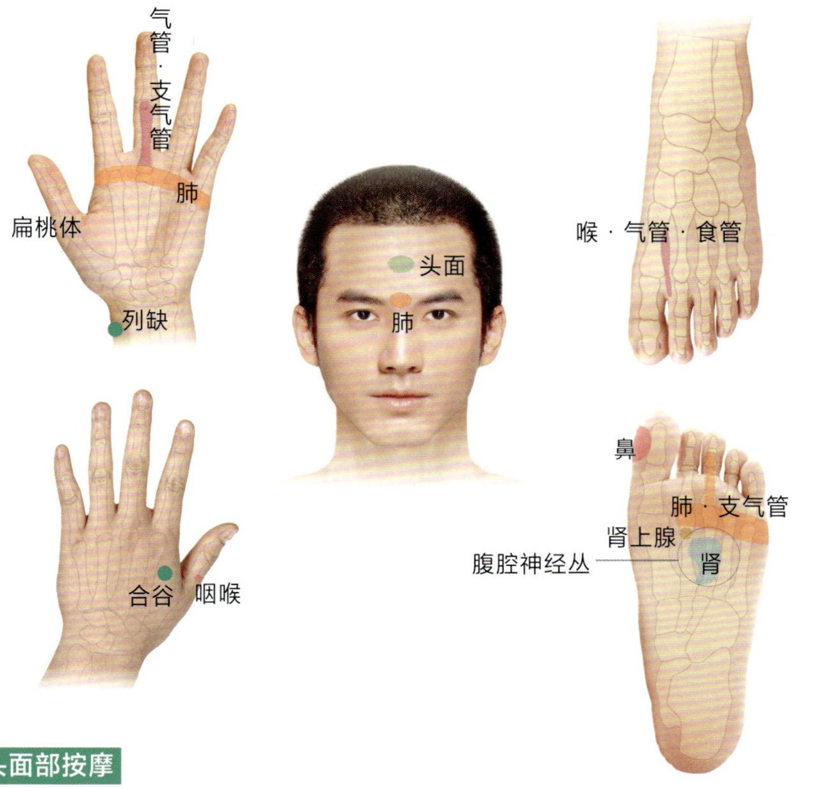

头面部按摩

1. 食指近侧指间关节点按头面反射区，以有轻微胀痛感为宜。
2. 拇指指腹强压肺反射区。

手部按摩

1. 拇指指腹按揉咽喉、扁桃体、气管·支气管、肺反射区各20~30次，以局部有轻度胀痛为宜。
2. 推按肺反射区20~30次，以局部有轻度胀痛为宜。
3. 拇指按揉列缺、合谷穴各3分钟，力度稍重，每分钟60下。同法按揉对侧。

足部按摩

1. 泡脚至全脚放松后操作，按摩喉·气管·食管反射区2分钟，以局部有酸胀感为宜。
2. 食指桡侧缘刮肺·支气管、鼻反射区各5分钟，以局部有酸麻胀感为宜。
3. 食指指间关节刮压肾上腺、腹腔神经丛、肾反射区，反复操作3~5分钟。

7 Strengthening Immunity

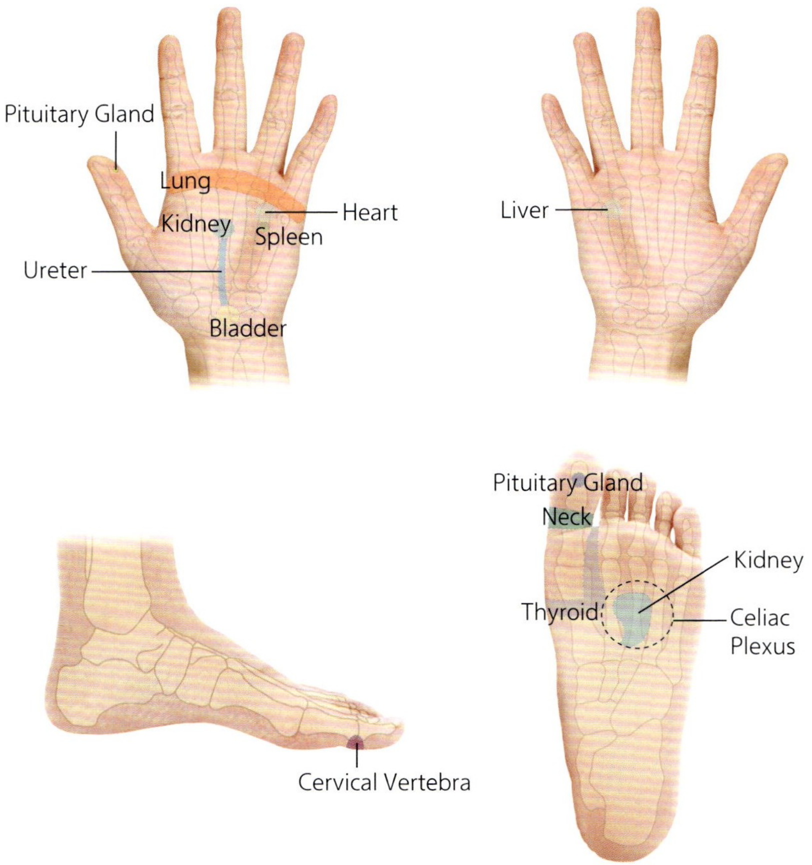

Hand Massage

1. Press the reflex zones of Kidney, Bladder and Ureter for 20 to 30 times and a slight local soreness is preferred.
2. Massage the reflex zones of Heart, Liver, Lung, Spleen and Pituitary Gland each for 20 to 30 times with thumbs. The strength should refer to the tolerance degree of the patient.

Foot Massage

1. Press and press the reflex zones of Thyroid and Celiac Plexus each for 10 times using interphalangeal joint at the proximal side of index fingers. It is preferred to have a local soreness.
2. Massage the Pituitary and Kidney reflex zones each for 20 times with finger pulp.
3. Press Cervical Vertebra and Neck reflex zones each for 10 minutes with interphalangeal joint at the proximal side of index fingers and middle fingers. There would be 20 to 40 times in each minute.

8 Cold

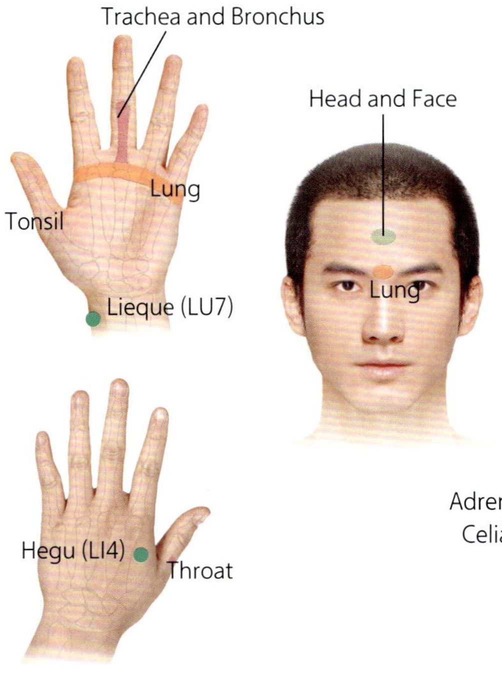

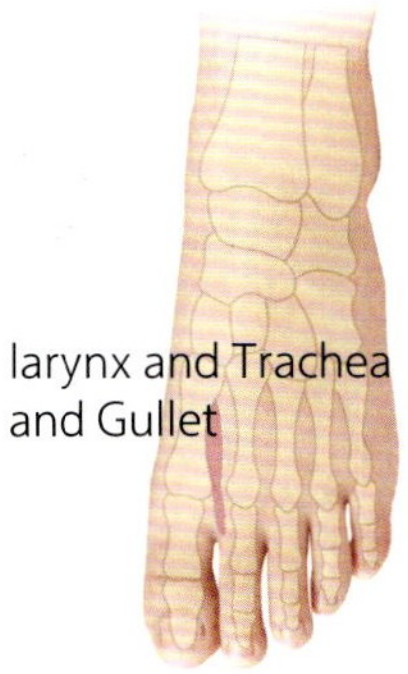

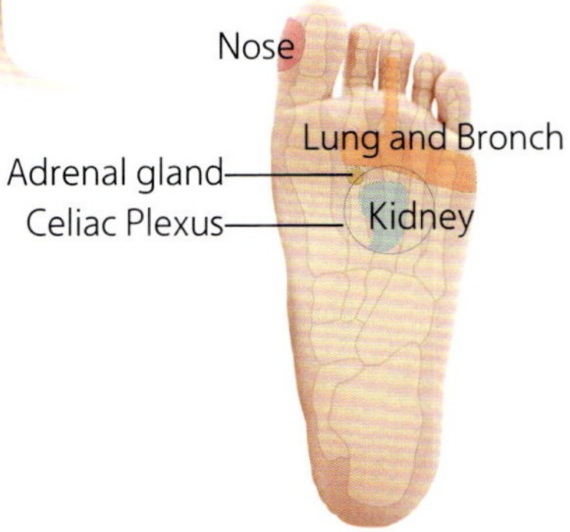

Head and Facial Massage

1. Press the Head and Facial reflex zones with interphalangeal joint at the proximal side of index fingers with proper slight distending pain.
2. Hard pressure on the Lung reflex zone with thumb pulp.

Hand Massage

1. Massage the reflex zones of Throat, Tonsil, Lung, Trachea and Bronchus with thumb pulp for 20 to 30 times. It is preferred to have slight local distending pain.
2. Press the Lung reflex zone for 20 to 30 times, and slight local distending pain is preferred.
3. Massage Lieque (LU7) and Hegu (LI4) each for 3 minutes, and it includes 60 times in each minute. The same manipulation should be applied to the other side.

Foot Massage

1. The manipulation should be after a overall relaxation with foot bath. Massage the reflex zones of Throat, Trachea and Gullet for 2 minutes. A local sense of soreness and distension is preferred.
2. Scratch the reflex zones of Lung, Bronchus and Nose each for 5 minutes with radical margins of index fingers. A local sense of soreness, numbness and distension is preferred.
3. Scratch and press the reflex zones of Adrenal Gland, Celiac Plexus and Kidney with interphalangeal joint at the proximal side of index fingers. The manipulation should be repeated for 3 to 5 minutes.

9 中暑

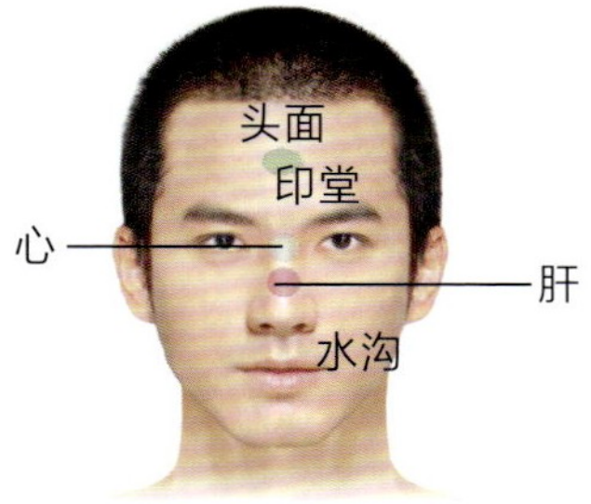

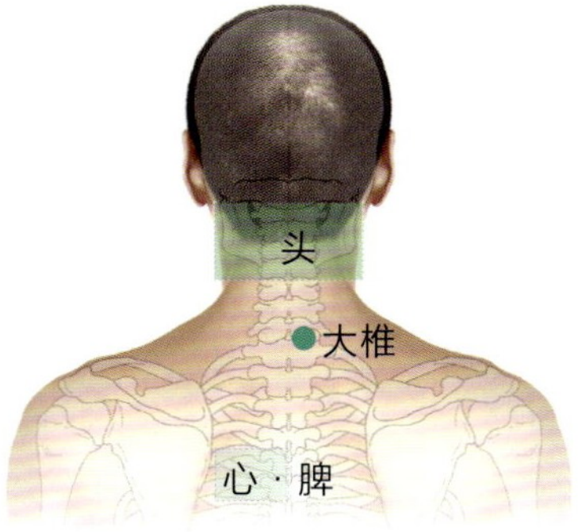

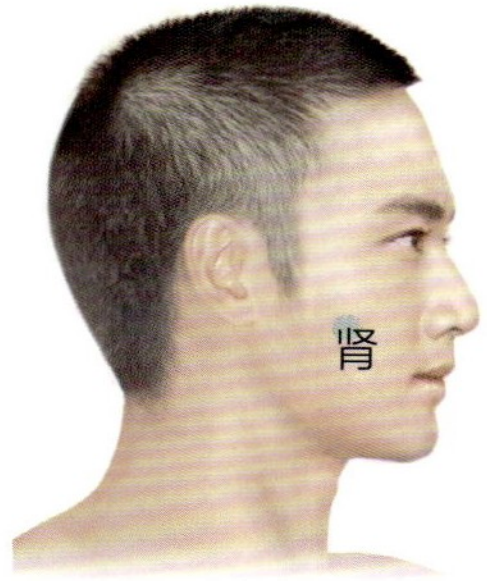

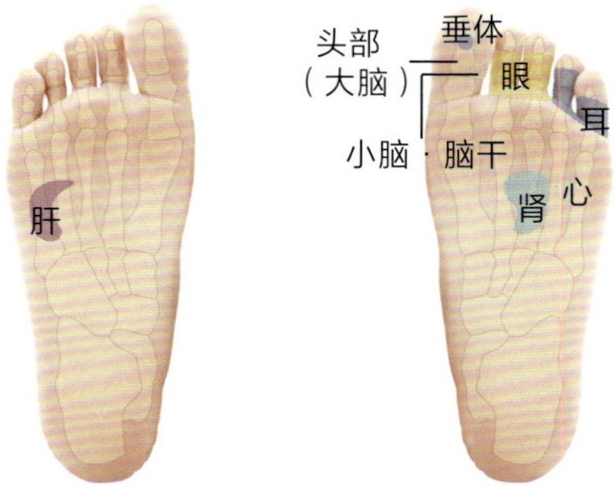

头面部按摩

1. 推压印堂穴数次。
2. 若有昏厥现象，快速重力掐压水沟穴。
3. 棒针点按头面、心、肝、肾反射区 3~6 分钟，以局部有轻痛感为宜。

脊背按摩

1. 掐压大椎穴 1~3 分钟，以局部皮肤呈现紫斑为度，酌情用力。
2. 拇指指腹点按头、心・脾反射区各 3 分钟，宜有节奏、用力均匀、力度适中。

足部按摩

1. 食指近侧指间关节点按心、肝、肾反射区各 5 分钟，用力均匀，力度适中。
2. 点按小脑・脑干、垂体、头部（大脑）、耳、眼反射区，力度以被按摩者耐受为度，以局部有酸胀感为宜。

10 发热

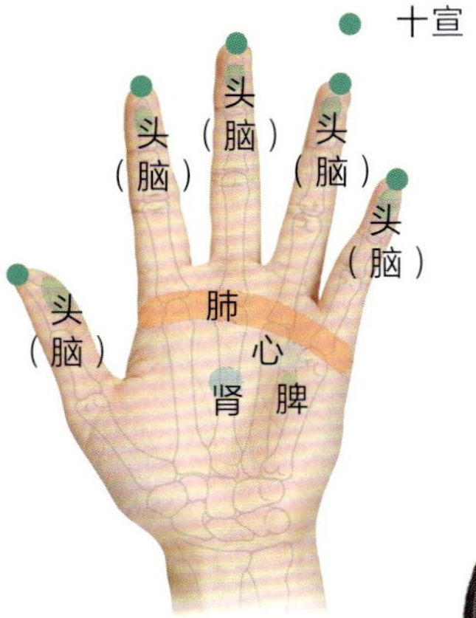

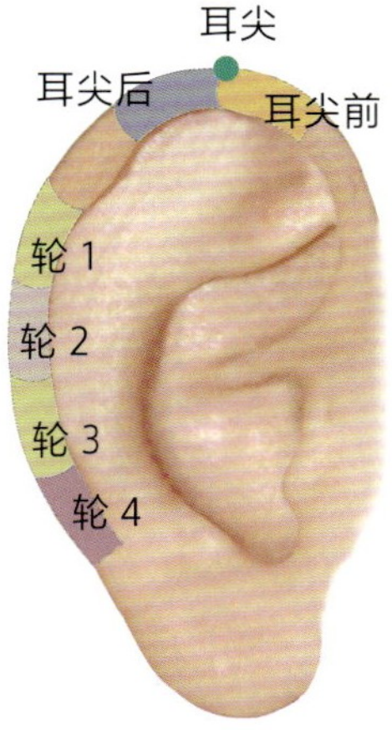

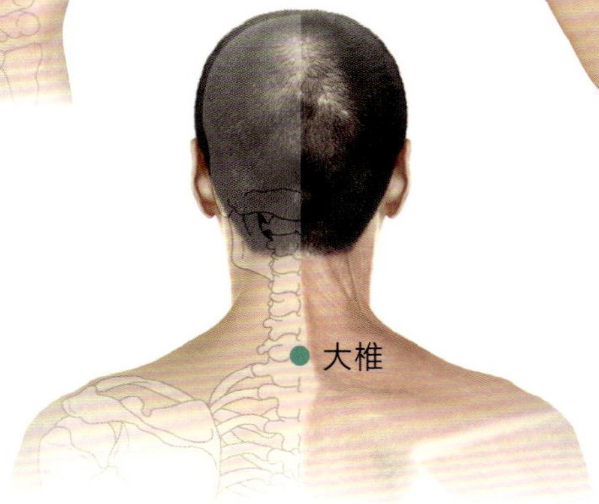

脊背按摩

两手食指重叠用力按压大椎穴，每次停留片刻后放松，重复 5~6 次。

耳部按摩

1. 拇指按摩耳尖前、耳尖、耳尖后反射区 3~5 分钟，每分钟 50~100 次，手法要由轻到重，再由重到轻，逐渐渗透。
2. 按摩棒点按轮 1、轮 2、轮 3、轮 4 反射区各 30~50 次，以局部有轻痛感为宜，切忌用力过度。

手部按摩

1. 拇指或牙签束点按头（脑）反射区 30~50 次，以局部有轻微胀痛为宜。
2. 拇指指腹按揉心、肺、脾、肾反射区各 20 次，以被按摩者能耐受为度。
3. 拇指指甲掐按十宣穴 30 下，掐后再按揉 30 下，力度稍重。

9 Heatstroke

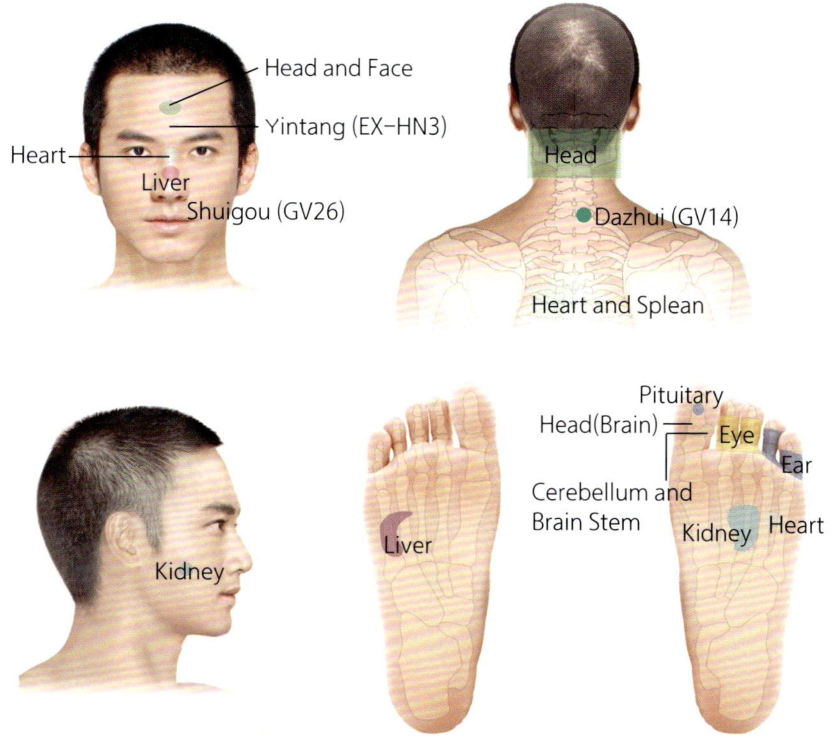

Head and Facial Massage

1. Press and press the acupoint of Yintang (EX-HN3) for several times.
2. Nip and press the acupoint of Shuigou (GV26) rapidly with great pressure once there appears syncope.
3. Press and press the reflex zones of Head, Face, Heart, Liver and Kidney with needles for 3 to 6 minutes. It is preferred to have a local sense of slight pain.

Back Massage

1. Nip Dazhui (GV14) for 1 to 3 minutes, and the strength should refer to the purple plague that locally appears on the skin.
2. Press the reflex zones of Head, Heart and Spleen each for 3 minutes with thumb pulp. The manipulation should be moderate with appropriate strength and rhythm.

Foot Massage

1. Press the reflex zones of Heart, Liver and Kidney with interphalangeal joint at the proximal side of index fingers each for 5 minutes with moderate strength.
2. Press the reflex zones of Cerebellum, Brain Stem, Pituitary, Head (Brain), Ear and Eye. The strength should refer to the tolerance degree of the patient and a local sense of soreness and distension is preferred.

10 Fever

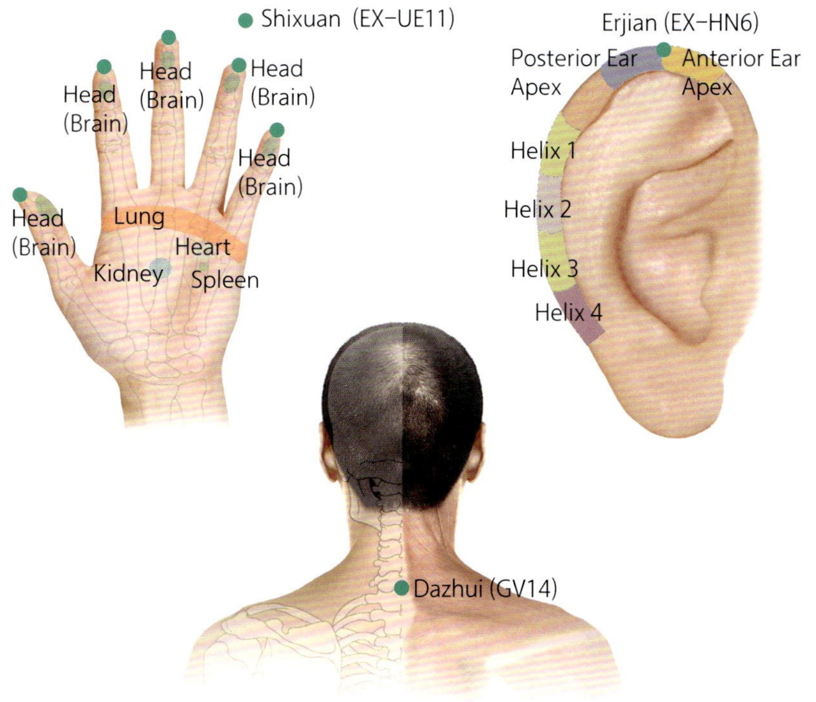

Back Massage

Press hard on Dazhui (GV14) with overlapped index fingers, and relax after each short stay. Repeat the manipulation for 5 to 6 times.

Ear Massage

1. Use thumbs to massage the reflex zones of Erjian (EX-HN6) and those before and after Erjian (EX-HN6) for 3 to 5 minutes, and there are 50 to 100 times of manipulations in each minute. The strength should penetrate gradually deriving from slight ones to heavy ones and then the opposite.
2. Press the reflex zones of Helix 1. 2. 3. 4 with massage stick for 30 to 50 times, and a local sense of slight pain is preferred without overexertion.

Hand Massage

1. Press the Head (Brain) reflex zones for 30 to 50 times with thumbs or a bundle of tooth pick, and a local sense of slight dissension is preferred.
2. Massage the reflex zones of Heart, Lung, Spleen and Kidney with thumb each for 20 times taking the tolerance degree of the patient into consideration.
3. Nip Shixuan (EX-UE11) with the nail of the thumb each for 20 times taking the tolerance degree of the patient into consideration.

11 咳嗽

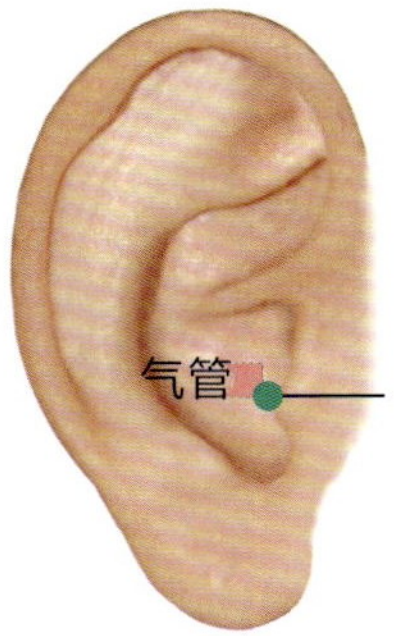

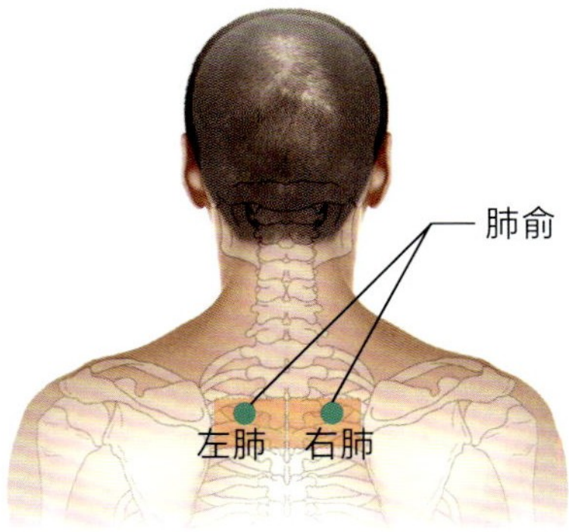

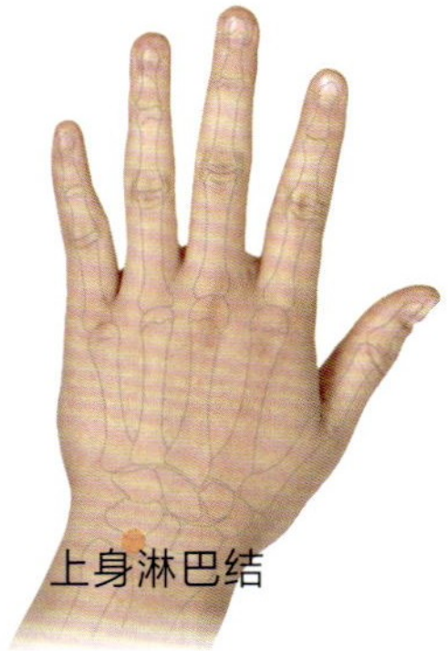

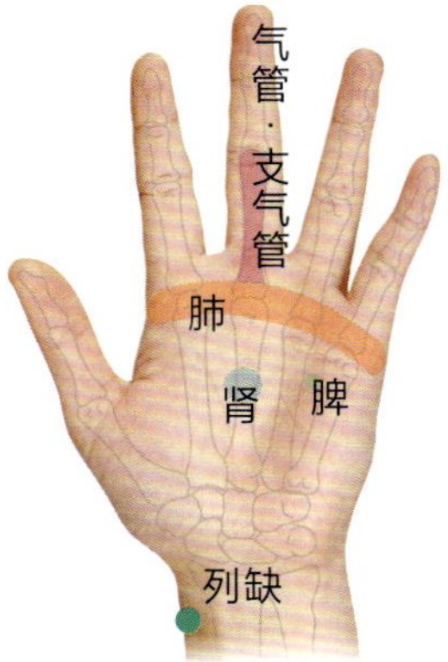

耳部按摩

按摩棒推气管、肾上腺反射区各 5 分钟，每分钟 90 次。

脊背按摩

1. 手指用力按压肺俞穴，每次停留片刻后放松，重复 5~6 次。同法按揉对侧肺俞穴。
2. 拇指指腹点按肺反射区 3 分钟，做到有节奏、用力均匀、力度适中。

手部按摩

1. 拇指或牙签束点按肺、脾、肾反射区各 3~5 次，以局部有轻微胀痛为宜。
2. 食指近侧指间关节点按气管·支气管、上身淋巴结反射区，各连续点按 5~10 次。
3. 拇指指腹用力按压列缺穴 2 分钟。同法按揉对侧。

12 哮喘

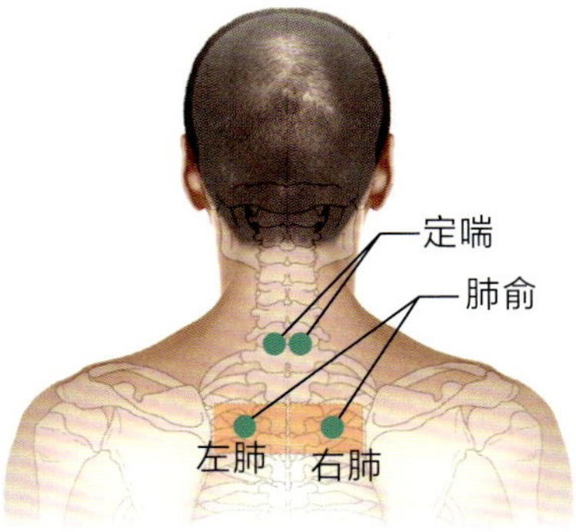

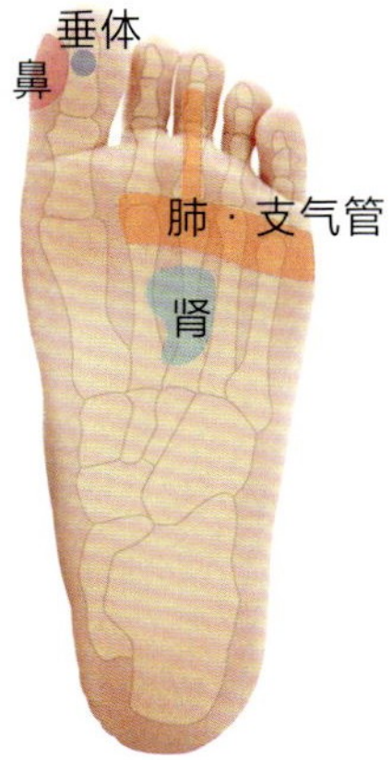

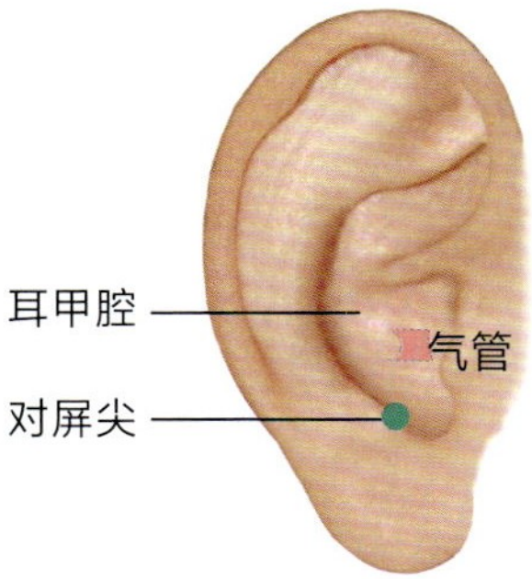

耳部按摩

1. 按摩棒揉气管、对屏尖反射区各 5 分钟，每分钟 90 次。
2. 食指指腹按揉耳甲腔部 5 分钟，每分钟 60 次。

脊背按摩

1. 拇指指腹按揉肺反射区，以局部有热胀感为宜。
2. 食指、中指重叠按压肺俞、定喘穴，重复 7~8 下。同法按揉对侧穴位。

足部按摩

1. 食指近侧指间关节点按肺·支气管、鼻反射区各 2~3 分钟，用力均匀，力度适中。
2. 拇指指腹按压肾、垂体反射区，以局部有轻度酸胀感为宜。

11 Cough

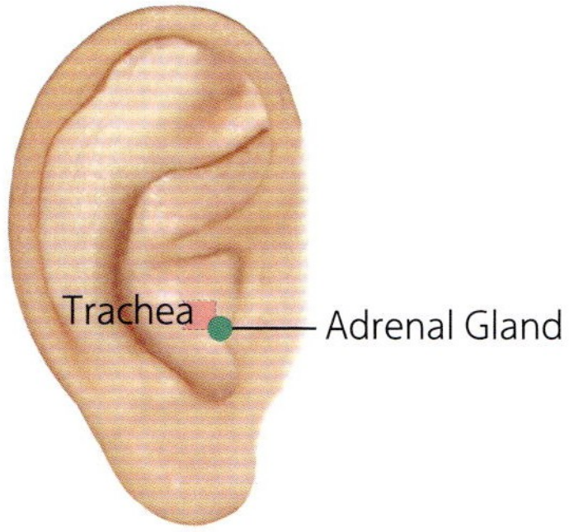

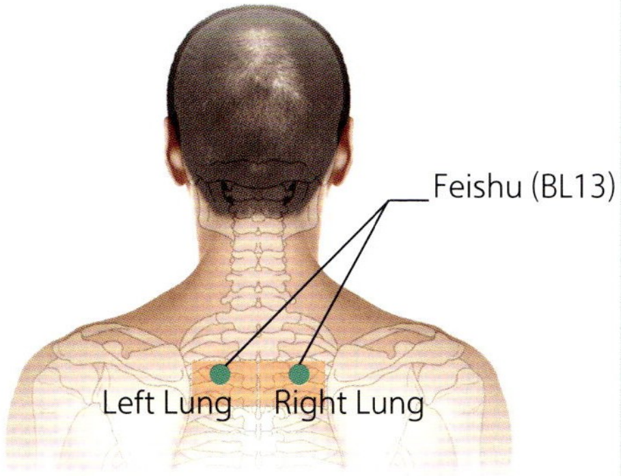

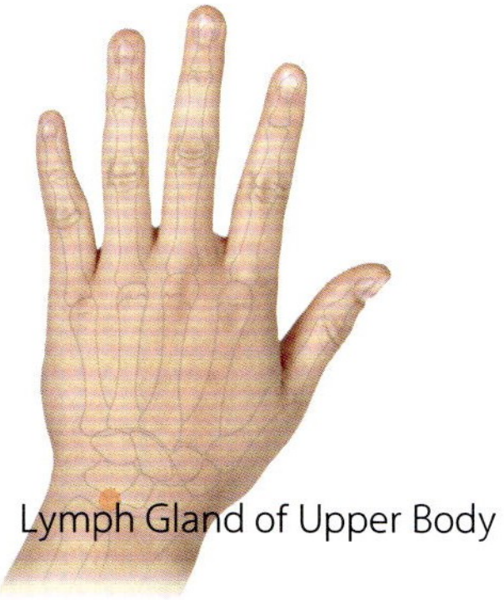

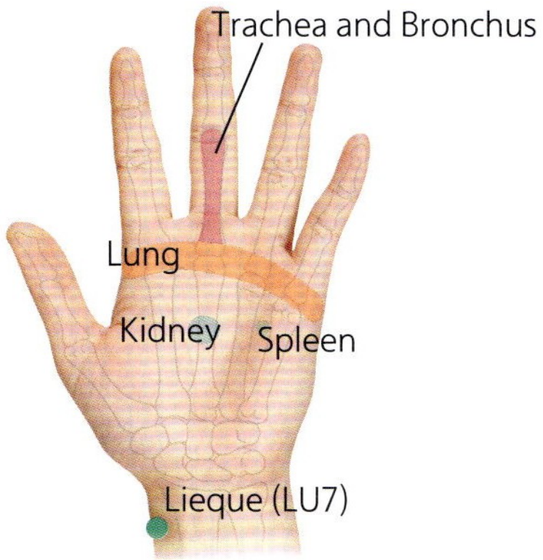

Ear Massage

Press the reflex zones of Trachea and Adrenal Gland with massage stick, each for 5 minutes, 90 times every minute.

Back Massage

1. Press hard on Shenshu (BL13) with fingers, and relax after each manipulation. Repeat 5 to 6 times and apply the same manipulation on the opposite side.
2. Press the reflex zone of Lung with finger pulp for 3 minutes with moderate strength and temple.

Hand Massage

1. Press the reflex zones of Lung, Spleen and Kidney with thumbs or toothpick each for 3 to 5 minutes. It is preferred to have a local sense of slight distension.
2. Press the reflex zones of Trachea, Bronchus and the Lymph Gland of Upper Body with interphalangeal joint at the proximal side of index fingers each for 5 to 10 times continuously.
3. Press hard on Lieque (LU7) with thumb for 2 minutes and apply the same manipulation on the opposite side.

12 Asthma

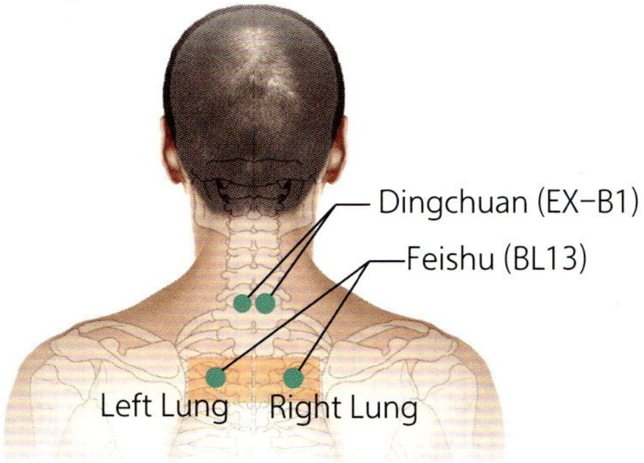

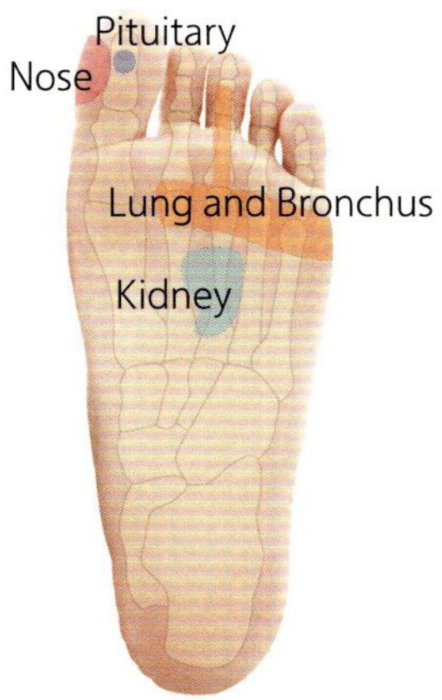

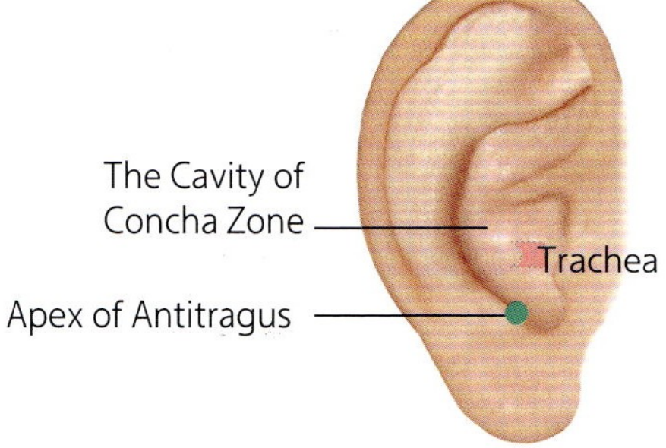

Ear Massage

1. Massage the reflex zones of Bronchus and Apex of Antitragus with massage stick each for 5 minutes, and every minute include 90 times.
2. Massage the cavity of concha zone with the finger pulp for 5 minutes and every minute cover 60 times.

Back Massage

1. Massage Lung reflex zone with thumb and a local sense of warmth and distension is preferred.
2. Overlap your index finger and middle finger to press Feishu (BL13) and Dingchuan (EX-B1) for 7 to 8 times repeatedly. Apply the same manipulation on the opposite acupoints.

Foot Massage

1. Press the reflex zones of Lung, Bronchus and Nose with interphalangeal joint at the proximal side of index fingers each for 2 to 3 minutes with moderate strength.
2. Press the reflex zones of Kidney and Pituitary with thumb and it is preferred to have a local sense of slight soreness and distension.

13 胃痛

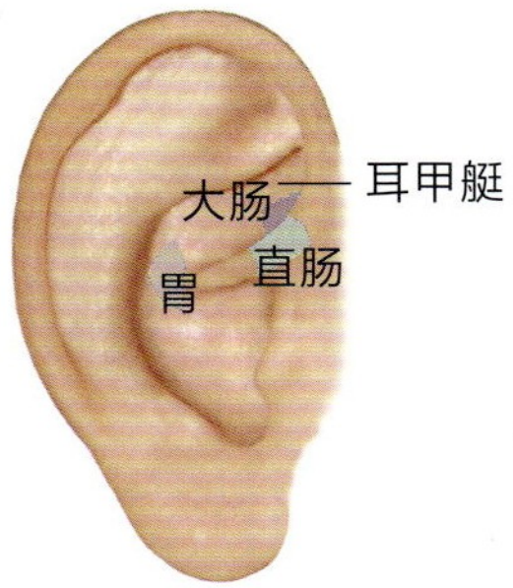

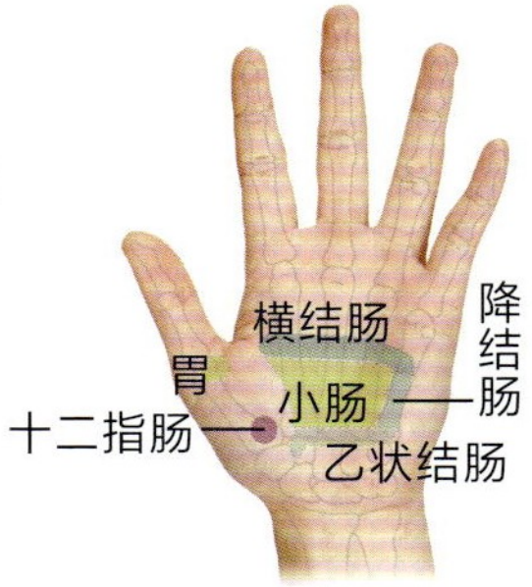

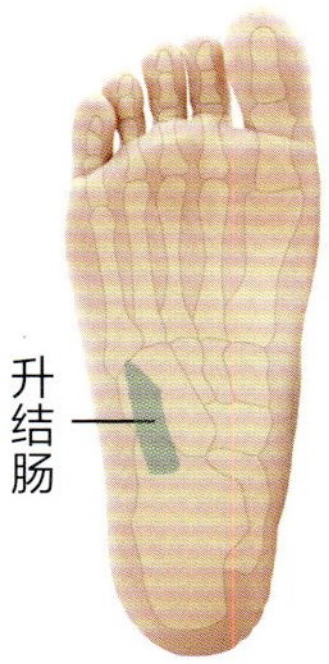

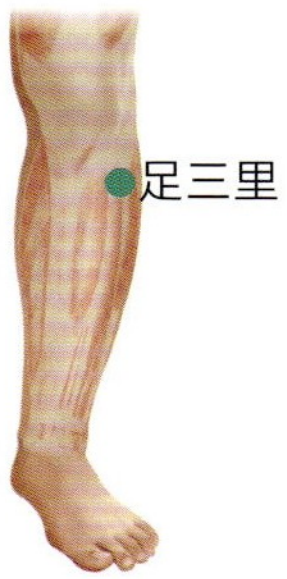

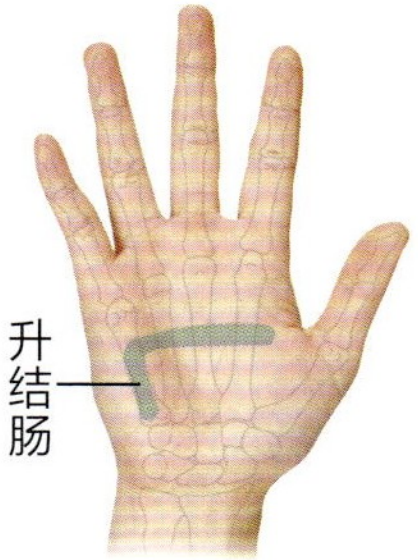

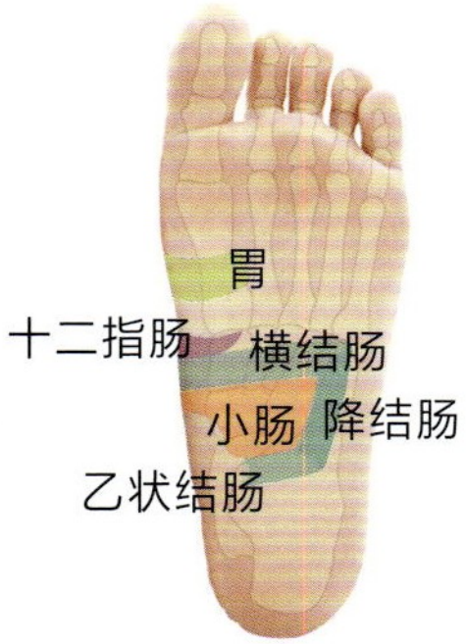

耳部按摩

1. 按摩棒推大肠、胃反射区各 5 分钟，每分钟 90 次。
2. 拇指按揉直肠反射区 5 分钟，每分钟 75 次。
3. 指揉耳甲艇部 5 分钟，每分钟 75 次。

手部按摩

1. 食指、中指近侧指间关节推压胃反射区各 1 分钟，每分钟 20~40 次。
2. 拇指指腹按揉十二指肠反射区 2 分钟，以被按摩者能耐受为度。
3. 拳刮小肠反射区 2 分钟。
4. 拇指推升结肠、横结肠、降结肠、乙状结肠反射区各 1 分钟。

足部按摩

1. 用拇指或牙签束点按胃、十二指肠反射区各 30~50 次，以局部有轻微胀痛为宜。
2. 用食指近侧指间关节点按升结肠、横结肠、降结肠、乙状结肠、小肠反射区，各连续点按 5~10 次。
3. 以拇指强压足三里 3~5 分钟，每分钟 60 次。

14 消化不良

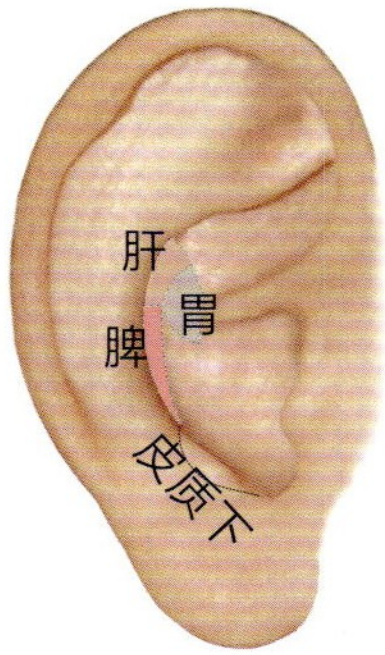

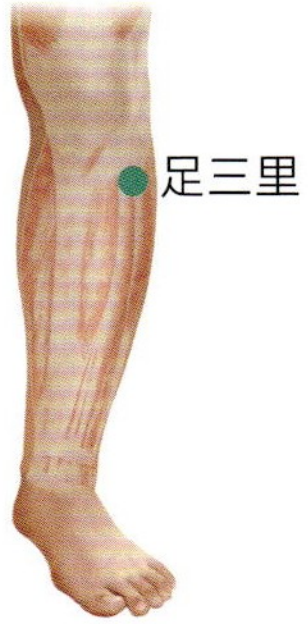

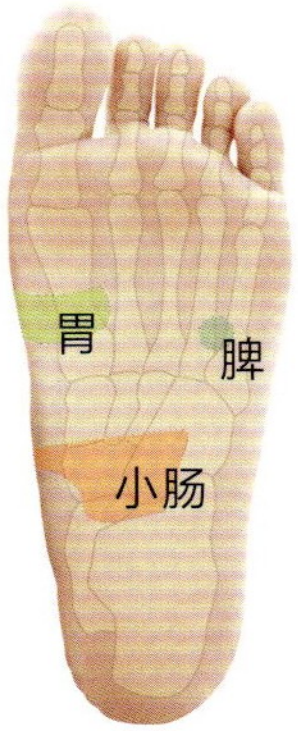

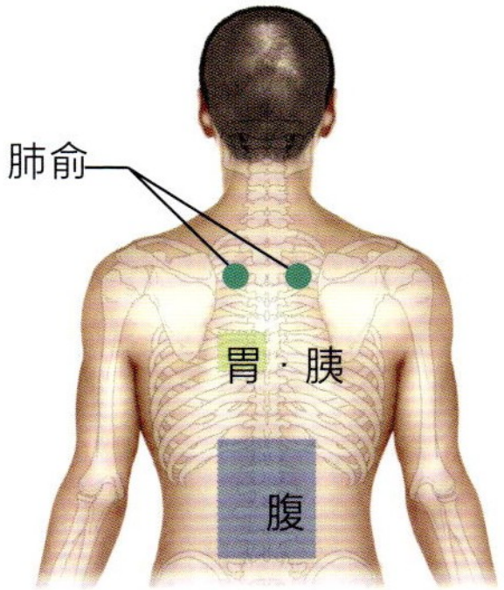

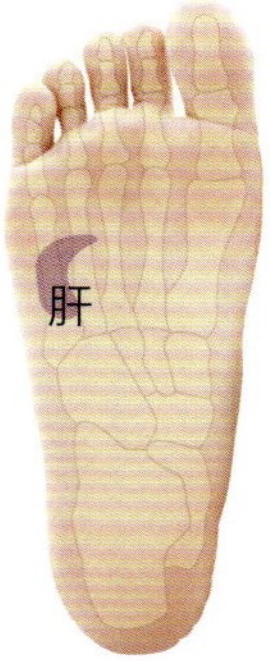

耳部按摩

1. 按摩棒点按胃、肝穴各 4 分钟，每分钟 90 次。
2. 食指按压脾、皮质下穴各 4 分钟，每分钟 90 次。

脊背按摩

1. 两手绕拳于背后，用关节处稍微用力按压两侧肺俞穴各 2 分钟，每次停留片刻后放松，重复 5~6 次。
2. 拇指指腹推按胃 · 胰、腹反射区，以局部有热胀感为宜。

足部按摩

1. 食指推压胃反射区 10~20 次。
2. 推按肝、脾、小肠反射区各 3~5 分钟，以局部有轻度胀痛为宜。
3. 拇指按揉足三里穴 2 分钟，力度稍重。同法按揉对侧足三里穴。

13 Stomachache

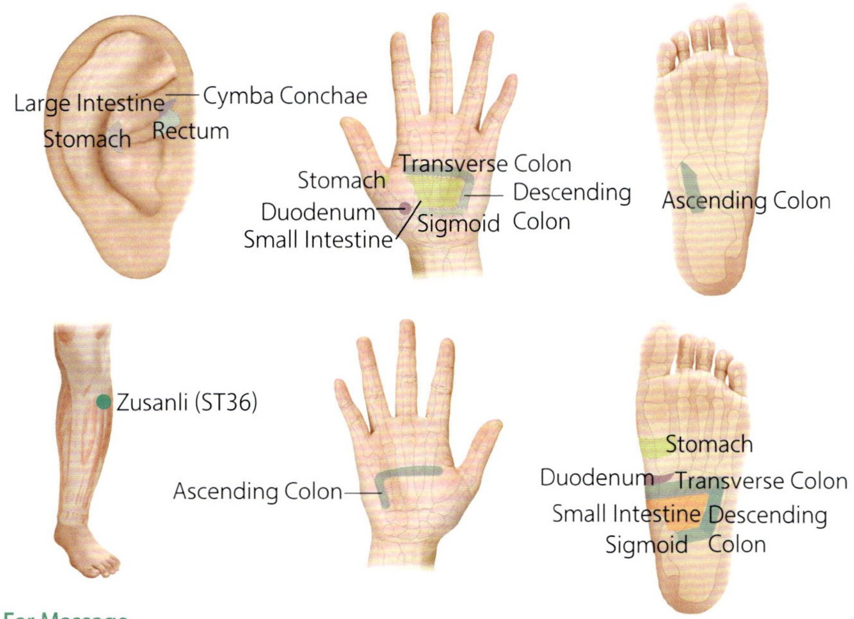

Ear Massage

1. Massage the reflex zones of Large Intestine and Stomach with massage stick each for 5 minutes with 90 times in each minute.
2. Massage the Rectum reflex zone with thumb for 5 minutes and it includes 75 times of manipulations in each minute.
3. Massage the Cymba Conchae for 5 minutes with 75 times in each minute.

Hand Massage

1. Press and press the Stomach reflex zone with interphalangeal joint at the proximal side of index fingers and middle fingers each for 1 minute, and it includes 20 to 40 times of manipulations in each minute.
2. Massage the Duodenum reflex zone for 2 minutes with thumb and you have to consider the tolerance degree of the ones being massaged.
3. Use fist to scratch Small Intestine reflex zone for 2 minutes.
4. Take advantage of thumbs to press the reflex zones of Ascending Colon, Descending Colon, Transverse Colon and Sigmoid each for 1 minute.

Foot Massage

1. Press the reflex zones of Stomach, Duodenum with thumb or toothpick each for 30 to 50 times, and it is preferred to have a sense of slight distending pain locally.
2. Press the reflex zones of Ascending Colon, Descending Colon, Transverse Colon, Small Intestine and Sigmoid with interphalangeal joint at the proximal side of index fingers. Press each zone for 5 to 10 times.
3. Press hard on Zusanli (ST36) with thumb for 3 to 5 minutes, and it includes 60 times in each minute.

14 Indigestion

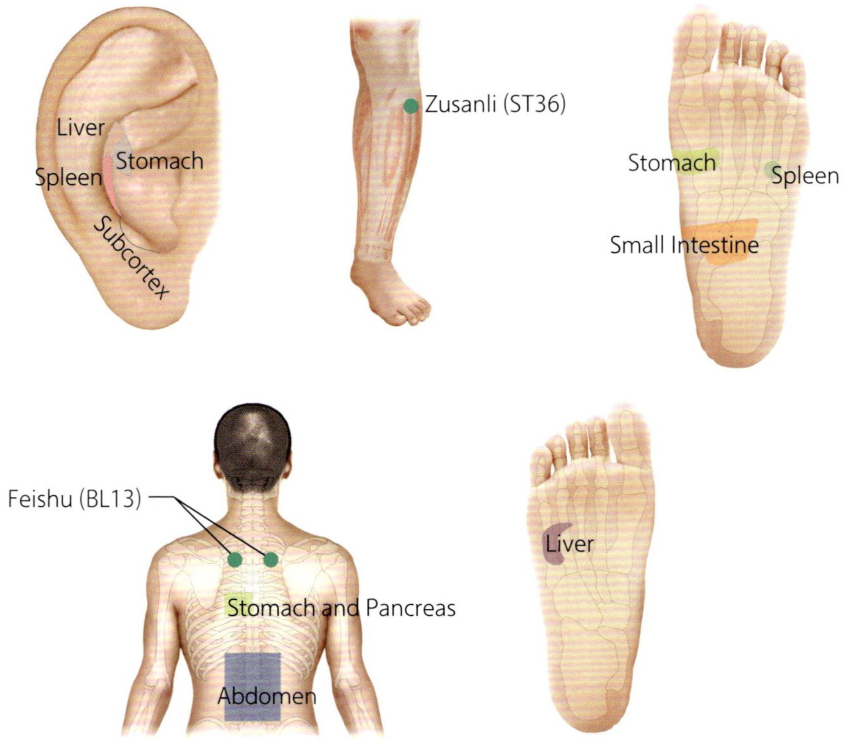

Ear Massage

1. Slightly press the acupoints concerning Stomach and Liver with massage stick each for 4 minutes and there are 90 times in each minute.
2. Press the acupoints of Spleen and Subcortex each for 4 minutes with 90 times in each minute.

Back Massage

1. Roll your fists and use the joints to press the Feishu (BL13) on both sides of the back each for 2 minutes and relax after every short stay. Repeat the manipulation for 5 to 6 times.
2. Press and press the reflex zones of Stomach, Abdomen and Pancreas and it is preferred to have a sense of warmth and distension.

Foot Massage

1. Press the Stomach reflex zone for 10 to 20 times with index fingers.
2. Press and massage the reflex zones of Liver, Spleen and Small Intestine each for 3 to 5 minutes with properly slight distending pain locally.
3. Massage the acupoint of Zusanli (ST36) using thumbs with a little pressure and apply the same manipulation at the opposite Zusanli (ST36).

15 腹泻

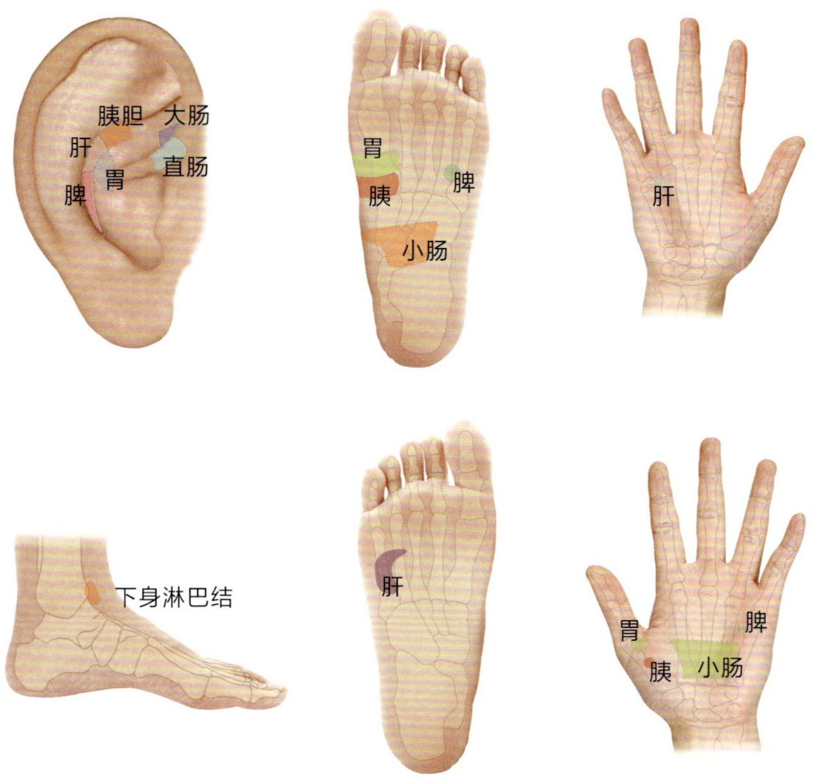

耳部按摩

1. 拇指指间关节轻轻揉压胃、胰胆、肝反射区。
2. 指甲刮直肠反射区 5 分钟，酌情用力，使局部皮肤潮红。
3. 按摩棒推大肠、脾反射区各 5~6 分钟，每分钟 90 次。

手部按摩

1. 食指近侧指间关节点按胃、胰、肝、脾反射区，胃反射区可以用双食指按压法。
2. 食指近侧指间关节点按小肠反射区，然后再用拳背叩击此反射区 2~3 分钟。

足部按摩

1. 拇指点按胃、胰、肝、脾反射区，力度以被按摩者耐受为度，以局部有酸胀为宜。
2. 拇指或牙签束点按小肠、下身淋巴结反射区。

16 便秘

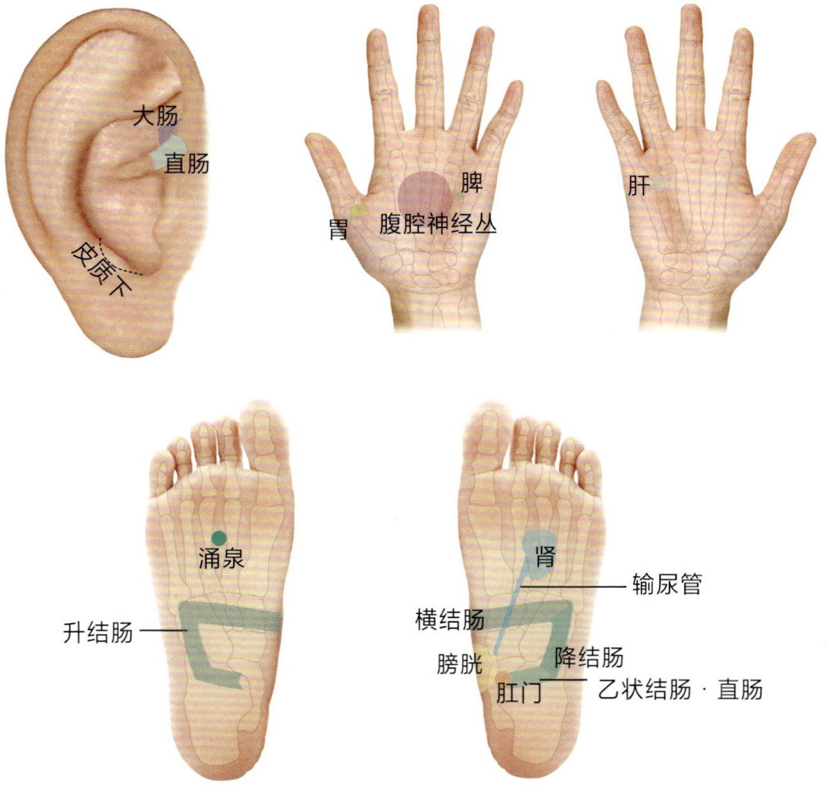

耳部按摩

1. 按摩棒轻按直肠反射区 5 分钟，配合腹式呼吸，尽量延长呼与吸时间，减少呼吸次数。
2. 食指指腹按揉大肠、皮质下反射区各 5 分钟，每分钟 60 次。

手部按摩

拇指指腹点按胃、肝、脾反射区各 3~5 分钟，然后按揉腹腔神经丛反射区 2~3 分钟。

足部按摩

1. 拇指推升结肠、横结肠、降结肠、乙状结肠 · 直肠反射区。
2. 拇指推肛门反射区，老年人可加按肾、膀胱、输尿管反射区。
3. 食指按揉涌泉穴 3~5 分钟。

15 Diarrhea

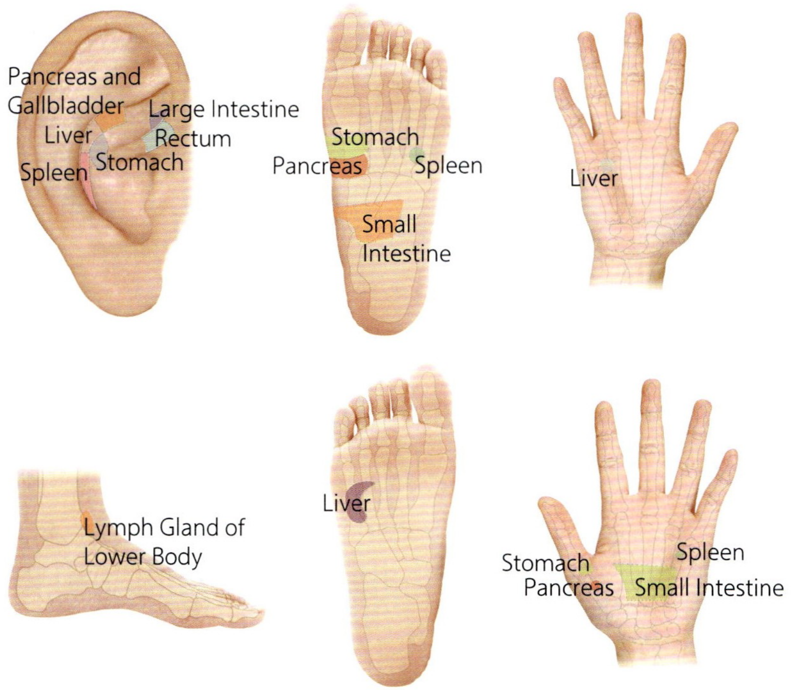

Ear Massage

1. Use interphalangeal joints of thumbs to gently massage the reflex zones of Stomach, Pancreas and Liver.
2. Scratch the Rectum reflex zone with nails with proper strength so to have a local blush on the skin.
3. Press the reflex zones of Large Intestine and Spleen with massage stick each for 5 to 6 minutes and there are 90 times in each minute.

Hand Massage

1. Press the reflex zones of Stomach, Pancreas, Liver and Spleen with interphalangeal joint at the proximal side of index fingers. It is allowed to use the pressing method of double index fingers at the Stomach reflex zone.
2. Press the reflex zones of Small Intestine with interphalangeal joint at the proximal side of index fingers, then rap this zone for 2 to 3 minutes with fists.

Foot Massage

1. Press the reflex zones of Stomach, Pancreas, Liver and Spleen with thumbs taking the tolerance degree of the patient into consideration. A local sense of soreness and distension is preferred.
2. Press the reflex zones of Small Intestine and Lymph Gland of Lower Body with thumb or a toothpick.

16 Constipation

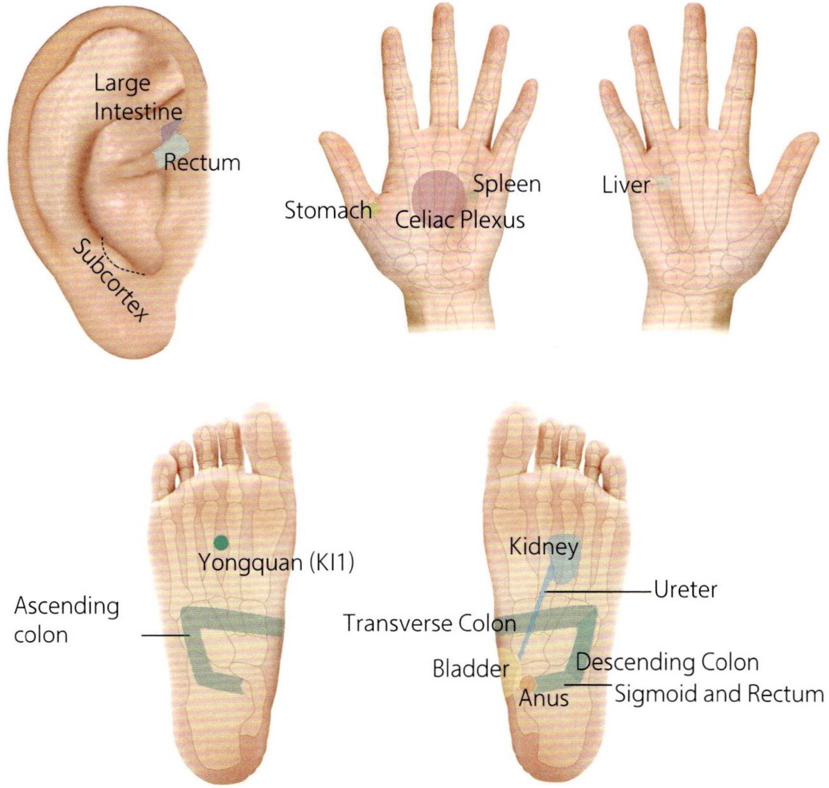

Ear Massage

1. Slightly massage the Rectum reflex zone for 5 minutes with massage stick combined with abdominal respiration in which the time of exhaling and inhaling is extremely prolonged so that the times of breath are reduced.
2. Massage the reflex zones of Large Intestine and Subcortex each for 5 minutes with index finger pulp, and there are 60 times in each minute.

Hand Massage

Press the reflex zones of Stomach, Liver, Spleen with thumbs each for 3 to 5 minutes, and then massage the Celiac Plexus reflex zone for 2 to 3 minutes.

Foot Massage

1. Massage the reflex zones of Descending Colon, Ascending Colon, Sigmoid and Rectum with thumbs.
2. Massage the Anus reflex zone with thumbs, and the reflex zones of Kidney, Bladder and Ureter could be added when the patients are the aged.
3. Massage the Yonquan (KI1) for 3 to 5 minutes with index fingers.

17 糖尿病

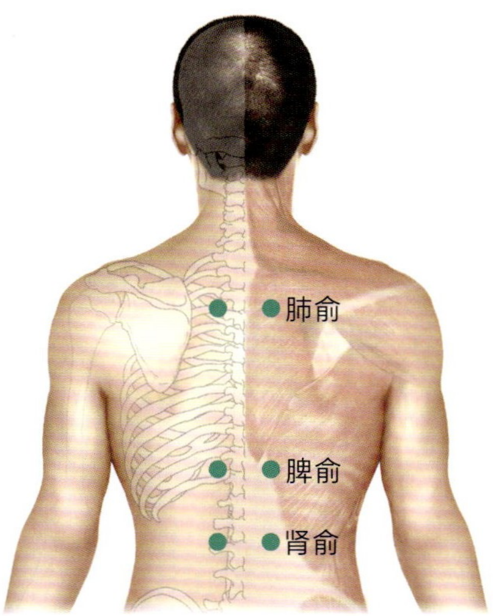

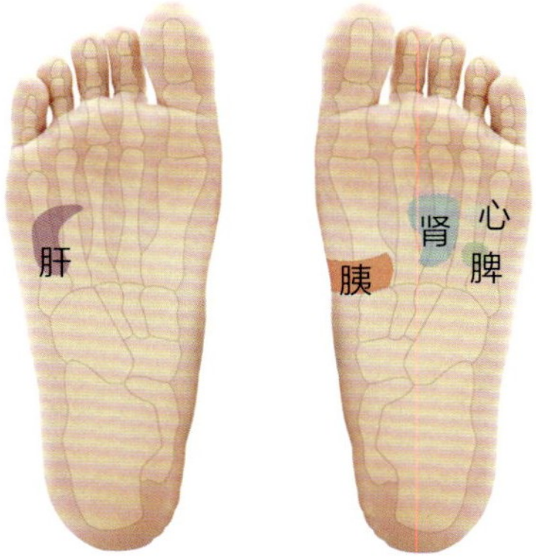

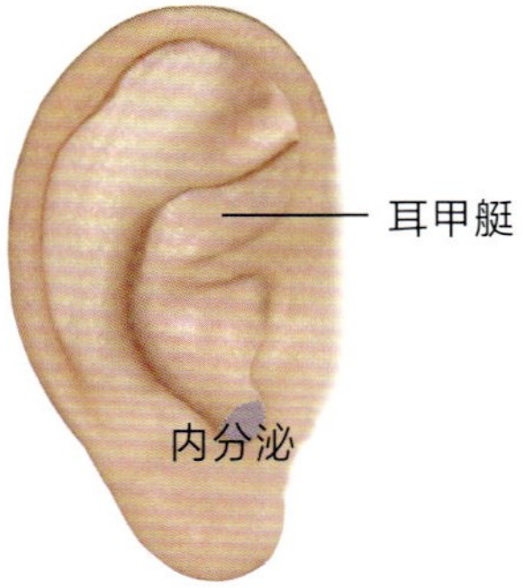

耳部按摩

1. 按摩棒按揉内分泌反射区 6 分钟，每分钟 90 次。
2. 拇指指腹稍用力按揉耳甲艇部 6 分钟，每分钟 60~70 次。

脊背按摩

1. 两手握拳置于背后，用关节处稍微用力分别按压两侧肾俞、脾俞穴各 2 分钟，每次停留片刻后放松，重复 5~6 次。
2. 将手抬起放于背后，用手指指腹稍用力按压肺俞穴，每次停留片刻后放松，重复 5~6 次。同法按揉对侧肺俞穴。

足部按摩

1. 拇指指腹点按肝、胰、脾反射区，力度以被按摩者耐受为度，以局部有酸胀感为宜。
2. 食指近侧指间关节分别点按肾、心反射区，动作均匀连贯，连续点按 5~10 次，持续 3 分钟。
3. 循序渐进按摩足拇趾内侧，使趾内侧到趾尖处硬块或条索状物逐渐变柔软至散开。

18 高血压

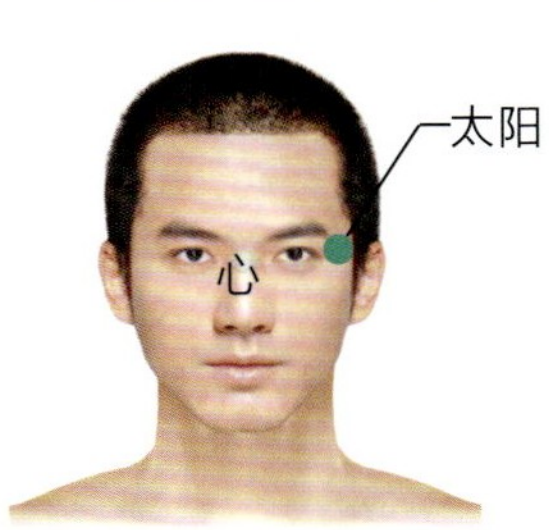

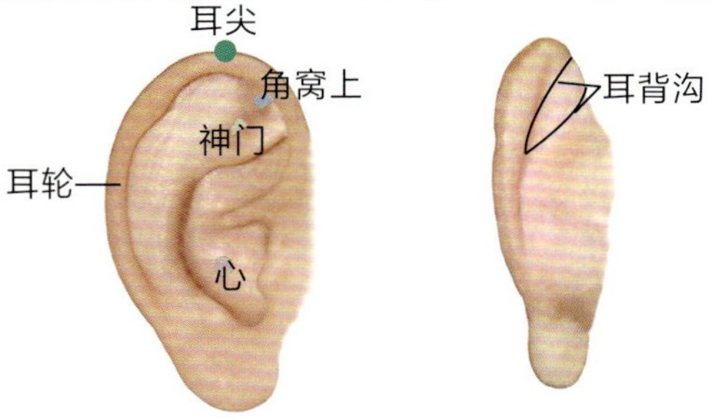

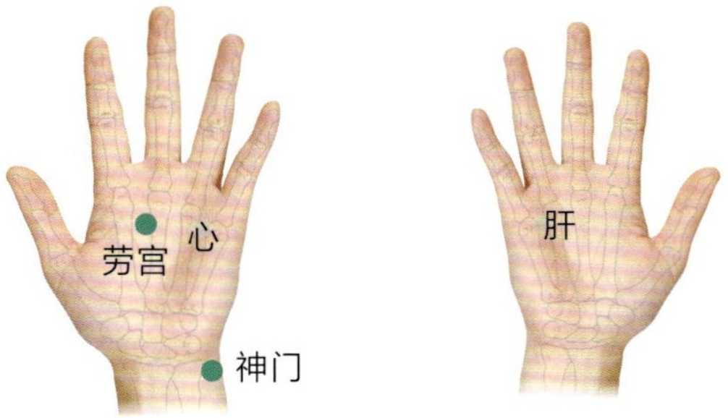

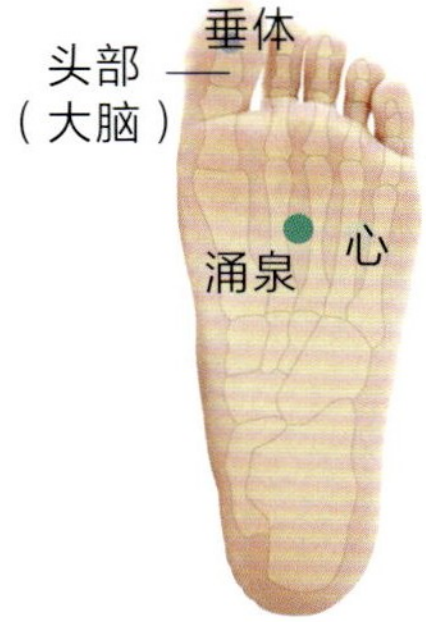

头面部按摩

1. 两手拇指勾揉两侧太阳穴 2 分钟，力度适中。
2. 食指近侧指间关节点按心反射区 2~3 分钟，力度适中，以局部有轻度胀痛为宜。

耳部按摩

1. 手指搓擦心、角窝上反射区及神门各 30 次，以有透热感为度。
2. 拇指轻推耳背沟、耳尖反射区各 6 分钟，每分钟 90 次。
3. 捻耳轮部 6 分钟，每分钟 90 次，重点捻耳尖。
4. 掌擦耳背部 3 分钟，酌情用力，每分钟 120 次。

手部按摩

1. 点按肝、心反射区 1~2 分钟。
2. 拇指指腹用力按压劳宫、神门穴，每次停留片刻后放松，重复 5~6 次。同法按揉对侧劳宫、神门穴。

足部按摩

1. 推按头部（大脑）、垂体反射区各 20~30 次，以局部有轻度胀痛为宜。
2. 食指近侧指间关节刮压心反射区 2~3 分钟，力度由轻到重，不可过重。
3. 拇指指尖掐揉涌泉穴，力度稍重，同法按揉对侧涌泉穴。

17 Diabetes

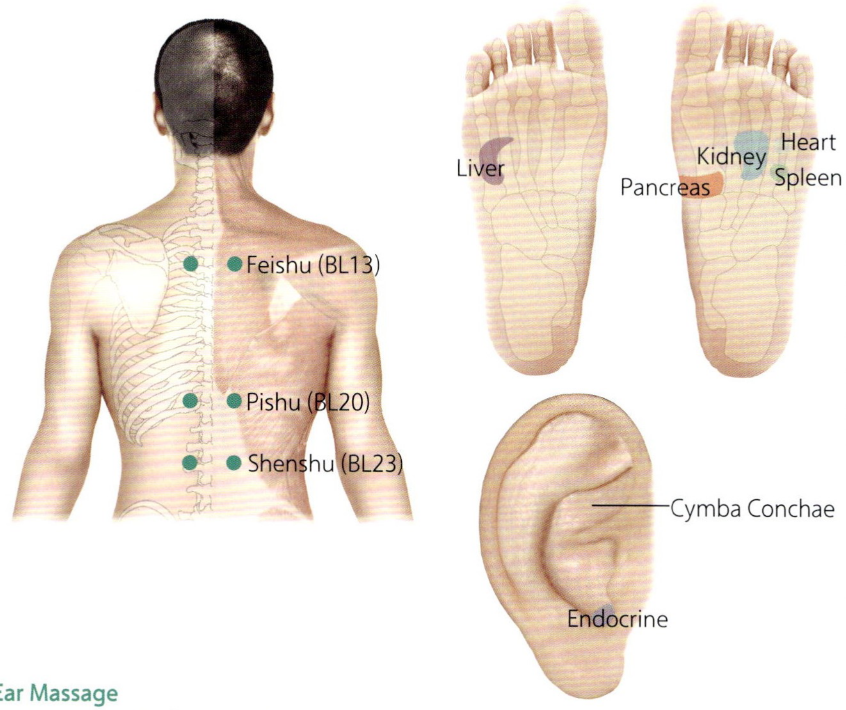

Ear Massage

1. Massage the Endocrine reflex zone with massage stick for 6 minutes, and there are 90 times of massage in each minute.
2. Massage the Cymba Conchae with a little pressure with thumbs for 6 minutes, it covers 60 to 70 times in each minute.

Back Massage

1. Fold your fists at one' s back and use the joints to press the acupoints of Shenshu (BL23) and Pishu (BL20) on either side with a little pressure each for 2 minutes. Relax after every short stay and repeat the manipulation for 5 to 6 times.
2. Raise your hands at the back and use the thumbs to press the acupoint of Shenshu (BL23) on both sides with a little pressure. Relax after every short stay and repeat the manipulation for 5 to 6 times.

Foot Massage

1. Press the reflex zones of Liver, Spleen and Pancreas with thumbs taking the tolerance degree of the ones being massaged into consideration. It is preferred to have a local sense of soreness and distension.
2. Press the reflex zones of Kidney and Heart with interphalangeal joint at the proximal side of index fingers with coherent movement and press 5 to 10 times continuously for 3 minutes.
3. Take massage progressive massage for the inner side of foot thumbs so that the hard and striped stuff from the inner side to the tip could be gradually softened and spread.

18 Hypertension

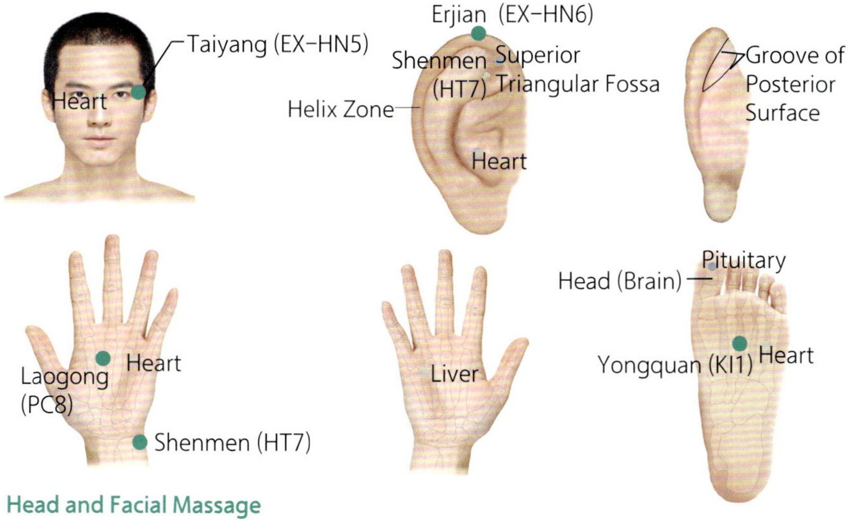

Head and Facial Massage

1. Massage the acupoints of Taiyang(EX-HN5) on both sides using thumbs with moderate strength.
2. Press the Heart reflex zone with interphalangeal joint at the proximal side of index fingers for 2 to 3 minutes with moderate strength and it is preferred to have a local sense of slight distending pain.

Ear Massage

1. Rub the reflex zones of Heart, Superior Triangular Fossa and Shenmen (HT7) each for 30 times, and it should refer to the heat degree.
2. Slightly press the reflex zones of the Groove of Posterior Surface and Erjian (EX-HN6) with thumbs each for 6 minutes with 90 times in each minute.
3. Twist the helix zones for 6 minutes with 90 times in each minute. Erjian (EX-HN6) holds the key to the manipulation.
4. Rub the posterior surface of ear with palm with relatively moderate strength with 120 times of manipulation in every minute.

Hand Massage

1. Press the Heart and Liver reflex zone for 1 to 2 minutes.
2. Press hard on the acupoints of Laogong (PC8) and Shenmen (HT7) with thumbs and relax after each short stay. Repeat the manipulation for 5 to 6 times and it is the same with the opposite side.

Foot Massage

1. Press the reflex zones of Head (Brain) and Pituitary each for 20 to 30 times and it is preferred to have a local sense of slight distending pain.
2. Scratch and press the Heart reflex zone with interphalangeal joint at the proximal side of index fingers for 2 to 3 minutes with gradually aggravated strength in case of overexertion.
3. Pinch rubbing Yongquan (KI1) using thumb tip with relatively strong strength and apply the same manipulation to the opposite acupoint.

19 冠心病

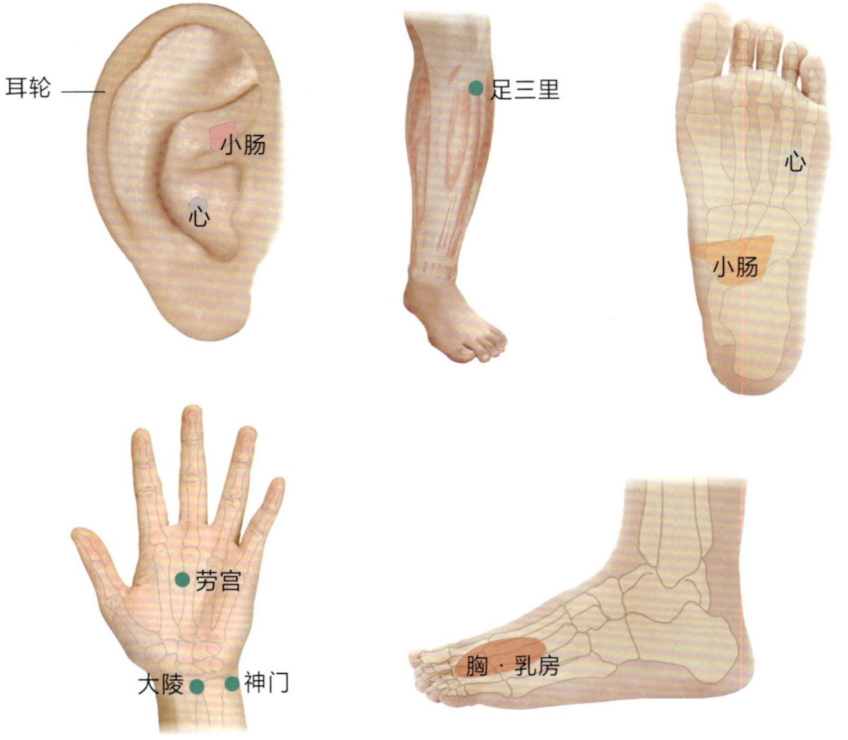

耳部按摩

1. 指推心、小肠反射区各 3 分钟，每分钟 60 次。
2. 指擦耳背部 3 分钟，酌情用力，每分钟 120 次。
3. 捻耳轮部 3 分钟，每分钟 60 次。

手部按摩

1. 轻揉劳宫穴 3~5 分钟，每分钟 90 次。
2. 重按大陵穴 3~5 分钟，每分钟 60 次。若有心悸，可加按神门穴。

足部按摩

1. 食指近侧指间关节依次刮压心、小肠、胸·乳房反射区各 30 次。
2. 双手拇指指尖放在一侧足三里穴上，其余四指置于小腿后侧，拇指适当用力掐按 1~2 分钟。同法按揉对侧足三里穴。

20 高脂血症

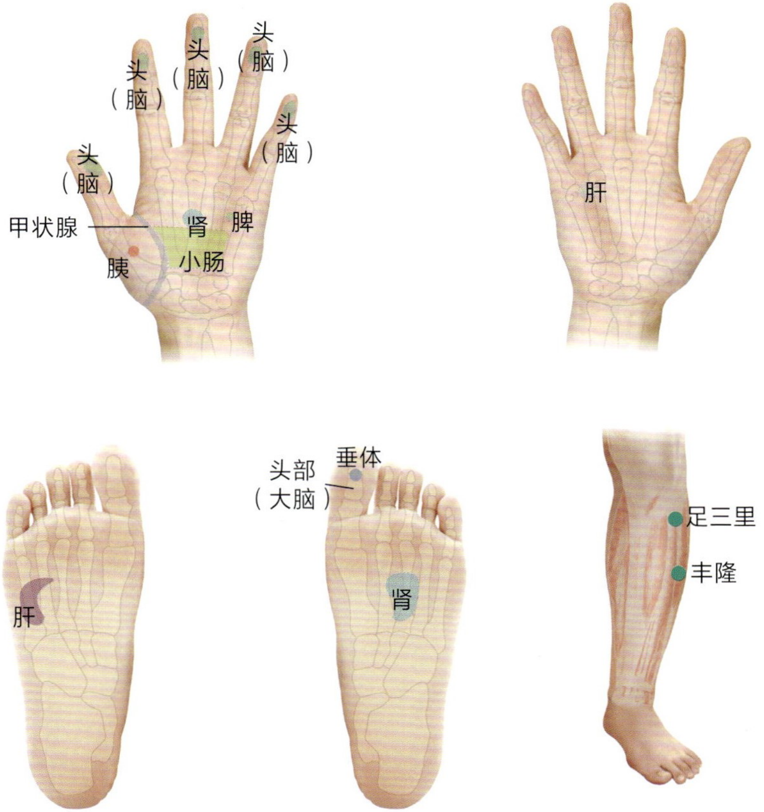

手部按摩

1. 食指近侧指间关节刮压头（脑）、胰、甲状腺反射区各 2~3 分钟。
2. 食指桡侧缘刮肾、肝、脾反射区各 3~5 次，以局部有酸麻胀感为宜。
3. 揉掐或推按小肠反射区 20~30 次，力度适中。

足部按摩

1. 泡脚至全脚放松后操作，按摩头部（大脑）、垂体反射区，以局部有热胀感为宜。
2. 食指近侧指间关节依次压刮肾、肝反射区各 3~5 次。
3. 拇指指腹按揉丰隆穴 2 分钟，力度稍重，同法按揉对侧丰隆穴。
4. 拇指按压足三里穴 2 分钟，每分钟 60 次，同法按压对侧足三里穴。

19 Coronary Heart Disease

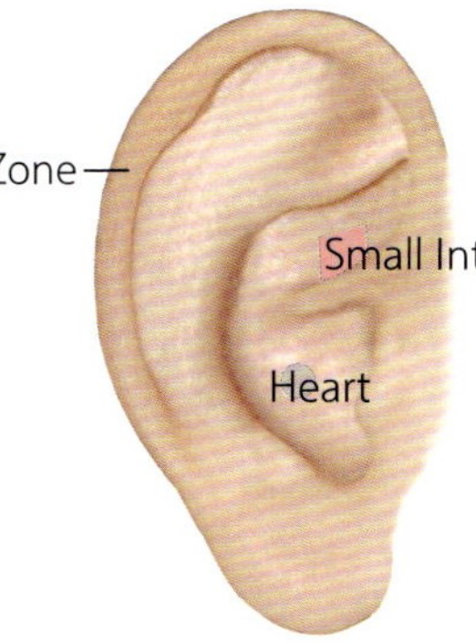

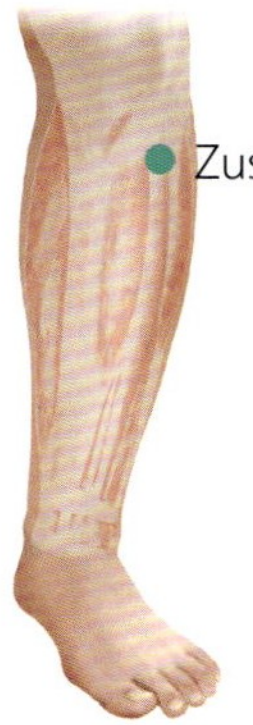

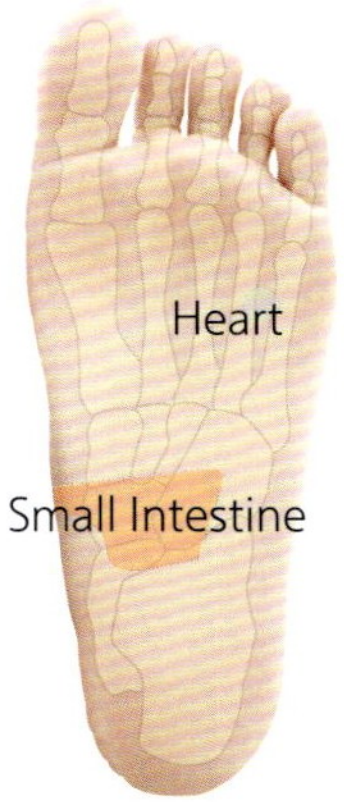

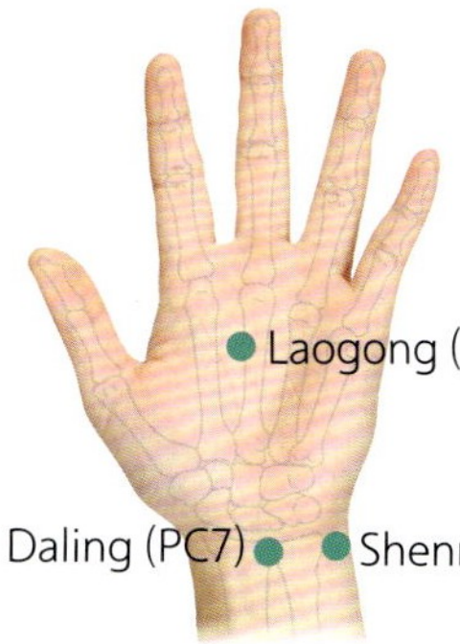

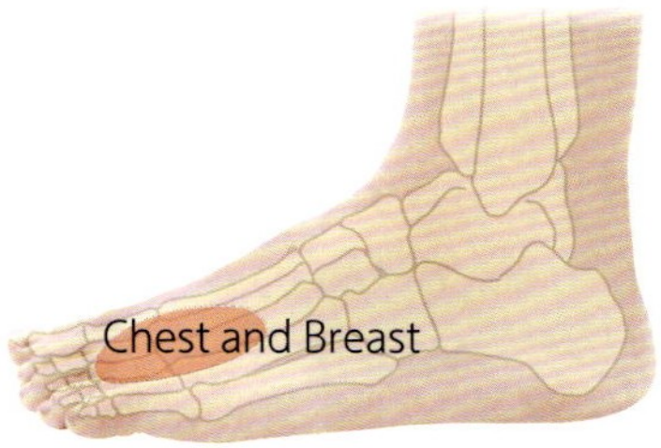

Ear Massage

1. Massage the reflex zones of Heart and Small Intestine each for 3 minutes with 60 times in each minute.
2. Rub the posterior surface of ear for 3 minutes with appropriate strength with 120 times in every minute.
3. Twist the Helix zone for 3 minutes with 60 times in each minute.

Hand Massage

1. Gently massage Laogong (PC8) for 3 to 5 minutes with 90 times in each minute.
2. Press hard on Daling (PC7) for 3 to 5 minutes with 60 times in each minute. You can add Shenmen (HT7) into the manipulation for palpitation.

Foot Massage

1. Scratch and press the reflex zones of Heart, Small Intestine, Chest and Breast successively each for 30 times with interphalangeal joint at the proximal side of index fingers.
2. Place both thumb tips on one of the acupoints of Zusanli (ST36) and the other 4 fingers at the rear side of crus. Nip with thumbs with appropriate strength for 1 to 2 minutes and apply the same manipulation at the opposite.

20 Hyperlipemia

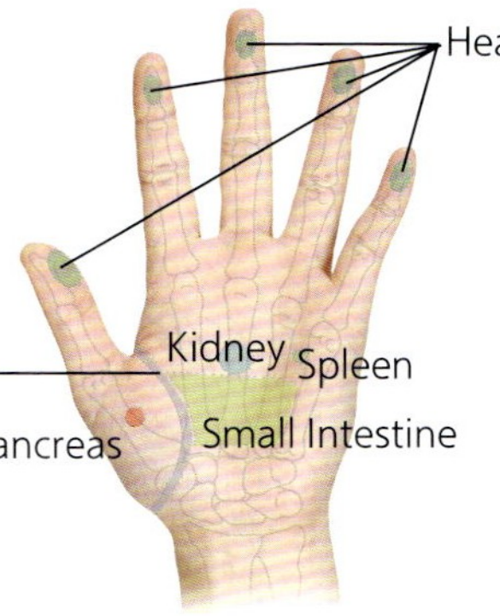

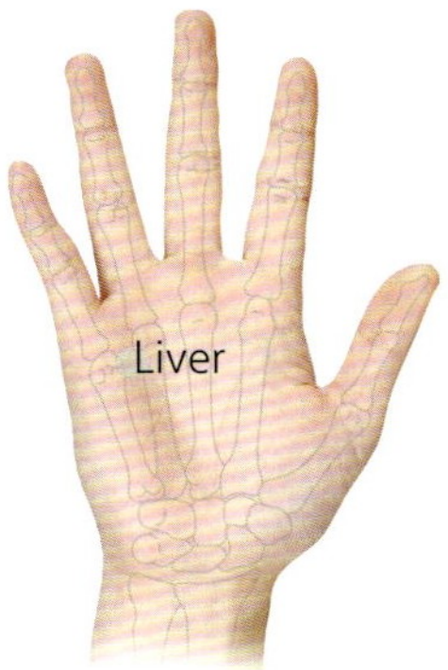

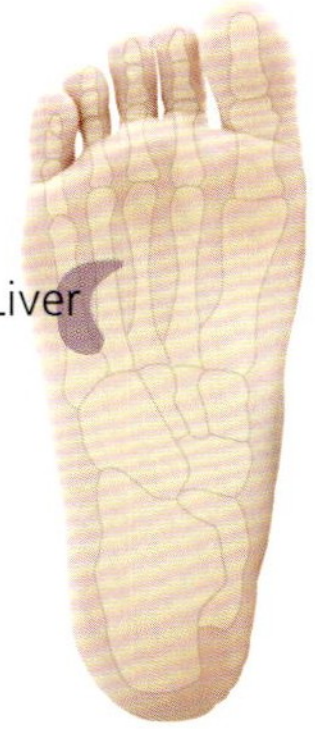

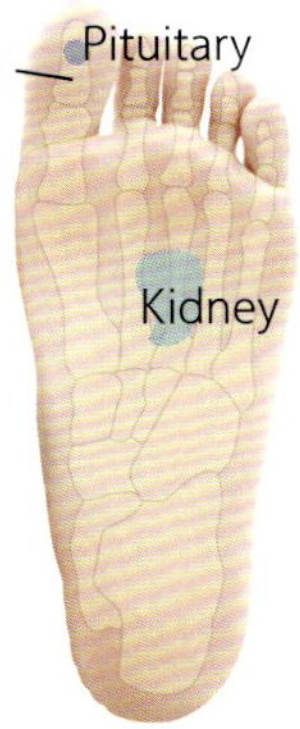

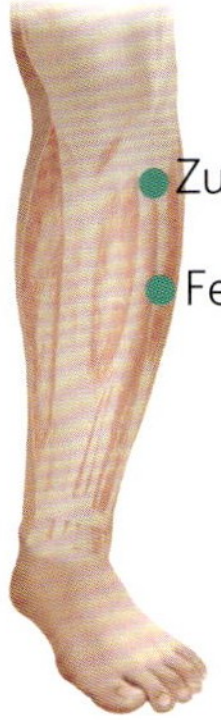

Hand Massage

1. Scratch the reflex zones of Head (Brain), Pancreas and Thyroid Gland with interphalangeal joint at the proximal side of index fingers for 2 to 3 minutes.
2. Scratch the reflex zones of Kidney, Liver and Spleen with the radical margin of index fingers each for 3 to 5 times and it is preferred to have a local sense of soreness, distension and numbness.
3. Massage or nip the Small Intestine reflex zone for 20 to 30 times with moderate strength.

Foot Massage

1. Take the massage after overall relaxation with foot bath. Massage the reflex zones of Head (Brain) and pituitary and a local sense of heat and distension is preferred.
2. Successively press and scratch the reflex zones of Kidney and Liver each for 3 to 5 times with interphalangeal joint at the proximal side of index fingers.
3. Massage the acupoint of Fenglong (ST40) with relatively strong strength on both sides.
4. Press the acupoint of Zusanli (ST36) for 2 minutes on both sides, and there are 60 times of massage in each minute.

21 心律失常

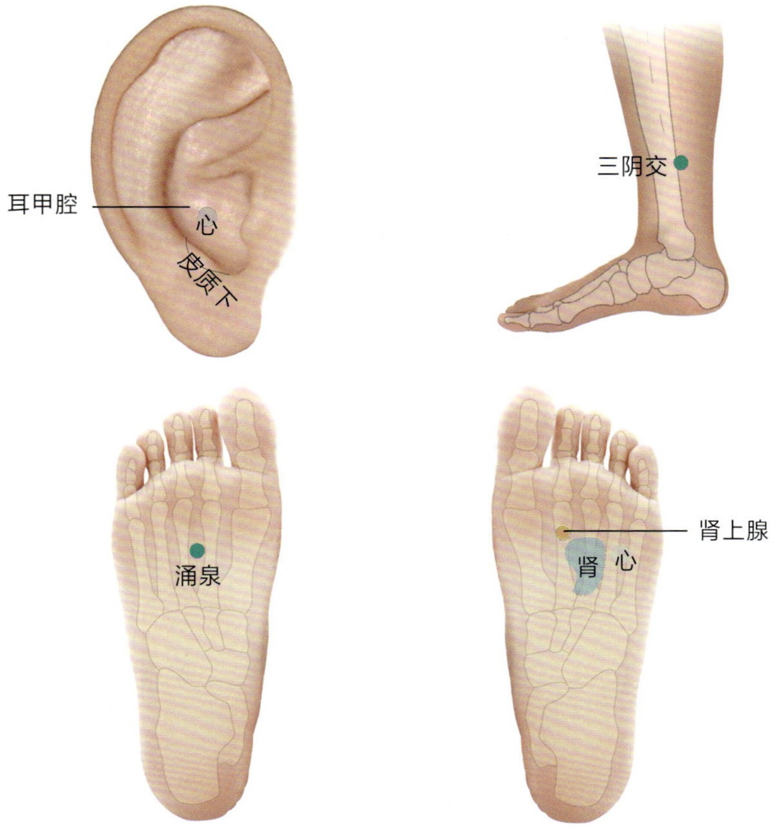

耳部按摩

1. 食指近侧指间关节点按心反射区 6 分钟，指力适中，被按摩者配合深度呼吸。
2. 指甲轻刮皮质下反射区 3 分钟，每分钟 60 次，以局部微痛、微红为宜。
3. 指腹轻按耳甲腔部 5 分钟，每分钟 60 次。

足部按摩

1. 手掌重擦足底，食指点揉足部心、肾、肾上腺反射区。
2. 拇指指腹稍微用力按压三阴交穴 2 分钟，每次停留片刻后放松，重复 5~6 次。
3. 按摩棒点按涌泉穴，力达深部。

22 中风后遗症

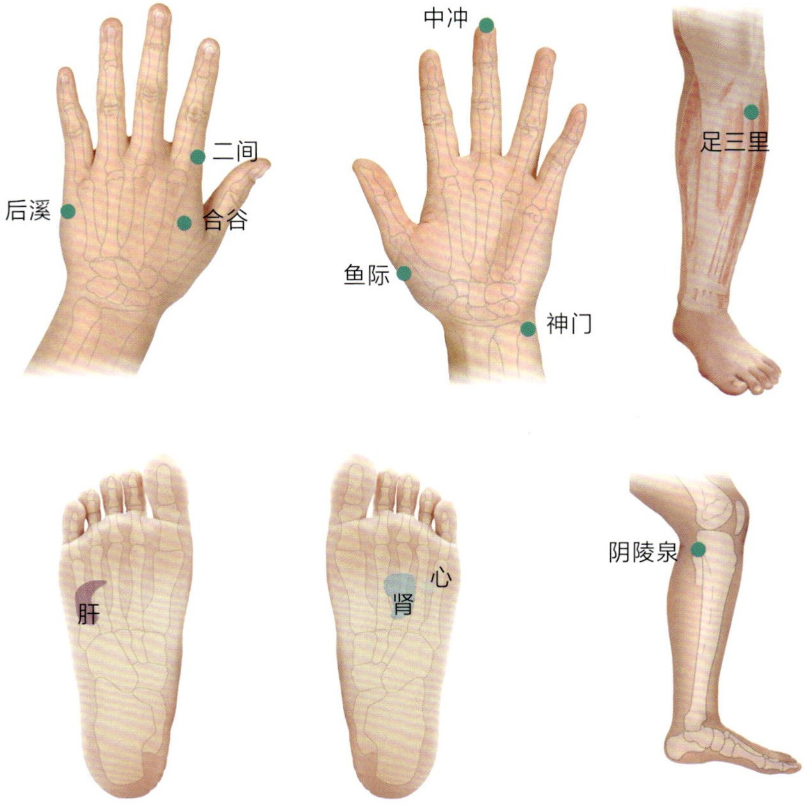

手部按摩

1. 按合谷穴，直至有酸胀和麻痛感为止。
2. 若有头晕目眩症状，加按后溪、二间、神门穴各 2 分钟。
3. 有失语症状，掐按鱼际穴，点按中冲穴。

足部按摩

1. 食指尺侧缘刮肾、肝反射区 5 分钟，以局部有酸麻胀感为宜。
2. 手指擦足部的心反射区。
3. 拇指指腹重压足三里、阴陵泉穴各 2 分钟。

21 Arrhythmia

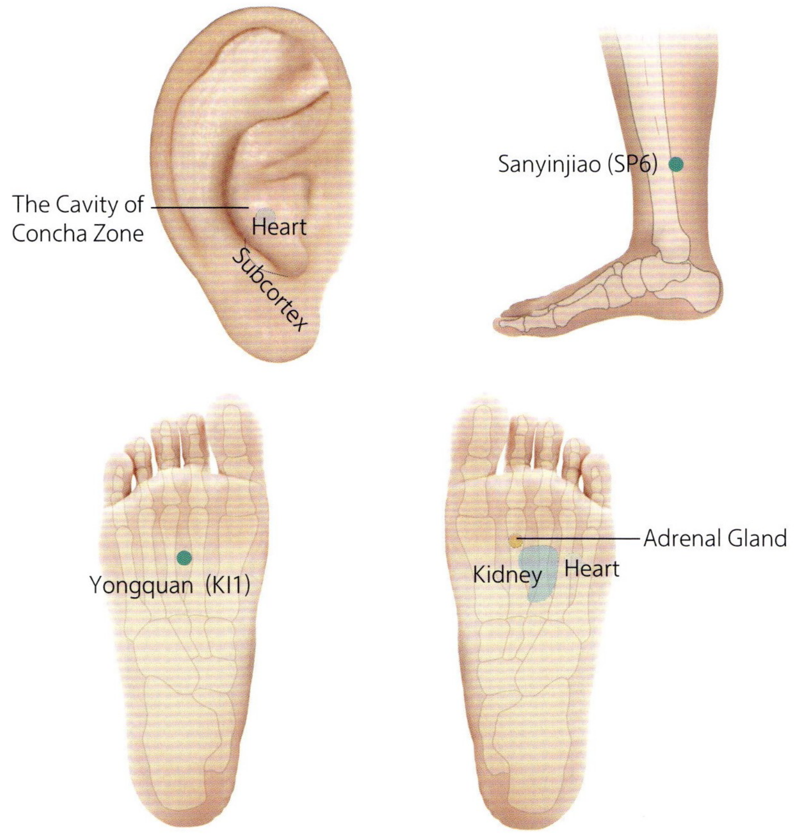

Ear Massage

1. Press the Heart reflex zone with interphalangeal joint at the proximal side of index fingers using moderate strength. Ask the patient to take a deep breath during the massage.
2. Slightly scratch the Subcortex reflex zone with nails for 3 minutes, with 60 times of scratch in each minute. It is preferred to have slight pain and blush locally.
3. Slightly press the Cavity of Concha zone with finger pulp for 5 minutes and there are 60 times in each minute.

Foot Massage

1. Hard rub the pelma with palm and press the reflex zones of Heart, Kidney and Adrenal Gland on foot with index fingers.
2. Press the acupoint of Sanyinjiao (SP6) with a little pressure using thumbs for 2 minutes and relax after each short stay. Repeat the manipulation 5 to 6 times.
3. Press the acupoint of Yongquan (KI1) to its deep section with a massage stick.

22 Sequela of Wind Stroke

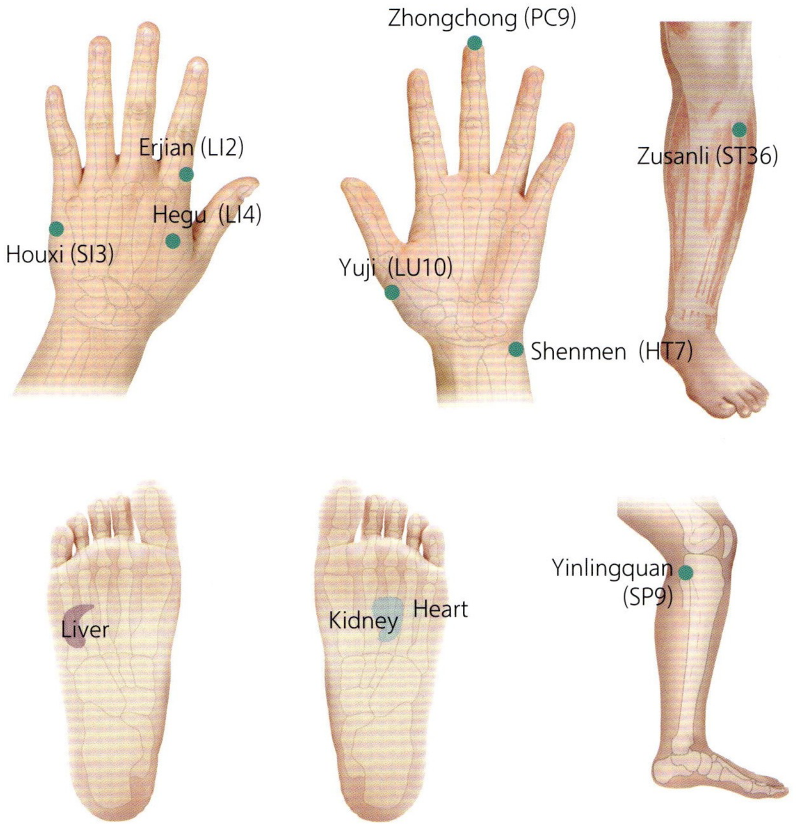

Hand Massage

1. Massage the acupoint of Hegu (LI4) until there appears a sense of soreness, distension and numb pain.
2. Only if there were dizziness, add the acupoints of Houxi (SI3), Erjian (LI2) and Shenmen (HT7) into the massage.
3. Nip the acupoint of Yuji (LU10) and press Zhongchong (PC9) for caught aphasia.

Foot Massage

1. Scratch the Kidney and Liver reflex zones with ulnar side of index fingers and it is preferred to have local soreness, numbness and distension.
2. Rub the Heart reflex zone on foot with fingers.
3. Press hard on the acupoints of Zusanli (ST36) and Yinlingquan (SP9) each for 2 minutes with thumbs.

23 胆囊炎

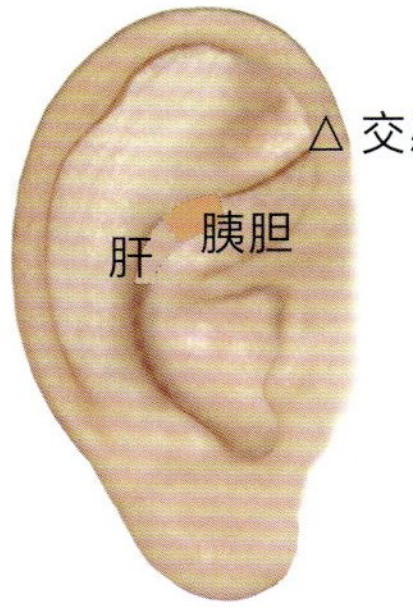

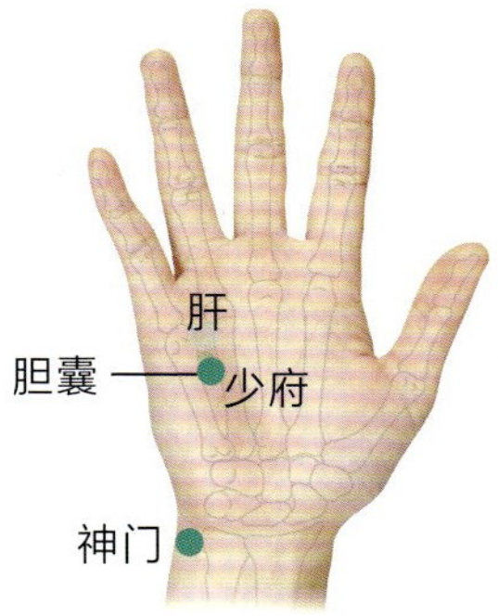

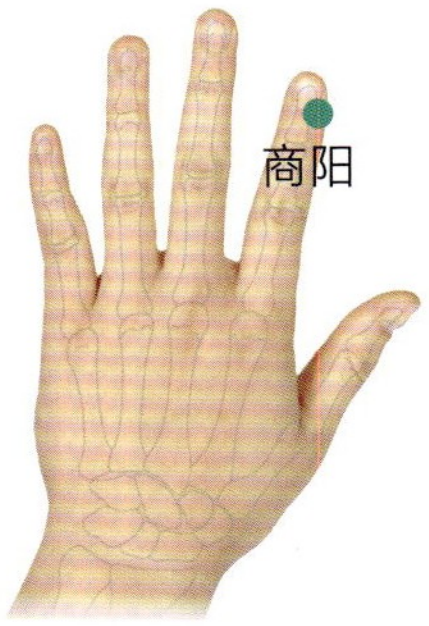

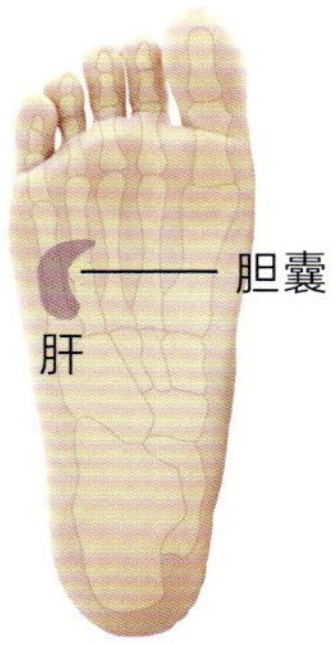

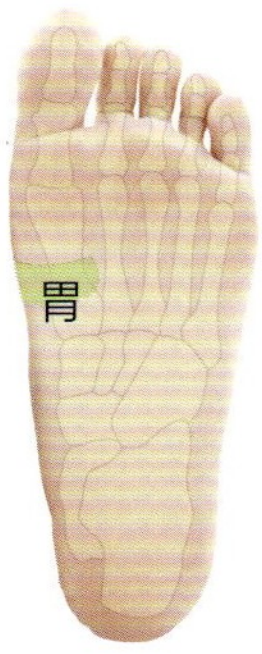

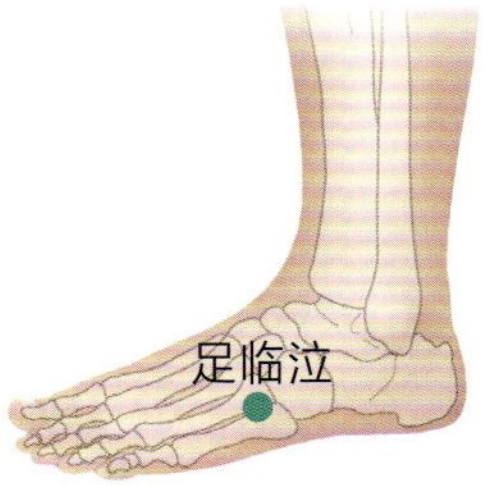

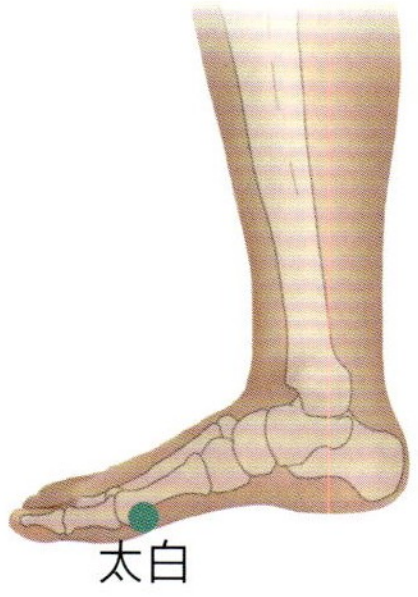

耳部按摩

1. 按摩棒推肝、胰胆反射区各 5 分钟，每分钟 20 次。
2. 食指轻压交感反射区 6 分钟，以压耳时感轻微刺痛、胀、耳郭灼热为宜。

手部按摩

1. 点按商阳穴，每次停留片刻后放松，重复 5~6 次。同法按揉对侧商阳穴。
2. 伴有胸胁头痛，可加按少府、神门穴。
3. 点按肝、胆囊反射区 30~50 次，力度适中。

足部按摩

1. 持续有力地点按足临泣、太白穴。
2. 揉擦或按压足部肝、胆囊、胃反射区各 3 分钟。

24 面瘫

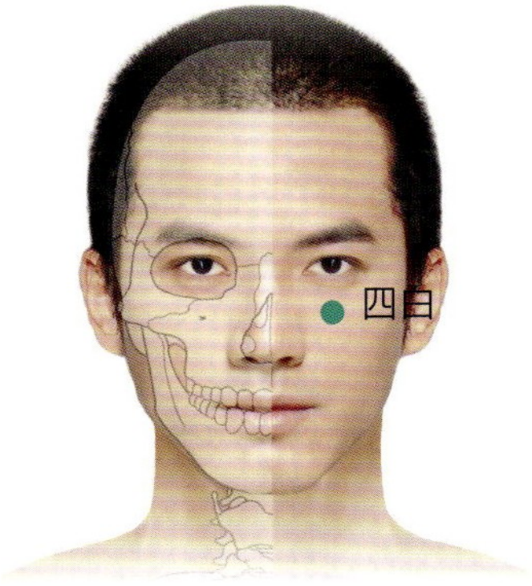

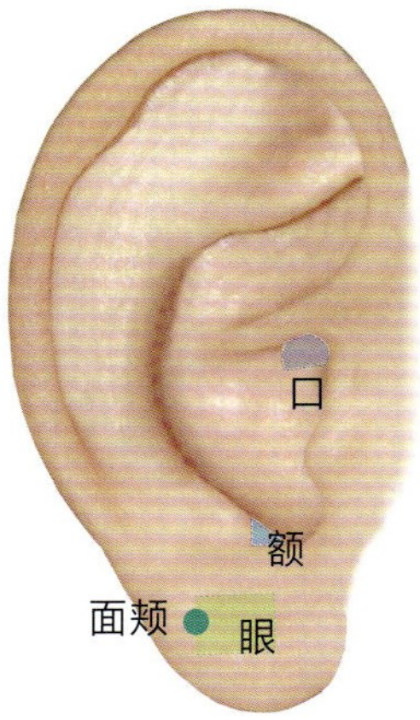

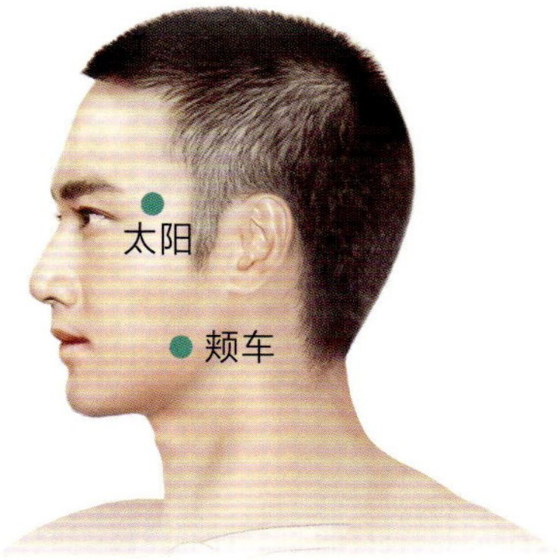

头面部按摩

1. 双手拇指按揉双侧太阳穴 2 分钟，力度适中。
2. 双手食指按压两侧四白穴，每次停留片刻后放松，重复 5~6 次。
3. 拇指指腹按压两侧颊车穴，力度适宜，每次停留片刻后放松，重复 5~6 次。

耳部按摩

1. 按摩棒揉眼、面颊反射区各 3 分钟，每分钟 90 次。
2. 三指拿耳垂部反射区 3 分钟，每分钟 90 次。
3. 将王不留行籽贴附于口、额反射区，每天按揉数次。

23 Cholecystitis

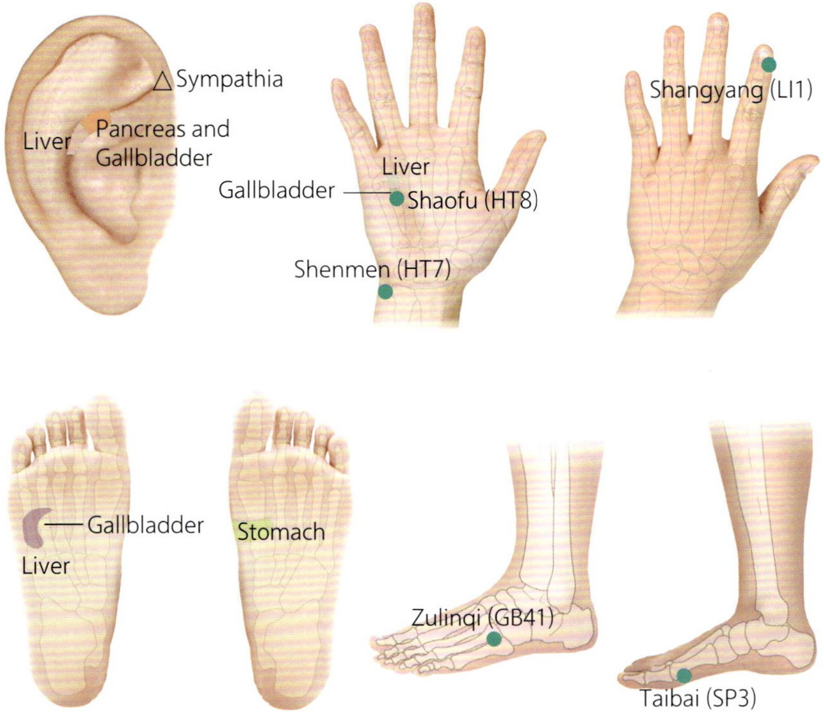

Ear Massage

1. Press the reflex zones of Liver and Pancreas and Gallbladder with massage stick each for 5 minutes with 20 times in each minute.
2. Slightly press the Sympathetic reflex zone with index fingers for 6 minutes and it is preferred to have a sense of slight stabbing pain, distension and burning heat of the ear while pressing the ear.

Hand Massage

1. Press the acupoint of Shangyang (LI1) and relax after every short stay. Repeat the movement 5 to 6 times and apply the same manipulation to the opposite acupoint.
2. Add the acupoints of Shaofu (HT8) and Shenmen (HT7) if accompanied with discomfort in the reflex zones of Chest and Hypochondrium or headache.
3. Press the Liver and Gallbladder reflex zones for 30 to 50 times with moderate strength.

Foot Massage

1. Continuously press hard on the acupoints of Zulinqi (GB41) and Taibai (SP30).
2. Rub or press the reflex zones of Liver, Gallbladder and Stomach on foot each for 3 minutes.

24 Facial Paralysis

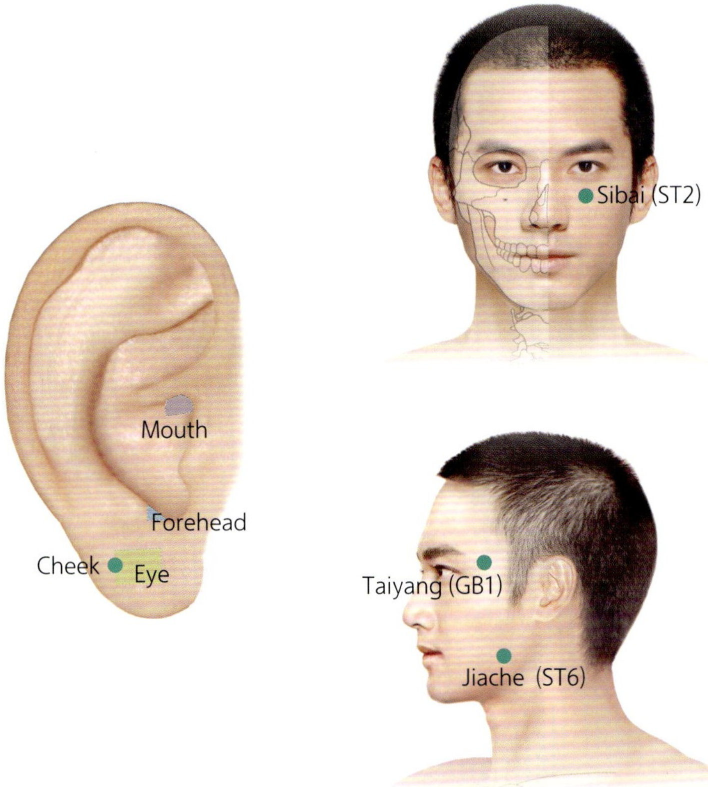

Head and Facial Massage

1. Massage Taiyang (GB1) on both sides with 2 thumbs for 2 minutes in moderate strength.
2. Press Sibai (ST2) on both sides with 2 index fingers and relax after each short stay. Repeat 5 to 6 times.
3. Press Jiache (ST6) on both sides with thumbs in moderate strength and relax after each short stay. Repeat 5 to 6 times.

Ear Massage

1. Massage the reflex zones of Eye and Cheek each for 3 minutes with massage sticks with 90 times in each minute.
2. Massage the Earlobe reflex zone with 3 fingers for 3 minutes with 90 times in each minute.
3. Attach cowherb seed to the reflex zones of Mouth and Forehead for several times every day.

25 头痛

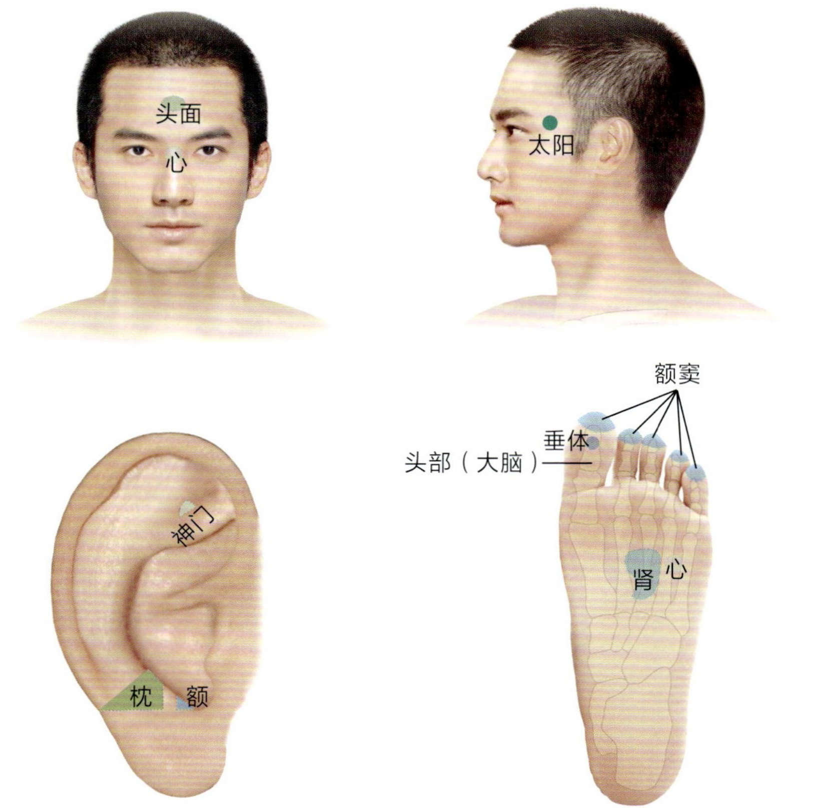

头面部按摩

1. 拇指指腹按揉太阳穴 3 分钟，每分钟 60 次。
2. 揉掐或推按头面、心反射区各 20~30 次，推按速度每分钟 20~40 次。

耳部按摩

1. 按摩棒推神门反射区 5 分钟，每分钟 90 次。
2. 食指近侧指间关节刮压额、枕反射区，反复操作 2~3 分钟。

足部按摩

1. 食指近侧指间关节点按垂体、肾、心反射区各 5 分钟，用力均匀，力度适中。
2. 拇指点按头部（大脑）、额窦反射区，力度以被按摩者耐受为度，以局部有酸胀感为宜。

26 失眠多梦

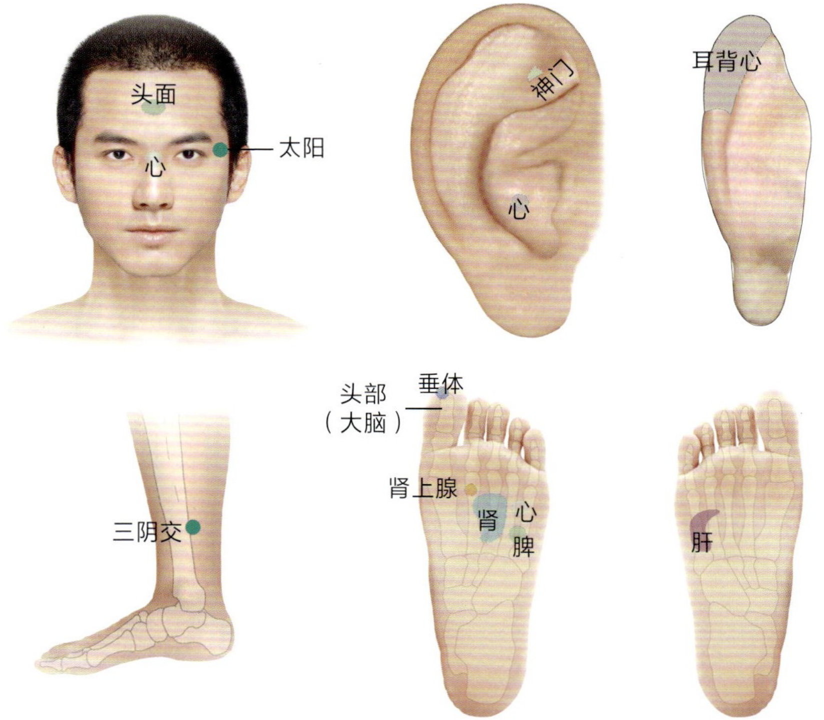

头面部按摩

1. 食指近侧指间关节点按头面、心反射区各 2~3 分钟，力度适中，以局部有轻度胀痛为宜。
2. 拇指指腹按揉太阳穴，力度以被按摩者耐受为度，以局部有轻度胀痛为宜。

耳部按摩

1. 按摩棒揉神门反射区 5 分钟，用力宜轻，每分钟 120 次。
2. 指振心反射区 3 分钟，每分钟 240 次。
3. 揉捏耳背心反射区 5 分钟，每分钟 90 次。

足部按摩

1. 拇指指腹推三阴交穴 4 分钟，用力稍重，每分钟 60 次。
2. 泡脚至全脚放松后操作，按摩头部（大脑）、垂体、肾、心反射区，以局部有酸胀感为宜。
3. 拇指压肝、脾、肾上腺反射区各 20 次，再次放松全足结束按摩。

25 Headache

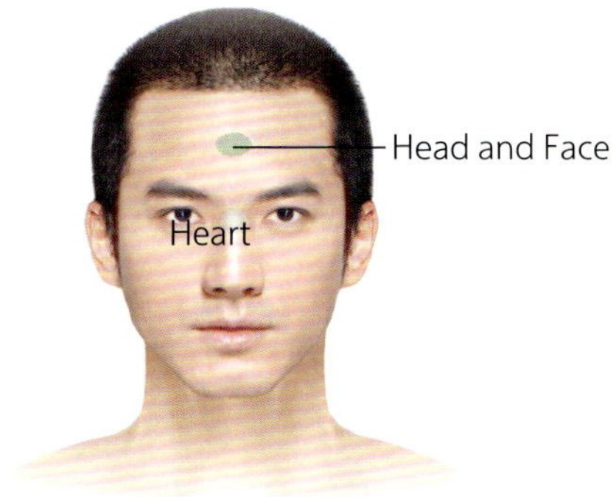

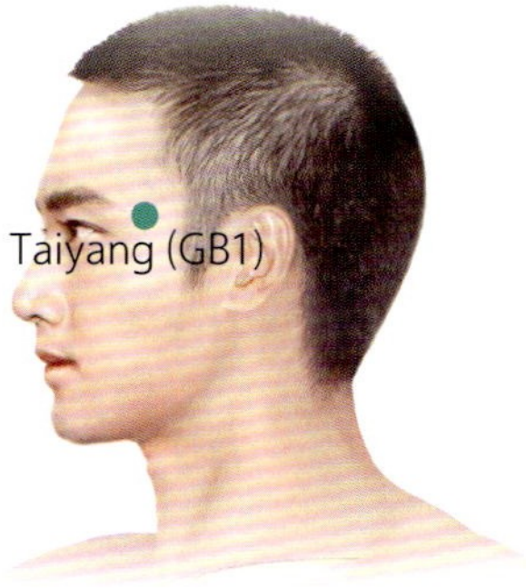

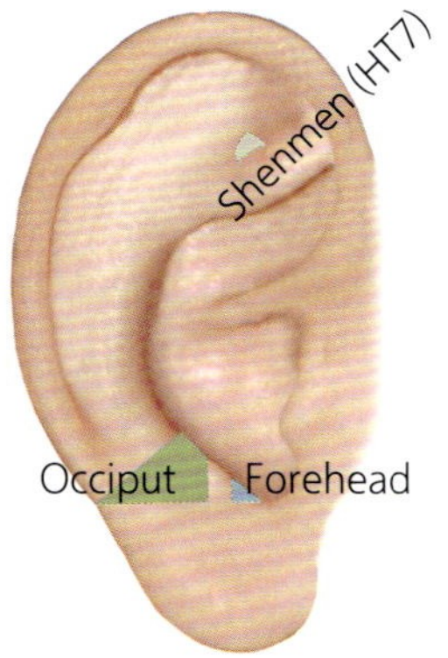

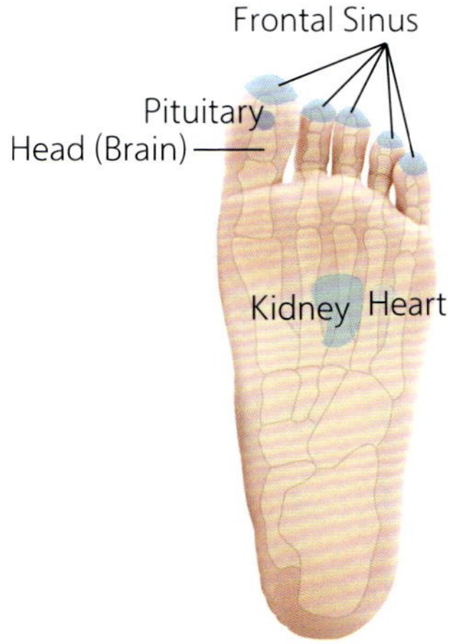

Head and Facial Massage

1. Massage Taiyang (GB1) with thumbs for 3 minutes and there are 60 times in each minute.
2. Nip or press Head and Face reflex zone and Heart reflex zone for 20 to 30 times and massage the zone 20 to 40 times in each minute.

Ear Massage

1. Press Shenmen (HT7) reflex zone with massage stick for 5 minutes and there are 90 times in each minute.
2. Scratch and press the reflex zones of Forehead and Occiput with interphalangeal joint at the proximal side of index fingers and repeat the massage for 2 to 3 minutes.

Foot Massage

1. Press the reflex zones of Pituitary, Kidney and Heart with interphalangeal joint at the proximal side of index fingers each for 5 minutes in moderate strength.
2. Press the reflex zones of Head (Brain) and Frontal Sinus with thumbs taking the tolerance degree of the ones being massaged into consideration. It is preferred to have a local sense of soreness and distension.

26 Insomnia with Abundant Dreams

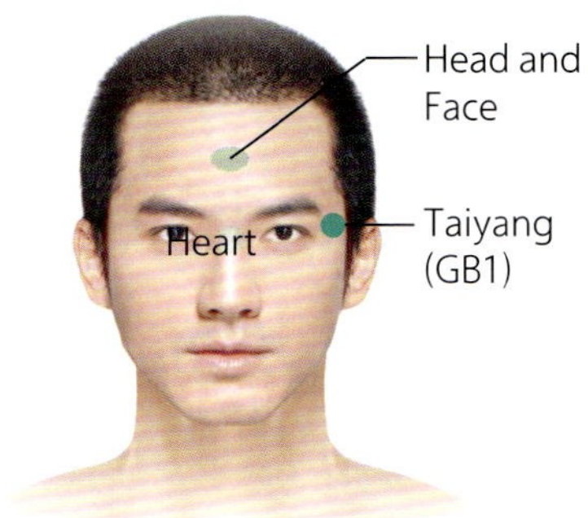

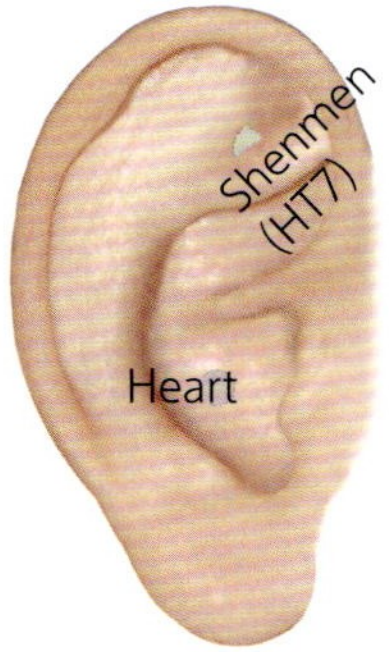

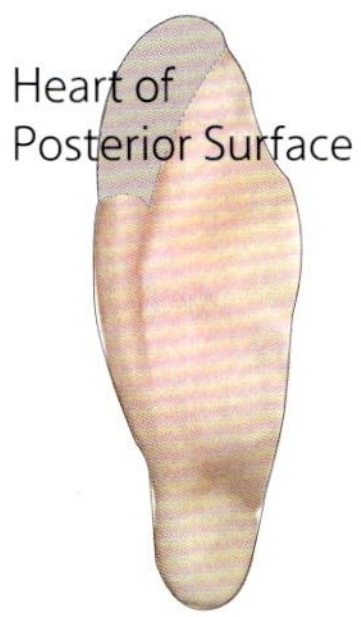

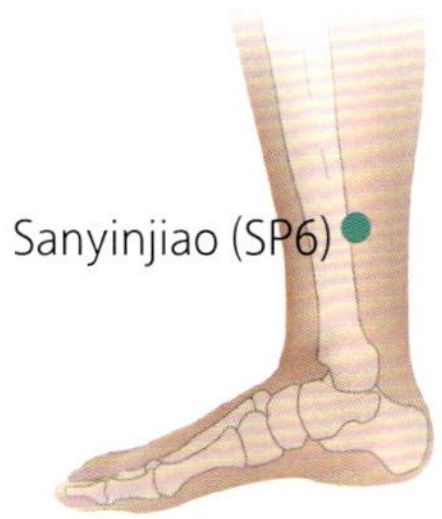

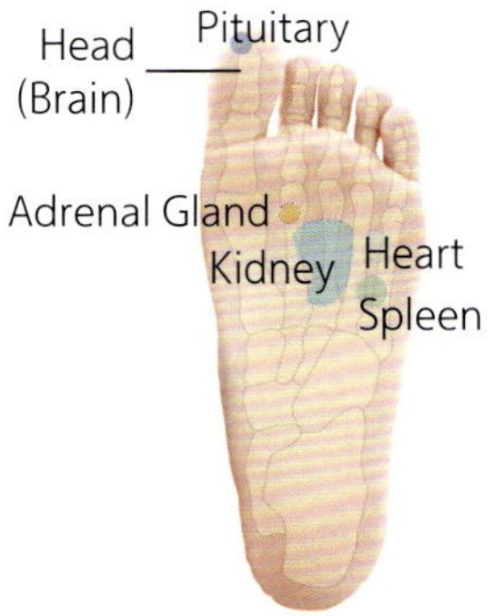

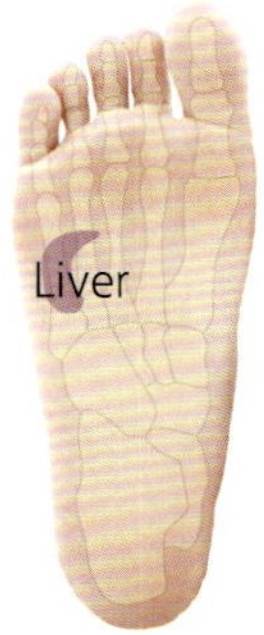

Head and Facial Massage

1. Press the Head and Face reflex zone and Heart reflex zone each for 2 to 3 minutes with interphalangeal joint at the proximal side of index fingers in moderate strength and it is preferred to have a local sense of slight distending pain.
2. Massage Taiyang (GB1) with thumbs in appropriate strength that the ones being massaged could tolerant and it is preferred to have a local sense of slight distending pain.

Ear Massage

1. Massage Shenmen (HT7) reflex zone for 5 minutes with massage sticks with gentle strength and there are 120 times in each minute.
2. Shake Heart reflex zone with fingers for 3 minutes in 240 times in each minute.
3. Massage the reflex zone of Heart of Posterior in 90 times in each minute.

Foot Massage

1. Massage Sanyinjiao (SP6) with thumbs for 4 minutes in relatively strong strength in 60 times in each minute.
2. Take the massage after a overall relaxation with a foot bath. Massage the reflex zones of Head (Brain), Pituitary, Kidney and Heart and it is preferred to have a local sense of soreness and distension.
3. Press the reflex zones of Liver, Spleen and Adrenal Gland with thumbs each for 20 times. Then end the whole foot massage with another relaxation.

27 慢性咽炎

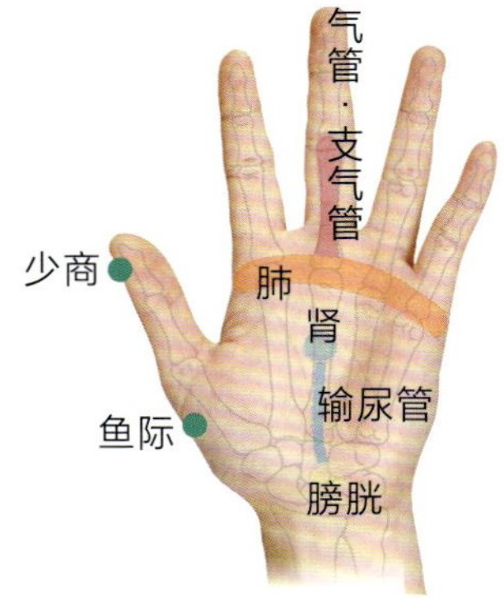

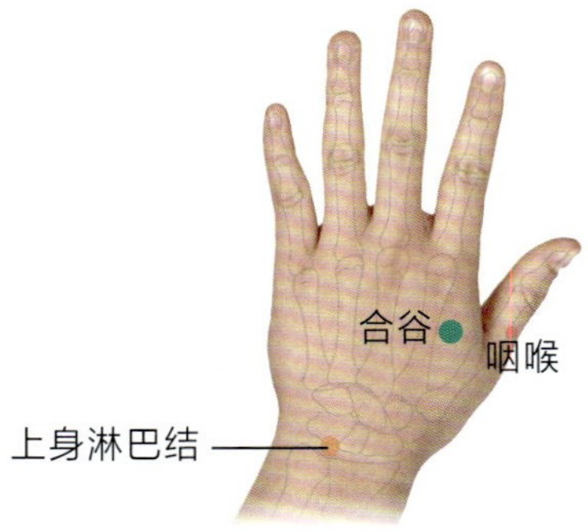

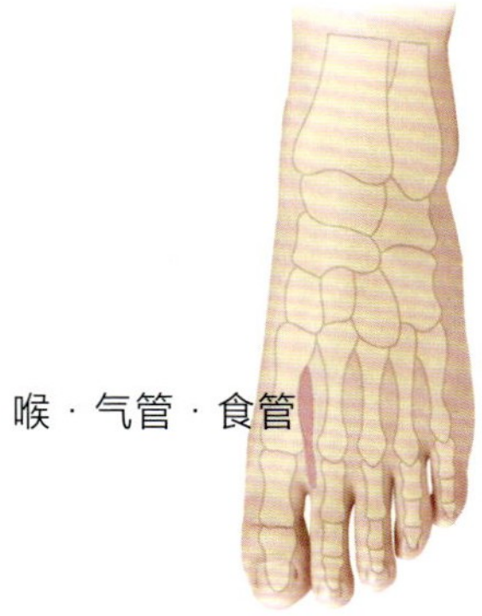

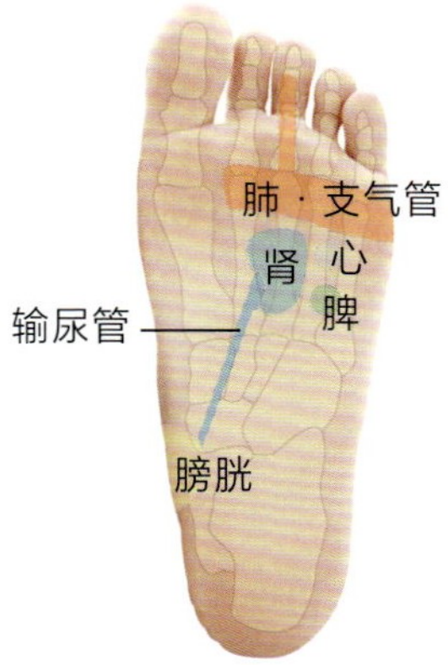

手部按摩

1. 放松手部，拇指轻轻按揉咽喉、气管·支气管、上身淋巴结反射区，以局部有酸痛感为宜。
2. 点按肺、肾、输尿管、膀胱反射区，力度以被按摩者耐受为度。
3. 食指近侧指间关节点按少商、合谷、鱼际穴，用力均匀，力度适中，重复 1 分钟。

足部按摩

1. 食指近侧指间关节刮压喉·气管·食管反射区，反复操作 2~3 分钟。
2. 泡脚至全脚放松后，按摩心、肺·支气管、脾、肾反射区各 2 分钟，以局部有酸胀感为宜。
3. 食指桡侧缘刮输尿管、膀胱反射区各 3~5 次，以局部有酸麻胀感为宜。

28 口腔溃疡

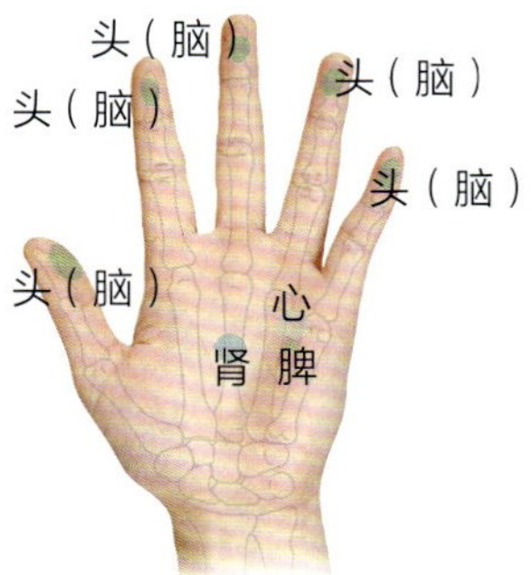

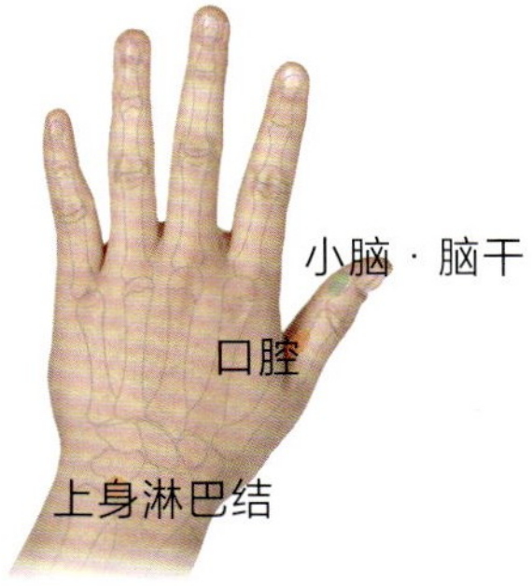

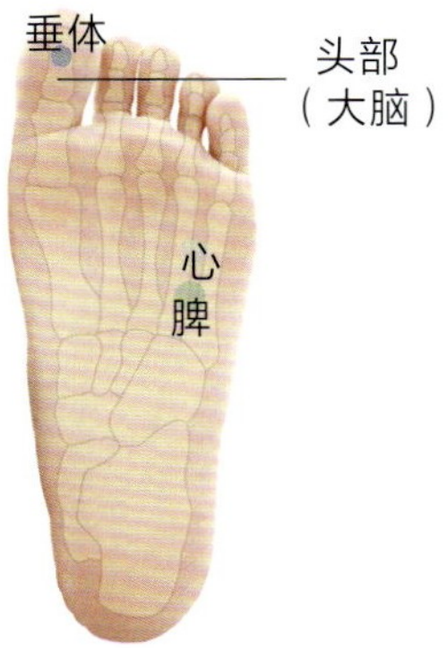

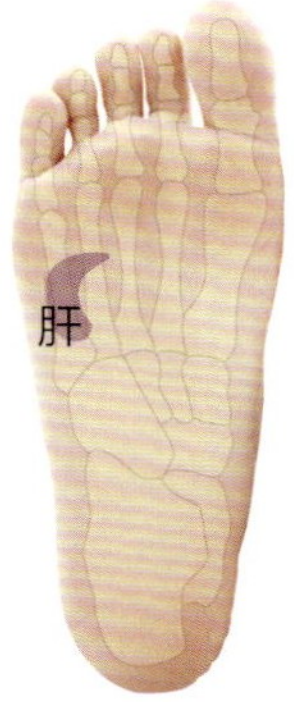

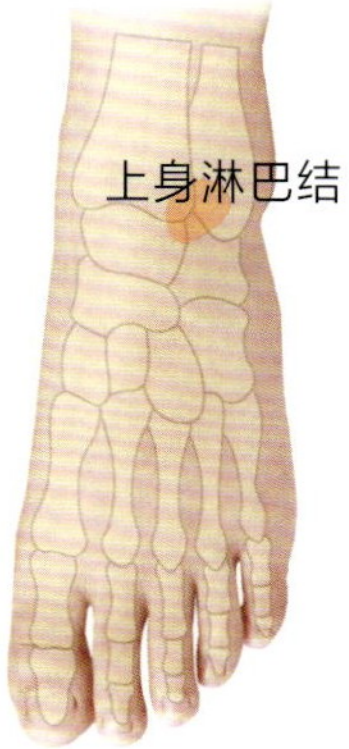

手部按摩

1. 拇指指腹按揉口腔反射区 5 次。
2. 放松手部，拇指轻轻按揉头（脑）、小脑·脑干、上身淋巴结反射区各 10 次。
3. 点按肾、心、脾反射区各 5~10 次，力度适中，手法要逐渐渗透。

足部按摩

1. 泡脚至全脚放松后，按摩头部（大脑）、上身淋巴结反射区，以局部有酸胀感为宜。
2. 食指近侧指间关节点按或用踩核桃的方式按压垂体、心、肝、脾反射区各 5~10 次。

27 Chronic Pharyngitis

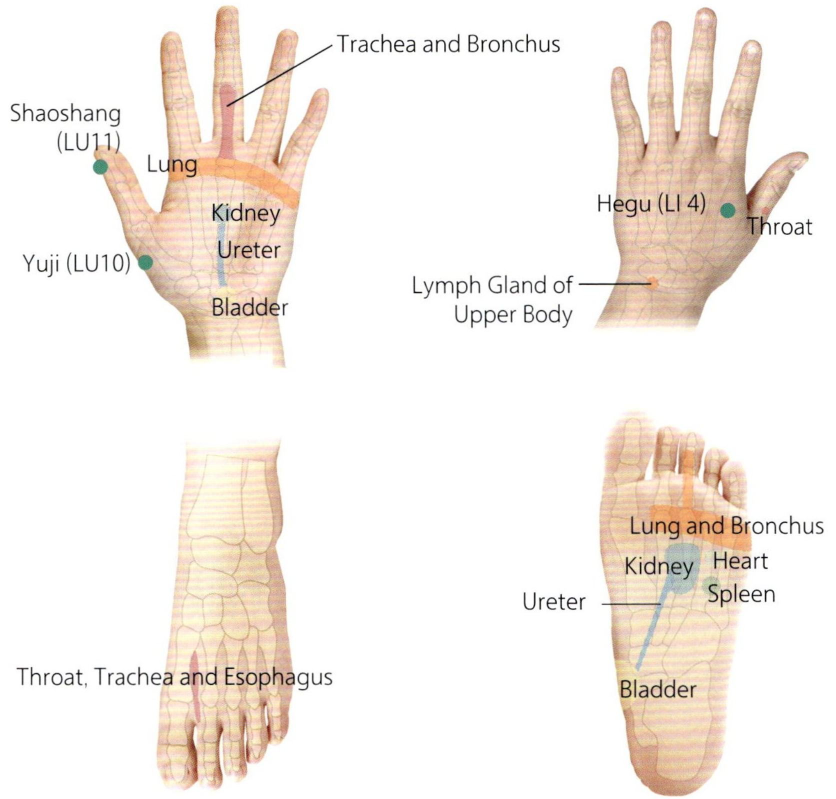

Hand Massage

1. Relax hands and gently massage the reflex zones of Throat, Trachea, Bronchus and Lymph Gland of Upper Body with thumbs. It is preferred to have a local sense of aching pain.
2. Press the reflex zones of Lung, Kidney, Ureter and Bladder and the strength should refer to the tolerance degree of the ones being massaged.
3. Press the acupoints of Shaoshang (LU11), Hegu (LI4) and Yuji (LU10) with interphalangeal joint at the proximal side of index fingers in moderate strength for 1 minutes.

Foot Massage

1. Scratch the reflex zones of Throat, Trachea and Esophagus with interphalangeal joint at the proximal side of index fingers repeatedly for 2 to 3 minutes.
2. After relaxing the feet with a foot bath, massage the reflex zones of Heart, Lung and Bronchus, Spleen and Kidney each for 2 minutes and it is preferred to have a local sense of aching pain.
3. Scratch the Ureter and Bladder reflex zones each for 3 to 5 minutes with radical margin of index fingers and it is preferred to have a local sense of soreness, numbness and distension.

28 Oral Ulcer

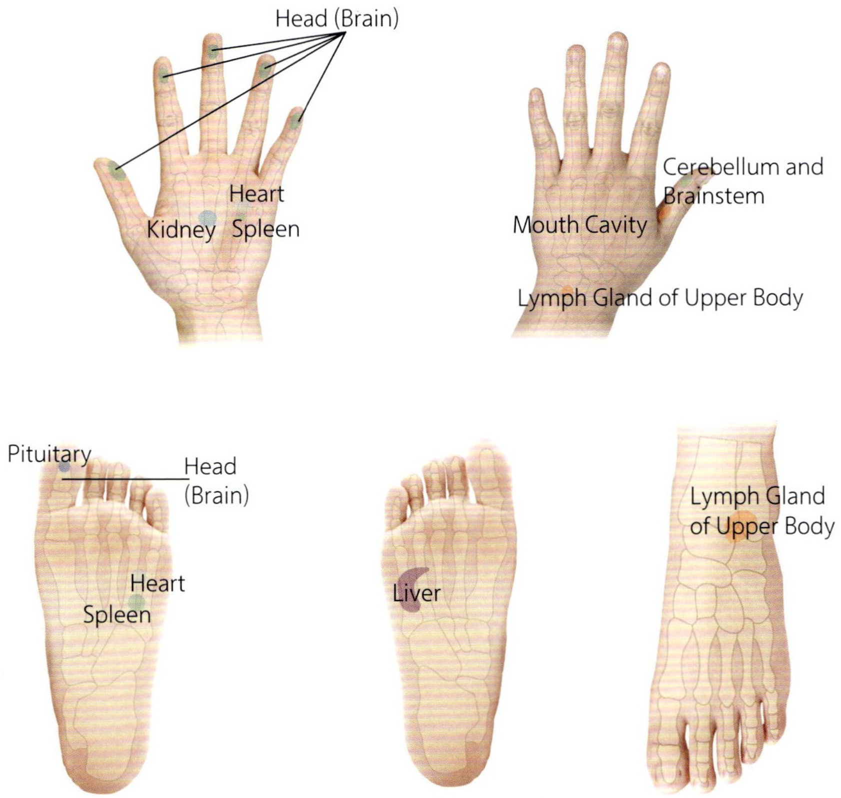

Hand Massage

1. Massage the Mouth Cavity reflex zone 5 times with thumbs.
2. Relax hands and gently massage the reflex zones of Head (Brain), Cerebellum, Brainstem and Lymph Gland of Upper Body each for 10 times.
3. Press the reflex zones of Kidney, Heart and Spleen each for 5 to 10 times with moderate strength and the manipulation should gradually penetrate into the skin.

Foot Massage

1. After relaxing the feet with a foot bath, massage the reflex zones of Head (Brain) and Lymph Gland of Upper Body and it is preferred to have a local sense of soreness and distension.
2. Use interphalangeal joint at the proximal side of index fingers to press the reflex zones of Pituitary, Heart, Liver and Spleen each for 5 to 10 times or you can take advantage of the method of pressing like treading on walnut.

29 鼻炎

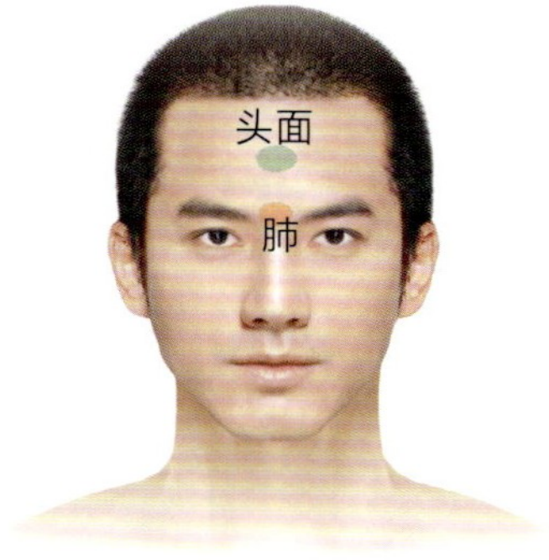

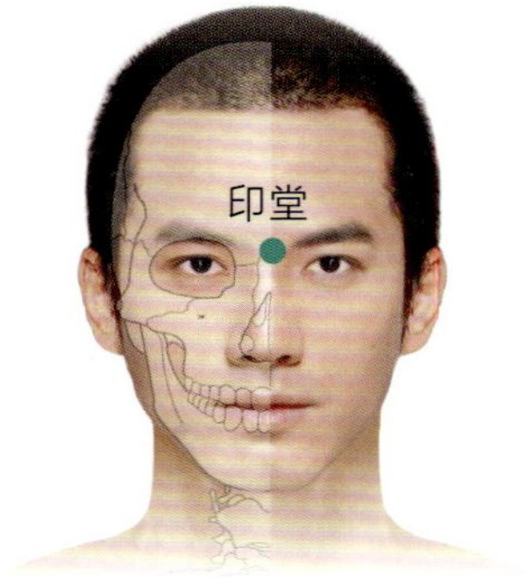

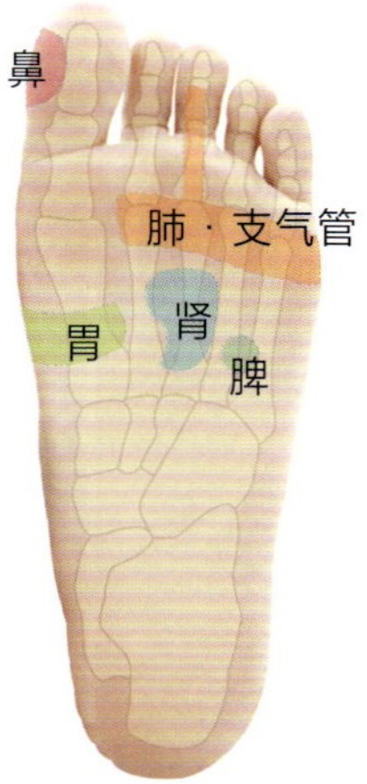

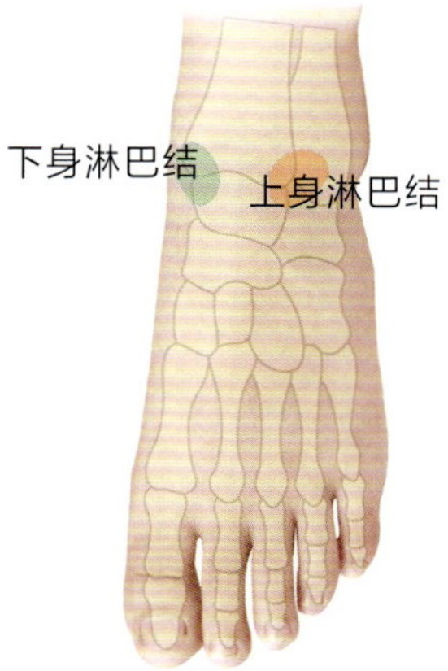

头面部按摩

1. 指推印堂穴 2 分钟，每分钟 90 次。
2. 用工具如铅笔点按头面、肺反射区各 10~15 次，以局部有酸胀感为宜。

足部按摩

1. 泡脚至全脚放松后操作，按摩鼻反射区，以局部有热胀感为宜。
2. 食指刮压或用尖状物点按肺 · 支气管、胃、肾、脾反射区各 30 次，以局部有热胀感为宜。
3. 按摩上身淋巴结、下身淋巴结反射区各 3~5 分钟，以局部有热胀感为宜。

30 耳鸣耳聋

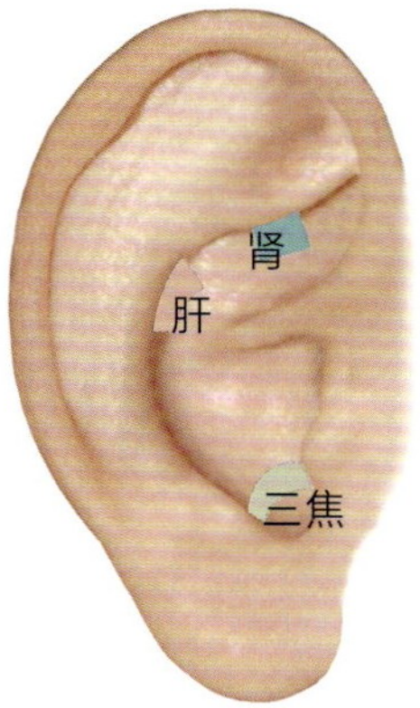

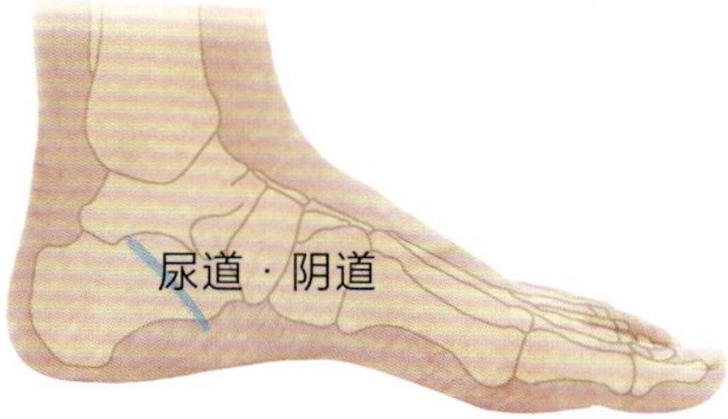

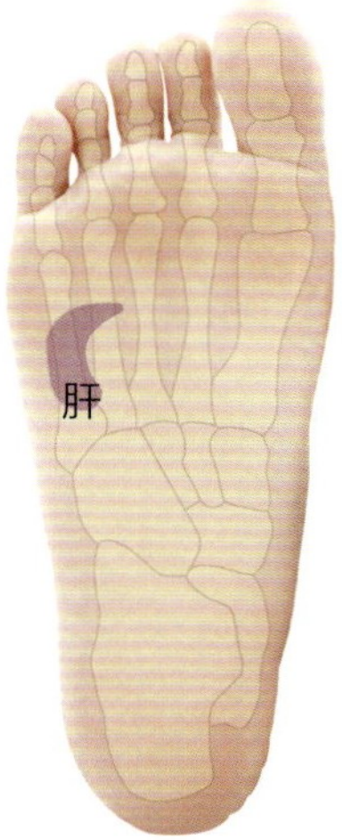

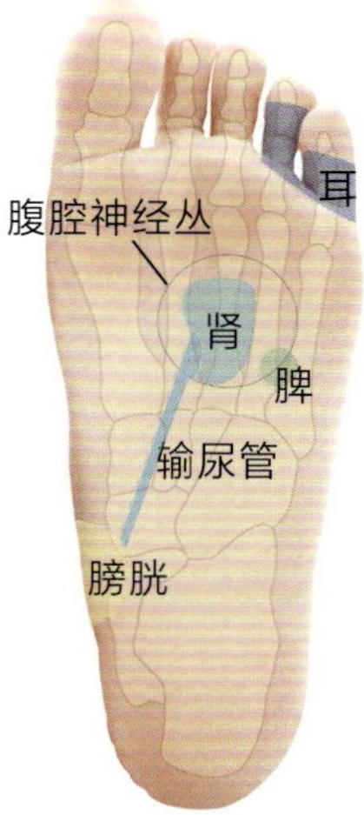

耳部按摩

1. 按摩棒揉肾反射区 3 分钟，每分钟 75 次。
2. 将王不留行籽贴附于肝反射区，点按 3 分钟，每分钟 90 次。
3. 拇指指腹揉三焦反射区，每分钟 120 次。

足部按摩

1. 泡脚至全脚放松后，按摩耳、肝、肾、脾反射区各 2 分钟，以局部有酸胀感为宜。
2. 食指近侧指间关节刮压腹腔神经丛、尿道 · 阴道、肾、输尿管、膀胱反射区各 3~5 次。
3. 左手掌搓摩右脚心，以透热为度，以局部有酸麻胀感为宜。

29 Rhinitis

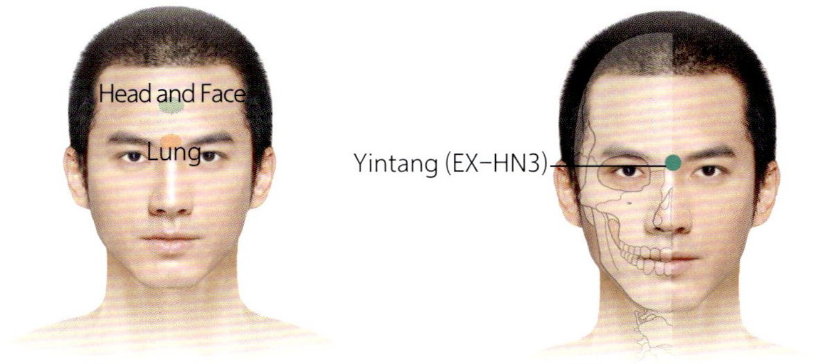

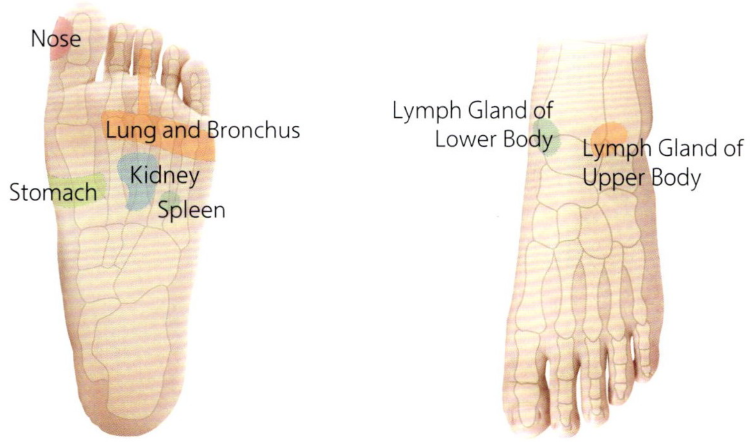

Head and Facial Massage

1. Press Yintang (EX–HN 3) with fingers for 2 minutes with 90 times in each minute.
2. Press the reflex zones of Face, Head and Lung with tools like pencils each for 10 to 15 times and it is preferred to have a local sense of soreness and distension.

Foot Massage

1. After relaxing the feet with a foot bath, massage the reflex zone of Nose and it is preferred to have a local sense of heat and distension.
2. Scratch with index fingers or press with pointed items the reflex zones of Lung, Bronchus, Stomach, Kidney and Spleen each for 30 times and a local sense of heat and distension is preferred.
3. Massage the reflex zones of Lymph Gland of Upper Body and Lower Body each for 3 to 5 minutes and a local sense of heat and distension is preferred.

30 Tinnitus and Deafness

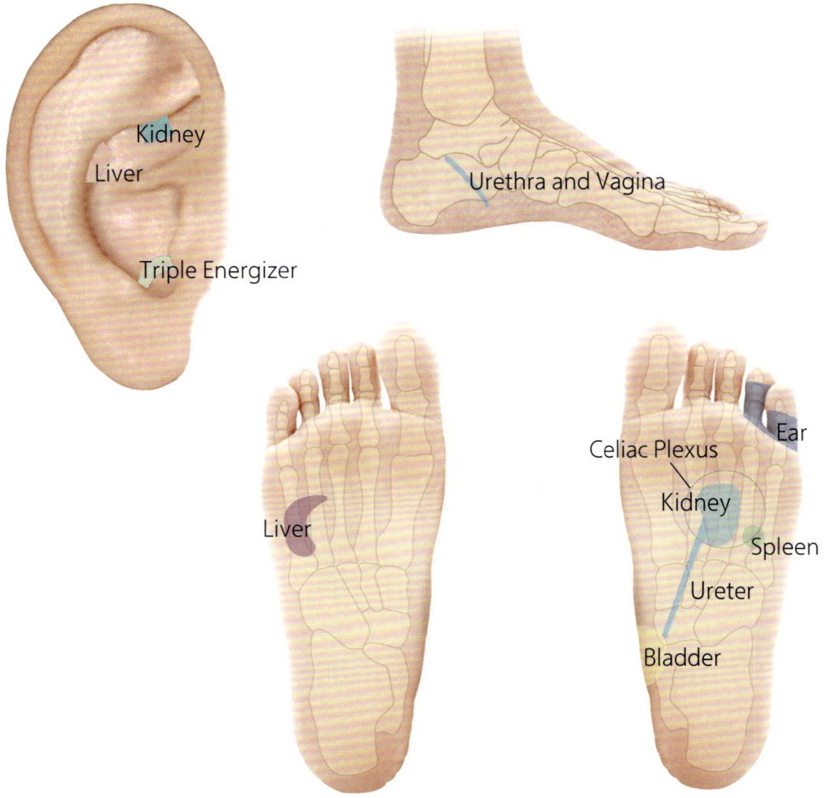

Ear Massage

1. Massage the Kidney reflex zone for 3 minutes with a massage stick with 75 times in each minute.
2. Attach cowherb seed to the reflex zone of Liver and press for 3 minutes with 90 times in each minute.
3. Massage the Triple Energizer reflex zone with thumbs with 120 times in each minute.

Foot Massage

1. After relaxing the feet with a foot bath, massage the reflex zone of Ear, Kidney, Liver and Spleen each for 2 minutes and it is preferred to have a local sense of soreness and distension.
2. Scratch the reflex zones of Celiac Plexus, Ureter, Vagina, Kidney, Urethra and Bladder each for 3 to 5 minutes with interphalangeal joint at the proximal side of index fingers.
3. Rub the right foot center with the left hand until there is appropriate heat degree and it is preferred to have a local sense of soreness, numbness and distension.

31 近视

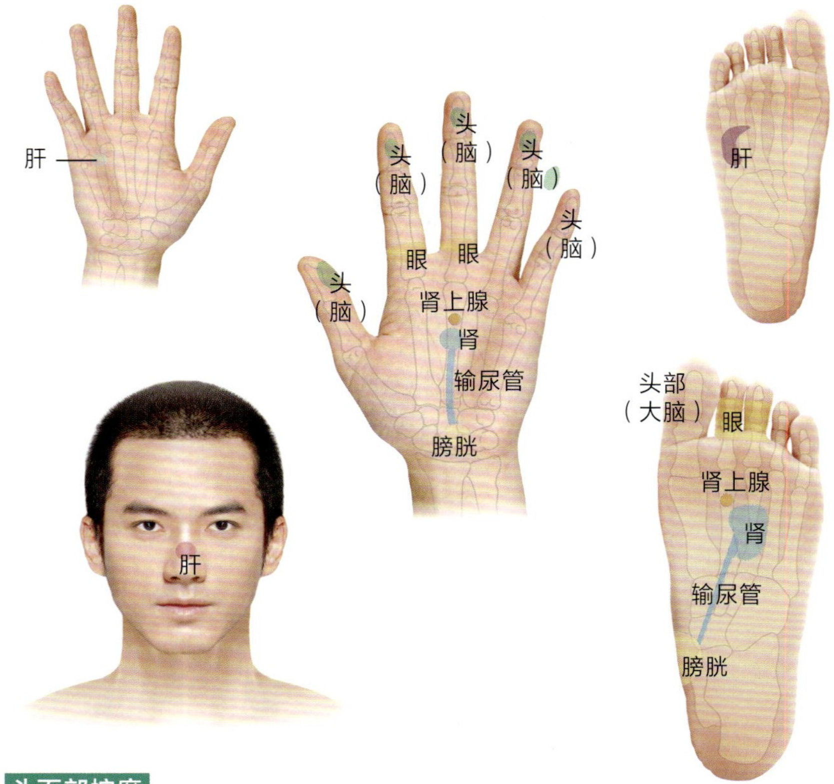

头面部按摩

1. 用工具如铅笔点按后头部，以局部有热胀感为宜。
2. 按摩肝反射区 3~5 分钟，以局部有热胀感为宜。

手部按摩

1. 放松手部，拇指轻轻按揉头（脑）、眼、肝反射区，以局部有酸痛感为宜。
2. 食指近侧指间关节点按肾、肾上腺、输尿管、膀胱反射区各 2~3 分钟，用力均匀，力度适中。

足部按摩

1. 用工具如铅笔点按眼反射区 30~50 次，以局部有热胀感为宜。
2. 按摩头部（大脑）、肝反射区 3~5 分钟，以局部有热胀感为宜。
3. 泡脚至全脚放松后，拇指点按肾、肾上腺、输尿管、膀胱反射区。

32 乳腺增生

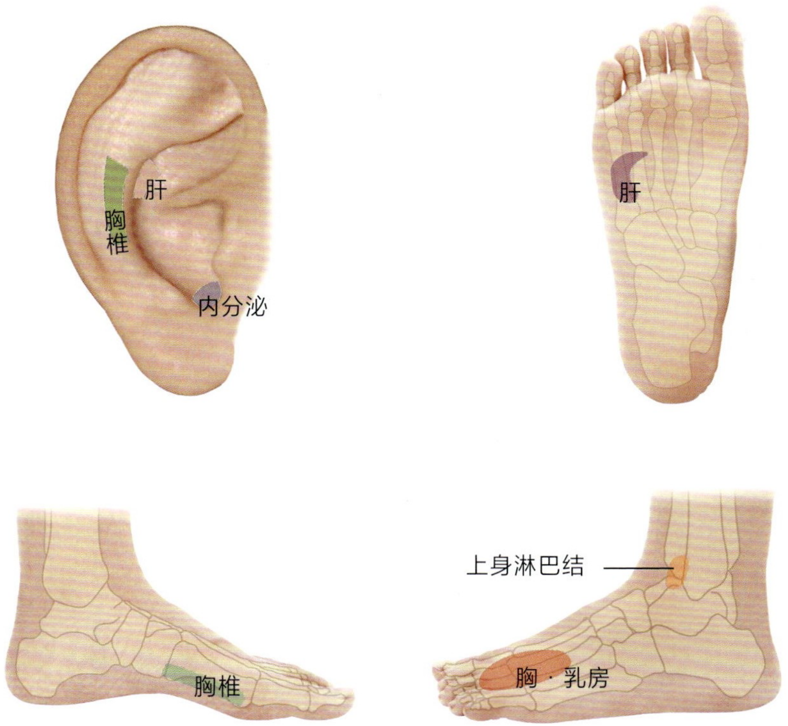

耳部按摩

1. 按摩棒揉胸椎反射区 5 分钟，压力适中，每分钟 75 次。
2. 将王不留行籽贴附于肝反射区，轻按 5 分钟，每分钟 75 次，被按摩者配合深呼吸。
3. 食指指腹按揉内分泌反射区 5 分钟，力度适中，每分钟 75 次。

足部按摩

1. 食指近侧指间关节刮压上身淋巴结反射区 2~3 分钟。
2. 泡脚至全脚放松后，掐按肝反射区 5~6 次，以局部有酸胀感为宜。
3. 食指桡侧缘刮胸椎、胸・乳房反射区各 5 分钟，以局部有酸麻胀感为宜。

31 Myopia

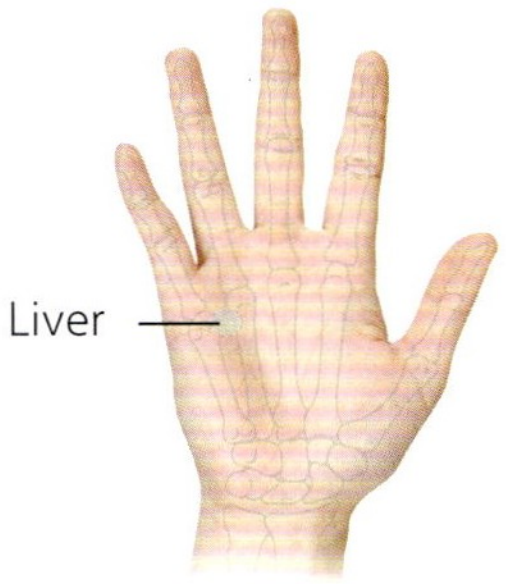

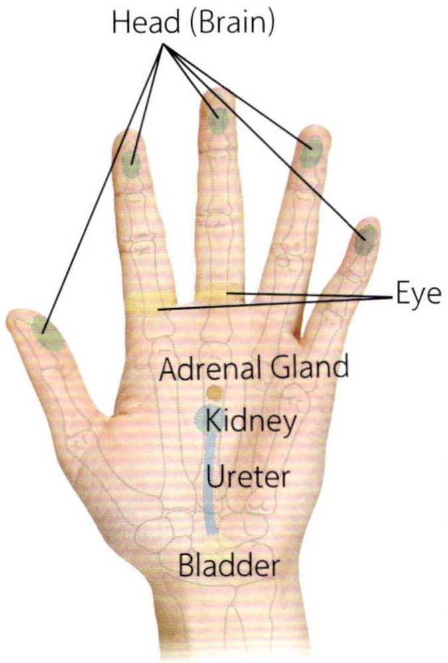

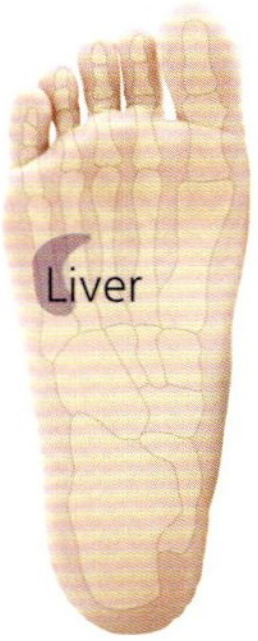

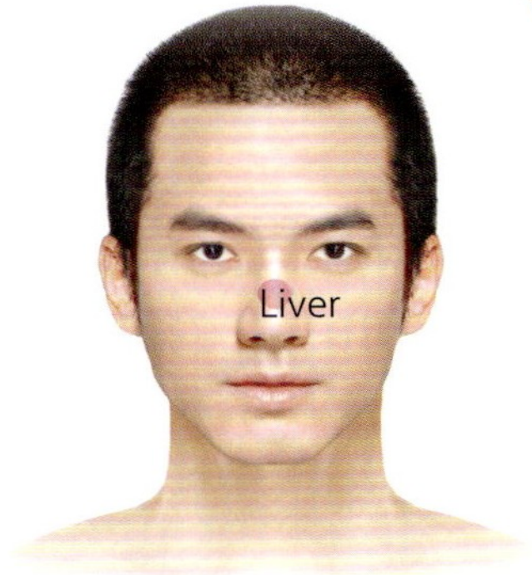

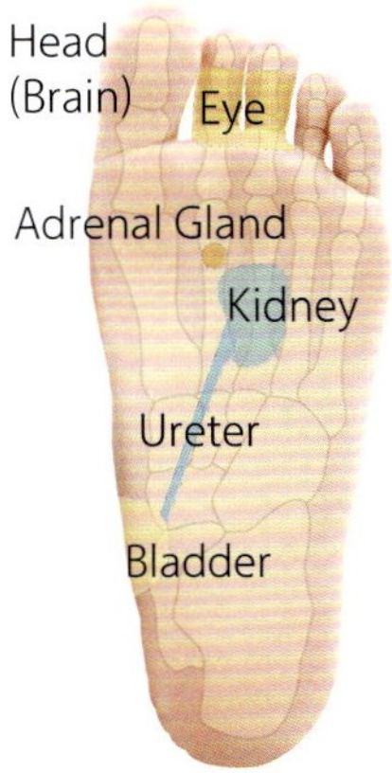

Head and Facial Massage

1. Press the reflex zones of Posterior Brain with tools like pencils and it is preferred to have a local sense of heat and distension.
2. Massage the Liver reflex zone for 3 to 5 minutes and it is preferred to have a local sense of soreness and distension.

Hand Massage

1. Relax hands and gently massage the reflex zones of Head (Brain), Eye and Liver with thumbs and it is preferred to have a local sense of aching pain.
2. Press the reflex zones of Kidney, Adrenal Gland, Ureter and Bladder each for 2 to 3 minutes with interphalangeal joint at the proximal side of index fingers in moderate strength.

Foot Massage

1. Use tools like pencils to press the Eye reflex zone for 30 to 50 times and it is preferred to have a local sense of heat and distension.
2. Massage the reflex zones of Head (Brain) and Liver for 3 to 5 minutes and it is preferred to have a local sense of heat and distension.
3. After relaxing the feet with a foot bath, massage the reflex zone of Ureter, Kidney, Adrenal Gland and Bladder with thumbs.

32 Breast Hyperplasia

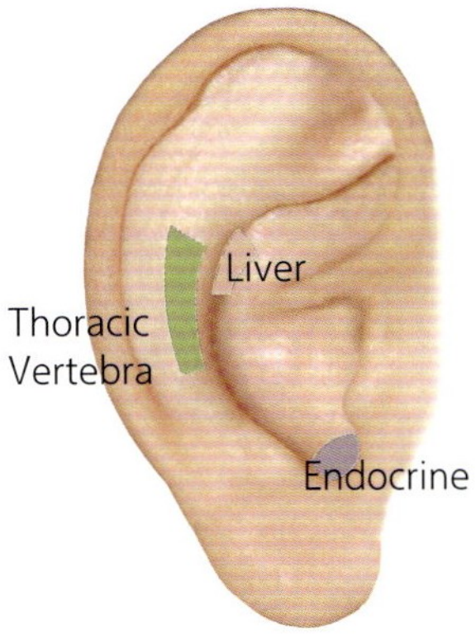

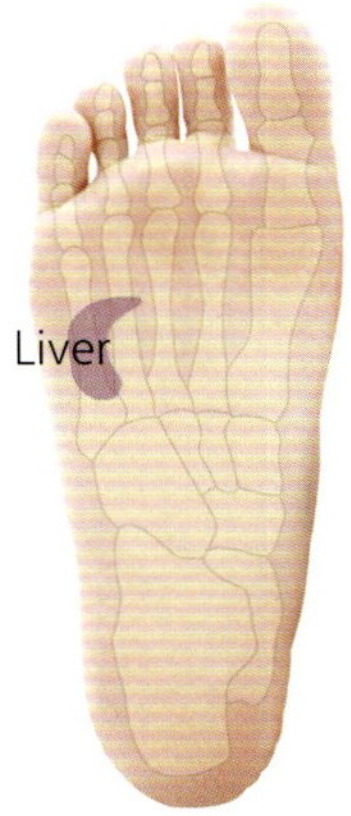

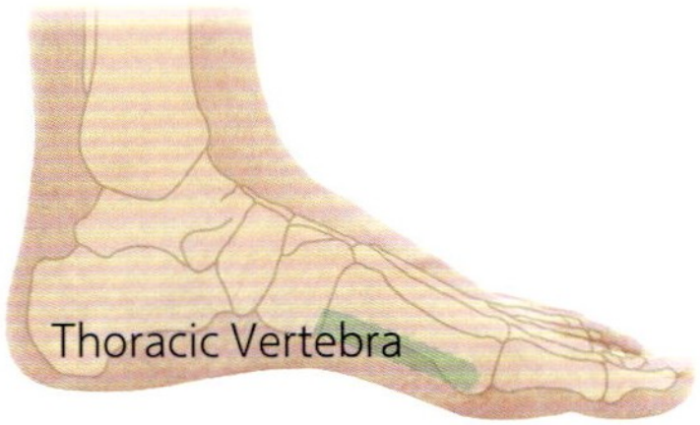

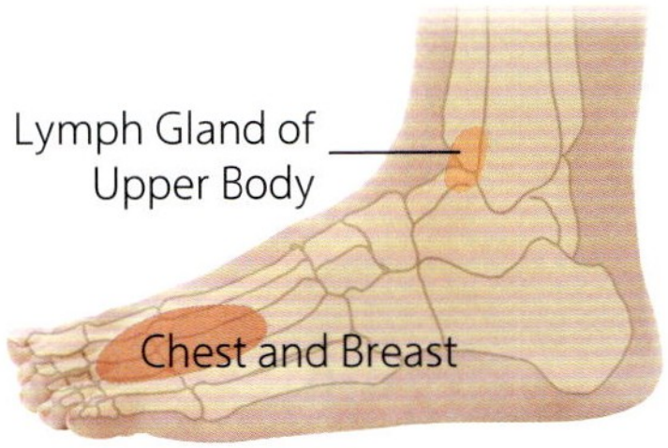

Ear Massage

1. Massage the Thoracic Vertebra reflex zone for 5 minutes with massage stick in moderate strength with 75 times in each minute.
2. Attach cowherb seed to the reflex zones of Liver and gently massage for 5 minutes with 75 times in each minute. Ask the ones being massaged to take a deep breath during the massage.
3. Massage the Endocrine reflex zone for 5 minutes with index fingers in moderate strength with 75 times in each minute.

Foot Massage

1. Scratch the reflex zone of Lymph Gland of Upper Body with interphalangeal joint at the proximal side of index fingers for 2 to 3 minutes.
2. After relaxing the feet with a foot bath, nip the Liver reflex zone for 5 to 6 times and it is preferred to have a local sense of soreness and distension.
3. Scratch the reflex zones of Thoracic Vertebra, Chest and Breast each for 5 minutes with radical margin of index fingers and it is preferred to have a local sense of soreness, numbness and distension.

33 月经不调

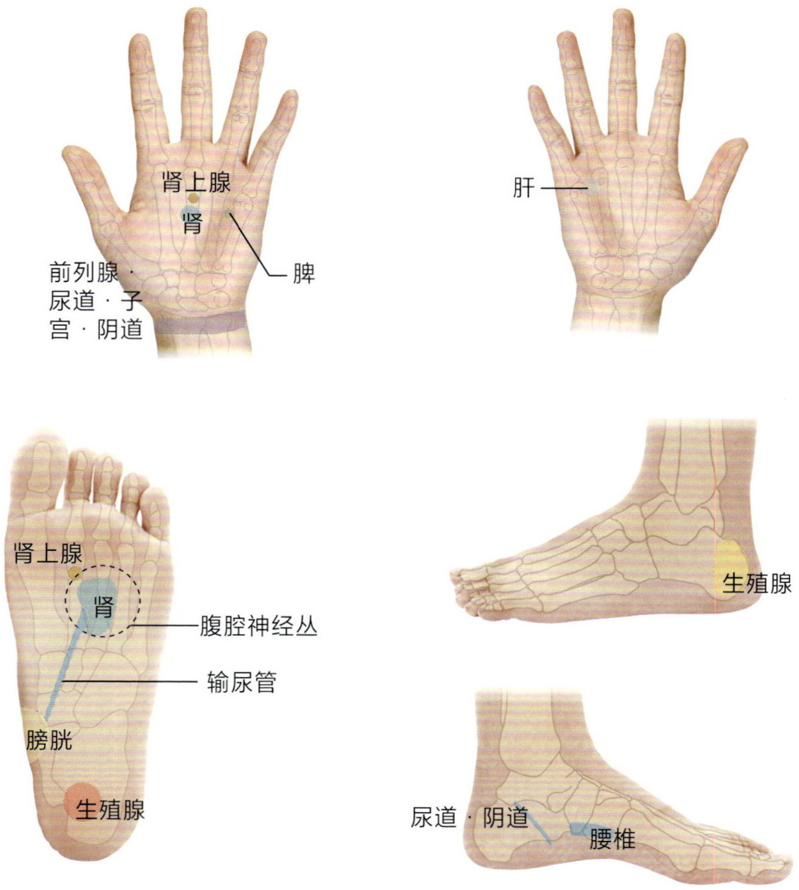

手部按摩

1. 点按或推按肾、肾上腺、肝、脾反射区各 20 次。
2. 揉掐前列腺·尿道·子宫·阴道反射区各 20 次，手法要由轻到重，再由重到轻。

足部按摩

1. 食指桡侧缘刮压腰椎、生殖腺、尿道·阴道反射区各 50 次，以局部有酸麻胀感为宜。
2. 食指近侧指间关节刮肾上腺、腹腔神经丛、肾、输尿管、膀胱反射区各 5 次。

34 痛经

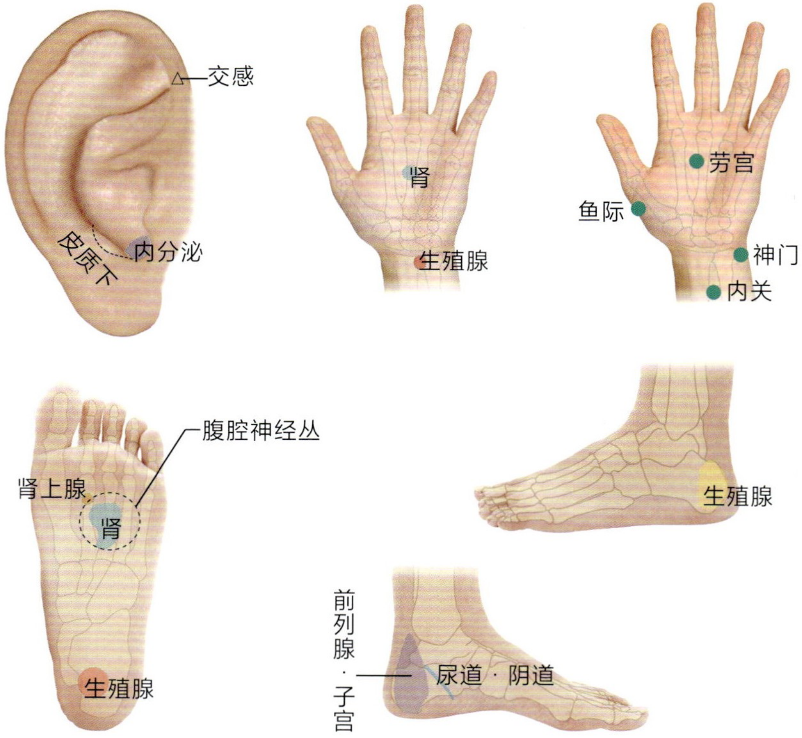

耳部按摩

1. 食指近侧指间关节按揉内分泌反射区 2 分钟，酌情用力，每分钟 75 次。
2. 将王不留行籽贴附于皮质下反射区，按揉 3 分钟，每分钟 60 次。
3. 用按摩棒揉交感反射区 3 分钟，酌情用力，每分钟 150 次。

手部按摩

1. 在肾、生殖腺反射区以重手法点、按、揉进行按摩，每个部位持续 1~3 分钟。
2. 用按摩工具推按鱼际穴 2 分钟。
3. 拇指尖揉掐神门、内关、劳宫穴各 2~3 分钟。

足部按摩

1. 双拇指推压或用电吹风吹生殖腺反射区 50 次，以局部有热胀感为宜。
2. 揉掐或推按肾上腺、腹腔神经丛、肾反射区各 3~5 次。
3. 拇指推压尿道·阴道、前列腺·子宫反射区各 20~30 次。

33 Irregular Menstruation

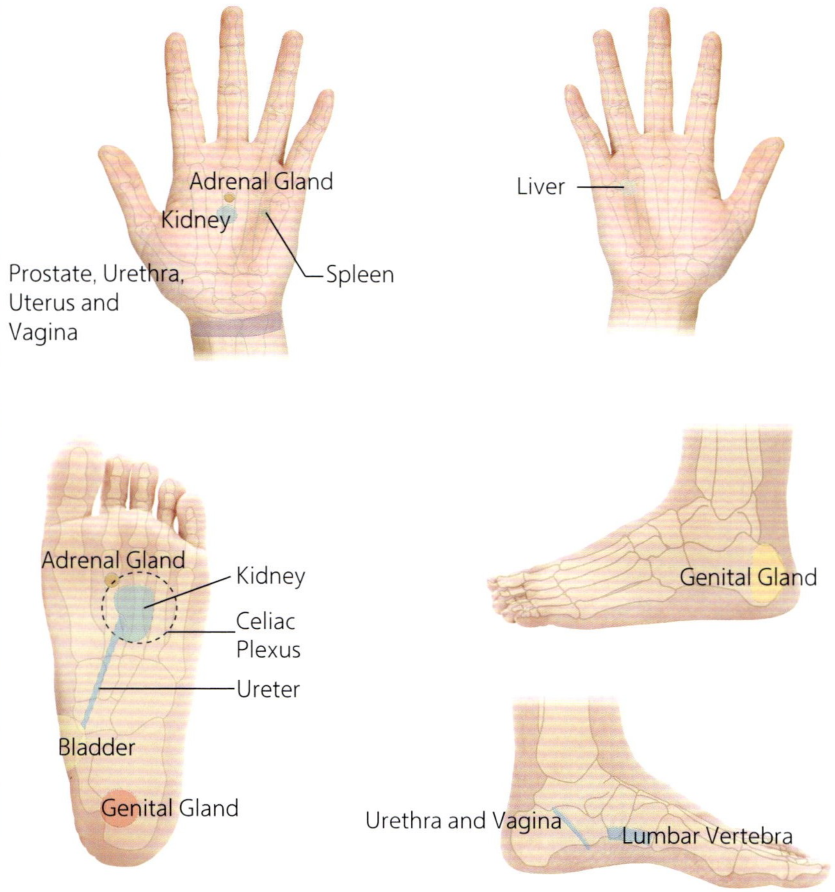

Hand Massage

1. Press or press the reflex zones of Kidney, Adrenal Gland, Liver and Spleen each for 20 times.
2. Nip the reflex zones of Prostate, Urethra, Uterus and Vagina each for 20 times with strength from slight to heavy and then heavy to slight.

Foot Massage

1. Scratch the reflex zones of Lumbar Vertebra, Genital Gland, Urethra and Vagina each for 50 times with radical margin of index fingers and it is preferred to have a local sense of soreness, numbness and distension.
2. Scratch the reflex zones of Adrenal Gland, Celiac Plexus, Kidney, Bladder and Ureter each for 5 times with interphalangeal joint at the proximal side of index fingers.

34 Dysmenorrhea

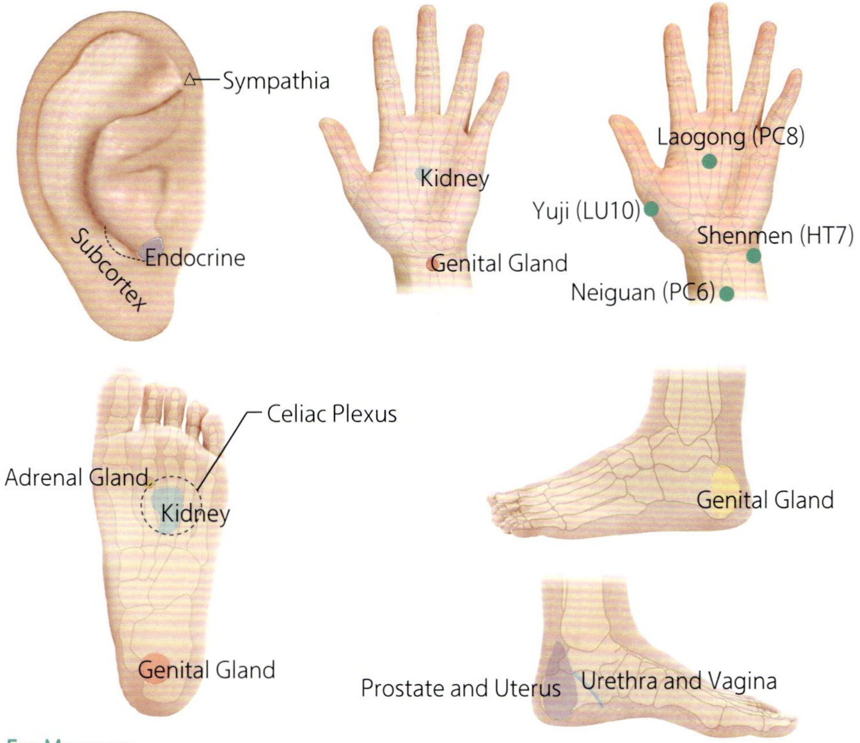

Ear Massage

1. Massage the Endocrine reflex zone for 2 minutes with interphalangeal joint at the proximal side of index fingers in moderate strength. It covers 75 times in each minute.
2. Attach cowherb seed to the subcortex reflex zone and massage for 3 minutes with 60 times in each minute.
3. Massage the Sympathetic reflex zone with massage stick in moderate strength with 150 times in each minute.

Hand Massage

1. Press or press the reflex zones of Kidney and Genital Gland with great pressure each for 1 to 3 minutes.
2. Press the acupoint of Yuji (LU10) with massage tools for 2 minutes.
3. Nip the Shenmen (HT7), Neiguan (PC6) and Laogong (PC8) with thumb tips.

Foot Massage

1. Press with 2 thumbs or blow with a electric hair drier the Genital Gland reflex zone for 50 times and it is preferred to have a local sense of heat and distension.
2. Nip or press the reflex zones of Adrenal Gland, Celiac Plexus and Kidney each for 3 to 5 minutes.
3. Press the Urethra, Vagina, Genital Gland and Uterus reflex zones each for 20 to 30 times.

35 围绝经期综合征

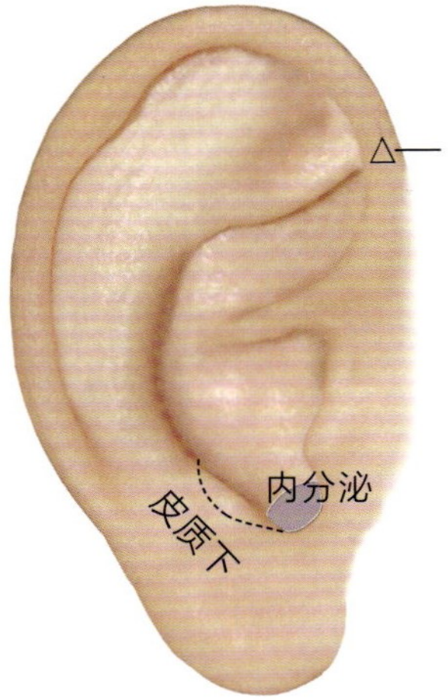

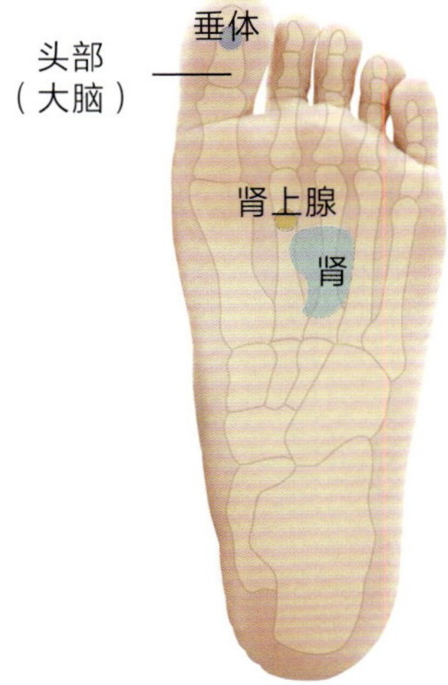

耳部按摩

1. 用按摩棒稍用力按内分泌反射区 3 分钟，每分钟 60 次。
2. 拇指指腹按揉皮质下反射区 3 分钟，力度适中，每分钟 75 次。
3. 将王不留行籽贴附于交感反射区，点按 3 分钟，每分钟 90 次。

足部按摩

1. 泡脚至全脚放松后，按摩肾、肾上腺反射区，以局部有轻度胀痛感为宜。
2. 用工具如铅笔点按头部（大脑）、垂体反射区各 30 次。

36 阳痿

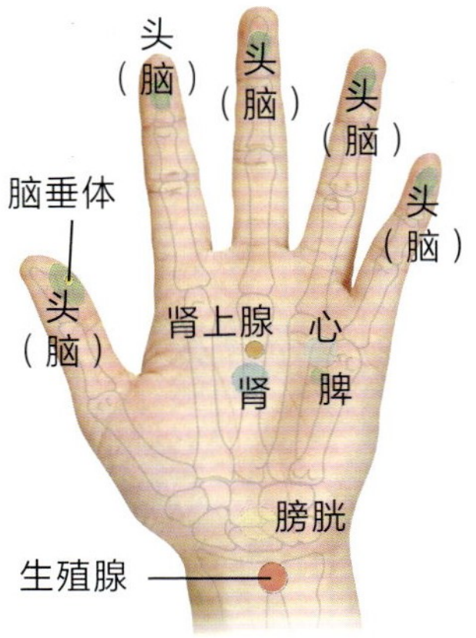

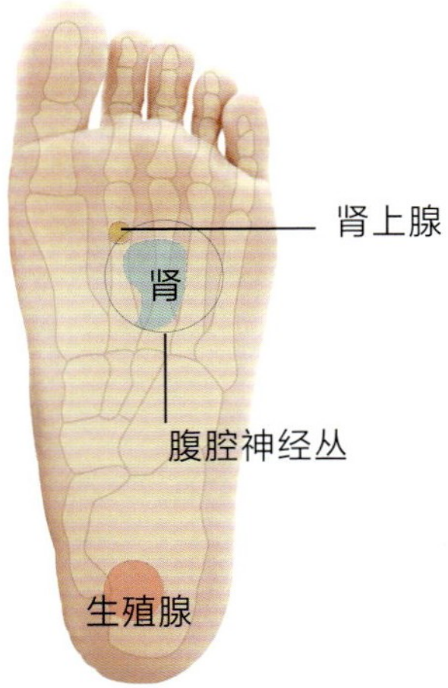

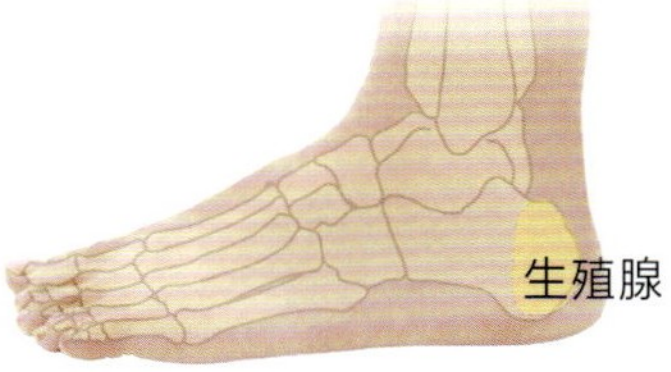

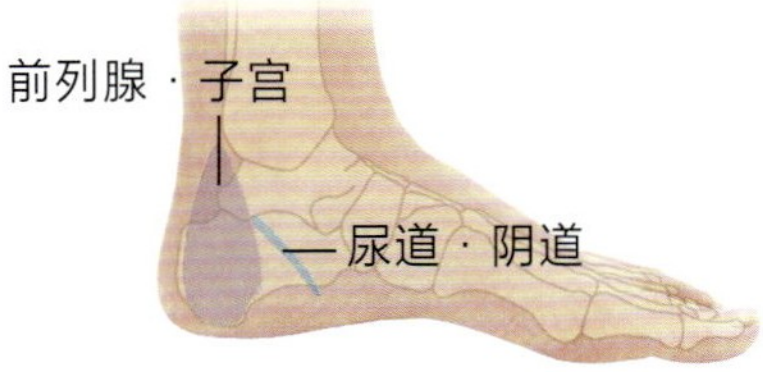

手部按摩

1. 食指近侧指间关节按揉头（脑）、脑垂体、肾、心、脾反射区各 10 次。
2. 揉掐或推按生殖腺反射区 10 次。
3. 揉掐或推按肾上腺、肾、膀胱反射区各 5 分钟，每分钟 20~30 次。

足部按摩

1. 食指桡侧缘刮压生殖腺、前列腺·子宫、尿道·阴道反射区各 50 次，以局部有酸麻胀感为宜。
2. 按摩肾上腺、肾反射区各 2 分钟。
3. 食指指尖推压腹腔神经丛反射区 10 次。

35 Perimenopausal Syndrome

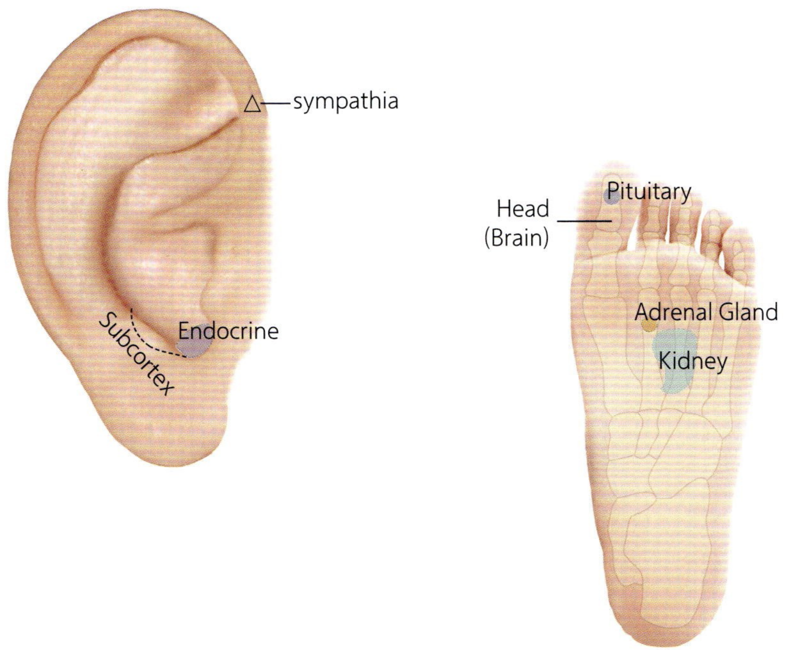

Ear Massage

1. Press hard on the Endocrine reflex zone with massage stick for 3 minutes with 60 times in each minute.
2. Massage the Subcortex reflex zone with thumbs for 3 minutes in moderate strength with 75 times in each minute.
3. Attach cowherb seed to the Sympathetic reflex zone and press for 3 minutes with 90 times in each minute.

Foot Massage

1. After having overall relaxation with a foot bath, massage the reflex zones of Kidney and Adrenal Gland and it is preferred to have a slight distending pain.
2. Press the reflex zones of Head (Brain) and Pituitary each for 30 times with tools like pencils.

36 Impotence

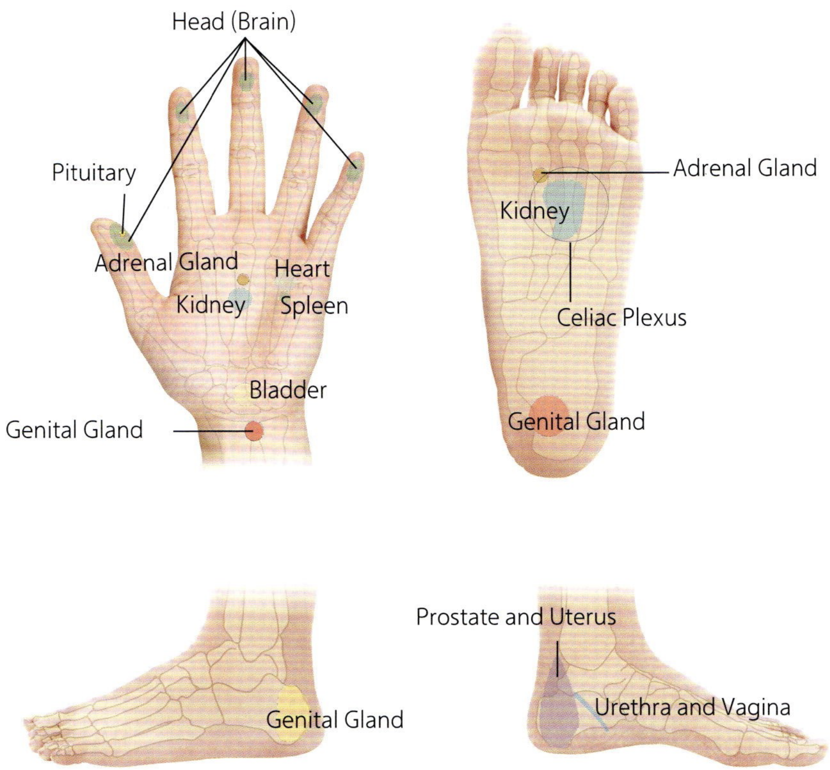

Hand Massage

1. Massage the reflex zones of Head (Brain), Pituitary Gland, Heart and Spleen each for 10 times with interphalangeal joint at the proximal side of index fingers.
2. Nip or press the Genital Gland reflex zone for 10 times.
3. Nip or press the reflex zones of Adrenal Gland, Kidney and Bladder each for 5 minutes with 20 to 30 times in each minute.

Foot Massage

1. Scratch the reflex zones of Genital Gland, Prostate, Uterus, Vagina and Urethra with radical margin of index fingers and it is preferred to have local sense of soreness, numbness and distension.
2. Massage the reflex zones of Adrenal Gland and Kidney each for 2 minutes.
3. Press the Celiac Plexus reflex zone with the tip of index fingers for 10 times.

37 早泄

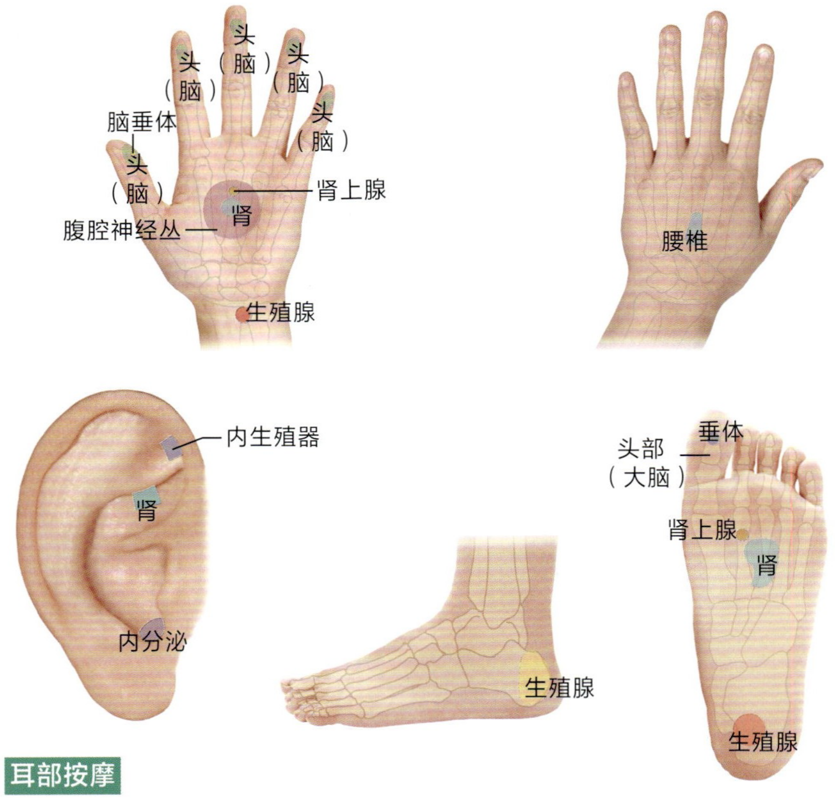

耳部按摩

1. 按摩棒揉内生殖器反射区 3 分钟，压力适中，每分钟 60 次。
2. 按摩棒推肾、内分泌反射区各 4 分钟，压力稍轻，每分钟 75 次。

手部按摩

1. 点按生殖腺、头（脑）、脑垂体反射区各 20 次，以被按摩者能耐受为度。
2. 放松手部，拇指轻轻按揉腰椎反射区 10 次。
3. 食指近侧指间关节点按肾上腺、腹腔神经丛、肾反射区各 5 次，用力均匀，力度适中。

足部按摩

1. 泡脚至全脚放松后操作，按摩生殖腺、肾上腺、肾反射区各 2 分钟，以局部有酸胀感为宜。
2. 拇指指腹按揉头部（大脑）、垂体反射区各 5 分钟。

38 遗精

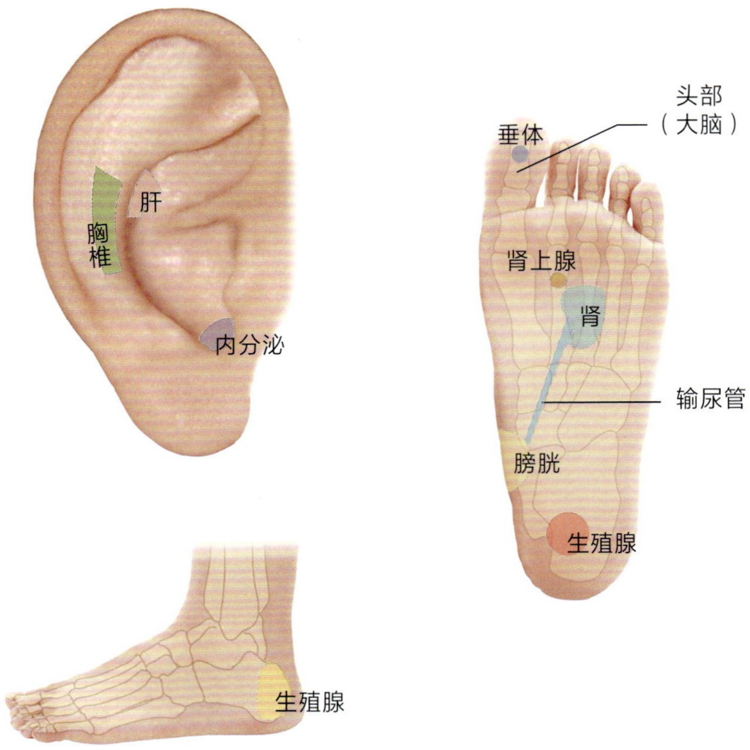

耳部按摩

1. 按摩棒揉胸椎反射区 5 分钟，压力适中，每分钟 75 次。
2. 将王不留行籽贴附于肝反射区，轻按 5 分钟，每分钟 75 次，被按摩者配合深呼吸。
3. 拇指指腹按揉内分泌反射区 5 分钟，力度适中，每分钟 75 次。

足部按摩

1. 食指桡侧缘刮生殖腺反射区 5 分钟，以局部有酸麻胀感为宜。
2. 泡脚至全脚放松后，按摩头部（大脑）、垂体反射区各 2 分钟，以局部有酸胀感为宜。
3. 食指近侧指间关节刮压肾上腺、肾、输尿管、膀胱反射区各 2~3 分钟。

37 Prospermia

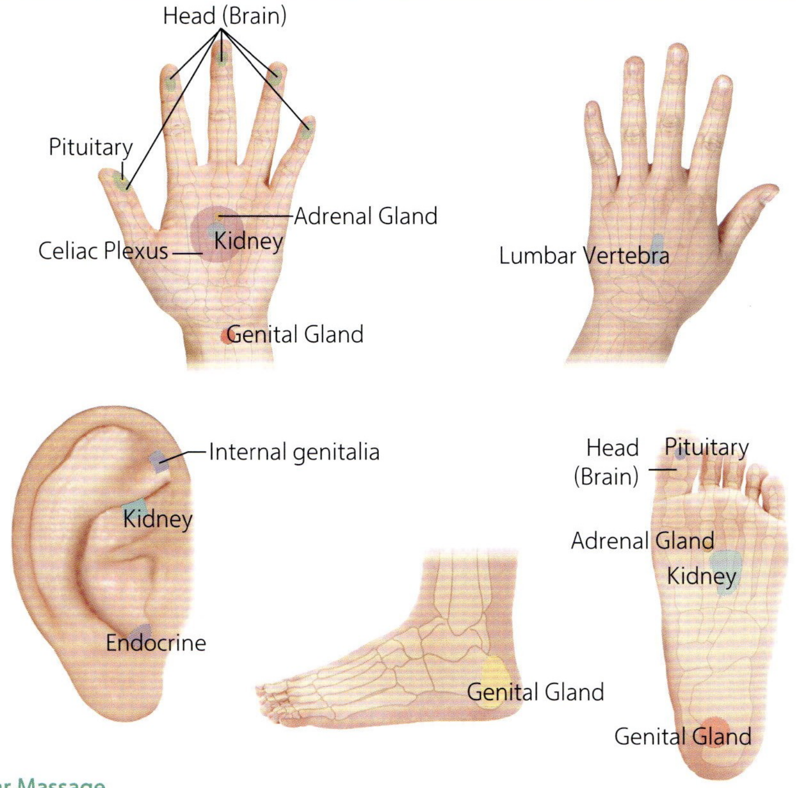

Ear Massage

1. Massage the Internal Genitalia reflex zone for 3 minutes with massage stick with moderate pressure in 60 times per minute.
2. Press the Kidney and Endocrine reflex zones each for 4 minutes with slight pressure in 75 times per minute.

Hand Massage

1. Press the reflex zones of Genital Gland, Head (Brain) and Pituitary Gland each for 30 times taking the tolerance degree of the ones being massaged into consideration.
2. Relax hands and gently massage the Lumbar Vertebra reflex zone with thumbs for 10 times.
3. Press the reflex zones of Adrenal Gland, Celiac Plexus and Kidney with interphalangeal joint at the proximal side of index fingers each for 5 times in moderate strength.

Foot Massage

1. After having overall relaxation with a foot bath, massage the reflex zones of Genital Gland, Adrenal Gland and Kidney each for 2 minutes and it is preferred to have a local sense of soreness and distension.
2. Massage the reflex zones of Head (Brain) and Pituitary each for 5 minutes with thumbs.

38 Spermatorrhea

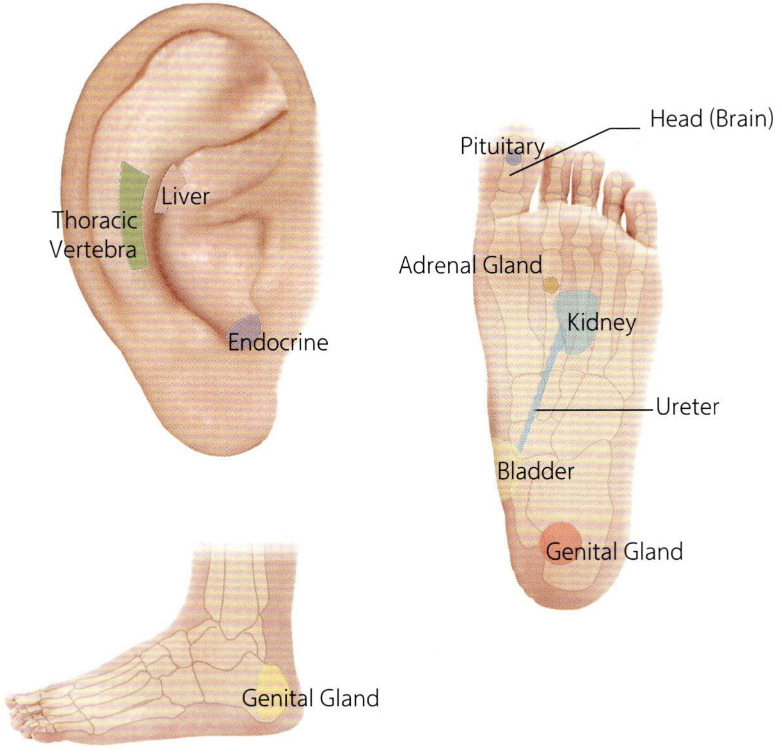

Ear Massage

1. Massage the Thoracic Vertebra reflex zone for 5 minutes with massage sticks in moderated strength with 75 times in each minute.
2. Attach cowherb seed to Liver reflex zone and slightly massage for 5 minutes with 75 times in each minute.
3. Massage the Endocrine reflex zone with thumbs for 5 minutes in moderate strength with 75 times in each minute.

Foot Massage

1. Scratch the Genital Gland reflex zone for 5 minutes with the radical margin of index fingers and it is preferred to have a local sense of soreness, numbness and distension.
2. After having overall relaxation with a foot bath, massage the reflex zones of Head (Brain) and Pituitary each for 2 minutes and it is preferred to have a local sense of soreness and distension.
3. Scratch the reflex zones of Adrenal Gland, Kidney, Ureter and Bladder with interphalangeal joint at the proximal side of index fingers each for 2 to 3 minutes.

39 前列腺炎

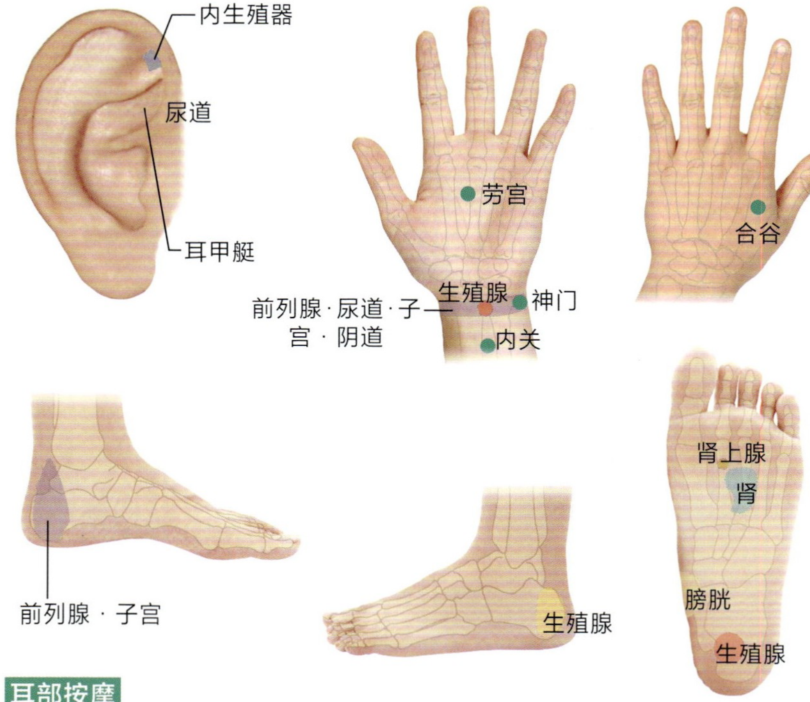

耳部按摩

1. 按摩棒揉内生殖器反射区 3 分钟，每分钟 75 次。
2. 食指指腹按揉尿道反射区 3 分钟，力度适中，每分钟 75 次。
3. 指揉耳甲艇部 3 分钟，酌情用力，每分钟 75 次。

手部按摩

1. 揉掐或推按前列腺·尿道·子宫·阴道、生殖腺反射区各 20~30 次，每分钟 30~60 次。以局部有热胀感为宜，手法连贯、均匀、柔和，要由轻到重，再由重到轻，逐渐渗透。
2. 点按合谷、神门、劳宫、内关穴各 2 分钟。

足部按摩

1. 食指近侧指间关节点按前列腺·子宫、生殖腺反射区各 5 分钟，用力均匀，力度适中。
2. 点按肾、膀胱反射区，力度以被按摩者耐受为度，以局部有酸胀感为宜。
3. 手指搓擦肾上腺反射区 30 次，以足有透热感为宜。

40 落枕

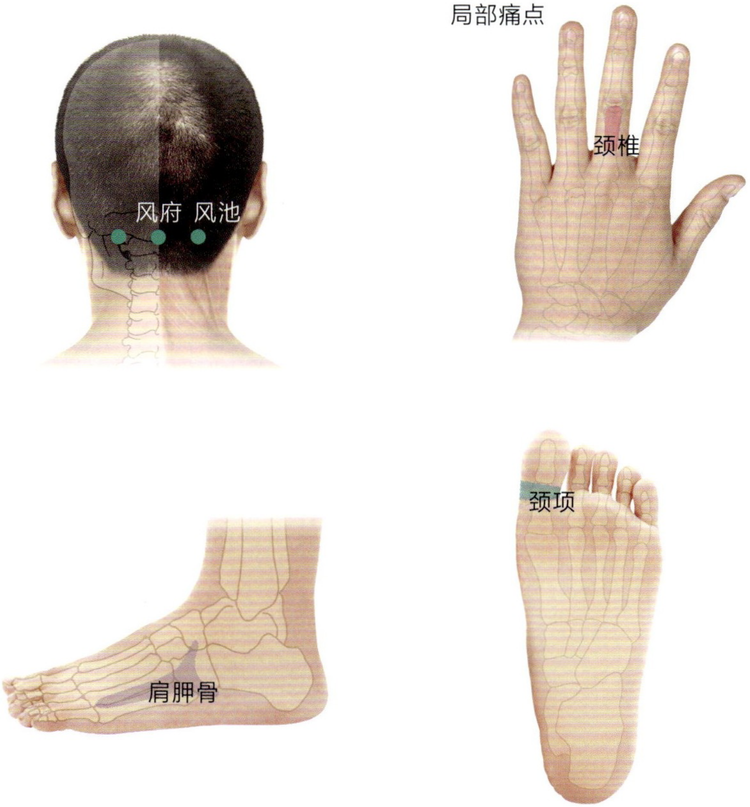

头面部按摩

1. 拇指重叠稍用力按压风池穴 5~6 次，每次停留片刻后放松。同法按压对侧风池穴。
2. 拇指指腹按揉风府穴和局部痛点各 2 分钟，力度适宜。

手部按摩

拇指从上到下推压颈椎反射区 5~7 次。

足部按摩

1. 手握住脚板固定，摇转足拇趾 10 次，顺时针和逆时针方向交替进行。
2. 拇指按压颈项反射区 10 次，由足小趾侧向足拇趾侧推压。
3. 双手拇指指腹从脚趾至脚跟方向推压肩胛骨反射区 5~7 次，以透热为度。

39 Prostatitis

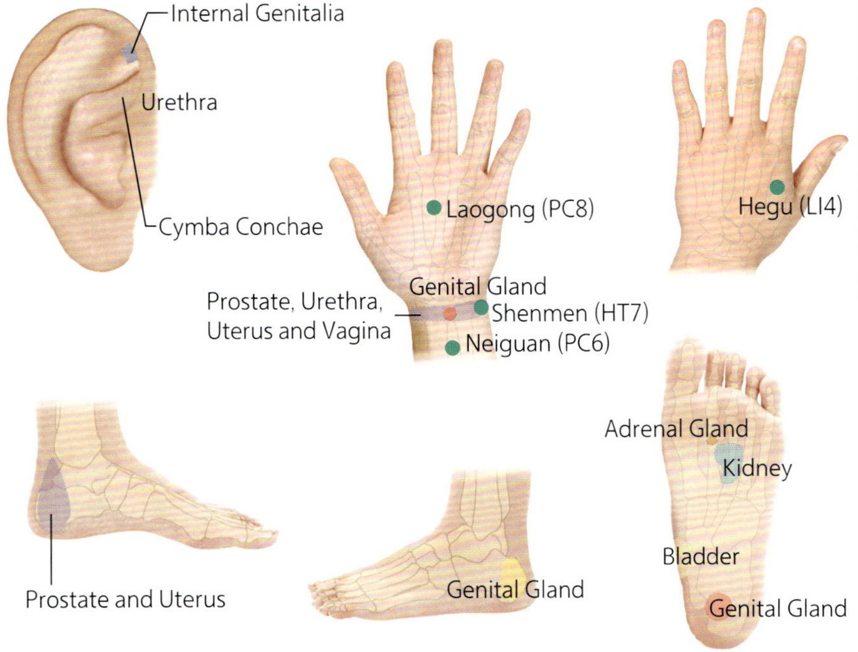

Ear Massage

1. Massage Internal Genitalia reflex zone for 3 minutes with massage stick in 75 times a minute.
2. Massage the Urethra reflex zone with index fingers for 3 minutes in moderate strength with 75 times in each minute.
3. Massage the cymba conchae for 3 minutes in appropriate strength with 75 times in each minute.

Hand Massage

1. Nip or press the reflex zones of Prostate, Urethra, Uterus, Vagina and Genital Gland each for 20 to 30 times in 30 to 60 times per minute and it is preferred to have a local sense of heat and distension. The manipulation is supposed to be coherent and gentle with strength from slight to heavy and then heavy back to slight.
2. Press the acupoints of Hegu (LI4), Shenmen (HT7), Laogong (PC8) and Neiguan (PC6) each for 2 minutes.

Foot Massage

1. Press the reflex zones of Prostate, Uterus and Genital Gland each for 5 minutes with interphalangeal joint at the proximal side of index fingers each for 5 minutes in moderate strength.
2. Press the Kidney and Bladder reflex zones and the strength should refer to the tolerance degree of the ones being massaged. It is preferred to have a local sense of soreness and distension.
3. Rub the Adrenal Gland reflex zone for 30 times with fingers until there is clear heat.

40 Stiff Neck

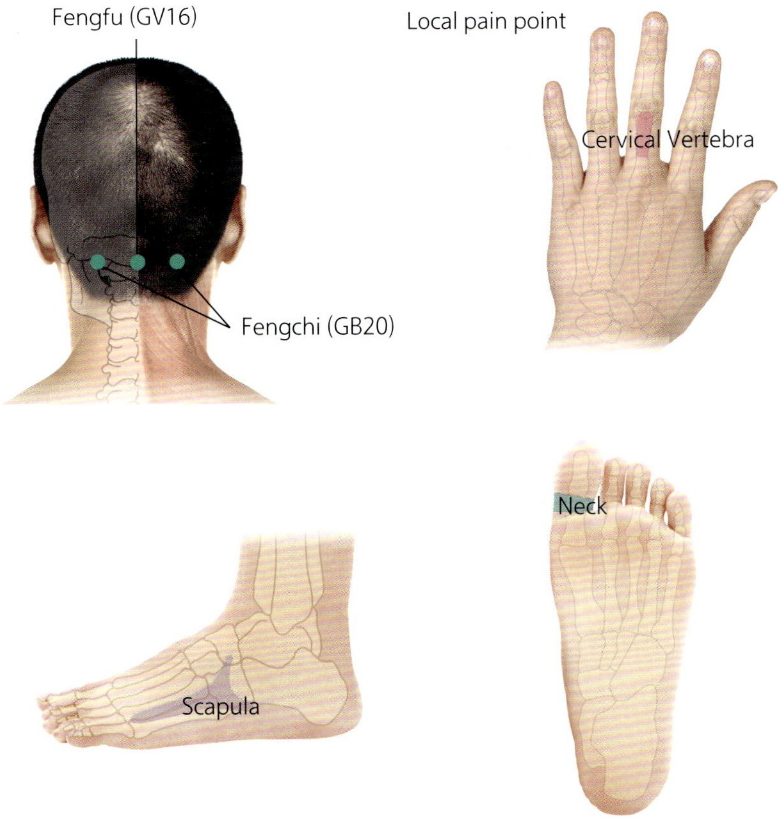

Head and Facial Massage

1. Use overlapped thumbs to press hard on Fengchi (GB20) and relax after each short stay. Apply the same manipulation to the opposite.
2. Massage Fengfu (GV16) and local pain points each for 2 minutes with thumbs in moderate strength.

Hand Massage

Press and press Cervical Vertebra reflex zone from top to bottom with thumbs.

Foot Massage

1. Fix the feet with hands and twist toes for 10 times alternately clockwise and anticlockwise.
2. Press the Neck reflex zone for 10 times with thumbs from the big toe to the little one.
3. Use 2 thumbs to press the Scapula reflex zone for 5 to 7 times from toes to heels with appropriate heat sensation.

41 颈椎病

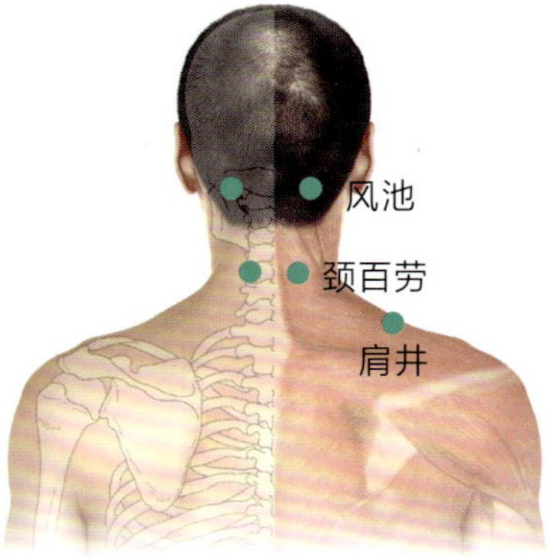

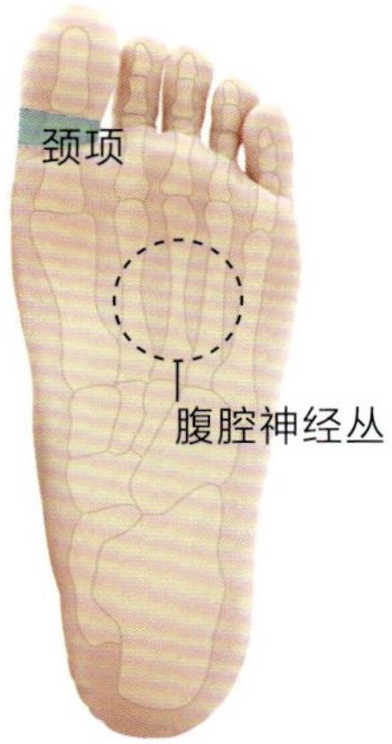

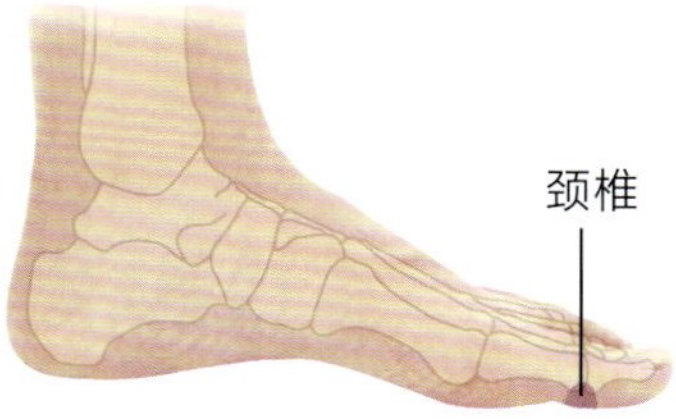

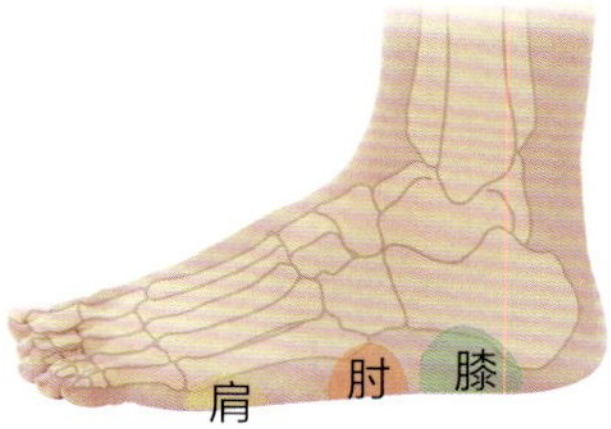

头面部按摩

两手食指、中指并拢按揉两侧风池穴，力度稍重，每次停留片刻后放松。

脊背按摩

1. 两手拇指交叉按揉肩井穴 5~6 次，每次停留片刻后放松。同法按压对侧肩井穴。
2. 拇指指腹按揉颈百劳穴 2 分钟，力度适宜。

足部按摩

1. 点按颈椎、颈项反射区各 5~10 次，按摩力度以局部胀痛为宜。
2. 食指推压或以双指钳按摩肩、肘、膝反射区各 10~20 次。
3. 食指刮压或拇指推压腹腔神经丛反射区 3~5 次。

42 肩周炎

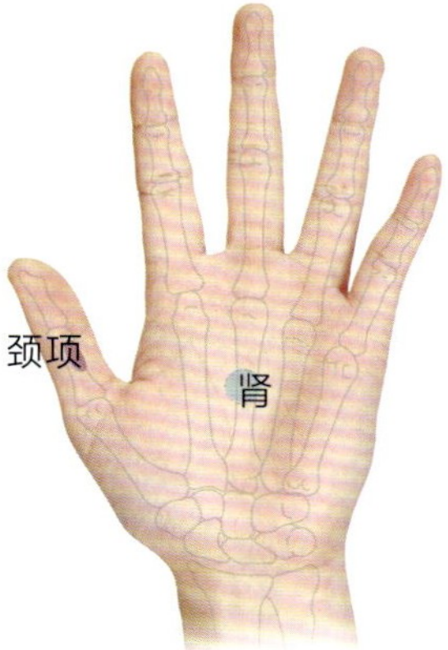

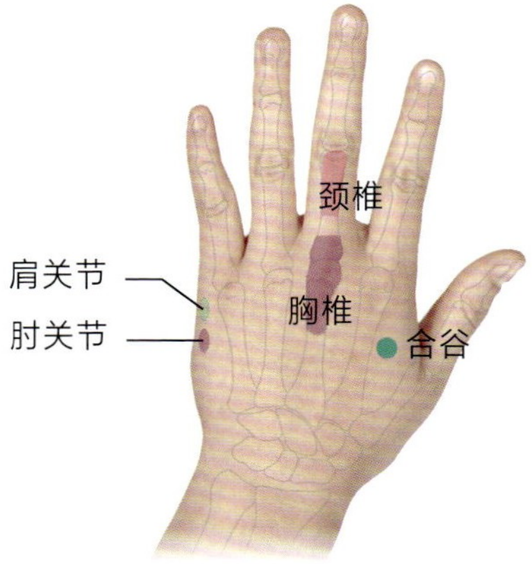

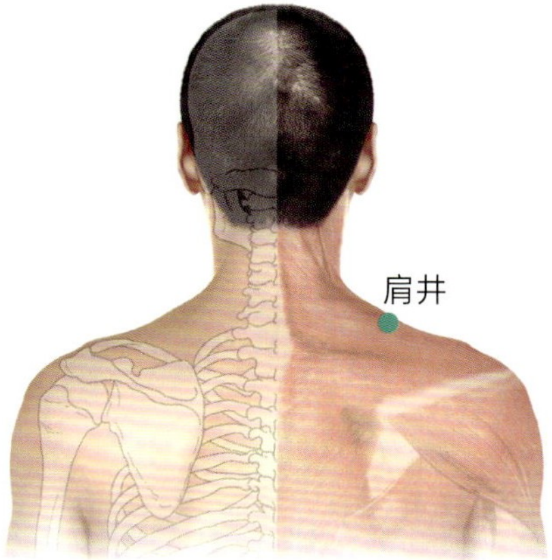

脊背按摩

1. 两手拇指交叉按揉肩井穴 5~6 次，每次停留片刻后放松。
2. 拇指指腹按揉肩关节周围痛点 2 分钟，力度适宜，边按边活动肩关节。

手部按摩

1. 用中等力度点按合谷穴，每穴 1~2 分钟，以局部有酸麻感为宜。
2. 点按后推按肩关节、肘关节、肾、颈项、颈椎、胸椎反射区各 1~2 分钟。

41 Cervical Spondylopathy

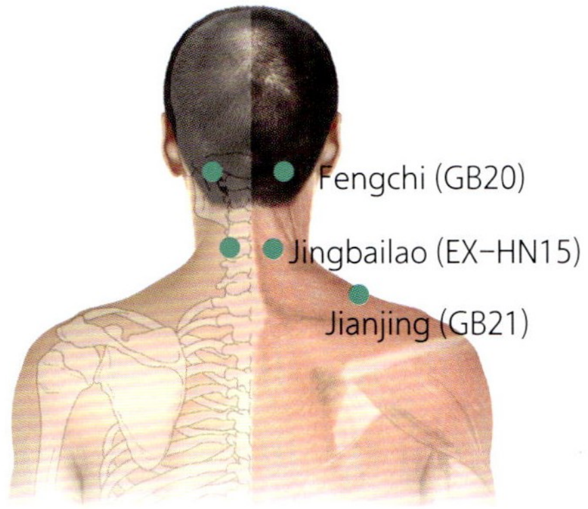

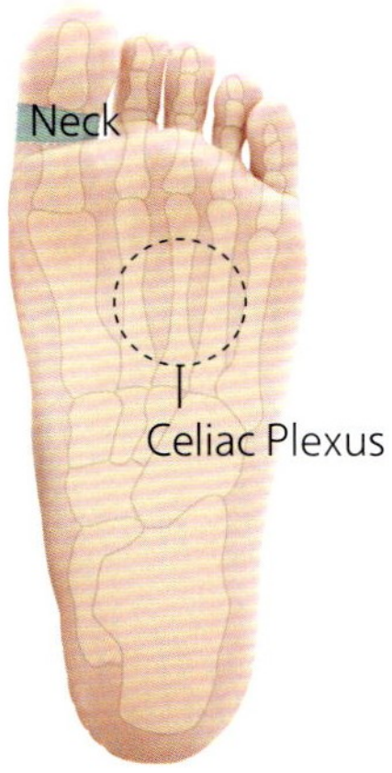

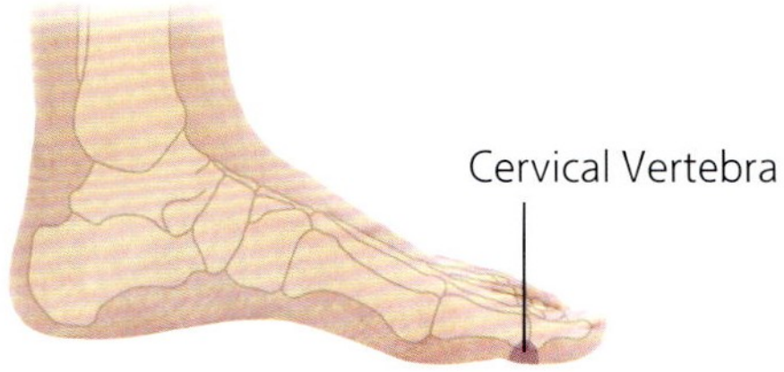

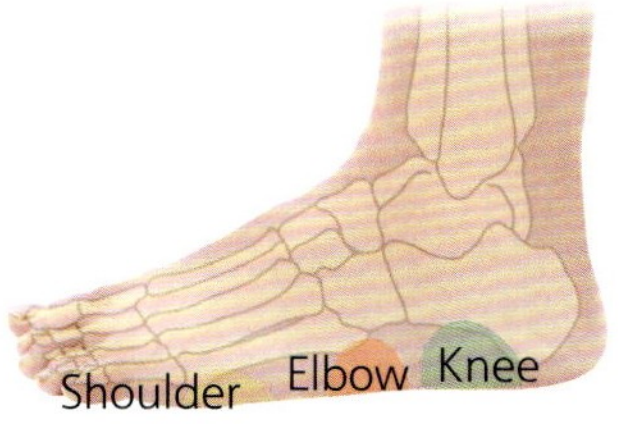

Head and Facial Massage

Fold 2 index fingers and 2 middle fingers to massage Fengchi (GB 20) on both sides with a little pressure and relax after each short stay.

Back Massage

1. Cross 2 thumbs to massage Jianjing (GB21) and relax after each stay. Apply the same manipulation on the opposite Jianjing (GB21).
2. Massage Jingbailao (EX-HN15) with thumbs in moderate strength.

Foot Massage

1. Press the reflex zones of Neck and Cervical Vertebra each for 5 to 10 times and it is appropriate to have local distending pain.
2. Press with index fingers or clamp with 2 fingers the reflex zones of Shoulder, Elbow and Knee each for 10 to 20 times.
3. Scratch with index fingers or press with thumbs the Celiac Plexus reflex zone for 3 to 5 times.

42 Shoulder Periarthritis

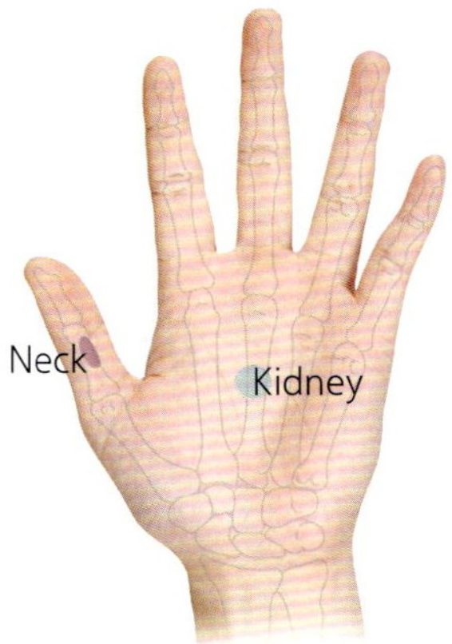

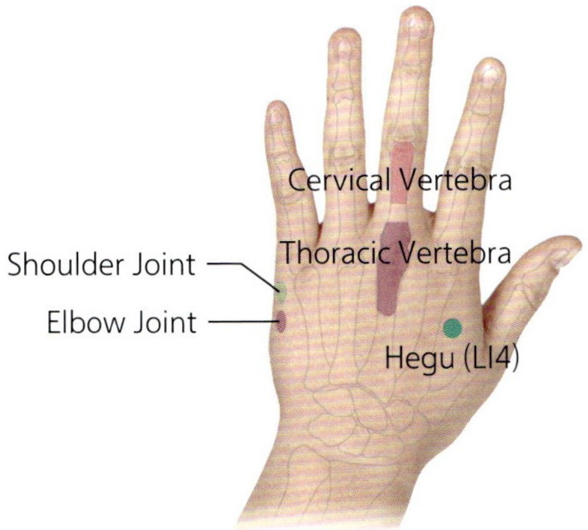

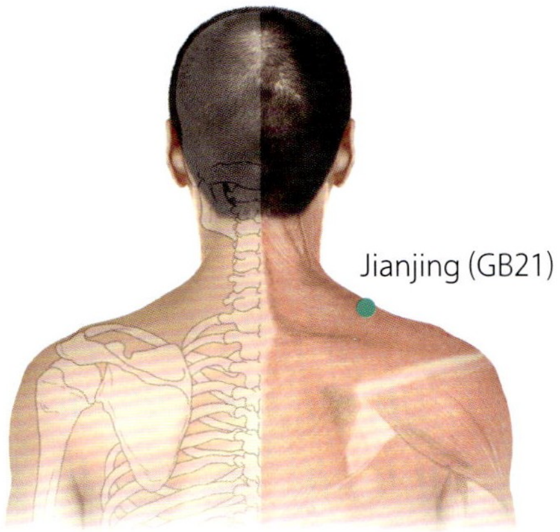

Back Massage

1. Massage the Jianjing (GB21) with folded thumbs for 5 to 6 times and relax after each short stay.
2. Massage the pain spots around shoulder joints with thumbs in moderate strength and activate the shoulder joints during the massage.

Hand Massage

1. Press the acupoints of Hegu (LI4) for 1 to 2 minutes and it is preferred to have a local sense of soreness and distension.
2. Press the reflex zones of Shoulder and Elbow Joints, Kidney, Neck, Cervical Vertebra and Thoracic Vertebra each for 1 to 2 minutes.

43 腰痛

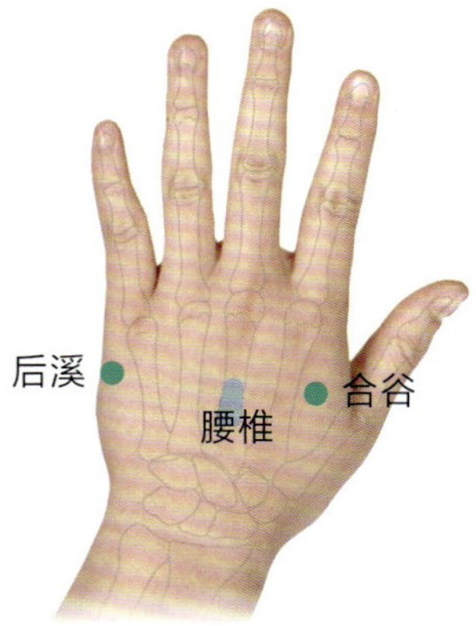

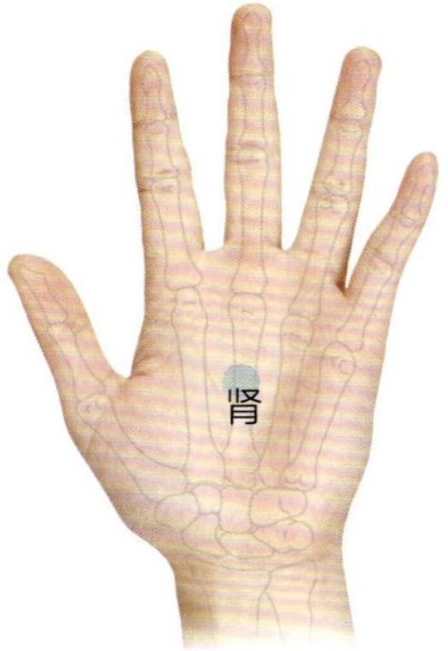

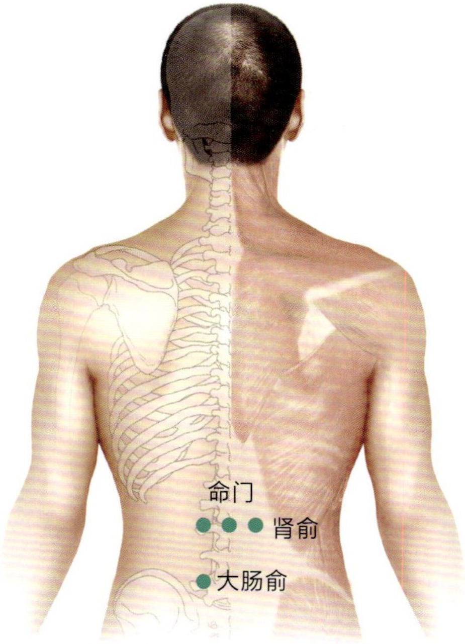

脊背按摩

1. 两手握拳绕于背后，用食指指腹稍微用力按压两侧大肠俞穴各 2 分钟，每次停留片刻后放松。
2. 两手握拳绕于背后，用关节处稍微用力按压两侧肾俞、命门穴各 2 分钟，每次停留片刻后放松。

手部按摩

1. 点按或推按肾反射区 1 分钟，以局部有胀痛感为宜。
2. 用按摩棒按揉腰椎反射区 2~3 分钟，每分钟 20~40 次。
3. 按揉合谷、后溪穴各 2~3 分钟，以局部有酸胀感为宜。

44 急性腰扭伤

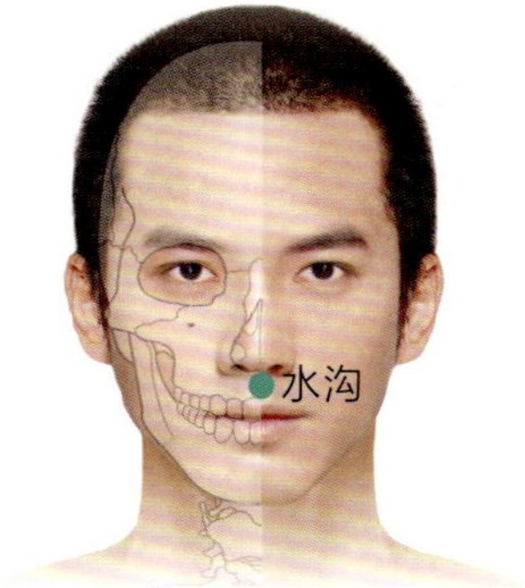

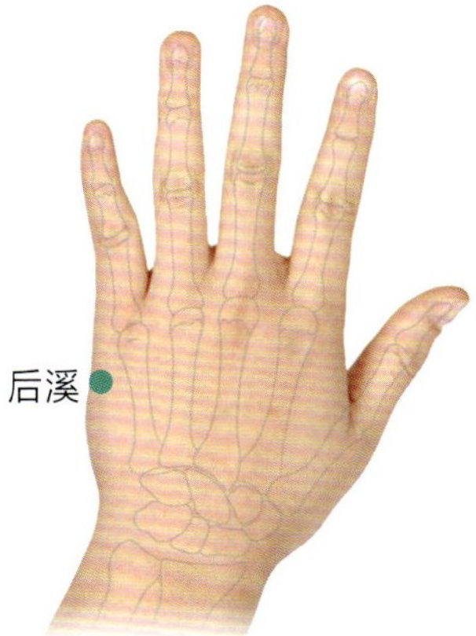

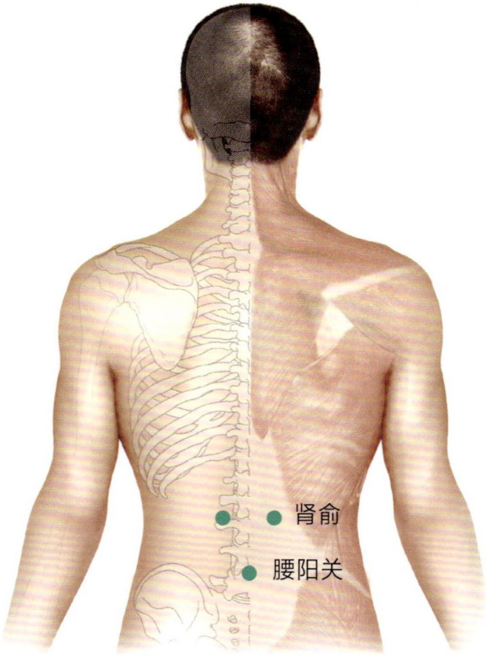

头面部按摩

拇指指甲掐按水沟穴 30 下，掐后再揉按 30 下，力度宜稍重。

脊背按摩

两手握拳绕于背后，用指关节稍微用力按压两侧肾俞、腰阳关穴各 2 分钟，每次停留片刻后放松，重复 5~6 次。

手部按摩

拇指稍用力按压后溪穴 5~6 次，每次停留片刻后放松。同法按压对侧后溪穴。

43 Lumbago

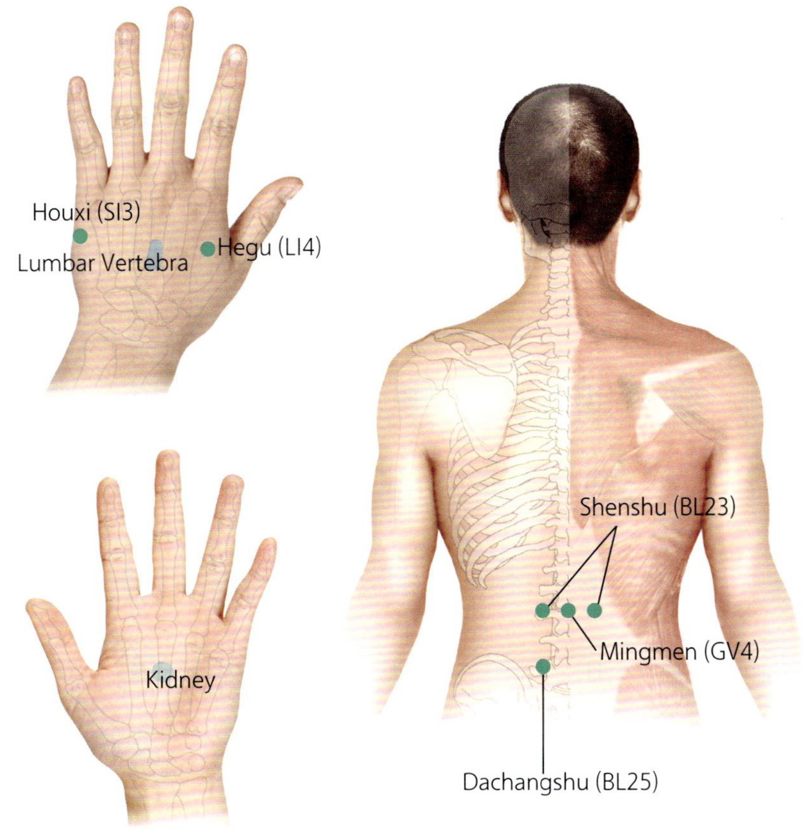

Back Massage

1. Fold the fists at the back and press Dachangshu (BL25) on both sides using index fingers with a little pressure each for 2 minutes and relax after every short manipulation.
2. Fold the fists at the back and press Shenshu (BL23) and Mingmen (GV4) on both sides using joints each for 2 minutes and relax after each short manipulation.

Hand Massage

1. Press or press the Kidney reflex zone for 1 minute with appropriate local sense of distending pain.
2. Massage the Lumbar Vertebra reflex zone for 2 to 3 minutes with massage stick in 20 to 40 times per minute.
3. Massage Hegu (LI4) and Houxi (SI3) each for 2 to 3 minutes and it is preferred to have a local sense of soreness.

44 Acute Lumbar Sprain

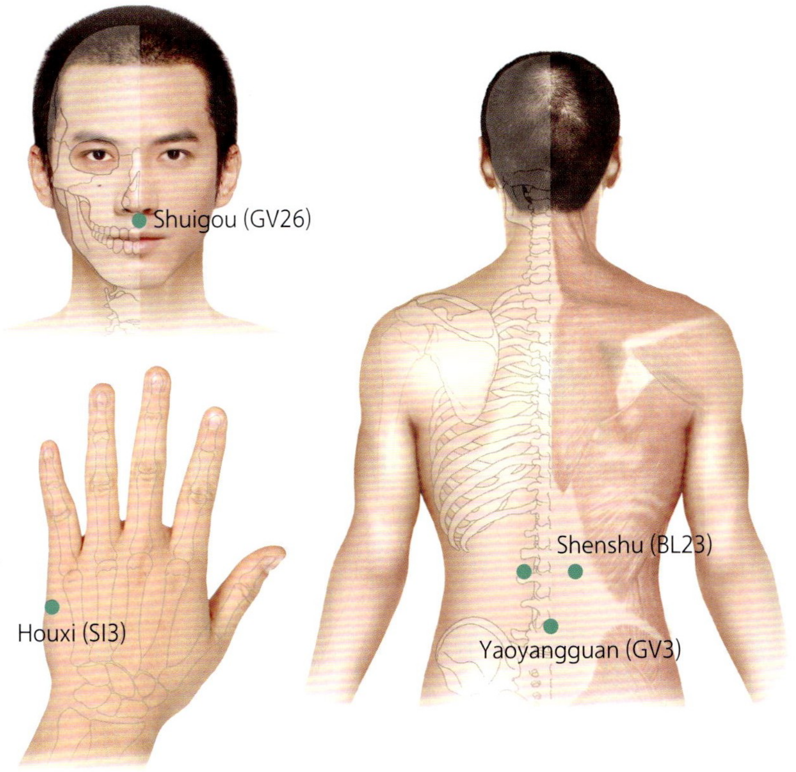

Head Facial Massage

Nip the Shuigou (GV26) with the nails of the thumbs for 30 times and then massage for 30 times with relatively heavy pressure.

Back Massage

Fold the fists at the back and press the Shenshu (BL23), Yaoyangguan (GV3) on both sides with finger joints each for 2 minutes. Relax for each short stay and repeat the massage 5 to 6 times.

Hand Massage

Press hard on Houxi (SI3) with thumbs for 5 to 6 times and relax after every short stay. Apply the same manipulation to the opposite Houxi (SI3).

45 膝关节炎

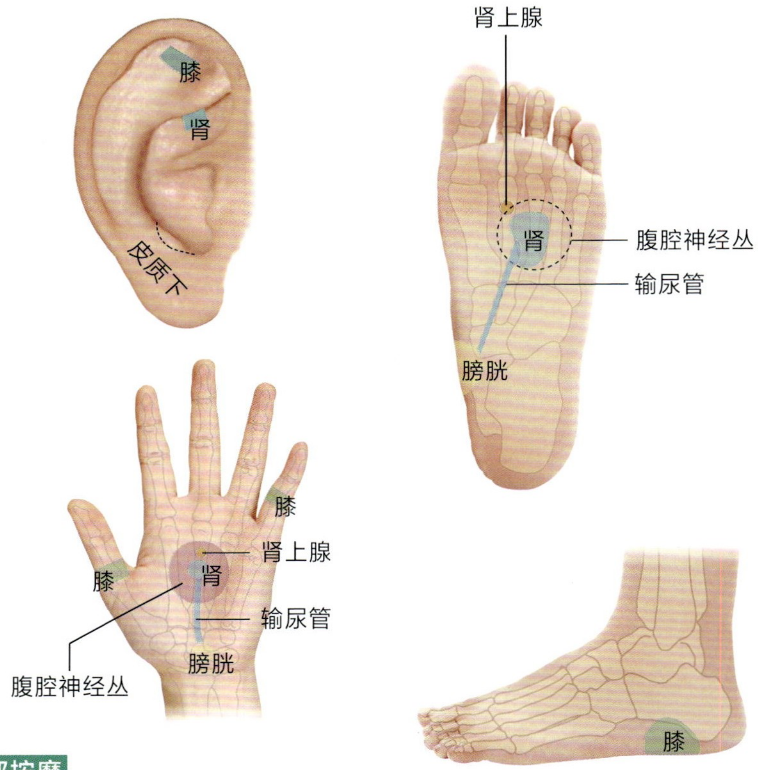

耳部按摩

1. 按摩棒推膝反射区 3 分钟，每分钟 120 次。
2. 将王不留行籽贴附于肾反射区，按压 2 分钟，每分钟 75 次。
3. 拇指指腹按揉皮质下反射区 2 分钟，力度适中，每分钟 75 次。

手部按摩

1. 食指近侧指间关节点按肾、肾上腺、输尿管、腹腔神经丛、膀胱反射区各 2~3 分钟，以局部有轻度胀痛为宜。
2. 拇指指腹点按膝关节对应的全息区，以被按摩者耐受为度。

足部按摩

1. 泡脚至全脚放松后，按摩肾、肾上腺、输尿管、腹腔神经丛、膀胱反射区，以局部有酸胀感为宜。
2. 用软毛牙刷刷膝反射区 2~3 分钟。

46 踝关节扭伤

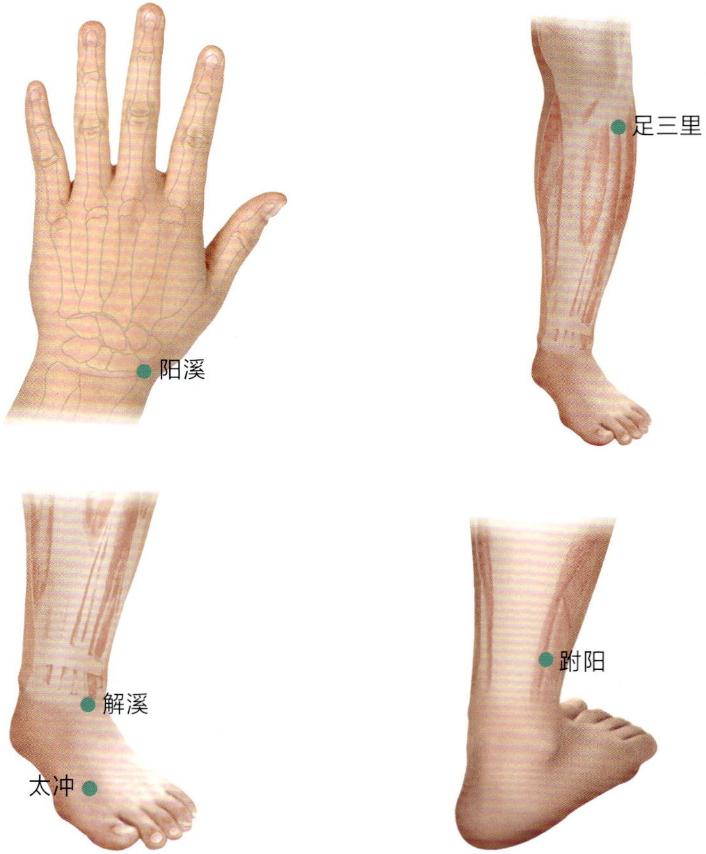

手部按摩

掐压阳溪穴，并活动踝关节，双手各 3 分钟。

足部按摩

1. 指推足三里、解溪、跗阳穴各 3 分钟，每分钟 75 次。
2. 拇指指腹按揉太冲穴 1 分钟，用力稍重，每分钟 75 次。
3. 指推踝部，分别沿以内踝和外踝为圆心的圆周逐点推动，每个着力点推 1 分钟，每分钟 75 次。

45 Gonarthritis

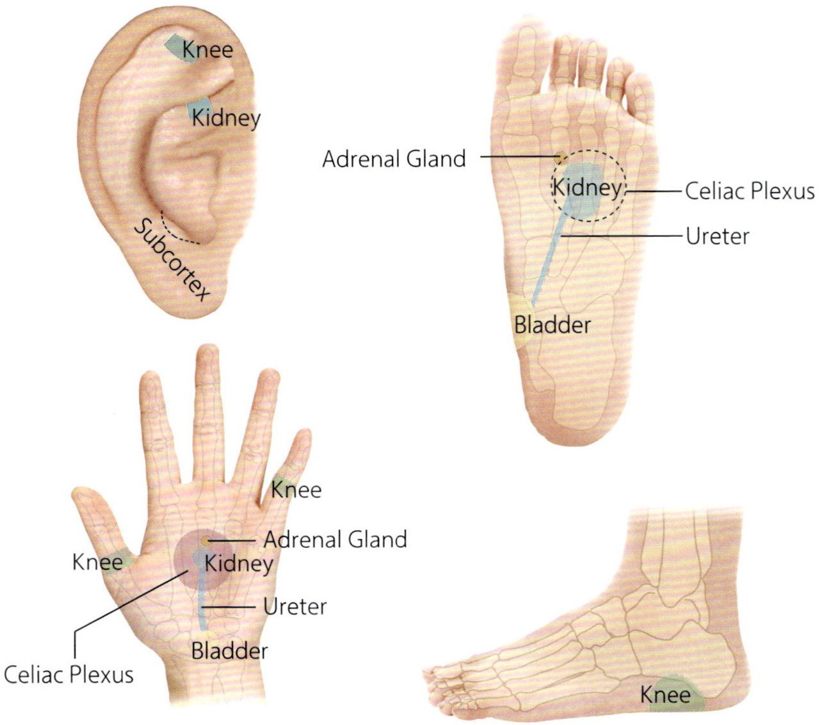

Ear Massage

1. Press the Knee reflex zone with a massage stick for 3 minutes and covers 120 times in each minute.
2. Attach the cowherb seed to the Kidney reflex zone and press for 2 minutes with 75 times in each minute.
3. Massage the Subcortex reflex zone with thumbs for 2 minutes in moderate strength with 75 times in each minute.

Hand Massage

1. Press the reflex zones of Kidney, Adrenal Gland, Ureter, Celiac Plexus and Bladder each for 2 to 3 minutes with interphalangeal joint at the proximal side of index fingers and it is preferred to have a local sense of slight distending pain.
2. Press the holographic zone correspondent to knee joint with thumbs and the strength should refer to the tolerance degree of the one being massaged.

Foot Massage

1. After overall relaxation with a foot bath, massage the reflex zones of Kidney, Adrenal Gland, Ureter, Celiac Plexus and Bladder and it is preferred to have a local sense of soreness and distension.
2. Use soft brushes to brush the Knee reflex zone for 2 to 3 minutes.

46 Ankles Sprain

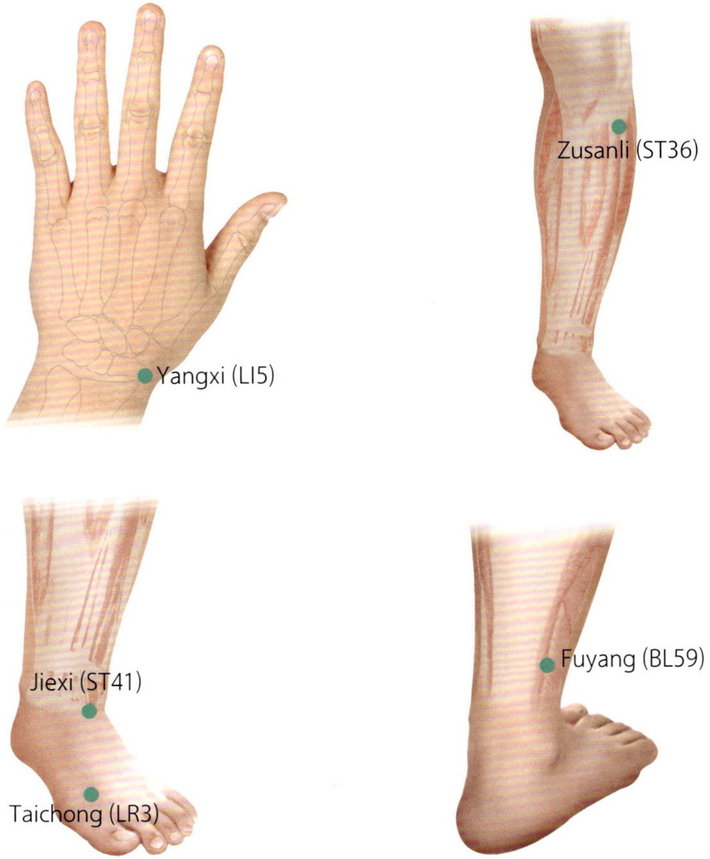

Hand Massage

Nip the acupoint of Yangxi (LI5) and activate the ankles with both hands for 3 minutes.

Foot Massage

1. Press the acupoints of Zusanli (ST36), Jiexi (ST41) and Fuyang (BL59) with relatively heavy pressure with 75 times per minute.
2. Massage the Taichong (LR3) for 1minute with pressure with 75 times per minute.
3. Massage the ankles point by point taking the inside and the outside of the ankles as the centers of 2 circles. It takes 1 minute on each point with the speed of 75 times per minute.

47 足跟痛

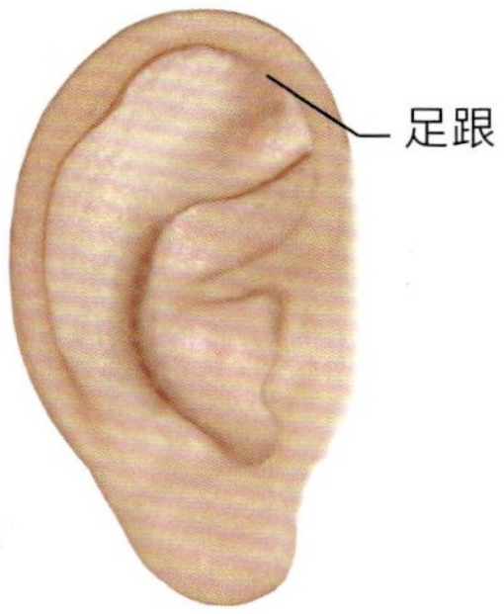

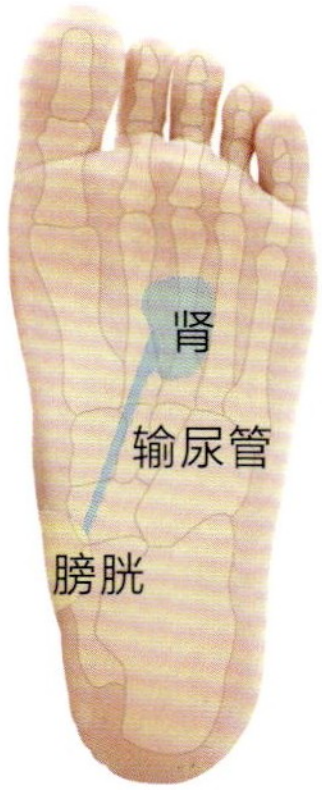

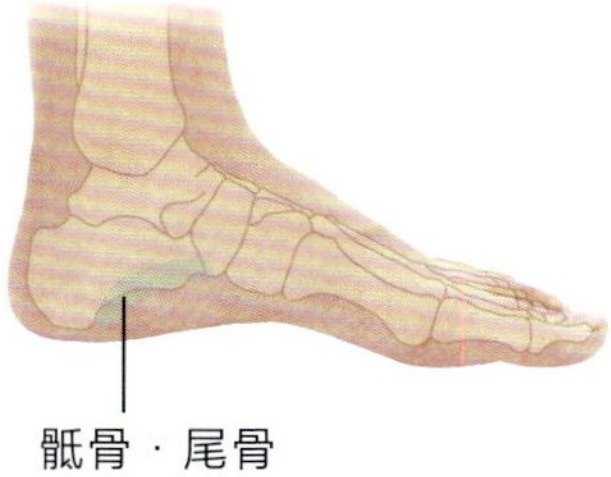

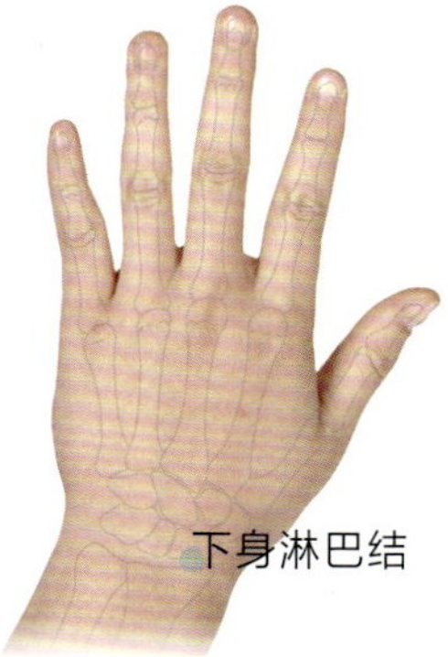

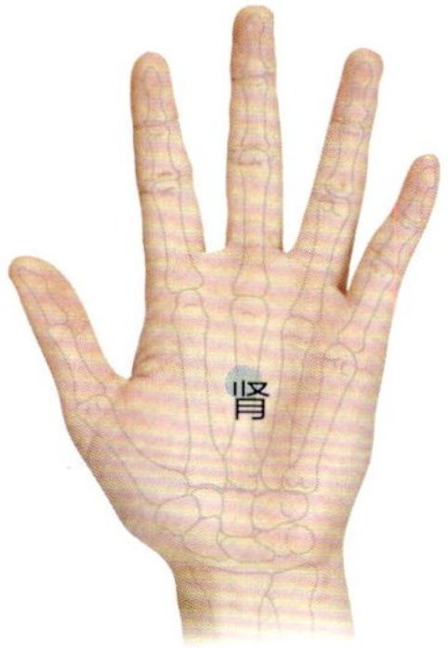

耳部按摩

用工具如铅笔点按足跟反射区 30~50 次，以局部有热胀感为宜。

手部按摩

1. 点按肾反射区，力度以被按摩者耐受为度，以局部有酸胀感为宜。
2. 食指近侧指间关节点揉下身淋巴结反射区 2~3 分钟，用力均匀，力度适中。

足部按摩

1. 泡脚至全脚放松后，按摩肾、输尿管、膀胱反射区各 2 分钟，以局部有热胀感为宜。
2. 拇指指腹推按骶骨・尾骨反射区，以局部有热胀感为宜。
3. 食指近侧指间关节按揉足跟的压痛点及其周围各 5~10 分钟，拿小腿后侧腓肠肌 3 分钟，擦热足跟并热敷。

48 痔疮

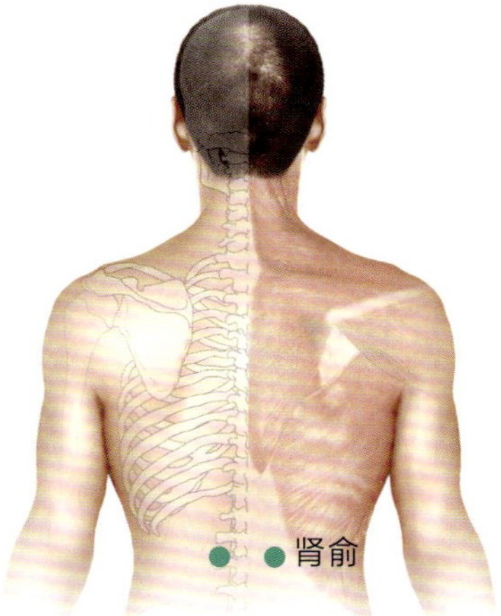

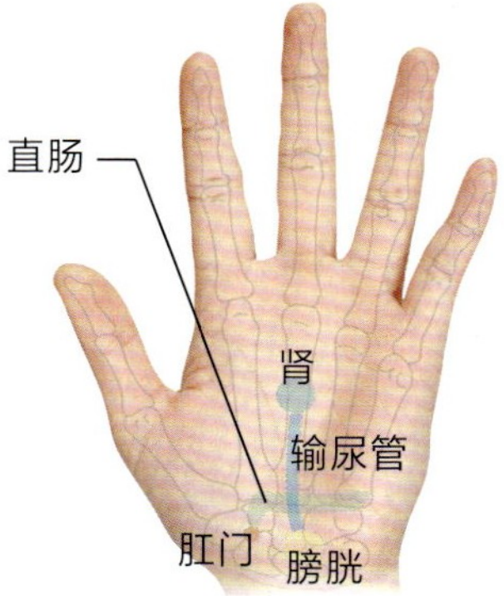

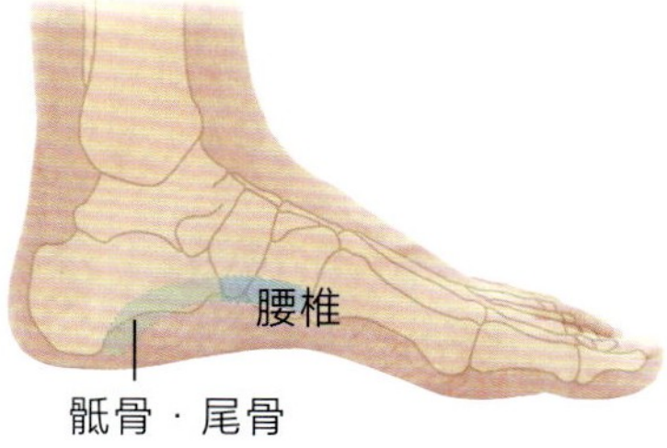

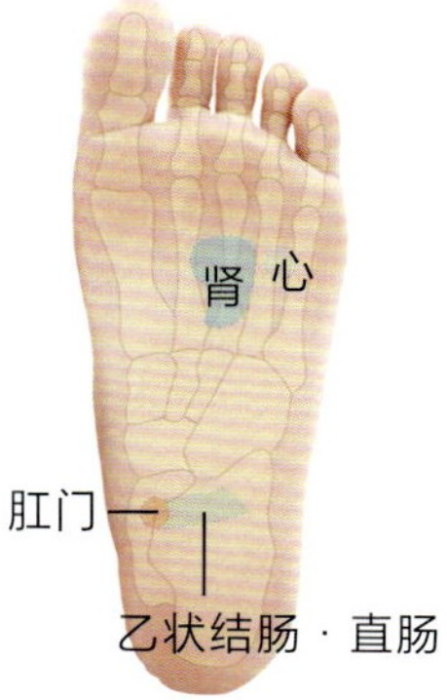

脊背按摩

两手握拳绕于背后，用食指指腹稍微用力按压两侧肾俞穴各 2 分钟，每次停留片刻后放松，重复 5~6 次。

手部按摩

1. 放松手部，拇指轻轻按揉肛门、直肠反射区，按摩的手法要柔和渗透。
2. 食指近侧指间关节点按膀胱、输尿管反射区 1 分钟，用力均匀，力度适中。
3. 点按肾反射区，力度以被按摩者耐受为度，以局部有酸胀感为宜。

足部按摩

1. 食指近侧指间关节刮压肛门、乙状结肠・直肠反射区各 2~3 分钟。
2. 泡脚至全脚放松后，按摩心、肾反射区各 2 分钟，以局部有酸胀感为宜。
3. 食指桡侧缘刮骶骨・尾骨、腰椎反射区各 3~5 次。

47 Heel Pain

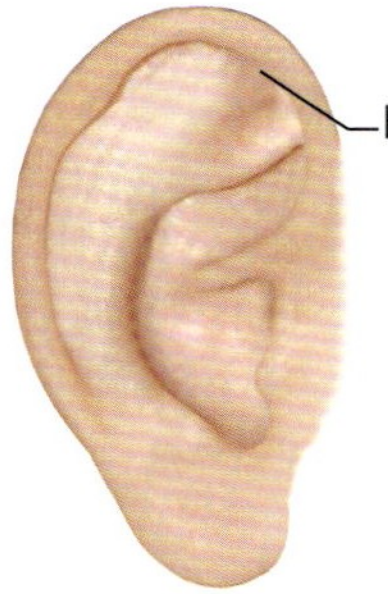

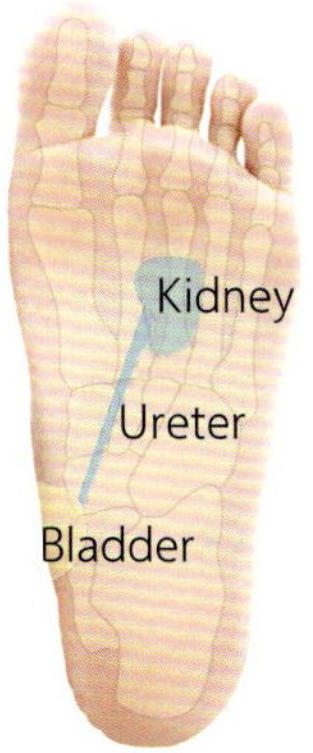

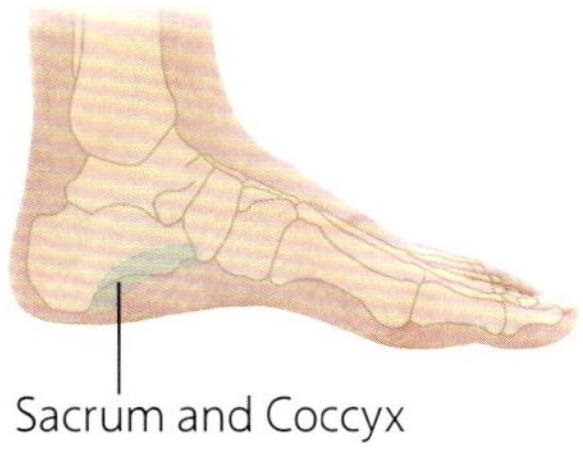

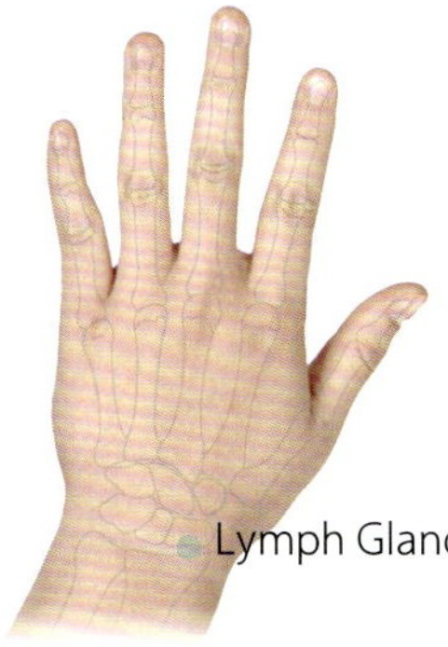

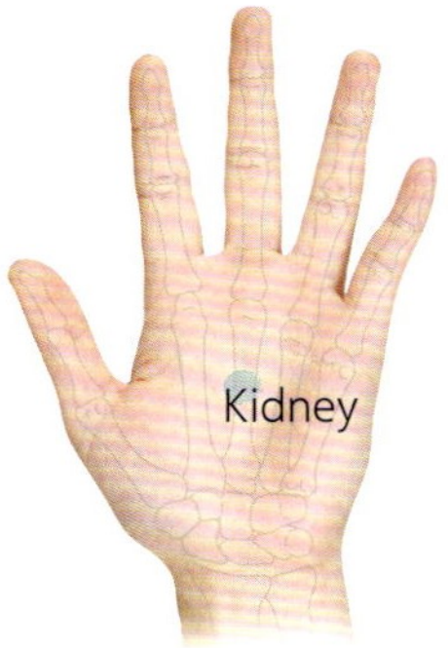

Ear Massage

Press the Heel reflex zone with tools like pencils for 30 to 50 times and it is preferred to have a local sense of heat and distension.

Hand Massage

1. Press the Kidney reflex zone and the strength should refer to the tolerance degree of the one being massaged with appropriate local soreness.
2. Massage the reflex zones of Lymph Gland of Lower Body for 2 to 3 minutes with interphalangeal joint at the proximal side of index fingers in moderate strength.

Foot Massage

1. After taking a foot bath to have overall relaxation, massage the reflex zones of Kidney, Ureter and Bladder each for 2 minutes. It is preferred to have a local sense of heat and distension.
2. Press and press the reflex zones of Sacrum and Coccyx with thumbs and it is preferred to have a local sense of heat and distension.
3. Massage the pain spots on heels and the zone around with interphalangeal joint at the proximal side of index fingers each for 5 to 10 minutes and then massage the gastrocnemius at the backside of the shank for 3 minutes. Chafe the heels and give them a hot compress.

48 Hemorrhoid

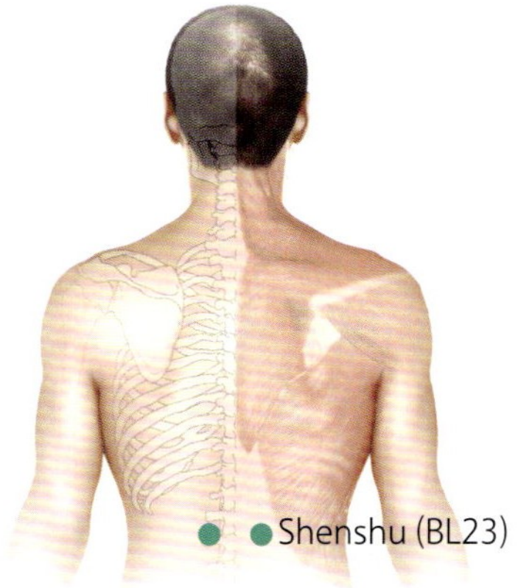

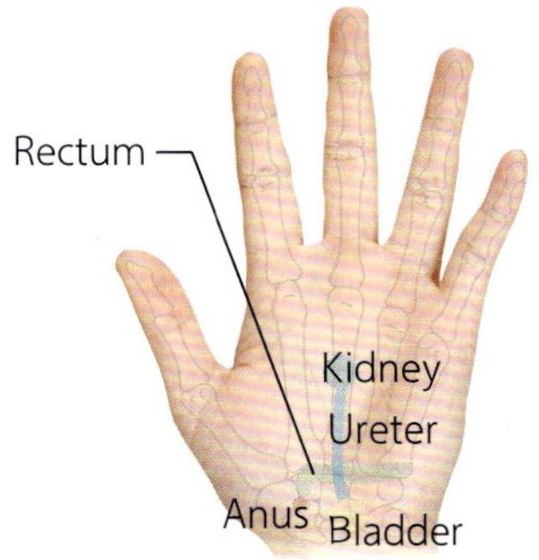

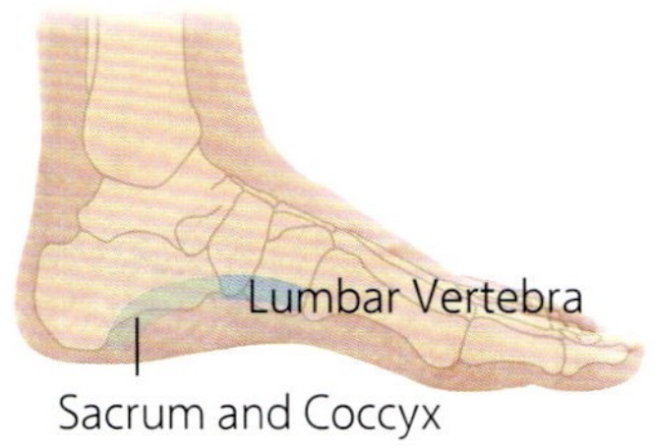

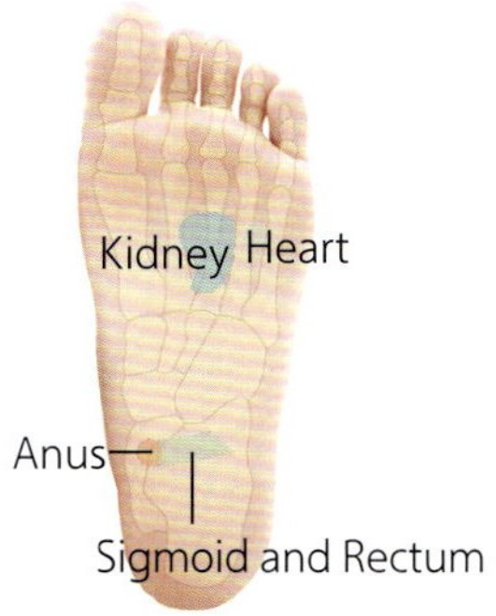

Back Massage

Fold your fists at the back and press Shenshu (BL 23) on both sides with a little pressure using index fingers each for 2 minutes and relax after each short stay. Repeat the massage for 5 to 6 times.

Hand Massage

1. Relax hands and gently massage the Anus and Rectum reflex zones with thumbs with gradually penetrating manipulation.
2. Press the reflex zones of Bladder and Ureter with interphalangeal joint at the proximal side of index fingers in moderate strength.
3. Press the Kidney reflex zone and the strength should refer to the tolerance degree of the ones being massaged. It is preferred to have a local sense of soreness and distension.

Foot Massage

1. Scratch and press the reflex zones of Anus, Sigmoid and Rectum each for 2 to 3 minutes with interphalangeal joint at the proximal side of index fingers.
2. After taking a foot bath to have overall relaxation, massage the reflex zones of Heart and Kidney each for 2 minutes and it is preferred to have a local sense of soreness.
3. Scratch the reflex zones of Sacrum, Coccyx and Lumbar Vertebra each for 3 to 5 times with the radical margin of index fingers.